Clinical Child Psychiatry, Third Edition

Clinical Child Psychiatry, Third Edition

Editors

William M. Klykylo, M.D.
Professor and Director, Division of Child and Adolescent Psychiatry, Wright State, University, Dayton, OH, USA

Jerald Kay, M.D.
Professor and Chair, Department of Psychiatry, Wright State University, Dayton, OH, USA

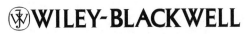

A John Wiley & Sons, Ltd., Publication

This edition first published 2012
© 2012 by John Wiley & Sons, Ltd

Wiley-Blackwell is an imprint of John Wiley & Sons, formed by the merger of Wiley's global Scientific, Technical and Medical business with Blackwell Publishing.

Registered office: John Wiley & Sons, Ltd, The Atrium, Southern Gate, Chichester, West Sussex, PO19 8SQ, UK

Editorial offices: 9600 Garsington Road, Oxford, OX4 2DQ, UK
The Atrium, Southern Gate, Chichester, West Sussex, PO19 8SQ, UK
111 River Street, Hoboken, NJ 07030-5774, USA

For details of our global editorial offices, for customer services and for information about how to apply for permission to reuse the copyright material in this book please see our website at www.wiley.com/wiley-blackwell.

The right of the author to be identified as the author of this work has been asserted in accordance with the UK Copyright, Designs and Patents Act 1988.

Library of Congress Cataloging-in-Publication Data

Clinical child psychiatry / editors, William M. Klykylo and Jerald L. Kay. – 3rd ed.
 p. ; cm.
 Includes bibliographical references and index.
 ISBN 978-1-119-99334-6 (pbk.) – ISBN 978-1-119-96221-2 (ePDF) – ISBN 978-1-119-96222-9 (oBook) –
ISBN 978-1-119-96770-5 (ePub) – ISBN 978-1-119-96771-2 (Mobi)
 I. Klykylo, William M. II. Kay, Jerald.
 [DNLM: 1. Adolescent Psychiatry–methods. 2. Child Psychiatry–methods. 3. Adolescent. 4. Child. 5. Developmental Disabilities.
6. Infant. 7. Mental Disorders. WS 350]

 616.8900835–dc23

2011038027

A catalogue record for this book is available from the British Library.

Wiley also publishes its books in a variety of electronic formats. Some content that appears in print may not be available in electronic books.

Set in 9/11pt Galliard by Thomson Digital, Noida, India
Printed and bound in Singapore by Markono Print Media Pte Ltd

First Impression 2012

DEDICATION

To our teachers, our students, our patients, and our families.

Contents

CONTENTS

Companion website

The book is accompanied by a companion resources site:

clinicalchildpsychiatry.com

With interactive multiple-choice questions for each chapter.

Contributors

Rick T. Bowers, South Community Behavioral Healthcare, 3095 Kettering Blvd, Dayton, OH 45439, USA

L. Lee Carlisle, Division of Child and Adolescent Psychiatry, Department of Psychiatry and Behavioral Sciences, University of Washington School of Medicine, Child Study and Treatment Center, 8805 Steilacoom Boulevard SW, W27-25, Lakewood, WA 98498-4771, USA

Christina C. Clark, Psy.D., LLC, 666 High Street, Suite 200D, Worthington, OH 43085-4135, USA

Barbara J. Coffey, Child Study Center, New York University School of Medicine, 577 First Avenue, New York, NY 10016, USA

Antoinette S. Cordell, PhD and Associates, 5045 N. Main Street, Suite 223, Dayton, OH 45415, USA

Jacqueline Countryman, Department of Psychiatry, Wright State University School of Medicine, 627 S. Edwin C Moses Blvd, P.O. Box 927, Dayton, OH 45401-0927, USA

Jennifer Couturier, Department of Psychiatry & Behavioural Neurosciences, McMaster University, 200 Main Street W., Hamilton, Ontario, L8N 3Z5, Canada

Sergio V. Delgado, Children's Hospital Medical Center, 3333 Burnet Avenue, Cincinnati, OH 45229-3039, USA

David Ray DeMaso, Department of Psychiatry, Children's Hospital of Boston, Hunnewell 121, 300 Longwood Ave., Boston, MA 02115, USA

Craig L. Donnelly, Section of Pediatric Psychopharmacology, Dartmouth-Hitchcock Medical Center, One Medical Center Drive, Lebanon, NH 03756-0001, USA

Martin J. Drell, LSUHSC, Department of Psychiatry, Room A 236, 1542 Tulane Avenue, New Orleans, LA 70112, USA

James H. Duffee, Rocking Horse Center, 651 South Limestone Street, Springfield, OH 45505, USA

Jennifer P. Edidin, Department of Psychiatry & Behavioral Neuroscience, The University of Chicago, 5841 S. Maryland Avenue., MC 3077, Chicago, IL 60637, USA

Sidney Edsall, Department of Psychiatry, Stanford University, 401 Quarry Road, Palo Alto, CA 94305

Dorothyann Feldis, College of Education, 600 E Teacher's College, University of Cincinnati, PO Box 210022, Cincinnati, OH 45221-0022, USA

Scott D. Grewe, Sage View Youth Psychology, 1950 Keene Road, Bldg. O, Richland, WA 99352, USA

Pamela A. Gulley, 640 Concord Village Circle, Johnston, OH 43031, USA

Julia Huemer, Department of Child and Adolescent Psychiatry, Medical University of Vienna, Waehringer Guertel 18-20, 1090 Vienna, Austria

Scott J. Hunter, Department of Psychiatry & Behavioral Neuroscience, The University of Chicago Medical Center, 5841 S. Maryland Avenue, MC 3077, Chicago, IL 60637, USA

Patricia I. Ibeziako, Department of Psychiatry, Children's Hospital of Boston, Hunnewell 121, 300 Longwood Ave., Boston, 02115, USA

Julia Jackson, Department of Psychiatry, Wright State University, School of Medicine, PO Box 927, Dayton, OH 45401-0927, USA

Niranjan S. Karnik, Department of Psychiatry and Behavioral Sciences, The University of Chicago, 5841 S. Maryland, MC 3077, Chicago, IL 60637, USA

Tejal Kaur, Division of Cognitive Neuroscience, Columbia University, 622 W. 168th Street, PH1291, New York, NY 10032, USA

Jerald Kay, Department of Psychiatry, Wright State University School of Medicine, P.O. Box 927, Dayton, OH 45401-0927, USA

Young Shin Kim, Associate Professor, Yale University Child Study Center, Nieson-Irving Harris Blvd., 230 S. Frontage Road, I-379, New Haven, CT 06519, USA

Bryan H. King, University of Washington and Seattle Children's Hospital, 4800 Sand Point Way, NE, PO Box 5371/M1-1, Seattle, WA 98105, USA

Bonnie Klimes-Dougan, University of Minnesota, N414 Elliott Hall, 75 East River Road, Minneapolis, MN 55455-0344, USA

William M. Klykylo, Department of Psychiatry, Wright State University School of Medicine, 627 S. Edwin C Moses Blvd, P.O. Box 927, Dayton, OH 45401-0927, USA

Kevin Lam, NYU Child Study Center and Bellevue Hospital Center, 577 First Avenue, New York, NY 10016, USA

Bennett L. Leventhal, Deputy Director, Nathan Kline Institute for Psychiatric Research (NKI), 140 Old Orangeburg Road, Bldg 35, Orangeburg, NY 10962, USA

James Lock, Department of Psychiatry and Behavioral Sciences, Stanford University School of Medicine, 401 Quarry Road, MC 5719, Stanford, CA 94305-5719, USA

Arthur Maerlender, Dartmouth-Hitchcock Medical Center, One Medical Center Drive, Lebanon, NH 03757, USA

Ryan C. Mast, Department of Psychiatry, Wright State University School of Medicine, 627 S. Edwin C Moses Blvd, P.O. Box 927, Dayton, OH 45401-0927, USA

Jill D. McCarley, East Tennessee State University, Quillen College of Medicine, PO Box 70567, Johnson City, TN 37614, USA

Brian J. McConville, Department of Psychiatry, University of Cincinnati College of Medicine, 2444 Madison Road, #1105, Cincinnati, OH 45208-1225, USA

Douglas Mossman, University of Cincinnati College of Medicine, Dept. of Psychiatry, 260 Stetson Street, Suite 3200, PO Box 670559, Cincinnati, OH 45267-0559, USA

Susan C. Mumford, Department of Psychiatry, Wright State University School of Medicine, 627 S. Edwin C Moses Blvd, P.O. Box 927, Dayton, OH 45401-0927, USA

Thomas B. Owley, Institute for Juvenile Research, Department of Psychiatry, University of Illinois at Chicago, 1747 W. Roosevelt Road, Chicago, IL 60608, USA

George Realmuto, Department of Psychiatry, University of Minnesota, F256/2B West, 2450 Riverside Avenue, Minneapolis, MN 55454-1495, USA

Jesse C. Rhoads, Section of Pediatric Psychopharmacology, Dartmouth-Hitchcock Medical Center, One Medical Center Drive, Lebanon, NH 03756-0001, USA

David M. Rube, Queen's Children's Psychiatric Center, 74-03 Commonwealth Blvd, Bellrose, NY 11426, USA

Lori A. Sansone, Wright-Patterson Air Force Base, 88 MDOS/SGOPC, 4881 Sugar Maple Drive, WPAFB, OH, 45433, USA

Randy A. Sansone, Sycamore Primary Care Center, 2115 Leiter Road, Suite 300, Miamisburg, OH 45342-3659, USA

Martin B. Scharf, Center for Research in Sleep Disorders, 1275 East Kemper Road, Cincinnati, OH 45237, USA

Andrew B. Smith, Department of Psychiatry, Wright State University School of Medicine, 627 S. Edwin C Moses Blvd, P.O. Box 927, Dayton, OH 45401-0927, USA

Jamie Snyder, Child and Adolescent Psychiatry and Post-Pediatric Portal Program, Creighton University/University of Nebraska Training Programs, 3500 S. 91st Street, Lincoln, NE 69520-1429, USA

Michael T. Sorter, Cincinnati Children's Hospital Medical Center, University of Cincinnati, 3333 Burnet Avenue, M.L. 3014, Cincinnati, OH 45229, USA

Hans Steiner, Department of Psychiatry and Behavioral Sciences; Child and Adolescent Psychiatry Clinic, Stanford University School of Medicine, 401 Quarry Road, MC 5719, Stanford, CA 94305-5719, USA

Russell Tobe, Medical Director, Outpatient Research Department, Nathan S. Kline Institute for Psychiatric Research, Orangeburg, NY, USA

Daniel A. Vogel, Cincinnati Children's Hospital Medical Center, 3333 Burnet avenue, MI 3014, Cincinnati, OH 45229-3014, USA

Christine V. Wellborn, Education Director, Tri-State Sleep Disorders Center, 1275 East Kemper Road, Cincinnati, Ohio 45246, USA

Christina G. Weston, Department of Psychiatry, Wright State University, School of Medicine, PO Box 927, Dayton, OH 45401-0927, USA

Keith Owen Yeates, Department of Psychology, The Ohio State University, and Center for Biobehavioral Health, The Research Institute at Nationwide Children's Hospital, 700 Children's Dr., Columbus, OH 43205, USA

Preface To Clinical Child Psychiatry, Third Edition

In the preface to the first edition of this work, we stated that the changes in child psychiatry occurring then would have been barely imaginable 15 years earlier. In the preface to the second edition, we remarked that we could not have predicted then how much the whole world would change thereafter. The subsequent world crises have only intensified the demands placed upon child and adolescent psychiatry. We have ever growing demands for service to our patients, whose stressors and pathology become more severe and pervasive. We are fortunate that our understanding of disease and our armamentarium of treatments also continue to increase. Regrettably, the resources allocated for those treatments have not always grown apace; so we must continue to do more with less and do so ever more quickly and efficiently.

The welcome growth of knowledge in our field continues to change clinical practice, creating a need for an update of this book. Like its predecessors, *Clinical Child Psychiatry, Third Edition* is presented neither as a comprehensive textbook covering the entire field, nor as a brief introduction. It still attempts to serve as a focused study of major problems, challenges, and practices commonly encountered in clinical work. It remains directed toward experienced clinicians encountering new areas of practice, as well as to students and residents entering the field. We especially hope that pediatricians and family physicians, who throughout the world provide the preponderance of child psychiatric services, will find this volume useful. We also wish it to be informative to professionals outside of medicine as an overview of what child psychiatry can – and should – do today. As always, but in these times especially, we must work together as best we can.

Whatever its merits, *Clinical Child Psychiatry, Third Edition* is the product of the individuals' efforts. We have been well served by our publisher John Wiley & Sons, Ltd, and especially by our Project Editor Fiona Seymour, our Associate Editor Robyn Lyons, and our Publisher Joan Marsh. They bring to their work an enviable combination of knowledge, experience, patience, and good humor that has encouraged and sustained us. We could not have assembled this book without the support of our staff at Wright State University Boonshoft School of Medicine, most notably Laura Johnson and Megan McKenzie. Our contributors are the ultimate source of this volume's content and value, and we are in their debt. Finally, our families continue to support us with their affection and patience.

William M. Klykylo
Jerald Kay

Section I
The Fundamentals of Child and Adolescent Psychiatric Practice

1

The Initial Psychiatric Evaluation

William M. Klykylo

This chapter is an introduction both to this textbook and to the approach of patients and families in child and adolescent psychiatric practice. Child and adolescent psychiatrists should be broadly trained clinicians able to address a variety of somatic, psychologic, and social needs of the patient and family. Their approach should combine the caution and competence required of a physician treating an individual patient with a broad concern for that patient's development in the context of family, school, and society. This textbook provides an overview of child and adolescent psychiatric practice while focusing on the more common areas of clinical practice. As such, it should serve the established practitioner as a rapid and accessible introduction to unfamiliar areas by taking into account the ever-expanding breadth of clinical practice. For general readers or students in professions other than medicine, this book will serve as an introduction to both the assessment and management of some commonly encountered clinical entities and to the range and standards of practice expected of a contemporary child and adolescent psychiatrist. There are currently about 6000 child psychiatrists in some sort of clinical practice in the United States, whereas there are between 7 and 12 million children with psychiatric illnesses, as identified by *Diagnostic and Statistical Manual,* Fourth Edition, Text Revision (DSM-IV-TR) criteria [1, 2]. The median prevalence estimate of functionally impairing child and adolescent psychiatric disorders is 12%, although the range of estimates is wide. Disorders that often appear first in childhood or adolescence are among those ranked highest in the World Health Organization's estimates of the global burden of disease [3]. Most of these children will not see a child and adolescent psychiatrist and, in many instances, the parents, teachers, and other professionals attempting to serve them may be unaware of the contribution that child and adolescent psychiatry can make to the child's care.

The traditional roles of child and adolescent psychiatrists are those of diagnostician, therapist, and consultant. First, child and adolescent psychiatrists should offer a child and family a comprehensive diagnostic assessment that addresses the medical condition of the child; delineates the child's emotional, cognitive, social, and linguistic development; and identifies the nature of the child's relationship with his or her family, school, and social milieu.

Second, child and adolescent psychiatrists as physicians treat illnesses, using an armamentarium of somatic treatments and the more traditional skills of individual, family, and group psychotherapists. Because of the breadth of training they receive, child and adolescent psychiatrists should have special skill in appreciating the interaction among these therapies and their effects on one another and on the child and family.

Finally, in many cases, child and adolescent psychiatrists will serve as consultants. This role is more developed in our specialty than in most other areas of medicine because of the constant disproportion between the number of patients and the number of clinicians. Inevitably, we consult and collaborate with parents, educators, and other professionals who may see the child and family more frequently and intensively than we do; because of the breadth of our training, we should offer a special competence in coordinating these efforts. Concurrent with this role, we often must serve as advocates for children and their families in today's environment of great clinical needs and comparatively limited resources.

Referral Sources

Because of the broad responsibility shared by child and adolescent psychiatrists, our evaluations must address not only a narrow consideration of clinical diagnosis but also a larger set of issues that are truly biopsychosocial

Clinical Child Psychiatry, Third Edition. Edited by William M. Klykylo and Jerald Kay.
© 2012 John Wiley & Sons, Ltd. Published 2012 by John Wiley & Sons, Ltd.

and require a more than casual competence in each of these areas. We must therefore address the specific needs and questions posed by each referral source. Children are today served by a variety of individuals and agencies, each possessing their own particular agendas and separately approaching physicians and other consultants. These agendas must be recognized and served, given today's consumer-oriented society. At the same time, we have a responsibility to those individuals seeking our professional services to educate them with the wider range of concerns that may be affecting a given child's or family's life.

In today's environment, we frequently receive referrals from, or may be employed in contractual relationships with, various social and legal agencies such as courts and departments of human services. Each of these agencies has a particular agenda, generally mandated by legislation or charter, to determine the eligibility of children for various services or proceedings. The agencies frequently approach their duties with an intense dedication to children but an incomplete familiarity with the knowledge and assumptions that inform our practice. Referrals may also come from teachers or schools. These referrals may be a result of the child's behavioral disruptions or eccentricities, his or her academic difficulties, or simply the distinct if sometimes uncertain perception of a dedicated teacher that something is wrong. Referrals may come to us from other physicians. In today's atmosphere of comprehensive primary practice, these physicians may have already begun the diagnosis and treatment of mental illness in a child, and established an ongoing relationship with this child and his or her family. Such referrals require a balanced response of both expertise and respect. Finally, many referrals come directly from parents, who are generally very concerned about their child's impaired functioning and suffering. They may bring to the process a mixed heritage of concern, guilt, and shame, frequently fearing that they will be judged as they seek help. Concurrent with this are often ambivalent feelings of love and frustration toward a difficult child. The task of child and adolescent psychiatrists is to recognize all these needs and address them in a fashion that is not only authoritative but also tactful and empathetic.

Elements of the Evaluation

This section provides an overview of the elements of a comprehensive child and adolescent psychiatric evaluation in the context of contemporary knowledge and patient needs. More detailed considerations of the process of the clinical interview are also available [4–8]. The assessment of particular disorders as well as laboratory, psychologic, and educational assessments is covered in other chapters of this book.

Collateral and Preliminary Information

Today, most children who are seen by child and adolescent psychiatrists have already received a great deal of attention from other professionals. To fail to gather information from these people prior to a formal evaluation is a serious mistake, leading to wasted time and frustrated relationships. If at all possible, it is usually most efficient to speak directly with a referring professional. This is especially true in the case of primary care physicians, who may have a long-standing relationship with the child and family. Other mental health professionals referring a child usually have conducted their own evaluation. Children's school records can be a rich source of information about their cognitive and emotional development. Examination of all these data can enrich an evaluation; similarly, failure to do so can lead to embarrassing lapses.

Clinicians in the past may have at times assessed a child while deliberately ignoring collateral information, presumably to evolve an unbiased assessment. There may be certain unusual situations in which this tactic is indicated. More often than not, however, this approach ignores the reality of the lives of children, who live in asymmetrical relationships with adults and agencies, all of whom have considerable knowledge and power over them. This approach is almost always a departure from best practice.

Encounters with Referring Professionals

Often a child and adolescent psychiatrist's first personal encounter in assessing a patient is with another professional – a clinician, educator, or case worker who has sought the evaluation. The enormous value of their information has already been addressed. The clinician must also recognize the sensitivities of these people: they may be grateful for the opportunity to meet with the psychiatrist and eager in their anticipation of the evaluation, perhaps even to an unrealistic degree. At the same time, the act of seeking a consultation may, at least unconsciously, signify to them a failure on their part. They may be concerned that their relationship with the child or family will in some way be disrupted or supplanted, or that they will be criticized by the psychiatrist.

Parents

Parents bringing their child to a child and adolescent psychiatrist come with a rich and often contradictory mix of feelings. Frequently they reach the psychiatrist at the end of a long, complicated process of evaluations and treatment attempts. They are almost invariably concerned and anxious over their child's condition and prospects. In a way that, for those who are not parents, may be difficult to understand fully, they may have many fears about the consequences of a psychiatric referral, as do referring professionals. They may feel that they will be judged or, in extreme cases, that their children will be removed from their care. In a more subtle way, they may also worry that their relationship with their child will be supplanted or superseded. They may be concerned about the moral and philosophic basis of the psychiatrist's approach, fearing that parental ethical standards and religious beliefs will in some way be contradicted. Sometimes, simultaneously, they may have unrealistically optimistic or hopeful fantasies of "absolution" of unconscious guilt, or of quick cures. More often than not, in my experience, parents have no idea of the specifics of psychiatric assessment or treatment. Their opinions may have been formed by mass media or public prejudice. Before any specific information can be gathered or plans made, the above issues must be addressed, in the interest of time and efficiency as well as of engagement. Simply put, the child and adolescent psychiatrist needs to understand how the parents feel about the referral and what they expect to gain from it.

A great deal of information should be collected from parents, since they know the child best. The details of this data collection, including various outlines for its organization, are described elsewhere in this book. Most child and adolescent psychiatrists today use a traditional medical format to organize their data, with headings such as Chief Complaint, History of Present Illness, Past Medical History, Family History, and Review of Systems. More often than not, the specifically medical aspects of these data are already available. Not infrequently, however, child and adolescent psychiatrists encounter families that have not received regular primary pediatric care. In these cases, it is incumbent on the psychiatrist as physician to take a comprehensive medical history in addition to acquiring other information. In all these areas of questioning, psychiatrists collect data as do all other physicians, usually attempting to delineate and organize the information in a chronological fashion. What is unique about a psychiatric evaluation is that physicians pursue not only the specific data but also their affective implications. In other words, they seek to find out not only what specifically happened but also how it made the child or family members feel and what consequences it had on their lives.

Another area of inquiry of particular importance to physicians treating children, and certainly to child and adolescent psychiatrists, is the developmental history. Child and adolescent psychiatrists must be absolutely familiar with normal developmental patterns, milestones, and expectations. Psychiatrists often approach these phenomena informed by traditional theories of psychosexual, social, and cognitive development. Although these theories frequently hold great importance for their heuristic value, the clinician must remember that they are, at best, models or theories and not immutable facts. Thus, the clinician must also be aware of contemporary empirical data about normal development and its variations. The developmental history secured by a child and adolescent psychiatrist should in many ways be similar in depth and breadth to that obtained by a developmental pediatrician. At the same time, as psychiatrists we should focus special emphasis on the social and affective consequences of developmental phenomena. In other words, we should be concerned about not only at what age a child reached a given milestone but also how the attainment of that milestone affected that child and his or her family. We must recognize that some developmental processes or stages may inherently be more or less comfortable for some parents, and that there is a wide range of variation in the degree of comfort and discomfort that development engenders. Finally, we must recognize the great variations in developmental patterns and expectations found among different cultures. Summaries of typical developmental sequences are found in Appendix 1.1.

A detailed consideration of family dynamics and therapeutics is beyond the scope of this textbook. We know from the contributions of clinicians with approaches as diverse as those of Satir [9], Whitaker [10], Minuchin [11], Haley [12], and cognitive therapists [13] that the family has an immense and profound influence on the development of each of its members and may be viewed as a distinct entity [14]. It is therefore invaluable, as part of a comprehensive psychiatric observation, to spend some time in the company of the entire family. Frequently, families referred to us have already been assessed in this fashion by competent family therapists, and the child and adolescent psychiatrist may not need or have the opportunity to pursue extensive family treatment. Nonetheless, the opportunity to observe firsthand how the members of a family act with each other can be enriching for a clinician attempting to understand the consequences of each family member's behavior on the others. In addition, if this observation is done early, it may serve as a more comfortable entrance to the evaluation process for a shy or otherwise recalcitrant child or other uncooperative family member.

Meeting the Child

In practice, most clinicians develop a somewhat personal style of interaction usually formed by psychodynamic and interactional approaches and also more structured, empirical techniques. Clinicians in any setting soon realize that, outside of the specific requirements of a structured interview instrument, they need to be flexible in their approach. The schemes that we use for reporting an interview are generally best conceived as devices for retrospective organization rather than templates for an interview. This is of particular importance with children. Any pediatrician knows that in the course of a physical examination one does what one can when one can. Similarly, in the psychiatric interview with the child, one must be flexible and mobile both verbally and physically.

The most important element of an initial psychiatric interview with the child is the establishment of a productive relationship – in other words, "making friends." The clinician must keep in mind how children feel in the context of an interview. Children may share or reflect the same complicated and ambivalent mixture of fear, shame, hope, and misapprehension that their parents bring to the process, and they often have not been fully prepared by the parents or others for the interview. Such preparation, if it can be done by parents prior to bringing the child in, can be helpful. Many children, in my experience, have been told nothing at all, other than "Come along, we are going to see someone." Or they may have been told that they are going to see a doctor, which can convey fears of injections and manipulations. Some children may have been led to assume that the evaluation is part of a punitive process. Others may feel that by virtue of referral they have been singled out in some way as "weird" or "crazy." Concurrently, the child may expect to see the physician as some sort of remote, distant, punitive, or bizarre figure. All these issues must be promptly investigated and addressed in a developmentally appropriate fashion for a productive interview to ensue.

How one deals with the above issues is affected by one's own personality and training, and by the circumstances of the child and family. Preschool children are seldom able to sustain any type of formal interview, although they may answer some questions during play activities or while "on the run." Their preoperational style of cognition makes the standard interview format, with its attention toward consequence and chronology, irrelevant. One assesses these children through observation and interaction. By contrast, the school-age child will have some comprehension of the psychiatrist's role. It may help to introduce one's self as a "talking doctor"

or "problem doctor" who deals with the problems that many children have (generalization may make the child feel less singled out) through conversation as well as traditional somatic treatments, and who does not give injections in the office setting. Older children and adolescents can often be asked directly about how they were brought to evaluation, as well as their opinions about its necessity and desirability. With school-age children, an initial request about what sort of problems they may have encountered in their life may be met with diffidence or avoidance. In this instance, simply playing together at some mutually acceptable activity may be an important first step. Older children and adolescents may at this time be able to tolerate tactful questions or the mention of other material or information. They will still benefit from the opportunity to talk or interact about areas that they like, perhaps later in the interview. A frequent icebreaker employed by child and adolescent psychiatrists is drawing. Children who are seated in the waiting room while their parents are being interviewed can be given the opportunity to draw a picture of their family or some other subject of interest to them. Such a drawing can serve as both a projective device and a conversation starter later in the process. Of course, children can also be encouraged to draw at other times during the interview.

In many instances, children do not respond to a standard, direct, complaint-centered line of questioning, even after several attempts by the clinician. The clinician is then best advised to relent and ask the child to talk about more general aspects of his or her life. The patient can be encouraged to tell the physician about his or her family, including each individual member and relationship, and school, including academic and social behavioral aspects and social life in general. In doing so, the clinician can often assemble a broad picture of the child's life as well as specific medical information about phenomenology. Some areas may need to be more directly pursued, usually later in the interview when a presumably more trusting relationship has been established. These include items that are considered part of the mental status examination, such as the presence of affective symptomatology (including suicidal ideation or plans) and psychotic phenomena (including hallucinations, delusions, or ideas of reference). Not every child needs to be asked about these things since for some children merely inquiring in an initial interview can be disruptive or fearful. Nonetheless, these issues must be pursued if there is any indication of a disorder in the given area. Suicidal ideation in particular must be pursued in the context of any affective disorder. Other important behavioral areas such as sexual behavior, using drugs, and health risk behavior may also need to be pursued.

The issue of confidentiality warrants special consideration. Child and adolescent psychiatrists must use their clinical skill to moderate two conflicting demands: the child's right to confidentiality as a patient versus the right of parents and, in some instances, agencies or institutions to be aware of the child's needs and requirements. In my experience, most parents want to know what their child is experiencing; concurrently, most children want their parents to understand them, although they may prefer to conceal some specific details. Younger children may be told they have a right to hold secrets, but that their parents also have a right to know what in general is going on in their lives. Adolescents and their parents may be told that in general they have a right to confidentiality, but that some information involving a serious risk to themselves or others could be shared. Conflicts over confidentiality often overlie larger family issues that, if addressed, make the confidentiality issues moot or irrelevant.

Child and adolescent psychiatrists have traditionally been encouraged to pursue children's fantasies in the course of an assessment. The various approaches to this tend to be highly personalized by each clinician and may include asking a child for three wishes, positive or negative animal identifications (what animal would you like or not like to be), story completion, response to fables, or other techniques. Few if any of these approaches, as used idiosyncratically in an unstructured interview, have ever been validated. They should not be treated as sources of empirical data in and of themselves. They can, however, be important probes to seek other information that can be validated and, more important, that relates to specific emotional concerns of an individual child or adolescent.

Frequently nonmedical professionals refer to the psychiatric evaluation as the "mental status exam," but in fact this examination is not always used in evaluating children and adolescents – certainly a formal mental status examination must be pursued when there is evidence of a thought disorder. In these instances, the type of examination used with adults generally suffices for adolescents as well. In younger children, the mental status examination is often a list of observations that is retrospectively organized from the content of the interview thus far described. (The outline of this examination is summarized in the article by Lewis and King [7], and in Table 1.1.) In most child and adolescent psychiatric assessments, these parameters are not all specifically cited but are mentioned as part of the narrative or may be drawn from inference by the reader. When the patient in question possibly has a major thought or affective disorder, however, specific adherence to this outline may be useful.

Table 1.1 Mental status examination outline.

1.	Physical appearance
2.	Separation from parent
3.	Manner of relating
4.	Orientation to time, place, and person
5.	Central nervous system functioning
6.	Reading and writing
7.	Speech and language
8.	Intelligence
9.	Memory
10.	Thought content
11.	Quality of thinking and perception
12.	Fantasies and inferred conflicts
13.	Affects
14.	Object relations
15.	Drive behavior
16.	Defense organization
17.	Judgment and insight
18.	Self-esteem
19.	Adaptive qualities
20.	Positive attributes
21.	Future orientation

Adapted from Lewis ME, King RA (2002), p. 531 [7].

Other Aspects of Psychiatric Evaluation

Standardized Assessment Instruments

Structured interviews, rating scales, and questionnaires have become increasingly used in child and adolescent psychiatry in recent years, although their primary venue remains in research settings. Angold and Costello, in their masterful review of the current state of nosology and measurement [15], state that a comprehensive and authoritative evaluation should include their use. Many clinicians believe that, in many cases, a useful evaluation can be conducted and reported without resort to these instruments; and some instruments may require a degree of time and expense unavailable outside a research setting. However, as diagnostic categorization under the DSM system has become more standardized and reproducible, clinicians are more frequently using validated instruments, at the very least to clarify or affirm impressions that come from their personal evaluations. Thienemann has produced a thoughtful commentary on the process of combining these elements in a fashion that is both dynamically sensitive and empirically valid:

Ideally, using intuition and experience, the psychiatrist bloodhound will use clinical senses to sniff out clues to diagnosis at first encounter. On picking up a diagnostic scent, he or she will doggedly follow it into a specific diagnostic room to gather details, thereby determining a diagnosis' presence and clarifying its severity. Integrating this reliable diagnostic information with clinical observations, the clinician will be better positioned to engage patients and their families with effective treatments [16].

Many clinicians use initial screening or parental report instruments such as the Achenbach Child Behavior Checklist (CBCL) [17] to aid in the early collection of data. Other instruments such as the Conners questionnaires used by parents or teachers [18, 19] may be useful in the ongoing assessment for management of specific disorders such as attention-deficit hyperactivity disorder (ADHD). The Vanderbilt ADHD Rating Scale (VARS) is frequently used in the early assessment of children with these disorders, and has been shown to be useful in ruling out the presence of comorbid reading or spelling learning disabilities [20].

The Children's Interview for Psychiatric Symptoms (ChiPS) [21] is a screening tool that addresses some 20 Axis I entities. Respondent-based instruments rely upon responders to identify the presence or absence of symptoms. Besides the Conners scales, these include the Diagnostic Interview Schedule for Children (DISC) [22], the computer-assisted (but not the live version) Diagnostic Interview for Children and Adolescents (DICA) [23], and the pictorial DOMINIC-R [24], which is used with children under age 11.The specific utility of these instruments is discussed in the references [25] and in Chapters 2 and 8.

Perhaps the most studied diagnostic interviews for children are the K-SADS array (Schedule for Affective Disorders and Schizophrenia for School-Age children, or "Kiddie-SADS"). These interviews are designed to be administered by clinicians to children and parents, and the clinician is given latitude in reconciling the separate accounts, according to clinical judgment. The original K-SADS was developed from the adult SADS, but was designed for use with children and adolescents. The K-SADS presently in use include a number of variants (K-SADS-P-IVR, -E, -PL, and others) [26, 27]. The K-SADS array is designed to correlate with DSM-IV. The instruments can provide useful diagnostic information for conditions beyond schizophrenia and depression, including ADHD [28].

Psychological and Educational Evaluation

Psychological and educational evaluation are both discussed in subsequent chapters. Along with psychiatric evaluation, they stand as distinct and useful procedures that cannot be substituted for each other. Today, many patients who come to a child and adolescent psychiatrist have already been given psychological testing; the

results, as noted, can be useful information. Far fewer of these children have received an educational evaluation or prescription, which may be an extremely useful part of the child's assessment and rehabilitation, especially as psychiatric treatment progresses. In both cases, psychiatrists should present these assessments as opportunities to better understand a patient's assets and liabilities. Parents should not be led to believe that either the psychological or educational assessment will produce some sort of miraculous answer to chronic problems or that seeking them implies some failure or inadequacy on the part of them or the physician. Rather, these assessments are specialized procedures that hold unique value in understanding a child's cognitive structure, learning style, and educational needs. Projective testing can be useful in obtaining a deeper understanding of the patient's emotional substrate, especially early in the treatment of withdrawn or verbally inhibited children.

Laboratory Assessment

Laboratory assessment has become a much more frequent part of psychiatric evaluation in recent years (see also Chapter 3). Many patients of child and adolescent psychiatrists will have already undergone a comprehensive laboratory assessment, even including neuroimaging, by their referring physicians; the burden of further assessment of these patients is thus not borne by the psychiatrist.

Conversely, some patients will have had little if any laboratory workup, and such assessments may be indicated in an orderly, stepwise fashion. For example, patients might receive standard hematological and chemical screenings prior to more exotic endocrinological and nutritional assessments. Similarly, it is seldom appropriate to seek an expensive and complicated neuroimaging procedure in a patient who has not yet received a neurological examination.

Given both the immense progress in neuroimaging and the intense media coverage devoted to this progress in recent years, some patients and families will assume that procedures such as computed tomography (CT) or magnetic resonance imaging (MRI) scanning are an essential part of the psychiatric examination. This, of course, is frequently not the case. Clinicians may be best advised to deal with these demands by recognizing the underlying motivations of concern, anxiety, or entitlement that evoke these requests. At the same time, as physicians, child and adolescent psychiatrists must be aware of the infrequent but poignant circumstances in which gross central nervous system pathology, such as vascular malformations and space-occupying lesions, may manifest themselves.

Outcome of the Evaluation

Presentation of Findings and Recommendations to Parents and Referring Sources

In the past, some psychiatrists, perhaps out of a specialized conception of confidentiality, have been reluctant or even reclusive in sharing their findings with others. In some instances, this practice has even been directed to parents, who may have been told merely to continue bringing their child for treatment. Such positions were, thankfully, relatively unusual, and current demands for consumer orientation and accountability have since made them utterly untenable. Parents or guardians and referring professionals or agencies are entitled to a concise and comprehensible statement of findings and recommendations. The manner in which this information is delivered depends on the needs of the child and the relationship of the child to these individuals or agencies.

As noted earlier, parents approach psychiatric evaluation with a rich mixture of concerns, hopes, and fears, which often come to a head at the time of the counseling or informing interview. I have met parents who could give me a verbatim account of their contact years earlier with a professional regarding their child's status; the affective intensity of this moment sears it into memory. The fashion in which this powerful circumstance is addressed can profoundly affect the subsequent conduct of the patient's treatment. It is a truism that at such moments, parents may hear only the first thing told them. Indeed, it often may be enough in one interview to convey a single major piece of information and attempt thereafter to address its affective consequences. If a diagnostic impression or therapeutic recommendations are at all complicated, parents may need a frequent restatement of this content, perhaps accompanied by written or audiovisual supplements and aids. Many parents may require a series of contacts to fully understand and process this information. Given the restrictions in contact imposed by some care-management agencies, it may be helpful to incorporate into this process case managers or other professionals who have a relationship with the family. In my experience, however, the ultimate responsibility as well as the ultimate effectiveness in dealing with these issues for families resides with the diagnosing physician. It is therefore absolutely incumbent on child and adolescent psychiatrists to deal first and foremost with the affective consequences of whatever information is being presented. To fail to do so is not only inhumane but is likely to seriously compromise the subsequent physician-family relationship and the family's compliance with treatment recommendations. It should go without saying that all these considerations must also be addressed, in a developmentally appropriate fashion, in explaining the findings and recommendations to the child or adolescent as well.

Many psychiatric disorders of children have been addressed with varying degrees of accuracy in the public media, for example, conveying both conscious and unconscious expectations to parents. The child and adolescent psychiatrist must thus explore the specific meaning and implication of any diagnosis for a given family. Specific treatment recommendations may carry with them certain implications, any or all of which may amplify or exaggerate a parent's feelings of inadequacy or incompetence. Fears may arise in connection with specific treatment recommendations. The use and misuse of psychopharmacology has been pursued in excruciating detail and with variable accuracy by the media. In addition, certain religious and political groups have publicly pursued an agenda opposing psychopharmacology, often in an ill-advised and misinformed fashion. All this information can be on parents' minds. Concurrently, however, they or their children may see medication as a means of control or as a source of some sort of magical improvement.

Although many parents may see psychotherapy as a more benign intervention than somatic treatment, they may still have concerns or misconceptions about it. The usual recommendation for family involvement or family therapy may be interpreted by some parents as an indictment of their own actions. Psychotherapy, and the fashion in which it helps or cures, may also be a mystery to parents. A careful, thoughtful, and concise explanation of the rationale for psychotherapy should always be given. The explanation should include the indications for psychotherapy, the options of therapeutic methods and approaches applicable to a given situation, the manner in which psychotherapy can be expected to help, the role of the family in this therapy, and an estimate of duration and cost.

Treatment Planning

Treatment planning is considered in greater detail in Chapter 6. It is informed by a variety of considerations, including the specific disorders of the patient or family; the preferences, hopes, fears, and fantasies of the patient or family; and systemic availability and limitation of resources. A treatment plan must be developed that is both appropriate for the disorder under treatment and realistic in the context of patient and family wishes and resource limitations. In today's environment of care management for fiscal ends and with limited resources, clinicians may frequently be tempted to offer treatment plans that are suboptimal or even inadequate for the patient's needs. It is the professional and ethical responsibility of any physician, certainly including child and adolescent psychiatrists, to provide patients and families with a clear indication of the most clinically effective treatment recommendations – even if they are not economically feasible. McConville (see Chapter 6) offers a model of treatment planning that places interventions on separate continua of directivity and restrictiveness and allows for a sequential arrangement of multiple interventions.

Sharing Information with Other Physicians, Schools, and Agencies

Since many patients seek child and adolescent psychiatrists as a result of a referral from physicians, schools, or other agencies, information must frequently be shared regarding the patient's condition, prognosis, and treatment. It is axiomatic that information on any patient cannot be released without the expressed (and usually written) permission of the patient or, in the case of a minor, the patient's parents or legal guardian. Both the content of shared information and the manner in which it is communicated are matters of clinical judgment and practical wisdom, and should be discussed in advance with patients, families, or guardians. Information should be distributed only as requested, and psychiatrists should avoid automatic release of entire reports or clinical notes. These issues of confidentiality are especially complicated by third-party reimbursement. Many patients and families routinely authorize unlimited release of clinical information for the purpose of reimbursement, and in fact may be forced to do so. Unfortunately, this information can then become accessible to an almost unlimited number of individuals and organizations.

In general, referring sources should not be given detailed information about members of the family other than the patient. This is especially critical in educational settings, since many school records are virtually public documents. Much of the time, these dilemmas can be claimed or resolved before any records or reports are released by conversing with the professional or agency requesting information. The type of information shared with a referring physician may be very different from that shared with the school, however, in both content area and detail.

Referral sources sometimes pursue psychiatric evaluation of a child or adolescent in a conscious or unconscious attempt to gain information about the parents or other family members. Such requests, even when made with good intentions, are usually ethically indefensible. They are also logically suspect, since they seek information that arises from hearsay and surmises. An extreme example of this situation is when the child and adolescent psychiatrist is asked to comment on the fitness for child custody of a parent whom the psychiatrist has never met. Complying with such a request can embroil the psychiatrist in conflicts that make further engagement with the family impossible, while the child has been done no substantive good: The psychiatrist should be ready to discuss the specific needs of a child, however, irrespective of the particulars of physical setting.

Consultation, Collaboration, and Advocacy

Children's needs are addressed in our culture by a wide variety of people: parents, professionals, and educators, among others. Even in the case of the child with a major mental illness whose psychiatric needs may be paramount, it is usually impossible for a child and adolescent psychiatrist to function alone. The psychiatrist will therefore be asked to consult with other professionals and educators. (The manner of these consultations is discussed in Chapters 4, 5, 29 and 30.) Such consultation may be an intermittent advisory relationship, or it may involve ongoing collaboration wherein child and adolescent psychiatrists and other professionals interact in discipline-specific roles.

In today's environment of competition for social and educational resources, and of active intervention in the lives of children and families who are in danger, the child and adolescent psychiatrist has a special role of advocacy. This role may develop as a result of a request by a patient and family or the psychiatrist's perception that some special intervention or communication is required. Despite the changing and challenged role of physicians in our society, the child and adolescent psychiatrist can still be an important and potent agent in the workings of educational, social, and legal systems.

Conclusion

The child and adolescent psychiatrist has a unique role within medicine, providing diagnostic assessment, therapeutic services, consultation, and advocacy for children and their families. In a broad biopsychosocial context, child and adolescent psychiatrists attempt to best meet the needs of children and families by providing these services in a fashion informed by scientific rigor, personal sensitivity, and social responsibility. An encounter with the child and adolescent psychiatrist should provide clinical clarification, personal reassurance, and practical direction.

Appendix 1.1

Biological Development
0–24 months

0–2 months

Increasing organization of sleep patterns
Quantitative changes in brain developmet

    2–6 months

    Rapid growth of synapses
    Rapid increase in cerebral glucose metabolism
    Social smiling emerges
    Diurnal sleep–wake cycles emerge

18–20 months

Density of dendritic spines
   dercreases
Cerebral glucose metabolic rates
   reach adult levels
Increasing lateral and anterior-
   posterior cerebral specialization
   of language centers

    7–9 months

    Growth in head circumference with rapid cerebral growth
    Myelination of limbic system
    Enhanced associative pathways
    Improved inhibitory control of higher centers

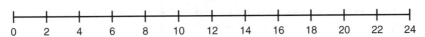

Figure 1.1 Biological development during the first two years of life.

Cognitive Development
0–24 months

0–2 months

Rapid development of olfactory and auditory recognition
Emergence of cross-modal fluency
Recognition of maternal face

    2–6 months

    Emergence of classical and operant conditioning
    Development of habituation

18–20 months

Development of
   symbolic representation
Emergence of personal pronouns
Pretend play is progressively
   other directed

    7–9 months

    Means-ends behavior develops
    Demonstration of object permanence
    Stranger reaction and separation protest appear
    Exploration of novel properties of objects
    Emergence of mastery motivation and symbolic play
    Emergence of the discovery of intersubjectivity

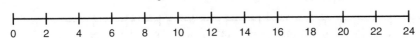

Figure 1.2 Cognitive development during the first two years of life.

Emotional Development
0–24 months

0–2 months

Maternal recognition of contentment
Maternal recognition of interest
Maternal recognition of distress

    2–3 months

    Differentiation of joy from contentment
    Differentiation of surprise from interest
    Differentiation of sadness, disgust, and anger

18–20 months

The Rapprochment crisis occurs
Emergence of embarrassment,
   empathy, and envy

        7–9 months

        Affect attunement
        Emergence of instrumental use of emotion
        Emergence of social referencing

          9–24 months

          Discriminates emotions by facial expressions
            and vocalizations

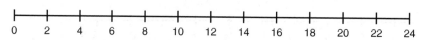

  0   2   4   6   8 10 12 14 16 18 20 22 24

Figure 1.3   Emotional development during the first two years of life.

Social Development
0–24 months

0–2 months

Interactive communication
   occurs
Stimulates social responses

7–9 months

Increasing evidence of intersubjectivity
Responds to caregiver empathy
Emergence of separation protest and
   stranger reactions

    2–3 months

    Vocalizations become social
    Emergence of turn taking in vocalizations
    Emergence of mutual limitation
    Emergence of sound localization
    Recognition of verbal affect

18–20 months

Words used for social functions
Language development
   enhances relatedness
Increased evidence of
   social relationships

    2–7 months

    Eye to eye contact begins
    Emergence of the social smile
    Emergence of social interaction
    Diminished crying

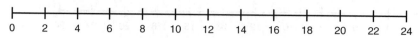

  0   2   4   6   8 10 12 14 16 18 20 22 24

Figure 1.4   Social development during the first two years of life.

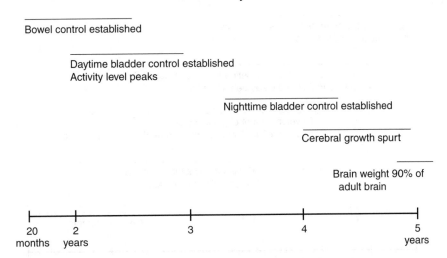

Figure 1.5   Biological development during the preschool years (20 months–5 years).

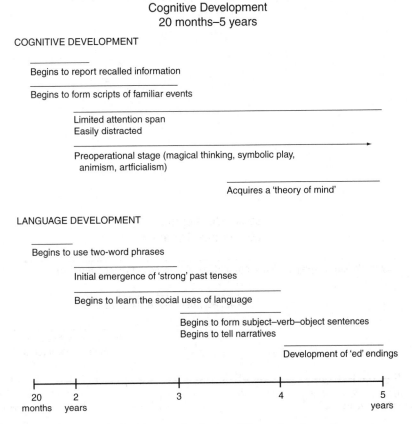

Figure 1.6   Cognitive development during the preschool years (20 months–5 years).

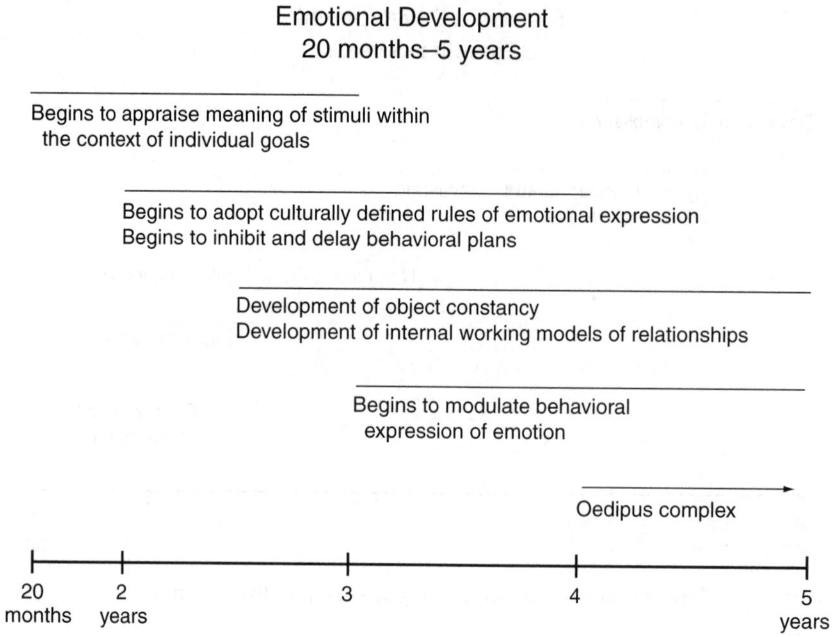

Emotional Development
20 months–5 years

Begins to appraise meaning of stimuli within
the context of individual goals

Begins to adopt culturally defined rules of emotional expression
Begins to inhibit and delay behavioral plans

Development of object constancy
Development of internal working models of relationships

Begins to modulate behavioral
expression of emotion

Oedipus complex

20   2   3   4   5
months   years   years

Figure 1.7   Emotional development during the preschool years (20 months–5 years).

Social Development
20 months–5 years

Play modalities develop (solitary, pretend, parallel, associative, cooperative)

Can act out role-specific behaviors

Social role behavior in
complementary roles

20   2   3   4   5
months   years   years

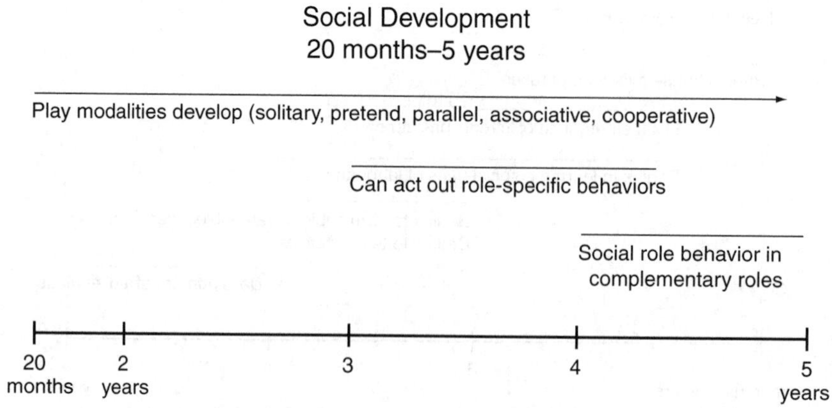

Figure 1.8   Social development during the preschool years (20 months–5 years).

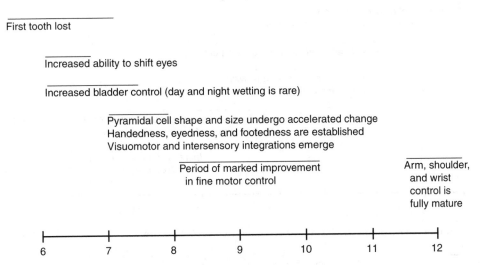

Biological Development
6–12 years

First tooth lost

Increased ability to shift eyes

Increased bladder control (day and night wetting is rare)

Pyramidal cell shape and size undergo accelerated change
Handedness, eyedness, and footedness are established
Visuomotor and intersensory integrations emerge

Period of marked improvement
in fine motor control

Arm, shoulder,
and wrist
control is
fully mature

6   7   8   9   10   11   12

Figure 1.9   Biological development in the school-age child (6–12 years).

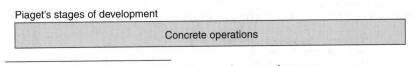

Cognitive Development
6–12 years

Piaget's stages of development

Concrete operations

Role learning, categorization, or elaboration to enhance performance

Switch from egocentric to social speech
Understanding of temporal sequences and the differences between
    day, time, and month emerges
Understanding of the conservation of material volume emerges
Make-believe play (role-playing)

Emergence of declarative memory
Ability to take another's point of view emerges
Shift from irreversible to reversible operations occurs
Ability to understand logical principles develops (e.g., reciprocity,
    classification, class inclusion, seriation, and number)

Increasing awareness of one's own abilities and
comprehension (or lack thereof)

Development of competence
motivation

6   7   8   9   10   11   12

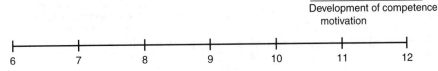

Figure 1.10   Cognitive development during the school-age child (6–12 years).

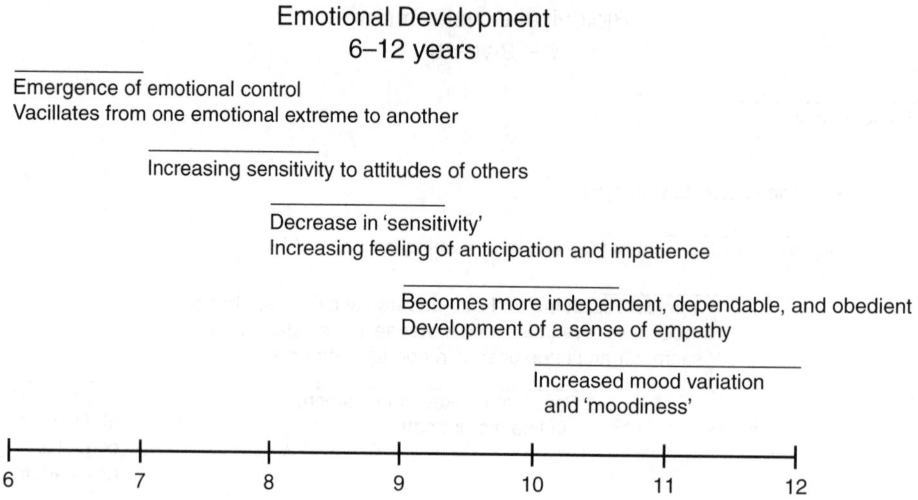

Emotional Development
6–12 years

Emergence of emotional control
Vacillates from one emotional extreme to another

Increasing sensitivity to attitudes of others

Decrease in 'sensitivity'
Increasing feeling of anticipation and impatience

Becomes more independent, dependable, and obedient
Development of a sense of empathy

Increased mood variation
and 'moodiness'

6   7   8   9   10   11   12

Figure 1.11   Emotional development during the school-age child (6–12 years).

Social Development
6–12 years

Understands that people can have multiple roles
Likes some social routines

Interested in secrets, collecting, and organized games and hobbies
Off-color humor emerges
Primarily unisex friendships
Explains actions by referring to events of immediate situation

Redefines status relationships with friends
Same-sex groupings prominent
Punchlines emerge in humor
Focus on peoples' physical appearances as opposed
     to their personality dispositions

Adoption of group's values, speech patterns, and manners
Strong peer group affiliation

Rise in social consciousness with
     respect to what is 'in'
Increased self-regulation
Best friends rise in importance

Understands that emotions have
     internal causes
Recognizes that people can have
     conflicting feelings and can sometimes
     mask true feelings

Relates actions to
     personality traits and feelings
Sees friends as people who
     understand each other and
     share thoughts and feelings

6   7   8   9   10   11   12

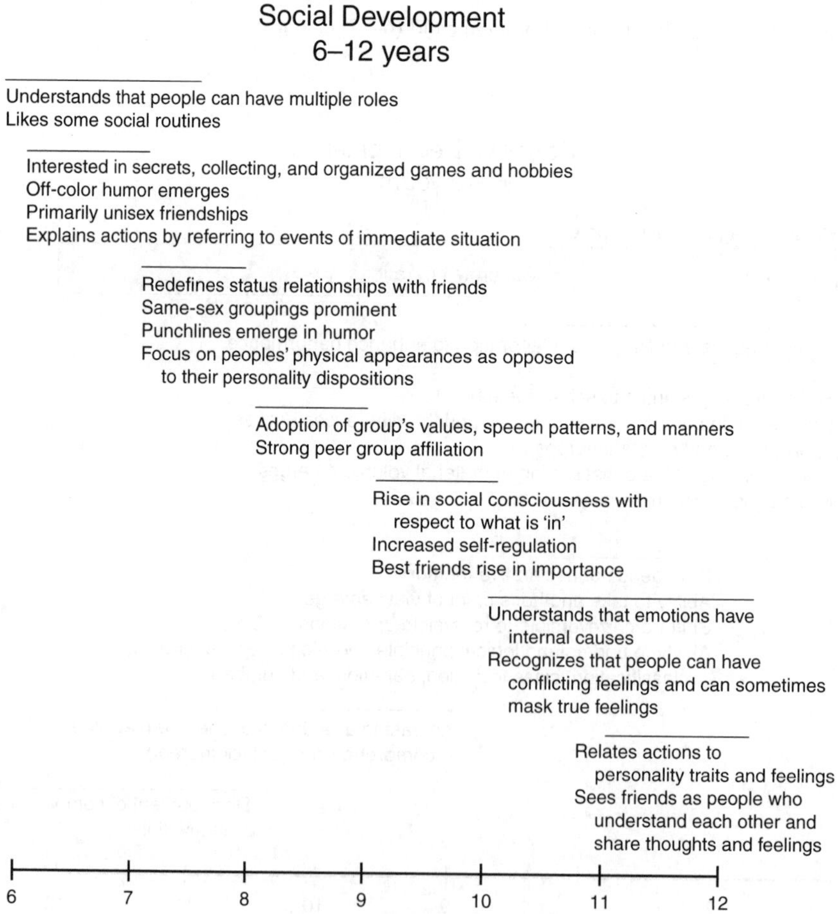

Figure 1.12   Social development during the school-age child (6–12 years).

Cognitive Development
13–18 years

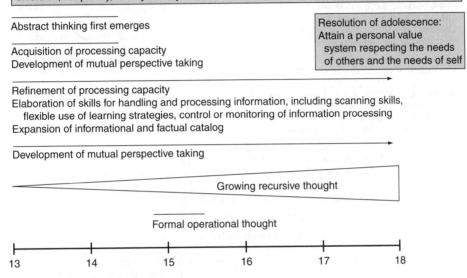

Figure 1.13   Cognitive development during the adolescent period (age 13–18 years).

Emotional Development
13–18 years

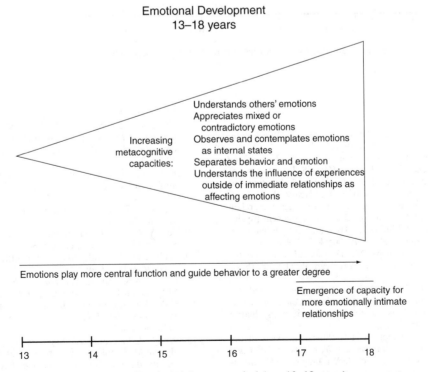

Figure 1.14   Emotional development during the adolescent period (age 13–18 years).

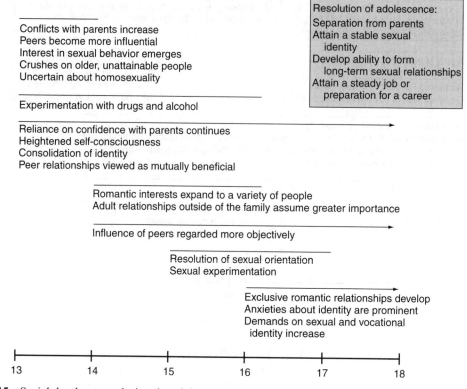

Social Development
13–18 years

Conflicts with parents increase
Peers become more influential
Interest in sexual behavior emerges
Crushes on older, unattainable people
Uncertain about homosexuality

Experimentation with drugs and alcohol

Reliance on confidence with parents continues
Heightened self-consciousness
Consolidation of identity
Peer relationships viewed as mutually beneficial

Romantic interests expand to a variety of people
Adult relationships outside of the family assume greater importance

Influence of peers regarded more objectively

Resolution of sexual orientation
Sexual experimentation

Exclusive romantic relationships develop
Anxieties about identity are prominent
Demands on sexual and vocational
identity increase

Resolution of adolescence:
Separation from parents
Attain a stable sexual
identity
Develop ability to form
long-term sexual relationships
Attain a steady job or
preparation for a career

13 14 15 16 17 18

Figure 1.15 Social development during the adolescent period (age 13–18 years).

References

1. Costello EJ, Pantino T. The new morbidity – Who should treat it? *Dev Behav Pediatr* 1987;**8**:288–291.
2. US Public Health, Service. *Mental Health: A Report of the Surgeon General.* Rockville, MD: US Department of Health and Human Services, National Institutes of Health, National Institute of Mental Health, 1999.
3. Costello EJ, Egger H, Angold A. 10-year research update review: the epidemiology of child and adolescent psychiatric disorders: I. Methods and public health burden. *J Am Acad Child Adolesc Psychiat* 2005;**44**:972–986.
4. Greenspan SI, Greenspan NT. *The Clinical Interview of the Child.* Washington, DC: American Psychiatric Press; 2003.
5. Kestenbaum CJ. The clinical interview of the child. In: Wiener JM (ed.) *Textbook of Child and Adolescent Psychiatry*, 2nd edn. Washington, DC: American Psychiatric Press, 1997; pp. 79–88.
6. King RA, Schowalter JE. The clinical interview of the adolescent. In: Wiener JM (ed.) *Textbook of Child and Adolescent Psychiatry*, 2nd edn.Washington, DC: American Psychiatric Press, 1997; pp. 89–94.
7. Lewis ME, King RA. Psychiatric assessment of infants, children. and adolescents. In: Lewis ME (ed.) *Child and Adolescent Psychiatry: A Comprehensive Textbook*, 3rd edn. Baltimore. MD: Williams & Wilkins, 2002; pp. 525–543.
8. Bostic JQ, King RA. Clinical assessment of children and adolescents: content and structure. In: Martin A, Volkmar FR (eds) *Lewis's Child and Adolescent Psychiatry: a Comprehensive Textbook*. Philadelphia: Lippincott Williams & Wilkins, 2007; pp. 232–343.
9. Satir V. *Conjoint Family Therapy: A Guide.* Palo Alto, CA: Science and Behavior Books, 1964.
10. Whitaker C. My philosophy of psychotherapy. *J Contemp Psychother* 1973;**6**:49–52.
11. Minuchin S. *Families and Family Therapy.* Cambridge. MA: Harvard University Press, 1974.
12. Haley J. Conducting the first interview. In: Haley J (ed.) *Problem-Solving Therapy.* San Francisco: Jossey Bass, 1976; pp. 9–47.
13. Wood JJ, Piacentini JC, Southam-Gerow M, Chu BC, Sigman M. Family cognitive behavioral therapy for child anxiety disorders. *J Am Acad Child Adolesc Psychiat* 2006;**45**:314–321.

14. American Academy of Child & Adolescent, Psychiatry. Practice parameter for the assessment of the family. *J Am Acad Child Adolesc Psychiat* 2007;**46**:922–937.
15. Angold A, Costello E. Nosology and measurement in child and adolescent psychiatry. *J Child Psychol Psychiat* 2009;**50**:9–15.
16. Thienemann M. Introducing a structured interview into a clinical setting. *J Am Acad Child Adolesc Psychiat* 2004;**43**:1057–1060.
17. Achenbach TM, Edelbrock CS. *Manual for the Child Behavior Checklist and Revised Child Behavior Profile*. Burlington, VT: University of Vermont Press, 1983.
18. Conners CK, Siarenios G, Parker JD, Epstein JN. The Revised Conners' Parent Rating Scale (CPRS-R): factor structure, reliability, and criterion validity. *J Abnorm Child Psychol* 1998;**26**:257–268.
19. Conners CK, Sitarenios G, Parker JD, Epstein JN. Revision and restandardization of the Conners Teaching Rating Scale (STRS-R): factor structure, reliability, and criterion validity. *J Abnorm Child Psychol* 1998;**26**:279–291.
20. Langberg JM, Vaughn AJ, Brinkman WB, Froehlich T, Epstein JN. Clinical utility of the Vanderbilt ADHD Rating Scale for ruling out comorbid learning disorders. *Pediatrics* 2010;**12**:e1033–e1038.
21. Weller E, Weller R, Fristad MA *et al.* Children's Interview for Psychiatric Syndromes (ChIPS). JT J Am Acad Child Adolesc Psychiat 2000;**39**:76–84.
22. Shaffer D, Fisher P, Lucas C, Dulcan MK, Schwab-Stone ME. NIMH Diagnostic Interview Schedule for Children Version IV (NIMH DISC-IV): description, differences from previous versions, and reliability of some common diagnoses. *J Am Acad Child Adolesc Psychiat* 2000;**39**:28–38.
23. Reich W. Diagnostic Interview for Children and Adolescents (DICA). *J Am Acad Child Adolesc Psychiat* 2000;**39**:59–66.
24. Valla JP, Bergeron L, Smolla N. The Dominic-R: a pictorial interview for 6- to 11-year-old children. *J Am Acad Child Adolesc Psychiat* 2000;**39**:85–93.
25. Myers K, Winters N. Ten-year Review of rating scales. I: Overview of scale functioning, psychometric properties, and selection. JT J Am Acad Child Adolesc Psychiat 2002;**41**:114–122.
26. Angold A, Costello EJ, Egger H. Structured interviewing. In Martin A, Volkmar FR (eds) *Lewis's Child and Adolescent Psychiatry: A Comprehensive Textbook*. Philadelphia: Lippincott Williams & Wilkins, 2007; pp. 344–357.
27. Birmaher B, Ehmann M, Axelson DA, *et al.* Schedule for affective disorders and schizophrenia for school-age children (K-SADS-PL) for the assessment of preschool children – A preliminary psychometric study. *J Psychiatr Res* 2009;**43**:680–686.
28. Rucklidge J. How good are the ADHD screening items of the K-SADS-PL at identifying adolescents with and without ADHD? *J Atten Disord* 2008;**11**:423–424.

2

Psychological Assessment of Children

Antoinette S. Cordell

Effective diagnosis and treatment planning requires a flexible approach to child assessment that includes data from multiple sources as well as parental involvement. Mooney and Harrison reported that those psychologists who see many children for school-related concerns address cognitive-academic or personalityissues but provide much less information on social influences and the context of the children's lives [1]. The most frequently used means of gathering information include the Wechsler, Rorschach, and Bender Gestalt tests, the Thematic Apperception Test (TAT), achievement tests, and drawings. There are limitations to the strictly intrapersonal perspective, however, since children should be understood within the context of their lives [1]. Assessment techniques should be broad and should include measures that draw on the child "in action." Psychological techniques suggested for this type of assessment include parent/teacher questionnaires, intelligence and achievement testing, drawings, projective testing, child questionnaires, behavioral assessment, play observations, and family interaction (see Appendix 2.1).

Parent/Teacher Questionnaires

The Eyberg Child Behavior Inventory is a straightforward 36-item questionnaire that can be completed by parents of children who are 2 to 7 years of age. The Eyberg is relatively simple to fill out and yields information on a wide variety of behavioral problems [2], including dawdling, defiance, and opposition, seeking attention and difficulty concentrating.

The Parenting Stress Index (PSI) by Abidin is filled out by parents of children ranging in age from 1 month to 12 years [3] (a short form is available). The PSI provides Child Domain scores for the following categories: distractibility/hyperactivity, adaptability, reinforcement of parents, demandingness, mood, and acceptability. In the Parent Domain, the categories include competence, isolation, attachment, health, role restriction, depression, and relationship with spouse. The Total Stress score combines both domains and allows for an analysis of the source of stress. This index, then, can be used to assess the degree to which the child's behavior is stressful versus the difficulty the parents have in adjusting to their parenting roles. PSI results are also helpful in communicating with parents; the clinician can report, for example, that the parents provided the information that they feel depressed or that they are experiencing communication barriers with their spouse. Parents are less likely to be defensive, and the clinician can be more reflective and understanding rather than intrusive (Figure 2.1).

The same authors headed by Sheras (1998) developed the Stress Index for Parents of Adolescents (SIPA), a questionnaire for parents that applies to teens aged 11 to 19 years [4]. Categories in the Adolescent Domain (AD) include: Moodiness/Emotional Lability (MEL); Social Isolation/Withdrawal (ISO); Delinquency/Antisocial (DEL); and Failure to Achieve or Persevere (ACH). In the Parent Domain, the following categories are assessed:Life Restrictions (LFR); Relationship with Spouse/Partner (REL); Social Alienation (SOC); and Incompetence/Guilt (INC). The Adolescent-Parent Relationship Domain (PRD) assesses the parent's view of the quality of the relationship that the parent has with the adolescent. Additional scales include the Life Stressors scale (LS) and an index of Total Parenting Stress (TS). Like the PSI, this tool is useful in assessing the parental perspective in raising an adolescent. The parent is able to provide information on their teen's behavior, their own assessment of their parenting, and the relationship between them.

The Child Behavior Checklist is completed by parents of children aged 4 to 16 years, and teachers complete the Teacher Report Form(TRF) for school-age children [5, 6]. The accompanying Youth Self-Report Scale is completed by youngsters aged

Clinical Child Psychiatry, Third Edition. Edited by William M. Klykylo and Jerald Kay.
© 2012 John Wiley & Sons, Ltd. Published 2012 by John Wiley & Sons, Ltd.

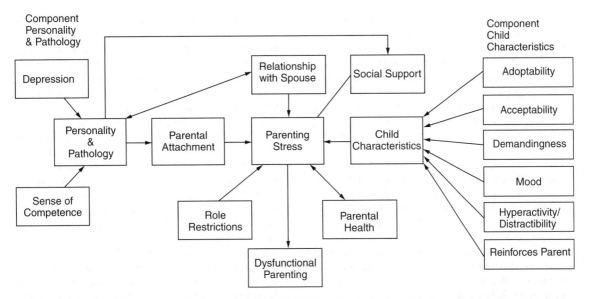

Figure 2.1 Reproduced by special permission of the Publisher, Psychological Assessment Resources, Inc., 16204 North Florida Avenue, Lutz, Florida 33549, from the Parenting Stress Index Professional Manual by Richard R. Abidin, Ed.D., Copyright 1983, 1990, and 1995 by PAR, Inc. Further reproduction is prohibited without permission of PAR, Inc.

from 11 to 18 years. These questionnaires have the advantage of providing a behavior profile that gives information on the following dimensions: Withdrawn; Somatic Complaints; Anxious/Depressed; Social Problems; Attention Problems; Delinquent Problems; and Aggressive Behavior. Separate forms are used for boys and girls in age groups 4 to 5, 6 to 11, and 12 to 16 years. The Children Behavior Checklist-Direct Observation form can also be used for structuring behavioral observations. There is also the Caregiver-Teacher Report Form for preschoolers aged 1½ to 5 years, to be filled out by the preschool teacher or caregiver in a daycare setting. This tool provides the clinician working with young children an additional perspective on the child's behavior and emotional needs in a structured setting outside of the home [7].

The Conners' Rating Scales-Revised provide teacher- and parent-rating scales and an adolescent self-report scale [8]. A new empirically based attention-deficit hyperactivity disorder (ADHD) index can be used to assess children at risk for ADHD. In addition, the McCarney Attention-Deficit Disorders Evaluation Scale condenses the three subscales of inattentiveness, impulsivity, and hyperactivity to two scales: inattentiveness and impulsivity/hyperactivity [9]. It is useful to have a measure of both of these characteristics in child evaluations since they have different implications for treatment. These

scales can also be used to assess improvements due to the use of psychoactive medication.

The Attachment Disorder Questionnaire developed by E.M. Randolph allows an assessment of the more problematic behaviors and traits of children who have reactive attachment disorder [10]. Items include statements such as "My child uses his/her 'cuteness' or charm to get others to do what he/she wants"; "My child goes up to strangers and becomes overly affectionate with them or asks to go home with them"; "My child is cruel to animals or other people." This questionnaire can be helpful in identifying the nature and severity of the child's symptoms.

Cognitive Assessment

Kaufman and Ishikuma presented a model for intelligence and academic testing that allows the clinician to combine test administration with an in-depth understanding of human development [11]. The goal is to assist individuals in addressing their problems and to improve their functioning, rather than to limit them via labeling or diagnosing.

Intelligence testing is both overrated and underrated. Many people place too much emphasis on intelligence quotient (IQ) scores per se. It is important to realize that psychological tests provide a wide range of information regarding strengths, weaknesses, learning style, and needs. There are many personal qualities that intelligence tests do not measure, however, such as creativity, determination, and persistence over a period of time. As a result, many individuals who score high on IQ tests perform below this level of expectation, and others who score at more modest levels nonetheless accomplish many fine and far-reaching goals. It has never been possible to capture the inventiveness of the human spirit on paper!

There are many factors other than difficulties with intellectual functioning that can lead to low IQ scores. Factors such as cultural or linguistic differences, distractibility or anxiety, refusal to cooperate, and disabling conditions such as autism and deafness can all limit a person's ability to perform the tasks on an IQ test. Research has shown that the norms for intelligence tests become dated over time and that IQ scores gradually drift upward. When current norms are used, a child's score may be slightly lower [12].

Intelligence tests give a wide range of information about children's abilities in several areas of functioning. Wechsler considered intelligence a combination of abilities reflecting an overall level of intellectual capability. The newly revised Wechsler Intelligence Scale for Children – Fourth Edition (WISC-IV) provides subtest and composite scores in specific areas as well as an overall cognitive score representing general intellectual ability (i.e., Full Scale IQ) [12]. This revised edition has updated norms, new subtests, and greater emphasis on discrete domains of cognitive functioning. It is easier to administer and score. The revisions were based on research findings on cognitive development and intellectual assessment. Ten subtests have been retained from the WISC-III, and there are five new subtests (Picture Concepts, Letter-Number Sequencing, Matrix Reasoning, Cancellation, and Word Reasoning). The subtests of the WISC-IV cover a wide variety of abilities that can contribute to successful performance in school. For a 16-year-old whose ability is above average, the Wechsler Intelligence Scale-IV test for adults may be most appropriate (http://www.pearsonassessments.com/HAIWEB/Cultures/en-us/Productdetail.htm?Pid=015-8980-808).

The Wechsler Preschool and Primary Scale of Intelligence-III (WPPSI-III) offers an assessment of the intelligence of children aged from 2 years 6 months through 7 years 3 months [13]. Like the other Wechsler tests, it provides an overall cognitive score as well as scores for verbal and performance abilities. A major advantage of the WPPSI-III is that it follows the same structural format and philosophy as the WISC-IV. The seven core subtests are: Block Design; Information; Matrix Reasoning; Vocabulary; Picture Concepts; Word Reason-

ing; and Coding. There are seven supplemental subtests: Symbol Search; Comprehension; Picture Completion; Similarities; Receptive Vocabulary; Object Assembly; and Picture Naming. For a 6-year-old child whose ability is below average, the best choice for intelligence testing may be the Wechsler Preschool and Primary Scale of Intelligence-III (WPPSI-III).

One of the advantages of ability testing is that it provides us with information on the pattern of strengths and weaknesses that can affect the student's ability to function in the classroom. It gives information to the educator about the special needs and learning style of the student. In clinical practice, several findings can be significant. When there is a low score on the Coding subtest relative to the other scores, for example, the child often has difficulty with handwriting and motor performance in the classroom. Some children may exhibit only this single deficit. These children struggle greatly to perform written work in the classroom, particularly in the primary grades, and are often labeled as "lazy," when in fact their neurological processing proceeds at a different rate than that of other children in the classroom. The Similarities subtest scores can be quite important, since they relate specifically to abstract reasoning and what we commonly consider overall intelligence. All of the areas assessed on the WISC-IV, however, are relevant for understanding the child's functioning in the classroom (Table 2.1 and Figure 2.2).

Children who have marked discrepancies between verbal and performance IQ scores can experience difficulty functioning in the classroom. Any child who has a severe deficit may be affected severely, even if many other subtest scores are average or above average. Children with high verbal scores but low performance scores struggle with the production of work in the classroom. Children with high performance scores and low verbal scores are often impulsive, action-oriented individuals who have difficulty reflecting or using language to process their experience. The psychologist should look for unique patterns of strengths and weaknesses and attempt to understand them in relation to the overall functioning and personality of the child.

Table 2.1 Abbreviations of composite scores.

Composite Score	Abbreviation
Verbal Comprehension Index	VCI
Perceptual Reasoning Index	PRI
Working Memory Index	WMI
Processing Speed Index	PSI
Full Scale IQ	FSIQ

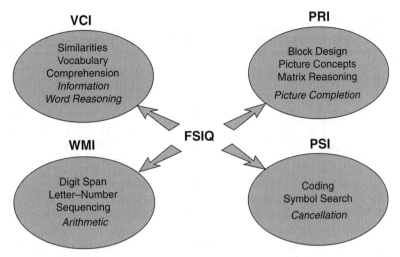

Note: Supplemental subtests are shown in italics

Figure 2.2 WISC-IV test framework.

Some children, such as the learning disabled (LD)/gifted child, have complex combinations of cognitive abilities. There appear to be multiple patterns of scores for LD/gifted students. One pattern involves high reasoning/verbal abilities with deficiencies in performance abilities or slow fine-motor coordination (shown by a low Coding score); there may also be difficulties with attention span and focusing. Another pattern is high performance abilities combined with a low verbal score; this pattern may be particularly difficult to identify, because we usually rely on children's verbal functioning as an overall indication of high intelligence. Another pattern is characterized by a relatively high overall IQ but a high degree of distractibility. In the classroom, several areas of special needs should be addressed, including distractibility, slowness in handling written work, difficulty with organization, emotional lability, and negative self-concept [14].

How does ADHD affect intelligence test results? No conclusive battery of tests exists for this disorder. ADHD children often score low on one or more subtests of the WISC-IV, including Arithmetic, Coding, Information, and Digit Span. The Freedom from Distractibility factor is not a pathognomonic indicator of ADHD, however. There is tremendous variability in the relative abilities of children with ADHD, and ADHD thus negatively affects performance on structured tests in varied ways. Further, ADHD symptoms present in several childhood disorders. Suggestions for diagnosis include using a variety of assessment instruments to improve convergent validity as well as taking a thorough history from multiple sources if possible.

Believe your data. Carefully review intratest and intertest scatter, behavioral observations as the child approaches tasks, and unusual errors; work hard to communicate to others the importance of your assessment data for intervention and treatment planning.

The Stanford–Binet Intelligence Scale–Fourth Edition yields scores for Verbal Reasoning, Abstract/Visual Reasoning, Quantitative Reasoning, and Short-Term Memory [15]. The current edition includes many performance items and so has addressed earlier criticism of the Binet that it was too verbally oriented. Using either the WISC-IV or the Binet to ascertain strengths can provide useful information for guiding an individual in school and in making later career choices. Our schools tend to be highly verbally and language oriented. Not all careers require such a strong emphasis in this area; some use performance abilities, for example. It is often difficult for the classroom teacher to realize the ability areas of children who exhibit low verbal and language abilities but stronger performance abilities.

The Leiter International Performance Scale-Revised has the strong advantage of being a nonverbal test of intelligence [16]. It can be used to evaluate children with sensory or motor deficits or language problems, or those who speak a different language from the examiner. It contains 54 tests from levels II to XIV and takes 30 to 45 minutes to complete. The tests involve arranging a series of blocks initially from pairings of colors, shapes, and objects to analogies, perceptual patterns, and concepts at later levels. Instructions are given in pantomime. The Leiter has recently been revised and may thus address uneven item difficulty at various levels. This test is certainly

Table 2.2 Comparison chart.

	Leiter-R	WISC-IV	WPPSI-III	SB-4	WJ-R
Completely nonverbal	Yes	No	No	No	No
Domains measured					
Visualization	Yes	Yes[1]	Yes[1]	Yes	Yes[1]
Reasoning	Yes	Yes[1]	Yes[1]	Yes	Yes[1]
Memory	Yes	Yes[1]	No	Yes	Yes
Attention	Yes	No	No	No	Yes[1,4]
'Growth' scores	Yes	No	No	No	Yes[6]
Age range	2–21	6–16	3–7	2–90	2–90
Appropriate for					
Cognitive delay	Yes	Yes[3]	Yes[3]	Yes[3]	Yes
ESL	Yes	No	No	No	No
Limited English	Yes	No	No	No	No
Learning disabilities	Yes	Yes	Yes	Yes	Yes
ADHD	Yes	Yes	No	Yes	Yes
Deafness	Yes	No[5]	No[5]	No[5]	No[5]
TBI	Yes	No[5]	No	Yes[4,5]	Yes[4,5]
Communication disorders	Yes	Yes[5]	No	No[5]	No[5]
Diverse cultures	Yes	No[5]	No[5]	No[5]	No[5]
Motor impaired	Yes	Yes[2,5]	Yes[2,5]	Yes[2,5]	Yes[2,5]
Fast screening	Yes	No	No	No	No

1 Some subtests measure related areas, but require hearing, language, reading or motor skills.
2 Verbal skills only.
3 Restricted lower bound of IQ ranges.
4 Some areas, but not the complete spectrum provided in Leiter-R.
5 Adjusted administration required.
6 Uses Rasch modeling to derive other special scores.
ADHD = Attention deficit hyperactivity disorder; ESL = English as a second language; Leiter-R = Leiter – Revised; SB-4 = Stanford–Binet – 4th Edition; TBI = traumatic brain injury; WISC-III = Wechsler Intelligence Scale for Children – 3rd Edition; WJ-R = Woodcock–Johnson – Revised; WPPSI-R = Wechsler Preschool and Primary Scale of Intelligence – Revised.
From Leiter RG: *Leiter International Performance Scale – Revised.* Wood Dale, IL: Stoelting; 1997.

less culturally loaded than other IQ tests, but there is no evidence on whether it is "free" of cultural bias (Table 2.2).

A quick assessment of intelligence is provided by the Kauffman Brief Intelligence Test (K-BIT) [17]. This can be used for children, adolescents, and adults from the ages of 4 to 90 years. The test has the advantage of taking between 15 to 30 minutes to administer with only two subtests including Vocabulary and Matrices. It appears to be useful for establishing a baseline of intelligence but does not provide in-depth information on strengths and weaknesses. Specifically, the many difficulties with cognitive functioning that a child or adult may show may not be revealed. The use of the K-BIT, therefore, is limited from a clinical perspective.

Another relatively brief assessment of capability is found in the Peabody Picture Vocabulary Test – Third Edition (PPVT-III) [18]. This test is designed to measure receptive vocabulary over a wide range using a friendly approach. The subject is shown four pictures and given a single word. The child then indicates either verbally or nonverbally which picture best represents that word. The simplicity of the test is useful in some situations when a more comprehensive assessment might not be possible, and it may enhance the likelihood of cooperation as well.

The Woodcock–Johnson-III Tests of Achievement (WJ-III) [19] and the Wechsler Individual Achievement Test – Third Edition [20] provide information on basic academic skills. Learning disabilities are defined as major discrepancies between IQ level and tested academic skills. Some children, however, experience significant learning problems in the classroom but do not show such severe discrepancies. The field of education is moving toward a team-based method of assessing learning problems and special educational needs, but individual psychoeducational testing should remain an integral part of this assessment process.

IQ scores should never stand alone in patients being diagnosed for developmental disabilities or mental retardation. Rather, clinicians should consider the pattern of strengths and weaknesses on IQ tests, assess adaptive and other behaviors, and use common sense.

When assessing a child, it is important to seek multiple sources of data, including information on the child's personal and social sufficiency at home, at school, and in the community. The Vineland-II Adaptive Behavior Scales can be used to measure communication, daily living skills, socialization, and motor skills in children from birth to 18 years 11 months of age or in low-functioning adults [21]. The scales can be used for handicapped individuals as well. The Vineland requires a respondent who is familiar with the individual's behavior. The survey form contains 297 items, although only those items necessary to establish basal and ceiling levels are used. The test takes 20 to 30 minutes to administer and yields useful information on strengths and weaknesses in adaptive behavior.

Two additional tools may be helpful. First, the Achievement Identification Measure by S. Rimm can be used to assess underachievement [22]. It identifies students who are performing in school below their ability level. Some may be sliding through on the basis of "brains," not effort, whereas others may be in the early stages of underachievement before it has been noted on their report card. The scale measures six dimensions of adaptive attitudes toward academic competition, responsibility, control, achievement, communication, and respect – as well as a total score that reflects a child's overall potential for success in school. Second, Light's Retention Scale can assist in objectifying the issues involved in retaining a child below his or her grade level [23]. This can be a difficult, emotional process of decision-making, so it helps to have a systematic method of weighing the facts. In addition, the book *Summer Children: Ready or Not for School* can be reviewed [24].

Neuropsychological assessment for children has recently been expanded (see Chapter 25). Such tests as the NEPSY-II (Developmental Neuropsychological Assessment) demonstrate enhanced clinical utility compared to some older instruments. The NEPSY-II provides useful clinical information on areas of deficit, for treatment plans and school interventions. Six domains can be assessed with the NEPSY-II: Attention and Executive Function; Language; Memory and Learning; Social Perception; Sensorimotor; and Visuospatial Processing [25].

Drawings

DiLeo acknowledged that interpreting children's drawings requires more than one approach to understanding [26]. In the correlational approach, data are collected and statistically analyzed to determine any correlation between a characteristic in the drawing and the significance that the clinician attaches to it. In the longitudinal approach, the clinician performs an in-depth study of the patient and examines the relationship between characteristics shown in the patient's drawings and the patient's behavior and overall development.

Clinicians use subjectivity as well as a backlog of clinical experience in interpreting children's drawings. This process involves generating hypotheses to be tested with the use of other data and behavioral observations. Drawings should never be used by themselves to establish clinical "facts."

The age and developmental level of the child need to be considered in the interpretation of drawings, and the clinician should be familiar with what is normative for specific developmental levels. Preschool children, for example, often fail to integrate parts into a whole, but this failure is abnormal in an older child. Developmental milestones and stage-dependent theories have been presented by Freud, Erickson, Piaget, and Gesell.

Drawing characteristics that have interpretive significance include the use of space; the quality of line; orientation; shading (as an indicator of anxiety); integration of the human figure drawings, symmetry, and balance; and style. Drawings are also reflective of cognitive development. The drawing of a person "yields an overview of intellectual maturity" [26]. House drawings give information about the change from an egocentric to an objective view (Table 2.3; see also Appendix 2.2).

DiLeo discussed several pitfalls in the analysis of drawings, including inconsistency in drawing performance [26]. When features appear consistently in several drawings, there is a great likelihood that they have been integrated into the child's concept. Particularly when working with young children, therefore, the clinician should obtain several drawing specimens. Another pitfall is to assign excessive weight to specific details. It is important to use a holistic approach and examine the overall impression of the drawing and to appreciate that environmental factors, such as the season of the year or specific holidays, influence the content of children's drawings. DiLeo cautions against overinterpreting ambiguous sexual symbols in the drawings of young children or using a mechanistic, point-by-point analysis [16]. It should be recognized that drawings can be misleading.

For the Kinetic Family Drawing (KFD), the child is asked to "draw a picture of everyone in your family,

Table 2.3   Development of drawing related to Piaget's stages of cognitive development – A synoptic view.

Approximate age (yr)	Drawing	Cognition
0–1	*Reflex response to visual stimuli.* Crayon is brought to mouth; the infant does not draw.	*Sensorimotor stage* Infant acts reflexively, thinks motorically.
1–2	At 13 months, the first scribble appears: zig-zag. Infant watches movement leaving its marks on a surface. Kinesthetic drawing.	Movement gradually becomes goala directed as cortical control is gradually established.
2–4	Circles appear and gradually predominate. Circles then become discrete. In a casually drawn circle, the child envisages an object. A first graphic symbol has been made, usually between three and four years.	The child begins to function symbolically. Language and other forms of symbolic communication play a major role. The child's view is highly egocentric. Make-believe play.
4–7	*Intellectual realism* Draws an internal model, not what is actually seen. Draws what is known to be there. Shows people through walls and through hulls of ships. Transparencies. Expressionistic. Subjective.	*Preoperational stage* (intuitive phase) Egocentric. Views the world subjectively. Vivid imagination. Fantasy. Curiosity. Creativity. Focuses on only one trait at a time. Functions intuitively, not logically.
7–12	*Visual realism* Subjectivity diminishes. Draws what is actually visible. No more X-ray technique (transparencies). figures are more realistic, proportioned. Colors are more conventional. Distinguishes right from left side of the figure drawn.	*Concrete operations stage* Thinks logically about things. No longer dominated by immediate Human perceptions. Concept of reversibility: things that were the same remain the same though their appearance may have changed.
12 +	With the development of the critical faculty, most lose interest in drawing. The gifted tend to persevere. concrete aspects of a situation.	*Formal operations stage* Views his/her products critically. Able to consider hypotheses. Can think about ideas, not only about.

From DiLeo JH: *Interpreting Children's Drawings.* New York: Brunner/Mazel; 1983:38.

including you, doing something. Try to draw whole people, not cartoons or stick people. Remember to make everyone doing something – some kind of action." [27]. The child is given a plain white $8\frac{1}{2} \times 11$-inch piece of paper with a No.2 pencil placed in the center of the paper and is seated individually in a chair at a table of appropriate height. The examiner leaves the room and checks back periodically. Noncompliance is extremely rare. If children say "I can't," they are encouraged periodically and left in the room until they complete the KFD.

Characteristics of individual figures that are analyzed in the KFD include arm extensions, elevated figures, erasures, figures on the back of the page, hanging, omission of body parts, omission of figures, eyes, and rotated figures. The action depicted is also analyzed in terms of intensity, symbolism, fixation, conflict, internal-

ization, avoidance, and harmony. The mean age for both boys and girls performing the KFD is about 10 years, and ages range from 5 to 20 years, skewed toward the "10 and below" age group. Data are also available elsewhere on the actions of individual KFD figures and the frequency of actions for various family members, including father, mother, and self [27]. One should also consider the type of action between KFD figures, such as throwing balls, and the existence of barriers, dangerous objects, or heat, light, and warmth. Drawing styles can be categorized as compartmentalization, encapsulation, lining at the bottom, underlying individual figures, edging, lining at the top, folding compartmentalization, and evasions.

In addition to the Draw-A-Person test (DAP) and the KFD, the House-Tree-Person test (HTP) developed by J. Buck in 1948 can also be revealing [28]. In this approach, the house is viewed primarily as a reflection of the home environment and family functioning, the tree is viewed as a reflection of psychosexual-psychosocial history, and the person is viewed as a reflection of interpersonal functioning and relationships with others. The HTP can be used for children aged 5 or 6 years, although some children of this age may not be mature enough in terms of their drawings skills. One major advantage of this test is that it uses a projective technique that taps into unconscious behavior and cannot be faked, except possibly to "fake bad." (It is considered unlikely that individuals can "fake good.")

Drawings are useful for children to express their feelings regarding their parents' divorce. Cordell and Bergman-Meador suggested that having children "draw a picture of [their] family divorcing" can help them express underlying attitudes regarding the divorce as well as their attitudes or misconceptions about the process [29]. The four rating scales are denial/acknowledgement, emotionality, aggression, and the use of people. Children's divorce drawings can be rated "0" or "1" for the absence or presence of each of these four items (Figures 2.3 and 2.4).

Characteristics of children's drawings can point to underlying fears and concerns that may be related to coping styles such as repression or sensitization. This technique can be used in initial assessments for treatment during the therapy process or for court-ordered evaluations regarding custody or visitation.

Projective Testing

Projective tests have received extensive criticism, because they are based on theories of unconscious internal processes and are therefore difficult to establish in terms of reliability and validity. According to Klein, the most commonly used projective tests are the following [30]:

- Rorschach
- Thematic Apperception Test (TAT)
- Children's Apperception Test (CAT)
- Blackey Pictures Drawings
- Bender Gestalt Test

Klein discussed the origin of projective tests from psychoanalytic theory, which interprets all human experiences as colored by unconscious repressed mental content [30]. More intrapsychic material can be expected during ambiguous tasks. Projective techniques provide the individual with an ambiguous stimulus, and the individual's response is thought to reflect underlying conflicts, needs, and features of personality. Klein argued that projective testing cannot pinpoint types of personality organization, specific personality characteristics, or the diagnosis of mental disorders [30]. Further,

the TAT has failed to show satisfactory validity, and in her view too little work has been done with the Rorschach to assess its validity with children. Given our state of knowledge, it is certainly not justified to rely on projective test results to rule out the presence of disorders when symptoms are evident, or to assume from the tests that personality deviance is present when it is not shown in the child's behavior. For diagnosis, Klein maintained that projective tests are not useful except in instances of mental retardation and specific developmental disorders. She maintained that when test results can be used accurately to diagnose, the deviance may already be obvious [30]. Similarly, it is unreliable to reconstruct the child's early developmental psychological history based on projective tests or to use projective tests to predict what is likely to happen to a child.

Despite the strength of the previous criticism, projective tests are used extensively. So what is the usefulness of these procedures? Projective tests can first and foremost provide a structured format for assessing a child's reactions and observing his or her behavior. It takes the focus off the child and the need for verbal response and instead allows the child to engage in action-oriented activity. Thus, the child can be more comfortable and spontaneous. Second, projective tests allow the psychologist to understand more about the individual child's worldview. The Rorschach provides information on processing, and the TAT provides information on interpersonal relationships. Third, the structural approach, as exemplified by Exner, fulfills criteria of the scientific method [31]. Projective information can be useful in planning the treatment process and in identifying important goals and effective strategies.

Projective tests appear to be particularly useful for children who are anxious or depressed or who have a history of abuse and neglect. One area in which projective tests can be quite misleading, however, is in the assessment of children with conduct disorders. From a clinical perspective, these children often have projective test responses that reflect a wide range of feelings and reactions and do not seem substantially different from those of children with other diagnoses. Their responses may not necessarily reveal the characteristics that could be considered indicators of conduct disorder. In fact, "projective techniques do not enjoy widespread use for conduct disorders" (ref. 32, p. 301) This may be unfortunate, because the child's worldview can still significantly affect the treatment process.

Exner and Weiner discussed the nature of the Rorschach test and on what basis Rorschach interpretations can be justified [33]. The Rorschach was developed as a psychodynamic reflection of personality. It is now viewed as a "perceptual-cognitive task," however, and

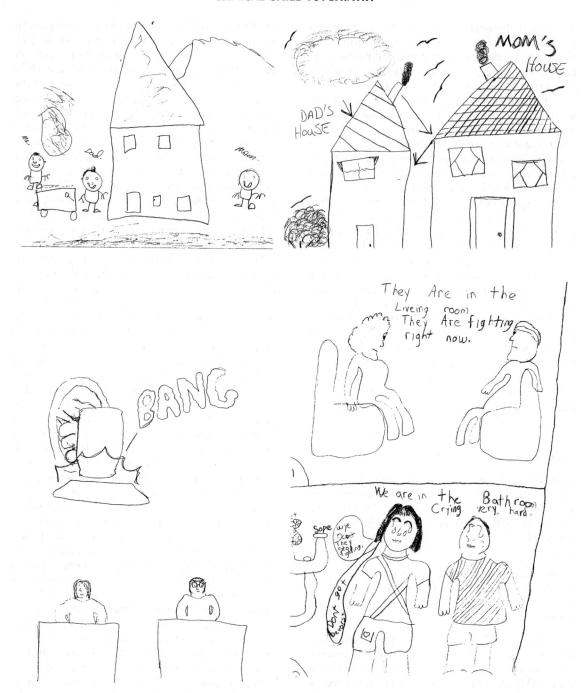

Figure 2.3 (a), seven-year-old boy, Scale I – acknowledgment, 0 = no direct reference to divorce; (b), 13-year-old girl, Scale I – acknowledgment, 1 = divorce clearly acknowledged; (c), 12-year-old boy, Scale II – emotionality, 0 = no emotion directly depicted; (d), seven-year-old girl, Scale II – emotionality, 1 = emotion shown.

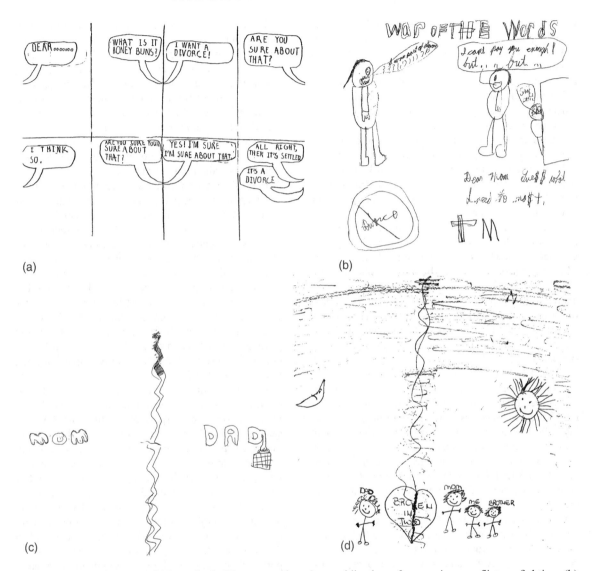

Figure 2.4 (a), nine-year-old boy, Scale III – aggression, 0 = no idication of aggression, conflict, or fighting; (b), 11-year-old boy, Scale III – aggression, 1 = aggression, conflict, or fighting depicted; (c), 12-year-old girl, Scale IV – use of people, 0 = no people pictured; (d), teenage girl, Scale IV – use of people, 1 = people pictured.

we can be more certain in our interpretation of the Rorschach results. When the Rorschach is viewed as a perceptual-cognitive task, the ink blots are considered an ambiguous source of stimulation on which the client imposes structure and organization; interpretations are based on the structure of how individuals process stimuli. Rorschach scoring allows us to derive data on how individuals perceive and respond to their environment. We can then draw inferences about personality functioning, including traits, dispositions, coping styles, and sources of concern that lend consistency to individual behavior.

When interpreting the Rorschach, clinicians need to be aware of situational and developmental factors that influence the stability of the Rorschach indices. Rorschach results generally give a picture of stable personality characteristics. The results are also representative of behavior; the task presented on the test is a sample of behavior, and behavior is the best predictor of future behavior. Interpretations of the Rorschach are reasonably certain and require "very few levels of inference" [33].

When the Rorschach is viewed as a stimulus to fantasy, different guidelines are applied in the analysis, and interpretations may be based on Rorschach content. What individuals say as they respond with images is particularly revealing. Content interpretations come from the language or words that the individuals use and can be used to address personality dynamics; in this sense, Rorschach responses can also be viewed as symbolic of behavior. Interpretations should be relatively speculative and phrased only as hypotheses. Interpreters should remember that the two forms of interpretation have differing levels of certainty.

Special consideration should be used to guide the evaluation of Rorschach records obtained from younger clients. Knowledge of the normative data is critical. The proper procedures must be used in collecting the data, and the interpreters working with children should have a solid understanding of developmental psychology and developmental psychopathology. (Exner and Weiner argued, however, that "Rorschach behavior means what it means regardless of the age of the subject" [33].)

The TAT requires patients to examine picture cards and then devise stories inspired by the cards. Henry's book *The Analysis of Fantasy* described how stories reflect thought processes as well as emotional functioning [34]. The interpretation of thematic apperception uses the overlapping frameworks of private, or less conscious, motives and the public, more conscious approach to social interactions. Thus, the stories are derived from personal experiences as translated into our social world [34].

Individuals learn societal expectations through a series of daily interactions in which skills and feelings are required. As individuals learn to conform to these expectations, they develop and organize their own personality. Their personality receives and processes the demands of social interaction and is also projected outward onto behavior, including responding to the TAT cards, for example. Telling stories is similar to the tasks involved in typical social interactions; in other words, the individual responds to the pictures in terms of both personal significance and "cultural training." People respond to the TAT pictures according to their own techniques of adapting to emotions and social demands as well as the manifest content and latent content of the pictures. For some people, the form and content of the picture draw emotional reactions that are termed the latent stimulus of the picture. Thus, the TAT is able to produce material that reflects the deeper emotional issues of the individual as stories are told.

Henry discussed analyzing TAT stories in terms of form, content, and dynamic structure, including the interpretation of symbolic content [34]. In the conceptual framework for individual case analysis, Henry considered several areas: mental approach, imaginative processes, family dynamics, inner adjustment, emotional reactivity, sexual adjustment, behavioral approach, and descriptive interpretive summary [34].

Children generally enjoy the TAT because they find it relatively undemanding and nonthreatening. Some 5- and 6-year-olds can handle the TAT cards, as opposed to the CAT. Stories are often a transparent reflection of a child's point of view. Occasionally, a child will exclaim, "This is just like me!" In these instances, children typically proceed comfortably with their storytelling. The TAT is a popular technique clinically. It may bias toward stimulating negatively toned stories, however, and the cards themselves are somewhat dated.

The Roberts Apperception Test for Children (RATC) is also a popular projective test to aid in assessing the psychological development of children [35]. The RATC was specifically designed for children aged 6 through 15 years and depicts children in all 16 of the cards. The current set of stimulus cards was drawn up in 1968 and later compared by Roberts to the Children's Apperception Test and the Thematic Apperception Test. The cards are realistic drawings of children and adults engaged in everyday interpersonal events. The RATC is easily scored with objective measures and a high degree of agreement between raters. Its goal is to assess children's perceptions of interpersonal situations. The scoring system assesses both adaptive and maladaptive traits. There is both qualitative and quantitative interpretation, so structural analysis is possible. There are normative data for a sample of 200 well-adjusted children aged 6 through 15 years. The categories depicted on the cards include: Family Confrontation; MaternalSupport; School Attitude; Support/Aggressions; Parental Affection; Peer/Racial Interaction; Dependency/Anxiety; Family Conferences; Physical Aggression toward Peer; Sibling Rivalry; Fear; Parental Conflict/Depression; Aggression Release; Maternal Limit-Setting; Nudity/Sexuality; and Paternal Support.

The CAT was designed for children aged 3 to 10 years and was inspired by the TAT [36]. It was hypothesized that children would identify easily with animal figures. A set of 10 pictures of animals in a variety of situations is used with an *apperception* method that studies personality by examining individual differences in response to standard stimuli and the dynamic significance of these differences. The CAT provides data on how children relate to the key individuals in their life and to their own needs. The cards stimulate issues related to eating, sibling rivalry, relationships to parents as individuals and as a couple, aggression, acceptance of the adult world, loneliness at night, and toileting.

Like the TAT, the CAT is concerned with content and what children see and think. The developers of the CAT acknowledge that it may not facilitate formal diagnosis like the Rorschach, but it is "better able to reveal the dynamics of interpersonal relationships, of drive constellation, and the nature of defenses against them" [36]. The animal pictures are equally applicable for all groups of children, so the CAT is "relatively culture free" [36]. The examiner tells the child, "We are going to engage in a game in which [you have] to tell a story about pictures; [you] should tell what is going on, what the animals are doing now." At suitable points, the child may be asked what went on in the story before and what will happen later (ref. 36, p. 2).

More recently, cards with human figures have been provided [37]. Some preliminary studies have indicated that human figures may have greater stimulus value than drawings of animals. Some children may do better with the animal cards and some with the human ones; the regular CAT is recommended for use first. The CAT-Human Figures, however, might be considered for children aged 7 to 10 years or those who are particularly bright; it is available when the CAT has not yielded satisfactory results. The Children's Apperception Test, Supplemental (CAT-S) is also available for exploring special circumstances such as physical disability, psychosomatic disorder, or the mother's pregnancy [38].

The Projective Storytelling Cards are useful in depicting a wide array of situations [39]. The 25 cards represent a variety of themes dealing with problems that children and teens face, with a focus on traumatic events, conflict in the family or social arena, and possible physical and sexual abuse. These cards can be used at any time during treatment, but they are especially useful for diagnosis and for establishing rapport. They have the goal of inspiring children to express their feelings, attitudes, and experiences in thematic form. The cards are particularly useful in helping children set goals to cope with physically or sexually abusive situations.

The Adoption Story Cards developed by R. Gardner can be used diagnostically as well as therapeutically to evoke issues relating to adoption [40]. This is a particularly difficult area to assess, since denial is often very strong. The cards were designed to provide the therapist with some access to information that children may otherwise be resistant to reveal.

Child Questionnaires

The Incomplete Sentences Blank forms are useful for young people in high school or college [41]. The Sentence Completion Test for Children has been used in this practice for the past 25 years (see Appendix 2.3). It is a simple, two-page sentence completion form with 25 items. It is useful for children aged 5 through 12 years. For some children, it may help if clinicians read the questions aloud and write down the child's responses. Other children, particularly older children or those who seem very private, might respond more openly by doing it themselves in their own handwriting. In one evaluation, an 11-year-old girl gave as little response as possible on all other assessment tools, including an interview. The sentence completions, however, were extremely revealing about the depth of feeling and dissatisfaction toward her parents and family. It was the only time in the entire evaluation process during which she shared these feelings.

The Child Anxiety Scale (CAS) can be useful in some instances for children aged 5 through 12 years [42]. It involves 20 straightforward questions in which a child marks on either a red circle or a blue circle. It can be administered through a tape or by the clinician. Children who are very anxious, however, may base their responses on denial. CAS users need to note extremely high or extremely low scores: high scores consistently reflect a high level of anxiety; and low scores could indicate a high anxiety level that is being systematically denied. Further, studies have shown that children may often resist reporting negative experiences and instead present a favorable view that may underestimate their actual anxiety levels.

The Children's Depression Inventory (CDI) is the most popular child questionnaire for assessing depression in children [43]. It was developed by Kovacs based on the Beck Depression Inventory for adults [44]. The long form has 27 items, and a short form (CDI-S) has 10 items. It is suitable for children aged 7 to 17 years, and requires only a third-grade reading level, the lowest of any childhood depression measure. For each item, children choose one of three statements reflecting minimal, moderate, or severe depression in the past 2 weeks. The items pertain to depressive symptoms such as a negative mood, a lack of pleasure, sleeping or eating disturbances, their self-image, and behavior with peers or at school. There are high positive correlations of test scores with self-reported anxiety and negative correlations of test scores with self-esteem. Self-esteem, defined as the "extent to which the individual believes himself to be capable, significant, successful, and worthy" (ref. 45, p. 5), is measured by items such as "I'm doing the best work that I can," "I'm pretty sure of myself," "I wish I were someone else," and "I often get discouraged in school." Self-esteem involves a *personal* assessment of worthiness and capability that is apparent in the beliefs and attitudes that children maintain toward themselves. Although the CDI has been shown to be a reliable measure of distress and depressive symptoms, it should not be used alone to diagnose depression.

Following a social learning analysis, Harter discussed how competence motivation leads children toward independent attempts at mastery [46]. They may receive positive or negative feedback from several sources, including their own assessment of the outcome as well as the reactions of others. Positive feedback leads to feelings of success, renewed efforts, an inner sense of capability, and worthiness or high self-esteem. Overly negative feedback can lead to a sense of failure and lower competence motivation. It can contribute to a tendency to avoid challenges, to depend on others to solve problems, and, ultimately, to fail more often – low self-esteem.

Among the self-esteem inventories, the Culture-Free Self-Esteem Inventory can be useful in assessment and preassessment for both individual and group treatment [47]. The Piers–Harris Self-Concept Inventory is also available. With self-esteem measures, however, there is a strong tendency for children to report what they think the adult wants to hear or they themselves want to believe [48]. Such inventories may be less revealing of deeper feelings than many other assessment tools.

Seligman and colleagues emphasized success at performance and accomplishment as a pivotal component of self-esteem [49]. They did not support the theory that we can "give" our children self-esteem by seeking only to help them "feel good" and instead designed a program for children to learn the skills of optimism. Their Children's Attributional Style Questionnaire measures aspects of self-esteem based on performance capability rather than the "feel good" school of thought. Attitudes toward self and events contribute to the experience of success.

Kurdek and Berg developed a helpful assessment tool for children of divorce who are 5 to 18 years of age [50]. The Children's Beliefs About Parental Divorce Scale has six scales that reflect peer avoidance, paternal blame, fear of abandonment, maternal blame, hopes of reunification, and self-blame, as well as a total score for maladaptive attitudes. The questionnaire allows questions to be structured around divorce and is therefore more revealing than generic questions that do not relate to divorce specifically, or questions that make children feel put on the spot or require them to "criticize" their parents. This scale has been used in our office since it was developed and has been found useful even when the divorce occurred at some considerable time in the past.

Behavioral Assessment

The behavioral assessment of children follows a problem-solving strategy. It is an empirical approach to clinical child assessment, utilizing what we know of child development and developmental psychopathology. Behavioral assessment allows for the evaluation of treatment outcome and can improve the effectiveness of services for children. Certain concepts are pivotal, such as the importance of situational influences, direct observation of behavior, and treatment evaluation. This is a rapidly emerging field that is still refining techniques for clinical practice. Accurate observations and objectivity in reporting are guiding principles. Behavioral assessment does not rely on inferences or underlying personality constructs but is instead concerned with the child's actual behavior in certain situations.

For example, in the behavioral assessment of enuresis, it is helpful to inquire whether children sleep in their own room or with siblings, where they sleep relative to their parents' bedroom(s), and the time at which the children and their parents go to bed. Further, it is important to assess what children know about the problem and the treatment. They may feel that the bedwetting is their fault. Do they realize that it is a common problem among other children? Projective assessment can be used to determine how concerned children are about bedwetting and how much they want to be cured. Sometimes embarrassment or denial can lead parents to feel that their children are indifferent to the symptoms. Also, when children are dry sleeping away from home, the parents might think that they are bedwetting on purpose at home. Usually, however, children simply sleep less soundly in an effort to prevent the bedwetting away from home.

When treating encopresis, the clinician should assess the frequency of the problem, when it occurs during the day or night, how much occurs, and variations in the pattern. The clinician should also ask who has the responsibility for the cleanup. Further, the clinician should inquire of the parents the exact words used in talking to the child as well as what the child actually does in response. The parents can keep a behavioral record for a week to answer some of these questions. Since this is an extremely frustrating symptom for parents, their tolerance level has usually been exceeded, and they may be extremely angry and frustrated. It is important for the clinician to be able to get past the emotional reactions into a more objective evaluation of what is actually occurring. In addition, it is important to assess how emotions are handled generally within the family. A merely mechanistic record of behavior cannot by itself be definitive.

Another symptom that can be usefully evaluated from a behavioral perspective is children's fears. One useful method with school-age children of 6 years and older, as well as teenagers, is to use systematic desensitization, beginning with constructing a rank ordering of fears. For older children, a 10-point scale can be used, with "10" indicating the situation in which they would feel the most fear and "1" the situation in which they would feel the most relaxed and comfortable. As children are selecting situations to put on their scale, their reactions and feelings in many situations can be effectively diagnosed. This simple assessment can then be used in a systematic desensitization routine in which the child is taught a method of relaxation and then imagines a situation on the scale and practices relaxing. This is an instance in which assessment and treatment are closely combined. Given the aversiveness of anxious reaction, this approach is often used immediately in treating an anxious child.

There are refined behavioral techniques for assessing obsessive-compulsive disorder (OCD) in childhood [51]. The Leyton Obsessional Inventory-Child Version and the 20-item Leyton Obsessional Inventory are extremely helpful in assessment and treatment planning [51]. In addition, the Yale–Brown Obsessive-Compulsive Scale has specific instructions for children [51]. There is also a National Institute of Mental Health (NIMH) Teacher Rating of OCD [51].

Behavioral assessment of conduct disorders in children has expanded rapidly in recent years (Table 2.4). Atkeson and Forehand discussed characteristics of conduct-disordered children, which include a high rate of

Table 2.4 Selected measures of antisocial behaviors for children and adolescents.

Measure	Response format	Age range[*]	Special features
Children's Hostility Inventory[†]	38 true–false statements assessing different facets of aggression and hostility.	6–13 yr	Derived from Buss-Durke Hostility Guilt Inventory. A priori subscales from that scale comprise factors that relate to overt acts (aggression) and aggressive thoughts and feelings (hostility).
REPORTS OF OTHERS			
Eyberg Child Behavior Inventory	36 items rated on 1 to 7 points scale for frequency and whether the behavior is a problem.	2–17 yr	Designed to measure wide range of conduct problems in the home.
Sutter-Eyberg Student Behavior Inventory	36 items identical in format but not content to the Eyberg Child Behavior Inventory.	2–17 yr	Measures a range of conduct problem behaviors at school.
Peer Nomination of Aggression	Items that ask children to nominate others who show the characteristics (e.g., 'Who starts a fight over nothing'?).	3rd through 13th grade	Items reflect the child's reputation among peers regarding overall aggression. Different versions of peer nominations have been used.
DIRECT OBSERVATIONS			
Adolescent Antisocial Behavior Checklist	57 items to measure antisocial behavior during hospitalization. Behaviors are rated as having occurred or not based on staff observations.	Adolescence	The items can be scored using different sets of subscales; one set focuses on the form of the problems (e.g., physical vs. verbal harm); another set focuses on the objects of aggression (e.g., toward self, others, property). Different versions are available and differ in scoring.

(*Continued*)

Table 2.4 (*Continued*)

Measure	Response format	Age range[*]	Special features
Family Interaction Coding System (FICS)	Direct observational system to measure occurrence or nonoccurrence of 29 specific parent–child behaviors in the home. Each behavior is scored within small intervals for an hour each day for a period of several days.	3–12 yr	Individual behaviors are observed but usually summarized with a total aversive behavior score. The general procedure can be adopted using some or all of the behaviors of the FICS.
Parent Daily Report	Parents identify symptoms of antisocial behavior. After symptoms are identified, the parent is called daily for several days. Each day the parent is asked if each behavior has or has not occurred in previous 24-hr period.	3–12 yr	Measure does not reflect a standardized set of items but rather refers more to an assessment approach for collecting date on behaviors at home.
SELF-REPORT			
Children's Action Tendency Scale	30 items in forced-choice format, child selects what he or she would do in interpersonal situations.	6–15 yr	Scores for response dimensions: aggressiveness, assertiveness, and submissiveness.
Adolescent Antisocial Self-Report Behavior Checklist	52 items, each of which is rated by the child on a 5-point scale (from never to very often).	Adolescence	The measure samples a broad range of behaviors from mild misbehavior to serious antisocial acts. The items load four factors: delinquency, drug usage, parental defiance, and assaultiveness.
Self-Report Delinquency Scale	47 items that measure frequency with which individual has performed offenses included in the Uniform Crime Reports. Responses provide frequency with which behavior was performed over the last year.	11–21 yr	Measure has been developed as part of the National Youth Survey, an extensive longitudinal study of delinquent behavior, alcohol and drug use, and related problems in American youths.
Minnesota Multiphasic Personality Inventory Scales	True–false items derived from Scales F (test-taking attitude), 4 (psychopathic deviate) and 9 (hypomania) are summed to yield an aggression/delinquency.	Adolescence	Part of more general measure that assesses multiple areas of psychopathology.
Interview for Aggression[†]	Semistructured interview, 30 items pertaining to aggression such as getting into fights, starting arguments. Each item rated on a 5-point scale for severity and 3-point scale for duration.	6–13 yr	Yields scores for severity, duration, and total (serverity + duration) aggression. Separate factors assess overt and covert behaviors.

[*]The age ranges are tentative and derived from the ages of cases reported rather than inherent restrictions of the measure.
[†]This measure has separate versions: (1) a self-report measure for children, and (2) a parent-report measure to evaluate children's behavior.
From Kazdin AE: Conduct disorder. In: Ollendick TH, Herson M, eds. *Handbook of Child and Adolescent Assessment*. Boston: Allyn & Bacon; 1993:295. Copyright ® 1993 by Allyn & Bacon. Reprinted by permission.

negative commands, disapproval, humiliation, non-compliance, negativism, teasing, physically negative acts, and yelling, as well as high-intensity deviant behavior such as destructiveness [52].

These children also exhibit a low frequency of positive behavior, such as approval expressed to others, positive attention, independent activity, laughing, and talking. Further, "in the negative reinforcement model, coercive behavior on the part of one family member is reinforced when it results in the removal of an aversive event being applied to another family member" (ref. 52, p. 188). Three strategies have been employed in the assessment process: behavioral interviews, behavioral questionnaires, and behavioral observations; see Holland's Interview Guide (ref. 52, p. 1951). Behavioral questionnaires have included the Becker Bipolar Adjective Checklist [52], Parent Attitude Test [52], Walker Problem Behavior Identification Checklist [52], and Behavior Problem Checklist [52]. Direct observations of parent–child interactions are considered the most valid source of data.

Researchers have developed elaborate coding systems for research in the home environment, such as the Family Interaction Coding System of Patterson and colleagues [53]. Since few clinical settings have the resources for this, structured clinical observations of parent–child interactions are instead recommended. One simple technique that can be used is the Behavior Management Questionnaire, completed by parents, which covers the activities and interests of the child and disciplinary practices of the parents. This was developed for use with autistic children [54].

Barkley presented an extensive training program for parents of children who have behavior problems, including ADHD and conduct disorders [55, 56]. Decreasing noncompliance, decreasing disruptiveness, and increasing independent play are major components of the program. Children are also taught a "think aloud-think ahead" self-control technique. Parents may be trained in the office, but in-home practice methods are also an integral part of the program.

Useful assessment tools of Barkley's program include the Parent–Child Interaction Interview Form, Home Situations Questionnaire, Parent's and Teacher's Questionnaire, and School Situations Questionnaire [56]. In addition, there are behavioral sheets for observing the parents and child together, which include Recording Observations of Parent–Child Interactions and Coding Form for Recoding Parent–Child Interactions. Barkley also assists parents in understanding their problems through the Profile of Child and Parent Characteristics and the Family Problems Inventory [56].

Kazdin stresses that the assessment of conduct disorders should be multimodal [32]. The process should include different methods (interviews and direct observations), perspectives (child, parent, and teacher), domains (affect, cognition, and behavior), and settings (home, school, and community). Further, prosocial behavior and adaptive skills should be assessed as well as the theory that "antisocial behavior is not merely the opposite of prosocial behavior" (ref. 32, p. 392).

Play Observations

The importance of play and the use of imagination in child development cannot be overstated. The use of fantasy enables children to delay gratification and to deal more effectively with frustration, which in turn has implications for their success in the classroom [57]. By studying preschool children, Parten identified five ways that children play:

(1) in solitary play, children are unaware of others and play alone;
(2) in onlooker play, children watch others play;
(3) in parallel play, children play side by side with little interaction;
(4) in associative play, children interact and share;
(5) in cooperative play, they relate to each other, helping and taking turns [58].

Piaget described three types of play – practice games, symbolic games, and games with rules – through which children learn the rules of social exchange and enhance their sense of competence and self-esteem [59].

It has long been recognized that children use play as their natural medium of self-expression and as an avenue for cognitive development. It can therefore be useful to incorporate some opportunity to observe unstructured play in child assessment procedures. Typically, a doll's house, large blocks, and trucks can be used. Children's personalities are revealed in the way that they approach these materials. Straightforward observation of their behavior can indicate how they typically behave in similar situations. Some children are quiet and resilient, seeking permission before beginning play, whereas others race rambunctiously into the thick of it, with nary a thought to protocol or manners. Some children play quietly without verbalization, whereas others talk constantly.

Clinicians can use some of their own feelings and reactions to the child to diagnose potential problem areas, as demonstrated by the following case study.

CASE STUDY

A 6-year-old girl was demanding and bossy with her therapist; she would sweetly ask the therapist to play with her and seemed dependent in this respect. Every time the therapist picked up a toy to begin to play or make some independent gesture, however, the girl would give orders for it to be done differently. The therapist, being very accommodating, tried to comply, only to find herself feeling irritated. Finally, the therapist identified that this little girl was likely to be bossy and demanding in a sweet way in her interactions with both peers and adults. This became a major focus of the treatment plan.

The themes of play can also be meaningful, although the style of approaching the play materials should be observed as well.

Many youngsters who come for assessment and treatment have difficulties engaging in pretend play. "Their play doesn't hang together; it may seem disconnected, a fragmented puzzle, hardly a way for them to learn about themselves and the world around them" (ref. 60, p. 153). Different ways of using play in diagnosis and treatment have been presented that offer observation of the child's verbal and nonverbal reactions, thought process and decision-making, style in using materials, nature and content of play, and interaction with the clinician. Children reveal individualized aspects of personality in their responses as well as in their interests and preferences.

Behar and Rapoport discussed the usefulness of summarizing play behavior of young children as a general clinical screening tool: "The diagnostic play interview seems particularly important for children before they have found more adult, or structured, outlets (ref. 61, p. 193). These authors recommended play assessment when (i) parents and teachers offer conflicting reports, (ii) reports and clinical observation differ, (iii) verbal communication is inadequate or the child is too young, or (iv) when there is shyness or withdrawal in the child's behavior. Children's play can reveal: (i) the style of interaction with a parent; (ii) the style of separation from the parent; (iii) the style of relating to the examiner; (iv) the use of toys in play; (v) spontaneous behavior; and (vi) play behaviors relevant to the diagnosis [52]. Play may be particularly useful in diagnosing young or nonverbal children.

In an extensive manual, Schaefer and colleagues presented a variety of uses for the assessment of play [62]. There are articles on scales for developmental play, diagnostic play, parent–child interaction, peer interaction, projective play assessment, and play therapy. As noted by Westby, the" evaluation of children's play skills permits assessment not only of the knowledge children have, but also of how they use this knowledge in a real-world context (ref. 63, p. 133). The Westby Symbolic Play Scale presents developmental levels for play shown by children from 8 months to 5 years of age [63].

Family Interaction

Family interaction should be considered in any assessment of children. Family sessions can be used for diagnostic purposes and are also particularly useful when working with children and their parents to teach child management techniques for externalizing disorders such as ADHD and oppositional defiant disorder (ODD). In all families, however, the child's role within the family strongly affects his or her feelings, attitudes, and behaviors, and clinicians should assess these characteristics when planning for treatment. Baumrind demonstrated that a child's characteristics are closely related to the structure of that child's family [64], and Hetherington and Parke compared parenting styles with children's behavior and self-esteem [65]. Clinicians often assess the child individually, although others advocate "incorporating family assessment into comprehensive child assessment" (ref. 66, p. 136). The latter approach may make it more difficult to develop a rapport with the child or teenager, however. Both approaches have their advantages and disadvantages. In general, it is important for the individual conducting the assessment to be aware of certain common family patterns that can influence a child's behavior.

It is important for clinicians to assess parental warmth, a factor important to the child in terms of seeking approval. Parents showing this warmth may be more likely to provide information about alternative social responses available to the child. "Warm" parents also frequently use reasoning and explanations that permit children to internalize social rules and to identify and discriminate situations in which a given behavior is appropriate. Warmth is likely to be associated with responsiveness to the child's needs. Warm parents do not have to resort to methods that are frustrating to the child, and children are less likely to avoid contact with the parents; this facilitates the socialization process.

Clinicians should also evaluate parental control. Parental restrictiveness or permissiveness can lead to problems in child functioning. A permissive family can cause problems of neglect and may also damage a child's adaptive ability. Authoritarian family approaches may have the advantage of preparing children to deal with rules and limits but the disadvantage of limiting overall competence.

In families of neglect, the mother often exhibits depression and detachment. Depressed mothers have difficulty finding the energy to take care of their children. Parental detachment may be encouraged by our narcissistic culture that gives permission for seeking personal gratification before the needs of others. Divorce also contributes to parental neediness.

Beavers and Hampson presented a paradigm for analyzing family interaction in terms of overall competence and family style [67]. Family style relates to the positioning of the family in the community: Centripetal families bind their members to the family, making any absence difficult; and centrifugal families expel the child from the family before individuation is complete. Family style and level of competence are used to classify families into types that may be relevant to the problems shown by offspring. For example, it is hypothesized that severely centrifugal families often have sociopathic offspring.

Beavers and Hampson developed a comprehensive scale to rate the nature of family interaction, termed the Beavers Interactional Scale: Family Competence and Family Style [67]. This scale is used by clinicians and allows ratings on the following dimensions: (i) structure of the family (specifically overt power, parental coalitions, and closeness); (ii) mythology; (iii) goal-directed negotiation; (iv) autonomy, including clarity of expression, responsibility, and permeability; and (v) family affect, assessed through range of feelings, mood and tone, unresolvable conflict, and empathy. In addition, the Global Health-Pathology Scale includes a Self-Report Family Inventory and an Individual Family Style Scale for family members to fill out, which can be useful in the assessment process [67]. The Self-Report Family Inventory (SFI) includes a scoring system for health/ competence, conflict, cohesion, leadership, and expressiveness [67]. A similar test that can be used in family sessions, called FACES II, was developed by Olson and colleagues at the Department of Family Social Science at the University of Minnesota [68]. It yields information on family cohesion and adaptability, indicating family type.

A discussion of family interaction would not be complete without considering the profound effect of extended family interaction, both for children who have an intact nuclear family and for those who are being raised by other family members including grandparents.

Further, extended family members may share in the upbringing of children significantly. These trends appear to be increasingly prominent. As clinicians, we see many children who are being raised by their grandparents. We also see many situations that are essentially shared parenting between parents and grandparents or other family members.

Grandparents may be raising children when they have little access to resources outside of their own family. In addition, in many US states there is no legal provision for grandparents to have parental rights or legal rights to parenting time. In some situations, it even makes sense for a parent and grandparents to have shared parenting with each other. This can be a useful arrangement, but Courts may be reluctant to encourage these arrangements without legal procedures that require cooperation between family members.

Special Issues

Social Skills and ADHD

It has recently been estimated that there are over 2 million school-age children in the United States alone with ADHD [69]. These are children who show significant behavioral problems that are very stressful for family life. There is often conflict over chores, homework, and getting along with siblings, with the ADHD child showing antagonistic behavior at school and in the neighborhood. Further, ADHD children typically have difficulties modulating their own emotional reactions. Such intense reactions create difficulties in social relationships. Children with ADHD tend not to see the connection between their behavior and the outcome, whereas other children learn this automatically. Low self-esteem results from the negative reactions of others, and specific social skills are lacking in children with ADHD.

There is a wide variety of social skills; these include: communication skills, sharing, social initiation, joining strategies, determining appropriate behavior for a given situation, listening and asking questions about ambiguous messages, smiling, sharing, positive physical contact, verbal complimenting, using instructions, modeling, praise, labeling emotions and facial expressions, referential communication accuracy, taking perspective, listening, making friends (including greeting), asking for information, including extension, giving information, giving help, and being observant of appropriate classroom behavior. Children with ADHD may be deficient in any number of these skills. Sometimes they have acquired certain steps but not the entire sequence of behaviors necessary for positive social exchange.

Fortunately, there has been great interest in developing procedures for enhancing children's interpersonal relationships with peers, since having well-developed social skills corresponds to fewer mental health problems. Popular children behave in specific ways, initiate interactions, smile, and make positive comments. The fact that children can be taught social skills has been applied to a wide variety of problems and disorders, including ADHD.

A variety of intervention strategies have been used to effectively teach social skills. These include contingent positive reinforcement, modeling, coaching and behavioral rehearsal, and peer initiation. The first step is to evaluate the strengths and weaknesses of each child individually, as there is a wide variety of specific deficits.

Social skills can be evaluated using the Social Skills Rating System for parents, teachers, and children [70]. Behaviors that influence a child's social capability and adaptive skills at home and school can be assessed systematically, which can help in further assessment and treatment planning as well as the outcome evaluation of individual or group intervention. Teacher and parent forms are available for preschool, kindergarten through grade 6, and grades 7 through 12. Separate self-rating forms are available for students in grades 3 through 6 and in grades 7 through 12. Prosocial behaviors that are assessed include cooperation, assertion, responsibility, empathy, and self-control.

Goldstein and colleagues' Skillstreaming material allows for the assessment of a wide variety of specific social skills [71]. There are 50 social skills that can be taught, and the curriculum even includes listening! The Structured Learning Skill Checklist is used in the assessment process.

Adolescents

Teens may be reluctant to sit and talk about their feelings and experiences with a grownup, particularly a professional. They generally respond well to structured assessment procedures, however, including drawings, projective tests, and sentence completions. Establishing rapport is possible by allowing teens "space" to express themselves in their own way.

The Millon Adolescent Clinical Inventory (MACI) for teens (13–19 years) is both useful and relatively short, consisting of only 160 items [72]. The recent revision gives information on borderline tendencies and abuse experiences. The four new personality scales for the MACI measure self-demeaning, forceful, doleful, and borderline tendencies. The majority of teens complete the MACI easily. Occasionally, a younger teenager makes a comment implying that they do not know how to answer the items relating to sex, such as "I enjoy thinking about sex," or "Sex is enjoyable." It is helpful to review the form carefully before sending it in for computer analysis, because some teenagers leave too many items blank. It is important for the teens to have a sense about why they are going through the assessment process. There will occasionally be difficulty with compliance, in which case it is best to move on to other assessment methods. We have found the narrative description of personality provided by the MACI to be accurate and useful in treatment planning. It includes a section on pointers for psychotherapy as well.

The preferred Millon assessment tool for younger preteens aged 9–12 years is the Millon Pre-Adolescent Clinical Inventory (M-PACI) [73]. It contains fewer than 100 questions and takes only 15–20 minutes for youngsters to finish. It has been validated and there are up-to-date national norms with a detailed interpretive report for the clinician. The M-PACI focuses on clinical problems comprehensively, not just a single issue, and identifies emerging personality styles that will aid the clinician in planning intervention and pinpointing effective methods.

Teens can be engaged in assessment and treatment if the goals are defined on their terms. Many teens like the idea of "learning more" about themselves. Psychoeducational assessment can also be interesting to them as a way of developing strategies for success in school and planning for college (viewed as a chance to be away from home!).

Of particular interest to teens are the personality styles of the Myers–Briggs Type Indicator [74]. This is a "nonpathologizing" measure of personality. Its analysis of personality types provides a comprehensive theory of personality functioning by describing four types of mental processes: sensing (S), intuition (N), thinking (T), and feeling (F). Sensing is the ability to understand through observation and the senses; intuition is the conceptualization of possibilities; thinking is the process of linking ideas together in a logical way; and feeling is a more subjective process based on values. There are four basic personality types and the possibility of 16 subtypes when two additional dimensions are added (Extrovert-Introvert and Judgment-Perception). The four basic types of individuals are as follows:

- ST – Sensing and thinking
- SF – Sensing and feeling
- NF – Intuition and feeling
- NT – Intuition and thinking

STs focus on facts and the use of interpersonal analysis. They tend to be practical and matter-of-fact and to develop technical skills with facts and objects. SFs focus on facts and the use of personal warmth. They tend to be sympathetic and friendly and emphasize practical help and services for people. NFs focus attention on possibilities and the use of personal warmth. They are enthusiastic and insightful and have strengths in understanding and communicating with people.

NTs focus on possibilities by using impersonal analysis. They are logical and ingenious and emphasize theoretical and technical developments. Teens can be intrigued with learning more about themselves and, without realizing it, may apply this information to help them cope with their own lives.

Although teens may be anxious and avoid responsibility for planning for the future, they also typically lack skills for systematically addressing these issues. They often respond favorably to discussions on this topic as well as to specific assessment procedures such as the Harrington–O'Shea Career Decision-Making System-Revised [75]. In their responses to the Survey Booklet, teens express their likes and dislikes for many activities, and Career Clusters that match their interests are then suggested to the teens. Their interests only suggest jobs that they might like, however. Teens also need to consider ability, values, training, and employment outlook to make career decisions.

Such nonpathologizing ways of working with teens can be surprisingly effective. They learn problem-solving skills that can help them overcome their difficulties. The process also emphasizes teens' independence from their family and their own responsibility for their futures.

It is easy for mental health clinicians to sidestep the issues of substance abuse as they are facing a young and seemingly healthy individual who does not as yet typically show the long-term effects of substance use. To aid in assessing teens for substance abuse issues, the adolescent form of the Substance Abuse Subtle Screening Inventory (SASSI) is available for ages 12 through 18 [76]. Many teenagers will give significant information regarding substance abuse habits on a questionnaire when they may volunteer no information in an interview. Teenagers may not spontaneously provide information but may provide information on their use if asked specific questions. However, the clinician may worry that it is easy to produce false positives by asking leading questions. Further, it is difficult to distinguish between the acting out adolescent who is chemically dependent and the acting out adolescent who is not.

Sexual Abuse

Evaluation for child sexual abuse should be comprehensive and cover all aspects of personality functioning. Such evaluations are extremely complex. Some of the following questionnaires may be useful as part of a comprehensive assessment.

Petty developed a Checklist for Child Abuse Evaluation [77]. This is an expansive questionnaire that covers all aspects of child abuse cases, including the following: the accuracy of validations by the reporter; interview with the child – physical or behavioral observations; interview with the child – disclosure; child psychological status; history and observed or reported characteristics of the accused; and credibility of the child – observed or reported. Conclusions cover the competence of the child as a witness, the level of stress on the child, and the protection of the child. Treatment recommendations are also included.

The Sex Abuse Legitimacy (SAL) Scale developed by Gardner attempts to differentiate between legitimate and fabricated child sexual abuse allegations [78]. It is most effective when the child, accuser, and accused all are interviewed. The scale is less valuable but may still be used, however, when the alleged perpetrator is unavailable. The SAL Scale was developed from studies conducted between 1982 and 1987 of children who made allegations of sexual abuse. It helps to organize data but does not produce a definitive conclusion and therefore should not be used as a questionnaire or a standardized psychological test. It can only be used as a guideline and should not be used as evidence in court proceedings.

Peterson [79]. proposed a child dissociation problem checklist to be used in diagnosing the dissociation identity disorder now included in the *Diagnostic and Statistical Manual for Mental Disorders,* Fourth Edition, Text Revision (DSM-IV-TR) [80]. The clinician may not be diagnosing this disorder in early childhood, because it is extremely rare and in fact may not exist in childhood. It may be misdiagnosed, exist along with another disorder, or have an atypical presentation in childhood (i.e., with fewer elaborate complex personalities and their alters). In addition, clinicians may not ask the appropriate questions to make an accurate diagnosis. For example, they should ask about missing blocks of time or other aspects of dissociation, and should also note if the child appears to be in a trance at any point. These experiences may not be discussed by children, owing to a fear of not being believed or being punished. There may be less differentiation between personality aberration and the age-appropriate behaviors of a child.

The presentation of multiple personality disorder (MPD) in childhood may be different than in adulthood, since the common characteristics of MPD in adults are not present in children. These characteristics in adults include persecutor personalities, inner self-helper personalities, and special-purpose fragments and systems of personalities. There may also be somatic complaints and severe headaches. Putnam and colleagues developed a child dissociation scale to be completed by the parents [81].

Conclusion

Psychological testing allows the clinician to collect a wide range of information about the child both efficiently and in a standardized way. The data that are generated have specific applications and usefulness for diagnosis and treatment planning. A broad approach that includes multiple sources of data and allows us to understand children in the context of their lives is recommended. Since children do not have the facility or experience to fully express themselves verbally, we as clinicians are interested in their worldview and how it can be revealed to us.

Appendix 2.1—Assessment Protocol

PSYCHOEDUCATIONAL TESTING

Cognitive Tests

Stanford–Binet
Wechsler Preschool and Primary Scale of Intelligence Wechsler Intelligence Scale for Children – 3rd Edition
Leiter-Revised
Peabody Picture Vocabulary Test

Achievement Tests

Woodcock–Johnson
Wechsler Individual Achievement Test

Note: The average psychoeducational assessment can be completed in two sessions. Exceptions include teenagers, very bright 10- to 12-year-olds, and children experiencing unusual emotional reactions to testing. Be sure to prepare the parents that a third session for psychoeducational testing may be necessary.

NEUROPSYCHOLOGICAL TESTING

NEPSY-II

PRESCHOOL (INFANCY TO 5 YEARS) ASSESSMENT

First Session

Background information from parents or guardian
Child Behavior Checklist and Caregiver-Teacher Report Form (C-TRF)
Parenting Stress Index (PSI)
VinelandII
Orientation

Second Session

Developmental measures
Bayley Scales of Infant Development Stanford-Binet
Wechsler Preschool and Primary Scale of Intelligence
Kaufman

Third Session

Personality assessment
Drawings
Rorschach (use *modified method* with no inquiry)
Children's Apperception Test

Play observation
Consider parent–child interaction

Fourth Session

Consultation with parents

Note: Assessment should be collapsed to three sessions when feasible.

SCHOOL-AGE (6 TO 12 YEARS) ASSESSMENT

First session

Background information from parents or guardian
Child Behavior Checklist (CBCL) and Teacher Report Form (TRF)
Parenting Stress Index(PSI)
Attention-Deficit Disorders Evaluation Scale (ADDES)
Orientation with child
Draw-A-Person (DAP)
Kinetic Family Drawing (KFD)
Sentence Completion Test for Children

Second Session

Personality testing
Rorschach
Thematic Apperception Test (TAT)
Interview

Third Session

Interview
Exploring treatment goals and possible intervention strategies and enlisting child'scooperation

Fourth Session

Consultation with parents and treatment planning

Note: Additional sessions are required for psychoeducational testing, but in this instance, another option is to collapse the second and third sessions into a one-hour session to reduce the number of sessions. A family interaction session frequently follows the consultation session with parents.

TEENS ASSESSMENT

First Session

Background information from parents
CBC and TRF
Orientation with teen
Millon Adolescent Clinical Inventory (MACI)
Draw-A-Person
Kinetic Family Drawing
Rotter Sentence Completions

Second Session

Personality testing
Rorschach
Thematic Apperception Test (TAT)
Interview

Third Session

Interview

Exploring treatment goals and possible intervention strategies (assess teen'spreferences)

Fourth Session

Consultation with parents and treatment planning (teen can be invited to participatein part of session)

Note: Modifying the protocol may be needed in crisis situations or with teens who are seriously uncomfortable. A family interaction session frequently follows the consultation session with parents.

Appendix 2.2 Interpretation of Drawings: Suggested Procedure

GLOBAL IMPRESSIONS (HOLISTIC VIEW)

Spontaneous selection of subject
Assigned topic

Pleasant effect of the whole
Unpleasant effect

Drawn from memory
Copied or imitating comic-stripcharacter

Freely drawn and bold
Tiny and at bottom or well away fromcenter

Elaborate
Limited

Vivid fantasy
Poor in content

Own sex drawn first in Draw-A-Person test
Other sex drawn first

Omission of self or other in familygroup
Inclusion of all members

Excessive shading
"Artistic" shading for modeling offigure

Static figures
Movement indicated

Full-face
Profile

Well-coordinated figure
Disjointed figure

Symmetry
    Preoccupation with perfectsymmetry
    Excessive disregard

Quality of line
    Broken
    Continuous

Pressure
    Barely visible figure
    Well defined
    Heavy, may punch holes throughpaper

Velocity
    Speedy and careless
    Exasperatingly slow

Mood
    Peaceful
    Turbulent

Organization
    Orderly
    Chaotic

Composition
    Simple
    Complex

CONTENT (ITEM ANALYSIS OF HUMAN FIGURE)

Head
    Huge
    Disproportionately small

Eyes
    Large
    Small
    Empty
    With pupils

Ears
    Prominent
    Absent

Hair
    Abundant, coiffured
    Scribbled
    Scant, absent

Fingers
    Five, supernumerary or absent
    Stick- or claw-like

Mouth
    Absent or emphasized
    Cosmetic or minimally represented

Arms
    Large, muscular
    Absent or stick-like
Legs
    Two or more
    Wide apart or close together
Crotch
    Excessive attention, erasures
    Shading, covered by hands
Trunk
    Absent or tiny, smaller than head
    Emphasized, organs or navel visible
Nose
    Absent or tiny
    Large, nostrils shown
Breasts
    Emphasized, firm or drooping
    Absent

Genitalia
    Suggested
    Explicitly shown, exaggerated
    Apparently ignored
    Concealed
Teeth
    Large, pointed
    Not visible
Clothing
    Appropriate
    Incongruous
    Profession or occupation shown
    Scant or absent
    Jewelry, ornaments

From DiLeo(1983), [26] pp. 217–220.

Appendix 2.3 Sentence Completion Test for Children

Name:

Date of Test:

(1) At times I feel
(2) At home
(3) Other kids
(4) My mother
(5) My biggest worry
(6) I feel happy when
(7) My dad
(8) What I like best is
(9) I cry
(10) I get mad when
(11) When I get mad, I
(12) If I could do anything, I would
(13) Boys
(14) Daddy gets mad when
(15) People are
(16) I feel sad when
(17) Girls
(18) What bothers me is
(19) Mommy gets mad when
(20) When I get nervous, I
(21) People think that I
(22) I cannot
(23) When I grow up
(24) In school I
(25) When I was little

References

1. Mooney KC, Harrison AJ. A content of analysis of child psychological evaluations. *J Child Adolesc Psychother* 1987;**4**:275–282.
2. Eyberg SM, Ross AW. Assessment of child behavior problems: The validation of a new inventory. *J Clin Child Psychol* 1978;**7**:113–116.
3. Abidin RR. *Parenting Stress Index: Professional Manual*, 3rd edn Odessa, FL: Psychological Assessment Resources, 1995.
4. Sheras PL, Abinin RR, Konold TR. *Stress Index for Parents of Adolescents: Professional Manual*. Odessa, FL: Psychological Assessment Resources, 1998.
5. Achenbach TM. *Manual for the Child Behavior Checklist/4-18 and 1991 Profile*. Burlington, VT: University of Vermont, 1991.
6. Achenbach TM. *Manual for the Teacher's Report Form and Profile*. Burlington, VT: University of Vermont, 1991.
7. Achenbach TM, Rescorla LA. *Manual for ASEBA Preschool Forms & Profiles*. Burlington, VT: University of Vermont, 2000.
8. Conners CK. *Conners' Rating Scales-Revised*. North Tonawanda, NY: MHS, 1997.
9. McCarney SB. *ADDES*, 2nd edn. Columbus, MO: Hawthorne Educational Services, 1995.
10. Randolph EM. *Attachment Disorder Questionnaire*, 1993. Call 910/674-8045 for information.
11. Kaufman AS, Ishikuma T. Intellectual and achievement testing. In: Ollendick H, Hersen M (eds) *Handbook of Child and Adolescent Assessment*. Boston, MA: Allyn and Bacon, 1993; pp. 192–207.
12. Wechsler D. *Wechsler Intelligence Scale for Children-Fourth Edition: Manual*. New York: Harcourt Brace Jovanovich, 2003.
13. Wechsler D. *Wechsler Preschool and Primary Scale of Intelligence-Third Edition: Manual*. San Antonio, TX: Harcourt Assessment, 2002.

14. Cordell AS, Cannon T. Gifted kids can't always spell. *Acad Ther* 1985;**21**:143–152.

15. Thorndike RL, Hagen EP, Sattler JM. *Stanford–Binet Intelligence Scale-Fourth Edition: Manual.* Chicago, IL: Riverside Publishing, 1986.

16. Leiter RG. *Leiter International Performance Scale-Revised.* Wood Dale, IL: Stoelting, 1997.

17. Kaufman AS, Kaufman NL. *Kaufman Brief Intelligence Test: Manual.* Circles Pines, MN: American Guidance Service, 1990.

18. Williams KT, Wang JJ. *Peabody Picture Vocabulary Test-Third Edition: Manual.* Circle Pines, MN: American Guidance Service, 1997.

19. Woodcock RW, McGrew KS, Mather N. *Woodcock-Johnson-III (WJ-III) Tests of Achievement.* Allen, TX: DLM Teaching Resources, 1989.

20. Smith D. et al. *Wechsler Individual Achievement Test-Second Edition: Examiner's Manual.* New York: Harcourt Assessment, 2002.

21. Sparrow SS, Cicchetti DV, Balla DA. *Vineland Adaptive Behavior Scales, Second Edition(Vineland-II)* Circle Pines, MN: American Guidance Service, 2005.

22. Rimm S. *Achievement Identification Measure.* Watertown, WI: Educational Assessment Service, 1985.

23. Light W. *Light's Retention Scale.* Novato, CA: Academic Therapy Publications, 1981.

24. Uphoff JK, Gilmore JE, Huber R. *Summer Children: Ready or Not for School.* Middletown, OH: J&J Publishers, 1986.

25. Brooks BL, Sherman EMS, Strauss E. NEPSY-II: A Developmental Neuropsychological Assessment, Second Edition. *Child Neuropsychol* 2010;**16**:80–101.

26. DiLeo JA. *Interpreting Children's Drawings.* New York: Brunner/Mazel, 1983.

27. Burns RC, Kaufman SH. *Actions, Styles, and Symbols in Kinetic Family Drawings (KFD)* New York: Brunner/Mazel, 1972.

28. Buck IN. *The House-Tree-Person Technique: Revised Manual.* Los Angeles: Western Psychological Services, 1970.

29. Cordell AS, Bergman-Meador B. The use of drawings. *J Div Remarr* 1991;**17**:139–155.

30. Klein RG. Questioning the clinical usefulness of projective psychological tests for children. *Dev Behav Pediatr* 1986;**7**:378–398.

31. Finch AJ, Belter RW. Projective techniques. In: Ollendick TH, Hersen M (eds) *Handbook of Childand Adolescent Assessment.* Boston, MA: Allyn and Bacon, 1993; pp. 224–236.

32. Kazdin AE. Conduct disorder. In: Ollendick TH, Hersen M (eds) *Handbook of Child and Adolescent Assessment.* Boston, MA: Allyn and Bacon, 1993; pp. 292–310.

33. Exner JE, Weiner IG. *The Rorschach: A Comprehensive System, vol. 3 Assessment of Childrenand Adolescents.* New York: John Wiley & Sons, 1982.

34. Henry W. *The Analysis of Fantasy.* New York: John Wiley & Sons, 1956.

35. McArthur D, Roberts G. *Roberts Apperception Test for Children: Manual.* Los Angeles: Western Psychological Services, 1982.

36. Bellak L, Bellak SS. *The Children's Apperception Test (CAT)* Larchmont, NY: C.P.S., 1976.

37. Bellak L, Hurvich MS. *Manual for the CAT-H.* Larchmont, NY: C.P.S., 1975.

38. Bellak L, Bellak SS. *Manual for Supplement to the Children's Apperception Test (CAT-S)* Larchmont, NY: C.P.S., 1978.

39. Caruso KR. *Basic Manual to Accompany Projective Storytelling Cards.* Redding, CA: Northwest Psychological Publishers, 1987.

40. Gardner RA. *The Adoption Story Cards.* Cresskill, NJ: Creative Therapeutics, 1978.

41. Rotter J. *Incomplete Sentences Blank.* New York: Harcourt Brace Jovanovich, 1977.

42. Gillis JS. *Child Anxiety Scale Manual.* Champaign, IL: Institute for Personality and AbilityTesting, 1980.

43. Ollendick TH, Hersen M (eds). *Handbook of Child and Adolescent Assessment.* Boston, MA: Allyn & Bacon, 1993.

44. Kovacs M. *Children's Depression Inventory (CDI)* New York: Multi-Health Systems, 1992.

45. Coopersmith S. *The Antecedents of Self-Esteem.* San Francisco: Freeman, 1967.

46. Harter S. Competence as a dimension of self-evaluation. Toward a comprehensive model of self-worth. In: Leahy R (ed.) *The Development of Self.* New York: Academic Press, 1983; pp. 51–121.

47. Battle J. *Culture-Free SEI: Self-Esteem Inventories for Children and Adults.* Seattle, WA: SpecialChild Publications, 1981.

48. Piers EV, Harris DB. *The Piers-Harris Children's Self-Concept Scale.* Los Angeles: WesternPsychological Services, 1969.

49. Seligman ME, Reivich K, Jaycox L, Gillham J. *The Optimistic Child: A Revolutionary Programthat Safeguards Children Against Depression and Builds Lifelong Resilience.* New York: Houghton Mifflin, 1995.

50. Kurdek LA, Berg B. The Children's Beliefs About Parental Divorce Scale: Psychometric characteristics and concurrent validity. *J Consul Clin Psychol* 1987; 55: 712–718.

51. Berg CZ. Behavioral assessment techniques for childhood obsessive-compulsive disorder. In: Rapoport JL (ed.) *Obsessive-Compulsive Disorder in Children and Adolescents.* Washington, DC: American Psychiatric Press, 1989; pp. 41–70.

52. Atkeson BM, Forehand R. Conduct disorders. In: Mash El, Terdal LG (eds) *Behavioral Assessmentof Childhood Disorders.* New York: Guilford Press, 1981; pp. 185–219.

53. Patterson GR, Reid JB, Jones RR, Conger RW. *A Social Learning Approach to Family Intervention.* Eugene, OR: Castalia, 1975.

54. Newsom C, Rincover A. Autism. In: Mash El, Terdal LG (eds) *Behavioral Assessment of Childhood Disorders.* New York: Guilford Press, 1981; pp. 414–415.

55. Barkley RA. *Defiant Children: A Clinician's Manual for Parent Training.* New York: Guilford Press, 1987.

56. Barkley RA. *Defiant Children: Parent-Teacher Assignments.* New York: Guilford Press, 1987.

57. Singer JL. *The Child's World of Make-Believe: Experimental Studies of Imaginative Play.* New York: Academic Press, 1973.

58. Parten MB. Social participation among pre-school children. *J Abnorm Soc Psychol* 1932;**27**:243–260.

59. Pulaski MA. Play symbolism in cognitive development. In: Schaefer C (ed.) *Therapeutic Use ofChild's Play.* New York: Jason Aronson, 1976; pp. 27–41.

60. Irwin EC. The diagnostic and therapeutic use of pretend play. In: Schaefer CE, O'Connor KJ (eds) *Handbook of*

Play Therapy. New York: John Wiley & Sons, 1983; pp. 148–173.

61. Behar D, Rapoport JL. Play observation and psychiatric diagnosis. In: Schaefer CE, O'Connor KJ (eds) *Handbook of Play Therapy*. New York: John Wiley & Sons, 1983; pp. 193–199.

62. Schaefer CE, Gitlin K, Sandgrund A (eds). Play Diagnosis and Assessment. New York: John Wiley & Sons, 1991.

63. Westby CE. A scale for assessing children's pretend play. In: Schaefer CE, Gitlin K, SandgrundA (eds) *Play Diagnosis and Assessment*. New York: John Wiley & Sons, 1991; pp. 131–161.

64. Baumrind D. Effective parenting during the early adolescent transition. In: Cowan PA, Hetherington EM (eds) *Family Transitions*. Hillsdale, NJ: Erlbaum, 1991; pp. 111–164.

65. Hetherington EM, Parke RD. *Child Psychology: A Contemporary Viewpoint*, 4th edn New York: McGraw-Hill, 1986.

66. Hughes IN, Baker DB. *The Clinical Child Interview*. New York: Guilford Press, 1990.

67. Beavers WR, Hampson RB. *Successful Families: Assessment and Intervention*. New York: W.W. Norton, 1990.

68. Olson DH, Portner J, Bell R. *FACES II*. St Paul, MN: Family Social Science, University of Minnesota, 1982.

69. Barkley RA. *Attention-Deficit Hyperactivity Disorder*. New York: Guilford Press, 1990.

70. Gresham FM, Elliott SN. *Social Skills Rating System*. Circle Pines, MN: American Guidance Service, 1990.

71. Goldstein AP, Sprafkin RP, Gershaw NJ. *Skillstreaming the Adolescent: A Structured LearningApproach to Teaching Prosocial Skills*. Champaign, IL: Research Press, 1980.

72. Millon T, Millon C, Davis R. *The Millon Adolescent Clinical Inventory*. Minneapolis, MN: Pearson Assessments, 2004.

73. Millon T, Tringone R, Millon C, Grossman S. *Millon Pre-Adolescent Clinical Inventory*. Minneapolis, MN: Pearson Assessments, 2004.

74. Myers IB, McCaulley MJ. Manual: *A Guide to the Development and Use of the Myers-BriggsType Indicator*. Palo Alto, CA: Consulting Psychologists Press, 1992.

75. Harrington TF, O'Shea AJ. *The Harrington-O'Shea Career Decision-Making System Revised*. Circle Pines, MN: American Guidance Service, 1992.

76. Miller GA. *The Substance Abuse Subtle Screening Inventory (SASSI) Manual: Chapter 8–The SASSI Adolescent Manual*. Addiction Research & Consultation. Call 1-800-726-0526 for more information, or visit www.sassi.com.

77. Petty J. *Checklist for Child Abuse Evaluation*. Odessa, FL: Psychological Assessment Resources, 1990.

78. Gardner RA. *The Sex Abuse Legitimacy Scale*. Cresskill, NJ: Creative Therapeutics, 1987.

79. Peterson G. *Diagnosis and Child and Adolescent Multiple Personality*. Chapel Hill, NC: Southeast Institute for Group and Family Therapy, 1989.

80. American Psychiatric, Association. *Diagnostic and Statistical Manual of Mental Disorder, Fourth Edition, Text Revision*. Washington, DC: American Psychiatric Association, 2000.

81. Putnam FW, Helmers K, Trickett PK. Development, reliability, and validity of a child dissociation scale. *Child Abuse Negl* 1993;**17**:731–741.

3

Neurobiological Assessment

George Realmuto, Bonnie Klimes-Dougan

Introduction

Neurobiological assessment for psychiatric disorders can't come along too quickly. Child mental health has several needs for such technology. The field needs to rapidly and easily measure the various capacities of the central nervous system (CNS) so that we can accurately evaluate cognitive, emotional, and behavioral variation. We need to go further and measure the genetic variation of these domains to understand risk and vulnerability prior to their developmental manifestations. The discovery, testing, validation, and dissemination of technological procedures to fill gaps in our assessment protocols could reshape our practice of patient care, standards of treatment, the scope of our intervention goals, and the direction in which resources are expended on mental health care. We currently face many problems with assessment that are still answered in ways based on decades-old approaches. What tools do we need, for example, that would allow us to know if a child with poor academic progress and identified dyslexia also had attentional problems that were consistent with attention-deficit hyperactivity disorder (ADHD) inattentive type? Or if an adolescent presented as withdrawn, isolated, and self-destructive, what neurobiological assessment would allow us to easily tell whether this was an acute reaction to significant loss, a major depressive disorder, or bipolar disorder? Could we use neuroimaging to separate very early prodromes of schizophrenia from Asperger's syndrome? Could we curtail the time burden of developmental, family, and medical history-taking by simply applying a piece of modern-day miracle technology? Do we have the neurobiological tools to refine diagnosis and treatment planning? At this point we do not. If we could, our entire nomenclature might need changing. For example, if neuroimaging provided enough information about brain–behavior relationships we might decide that disorders of the frontal cortex should be a major DSMx (*Diagnostic and Statistical Manual*) category. Limbic system disorders might encompass depression, anxiety, and adjustment disorders if assessment techniques could discriminate among them. New categories would group global brain problems such as mental retardation and autism together. Specific brain region disorders would be a collection of problems such as simple motor tic disorder, habit disorders, and blepharospasm. Rapid neurobiological assessment using one of the many forms of imaging such as positron emission tomography (PET), single-photon emission computed tomography (SPECT), and the various forms of magnetic resonance imaging (MRI) would improve identification and move treatment to early onset or even prodromal stages. We now have these technologies but they have not revolutionized the way we work with patients, and it may be time to hope the next generation of technologies will create these opportunities. An alternative is to start to look elsewhere for technologies that are waiting to be brought to clinical practice.

Pharmacogenomics

Pharmacogenomics may be a new place to start. It is a field that is as new as the effort to completely sequence the human genome. Only in 2001 was a first draft sequence of the entire human genome made available to the public by Lander and Venter. The human genome includes 22 pairs of autosomal chromosomes and an additional pair of sex chromosomes. The entire cellular DNA consists of approximately three billion base pairs that may encode 30 000–70 000 genes. One way of inquiring into this massive storehouse of our potential is the field of pharmacogenomics. What is pharmacogenomics not? It is not pharmacogenetics. Pharmacogenetics is the study of inheritance (a gene) and its interactions with medications. Pharmacogenomics is the convergence of advances in pharmacology and genomics. Pharmacogenomics is a scientific body of

Clinical Child Psychiatry, Third Edition. Edited by William M. Klykylo and Jerald Kay.
© 2012 John Wiley & Sons, Ltd. Published 2012 by John Wiley & Sons, Ltd.

knowledge and procedures that allows for genotypic screening to arrive at an informed clinical choice for psychotropic medication. Genomics is the study of whole sets of genes, gene products, and their interactions. Pharmacogenomics then asks questions about medications as they relate to an array of genes that influence those medications. In some sense pharmacogenomics is a study of the heritability of the variance that exists in drug effect. The implications of utilization of this expertise are enormous as it applies to medicine. One example is the choice of a chemotherapeutic agent for the treatment of cancer. One treatment may be intolerable for a particular cancer patient because drug metabolic processes cause intolerable side effects for that individual, and the full dosage cannot be applied. Another example is the widespread use of an effective analgesic medication. While analgesics are safe and effective in most patients, popular accounts suggest that in a very small group they can have very serious and life-threatening adverse effects. One such drug had a variant of a metabolic pathway that caused large accumulations of the drug leading to near fatal consequences. A simple test was devised to identify patients belonging to this group. Physicians were warned of this potential hazard, educated about identification procedures and screening, and at-risk patients were excluded from treatment with the drug. As compelling as these scenarios may seem in general medicine, in order for mental health to adopt pharmacogenomics a clear application needs to be found. Then why should pharmacogenomic technology become part of a practical and effective neurobiological assessment?

There is significant variation among individuals in the way they metabolize medications. For example, among individuals of European origin, 1 in 10 metabolize certain antidepressants poorly. A much smaller subset of Europeans metabolize the same drugs rapidly. If the clinician knew the status of a particular patient would that clinician make a more informed choice and reduce the risk of adverse side effects – i.e., slow metabolism and adverse effects or rapid metabolism and poor response?

Fluorescence *In Situ* Hybridization

Genetic testing is not new to psychiatry. We may not think too much about the procedure that we choose when a genetic disorder with significant behavioral and cognitive features is suspected. Fluorescence *in situ* hybridization (FISH) is a method of creating a sequence of DNA (the probe), attaching an identification tag on it, called a fluorophore, and incubating it with the genetic material in question. If the complementary sequence of genetic material to be tested is present, the probe will stick and the fluorophore will mark its presence through a light-emitting signal. FISH was developed in 1986 by Pinkel *et al*. His group found a method to visualize chromosomes using fluorescent-labeled probes. The procedure involves the annealing of the FISH probe DNA with complementary DNA sequences in the chromosomes. The presence or absence of the signal is observed with a fluorescence microscope. FISH probes have been developed for many disorders of interest to psychiatry. These include fragile X, velocardiofacial syndrome, Smith–Magenis syndrome, Prader–Willi and Angelman syndromes, and Williams syndrome. New tests could be developed at any time. A psychiatric researcher who had reason to believe that a specific sequence of DNA was responsible for a product that affected CNS functioning could develop a systematic test for that DNA sequence. FISH is less useful when variation in gene sequence is the issue, but it is very suitable for any application in which the presence or absence of a known DNA base pair sequence is to be determined.

Polymerase Chain Reaction

An important procedure that underlies the incredible advances that have taken place in DNA sequencing is the polymerase chain reaction (PCR). It is the most widely used molecular procedure and is part of most genetic testing strategies. PCR permits the copying of pieces of DNA multiple times to produce exact replicas of the original. The procedure begins with the identification of the double-stranded DNA template to be copied. The double-stranded DNA is heated to break the hydrogen bonds between the base pairs and separate the DNA into two complementary single strands. Other ingredients required include a synthetic or laboratory-constructed version of DNA sequences called oligonucleotide primers. These primers are complementary to a short segment of DNA sequence at either end of the template to be replicated. They serve as starting points for the replication. In addition the building blocks – nucleotide triphosphates – for DNA construction must be present. There are four types of nucleic acid, adenine, guanine, thymine, and cytosine, which are subsequently attached to a sugar–phosphate backbone. Finally, the reaction is catalyzed by DNA polymerase. This is an enzyme that synthesizes DNA by successively adding nucleotides to the free 3'-hydroxyl group of the growing strand. This enzyme is heat stable allowing for cooling and heating cycles. Each cycle involves binding of the primer to the DNA sequence that is immediately adjacent to the target sequence to be replicated; this enables the extension of the bound oligonucleotide primer by adding free nucleotides. Each cycle results in doubling of the number of target DNA regions, with a final target amplification of approximately more than a million copies.

Microarray Analysis

Microarray technology is a novel tool to evaluate many genes and gene products en masse with high efficiency. Microarray analysis, as its name suggests, is possible with the availability of miniaturized, computer-assisted imaging systems. If an investigator thought that a disease state was caused by or associated with a particular gene polymorphism or cluster of genes, multiple patients with this disorder could have this combination of genes evaluated and commonalities of specific polymorphisms could be determined. For the clinician, once this grouping is identified treatments could be devised to alter gene expression. The possible applications of DNA microarray analysis include identification of a specific gene of interest, screening for mutations or polymorphisms, and comparative genomic hybridization.

The physical features of a microarray chip might be consistent with a view of computers in general. The chip is made of chemically coated glass to which a nylon membrane is attached. A coating of polylysine or silane allows for the adhesion of the test probes. The cells are small, less than 250 nm in diameter (Figure 3.1a), and are topographically organized into an array of columns and rows capable of being assessed by computer-directed robotic readers with the input being systematically recorded. A place on the microarray at the intersection of a column and a row, known as an address, designates the location for the quantification of the expression of a

(a)

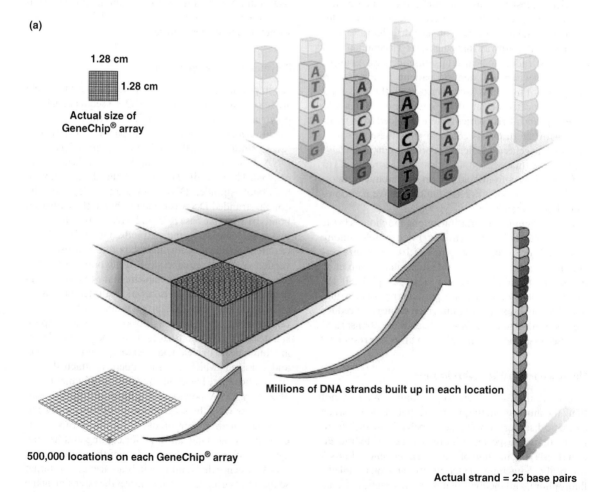

1.28 cm

1.28 cm

Actual size of GeneChip® array

Millions of DNA strands built up in each location

500,000 locations on each GeneChip® array

Actual strand = 25 base pairs

Figure 3.1a GeneChip™; cartoon depicting a single feature on an Affymetrix GeneChip™ microarray. (Image courtesy of Affymetrix.)

(b) **RNA fragments with fluorescent tags from sample to be tested**

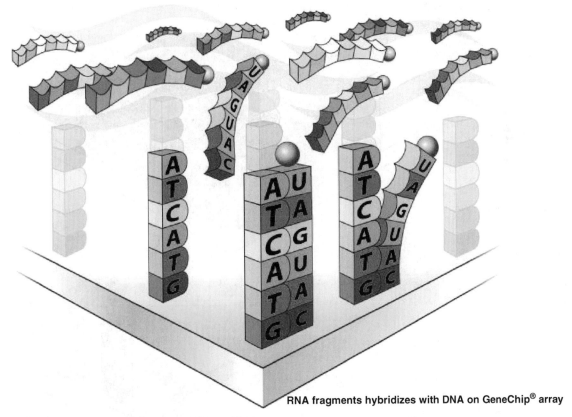

RNA fragments hybridizes with DNA on GeneChip® array

Figure 3.1b GeneChip™; cartoon depicting hybridization of tagged probes to Affymetrix GeneChip™ microarray. (Image courtesy of Affymetrix.)

gene for a particular subject or patient. The microarray chip containing these cells is embedded with a small fragment of DNA (Figure 3.1b). The DNA molecule that is attached to each cell on the chip is referred to as a probe. Probes are used to detect targets. The target is usually complementary DNA, made by synthesis using an RNA sequence as the template. The advantages of complementary DNA is that it is devoid of introns, sequences that are not represented in the product sequence of a gene. Introns are removed by a process known as intron splicing. The probes bind to their target sequences through hybridizing, involving alignment and base pairing. However, some experimental tasks require the use of genomic DNA. If a single DNA base pair distinguishes the subject from the norm, genomic DNA rather than expressed DNA or DNA made from RNA would be the target of choice. Then, the search is for single nucleotide polymorphisms (SNPs). A particular gene's activity or efficiency, or the developmental timing

of its expression, may be influenced by a SNP. A SNP requires very fine-scale detection procedures, and preparation of the probes needs to be carefully considered.

As mentioned above PCR techniques can produce large quantities of DNA products or probes. Where should one choose to obtain these probes? When looking for the variant it may be best to have probes of the wild-type or most common genetic variation. The absence then of a match between probe and target would indicate that a difference had been detected. Databases now detail extensive information about each probe at each cell location.

How are Matches and Nonmatches Detected?

During manufacture of a microarray, complementary DNA is deposited on the microarray cells by a computer-assisted high-speed robot. The number of cells on a chip depends on the manufacturer of the chip; some

(a)   **Shining a laser light at GeneChip® array causes tagged DNA fragments that hybridized to glow**

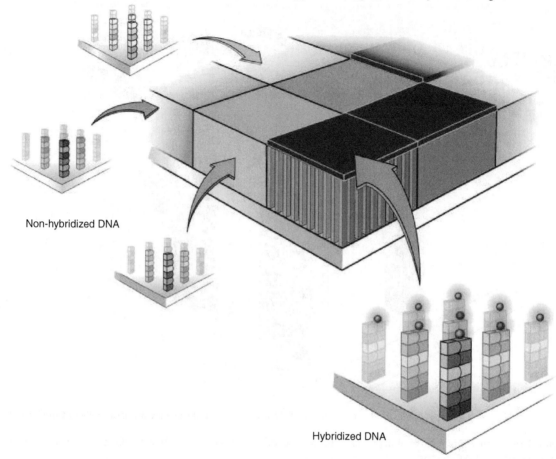

Non-hybridized DNA

Hybridized DNA

Figure 3.2a   Hybridized GeneChip™; cartoon depicting scanning of tagged and untagged probes on an Affymetrix GeneChip™ microarray. (Image courtesy of Affymetrix.)

chips carry as many as 65 000 cells. The probes are then processed with a fluorochrome dye, which is applied to the probes so that they can report the presence or absence of a target match. When a laser is focused onto a cell, light is emitted and each lit cell is detected and computer coded. The laser beam excites the fluorescent dye linked to the probe that has been hybridized with the target DNA (Figure 3.2a). A scanner monitors the fluorescence from each cell. The degree of fluorescence correlates with the abundance of target molecules at a specific cell (Figure 3.2b).

Clinical Applications of Microarrays

While the technology and processes are very sophisticated, the advantage for clinical practice can be exciting

and practical. One application already past the pilot stage is the identification of differences in enzyme systems that influence psychoactive drug metabolism. Of special interest to child and adolescent psychiatry is the P450 group of enzymes expressed in the liver. This family of enzymes is responsible for the metabolism of all currently available selective serotonin reuptake inhibitors (SSRIs), tricyclic antidepressants, and some antipsychotics. There are 10 enzyme systems in this family and each of the genes has an array of alleles that confer variability of metabolic rate. Within different ethnic groups there may be less heterogeneity. One of these is the *CYP2D6* allele. Humans have two copies of this allele. Since this enzyme is responsible for the metabolism of some antidepressants, the activity of a particular inherited variant may influence the effectiveness of treatment. The version of

(b)

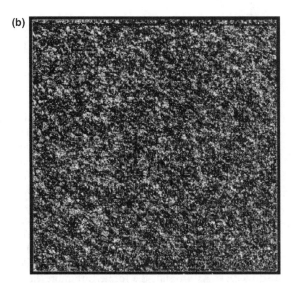

Figure 3.2b GeneChip™; array output data from an experiment showing the thousands of genes detected by a single GeneChip™ probe array. (Image courtesy of Affymetrix.)

the gene inherited will be demonstrated by a specific expression of metabolic activity. The kinds of gene differences that might lead to different outcomes could include a deletion of the allele, a redundant version due to duplication of the gene, or SNPs, which have a spectrum of effects. *CYP2D4* has 12 known variants; the variations are produced by different kinds of base pair alterations including shifts, additions, deletions, or single nucleotide substitutions. The consequences for metabolic activity range from slow metabolism to ultra-rapid. The slowest activity may be due to deletion or inactivation of both copies of the gene, whereas the heterozygous variant, with one inactive gene, results in an intermediate level of metabolism. The most common variant metabolizes some drugs fairly extensively. Finally there is a very rapid metabolic type that is due to multiple duplications of the gene. It is not uncommon for individuals with the highest level of metabolism to be unresponsive to treatment.

In clinical practice, a sample of the patient's blood is taken and DNA extracted from the white cells. Multiple copies of complementary DNA (cDNA) that is representative of this allelic site can be produced by PCR. A specific chip with probes for each variant can be prepared, and depending on the hybridization that occurs on the chip and the detection of target-probe matching through fluorescence emission, information about that individual's genetic variant can be determined.

This may be very useful for clinical decision-making. Since different SSRI antidepressants have a different profile of P450 enzyme metabolism, a specific choice of SSRI might be made on grounds other than "best guess." Paroxetine and fluoxetine are metabolized by the CYP2D6 enzyme system. This family is even more genetically diverse than the CYP2D4 family. It has been shown to have more than 50 allelic polymorphisms. As noted above, different ethnic groups have different profiles of polymorphisms, which in some cases can increase the accuracy of clinical guessing about the possible success of an antidepressant in a member of that group. However, we now have the laboratory capacity to determine in any individual the specific polymorphism of each of the P450 enzyme families. Therefore with a high degree of certainty, a laboratory test can determine the rate of metabolism and clearly indicate which antidepressant is likely to be effective or produce side effects, according to the presence of particular polymorphisms.

There are several implications of these procedures. Genetic profiling may identify patterns of gene variants that at some point in time may be linked to risk for disease. Informing a patient about their genotype in relation to clinical decisions about medication choice today may expose them to knowledge about their risk for disease in the near future. Such knowledge may not have been included in the informed consent that accompanied their decision to obtain information for medication decision-making. Therefore additional consent about the possible use of genetic testing would need to include a discussion about how the information would be documented and to whom the information would or would not be transferred now and in the future. Another implication is the role of pharmacogenomic testing for practice standards. If there is a way to choose a medication that will have fewer side effects and better efficacy should we not adopt such a test?

These tests are really here now. A well-known medical clinic in the US Midwest is already making a cytochrome P450 test available for a small sum of about $300 (David Mrazek, personal communication). The test will provide the clinician with a profile of a patient's cytochrome P450 2D6 genotype with information about the activity of each of the identified variants. The laboratory can be reached at 800 533 1710 or mayomedicallaboratories. com. Matching these genetic determinants with a drug's preferred metabolic pathway can be lifesaving: for example, a patient is admitted to an inpatient unit for continued suicidal ideation and attempt, and it is determined that the current SSRI is ineffective; making a wrong therapy choice could lead to a lengthy hospitalization whereas cytochrome P450 information could lead to an informed choice. The costs of the tests would quickly be recouped through shorter length of stay. We have been disappointed by the contributions that imaging and other technologies were expected to make to child and adolescent psychiatry. Although pharmacogenomic testing is new, it would seem to fulfill a need and fit a rationale. So will we adopt it?

Promising Technologies for Neurobiological Assessments

Many tools currently used for research show promise of making their way into clinical practice. These technologies depend on sophisticated computer hardware and software. In some cases, scientists with special expertise are needed beyond the highly trained technicians who prepare the patient and operate the equipment. However, the costs of individual examinations have fallen, bringing such methods of examination closer to clinical practice than ever before.

What follows is a brief description of the methods and principles of experimental neurobiological assessment techniques (Table 3.1).

Single-Photon Emission Computed Tomography

The technique of single-photon emission computed tomography (SPECT) detects and images gamma rays produced by radioactive isotopes. These gamma-emitting radiolabeled substances produce a single photon of energy that is detected by single-crystal scintillation instruments external to the subject. The radioactive distribution is analyzed by a computer and displayed as an image based on the energy produced and the position of the source of the energy (Figure 3.3). The procedure has gone through several refinements, including improved detection of photon emissions of newer radiopharmaceuticals.

There are several important differences between SPECT and positron emission tomography (PET). SPECT radioisotopes produce lower-energy gamma rays than the photons produced by the radionuclides used in PET. As a result, the former are more easily absorbed by the body and therefore require longer scanning sessions for adequate resolution. In addition, lower-energy isotopes result in deeper structures of the brain absorbing or attenuating emitted radiation, which requires some adjustment of the signal to decrease artifact.

Table 3.1 Potential neurobiological techniques.

Technique	Description	Potential application	References
Event-related potential	Summed electrical activity from groups of neurons responding to a time-locked stimulus	Neurodevelopmental disorder, early identification, and qualification of impairment	[1–3]
Magnetic resonance imaging (MRI)	Detection of radio waves from atomic particles and translation into computerized images	Brain-behavior correlations; identification of structures abnormal for volume and blood flow	[4,5]
Single-photon emission computed tomography (SPECT)	Radioactive substance produces an emission that can be detected and visualized	Identification of subgroups within diagnostic groups that may have different pathophysiological processes requiring different interventions	[6,7]
Positron emission tomography (PET)	Radioactive substance emits protons that produce photons that are detected and imaged, creating maps of activity or localization	Anatomical localization of important brain events or locales that underlie disorders or responses to treatments	[8–12]
Functional magnetic resonance imaging (fMRI)	$T2^*$, the modified time constant for transverse relaxation, is measured in various tissues whose differences emerge as a result of the imposition of a field magnet	Structure-function relationships of the central nervous system	[13]

Right **Anterior** **Left**

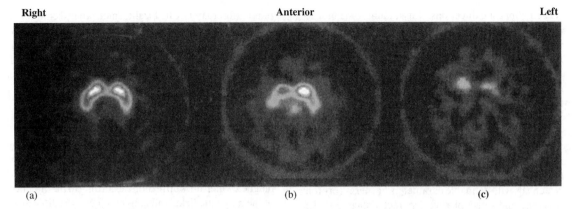

(a) (b) (c)

Figure 3.3 Transaxial single-photon emission computed tomography (SPECT) images at the level of the striatum in a healthy subject (a) and two patients with Parkinson's disease (b, early stage; c, late stage). The ^{123}I-labeled radiopharmaceutical b-CIT binds to dopamine transporters on the presynaptic terminals of dopamine neurons. The SPECT images demonstrate that patients with Parkinson's disease have fewer striatal uptake sites than healthy subjects, with greater loss in the putamen (posterior) region than in the head of the caudate. (Images courtesy of John Seibyl MD, Ken Marek MD, and Robert Innis MD, New Haven, CT.)

SPECT has been successfully used in the study of patients with ADHD. In a series of studies in which children and adolescents with ADHD inhaled radiolabeled xenon, results were consistent with other evidence for hypofrontality as well as hypoperfusion of the caudate nuclei. Administration of methylphenidate to a subgroup of these patients had a normalizing effect on brain activity as shown after rescanning [6]. Another center studied a larger and better-described group of children and adolescents with ADHD under resting and stress conditions. Again, prefrontal problems were noted [2].

There have been advances in the radiolabeling of a variety of pharmaceutical antagonists whose application is important to psychiatry, such as radiolabeled probes for D1 and D2 dopamine receptors [14, 15]. Poor morphological resolution and the use of radioactive substances that convey some small risk in children, whose nervous systems are developing rapidly, may limit the overall potential for child psychiatry. However, enhanced detection through computer software and other technical improvements as well as targeted probes identifying neurotransmitters and receptors may improve this technique to the point that SPECT closely rivals PET.

Positron Emission Tomography

PET permits measurements of the rate of radioactive substrate consumption. If the radioactive substrate collects at points of increased neural activity, the decay of the substrate at that locale will identify such processes.

If the substrate binds to a particular receptor, then the receptor will be localized during the degradation of the radioactive substrate.

The physics of PET scanning are founded on principles governing the emission of protons from nuclei during radioactive decay. The emitted proton inevitably collides with an electron, resulting in two photons traveling in almost opposite directions. The PET scanner can record these photons with scintillation detectors using sodium iodide or bismuth germanate crystals. The scintillation detectors convert the photon energy into visible light that can be recorded on film. Only those photons traveling in linear but opposite directions are saved as data points through the encircling array of scintillation detectors. The activity produced by the radioactive nuclei can be pinpointed in two-dimensional space and reorganized spatially to produce a graphic representation of the photons.

The advantages of PET over SPECT include higher-energy reactions and thus the emission of higher-energy protons with less attenuation from surrounding tissue, which produces cleaner images. Also, PET does not use collimators or parallel filters to focus photons, which may compromise the resolution of SPECT technologies.

There are limitations of PET, however. First, the energy of the radioactive substance used to generate protons is considered more hazardous to the host than that of the lower-energy chemicals used in SPECT, and this is an important factor in limiting the recruitment of children for PET studies. Second, the collision of proton and electron does not always produce photons traveling in exactly opposite directions, thus adding some blur to the image. Third, the scintillation detectors themselves have physical limits that affect clarity. What begins as a single point of activity in the brain may ultimately emerge as a 10 cm image. Fourth, the mathematical modeling methods used to extract absolute measurements are highly controversial. Because of differences between imaging centers' methods and equipment and mathematical algorithms, results might best be considered relative rather than absolute quantities. Finally, a unique requirement for PET scanning is the production of a radioactive tracer. High-energy radiolabeled pharmaceuticals with definable parameters of energy, proton emissions, and other physical characteristics must be created in a cyclotron. The substrates are bombarded with protons in the cyclotron to produce the desired probe. Since the probe decays rapidly, this technique requires on-site facilities to create tracer substances along with the personnel and capacity to deal with the spent low-level radioactive waste [16].

PET scan studies of interest to child and adolescent psychiatry were begun in 1990 by Zametkin and colleagues, using a sample of adults with ADHD [8]. In 1993, 10 adolescents with ADHD were studied, and six brain regions showed differences in activity when compared to controls. These included frontal, thalamic, hippocampal, and temporal areas with findings distributed by both hemisphere and rate (increase or decrease in brain metabolic activity) [9].

These studies were pursued to evaluate the metabolic activation of brain areas stimulated by dextroamphetamine (dexamfetamine) and methylphenidate [11, 17]. Unfortunately, the findings about the action sites of drugs did not give clear inferences about brain response to medication in regions specific to ADHD. A more promising study published by Matlay and colleagues used PET to view the action of medication in adults [12]. In this study, cognitive tasks of executive brain function were administered to subjects to stimulate metabolism in brain regions subserving those functions. Differential oxygen uptake enhancement by stimulant drug was observed in the prefrontal cortex and hippocampus.

In summary, although PET methodology was applied in a research setting to differentiate ADHD subjects from controls and to evaluate drug treatment effects, the results were disappointing. Few adolescents and no children participated in the studies because of concerns about the protection of human subjects, thus significantly limiting application to the patients of prime interest. Also, the results were neither anatomically specific nor, for the most part, consistent with hypothesized defects derived from other sources. The long-term prospect of PET scanning for the child and adolescent

population may not be bright, since other technologies subserve similar goals. Functional MRI (fMRI) has several advantages over PET and obtains similar information (see next section). Competition among technologies is good for the field, improving the time, convenience, cost, and information delivered.

Magnetic Resonance Imaging (MRI)

The technological procedure that appears to have the easiest entry into child and adolescent mental health is MRI. The equipment required includes a high-powered magnet, which lines up protons according to the direction of the magnetic field, and coils conducting radio waves. Radio waves alter the alignment of the protons, and the resulting signal produced from this realignment can be detected and fashioned into images using computer software. Stronger magnets, better software, and more experience with the location and pulse frequency of coils have improved the quality of the images (Figure 3.4).

Interesting work with MRI has elucidated the size of important brain structures and allowed clearer correlations between structure and function. For example, one report contributed to a better understanding of the basal ganglia in patients with obsessive-compulsive disorder (OCD). Basal ganglia volumes measured with MRI were compared with symptom severity at different times, and as treatment removed antistreptolysin O antigens, caudate size diminished and symptoms decreased [4]. In the future, an evaluation of structures such as caudate size may be useful in differential

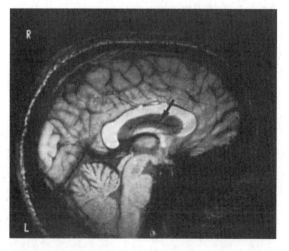

Figure 3.4 Sagittal view of the human brain at 4.1 tesla demonstrating exquisite neuroanatomical resolution. (Image courtesy of Dr Julie W. Pan and Hoby Hetherington PhD, Birmingham, AL.)

diagnosis and the evaluation of treatment response. Defining caudate volume may be useful in differentiating habit disorders from adjustment disorders, and neurobiological phenomena such as Tourette's syndrome and OCD, and may also give specific direction to treatment interventions and permit clearer measures of treatment response.

Limitations to this procedure are minimal. Contraindications include mainly the presence of ferrous metals in the body, although this is probably not a significant problem in the child and adolescent population. Multiple exposures were originally a concern, but these are now being permitted when clinically indicated, with few adverse experiences. Rapidly changing the direction of the magnetic field potentially produces electric shock and tissue damage, and alternations in magnetic polarity that are too rapid may induce electric currents within the body and may thus produce an activation of peripheral nerves that the patient may feel. In addition, tissues that have few ways to dissipate heat can be exposed to the hazard of energy produced by a rapidly changing magnetic field. The Food and Drug Administration has set limits on these parameters, and most MRI scanners have these upper limits built into the system software to prevent untoward events. Another limitation of use has been cost, particularly in setting up such equipment, but competition and the portability of the equipment have made MRI virtually universally available.

Given the opportunities for better definition of CNS substrates of psychopathology, it behooves the profession to develop medical necessity guidelines and criteria so that this and other technological procedures will be approved for use in children and adolescents as a standard of care.

Functional Magnetic Resonance Imaging (fMRI)

Mapping of physiological activity is a capability of MRI technology shared with PET, SPECT, and evoked potentials. However, high temporal and spatial resolution and the ability to repeatedly scan subjects give fMRI an advantage over other imaging techniques. Although this technique may circumvent many of the hazards that have precluded children from entering research protocols, fMRI has arrived only relatively recently, and there is little in the literature to demonstrate its superiority over other methods [18].

As described for MRI (see previous section), the physical basis of fMRI is the systematic manipulation of changes to the precession of atomic nuclei around their axes. The activity of spinning atomic nuclei results in minute magnetic fields, and anatomical structures differ in their chemical composition and thus magnetic characteristics. Differences in the magnetic susceptibility of these anatomical structures make it possible for these magnetic dipoles to be manipulated to produce radio frequencies that can be detected by specialized receiver coils. Using sophisticated computer technology, these differences are then spatially arranged into images. The largest magnetic fields are produced at the boundaries of volumes with the largest differences in magnetic susceptibility.

Magnetic susceptibility is caused by the propensity of a material to develop an internal magnetic field in response to one applied from the outside. In the case of fMRI, the field applied is the large magnetic field applied to the body [19]. Of particular importance in fMRI are the physiological changes that occur in the blood as it perfuses neural tissue. Activated tissue deoxygenates blood, and thus maps can be produced of localities in the brain where oxygen is being consumed at rates statistically different from baseline. Oxygen changes the magnetic properties of hemoglobin, and deoxygenated blood has very different magnetic properties from surrounding brain parenchyma, which can be detected as differences in magnetic field frequencies.

The specific type of MRI frequency that is measured in fMRI is the $T2^*$. When a static magnetic field is applied to a volume of tissue, atomic nuclei can respond by developing a magnetic field and thus magnetic susceptibility. However, the random directions of the magnetic fields of surrounding nuclei result in the neutralization of any particular summed field strength. These events are generated in the direction transverse to the static magnetic field. This equilibration of the magnetic field is called relaxation and it occurs over a specific time course. $T2^*$ therefore represents the modified time constant for transverse relaxation (Figure 3.5).

Little work has been done with fMRI in any population. Teicher and colleagues reported the effects of methylphenidate on ADHD symptoms and fMRI in children, and showed a strong correlation between the number of child movements on placebo and $T2^*$ relaxation times of the right caudate [13]. The optimal dose of methylphenidate exerted significant effects on frontal and caudate $T2^*$, which affected the right hemisphere more than the left. Another publication investigating the neuroanatomy of OCD symptoms in adults showed the activation of specific brain regions, including limbic structures that had been identified previously for subjects but not controls [20].

Conceptually, fMRI is more complicated than other imaging techniques. The master of fMRI requires skills in many technical and clinical areas. The first wave of studies to be published will likely be a replication of studies that have previously used other imaging

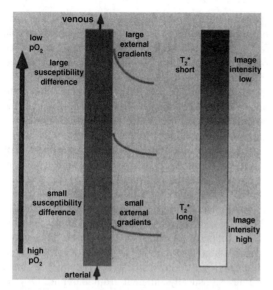

Figure 3.5 The physical basis of functional magnetic resonance imaging (fMRI) signal changes. From left to right, decreasing blood oxygenation increases field gradients surrounding vessels, which in turn decreases T2* and image intensity. Neuronal activity increases capillary level oxygenation, which is detected as an increase in T2*-weighted image intensity. (From Anderson and Gore [16].)

procedures. These replication studies may allow fMRI to quickly emerge as the imaging standard, and studies of all ages and conditions will likely follow (Figure 3.6).

Magnetic Resonance Spectroscopy

Preceding the more widely used imaging techniques of MRI was magnetic resonance spectroscopy (MRS), a novel investigative tool developed to understand the functional basis of disease [21]. MRS is capable of identifying important events in cell metabolism such as energy production and dissipation through the identification of chemicals that are produced or consumed by these processes.

The basic principles of MRS and MRI are identical. MRS, however, records differences in activity based on the detection of chemical shift. As described previously, atomic nuclei possessing magnetic properties rotate around an axis depending on the strength of the magnetic field applied. For MRS, however, detection of the differences in chemicals is based on the magnetic properties of atomic nuclei as they are influenced by the quantity of electrons possessed by a given chemical. This is the key point of the technique. Hydrogen protons may

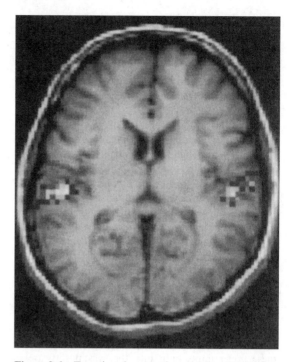

Figure 3.6 Functional magnetic resonance (MR) map of the primary auditory cortex. Pixels with significant signal changes associated with the presentation of sounds are shown in color (greater significance in lighter shades), superimposed on a conventional MR scan of the same slice through the brain. (Courtesy of Rene Marois, Yale University, New Haven, CT.)

precess at a certain frequency, but differences exist if the hydrogen atom is part of water, with an electrical cloud produced by two oxygen atoms, or if it is a hydrogen atom that is part of a methane moiety of a large organic molecule. Since each hydrogen atom experiences a slightly different local magnetic field owing to shielding by different clouds of electrons, each chemical shift is the difference in resonance frequency caused by the characteristics inherent in a particular nucleus. Detection of these differences is similar to procedures described for MRI and includes tipping the axis of the spinning atomic nuclei with a specific radio frequency and recording changes in magnetic field. Relaxation time as nuclei re-equilibrate is transformed into frequency values and displayed as unique frequency spectra [22].

MRS can detect cellular activity involving phosphorylated compounds including adenosine triphosphate (ATP) and its phosphorylated intermediates. Chemical products available for measurement with this technique include choline and lactate. Further extension of this technology includes quantitative measurement of neurotransmitter and neurochemical levels. Limitations that are generic to magnetic resonance technologies are also present with spectroscopy, including slow acquisition time, artifact created by patient movement, and relatively poor spatial resolution. However, more powerful computer software, higher field strengths of the magnet, and creative ways of improving patient cooperation may allow the detection of chemical events related to specific psychopathological processes [22].

Electrophysiological Procedures: Event-Related Potentials

The event-related potential is a neural phenomenon captured with a relatively noninvasive procedure, and some applications are not particularly demanding of a child's attention or self-discipline. Brain electrical activity can be recorded through the placement of electrodes on the skull in a system similar to that of electroencephalogram electrode placement. The brain produces a sequence of positive and negative deflections that are consistently observed as a consequence of auditory, visual, or somatosensory stimuli. These waves are generated by groups of aligned cells that together reach a state of depolarization or hyperpolarization that is detected by electrodes – in much the same way the center of an earthquake is detected by seismological instruments distributed across the Earth's crust. Courchesne and colleagues have done considerable work using this technique to further our understanding of autistic disorder [2]. It is with such neuropsychiatric conditions that organ level measurements become most useful, because of the significant communicative disability that makes direct inquiry difficult, if not impossible. One of the many findings contributed by a series of studies with autistic subjects was the reduction of amplitude of the P300 waveform. The P300 waveform is a characteristic positive deflection occurring approximately 300 milliseconds after the onset of a stimulus. The P300 response is generally evoked by target- or task-related events and may be influenced by the relevance of the stimuli, the motivation of the subjects, and other subject and stimuli variables. This late-appearing wave may therefore have something to do with cognitive processing as compared to earlier-appearing waves that may measure the "hard wiring" of the CNS. The subject is asked to complete a cognitive task that is reflected in the P300. The finding that nonretarded adolescent autistic subjects demonstrate smaller P300 amplitudes as well as other parameters suggests that autism is a disorder of focused attention in which novel and common stimuli are perceived with equal relevance [2]. Evoked potential procedures have been applied to infants and very young children who have experienced prenatal

or perinatal insults [23], and in a growing body of work, the examination of risk for chemical dependency has been quite fruitful [1].

Current limitations of this procedure include costs for computer hardware and software and ongoing technical support as well as the time and energy consumed by technical and computer glitches that appear to be a by-product of cutting-edge technology.

Electroencephalography

Old technology, namely the electroencephalogram (EEG), continues to have a place in the neurobiological assessment of children and adolescents. The earliest work on electroencephalography dates to the German psychiatrist Hans Berger, who published the EEG of his son in 1929. He showed that changes occurred in his son's alpha rhythm due to mental activity. EEG instrumentation identifies changes in direction of the flow of electrons as detected by electrodes placed on the patient's scalp. As groups of neurons depolarize an electrical field is developed, the direction of which can be detected by the electrodes. Fluctuations in field strength for each electrode are recorded on paper or captured by sophisticated computer software.

Among the disorders relevant for EEG assessment is autism. Differentiation of a disorder such as Landau–Kleffner syndrome, which has a specific treatment, from autism is very important. Also since autism has an incidence of seizures of about 20–30% with a peak risk for onset in early adolescence, the clinician should consider ordering an EEG as part of a work-up for any unusual change in the adolescent's clinical condition. EEG differences from normal have been noted for ADHD, conduct disorder, and learning disorders but the findings are nonspecific and may not be helpful for guiding treatment. Medication monitoring for drug treatments that lower seizure threshold may continue to define a use for EEG testing.

Measurement of Cortisol and its Importance in Mental Health Disorders

The Hypothalamic–Pituitary–Adrenal Axis

The Hypothalamic–Pituitary–Adrenal (HPA) axis serves to regulate basal body functions via a critically important neurohormonal cascade. The process is initiated in the brain and the end products, glucocorticoids (referred to as cortisol in humans), are secreted from the adrenal cortex in the abdomen. Healthy adaptation and, indeed, survival relies on an individual's ability to produce appropriate levels of neurohormones [24].

Under conditions of stress, key limbic structures, including the amygdala, serve to detect threat and initiate the HPA axis cascade. Prefrontal-amygdala and thalamic-amygdala neurocircuits are critical for providing, respectively, cognitive mediation and more reflexive processing of threat stimuli [25]. The resulting stimulation of the HPA axis serves to marshal the physical and cognitive resources of the individual. Negative feedback serves to abate the production of these neurohormones once the stressor has diminished. Advances in our understanding of HPA axis functioning have important implications for the field of child psychiatry.

Early life stress has been found to alter the functioning of the HPA axis. Seymour Levine in *Science* was the first to document that simply removing rat pups from their mother and handling them for a few moments daily had lasting effects of modifying the functioning of the HPA axis [26]. Subsequent work has clarified that there is a critical period in early development that influences programming of the HPA axis. Also, deprivation experiences have been found to reduce neural plasticity to stress experienced later in life [27]. Although in humans the developmental window for a "sensitive period" is likely to be more protracted, evidence is accumulating that early childhood and adolescent years provide key windows of potential vulnerability [28, 29]. There is also evidence that poorly regulated stress hormones may be implicated in brain degeneration and other long-term negative outcomes [30]. Due to the concentration of glucocorticoid receptor sites in the fronto-limbic neurocircuitry, the neuro-degenerative effects associated with HPA dysregulation selectively correspond with impairments in these regions including the hippocampus [31, 32].

Perhaps one of the most significant scientific breakthroughs implicating the high relevance of the HPA axis to the field was the discovery that stressful experiences could silence genes critical to the regulation of stress responses. This evidence for epigenetic effects was supported for the first time in animal studies, showing that early life stress alters the epigenetic status of the glucocorticoid promoter region [33]. The products of the HPA axis serves as a gene transcription factor, permitting sculpting of the neural systems involved in learning, memory, and emotion [34], and potentially altering the way the organism responds to a stressor the next time it is encountered [35]. Of importance to intervention efforts, not only is the epigenetic state of the gene capable of being programmed, but also that programming is potentially reversible [33].

Advances in understanding HPA axis functioning in humans have been facilitated by increased availability of assessment methodologies. Considerable efforts to control extraneous factors (e.g., time of day) are needed when assessing byproducts of the HPA axis. Cortisol circulates throughout the body and can be measured in any body fluid including cerebral spinal fluid, blood, saliva, urine, etc. While cortisol represents a limited index of neurohormonal functioning in the HPA axis, the feasibility and utility of obtaining salivary samples accounts for the recent surge in cortisol research with child and adolescent research participants. Salivary cortisol assays have numerous advantages. Not only is this approach likely to minimize selection biases for participants who may find other invasive procedures aversive (e.g., blood draws), they also enhance the ease with which repeated samples may be obtained and the potential use of more ecologically valid settings that do not require visits to the laboratory. Salivary cortisol assays are generally comparable to and even advantageous over other extraction methods (e.g., plasma, serum), and may represent a useful biomarker [36].

Not only should abnormalities in cortisol levels be noted, but also the pattern of secretion needs to be considered. Protracted hyperarousal of the HPA, as well as hypoarousal of the HPA axis, may be associated with a host of deleterious effects [37]. Disruptions in the HPA axis have been characterized by atypical diurnal patterns, including: a failure to mount a cortisol awakening response (CAR); flattened diurnal cycle across the day; elevated secretion at the nadir (just before going to sleep); or heightened day-to-day variability. While it is useful for the child to be able to mount a stress response in the face of a perceived threat, exaggerated levels of anticipatory stress, failure to accommodate to a stress, heightened stress responses (response), longer delays in returning to baseline (recovery), or a failure to mount a response to known stressors have all been considered disruptions of the expected HPA axis response. Laboratory paradigms initially used to investigate the stress response with adults have been adapted for use with children and adolescents, including the procedures used to evaluate the effects of psychological stress such as the Trier Social Stress Test [38], and pharmacological probes such as the dexamethasone suppression test (DEX) or corticotropin releasing hormone infusion test (CRH test). Also, stressors within the context of daily life have been utilized, such as the first day of kindergarten [39].

The significance of the measurement of cortisol as a neurobiological assessment tool has been demonstrated by disruption of the HPA axis in depression. Despite the evidence that HPA axis disruptions are represented in a host of child and adolescent behavioral and emotional problems that may be comorbid with depression, including anxiety disorders, conduct disorder [40], and even autism [18], our subsequent discussion focuses on addressing HPA axis functioning in children and adolescents with depression. Indeed, hyperarousal of the HPA axis in depressed adults is one of the most reliable phenomena associated with depression in biological psychiatry [41, 42], and pioneering work in this field of child and adolescent depression was conducted by researchers at the Western Psychiatric Association [43]. Several more recent reviews, including a recent meta-analysis, concluded that the HPA axis tends to be dysregulated in depressed youth as evidenced by biological probes, baseline cortisol values, and in response to psychological stressors [44–47]. Consistent with adult research that has specifically implicated disruptions in stress recovery [48], preliminary evidence suggests impairment in stress recovery in adolescents with internalizing problems and/or clinically depressed adolescents [49, 50]. Recent studies employing the Trier Social Stress Test (TSST) with depressed adolescents have documented more prolonged elevations of cortisol levels following psychosocial stress induction as compared to controls [51, 52].

Premorbid differences in the HPA axis precede and predict the development of depression in high-risk samples. Dysfunction of the HPA axis has been proposed as a biomarker [36, 53], and family risk models provide growing evidence of disruptions in the HPA cascade. Unaffected twins, discordant for affective disorder, have been found to exhibit elevated basal cortisol levels [54]. To date there has been some evidence of increased elevation in basal cortisol levels, higher variability in cortisol levels, and atypical responses to pharmacological probes in offspring of depressed parents [55–59].

Emerging evidence suggests that a poor prognosis may result when depression is accompanied by hyperarousal of the HPA axis. While the findings regarding HPA anomalies and the links with depression are more variable in adolescents, hyperarousal of the HPA axis in adolescence has been found to predict a more severe course of depression and an increased suicide risk [48]. For example, Mathew et al [60]. assessed 24-hour basal cortisol in normal controls and depressed adolescents. They followed these participants for up to 10 years later in young adulthood to determine that early patterns of HPA axis functioning were associated with later depressive and suicidal symptoms as young adults. As predicted, HPA axis activation in the late evening (a time when the normal HPA axis is at its nadir) predicted reports of suicide attempts during the follow-up assessment.

Disruptions in the stress regulatory systems may also predict response to intervention. A recent prevention study with young children suggested that atypical patterns of salivary cortisol production in response to a standard psychological stress paradigm predicted who would show behavioral improvements in the Early

Risers Skills for Success prevention program [61]. In a recent study with depressed adolescent patients, higher cortisol levels in combination with recent stressful experiences predicted recurrence of depression whereas social support was protective against recurrence [62]. Hyperarousal of the HPA axis has been found to be more prevalent in treatment-resistant depressed adults and predicts a poor response to standard interventions [63]. Adolescents with treatment-resistant depression should be assessed for events that may have permanently altered this system. For example, when children experience deprivation, trauma or disruption (e.g., being raised by a depressed mother, being sexually abused or experiencing circumstances surrounding adoption) the result may be a dysregulation of the HPA axis. Furthermore, several prospective longitudinal studies have documented that suicide completers are more likely to be DEX nonsuppressors than suppressors [64]. For example, Coryell and Schlesser [65] followed up on 78 affectively ill subjects 8 years after they underwent the DEX test. The suicide prevalence was 27% for nonsuppressors and 3% for suppressors.

Promising evidence suggests that HPA axis activity may be modified. As noted previously, the most solid evidence comes from animal research, which shows that early programming effects in rodents may be modified by maternal care. Work with foster preschoolers has documented that alterations in environment normalized diurnal stress production [66]. There is growing evidence that functional adaptation of the neurobiological stress system may be restored through psychotherapeutic processes including cognitive-behavioral stress management [67], social support [68] (which may have sex-specific effects [69]), psychopharmacological intervention [70], and potentially psychosurgery [71]. While some of the intervention approaches noted here are yet to be implemented with children and adolescent populations, and some are not relevant to these populations, the findings suggest that tremendous opportunities for intervention still await.

Conclusion

Neurobiological assessment has a bright future in identifying clinically significant differences in activation levels of specific brain regions, in measuring neurohumoral proclivities associated with fundamental biological activities, and in parceling out genetic and environmental endowment associated with diagnostic entities and behavioral, emotional, and ideational symptoms. Further, the wedding of information generated by these laboratory procedures to biological responses from the next generation of psychopharmacological agents may bring new insights into neurochemical brain–behavior relationships. These insights may provide the child and adolescent psychiatrist with powerful technologies to explore symptoms as well as comprehensive and integrative techniques that allow for predictive statements about disease progression and outcome. How this is to evolve is unclear. As with many challenges, the conquerors may already be staging an assault. It was premature a decade ago to assume that the dexamethasone suppression test would provide diagnostically useful information. We now know much more about cortisol and its relationship to acute and chronic stress and psychiatric disorders. That experience should have taught us that we cannot clearly predict the utility of our enhanced neurobiological assessment tools. We must also be concerned that, at this point in the evolution of managed care, investment in these approaches may be minimal. As with all leaps forward, all the right ingredients need to come together. Economic advantage, charismatic spokespersons, and a critical event are at least three of the requisite components to fuel this leap.

Glossary

allelic polymorphism
One of a pair or series of genes that occupy a specific position on a specific chromosome [72].

Angelman syndrome
A genetic disorder with developmental and neurological symptoms including severe mental retardation, seizures, ataxic gait, jerky movements, lack of speech, microencephaly, and frequent smiling and laughter [73].

complementary DNA (cDNA)
DNA whose base sequence is complementary to that of RNA. The RNA serves as a template for synthesis of the complementary DNA in the presence of the enzyme reverse transcriptase [73].

DNA polymerase
Any of various enzymes that function in the replication and repair of DNA by catalyzing the linking of dATP, dCTP, dGTP, and dTTP in a specific order, using single-stranded DNA as a template [72].

fluorescence *in situ* hybridization (FISH)
A process that vividly paints chromosomes or portions of chromosomes with fluorescent molecules [74].

fluorophore
An atomic group with one excited molecule that emits photons and is fluorescent; also written fluorophor [75].

fragile X syndrome
A hereditary condition that causes a wide range of mental impairment, from mild learning disabilities to severe mental retardation. It is the most common cause of genetically inherited mental impairment and is associated with a number of physical and behavioral characteristics [76].

genome
All the DNA contained in an organism or a cell, which includes both the chromosomes within the nucleus and the DNA in mitochondria [74].

(comparative) genomic hybridization (CGH)
A powerful molecular and cytogenetic technique that provides an overview of genetic imbalance within the entire genome [77].

genomics
The study of all of the nucleotide sequences, including structural genes, regulatory sequences, and noncoding DNA segments, in the chromosomes of an organism [72].

genotype
(i) The genetic makeup, as distinguished from the physical appearance, of an organism or a group of organisms. (ii) The combination of alleles located on homologous chromosomes that determines a specific characteristic or trait [72].

microarray analysis
A way of studying how large numbers of genes interact with each other and how a cell's regulatory networks control vast batteries of genes simultaneously [74].

oligonucleotide primers
Short sequences of single-stranded DNA or RNA, often used as probes for detecting complementary DNA or RNA because they bind readily to their complements [74].

pharmacogenetics
The study of genetic factors that influence an organism's reaction to a drug [72].

pharmacogenomics
A biotechnological science that combines the techniques of medicine, pharmacology, and genomics and is concerned with developing drug therapies to compensate for genetic differences in patients that cause varied responses to a particular therapeutic regimen [73].

polymerase chain reaction
A fast, inexpensive technique for making an unlimited number of copies of any piece of DNA [74].

polymorphism
The regular occurrence of two or more alleles of a gene. [73]

Prader–Willi syndrome
A syndrome characterized by severe hypotonia and feeding difficulties in early infancy, followed in later infancy or early childhood by excessive eating and gradual development of morbid obesity, unless externally controlled. All patients have some degree of cognitive impairment; a distinctive behavioral phenotype is common. Hypogonadism is present in both males and females. Short stature is common. Accurate consensus clinical diagnostic criteria exist, but the mainstay of diagnosis is DNA-based methylation testing to detect the absence of the paternally contributed Prader–Willi syndrome/Angelman syndrome (PWS/AS) region on chromosome 15q11.2-q13. Such testing detects over 99% of patients. Methylation-specific testing is important to confirm the diagnosis of PWS in all individuals, but especially those who are too young to manifest sufficient features to make the diagnosis on clinical grounds or those individuals who have atypical findings [78].

single nucleotide polymorphism (SNP)
Any of numerous single base pair variations that occur in human DNA at a frequency of 1 in every 1000 bases. These variations can be used to track inheritance in families [74].

Smith–Magenis syndrome (SMS)
A syndrome characterized by distinctive facial features, developmental delay, cognitive impairment, and behavioral abnormalities. The facial appearance is characterized by a broad, square-shaped face, brachycephaly, prominent forehead, synophrys, upslanting palpebral fissures, deep-set eyes, broad nasal bridge, marked mid-facial hypoplasia, short, full-tipped nose with reduced nasal height, micrognathia in infancy changing to relative prognathia with age, and a distinct appearance of the mouth, with fleshy everted upper lip with a "tented" appearance. Individuals with SMS function in the mild-to-moderate range of mental retardation. The behavioral phenotype includes significant sleep disturbance, stereotypies, and maladaptive and self-injurious behaviors. Childhood and adulthood are characterized by inattention, hyperactivity, maladaptive behaviors including frequent outbursts/temper tantrums, attention seeking, impulsivity, distractibility, disobedience, aggression, toileting difficulties, and self-injurious behaviors (SIB) including self-hitting, self-biting, and/or skin picking, inserting foreign objects into body orifices (polyembolokoilamania), and yanking fingernails and/or toenails (onchyotillomania). Two stereotypic behaviors, spasmodic upper-body squeeze or 'self-hug', and hand-licking and page flipping ('lick and flip'), seem to be specific to SMS.

Diagnosis/testing.
The diagnosis of SMS is confirmed either by detection of an interstitial deletion of the short arm of chromosome 17 band p11.2 (del17p11.2) by G-banded cytogenetic analysis and/or by fluorescence *in situ* hybridization (FISH) [79].

velocardiofacial syndrome (VCFS)
A syndrome whose common features include cleft palate, heart defects, characteristic facial appearance, minor learning problems, and speech and feeding problems. The gene or genes that cause VCFS have not been identified; most children who have been diagnosed with this syndrome are missing region 22q11 of the genome. VCFS is an autosomal dominant disorder; in most cases neither parent has the syndrome or carries the defective gene. The cause of the deletion is unknown [80].

Williams' syndrome
A rare genetic disorder characterized especially by hypercalcemia of infants, heart defects (as supravalvular aortic stenosis), characteristic facial features (as an upturned nose, long philtrum, wide mouth, full lips, and pointed chin), a sociable personality, and a high verbal aptitude, but with mild to moderate mental retardation [77].

References

1. Begleiter H, Porjesz B, Bihari B, Kissan B. Event-related potential in boys at risk for alcoholism. *Science* 1984;**225**:1493–1496.
2. Courchesne E, Lincoln AJ, Yeung-Courchesne R, *et al.* Pathophysiologic findings in nonretarded autism and receptive developmental language disorder. *J Autism Dev Disord* 1989;**19**:1–17.
3. de Regnier RA, Georgieff MK, Nelson CA. Visual event-related brain potentials in 4-month-old infants at risk for neurodevelopmental impairments. *Dev Psychobiol* 1997; **30**:11–28.
4. Giedd JN, Rapport JL, Leonard H, *et al.* Case study: Acute basal ganglia enlargement and obsessive-compulsive symptoms in an adolescent boy. *J Am Acad Child Adolesc Psychiat* 1996;**35**:913–915.
5. Piven J, Arndt S, Bailey J, Andresen N. Regional brain enlargement in autism: A magnetic resonance imaging study. *J Am Acad Child Adolesc Psychiat* 1996;**35**: 530–536.
6. Lou HC, Henricksen L, Bruhn P. Focal cerebral hypoperfusion in children with dysphasia and/or attention-deficit disorder. *Arch Neurol* 1984;**41**:825–829.
7. Amen DG, Paldi JH, Thisted RA. Brain SPECT imaging. *J Am Acad Child Adolesc Psychiat* 1993;**32**:1080–1081.

8. Zametkin AJ, Nordahl TE, Gross M, *et al.* Cerebral glucose metabolism in adults with hyperactivity of childhood onset. *N Engl J Med* 1990;**323**:1361–1366.

9. Zametkin AJ, Liebenauer LL, Fitzgerald GA, *et al.* Brain metabolism in teenagers with attention-deficit hyperactivity disorder. *Arch Gen Psychiat* 1993;**50**:333–340.

10. Matochik JA, Nordahl TE, Gross M, *et al.* Effects of acute stimulant medication on cerebral metabolism in adults with hyperactivity. *Neuropsychopharmacology* 1993;**8**:377–386.

11. Matochik JA, Liebenauer LL, King AC, *et al.* Cerebral metabolism in adults with attention-deficit hyperactivity disorder after chronic stimulant treatment. *Am J Psychiat* 1994;**151**:658–664.

12. Matlay VS, Berman KF, Ostrem JL, *et al.* Dextroamphetamine enhances "neural network-specific" physiological signals: A positron-emission tomography rCBF study. *J Neurosci* 1996;**16**:4816–4822.

13. Teicher M, Polcare A, Anderson C, *et al.* Methylphenidate effects on hyperactivity and fMRI in children with ADHD. *Sci Proc Am Acad Child Adolesc Psychiat* 1996;**12**:120.

14. Mozley PD, Zhu X, Kung HF. The dosimetry of iodine-123 labeled TISCH: A SPECT imaging agent for the D1 dopamine receptor. *J Nucl Med* 1993;**34**:208–213.

15. Seibyl JP, Woods SW, Zoghbi SS, *et al.* Dynamic SPECT imaging of dopamine D2 receptors in human subjects with iodine-123-IBZM. *J Nucl Med* 1992;**33**:1964–1971.

16. Anderson AW, Gore JC. Neuroimaging. *Child Adolesc Psychiatr Clin North Am* 1997;**6**:213–264.

17. Ernst M, Zametkin AJ, Matochik JA, *et al.* Effects of intravenous dextroamphetamine on brain metabolism in adults with attention-deficit hyperactivity disorder: Preliminary findings. *Psychopharmacol Bull* 1994;**30**:219–225.

18. Belliveau JW, Kennedy DN, McKinstry RC, *et al.* Functional mapping of the human visual cortex by magnetic resonance imagining. *Science* 1991;**254**:716–719.

19. Lim KO, Tew W, Kushner M, *et al.* Cortical gray matter volume deficit in patients with first-episode schizophrenia. *Am J Psychiat* 1996;**12**:1548–1553.

20. Breiter H, Rauch S, Kwong K, *et al.* Functional magnetic resonance imaging of symptom provocation in obsessive-compulsive disorder. *Arch Gen Psychiat* 1996;**53**:595–606.

21. Lauterbur PC. Image formation by induced local interactions: Examples employing nuclear magnetic resonance. *Nature* 1973;**242**:190–191.

22. Dager RS, Steen G. Applications of magnetic resonance spectroscopy to the investigation of neuropsychiatric disorders. *Neuropsychopharmacology* 1992;**6**:249–266.

23. DeRegnier RAO, Georgieff MK, Nelson CA. Visual event-related brain potentials in four-month-old infants at risk for neurodevelopmental impairments. *Dev Psychobiol* 1997;**30**:11–28.

24. Selye H. A syndrome produced by diverse nocuous agents. *Nature* 1936;**38**:32.

25. LeDoux J. *The Emotional Brain.* New York: Simon and Schuster, 1996.

26. Levine S. Infantile experience and resistance to physiological stress. *Science* 1957;**126**:405–406.

27. Mirescu C, Peters JD, Gould E. Early life experience alters response of adult neurogenesis to stress. *Nat Neurosci* 2004;**7**:841–846.

28. Heim C, Newport DJ, Metzko T, Miller AH, Nemeroff CB. The link between childhood trauma and depression: Insights from HPA axis studies in humans. *Psychoneuroendocrinology* 2008;**33**:693–710.

29. Romeo RD, McEwen BS. Stress and the adolescent brain. *Ann N Y Acad Sci* 2006;**1094**:202–214.

30. Bremner JD. Does stress damage the brain? *Biol Psychiatry* 1999;**45**:797–805.

31. Sapolsky RM, Krey LC, McEwen BS. The neuroendocrinology of stress and aging: The glucocorticoid cascade hypothesis. *Endocrinol Res* 1986;**7**:284–301.

32. Sapolsky RM. *Stress, the Aging Brain, and the Mechanisms of Neuron Death.* Cambridge, MA: MIT Press, 1992.

33. Weaver ICG, Cervoni N, Champagne F, *et al.* Epigenetic programming by maternal behavior. *Nat Neurosci* 2004;**7**:847–854.

34. de Kloet ER. Hormones, brain and stress. *Endocrine Regulations* 2003;**37**:51–68.

35. Sapolsky RM. Social status and health in humans and other animals. *Ann Rev Anthropol* 2004;**33**:393–418.

36. Hellhammer DH, Wust S, Kudielka BM. Salivary cortisol as a biomarker in stress research. *Psychoneuroendocrinology* 2009;**34**:163–171.

37. O'Connor TM, O'Halloran DJ, Shannahan F. The stress response of the hypothalamic-pituitary-adrenal axis: From molecule to melancholia. *Q J Med* 2000;**93**:323–333.

38. Kirschbaum C, Pirke KM, Hellhammer DH. The 'Trier Social Stress Test' – A tool for investigating psychobiological stress response in a laboratory setting. *Neuropsychobiology* 1993;**28**:76–81.

39. Smider NA, Essex MJ, Kalin NH, et al. Salivary cortisol as a predictor of socioemotional adjustment during kindergarten: A prospective study. *Child Dev* 2002;**73**:75–92.

40. van Goozen SH, Matthys W, Cohen-Kettenis PT, Buitterlaar JK, van Engeland H. Hypothalamic-pituitary-adrenal axis and autonomic nervous system activity in disruptive children and matched controls. *J Am Acad Child Adolesc Psychiat* 2000;**39**:1438–1445.

41. Jensen J, Realmuto GM, Garfinkel B. The dexamethasone suppression test in infantile autism. *J Am Acad Child Adolesc Psychiat* 1985;**24**:263–265.

42. Chrousos GP, Gold PW. The concepts of stress and stress system disorders. Overview of physical and behavioral homeostasis. *JAMA* 1992;**267**:1244–1252.

43. Pariante CM. Depression, stress and the adrenal axis. *J Neuroendocrinol* 2003;**15**:811–812.

44. Dahl RE, Puig-Antich J, Ryan NE. Cortisol secretion in adolescents with major depressive disorder. *Acta Psychiat Scand* 1989;**80**:18–26.

45. Adam E, Klimes-Dougan B, Gunnar MR. Emotional and social regulation of the adrenocortical response to stress. In: Coch D, Dawson G, Fischer K (eds) *Human Behavior and the Developing Brain,* 2nd edn. New York: Guilford Publications, Inc., 2007.

46. Guerry JD, Hastings PD. In search of HPA axis dysregulation in child and adolescent depression. *Clin Child Fam Psychol Rev* 2011;**14**:135–160.

47. Lopez-Duran NL, Kovacs M, George CJ. Hypothalamic-pituitary-adrenal axis dysregulation in depressed children and adolescents: A meta-analysis. *Psychoneuroendocrinology* 2009;**34**:1272–1283.

48. Zalsman G, Brent DA, Weersing VR. Depressive disorders in childhood and adolescence: an overview: epidemiology, clinical manifestation and risk factors. *Child Adolesc Psychiat Clin N Am* 2006; **15**:827–841.

49. Burke H, Davis M, Otte C, Mohr D. Depression and cortisol responses to psychological stress: A meta-analysis. *Psychoneuroendocrinology* 2005;**30**:846–856.

50. Klimes-Dougan B, Hastings PD, Granger DA, Usher BA, Zahn-Waxler C. Adrenocortical activity in at risk and normally developing adolescents: Individual differences in salivary cortisol response to social challenges, basal levels, and diurnal variation. *Dev Psychopathol* 2001; **13**:695–719.

51. Klimes-Dougan B, Cullen K, Kumra S, Klingbeil DK. HPA axis functioning in adolescents with major depressive disorder. International Society for Psychoneuroendocrinology, Dresden, 2008.

52. Rao U, Hammen C, Ortiz LR, Chen L, Poland RE. Effects of early and recent adverse experiences on adrenal response to psychosocial stress in depressed adolescents. *Biol Psychiat* 2008;**64**:521–526.

53. Hasler G, Drevets WC, Manji HK, *et al.* Discovery of endophenotypes for major depression. *Neuropsychopharmacology* 2004;**29**:1765–1781.

54. Vinberg M, Bennike B, Kyvik KO, *et al.* Salivary cortisol in unaffected twins discordant for affective disorder. *Psychiat Res* 2008;**161**:292–301.

55. Ellenbogen MA, Hodgins S, Walker C. High levels of cortisol among adolescent offspring of parents with bipolar disorder: A pilot study. *Psychoneuroendocrinology* 2004;**29**:99–106.

56. Halligan SL, Herbert J, Goodyer I, Murray L. Exposure to postnatal depression predicts elevated cortisol in adolescent offspring. *Biol Psychiat* 2004;**55**:376–381.

57. Lupien SJ, King S, Meaney M, McEwenB. Child's stress hormone levels correlate with mother's socioeconomic status and depressive state. *Biol Psychiat* 2000;**48**:976–980.

58. Mannie Z, Harmer NC, Cowen P. Increased wakening salivary cortisol levels in young people at familial risk of depression. *Am J Psychiat* 2007;**164**:617–621.

59. Young EA, Velaquez D, Jiang H, Pfeffer C. Salivary cortisol and response to dexamethasone in children of depressed parents. *Biol Psychiat* 2006;**60**:831–836.

60. Mathew SJ, Coplan JD, Goetz RR, *et al.* Differentiating depressed adolescent 24h cortisol secretion in light of their adult clinical outcome. *Neuropsychopharmacology* 2003;**28**:1336–1343.

61. Klimes-Dougan B, Houri A, Lee C-YS, Klingbeil D, August G. HPA axis functioning of children enrolled in Early Risers Prevention Program. Society for Prevention Research, Washington, DC, 2009.

62. Rao U, Hammen C, Poland RE. Longitudinal course of adolescent depression: Neuroendocrine and psychosocial predictors. *J Am Acad Child Adolesc Psychiatry* 2010; **49**:141–151.

63. Binder EB, Kunzel HE, Nickel T, *et al.* HPA-axis regulation at in-patient admission is associated with antidepressant therapy outcome in male but not in female depressed patients. *Psychoneuroendocrinology* 2009;**34**:99–109.

64. Jokinen J, Carlborg A, Martensson B, Forslund K, Nordstrom A-L, Nordstrom P. DST non-suppression predicts suicide after attempted suicide. *Psychiat Res* 2007;**150**: 297–303.

65. Coryell W, Schlesser M. The Dexamethasone Suppression Test and suicide prediction. *Am J Psychiat* 2001;**158**: 748–753.

66. Fisher PA, Stoolmiller M, Gunnar MR, Buraston BO. Effects of a therapeutic intervention for foster preschoolers on diurnal cortisol activity. *Psychoneuroendocrinology* 2007;**32**:892–905.

67. Gaab J, Blattler N, Menzi T, Pabst B, Stoyer S, Ehlert U. Randomized controlled evaluation of the effects of cognitive-behavioral stress management on cortisol responses to acute stress in healthy subjects. *Psychoneuroendocrinology* 2003;**28**:767–779.

68. Heinrichs M, Baumgartner T, Kirschbaum C, Ehlert U. Social support and oxytocin interact to suppress cortisol and subjective responses to psychosocial stress. *Biol Psychiat* 2003;**54**:1389–1398.

69. Kirschbaum C, Klauer T, Filipp SH, Hellhammer DH. Sex-specific effects of social support on cortisol and subjective responses to acute psychological stress. *Psychosom Med* 1995;**57**:23–31.

70. Schule C. Neuroendocrinological mechanism of actions of antidepressant drugs. *J Neuroendocrin* 2006;**19**: 213–226.

71. Mayberg HS, Lozano AM, Voon V, *et al.* Deep brain stimulation for treatment-resistant depression. *Neuron* 2005;**45**:651–660.

72. *The American Heritage Dictionary of the English Language*, 4th edn. Boston, MA: Houghton Mifflin Company, 2000.

73. *Merriam-Webster Medical Dictionary*. Springfield, MA: Merriam-Webster Inc., 2002.

74. National Human Genome Research Institute. Talking Glossary of Genetic Terms. Available at: http://www.genome.gov/10002096.

75. *Webster's New Millennium Dictionary of English, Preview Edition (v 0.9.5)*. Lexico Publishing Group, LLC, 2003, 2004.

76. Fast D. The National Fragile X Foundation: What is Fragile X Syndrome? Available at: http://www.fragilex.org/html/what.htm.

77. Corso C, Parry EM. The application of comparative genomic hybridization and fluorescence *in situ* hybridization to the characterization of genotoxicity screening tester strains AHH-1 and MCL-5. *Mutagenesis* 1999;**14**: 417–426.

78. Cassidy SB, Schwartz S. Prader–Willi syndrome. 1998–2004. Available at: http://medical-dictionary.thefreedictionary.com/Prader-Willi + Syndrome.

79. Smith ACM, Allanson JE, Allen AJ, *et al.* Smith–Magenis syndrome. 2001–2004. Available at: http://ghr.nlm.nih.gov/condition/smith-magenis-syndrome.

80. National Institute on Deafness and Other Communication Disorders. 2005. Health Information: Voice, Speech, and Language. URL: http://www.genome.gov/25521139.

4

Educational Assessment and School Consultation

Dorothyann Feldis

School is an environment in which children are asked to learn certain basic academic and social skills and in which their performance is judged and compared with that of other children. If children perform well, they learn that success provides opportunities and social status. If, on the other hand, they perform poorly for whatever reasons, they learn about failure and restricted opportunities. It is demoralizing to try to maintain a sense of self-worth and enthusiasm for learning within the confines of educational expectations that are impossible to achieve. Very early in their school careers, children essentially learn whether they are to be a success or a failure. The dilemma of failure is exacerbated by the fact that children are powerless to change their environment; they need adult support to identify learning problems and effective solutions to these problems. Child and adolescent psychiatrists and other professionals involved with children who are experiencing difficulty in school must understand the devastating impact that school failure has on a child's life, and must act swiftly to resolve the situation.

The firsts step in understanding a child's learning problems in school is devising some method of gathering information to help us understand the factors influencing the student's performance for the purpose of generating a solution. Historically, assessmenthas been used as amethod of sorting studentsto be channeled into "various segments of our social and economic system" rather thana method of tracking and enhancing "growth toward standards" as well asa method of motivating students "to strive for academic excellence" (ref. [1], p.15). Classroom teachers are quick to state that assessment is effective only if used as a problem-solving mechanism; data not directly related to improving school performance have little value to the classroom teacher.

The educational assessment of children is a specialized process that directly addresses overall achievement in school. Generally, success in school is based on academic performance. Students who achieve well academically are usually considered successful and those who perform poorly are targets for academic assistance and adjustments. However, variables considering students' dispositions "motivations, feelings and desires" must be included in that they "directly influence academic achievement" (ref. [1], p.199). This, of course, implies that the assessment process must have a collaborative approach: one that includes not only teachers, parents, and diagnosticians but also the child. The child must be more than the object of the process but a part of the process. Stiggins [1] asks us to consider the child as a "consumer of assessment results" (ref. [1], p.19). Positive, constructive results of continuous assessment build self-esteem along with feelings of "hopefulness" andthe "expectation of more success in the future" (ref. [1], p.19). The outcome of any assessment process should provide information that allows teachers, parents, and others to better create effective positive learning environments: environments that allow students to assume control of their own destiny in school. The performance of the child is not viewed in isolation but as part of a large ecosystem containing numerous interdependent variables. This approach acknowledges that factors other than ability affect learning and therefore requires that theenvironment as well asinstructionadjust to accommodate thelearning needs ofthechild.

The Evaluation Process

The educational evaluation is usually part of a multidisciplinary evaluation conducted by schools when a child is suspected of having a disability that is impacting his or her classroom performance. The purpose of the multidisciplinary evaluation is to determine if the child has a disability and is eligible for special education services.

Clinical Child Psychiatry, Third Edition. Edited by William M. Klykylo and Jerald Kay.
© 2012 John Wiley & Sons, Ltd. Published 2012 by John Wiley & Sons, Ltd.

This evaluation must be conducted by licensed professionalsoften employed by the school including theschool psychologist, speech and language therapist, physical therapist, occupational therapist, school nurse, and others who might contribute to the presenting problem. It can also include data from medical professionals including the pediatrician and child psychiatrist as well as other community professionals who have worked with the child and his or her family. An educational diagnostician or special educatortogether with the classroom teachercomplete the academic portion of theassessment focusing on the child's classroom performanceand learning needsSometimes schools do not havea diagnostic educator available to complete thiscomponent of the evaluation, and different portionsof this material are collected byother members of the interdisciplinary team. If this is the case caution must be takennot toomit consideration of a child's specific learning needs and performance within the classroom setting.

While the diagnostic educator contributes specific test results pertaining to academic and classroom performance, he or she also collaborates closely with the classroom teacher in combining diagnostic data with classroom performance assessment. Diagnostic data often include results from various norm-referenced and criterion-referenced tests usually identifying deficits in learning and the learning process. Performance assessment refers to the teacher's assessment ofstudent ability in theclassroom "to interact (perform) appropriately with relevant instructional materials, and the content of instruction" (ref. [2], p.283). Teachers are expected to understand andmeet the learning needs of a wide variety of learners who bring different cultural, language, and-ability levels to the classroom. Effective learningrequires teachers to assess student performance on a regular basis and adjust pedagogy to meet a variety ofstudent learning needs.

In addition to collecting and analyzing testing and performance data,the diagnostic educator must be a collaborator able to bring together all stakeholders including the child,school administrators, classroom teacher, parents, and others involved in the child'slife, into the process ofadjusting the learning environment to meet specificlearning needs.

When Should a Referral be Made?

A referral for a multidisciplinaryevaluation should be made when the child is suspected of having a disability that is impacting hisor her performance in school. Usually the childis experiencing behavioral and/or academic difficulties in the classroom. The child psychiatrist may contribute to thereferral and evaluation process based on their knowledge and interactions with the child and his/her family. The problem may be a new development, a chronic or crisis situation, or the result of cultural differences and language barriers. A *new problem* is a recent situation without an identified history, for example, a child in kindergarten or first grade for whom the teacher has expressed concerns about progress. Problems such as these might be considered "developmental," and teachers and other professionals might choose to take the "wait and see" approach. Many of these issues, however, often materialize into significant learning problems in the second or third grade, when the child actually begins to fail. Serious consideration should therefore be given to early concerns about a child's progress, before school expectations begin to appear insurmountable to the child and his/her family. Other new problems might be caused by illness or other family trauma that has affected school performance for a child who historically has been considered a typical learner.

In some *chronic situations* children may have received some form of assessment or intervention, and in other cases they may not have received any consideration. An example of the former would be a sixth-grade child with a history of reading problems who has received some individual tutoring but whose report cards continue to indicate little or no improvement. An example of the latter would be a ninth-grader with a history of learning problems who has managed to perform adequately through elementary and junior high school, but who has significant difficulty adjusting to the expectations of the secondary school environment.

A *crisis situation* needs immediate action and has the potential for seriously compromising the future academic progress of the child. There are various circumstances that might generate a crisis, but two situations should be addressed without hesitation: grade retention and school suspension or expulsion. In the case of grade retention, one ground rule exists: No decision should be made until the child receives an interdisciplinary evaluation that includes an educational, psychological, psychiatric, and speech and language assessment. The reason for failure must be specifically identified and a plan for intervention designed; the child deserves every resource available to resolve the problem. In the case of school suspension or expulsion, the child also needs an interdisciplinary evaluation to determine the variables affecting behavioral issues, and to rule out other contributing factors such as learning disorders and psychiatric illness. If the child has been assessed in the past, these reports need to be reviewed and updated. If the child has been suspended, the present education program is not helping him or her adjust to the expectations of the learning environment, and the child's situation needs to be reconsidered. The cause of problematic behavior must be identified and an intervention plandeveloped, if re-entry is to be successful. In these cases the psychiatrist needs the educator to assess academic performance and identify learning needs and the necessary accommodations required for successful progress to occur.

Cultural differences and language barriers must also be considered when assessing a child's performance in school. Many children live in families where English is not the primary language and wherecultural standards interpret interaction with schools and teachers differently. These children must adjust to school standards without clarification usually supplied to them by parentsand other caretakers in the home environment. Often, the result is "an achievement gap between these students and European American students" (ref. [3], p.58),which complicates the identification and impact of specific learning problems on classroom performance. Whatever the problem, it is important to remember that children cannot usually develop coping mechanisms on their own or adjust their school environment to help them better meet expectations. If professionals hesitate in obtaining an assessment there can be misdirected, inefficient, and often disappointing results for all.

Legislation and Rights

Historically, classroom teachers have assessed children by trying to discover what they do or do not know and why they have learned some things and not others. If a teacher is skilled and the system supportive, this method can be effective. The individual skill of the teacher and the random sensitivity of the system, however, do not ensure that all children experiencing problems in school will be appropriately identified and provided with the adaptations necessary for learning to occur. The enactment in the United States of Public Law (PL) 94-142, the Education of Handicapped Children Act (1975), changed this process. Instead of depending on good teachers and interventions, the law mandated that all children aged 5 to 21 years with an identified handicap will have a free and appropriate education. It also provided procedures to determine eligibility for special education services and appropriate programming. This legislation was revised in 1990 (PL 101-476) and renamed the Individuals with DisabilitiesEducation Act(IDEA), recognizing the concept of considering theindividual first, then identifying their characteristics; it also extended the mandate to serve children aged 3 to 21 years. The most recent revision, Individuals with Disabilities Education Improvement Act of 2004(IDEA 2004),includes raising expectations for children with disabilities, ensuring that children with disabilities have increased access to the general education curriculum, and strengthening the role of parents. The statutory requirements of this legislation are elaborated in Chapter 30 of this book.

This legislation emphasizes educating children in the least restrictive learning environment as possible, one that can provide inclusion in the general curriculum. Good program decisions usually consider the child's educational needs, the support services needed to accommodate those needs, and methods of embedding supports into the general curriculum. It also emphasizes nondiscriminatory evaluation including testing materials in the child's primary language.

The legislation provides a specific set of procedures for identifying a child's disability and determining anappropriate educationalprogram. These procedures ensure the right of all children to receive services for which they are eligible. Any child suspected of a disability must have an initial eligibility ormultidisciplinary evaluation, which assesses all areas related to the suspected disability. This evaluation must include a variety of professionals qualified to assess specific areas of development. Following completion of all parts of the evaluation the evaluation team meets to determine if the child is eligible for special education programming. If eligible, an individualized education program (IEP) conference is convened to define the least restrictive learning environment and other support systems necessary to provide an appropriate and effective learning environment for the child. Because of the school's obligation to determine an IEP for each identified child and to define educationalgoals and instructional strategies, educators have begun to perfect the educational assessment as a means of providing data pertinent to classroom learning and curricula.

Schools must by law provide anondiscriminatory multidisciplinaryevaluation for any child suspected of having a disability. The referral may be made by the parents or school personnel. Community professionals like child psychiatrists, pediatricians, social workers, and others can be instrumental in assisting parents to pursue a referral. They can also provide initial documentation pertaining to the suspected disability. If parents are making the referral, they should do so in writing, indicating that they suspect that their child has a disabilitythat is impacting their school performance and requires a full evaluation of the child's learning needs. Prior to referral manyschools attempt prereferral interventions to address behavior and academic difficulties. If these strategies are not effective within a designated period the child isreferred for a multidisciplinaryevaluation. Schools sometimes ask professionals outside the school team, including child psychiatrists or pediatricians, to contribute diagnostic information to the evaluation process. If the school requests this assistance, it is obliged to pay for the service. If there is a disagreement over the evaluation, the parent has the right to an independent evaluation at the school's expense. Sometimes parents decide to pursue an independent multidisciplinary evaluation rather than using services provided by the school. This is a legitimate choice for parents, and the results must be considered by the school, as long as the professionals have the appropriate certification or license in their specific discipline. In this situation, however, the parents are obliged to cover the cost.

When the evaluation is completed, the school is required to hold a meeting, including the professionals involved in the evaluation process as well as the parents, to review the results of the evaluation and determine eligibility for services. If the child is eligible an initial IEP must be developed including a plan for an appropriate education program. This meeting must include parents as joint decision-makers. Parents may request other individuals to attend this meeting. These individuals may include professionals from outside the school who may have contributed assessment data to the evaluation or who were involved in implementing treatment programs – namely tutors, child and adolescent psychiatrists, occupational or physical therapists, and speech and language therapists. Parents may also invite an advocate or mentor to help them deal with the educational system on behalf of their child. Advocates or mentors are usually available through parent or child advocacy programs in the community. Many school districts are instituting parent mentor programs to help parents understand and effectively access the IEP process.

Once a child is enrolled in special education, the school district is obliged to conduct an annual review of the child's progress and notify parents of current IEP goals. A re-evaluation by the school district is required every 3 years. Parents should be notified of and informed about this process.

In summary, children with disabilities have a legal right to a free and appropriate education, and schools are legally obligated to meet these needs. Parents often require the support of mentors and professionals to ensure that their children's needs are in fact met. The National Dissemination Center for Children with Disabilities (NICHCY) provides more information regarding IDEA 2004, the multidisciplinary evaluation, the IEP process, and effective educational practices, besides other information about disabilities (www.nichcy.org).

The Educational Evaluation

The educational (academic) evaluation is part of the total multidisciplinary (eligibility) evaluation and re-evaluation process. The purpose of a specific educational

evaluation is to collect the data necessary to identify specific learning needs and effective instructional strategies as well as to contribute data to determine eligibility for special education programming. Eligibility is ultimately a procedural and legal decision that depends on present levels of performance in a variety of different areas as well as standardized test data; the identification of specific learning needs requires additional data emphasizing an analysis of the student's learning patterns, the school environment, and other social and cultural influences. Each component of an educational evaluation should contain information necessary to determine eligibility but also to identify evidenced-based instructional approaches. "Evidenced-based methods are those that are supported by scientific research and have been shown to demonstrate a relatively high degree of success in terms of student learning outcomes" (ref. [3], p.18). These components usually include background information, descriptive data, test data, and the educational plan.

Background Information

The background information in an evaluation includes school history, relevant medical history, the presenting problem, the duration of the problem, and the effect the problem has had on the child's development at home and in school. This information may be collected from parents, teachers, and other professionals and individuals involved in the care of the child. At this point in the process, the educational diagnostician's role is to determine how parents, teachers, and the child each perceive the child's difficulties in school. Do teachers perceive parents as helpful and supportive to the child and his or her learning process? Do parents view the teachers and other school personnel as willing to adjust teaching strategies to accommodate the child? How does the child perceive his/her performance? Can the child identify problems and possible solutions? How have teachers and parents responded to the child's school failure? Does the child view him/herself to be in a hopeless situation? Differences in these perceptions may have a significant impact on the resolution of the problem.

Test Data

An educational assessment usually includes both norm- and criterion-referenced testing of academic achievement, general knowledge, and specific skill mastery. Most tests divide the academic areas of reading, mathematics, and written language into different components to allow a more thorough analysis of the child's abilities.

In addition to providing information about what the child knows the educational assessment also needs to focus on how the child learns. This requires a careful analysis of the results including the child's responses to content as well as different test requirements. For example, some students do better on items that require a verbal response rather than timed, written responses. If these types of responses are a theme throughout the assessment process and also evident in the classroom, the educator can begin to identify effective learning strategies. This, of course, is the ultimate goal of the educational evaluation.

Depending on the presenting problem, information required for eligibility for special education services emphasizes test performance in specific areas of academic, cognitive, language, and behavioral development. This information compares the child with others and is called *norm referenced*. Information generated from norm-referenced tests compares the child's performance with a group of children similar in age, grade, and sometimes other characteristics. Criterion-referenced tests, also standardized, identify a student's mastery of specific skills based on an established criterion usually aligned with the classroom curriculum. Criterion-referenced tests do not compare the child with a group of peers.

Because criterion-referenced tests tend to be more closely aligned with classroom curricula they allow for a more detailed interpretation of the child's performance than do norm-referenced tests. A norm-referenced test in reading and written language, for example, may indicate that a child's performance in reading comprehension and written language is within two standard deviations below the mean. This information probably confirms the teacher's concerns that the child can read but does not comprehend or express thoughts well; it does not, however, identify learning processes that might help the child or teacher to better understand their performance. More specific analysis of reading comprehension and written language is necessary. In this instance, criterion-referenced tests can help the educator to better analyze the child's ability to manage specific aspects of the learning process required in the classroom.

Although criterion-referenced tests do allow a more specific analysis of a child's performance, they may also suggest solutions based on isolated skill deficits, thus neglecting the effect of other variables within the learning environment. Additional data from the classroom teacher analyzing daily work performance is also necessary to adequately characterize a student's learning and to provide a more detailed analysis of the learning process. Teachers need to track not only student grades but also performance as a learner in the classroom. Often children with specific learning problems exhibit consistency in performance associated with specific types of instruction, testing, and classroom environment. Classroom instruction focused on the lecture and dependent on independent reading and note taking is frequently associated with poor performance on classroom tests and other evaluative measures. Whereas classroom instruction using multidimensional teaching strategies providing students the opportunity to practice and interact with concepts in the classroom often promotes more successful learning.

In addition the educational diagnostician must be sensitive to cultural differences and consider student progress in a culturally responsive manner. Turnbull *et al* [4]. caution teachers to avoid using standardized assessment measures "to dominate the assessment process" (ref. [4], p.74). Teachers should review student performance on an ongoing basis to determine student strengths as well as weaknesses and also "to assess the efficacy of their instructional approaches and processes" (ref. [4], p.74).

Descriptive Data

Descriptive data help to identify the environmental variables, teaching approaches, and other factors that might be affecting a child's progress in school. The data are usually collected via classroom observation and interviews with teachers, parents, and other specialists involved in the child's educational program. The child should also be included in this process and be given the opportunity to contribute their perception about the problem, its cause, and even possible solutions.

Classroom observation can provide information about a child's behavior, attention, and general ability to adapt to school expectations. The educational diagnostician is interested in the child's ability to learn in the classroom. Understanding how material is presented to the child, how the child is requested to respond, how the child responds, and the attitudes attached to the child's performance are all indicators of overall performance. For example, a child with a written language problem might be required to answer essay questions to pass tests in social studies. As a result of this testing procedure, the child will probably fail. To generate effective intervention strategies, the educator must not only identify the child's ability in social studies and written language but also understand the relationship between the two within the structure of the classroom. All this may become apparent only after classroom observation and discussion with the teacher, the child, and the parents. Descriptive data help to answer the following questions:

• Is the child motivated and interested in school?
• Is the child attentive in the classroom?
• Is homework and/or organization a problem?

- What is the child's attitude about school?
- How does the child respond to discipline?
- What are peer interactions like in the school environment?
- How do other students and the teacher respond to the child's performance?
- How is the child recognized in the classroom? Is the child regarded as a successful or unsuccessful learner?
- What types of instruction seem to be most effective for the child?
- What types of instruction seem to be least effective for the child?
- How frequently does the child receive positive feedback in the classroom?

Each source of information provides a different perspective of the problem, and information from all these sources needs to be analyzed to identify the child's learning problems and pedagogical strategies that might enhance or obstruct learning. The expectations and responses of all individuals involved with the child's learning must be understood if adjustments in the educational program are to be successful.

Educational Plan

The final component of an educational evaluation is the educational plan, which provides a framework for generating solutions. In the case of a child with written language problems, for example, the educational diagnostician and the teacher must generate two solutions: (i) a way to evaluate the child's knowledge of content that does not employ a weak skill as the vehicle for testing, and (ii) a plan to improve knowledge and, where possible, deficient skills. In the past, solutions have focused on requiring the child to improve performance through remediation and, of course, "try harder" without any significant environmental adjustments. Creating a more accessible learning environment that emphasizes strengths and decreases negative outcomes is crucial, however, if children with learning problems are to succeed. Even with the appropriate intervention, some children will never totally correct these weaknesses and must instead learn how to compensate. Although children may have some ability to identify stumbling blocks in their learning environment, they are almost always powerless to change them. Adults must ensure that the necessary adjustments occur.

When a child is referred for educational testing, the problem has already been identified. Assessment should do more than confirm the referral question; it should identify *skills* or learning behaviors that are interfering with learning, as well as a set of effective learning strategies. The educational plan should identify ways to adjust negative variables, introduce remediation, and emphasize possible variables to enhance learning. This purpose implies that intervention will focus on implementing changes in the environment and in instruction. The most difficult aspect of this approach is that persons other than the child may be expected to change and, consequently, that the child's progress may be dependent on changes in the environment.

Consultation, Collaboration, and Educational Planning

Historically, the medical literature has described consultation as a process by which one physician requests expert advice from another, usually pertaining to the condition or situation of a patient [5]. In these situations the consultant providing the advice has assumed no responsibility for the outcome but has merely shared knowledge. Although this is an accepted practice in medicine, educators are attempting to approach consultation as a process wherein teachers, parents, and others involved with a child work jointly to solve a problem. This usually involves adapting the learning environment to better meet the specific needs of the child. It also emphasizes the need for professionals to collaborate as a team to generate workable solutions that involve joint responsibility for implementation and outcome – a process called *collaborative consultation.*

School Dynamics and Collaborative Consultation

The Individuals with Disabilities Education Act assures the right for individuals with disabilities to receive a free and appropriate public education. It also assures that an individual be afforded due process in determining eligibility for special education services. However, for successful implementation of the provisions of the law "constructive and collaborative partnerships must be established among parents, teachers, school specialists, school administrators, and community agencies" (ref. [2], p. 25). Parents, administrators, support services, and teachers must assume responsibility for the outcome and work together with the student to create a more effective and productive learning environment.

West and Idol defined consultation as "a term used across various disciplines to refer to some type of triadic relationship among consultants, consultees, and clients or problems" (ref. [6], p.395). The expert consultation model may be distinguished from the collaborative consultation model: the former refers to a type of consultation in which an "expert," usually a school support professional such as a school psychologist, analyzes the problem, evaluates options, and prescribes interventions for the teacher to implement [7]. While thismodel has been replaced by more collaborative approaches, at times teachersstill experience situations where they are givenlittle opportunity for input but all the responsibility for change.

Child psychiatrists must understand that teachers regard collaboration as partnerships with shared decision-making. Prescribing classroom interventions for the teacher will be received negatively; sharing knowledge and partnering with the teacher to improve the learning environment for the child will be regarded as supportive and helpful. The child psychiatristmust also understand the process of collaboration is complicated when professionals from outside the school become involved in the process. Although these individuals may have crucial information that needs to be incorporated into the educational plan, effective results are dubious unless professionals understand teacher expectations and roles within the configuration of the school. In the hierarchy of professional competence, physicians have historically been rated higher and teachers lower than most other professionals. Teachers, of course, have resented interference by physicians and other professionals, who are viewed as more knowledgeable than themselves and whooften oversimplify the task of teaching. Teachers are expected to differentiate instruction to meet specific learning needs of all students. However, nonteacher professionals must rememberthat teachers interpret all diagnostic information into behavioral or academic instructionalintervention in the context of a group setting.

Many teachers return to their classrooms after planning meetings mumbling, "I'd like to see them manage a class like this alone for just one day." The lack of support and professional respect has promoted in teachers an attitude of suspicion of "outsiders." The psychiatrist must understand the process of collaboration in schools as well as the various levels of competence that exist. Some schools have established effective collaborative intervention models, some are in the process of developing these models, and some have not yet begun. Whatever the status of a school, the model of consultation used must be collaborative. IDEA, as well as good educational practice, expects team collaboration as well asteamresponsibility for outcomes.

To begin the process of collaboration, US schools are required by law to hold a meeting where the multidisciplinary team reviewsthe results of a multidisciplinary evaluation. Many schools also establish teams to address the needs of a child who may not yet have been referred for a multidisciplinary evaluation but who is experiencing learning or behavioral problems. These teams are called prereferralor early intervening services,and provide a mechanism for teachers to discuss a child's learning problems with support personnel, parents, and other teachers, and to collaboratively plan intervention strategies. It is fair to expect, with parent consent, the child's psychiatrist to become a part of these problem-solving teams. Although thesemeetingsinvolve time, the therapeutic process is augmented by establishing acollaborative relationship with the teacher and other team members as well as a formal method for problem-solving in the school.

Psychiatry, particularly child and adolescent psychiatry, is mysterious to the general public. Unlesspersonally faced with a child who requires the services of a child and adolescent psychiatrist, most people are unfamiliar with the psychiatrist's role in the care of children. As psychiatrists begin to interact collaborativelywith schools, they may need to explain to school personnel their perspective of the child's difficulties, their goals for the child and his or her family, and their current treatment plan including strategies such as therapy and medication. If medication is being considered as part of treatment, psychiatrists should explain the medication and the expected outcome as they relate to the overall treatment goals. They should emphasize the need for teachers to report behavioral changes in order to help determine the effectiveness of the medication. It may help to provide teachers with a specific format or behavior checklist for collecting this information and to periodically contact them by phone. Establishing clear avenues of communication is crucial; whatever method is chosen, psychiatrists should be proactive in establishing communication with teachers and other school personnel. Often, the most efficient way of achieving these goals and providing the family with the appropriate support is to attend the IEP and other team planning meetings.

The family as well as the child should play a part equal to that of the psychiatrist and the teacher in the collaboration process. The IDEA actually requires that parents and the child become involved in the IEP assessment process. This process is effective only if all members of the team appreciate the contribution of the family members and are skillful in including their participation. Many parents are proactive and aggressively solicit intervention for their child; others, however, are timid and unfamiliar with their rights as parents and the capacity of their influence. Whatever the circumstances, the psychiatrist should facilitate the process of collaboration by helping parents understand their child's needs, as well as the roles of parents and the process of collaboration in the problem-solving process.

Whereas parents, teachers, and other professionals join together to plan educational programs for children, the child is often absent from the discussions. This is an interesting situation, since most professionals and parents believe that they are acting on behalf of the child but may in fact have other agendas. Schools are affected by financial limitations and legislative mandates as well as their responsibility to accommodate the needs of an individual child. Accommodations to the learning environment may require financial commitment and a change in the school's perception of its responsibilities. Parents make requests influenced by their perception of the child's problem in school, the school's legal responsibilities to assist the child, the developmental issues affecting the child's performance, and their ultimate goals for the child. Conflict arises when perceptions of the school and the family differ; resolution, then, can occur only if both sides are able to jointly address the child's learning needs and adjust environmental variables accordingly.

The planning process can sometimes be augmented by inviting children to participate. Their interpretation of the situation should be considered, even if they are not present at the meeting, and their capacity to state their own educational needs should not automatically be dismissed. Children can often be helped in focusing on their school problems and beginning to identify intervention strategies that will help them succeed. If the child does not wish to be present or is too young to understand the purpose of the meeting, the child psychiatrist can be helpful in articulating the child's perceptions of the problem and possible ideas about the solution. Adolescents should definitely be given the option to contribute to the planning process and, if comfortable, to be present at planning meetings. If the adolescent is embarrassed to go to the office to be given medication, or if the adolescent is teased about leaving class for tutoring, there is a good chance that he or she will not cooperate and the plan will fail. These procedures should be adjusted whenever possible to preserve the child's dignity among his or her peers, because the success of any intervention program depends on the cooperation of the child or adolescent.

Techniques of School Collaboration

Successful communication with schools, *particularly for professionals outside the school domain*, depends on understanding the general administrative structure of schools as well as the function of individuals in the schools. Different problems require different administrative authority, and knowledge about these lines of authority can be important. Issues that focus on curriculum and adjustment in the classroom or school are generally managed by the teacher and the principal. If a teacher is resistant to adjusting classroom procedures or using a curriculum agreed on by the planning team, this problem becomes the principal's responsibility. Issues involving finances or the implementation of legislative mandates, including referral, evaluation, and eligibility for services, are responsibilities of the director of special education and the superintendent. Principals control building issues and the functions of school intervention; the director of special education, however, becomes involved when a child is suspected of having a developmental disability that would qualify him or her for special education services.

Contact with the school should generally begin with the school principal. The principal should introduce professionals from outside the school to the teacher, clarify the role of these professionals, and ensure that communication with the teacher has been authorized by the parents or guardian. It is important for "outsiders" to understand that the principal establishes the culture of the school building. This does not mean that the principal obstructs contact between teachers and outside professionals; rather that he or she is aware of individuals contacting teachers and monitors these contacts, particularly if he or she is concerned about the ability of a teacher to interact appropriately. Thus failure to contact the principal before communicating with a teacher can be an irreparable mistake. The principal also arranges for the involvement of the director of special education and other school support personnel (e.g., the school psychologist or a speech and language pathologist). If a principal does not appear to be knowledgeable about special education procedures and services, including the referral process and legislative mandates, the director of special education may need to be contacted directly. The superintendent is, of course, responsible for all activities in the school district and should be contacted if other administrators are unresponsive to the educational needs of a child. In practice, collaboration with a school is seldom successful without the wholehearted support of the principal.

For child psychiatrists, the most important part of collaboration with schools is to participate as much as possible. Whatever the situation, open communication with the school is important. Schools should be aware of the psychiatrist's involvement with the child, and the psychiatrist should be aware of the child's performance and adjustment to the school environment. The psychiatrist must willingly share information with the school but at the same time help the child and his or her family separate those issues that should be discussed with the school and those that should remain confidential. Children often have a clear perception of the things they would like teachers to know or not know about them. The psychiatrist can become an important conduit between the child, family members, and the school. This role, if supportive to all people involved, can have a positive effect on the problem-solving process.

The child psychiatrist should remember the following rules when collaborating with schools:

Always. . .

Initiate contact with the school

Share information

Explain your role

Represent the child's perspectives

Request school evaluation data

Expect team effort in problem-solving

Expect parents to collaborate as team members

Be a team member

References

1. Stiggins R. *Student-Involved Assessment For Learning*. Upper Saddle River, NJ: Pearson Merrill Prentice Hall, 2005.
2. Mastropiere MA, Scruggs TE. *The Inclusive Classroom – Strategies for Effective Differentiated Instruction*, 4th edn. Upper Saddle River, NJ: Merrill, 2010.
3. Rosenberg MS, Westling DL, McLeskey J. *Special Education for Today's Teachers – An Introduction*. Upper Saddle River, NJ: Pearson Merrill Prentice Hall, 2008.
4. Turnbull A, Turnbell R, Wehmeyer ML. *Exceptional Lives – Special Education In Todays' Schools*. Upper Saddle River, NJ: Pearson Merrill Prentice Hall, 2007.
5. Caplan G. *The Theory and Practice of Mental Health Consultation*. New York: Basic Books, 1970.
6. West FJ, Idol L. School consultation. Part 1: An interdisciplinary perspective on theory, models, and research. *J Learn Disab* 1987;**20**:388–408.
7. Reeve PT, Hallan DP. Practical questions about collaboration between general and special educators. *Focus Except Child* 1994;**26**:1–11.

5

Psychiatric Assessment in Medically Ill Children

James H. Duffee, William M. Klykylo, David M. Rube

Introduction

One-third to two-thirds of inpatient pediatric patients have to cope with psychological issues [1, 2] and could potentially benefit from psychiatric consultation.

Chronic physical illness appears to be a significant risk factor for emotional and behavioral difficulties, while emotional, behavioral, and family difficulties can negatively affect the course of physical disease [3]. In addition, comorbid psychiatric and pediatric medical problems contribute to increased health-care costs, less satisfactory outcomes, and increased diagnostic uncertainty [4]. In this age of children who survive severe medical illnesses such as leukemia, who undergo transplantation (e.g., cardiac, liver, lung, bone marrow), and who live with chronic illnesses for much longer than previously (e.g., cystic fibrosis, diabetes mellitus, infection with the human immunodeficiency virus [HIV]), psychiatric sequelae are common. Child and adolescent psychiatrists must work in collaboration with pediatricians to provide comprehensive care for these children.

Traditionally, consultation-liaison child psychiatry has taken place on pediatric wards and in hospital units. The influence of managed care, however, has shortened hospital stays, and more care is now being provided in the outpatient setting as well as in the home or day hospital. Consequently, consultation-liaison must adapt to the outpatient and homecare setting. In this chapter, we discuss the epidemiology and characteristics of psychiatric disorders and diagnostic dilemmas in the medically ill child. We follow this with discussions of the consultation and assessment process and the psychiatric sequelae of chronic medical problems. We conclude with a consideration of mental health care and the role of the psychiatrist in the fully integrated model of the medical home.

Epidemiology

Consultation-liaison child psychiatrists work with their pediatric colleagues to convey to them the importance of psychiatric consultation. When we assume the role of a consultant, we should help our pediatric colleagues by informing them of the data that exist regarding the comorbidity of medical and psychiatric disorders. The majority of children with chronic medical problems do not have a psychiatric illness. Reports indicate, however, that the risk for psychological and social adjustment problems in children with chronic medical problems is about twofold compared with the risk of healthy children [5–7]. Emotional and behavioral problems have been found to affect 18–20% of children in pediatric primary care practice [8], while estimates of psychological morbidity associated with chronic illness in childhood range from 10% to 30% [1]. Chronic medical problems affect 10–15% of the population under 18 years of age. A Swedish primary care district, however, estimated the prevalence of chronic illness in childhood to be 6% [9]. In the Isle of Wight Survey, 6% of the population had chronic physical illnesses [10]. In the latter study, Rutter and colleagues found that the prevalence of child psychiatric disorders in the general population was 7%, and that the prevalence of psychiatric conditions in children with chronic physical illnesses was 12% (illnesses without brain lesions) and 34% (illnesses with brain lesions).

The National Survey of Health Development in England, Wales, and Scotland and the Rochester Child Health Survey showed that the prevalence of chronic medical problems ranges from 10% to 20% [11]. The former survey observed that 25% of physically ill children below 15 years of age had two or more symptoms of behavior disorder, compared to 17% of the healthy population [11]. Similarly, the Rochester survey showed

Clinical Child Psychiatry, Third Edition. Edited by William M. Klykylo and Jerald Kay.
© 2012 John Wiley & Sons, Ltd. Published 2012 by John Wiley & Sons, Ltd.

that the rates of behavior problems in the chronically ill children were consistently higher than in healthy children and were reflected in behaviors such as a poor attitude toward school and truancy [12 and 13]. Additionally, studies showed higher frequencies of oppositional disorder and conduct disorder in children with cystic fibrosis compared with children with sickle-cell disease. The treatment regimen for cystic fibrosis, being highly demanding and involving numerous daily medications and chest physical therapy, may contribute to this difference [14].

Different theories attempt to explain this comorbidity and to identify factors that account for the variability in the psychological adjustment of children with chronic illness. Reports have described risk factors at multiple levels that can impede the psychological adjustment to chronic illness (Table 5.1). In this regard, studies suggest that severe asthma, inflammatory bowel disease (Crohn's disease or ulcerative colitis) and diabetes may have specifically elevated rates of depression [15]. Additionally, a meta-analysis of depression in children with chronic medical conditions showed higher rates of depression in children with asthma and sickle-cell anemia as compared with children with cancer. The unpredict-able and long-term course of those illnesses may potentially explain the difference [16].

Adolescent females with chronic medical conditions were found to have greater emotional problems, depression, sadness, anhedonia, and suicidal thoughts than were adolescent males with chronic medical conditions [17]. However, male gender may potentially pose a higher risk of emotional problems as suggested by the immunoreactive theory [8]. It is hypothesized that males are selectively afflicted with neurodevelopmental and psychiatric disorders of childhood and this may relate to the relative antigenicity of the male fetus, which may induce a state of maternal immunoreactivity leading to fetal damage. 57. There are protective factors as well. Children's personal strengths, whether in academic life, sports, music, or interpersonal skills could help maintain self-esteem and build important relationships [1]. The coping style confrontation, characterized by active and purposeful problem-solving along with seeking social support, was found to be related to positive psychosocial functioning [18]. Additionally, family flexibility, positive meanings ascribed to the condition, social integration, good communication, clear boundaries, and a support network in the community also appear to be protective [19].

Table 5.1 Risk factors affecting psychological adjustment in medically ill children.

Illness-related factors [1, 8, 14, 19, 20]
  1. Frequent or chronic pain (e.g. sickle-cell disease)
  2. Brain dysfunction as a result of illness or treatment
  3. Physical disability (e.g. decreased exercise endurance in advancing cystic fibrosis)
  4. Invisible condition
  5. Uncertain prognosis
  6. Multiple hospitalizations
  7. Intrusive care routines (e.g. numerous medication and chest physical therapy in cystic fibrosis)
  8. Dietary restrictions (e.g. diabetes)
Patient-related factors [8, 18–20]
  1. Young age
  2. Male gender (immunoreactive theory)
  3. Genetic loading
  4. History of psychiatric illness
  5. Insecure attachments
  6. Difficult temperament
  7. Low self-esteem
  8. Coping style with depressive behavior in reaction to daily problems
Family-related factors [1, 8–20]
  1. Single parent
  2. Low family income
  3. Parental anxiety, anger, sadness, guilt, blame
  4. History of psychiatric illness
  5. Poor family support
  6. Inadequate parenting

The above epidemiological evidence indicates a role for liaison with medical subspecialties to educate other physicians about psychiatric disturbances that may become evident in their patients. Since not all children develop psychiatric symptoms, baseline evaluations or screening devices are needed to clarify which children and families are at risk. The Pediatric Symptom Checklist developed by Jellinek and Murphy has been shown to be a helpful, user-friendly screening device for pediatricians and pediatric residents [21]. Jones and colleagues recommend the Pediatric Symptom Checklist to routinely screen all pediatric patients and, for those patients who meet the cutoff criteria, then using the Child Behavior Checklist [22]. This approach therefore provides an efficient means of screening for and then identifying child psychosocial problems in general pediatric populations.

The Consultative Process and Assessment

Reasons for Consultation

Consultation-liaison child psychiatrists, like other pediatric subspecialists, are called to consult on challenging or difficult cases. The most common reasons for psychiatric consultation encountered in major academic centers and tertiary care hospitals are presented in Table 5.2.

Five Fundamental Questions

Question 1

Is this patient safe to himself or herself or others in the current treatment setting?

The issues that may drive this question arise from individuals who attempt suicide and who may then need to be hospitalized for medical treatment in the intensive care unit (ICU) or on the general pediatric unit and may also require one-on-one intensive supervision. Other examples of this question may be the child who develops delirium and has visual or auditory hallucinations.

Another example in which this question is pertinent is with a child who in the hospital manifests severe behavioral dyscontrol that interferes with his or her treatment. This often takes the form of hyperactivity and aggressive behavior to the staff and other patients. A corollary to this question is, "What is the next treatment setting for this patient?" This latter question is particularly important for individuals who have attempted suicide. Referral to an inpatient psychiatric setting, an outpatient mental health agency, or private psychiatric practice depends on the nature and the assessment of the child's suicide attempt, as well as the presence of a major psychiatric disorder.

Question 2

Why is our patient not cooperating with treatment?

This consultative question is seen in numerous areas, for example, the cancer patient who is extremely anxious and fearful around medical procedures, the diabetic child who is noncompliant, and the depressed mother who has trouble following directions from the nursing staff. The differential diagnosis of noncompliance with treatment is broad and includes the following behaviors or characteristics:

(1) Inability to understand directions.
(2) Lack of education.
(3) Opposition and defiance.
(4) Developmental issues (IQ, Pervasive Developmental Disorder, etc.).
(5) A passive wish to die.
(6) Anxiety.
(7) Depression.
(8) Denial of illness.

Table 5.2 Common reasons for child and adolescent psychiatric consultation [23, 24].

1. Emergencies (e.g., suicide attempts, mental status changes)
2. Differential diagnosis of somatoform symptoms
3. Collaborative care of children with stress-sensitive illnesses
4. Diagnosis and care of children with psychiatric symptoms following a somatic illness
5. Chronic illness (e.g., major depression in a patient with cystic fibrosis)
6. Reactions to major pediatric treatment techniques (e.g. post-traumatic stress disorder following stem cell transplantation)
7. Reactions to pediatric illnesses
8. The child's reaction to his or her illness and hospitalization
9. Nonadherence to medical plan
10. Family assessments
11. Pretransplant (e.g., cardiac, liver, bone-marrow) psychiatric evaluation

(9) Passive vs active coping style [1].
(10) Embarrassment vs pride with respect to self-care [1].
(11) Limited family or peer support [1].
(12) Relationship with medical providers [1].

All of the above phenomena confront general pediatricians in their practice on a daily basis. Our liaison work, therefore, must focus increasingly, in view of the shorter hospital stays, on teaching our pediatric colleagues to ask the appropriate questions to achieve the right answers.

Question 3

This patient has had an extensive and expensive medical workup that has yielded no findings. Is there a psychological or psychiatric reason for the patient's medical symptoms?

Studies of somatization in children showed that medically unexplained physical symptoms are common in childhood and include in descending order of frequency:

- headaches;
- recurrent abdominal pain;
- limb pain;
- chest pain;
- fatigue [8].

Additionally, patients could present with complex syndromes involving both medical or neurological and somatoform symptoms (e.g., a patient with both seizures and pseudoseizures). Many parents with children presenting with these medical complaints are fearful of possible psychiatric consultation. As a result, there can be a relentless and aggressive medical workup. The primary fear of the child or family is that they are not being taken seriously or that nobody believes them. The fear of calling a psychiatric consultation is that the physician might think, "It is all in your head" or, "I think you're crazy." The primary care physician fears losing the alliance developed with the family.

The consultant's goal is twofold: to consult with the primary care physician on how best to approach the patient, and to be empathetic with the patient and his or her family in their frustration at not getting answers. A common approach is to present the psychiatric consultant's role as an adjunct to ongoing medical care, to help the child cope with the chronic symptoms interfering with his/her functioning, the stress of being in the hospital, or the frustration of "not finding the answer." Interaction with families should be supportive and non-confrontational, hopefully to begin the process of forming a therapeutic alliance that will allow the consultant to make recommendations to the family and primary

care physician. It is essential in the assessment of such cases to view the physical symptoms as real even if they seem to be occurring in the context of stress or psychiatric illness. These children are generally not faking or malingering and the symptoms are as real to them as the physical symptoms from a medical illness [25].

The above question is also relevant to cases in which both psychiatric treatment and medical treatment are necessary, as in diseases such as anorexia nervosa or bulimia nervosa. With the number of eating disorder units decreasing, hospitals are administering more medical and psychiatric care for anorexia and bulimia nervosa on the general pediatric unit. Medical hospitalization is usually prompted by a rapid or profound weight loss, cardiovascular abnormalities, electrolyte imbalance, and hypothermia, and may represent a failure of outpatient psychotherapy [1]. The psychiatric consultant's role is to "jump start" the psychiatric treatment for these patients and make recommendations regarding the level of psychiatric intervention after medical stabilization.

Question 4

I think my child is having a hard time since her diagnosis. Can you please send someone to talk with her?

This question is generally posed by parents to their primary care physicians, especially in the face of chronic illness. At times, parents will state that they are concerned that their child is having difficulty adjusting to a new diagnosis or may be suffering from depression as a result of treatment or the news of the diagnosis of a chronic illness. Or it may be a subtle request for the parents or other family members themselves, who may be experiencing difficulty adjusting to their child's chronic illness. Often, parents request that the patient's siblings or other family members be informed about their loved one's medical problems. As previously noted, disturbances requiring psychiatric attention are manifest in a greater proportion of chronically medically ill patients and their families than in healthy children. This is extremely important in the context of managed care, in which sicker and more unstable patients are at times the only patients on a hospital unit or ICU.

Parents sometimes request a psychiatric consultation to discuss how to tell their child bad news, or to prepare the child for medical procedures. The child psychiatric consultant is uniquely qualified to give the parents developmental guidelines about how to discuss these issues with their children.

Question 5

This patient has an end-stage organ or other serious disease and would require a pre-transplant psychiatric evaluation as part of the multidisciplinary transplantation assessment.

Solid organ and bone marrow transplantation have become recognized as legitimate treatments for many types of end-stage organ failures and hematologic/oncologic disorders. Hence, this question is frequently encountered by the psychiatric consultant in major academic centers where he or she is a member of the multidisciplinary transplantation team. The consultant's role is to conduct a thorough evaluation of the child and family with an emphasis on identifying psychopathology, potential risk factors for adjustment reactions or nonadherence to treatment, and the adequacy of social supports [26].

Assessment

1. Consultative Question

A significant challenge for the consultant is determining and often narrowing the question raised by the primary care team – i.e., framing the consultative question. When training for this specific task, the students and residents can be given clinical vignettes and asked to arrive at the consultative question. Training our future colleagues to ask appropriate consultative questions will help teach them how best to work with their consultants, and it will help us as psychiatric consultants to best fulfill our responsibilities to the treatment team and to the patient and family. An important component of an appropriate consultative request is to ascertain who is asking the question. This helps focus the intervention and recommendations of the consultant.

In addition, it is helpful to clarify who the "identified patient" and who the "real patient" are. For example, this question is critical when diagnoses such as a failure to thrive or Munchausen syndrome by proxy are being considered in the differential diagnosis of the consultative request.

2. Consent of the Parent and "Assent" of the Child

It is imperative that the team requesting the consultation notify the family (in the form of a request) of the need for psychiatric consultation and also inform the child that someone will be coming to talk with him or her. This is an area in which residents and medical students are fearful of patient reactions and need help in being able to discuss the potential for psychiatric problems with the parents of their patients. An appointment is scheduled with the parents so that the consultation can be completed, as quickly as possible. At this stage of clinical practice, the primary care team's responsibility is to inform the patient and help the family obtain authori-

zation for a mental health consultation through third-party carriers.

3. Medical Record Review

It is imperative that the consultant be thoroughly informed about the child's medical condition, the treatment of this condition, and the related side effects of treatment. The patient's laboratory values, electrocardiograms, and medications, etc. need to be reviewed thoroughly. A major component often lacking in psychiatric-pediatric collaboration has been communication. Stereotypes of psychiatrists depict them as impractical, unavailable, and not knowledgeable about medical illnesses and their treatment [27]. As psychiatrists, we can debate whether this is appropriate or not; however, these are the impressions that consultation-liaison psychiatrists face every day. Being aware of all the medical issues ensures that the pediatrician and the consulting psychiatrist speak the same language and thus provide the patient with the best service. In addition, the best way to collaborate is to be familiar with each other's work. An important finding is that child psychiatrists and pediatricians are better able to collaborate when they have been trained in a setting in which they worked together [28].

4. Psychiatric Interview

In Chapters 1 and 2, the details of the psychiatric and psychological assessments are discussed; however, the special considerations needed to evaluate a child with a medical condition are highlighted here. First, the psychiatrist should directly observe the patient and conduct an initial observation of the patient's status, regardless of whether his or her family members are staying overnight or are available for the appointment or where the patient is located (such as the day hospital, inpatient unit, ICU step-down unit, or burn unit). This provides a rapid assessment of the patient's medical needs at the time of consultation. Is the patient in bed, awake, alert, interacting with staff, watching television, playing games, or engaging in childlike activities? Is the child demonstrating that he or she is in pain? In general, for school-age children up to age 11 years, the consultant should meet with the parents first. The parents should be asked if their physician or treatment team requested this consultation and whether they were aware of it, or whether they requested the consultation themselves. It is important to ascertain the goals of the evaluation early in the process. A full history of the medical episode as well as a psychiatric review of systems, family history, social developmental history, current living situation, and school performance is obtained from the parents.

Based on the information gathered from the treatment team and the parents, the next step in the consultation is interviewing the child. The interview is generally briefer as the child could be too weak or irritable due illness to tolerate a lengthy examination [29]. In addition to conducting the general child psychiatric evaluation and mental status examination, the physician should direct special attention to the family's feelings and reactions toward the child (such as overprotective, distant, or fearful) and the child's understanding of his or her own illness; identification of any fantasy about the cause of illness is critical. It is important to know what the child experiences and their perceptions of their medical condition. The child may have fantasies of what caused their illness (i.e., punishment, etc.), which would be important in assessing the patient. Assessing how well family members are coping with the child's illness is also significant. Studies have measured the child's ability to cope and assessed what type of coping strategies children use to deal with their illnesses [30, 31]. This coping ability is especially important for children with chronic illness and their families. A thorough understanding of the patient's and family's coping strategies and defense mechanisms yields important information on how they cope with ongoing treatment and improvement or worsening of the medical condition.

5. Discussion of the Findings with the Referring Team

Once the assessment is completed it is helpful for the consultant to discuss the findings directly with the team or physician calling the consultation. This allows the consultant to fill in the gaps between the parental and the child interview. This will also allow the consultant to tailor psychiatric interventions that may be necessary and that are practical for this particular patient, family, and treatment team and the medical setting in which the patient is found.

Report and Recommendations

Our general medical and pediatric colleagues have reported over time that, although they appreciate detailed psychological and psychiatric reports, they find practical and concrete suggestions and recommendations for their patients to be the most helpful. It is not helpful, then, to submit a long report with only short, possibly unclear, recommendations. With those considerations in mind, a consultation report could be designed as follows:

(1) Reason for consultation.
(2) Patient's identifying data (age, gender, race, level of education, living arrangements, household and family structure).

(3) Sources of information (e.g. patient, family members, friends, medical records).
(4) History of present illness:
  – brief summary of the current medical condition and treatment;
  – psychiatric review of systems with pertinent positives and negatives; onset, duration and course of the psychiatric symptoms relative to the course of the medical condition;
  – recent psychosocial stressors.
(5) Past psychiatric history.
(6) Family history.
(7) Social/developmental history.
(8) Medical/surgical history.
(9) Current medication, laboratory data, vital signs.
(10) Mental status examination, including the assessment of cognitive function.
(11) Assessment and diagnosis.
(12) Plan and recommendations: will address the specifics of the consultation request and will include specific, concrete recommendations in nonpsychiatric jargon and followup, presented in list form and in decreasing order of importance; the patient's safety must be addressed first.

The psychiatric consultant must remain involved with the patient's care throughout both hospitalization and follow-up to the outpatient setting, if indicated. The psychiatric consultant should keep the patient's primary care physician informed of the type of treatment and its specific mode and goals. In our experience, pediatricians rarely receive these types of calls. The parents of the children appreciate that their child's psychiatric care is being discussed with their primary care physician. Table 5.3 summarizes the characteristics of an effective consultant and consultation.

Psychiatric Aspects of Chronic Medical Illness

The psychiatric aspects of chronic medical illnesses are well documented [20, 32–34]. A few additional points need to be made, especially for the child psychiatry/psychology trainee, that must be assessed.

Table 5.3 Characteristics of an effective consultant and consultation.

1. Available
2. Knowledgeable regarding medical issues
3. Communicative
4. Gives practical recommendations in nonpsychiatric jargon!!
5. Provides or arranges outpatient or ongoing follow-up

(1) *Does the illness or its treatment, such as brain tumor, diabetic ketoacidosis, or steroids, affect the brain? What is the patient's knowledge and information*

(2) *Regarding his or her illness?.* The consultation-liaison psychiatrist may help the treatment team explain and educate about a newly diagnosed illness. A psychiatric consultation may be called to evaluate the educational level or developmental level of a family, patient, or child and to assist the treatment team in explaining the child's illness in a way that can be more easily understood.

(3) *Developmental sequelae of chronic medical illness.* Children need to be children. The goal of treating pediatric illnesses is to keep or return a particular child and family to their normal developmental trajectory. Having an illness that results in multiple hospitalizations, clinic visits, injections, breathing treatments, physical changes such as hair loss, and other effects of medical problems or their treatments can change the way a child views his or her body and his/her self-esteem. It can also alter academic potential because of absence from school or cognitive changes. Sometimes these children have difficulty with peers who lack understanding about them and their medical problem.

(4) *Family dynamics.* As is true with all child psychiatric assessments, careful attention must be directed to the family, both immediate and extended, of a child with a chronic medical illness. Illness can change the family milieu, due to parents staying with the child, possibly taking time off from work and losing income. Family sessions may be needed to help a family adjust. Marital issues may arise owing to the extra strain of caring for a medically ill child. At times it is up to the psychiatric consultant to remind these parents to spend time together to keep the marriage and family functioning. Siblings also need attention from the treatment team and the psychiatric consultant to discuss issues about their ill brother or sister and their feelings regarding family changes.

(5) *Education of allied professionals.* In these days of managed care and short hospital stays, it is imperative that treatment teams have in-services regarding "the psychiatric review of systems." As previously mentioned, medically ill children report more psychiatric symptoms than do well children [10–12]. It is important to have refresher courses in psychiatric signs and symptoms to enable the staff to identify children who may have developed new psychiatric symptoms.

Medical illnesses may present as psychiatric illnesses. Children with brain disorders report psychiatric symptoms four to five times more than do well children [10]. At times, a change in mental status may be the first sign of a medication side effect, a recurrence of cancer, connective tissue diseases, or HIV. It is incumbent on consultation-liaison psychiatrists to work closely with residents and the nursing staff to observe and identify subtle mental status changes.

Psychiatric conditions may present as medical illnesses. In one study, psychosomatic disorders accounted for 28% of all child psychiatric consultations [24]. The Ontario Child Health Study estimated a prevalence rate of somatization syndromes of 4.5% for boys and 10.7% for girls aged 12 to 16 years [8]. These children had medical workups that were negative, and the presenting problems included failure to thrive, abdominal pain, headache pain, and eating disorders. In our hospital, GI complaints by far constitute the majority of consultation requests in this area. As mentioned previously, one of the difficulties the house staff tend to have with these patients is telling a parent that a psychiatric consultation is needed; they are fearful of parental reaction. We suggest the following approaches for house staff to deal with these issues:

(1) Emphasize the need for multiple team members on the treatment team, including mental health professionals.

(2) Do not imply that you are giving up on the patient and his or her problem.

(3) Feel free to express frustration at not being able to arrive at a medical diagnosis.

(4) At times, request a consultation for the purpose of offering support to the patient and family in dealing with medical complaints.

These suggestions may help patients accommodate to the possibility that a psychiatric component may have initiated or maintained their ongoing medical problem.

Pediatric Hospital Consultation Today

The role of the child and adolescent consultation in liaison psychiatry in acute settings is currently in a state of flux, as both the mode of health-care delivery and the patterns of reimbursement for consultation are changing. When evaluating many perplexing and difficult patients, liaison psychiatrists find themselves needing to adapt to various settings and lengths of time given for assessments. Acute hospitalizations are frequently very brief. The opportunity to interact with our colleagues is also lessened because, to keep up with demand, the work load of primary care physicians and pediatric specialists and hospitalists has increased. Nevertheless, the need for child and adolescent psychiatrists for consultation in hospitals continues to be high. In this context, the consultation-liaison child psychiatrist's task is to help educate pediatric colleagues about the comorbidity of medical and psychiatric disorders and the importance of psychiatric consultation, and to work as part of the multidisciplinary team in order to provide comprehensive care for these children. Additionally, with advances in HIV treatment making HIV infection more a sub-acute, chronic disease, the child psychiatrist is being called upon to help address the newly posed challenges to the neurocognitive and psychosocial development of children and families [35].

The liaison child psychiatrist has the additional important task of educating the patients and their families, in a developmentally appropriate way, about medical procedures, medical illness, and its potential psychological consequences. Additionally, in working with adolescent patients, the educative role with a focus on the risks for HIV infection and other sexually transmitted diseases (STDs) is essential, given their especially increased risk.

Using the clinical skills and research in our field, child and adolescent psychiatrists are well prepared to deal with the complex psychological and social consequences of chronic medical illness. While there is a growing body of literature on the psychosocial adjustment in children with chronic medical illness, more work is needed especially in the area of treatment interventions, both nonpharmacological and psychopharmacological. Additionally, collaboration between child psychiatrists, primary care physicians, and pediatric specialists will require ongoing attention and research in order to optimize the multidisciplinary approach to chronically ill pediatric patients.

Integrated Mental Health Care in the Medical Home

The Institute of Medicine in the Quality Chasm series challenged the health-care community to improve the quality of general health care by effective collaboration of all mental, substance abuse, general health care and other human service providers in coordinating the care of their patients [35]. Integrated primary care is a strategy in which behavioral health and medical care are rendered simultaneously and fluidly so that the patient experiences a holistic approach to wellness and chronic condition management. Most of the research documenting the need and potential benefits of primary care integration has concentrated on family practice or adult medicine. For instance, people with serious mental illness die on average 25 years earlier than the general population. Sixty percent of premature deaths of people with schizophrenia are caused by medical con-

ditions such as cardiovascular, pulmonary, and infectious diseases. When treating a young depressed woman, effective care of depression and marital problems improves physical health and reduces unnecessary or poorly understood medical visits for vague somatic symptoms.

However, the concept is also applicable to children in a medical home. As an example, low estimates for maternal depression range from 5% to 25%. In high-risk mothers, low-income or adolescent women, the rates are more in the range of 40–60% [36]. The deleterious effect of maternal depression on the development, both physical and social-emotional, of the child has been well documented. One valuable treatment strategy might be a dyadic intervention involving both the mother and infant within the medical home. In a familiar therapeutic environment such as a medical home, a family-based intervention could promote attachment between the mother and infant and link the family to other community support services.

Partnerships between child psychiatrists and primary care providers are "crucial to the integration of mental health into pediatric primary care [37]." This section will concentrate on the role of the child psychiatrist interacting with, or preferably integrated into, a pediatric medical home. In this setting, the child psychiatrist brings the clinical knowledge and skill set described above into a coordinated outpatient setting. The section will begin with a discussion of some characteristics of the medical home as it has developed particularly for children with special health-care needs. Then some aspects of behavioral health integration will be outlined from the perspectives of both pediatricians and child psychiatrists. Finally, the application of integrated primary care will be illustrated by discussing the special needs of children in foster care as encountered in an advanced medical home.

What is a Medical Home?

Although a medical home may be bricks and mortar, it is usually thought of as a philosophy of care. The concept developed as an attempt to improve the quality of care for children with special health-care needs (CSHCNs) [37]. Initially, it was thought that the children who might benefit most from comprehensive care in a medical home were defined by the Maternal and Child Health Bureau as those who have, or are at risk for, chronic physical, developmental, behavioral, or emotional conditions and who require health and related services of a type or amount beyond that required by children generally. In recent years, the concept has expanded to include health maintenance as well as chronic condition management, and also adults as well as children with special health-care needs.

Following current thinking, care in a medical home should be delivered or directed by well-trained practitioners who provide health maintenance, acute care, and chronic condition management. As defined by the American Academy of Pediatrics (AAP), the medical care of infants, children, and adolescents and young adults should be collaborative, comprehensive, family centered, coordinated, compassionate, and culturally appropriate [37]. For many pediatricians in the 1980s and 1990s, this paradigm shift was somewhat difficult to accept. Physicians in training did not receive guidance about how to be the head of the treatment team. They also were not trained in how to integrate social emotional care with traditional pediatric medicine.

In the first decade of the twenty-first century, the concept of a medical home for children with special health-care needs was expanded by internists and family practitioners to describe a philosophy or strategy for chronic condition management. The terminology changed somewhat to include "person centered medical home," "primary care home," or, most recently, "health home." These terms designate similar but not identical ideas.

The multidisciplinary team in a pediatric medical home often includes pediatricians, a child psychiatrist, and nurse practitioners, nurses, and clinical assistants. Additional professionals in more advanced team models include care coordinators, developmental specialists, and social workers. Family support team members comprise child and family therapists, home visitors, and eligibility specialists. Community partners often include representatives from health departments and public health agencies directed toward care for CSHCNs. Applying the team approach, a fully developed medical home offers chronic condition management with services for children and families who use the health-care system most often. Especially eligible children include those with emotional disorders such as those resulting from parental separation and divorce as well as neurodevelopmental disorders including the autistic spectrum disorder and fetal alcohol spectrum disorder. In addition, children who have emotional responses to chronic medical illness such as childhood cancer, cystic fibrosis, or diabetes will particularly benefit from primary care integration and medical home services. The medical home should be able to form active and lasting partnerships with families, identify and monitor children with special needs, coordinate care in a systematic manner, and communicate with other community resources including schools and juvenile court services.

Degrees of Integration

Concurrent with the emergence of the medical home as a health-care delivery ideal, pediatricians were grappling with a dramatic shift in the care needed by a routine pediatric practice. A new morbidity developed that was social and emotional in nature. School problems as well as minor psychiatric disturbances of childhood became part of the scope of practice. The shift in morbidity was complicated by the relative lack of access to child psychiatry. Pediatricians and to a lesser extent family practitioners, took on the care (including psychopharmacology) of learning disabilities and attentional problems. Pediatricians became very adept at the prescription of stimulants as well as adrenergic medications although, in general, were not comfortable with antidepressants or antipsychotics.

However, in the most recent years, pediatricians have started to assume primary care for fairly complicated psychiatric disorders. In the words of one pediatrician, "I used to be a Ritalin doctor but now I am a Risperdal doctor." As a consequence, a number of strategies have developed to address the shortage of primary care child psychiatrists as well as the need for primary care pediatricians to acquire a different skill set to take care of children with behavioral and developmental disorders of moderate severity.

Sadly, one of the most usual strategies to access behavioral health is what might be referred to as a "Hail Mary pass" (in American football, a long, forward pass thrown in desperation with little chance of completion). That is, a situation in which a pediatrician encounters a child in emotional or relationship-related stress and wants to make a referral to either a child psychiatrist or an appropriate therapist. When the channels of communication are not well established the pediatrician merely says to a family something like: "Your child needs therapy; here are some telephone numbers you might call." There is no certainty that this strategy will work. In many communities, substantial barriers exist, including financial limitations and extended wait lists, that reduce the likelihood that a first visit will be made.

The next level of continuity might be considered a facilitated referral. An example of this might be the referral of a patient to a therapist with whom a pediatrician has an existing relationship. A phone call might even be made from the pediatrician's nurse to the therapist's or child psychiatrist's office but little or no information is passed other than demographics sufficient to complete an appointment. If child psychiatry is the object of referral, it is hit or miss whether a return communication arrives to inform the pediatrician of the diagnosis or treatment plan. Many hazards remain in this model since the behavioral health provider remains isolated from the pediatric caregiver. It is very frustrating for a pediatrician to be asked, for instance, to renew medications with no documented justification for their prescription, or to struggle with the possibility of untoward effects of psychiatric medications presenting as occult signs and symptoms in the clinic. Conversely, the child psychiatrist may not be aware of the complexities of family adaptation in the context of medical illness and consequently either over- or under-diagnose. The lack of continuity is confusing for families and places the child at risk for inappropriate treatment.

A somewhat more advanced strategy is to co-locate behavioral health practitioners in the medical office. The benefits of this model include the opportunity for improved communication and continuity of care between the behavioral health provider and the pediatrician. Often this might occur in the hallway or lunchroom and may consist of a few quick words that will clarify the interaction between physical and emotional health. The financial arrangements can be various. The pediatrician, in some circumstances, may have the capacity to hire a therapist. As an alternative, the pediatrician may lease space to an outside agency that places a therapist or psychiatrist in office space adjacent to the pediatric provider. Conversely, some community mental health centers have experimented with placement of pediatric providers (usually mid-levels) within the mental health clinic. The drawback of these partial models is that some objectives central to the medical home philosophy are more difficult to attain and are often lost in misunderstandings and conflicting paradigms typically between pediatricians and psychotherapists.

Full integration provides the most comprehensive and holistic care, addressing emotions, mind, and body. Characteristics of behavioral health in a medical home include formal scheduled screening in the primary care of children for social and emotional development in addition to the usual domains of communication, motor coordination, and problem-solving. Minor variations in behavioral development can be addressed during usual well-child visits long before a problem develops to the degree consistent with the need for a diagnosis. There is on both sides, behavioral and medical, recognition of the interconnectedness among physical, social and emotional, and behavioral functioning. In the primary care team approach, the behavioral health consultant or practitioner is an integral part of a multidisciplinary team. The team leader is usually a pediatric physician but other team members include nurse practitioners, care coordinators, nurses, and ancillary care providers such as social workers and pediatric rehabilitation therapists. Essential to the functioning of a primary care team are

care conferences, during which families and children are discussed and an integrated plan of care is developed. These care conferences may also include representatives from outside agencies such as foster care workers or special education teachers.

A final level of primary care integration involves embedding behavioral health providers into the well-child clinic. In one evidence-based primary care model, Healthy Steps for Young Children [38], a developmental specialist accompanies the pediatric practitioner during health maintenance or well-child visits and is available to perform socio-emotional assessments and to counsel parents and families on appropriate management of minor developmental and relationship-based problems encountered during the child's earliest years. The program evaluation of Healthy Steps has revealed that both the parent and the pediatric provider are more satisfied with the encounters and that relatively minor interventions applied in the early stages of development can reap long-term benefits and improved attachments and understanding of temperament mismatches.

Although treatment plans are always individualized, evidence-based practices should be preferred for both medical and behavioral interventions. On the pediatric side, treatment of psychosomatic illness such as abdominal pain or headache should follow recognized practice guidelines. Conversely, behavioral health interventions and a medical home should be of the same rigorous quality. Some examples of evidence-based programs that are completely consistent with a primary care practice include Positive Parenting Program (Triple P) [39], Incredible Years [40], and Parent–Child Interaction Therapy [41]. All three are examples of primary or secondary interventions that reap full benefit from the enhanced surveillance and formal screening present in the pediatric medical home to identify parents, children, and families who are at high risk of developing serious emotional and behavioral problems. A clear advantage of integrated care is early detection of incipient disorders even in the preschool era when children are seen most often by pediatricians.

The role of care coordination and the care coordinator requires special comment. In the pediatric setting, care coordination involves collating the medical record and coordinating activities and recommendations of specialists in addition to the usual activities of case management often associated with a social worker. The behavioral health-care coordinator should be well acquainted with community resources and other agencies along the continuum of care including the need for involvement of juvenile corrections or partial hospitalization. The medical care coordinator needs to communicate regularly with other pediatric consultants such as the neurologists, developmental pediatricians, or oncologists. Obviously, the special needs care coordinator and the behavioral health coordinator should engage in a lively partnership so that the overall treatment plan is consistent with both the pediatric provider and the psychiatrist.

The Benefits of and Obstacles to Integrated Primary Care

The benefits of an integrated treatment plan addressing the whole child in the family living in a community consist of improved medical care, improved access to behavioral health practitioners, reduced stigma of psychiatric illness, and, from the health policy perspective, reduced expenditure for unnecessary and duplicative care. Consultation with families in a medical home most benefits those who have children with chronic illness, medical illness complicated by socio-emotional factors, and families with children with special health-care needs. The enhanced care coordination improves utilization of both medical and behavioral services. There is facilitated collaboration among practitioners with a system-wide consultative role of the therapist so that the pediatric provider is empowered to care for minor behavioral and social emotional problems without unnecessary referrals to busy therapists. On the organizational level, more efficient administration of unified programs is possible, especially with shared information systems.

There are, however, many obstacles to integration, some of which have to do with the differences in vocabulary and perspectives of medical providers and behavior health practitioners. Even the formation of multidisciplinary teams is difficult in a relationship-based organization and is fraught with unanticipated perils. Both pediatric providers and therapists may experience role confusion and blurred boundaries resulting in serious miscommunication. The establishment of a therapeutic environment may be sabotaged by various cultural norms and expectations of the different professional groups such as nursing staff, therapists, medical providers, and administrators. There may be conflicting priorities (both interdisciplinary and inter-agency) when outside agencies are involved. Difficulties with confidentiality may arise since releasing information from the pediatric record may have very different implications than those of releasing the records of therapy for a child who has been a victim of domestic violence or abuse.

Administrative obstacles to integration also exist. Particularly with integrated or embedded primary care, scheduling and record-keeping requirements are both significant challenges. Certification and accreditation requirements are peculiar to state boards, and paneling with managed care organizations is often a huge challenge. Reimbursement strategies vary from state to state and unintentionally may limit efforts to integrate care. Finally, in the age of the electronic health record, templates for behavioral health as well as medical encounters are necessary and, in general, subject to different quality review and confidentiality measures.

Psychiatric Consultation in the Medical Home

The psychiatrist may have a number of roles in community pediatric care as in other settings such as school consultation. The most common and perhaps the most comfortable role is to operate in the usual manner of an outpatient practice. In that model, the psychiatrist receives a referral from a pediatrician with or without medical history. The psychiatrist engages in an evaluation and makes a diagnosis that may or may not be communicated effectively to the pediatrician. The prescription of medications and a brief visit may be all that the psychiatrist can provide under the limitations of managed-care. Sadly common, this model of mental health delivery has little to do with care in a functioning, integrated medical home.

Taken from the perspective of the least intensive involvement, the psychiatrist may be called upon to provide consultation to the functioning of the primary care team. Pediatricians, in general, are not trained to be leaders of the treatment team. The modeling provided by a child psychiatrist, particularly in the arena of reflective supervision, can be immeasurably beneficial to the functioning of a primary care team. The child psychiatrist may be aware of boundary issues, jealousies, and blindspots in the treatment team that make it difficult for the team to provide the best care possible for children and families. The psychiatrist can gently mentor the pediatrician in the role of the head of the team as well as address dysfunctional elements within the treatment team related to blurred boundaries and particularly issues with confidentiality [42].

The role of reflective supervision is most important during the scheduled care conferences in which the primary care team gathers to discuss difficult patients or family situations and to develop an integrated treatment plan. The next level of consultation to the team is particular to the care of a family or patient. When the case presentation is by a therapist, the child psychiatrist may provide insight about the use of medications and interaction of the medications with potential medical illness or symptomatology. When the case presentation is made by the pediatrician or one of the nurse practitioners, the child psychiatrist may help with the management of the child by the pediatric health provider rather than assuming any other direct care role. In this circumstance, the child psychiatrist expands the skill set of the pediatric provider to intervene in a sensitive and compassionate way to help families adjust to minor deviations of socio-emotional development. An example might be the detection of a temperament mismatch between an infant and a mother at the four-month visit. In the enhanced medical home, temperament scales are often used at this age to provide some insight into the attachment patterns as well as to detect the potential for difficulties and mismatches between the mother and the infant. The child psychiatrist may help the nurse practitioner or physician to understand how to help the mother-child dyad without a formal referral or evaluation.

Another example of how the child psychiatrist may provide a broad and rich benefit for the treatment team involves the all too frequent behavioral disturbance in children when parents separate. Not all these families will require psychotherapy or psychiatric consultation. The psychiatrist may advise the pediatrician either specifically or generally about how to speak with the family to support them through a difficult transition and to understand the reaction of the child. The pediatrician may be generally but not deeply aware of how children may respond to the loss of a parent depending on their emotional development. For instance, it may be easy for a person not trained in therapeutic neutrality to take sides in parental conflict or to develop rescue fantasies that interfere with the objective and effective care of the child. The role of the child psychiatrist may be to help the pediatrician understand how the child might be feeling in the context of parental separation and to suggest advice to be given to the parents as well as guidance for developmentally appropriate interviewing of the child.

In addition to consultation with the treatment team about the team function as well as consultation regarding a particular case, the child psychiatrist may decide to evaluate the child personally and to report back to the team. An example of this function is the evaluation and diagnosis of autistic spectrum disorders. With the increased frequency of referral for diagnosis and the potential implications for school programs, it is important to develop local capacity for specific diagnosis and recommendations. In an advanced medical home, the pediatric developmental screening may identify a child at risk by using an M-Chat or other accepted screening instrument [43] at prescribed ages such as a 30-month visit. The psychiatrist may wish to see the child in consultation to the pediatrician in lieu of referral to

regional centers, particularly when there is a significant delay to obtain an appointment. In this strategy, the psychiatrist helps make a diagnosis and reports back to the treatment team without necessarily taking the patient on for regular visits.

The next level of consultation involves liaison treatment. With the frequent diagnosis of attention-deficit hyperactivity disorder (ADHD) in a usual pediatric practice, it is definitely not necessary for the child psychiatrist to take on all patients with that diagnosis. The pediatrician rightly believes the treatment and management of children with ADHD is within the scope of practice of a general pediatric provider. The child psychiatrist's role in this may be to refine the diagnosis, particularly when comorbidities are present, and to make suggestions about pharmacotherapy. There may also be an opportunity to elucidate family dynamics that need to be addressed in the holistic care of children with learning and attentional problems. However, once the treatment is refined, the child can be referred back to the pediatrician for ongoing care only to return to the child psychiatrist if the treatment plan is unsuccessful or some other problem develops that requires further diagnosis and treatment planning.

Finally, it is very reasonable to assume that a child psychiatrist will carry a caseload of children with moderate to severe mental illness. These are children who may have been identified during pediatric care but have the intensity or severity of illness that makes a relationship with a psychiatrist appropriate.

In summary, children who have a low to moderate risk for both behavioral and physical health complexity can be managed by the pediatrician with only minimal consultation with a psychiatrist. Children with a high risk for behavioral problems but a low to moderate risk for physical health complexity should be managed by the child psychiatrist with pediatric consultation. Those with a low to moderate risk for behavioral health complexity but high risk for physical health complexity should be managed in a liaison fashion with the pediatrician. The few children with a high risk and complexity for both behavioral and physical health likely would require intensive treatment by both the pediatric and behavioral health services, including care coordination and multidisciplinary team involvement.

The Foster Care Medical Home

Although a number of examples could be chosen, integrated primary care works extremely well for foster children. At any time in the United States, there are about half a million children in out-of-home care. An excess of health disparities exist in medical conditions, developmental disorders, and psychiatric disturbances compared to any other population. Children may enter care with poorly controlled chronic conditions because of neglect. Children often come from families that are poor, disorganized, drug-involved, and violent [44]. These adverse childhood experiences and frequent congenital biological risks compound the trauma of separation and loss magnifying the need for integrated mental health services.

The reaction of the child to placement in out-of-home care varies along the continuum of shock, grief, and loss. Often, the child longs for the biological family even if deeply dysfunctional. Some children respond with dramatic externalizing oppositional behavior. Others internalize and withdraw. Still others are chaotic or near psychotic. Long-term problems include personality disturbance similar to chronic post-traumatic stress disorder (PTSD; see Chapter 29).

These children are at risk for many medical problems. Nine of ten children in foster care have at least one physical health problem, while more than half have more than one problem. Developmental delays occur in about half and include language disorders, delayed motor skills, learning disabilities, and cognitive impairments [45]. Malnutrition and anemia are common in addition to growth failure. One in five children entering foster care is an infant. Eighty percent of infants are at risk for medical and developmental problems related to intrauterine exposure to substances of abuse. Forty percent are born preterm or with low birthweight. Long-term sequelae of physical abuse such as shaken impact syndrome may complicate neurodevelopmental progress.

About 80% of children in foster care require mental health services, compared to approximately 20% of the general child population [46]. There is a disproportionate prescription of psychotropic medication among foster care youth and a high utilization of inpatient services. Children in out-of-home care are three to ten times more likely to have psychiatric diagnoses, over seven times more likely to be hospitalized for mental health issues, and have over ten times more mental health expenditures compared to children not in foster care.

The medical home for children in foster care must assure developmentally appropriate and comprehensive health care. Formal screening for physical, cognitive, social, and emotional disturbances should be more common. Care coordination, including the establishment of portable medical records, is essential for continuity of care for the variety of services, specialists, and agencies that are involved with the child. The medical home should also ensure that infants in foster care have access to quality early care and education.

The guidelines for health care for children in foster care promulgated by the AAP include a comprehensive physical, developmental, and mental health evaluation within one month of placement [46]. The initial assessment can certainly be done by a pediatrician, but a child psychiatrist or mental health provider is able to more adequately understand the social and emotional development of the child in the context of the history of trauma in the family of origin and to contribute to a comprehensive treatment plan to address the initial reactions and the long-term sequelae of foster placement. In addition, the mental health specialist might address special challenges for foster parents of infants. A child psychiatrist may be in a unique position to advise a multidisciplinary team in the establishment of a many-faceted intervention strategy to address the developmental, relational, and emotional disturbances that complicate medical care. The psychiatrist also will contribute to a reunification plan if appropriate.

An additional role of the child psychiatrist is to promote the inclusion of mental health assessments and recommendations in court-approved social service plans [47]. The psychiatrist may be called upon to be a member of a core team that brings child development expertise to the judge, the guardian *ad litem*, or to social agencies (see Chapter 30). In addition to providing consultation to the multidisciplinary team within the medical home, the psychiatrist may be in a position to provide reflective supervision to foster care workers and other community-based agency representatives in order to extend the therapeutic environment from the medical home to the foster home and out into the community.

A recent development involves the integration of early childhood mental health consultation into child welfare agencies. Under direction of a child psychiatrist, early childhood mental health specialists may train and mentor foster care workers and foster parents in behavioral management techniques. As in consultation to the medical home multidisciplinary team, the consultant may influence the functioning of the team as a primary concern or may consult directly about a particular child after a comprehensive mental health evaluation. The psychiatrist may also take on the child as an individual patient and consult with the team after gaining special knowledge about the particular circumstances of the patient. The use of medications also may be necessary to address either acute or chronic problems.

In all these ways, a multidisciplinary team in a medical home that includes integration of mental health care is an ideal environment to care for foster children. The psychiatrist, although not head of the treatment team, may be absolutely essential in making sure the team functions well to address the many problems of foster children, especially those placed in infancy. Not all children need to become patients of the psychiatrist nor should all children require medications. However, all children will benefit from an in-depth social and emotional evaluation performed by a child psychiatrist and the inclusion of social and emotional factors into the foster care case plan.

Summary

This chapter provides an introduction to the variety of roles and responsibilities that may be assumed by a child psychiatrist functioning within an advanced primary care home with integrated mental health services. The need for improved mental health care in the medical home has arisen from a variety of social and public health changes in the past few decades. At the same time, the child psychiatry workforce has not kept up with demand and is frequently concentrated in academic centers. The inclusion of a child psychiatrist in a medical home multidisciplinary team provides the opportunity to promulgate the knowledge and treatment techniques to pediatricians, mid-level practitioners, therapists, and representatives of community-based service agencies. The example of foster children coping with early adversity and finding care in a medical home that includes mental health services provides a promising strategy to ensure that the child receives developmentally appropriate comprehensive care. An integrated primary care home can provide universal screening for emotional and social development, based on recognition of the interconnectedness among physical, relational, and behavioral functioning. The inclusion of child psychiatrists and evidence-based therapy represents an important step towards the delivery of comprehensive, coordinated, and community-based health care for all children and families.

Appendix 5.1—Case Studies

CASE ONE

A psychiatric consultation was received for Stephen, a nine-year-old boy with stomach cancer. The hematology/oncology team and the nursing staff found Stephen to be belligerent and aggressive during medical procedures. During 'off hours' he would be found in his room in the dark with the shades pulled, refusing visitors. He was belligerent throughout the day and consistently removed IVs. The consultation was held to evaluate Stephen's behavior. On examination, Stephen met criteria for a depressive disorder with associated anxiety symptoms. Individual psychotherapy and a trial of fluoxetine were initiated. Psychotherapy entailed play, drawing, storytelling and also distraction and relaxation techniques to help him cope with the procedures. Areas of focus included: education about his illness, the effects of his cancer and its treatment on body image, issues of life, death and grief, at a developmentally appropriate level. Gradually, Stephen was noted to be more upbeat, cooperative, pleasant, more open to procedures, and more emotionally open to discuss his medical condition. He started to interact more appropriately with physicians and staff and was more able to talk about death and dying to his parents and family.

CASE TWO

During her second hospital admission for an evaluation of abnormal wheezing, Sarah, a 12-year-old girl, underwent a psychiatric consult. An extensive workup for wheezing, including X-rays, sweat tests, and a computed tomography (CT) scan, all proved negative. The only procedure that helped Sarah not wheeze was lying recumbent. A psychiatric consultation was requested to elucidate any psychiatric factors that might be contributing to Sarah's medical condition. After interviews with Sarah and her parents, the physician found no evidence of depression, hypochondriasis, or any reported anxiety symptoms. During the interview, Sarah described an adult supervisor at recess who had been harassing her on the playground. This harassment consisted of teasing as well as telling other girls not to play with Sarah. The parents had brought this issue to the local school board but had received little assistance. Sarah had made a presentation and written a letter to the school board herself describing this harassment. It was about that time that Sarah's wheezing began. A school consultation was initiated by Sarah's psychiatric consultant. The harassment ended and so did Sarah's wheezing.

CASE THREE

Nancy is a 12-year-old girl with a previous medical history of Burkitts' lymphoma, which was treated approximately three years prior to the consultation and was currently in remission. She came to the children's hospital emergency department (ED) after having a seizure. She was loaded with phenytoin in the ED and became highly agitated and needed restraints. She professed to see airplanes going through her room and stated that she had to follow them, even if it meant jumping out the window to get them. A psychiatric consultation was called to best evaluate where in the hospital this patient should be placed and to help manage her delirium.

CASE FOUR

Amber was a 16-year-old girl who was admitted to the diabetic service in a coma caused by diabetic ketoacidosis. Five days prior to admission she had refused all laboratory tests during a clinic visit when she stated, 'I'm fine and I don't care.' The patient had a long history of noncompliance with her diabetic regimen. A psychiatric consultation was requested to evaluate Amber's noncompliance. During the assessment Amber admitted to being embarrassed by her illness and avoiding social contact. She stated that she slept most of the day, was truant from school, couldn't concentrate, had little energy, and was anhedonic. Although she was not actively suicidal, she was aware that noncompliance could lead to death. A diagnosis of major depression was made, with a recommendation for antidepressant medication and a trial of brief psychotherapy. The patient was agreeable to this plan. Psychotherapy sessions focused on psychoeducation regarding diabetes and its treatment and the impact of illness on her social, academic and family functioning. Cognitive behavioral interventions were employed to address her depressogenic cognitions and promote behavioral activation. Her mood symptoms gradually improved and there was subsequent improvement in her diabetic symptoms.

CASE FIVE

Aseven-year-old hyperactive child had a joint in his toe removed due to osteomyelitis and appeared despondent. The mother refused a psychiatric consultation but agreed to let a third-year medical student pediatric clerk work with the boy. The clerk was supervised on various techniques to engage the child and establish rapport with the mother. On discharge, the mother arranged an appointment with a child psychiatrist.

CASE SIX

Jane is a 15-year-old girl diagnosed as idiopathic pain syndrome fibromyalgia at age 11, readmitted to the pediatric ward for further assessment and recommendations. The presentation at age 11 included abdominal and joint pain, migraines and fever followed thereafter by multiple episodes of joint pain of increasing severity and duration. The current episode of one year includes right leg pain and shakiness, only present upon weight bearing and absent when lying down, leading to a significant walking impairment and a subsequent need to use a walker for assistance. For the last year she has been home schooled. There is a history of multiple failed treatment interventions including medication trials (e.g., analgesics, antidepressants), inpatient and outpatient rehabilitation, homeopathic treatment with acupuncture. A psychiatric consultation was requested to evaluate the underlying psychosocial factors for Jane's presentation and rule out the presence of a depressive condition.

CASE SEVEN

Mark was a six-year-old boy who was admitted to the burn unit after spilling hot water on most of his body. Prior to this hospitalization, Mark was completely toilet trained and was progressing in his development. During his hospitalization on the burn unit, he received numerous procedures and operations, including skin grafts. He became enuretic and encopretic in his bed. A psychiatric consultation was ordered when the patient became encopretic in the middle of the hospital unit.

It became clear throughout the consultative process that the consult was requested by the charge nurse and the nursing staff, for they had to clean up after the child. The consultant worked with the staff to institute a behavioral program to help the child regain control and limit his regression.

CASE EIGHT

A psychiatric resident was called to the ICU to evaluate a schizophrenic teenager who was still psychotic, despite what appeared to be adequate antipsychotic treatment. The patient was being treated for multiple infections and was intermittently in septic shock. On review of the patient's chart, the consultant noticed that the patient's blood cultures revealed that her current antibiotic therapy was inadequate. A recommendation was made that the antibiotics be changed and psychiatric follow-up conducted as needed.

CASE NINE

Anna was an 18-year-old female who had had diabetes mellitus since the age of eight years. She had been repeatedly hospitalized for noncompliance. During the evaluation, the psychiatry resident discovered that the patient had little knowledge and understanding of her illness. During the consultation and therapy sessions, the resident explained in detail about diabetes, insulin, the pancreas, hormones, and other aspects of the illness. The patient began to show more interest in caring for herself after these sessions. She actively sought out the diabetic educator as well as other patients who had diabetes and began to take an active interest in diabetic control.

CASE TEN

Billy was an eight-year-old boy diagnosed with rhabdomyosarcoma of his finger, which required amputation. He did not want to leave the hospital

on discharge, and a psychiatric consultant was called. During the evaluation, it became clear that the patient was fearful of leaving the hospital because he did not know how to hold a baseball bat after his surgery. He was afraid that other kids would make fun of him. The consultant worked with the child and his father, as did physical and occupational therapists, to show Billy how to hold a baseball bat.

References

1. Rauch P. Paediatric consultation. In: Rutter M, Taylor E (eds) *Child and Adolescent Psychiatry*, 4th edn. Blackwell Science, 2002; pp. 1051–1066.
2. Shugart MA. Child psychiatry consultations to pediatric inpatients: A literature review. *Gen Hosp Psychiat* 1991;**13**: 325–336.
3. Campo JV, Kingsley RS, Bridge J, Mrazek D. Child and adolescent psychiatry in general children's hospitals. A survey of chairs of psychiatry. *Psychosomatics* 2000;**41**: 128–133.
4. Steiner H, Fritz GK, Mrazek D, *et al.* Pediatric and psychiatric comorbidity. Part I: The future of consultation-liaison psychiatry. *Psychosomatics* 1993;**34**: 107–111.
5. Pless IB, Roghmann KJ. Chronic illness and its consequences: Observations based on three epidemiologic surveys. *J Pediatr* 1971;**79**:351–359.
6. Cadman D, Boyle M, Szatmari P, *et al.* Chronic illness disability and mental and social well-being. *Pediatrics* 1987;**79**:805–813.
7. Gortmaker SL, Walker DK, Weitzman M, *et al.* Chronic conditions, socioeconomic risks, and behavioral problems in children and adolescents. *Pediatrics* 1990;**85**:267–276.
8. Knapp PK, Harris ES. Consultation-liaison in child psychiatry: a review of the past 10 years. Part I: Clinical findings. *J Am Acad Child Adolesc Psychiat* 1998;**37**: 17–25.
9. Westborn L. Well-being of children with chronic illness: A population-based study in a Swedish primary care district. *Acta Paediatr* 1992;**81**:625.
10. Rutter M, Tizard J, Whitmore K. *Education, Health and Behavior.* New York: Wiley, 1970.
11. Douglas JWB, Blomfield JM. *Children Under 5.* London: Allen & Unwin, 1958.
12. Haggerty RJ, Roghmann KJ, Pless IB. *Child Health and the Community.* New York: Wiley Interscience, 1975.
13. Pless IB, Douglas JWB. Chronic illness in childhood. Part I: Epidemiological and clinical characteristics. *Pediatrics* 1971;**47**:405–414.
14. Thompson RJ, Gustafson KE, Gil KM, Godfrey J, Murphy LM. Illness specific patterns of psychological adjustment and cognitive adaptational processes in children with cystic fibrosis and sickle cell disease. *J Clin Psychol* 1998;**54**:121–128.
15. Burke P, Elliott M. Depression in pediatric chronic illness. A diathesis-stress model. *Psychosomatics* 1999;**40**:5–17.

16. Drell MJ, Hanson White TJ. Children's reaction to illness and hospitalization. In: Sadock B, Sadock V (eds) *Kaplan & Sadock's Comprehensive Textbook of Psychiatry*, 7th edn.Lippincott Williams &Wilkins, 2000; pp. 2889–2897.

17. Suris JC, Parera N, Puig C. Chronic illness and emotional distress in adolescence. *J Adolesc Health* 1996;**19**:153–156.

18. Meijer SA, Sinnema G, Bijstra JO, Mellenbergh GJ, Wolters WHG. Coping styles and locus of control as predictors for psychological adjustment of adolescents with a chronic illness. *Soc Sci Med* 2002;**54**:1453–1461.

19. Huurre TM, Aro HM. Long-term psychosocial effects of persistent chronic illness. A follow-up study of Finnish adolescents aged 16 to 32 years. *Eur Child Adolesc Psychiat* 2002;**11**:85–91.

20. Mrazek DA. Psychiatric aspects of somatic disease and disorders. In: Rutter M, Taylor E, Hersov L (eds) *Child and Adolescent Psychiatry: Modern Approaches*. London: Blackwell Scientific Publications, 1994; pp. 697–710.

21. Jellinek MS, Murphy M. Use of the Pediatric Symptom Checklist in outpatient practice. In: Jellinek MS (ed.) *Current Problems in Pediatrics: Psychosocial Aspects of Ambulatory Pediatrics*. Littleton, MA: Mosby-Year Book, 1990; pp. 602–609.

22. Jones RN, Latkowski ME, Green DM, *et al*. Psychosocial assessment in the general pediatric population: A multiple-gated screening and identification procedure. *J Pediatr Health Care* 1996;**10**:10–16.

23. Lewis M. The consultation process in child and adolescent psychiatric consultation-liaison in pediatrics. In: Lewis M (ed.) *Child and Adolescent Psychiatry: A Comprehensive Textbook*. Baltimore, MD: Williams & Wilkins, 1996; pp. 935–939.

24. Jellinek MS, Herzog DB, Selter LF. A psychiatric consultation service for hospitalized children. *Psychosomatics* 1987;**22**:29–33.

25. Slater JA. Deciphering emotional aches and physical pains in children. *Pediatrics Annals* 2003;**32**:402–407.

26. Slater JA. Psychiatric issues in pediatric bone marrow, stem cell, and solid organ transplantation. In: Lewis M (ed.) *Child and Adolescent Psychiatry: A Comprehensive Textbook*, 3rd edn.Philadelphia: Lippincott Williams & Wilkins, 2002; pp. 1147–1174.

27. Granger RH, Stone EL. Collaboration between child psychiatrists and pediatricians in practice. In: Lewis M (ed.) *Child and Adolescent Psychiatry: A Comprehensive Textbook*. Baltimore, MD: Williams & Wilkins, 1996; pp. 940–943.

28. Fritz GK, Bergman AS. Child psychiatrists seen through pediatricians' eyes: Results of a national survey. *J Am Acad Child Adolesc Psychiat* 1985;**24**:81.

29. Slater JA. The medically ill child or adolescent. In Scahill L, Martin A (eds) *Textbook of Pediatric Psychopharmacology*. New York: Oxford University Press, 2003; pp. 631–641.

30. Milousheva J, Kobayashi N, Matsui I. Psychosocial problems of children and adolescents with a chronic disease: Coping strategies. *Acta Paediatr* 1996;**38**:41–45.

31. Ryan-Wenger NA. Children, coping, and the stress of illness: A synthesis of the research. *J Soc Pediatr Nurs* 1996;**1**:126–138.

32. Krener PKG, Wasserman AL. Diagnostic dilemmas in pediatric consultation. *Child Adolesc Psychiatr Clin North Am* 1994;**3**:485–512.

33. Stuber ML. Psychiatric sequelae in seriously ill children and their families. *Psychiatr Clin North Am* 1996;**19**: 481–493.

34. Rubinstein B. Psychological factors influencing medical conditions. In: Kestenbaum CJ, Williams DT (eds) *Handbook of Clinical Assessment of Children and Adolescents*. New York: New York University Press, 1988; pp. 771–799.

35. American Academy of Pediatrics, Medical Home Initiatives for Children with Special Needs Project Advisory Committee. The medical home. *Pediatrics* 2002;**110**:184–186.

36. American Academy of Pediatrics, Committee on Psychosocial Aspects of Child and Family Health. Incorporating recognition and management of perinatal and postpartum depression into pediatric Practice. *Pediatrics* 2010;**126**: 1032–1039.

37. American Academy of Child and Adolescent Psychiatry, Committee on Collaboration with Medical Professionals. *A Guide to Building Collaborative Mental Health Care Partnerships in Pediatric Primary Care*. Washington, DC: AACAP, 2010.

38. Healthy Steps for Young Children (www.healthysteps. org).

39. Triple P (www.triplep.net).

40. The Incredible Years (www.incredibleyears.com).

41. Eyberg SM. Parent-child interaction therapy: Integration of traditional and behavioral concerns. *Child Fam Behav Ther* 1988;**10**:33–46.

42. The Zero to Three Institute promotes a useful model of reflective supervision. See Parlakian R. *Look, Listen, and Learn: Reflective Supervision and Relationship–Based Work*. Washington, DC: Zero to Three, 2001.

43. First Signs (www.firstsigns.org).

44. American Academy of Pediatrics District II, New York State Task Force on Health Care for Children in Foster Care. *Fostering Health: Health Care for Children and Adolescents in Foster Care*. Elk Grove, IL: American Academy of Pediatrics, 2005.

45. American Academy of Pediatrics, Committee on Early Childhood, Adoption and Dependent Care. Developmental issues for young children in foster care. *Pediatrics* 2000;**106**:1145–1150.

46. American Academy of Child and Adolescent Psychiatry Policy Statement. *Psychiatric Care of Children in the Foster Care System*. Washington, DC: AACAP, 2001.

47. Zero to Three. Court teams for maltreated infants and toddlers (http://www.zerotothree.org/about-us/funded-projects/court-teams/) [for a description of and resources for court team projects].

6

How to Plan and Tailor Treatment: An Overview of Diagnosis and Treatment Planning

Brian J. McConville, Sergio V. Delgado

The purpose of this chapter is not to describe the process of clinical evaluation of the child, adolescent, or family, since this was covered in Chapter 1. Rather, it is to address the increasing imperative in child and adolescent psychiatry to form a coherent diagnostic and initial treatment plan for a child, adolescent, or family, and to do it in such a way that this plan will be logical and agreed on by the consumers of mental healthcare – including the insurers. It is also important to be flexible, so as to alter treatment approaches with evolving clinical realities. As in the rest of medicine, evidence-based guidelines increasingly apply to child and adolescent psychiatry [1]. The precision of psychiatric assessment measures is comparable to that of physical diagnoses, and the overall results of treatment in child and adolescent psychiatry, especially for the Axis I diagnoses, are comparable to those in adult psychiatry [2]. The American Academy of Child and Adolescent Psychiatry has developed practice parameters, which continue to evolve in tandem with research [3–5]. This degree of precision is particularly true with pediatric pharmacotherapy, where the results for treatment of attention-deficit hyperactivity disorder (ADHD), obsessive-compulsive disorder (OCD), bipolar disorder, depressive disorder, and other conditions are extremely promising [6–9]. Equally promising results occur for pediatric psychotherapy research [10].

In the following sections, general principles of diagnosis and modes of therapy will be summarized, leading to schemata about how to select and alter modes of therapy as needed. Following this, brief descriptions of the different therapies will be given. Finally, combinations of therapies will be discussed, and clinical vignettes will be given.

Models of Diagnostic Classification

There are three common models for classifying disorders: *categorical*, *dimensional*, and *ideographic* [11]. This distinction is important because it is tempting to believe that the ordinary method of classification used, the clinical-categorical approach, is the only feasible one.

The categorical approach, which is similar to the general medical model of classification, is dichotomous in that it views a particular disorder as either present or absent. Comorbidity of diagnoses is not always assumed, even though this is common [12]. This approach implies that cases of a particular disorder show certain characteristic symptoms, which in turn suggests an underlying pathophysiology, or cause of disorder and treatment. But even in such systems as the *Diagnostic and Statistical Manual of Mental Disorders*, Fourth Edition, Text Revision (DSM-IV-TR) [13] or the still-evolving (in the United States) *International Classification of Diseases* (ICD-10) [14, 15], this approach is not always followed. Some disorders, such as depressive disorders, require cardinal features such as anhedonia, dysphoria, or irritability as cardinal symptoms, as well as a number of other symptoms for full diagnosis. In other disorders, such as ADHD, six of nine symptoms of inattention or hyperactivity/impulsivity or a combination of both allow for the diagnosis. Hence, disorders are diagnosed on the "Chinese menu" style of diagnosis, rather than with a strictly convergent system where a given number of symptoms always indicates a particular diagnosis [16].

The most commonly used pattern of categorical diagnosis in child psychiatry in North America is the DSM-IV-TR [13]. This consists of a number of axes:

Clinical Child Psychiatry, Third Edition. Edited by William M. Klykylo and Jerald Kay.
© 2012 John Wiley & Sons, Ltd. Published 2012 by John Wiley & Sons, Ltd.

- Axis I: Major clinical diagnoses
- Axis II: Developmental disorders and personality disorders
- Axis III: Physical disorders
- Axis IV: Psychosocial stressors
- Axis V: Global assessment of functioning

This concept of careful consideration of individual symptoms of particular disorders, often based on clinical categorical diagnostic categories, and often using multiple informants as well as inter-rater reliability, is now widely used in child and adolescent clinical psychiatry research, using such well-validated instruments as the KIDDIE-SADS Interview [17] and the Diagnostic Interview for Children and Adolescents (DICA) [18].

In addition, a number of recent rating systems also use this concept for particular disorders, as in the Children's Yale–Brown Obsessive-Compulsive Scale (C-YBOCS) [19], the Children's Depression Rating Scale [20], and the Young Mania Rating Scale [21], which measure the number and nature of particular symptoms of a disorder, but then use the degree of functional impairment in particular, and summed symptoms as an important component.

More recently, diagnostic systems have attempted to avoid theoretical or etiological considerations [11] and instead have widely used the phenomenological approach that operated in the original definition of Research Diagnostic Criteria [22]. Even under these conventions, however, disorders such as post-traumatic stress disorder or reactive attachment disorder of childhood clearly imply etiology. It does not necessarily follow that the disease concept is the most useful one to employ. An approach favoring an extension of the DSM-IV Axis V and stressing functional impairment, may at times be more generally useful [23], as in patients with mental retardation or autism.

In contrast, the *dimensional* or *multivariate statistical system*, such as that used in the Child Behavior Checklist of Achenbach and colleagues [24], uses the convention that symptom groups indicate the universe of behaviors in a given population. These symptom groups are selected from a fixed group of behavioral symptoms derived from factor analysis and varying with age and sex. Those cases that occur above a given cutoff point (usually the 98th percentile) are abnormal. Individual symptoms and particular "narrow band" syndromes may therefore occur or disappear at different ages and also differ between sexes. Comorbidity is a usual part of the diagnostic process, and rarer disorders such as autism do not emerge in the usual analyses of normative or clinical populations. In addition, using the list of symptoms found at the predetermined cutoff point

for abnormality may predetermine the frequency of the disorder (J. Anderson, personal communication, 1995). This system has been widely used in epidemiological studies, including international studies in which the general nature of the questions tends to minimize cultural differences in syndrome expressivity [25, 26].

A third system, *ideographic diagnosis*, uses an approach that focuses on the totality of the individual child's life and circumstances and avoids simple descriptive labels. Despite the seeming inherent validity of this approach, the lack of labels makes it difficult for clinicians to communicate with each other regarding such studies of unique individuals. Moreover, proponents of this approach usually operate from some theoretical framework that slants their clinical approach, as in psychoanalytic, behavioral, family, sociologic, or psychopharmacological viewpoints.

Other diagnostic systems can be used, including psychodynamic diagnosis. This has been proposed in the past for inclusion in the DSM system of classification, and family diagnosis [27]. The psychodynamic diagnosis approach has been implicit in a number of systems, such as that espoused by Freud [28] and by Nagera [29]. A later *Psychodynamic Diagnostic Manual* begins with the description of healthy mental functioning, involving cognitive, emotional, and behavioral patterns, on the basis that mental health comprises more than simply the absence of symptoms [30]. In the child and adolescent section, psychodynamic understandings are based on seven categories of mental functioning unique to each age: regulation, attention, and learning; affective experience of others; defensive patterns; internal representations; capacity for differentiation and integration; self-observing capacities; and internalizing standards and ideals.

Other Considerations in Child Psychiatric Diagnosis

A further aspect is to consider the question of what is being classified. Cantwell noted that diagnoses classified disorders, but not individual children [31]. Diagnosis refers to a process of assigning a label to a particular problem or a group of problems to allow for greater precision about treatment, prognosis, and possible etiology. But the diagnosis given to a child may vary from time to time, or be relatively fixed, depending on whether the disorder is an adjustment to some external stressor or a more internalized disorder following prolongation of a particular stressor, or the emergence of other internal and probably neuropathological factors, as in schizophrenia.

In contrast to adult psychiatry, where the opinions of various informants about a person's degree of impairment are often overlooked, child and adolescent diagnosis implies the gathering of information not only from the child but also from parents, teachers, and others. One of the earliest studies in this area, Rutter's Isle of Wight Epidemiologic Study [32], focused on the number of behavior problems shown in children in a particular village, as determined by different informants. When a group of village members was asked to name those children who had the most problems, the group of children selected showed a high degree of reliability among informants. Similarly, when the children's teachers were asked to name their problematic children, they replied with a high degree of inter-rater reliability about their chosen group. All the children came from the same pool of children in the village; however, there was little overlap between the two groups selected by village members and teachers, respectively. There was not only a difference in perceived behavior between informants, but also a difference in particular situations (as in school and home).

There are also times when the existence of problems relates more to "goodness of fit" between parents and the infant rather than to a uniformly recognized disorder in the child [33]. The child's and the parents' temperamental characteristics may interact negatively. In 1960, Kanner commented that behaviors thought of as disturbing by one set of parents were not necessarily thought of similarly by other parents; he made a distinction between the "disturbing" and the "disturbed" child [34]. The work of Werner and Smith showed that the prognosis of children with behavior disorders was dependent both on parenting techniques and social support [35]. LaRoche indicated that children of parents who were depressed were particularly at risk of perceiving their children as having behavioral problems, and that those parents who had violent and abusive parents were in turn likely to be abusive [36].

Diagnosis in children, therefore, relates largely to the issue of social context and also to factors of tolerance, parenting skills, temperament, and economic disadvantage [37]. There are also reasons to believe that cultural factors may determine what is seen as problematic in children.

Patterns of Child and Adolescent Psychotherapy

In child and adolescent psychotherapy, the basic patterns of psychodynamic psychotherapy, as Kay indicated in his clinical synthesis, are also true [38]. It is also possible to integrate increasing awareness of thoughts and feelings while supporting ego functions in a supportive expressive continuum [39]. But there has also been a significant addition of other psychotherapies,

along with an emphasis on evidence-based practice based on effect sizes in particular diagnoses including use of medications, cognitive behavior therapy (CBT), interpersonal psychotherapy (IPT), short-term psychotherapy (STPP), and behavioral activation and emotion-focused therapy [40]. For personality disorders in older children with borderline personality disorder, dialectical behavior therapy (DPT), which includes techniques from CBT and mindfulness, has been useful [41], as has attachment-based family therapy (ABFT), a family-based therapy that addresses these issues [42]. With the rapid evolution of more disorder-, family-,and community-directed approaches, there is a need for formal training in more disorder-directed types of therapy, especially those directed toward specific diagnoses (such as affective disorders or OCD), or specific family and social situations and modes of community intervention. Psychopharmacological and psychotherapeutic approaches are often used together, and need to be so, since pharmacotherapy aims to reduce or suppress problematic symptoms, and does not directly lead to new behavior.

The usefulness of such combination approaches has been recently demonstrated in the MTA study of the combination of behavior therapy and psychostimulants [43], and even more so in the TADS study for CBT and antidepressants for child and adolescent depression; here the combination showed clear improvement over the use of either medication or CBT alone [44]. However, the lack of clear separation between those treated with antidepressant medication and those on placebo, as well as the inadequate capture of initial and/or emerging suicidality during these studies, has led in part to recent concerns about the use of antidepressants and suicidality in children and adolescents [45, 46]. There is an emerging consensus about the need to combine pharmacotherapy and psychotherapy, and a need for collaboration between the pharmacotherapist and the psychotherapist, who should work closely together. Ideally these should be contained in the same person, since otherwise it is very difficult for either therapist to know what the other is doing [47].

Commonly Described Forms of Psychotherapy

The following sections expand on the most commonly described forms of psychotherapy, including pharmacotherapy. Basic underlying concepts in each form of therapy will be outlined; and it will be noted that there are frequently a number of different strategies and even schools of thought in each general form of therapy. Usually, these concepts and strategies overlap with those described above under the general model, although the jargon associated may be different. The primacy of a particular approach may at times be vehemently defended by its proponents, and lively and at times entertaining feuds may occur between disciples of different forms or sub-forms of therapy. But the important clinical fact remaining is the utility of a particular approach or strategy combination for the child at any time.

Child and Adolescent Psychopharmacotherapy

Recently, there has been a rapid evolution in the psychopharmacotherapy of children and adolescents, as Green has noted [48]. Given the recent changing patterns of psychiatric practice, there is now great emphasis on this mode of therapy.

The ordinary purpose of pharmacotherapy is to reduce the severity of target symptoms that are selected following the process of diagnosis. Maturational and developmental issues may influence physiologic, cognitive, psychological, and experiential factors. The provision of pharmacotherapy is part of an overall treatment plan that includes other diagnostic formulations as well as the involvement of the family. Compliance with medication is an issue of particular importance.

Each medication and its effects need to be explained fully to the child and adolescent. Because of medicolegal aspects, the adult or guardian also needs to understand the medication and its effects. In addition, several issues concerning informed consent will require discussion. There may be unknown risks when taking medication, especially when novel psychopharmacological treatments are used or when the risks versus benefits are uncertain. Since some medications are not specifically designated by the Food and Drug Administration (FDA) as being safe or effective for children, many are used in an off-label (non-FDA-approved) fashion. In all cases, however, the use of such medication should be consistent with ordinary clinical practice, and there should be some notation in the chart that the available literature has been studied.

Medication should continue to be monitored using the appropriate physical examination and laboratory tests and procedures, such as complete blood count with differential, urinalysis, liver, renal, and thyroid profiles, and electrocardiograms (ECGs) and electroencephalograms (EEGs) as required. Baseline clinical observations may include standard rating scales such as the Conners Parent/Teacher Scale and the Abnormal Involuntary Movement Scale. And because of recent concerns about antipsychotic weight gain, leading to predictable increases in insulin resistance, and risk for hyperglycemia, hypertension, dyslipidemias, and cardiovascular

disease, monitoring guidelines have recently been issued. These include personal/family history, weight, waist circumference, blood pressure, and fasting glucose and lipid profiles during antipsychotic therapy [49].

In this age of cost-consciousness, the clinician will often be required to distinguish between generic and brand-name preparations. In general, it is probably wise to start off with the brand name and then see whether the patient can be switched to a generic preparation without loss of effect or the development of unknown side effects due to the congeners found in some generic preparations.

Since some children may require more than one drug, they may experience significant drug interactions, particularly interactions involving the cytochrome P450 isoenzyme systems [50]. The drug dosage varies with age, with younger children often requiring larger doses proportional to age. Pharmacokinetics and pharmacodynamics (the interactions of one drug with another) are seldom fully studied in children, and much additional research is needed in this area [51]. Some drugs and/or their metabolites require monitoring, particularly those drugs used for bipolar disorders, such as lithium, valproic acid, and carbamazepine. Blood methylphenidate levels are not clearly related to clinical response.

Other than for finite problems, it is customary to continue psychotropic medication for a considerable time, with periodic withdrawal and tapering of medications to determine if it is possible for the child or adolescent to discontinue such medications. In the case of methylphenidate or other psychostimulants, cessation during the weekends or summer is important because of possible adverse effects on growth and height. In disorders such as bipolar disorder and schizophrenia, however, it may be difficult to reduce the dosage of medication, especially in those medications that require an adequate blood level. When drugs are withdrawn or tapered, withdrawal effects may occur.

In summary, pharmacotherapeutic agents are essentially suppressive, in that they reduce unwarranted symptoms or behaviors but by themselves may also allow for the development of new behavior, as in the results following reduced distress following treatment for OCD.

The Verbal Psychotherapies

Verbal psychotherapy, in contrast to pharmacotherapy, usually aims to change behavioral maladaptive patterns and may allow for longer-term remissions than pharmacotherapy, in which stopping medication usually results in the return of symptoms. This section outlines the more common child and adolescent psychotherapies.

Psychodynamic Psychotherapy

As noted, child and adolescent psychotherapy has tended to focus on intensive individual psychodynamic psychotherapy [52]. The approach is to form a trusting relationship between the therapist and the patient and to allow the verbal expression of feelings with increasing self-knowledge and self-mastery [53]. Formation of the therapeutic alliance is fundamental, especially in the initial phase when children are told that they will have a series of times set aside to begin to understand their problems. Children may indicate particular problems through play and with defensive structures. Following the initial phase, the therapist moves into the middle phase of psychotherapy, whose goals are to work through problems and also interpret the transference by which conflicts and associated symptoms experienced by the child are passed on to the therapist. As Delgado pointed out, the normal dependent development of the child throughout therapy may modify the transference [53].

Linking the child's behaviors with fantasies may be helpful, especially in the context of a personal myth held by the child. This myth may be used to link current and earlier behavior and to help uncover defenses. During the interpretative process, the therapist may place observations in the context of what has previously taken place or what is happening during the relationship between the child and the therapist. This process models that of the observing ego initially in the adult therapist, and then in the child. In the case of child therapy, this needs to be spelled out in a relatively concrete way, given the child's relative inability to abstract [54]. The process of working through requires a sustained therapeutic effect, since repetitive defensive conflicts will remain relatively unchanged unless the affects contained by such conflicts are able to be expressed. There is often a process of mourning when letting go of worked-through material, and also during the subsequent formation of alternate modes of coping. The process of gaining insight gradually leads to change of thought and behavior.

During the termination phase, the goals of therapy are to reduce anxiety, increase frustration tolerance, and improve relationships and the capacity for pleasure. The termination phase often brings up issues of separation and loss, relating both to previous experiences and the loss of the therapist.

Play is a frequent feature of psychodynamic psychotherapy [55]. Anna Freud [56] and Melanie Klein [57] initially provided principles for the use of play in child therapy as well as the understanding that play had unconscious meaning. Winnicott [58] expanded these concepts, using play as an intermediate or transitional object between fantasy and reality. Currently the techniques in psychodynamic psychotherapy are modified to meet the developmental needs of the child and there is active involvement of the parents in the process. Other aspects of play therapy include the mastery of conflictual situations, with the therapist suggesting alterations in repetitive or nonproductive play sequences, even in children with ADHD [59]. Alternatively, the therapist may remain an observer, while the child seeks his or her own solutions. Coppolillo indicated the powerful effects of play therapy, including the child's immersion into play and how possible affects are offset by the reality of the therapist's presence and his or her capacity to tolerate the child's impulses [55].

The effectiveness of psychodynamic therapy is unclear, since most therapies are used by individual clinicians. Weiss and Weisz [60] and Weisz and colleagues [61] indicated that psychodynamic therapies hadless measured therapeutic effect than behavioral treatments. On the other hand Fonagy and Target found that of children with disruptive behavior who remained in psychodynamic psychotherapy for more than a year "69% were no longer diagnosable on termination" [62].

Behavior Therapy

As described by Wolpe and Plaud [63] behavior therapy originated from the well-known experiments of Pavlov, who found that when an unconditioned stimulus appeared repeatedly with a previously neutral stimulus, this neutral stimulus would eventually elicit a conditioned response that resembled the unconditioned reflex [64]. For example, Pavlov's dogs, who initially salivated at the presentation of food, eventually salivated at the sound of a bell. Similarly in humans, a young boy named Albert heard a loud noise when he began to play with a rat and subsequently became fearful of the rat and other "furry animals," illustrating stimulus generalization [65]. A more flexible pattern of conditioning identified by Skinner as operant conditioning involved behaviors that could be modified or maintained by their consequences [66]. Behavior followed by pleasant consequences was likely to increase in frequency, whereas that followed by unpleasant consequences was likely to decrease.

A third development was cognitive behavior therapy, which has been widely used in both adult and child psychiatry [67]. The basic assumption is that cognitive processes, including expectations, beliefs, or attributions, influence behavior and affect. Irrational and faulty cognitive processes foster maladaptive behaviors, which can be reversed by modification of this cognition.

The cognitive behavioral approach is therefore less concerned with the influence of affect. In contrast, social learning theory, developed by Bandura, includes observational learning, in which behaviors change as a result of observing a model [68]. A child who views another child being rewarded for a particular behavior is more likely to perform similar behavior. Hence, the child is able to effect change by himself or herself.

Concepts that arise from observed behaviors rather than subjective experiences should indicate the success of the therapy, and all treatment techniques should be based on clinical applied science. Other individuals in the child's environment should be enlisted in the treatment of the child.

Behavior Therapy Techniques Particularly Used for Disruptive Behavior Disorders There are several terms used in the behavioral literature, many of which refer to the treatment of disruptive behavior disorders. General techniques of behavior therapy include *reinforcement*, in which behavior is strengthened by its consequences, as in *operant conditioning*. In *positive reinforcement* the reward is presented after the occurrence of a desired behavior, and in *negative reinforcement* the reward involves the removal of an aversive stimulus after the desired behavior happens. *Continuous reinforcements* are administered each time a response occurs, in contrast to *intermittent reinforcement*: in a *fixed interval* schedule, a child is reinforced after a specific time period regardless of the response, whereas in a *variable interval* schedule, the rate of reinforcement varies randomly. A *fixed ratio* technique administers reinforcement after a specific number of the child's responses, whereas a *variable ratio* technique reinforces randomly around a specific average of desired responses by the child. Intermittent reinforcement responses may be difficult to change; compulsive gambling, for example, indicates how intermittent reinforcement can lead to high rates of response. Parents who are inconsistent and variable in their responses to a child may reinforce the behaviors they wish to extinguish.

Other techniques include reinforcing a particular response in the presence of one stimulus but not in the presence of another. Common examples include *shaping,* in which closer and closer approximations of behavior produce a final desired behavior. In this approach, rewarding and reinforcing initially occur for small changes of behavior, and as the behavior becomes closer to the goal, the rewards continue but the tasks and standards of behavior become more stringent. In contrast, *fading* involves changing a stimulus so that a new stimulus eventually produces the same response. *Chaining* involves reinforcing more and more links to produce a complex chain of behavior, as in teaching an autistic child the sequence of dressing. *Contracting* is primarily used to increase specific behaviors or eliminate unwanted behavior. Contracts for particular patterns of performance commonly involve sequences about what the child and the parents should do. They are used especially with adolescents and have the advantage of *distancing*: the contract involves a relatively neutral, agreed-on interchange that is distinct from high-level arguing. Finally, *modeling* is clearly indicated in many parent–child or other adult–child interactions at home or at school.

Several suppressive techniques in behavior therapy are used to reduce or eliminate behavior; some of these techniques have achieved a degree of notoriety [69]. For example, the use of massive negative stimuli such as cattle prods to change the behavior of autistic children gave rise to justifiable concern. More generally, *extinction* occurs when reinforcement is withheld after an offered response in order to reduce the frequency of this response. For example, parents may be taught to respond to a child's crying at night by not going into the room immediately and to progressively increase the length of time before they go in. A similar response is that of *differential reinforcement*, in which reinforcement is given for nonoccurrence or low rates of occurrence of a problem behavior, such as hitting teachers or other children.

Punishment such as scolding, spanking, or removing privileges is used to reduce undesirable behavior through the introduction of an aversive stimulus or the removal of a positive stimulus. Punishment is able to elicit a rapid decrease in problem behaviors and may be useful for some self-injurious or aggressive behaviors. The behaviors usually change only temporarily, however, and may be associated with fear or escape responses, or even by reinforcement due to the negative attention the child receives during punishment (as distinct from the lack of attention otherwise received from the parent). The behavior may simply be displaced. Parental commands such as "Don't let me see you hit your sister" may lead to the child hitting his or her sister somewhere else; the parent who punishes may in turn model aggressive physical or verbal behavior as well as a lack of respect for the rights of others. Children who are physically aggressive have often seen such behavior modeled by others; similarly, those who have been severely beaten will frequently continue this behavior as they grow older.

Punishment procedures that appear to be effective include *time-out*, in which the child is removed from the setting where the behavior occurred and is placed in a restrictive environment such as his or her room for a brief period, and *response cost,* in which a reinforcer is removed because of misbehavior. In the latter case, a child may have privileges such as the use of a television or telephone temporarily removed, with the opportunity to earn back these privileges. In *over-correction,* the child may be required to negate the effects of his or her actions, for example in cleaning crayon off the walls or contributing toward the cost of repairing damage in the house. Alternatively, the child may be required to practice *positive behavior incompatible with misbehavior*; for example, a child who leaves his or her books around in a messy fashion may be required to line up the books in a particularly neat fashion.

Conduct disorder and antisocial behavior may be approached by *problem-solving skills training* (PSST) or *behavioral parent training* [70]. Kazdin and colleagues showed that a combined approach of PSST and parent training is effective in treating antisocial behavior in children [71]. Those children who respond best, however, may have more internal motivation and more motivated parents.

Behavior therapy for ADHD has been shown to enhance learning and improve academic performance, although the usefulness of such techniques in the absence of psychostimulant medication is still a matter of discussion [72]. This issue has been clarified by results of the National Institute of Mental Health multimodality treatment study of children with ADHD [73]. In this large study, subjects were randomly assigned to one of three manually based protocols – medication only, psychosocial therapy only, or combined medication and psychosocial therapy – versus a community standard treatment.

Other areas for behavioral techniques include pervasive developmental disorders, autism, and mental retardation, all of which focus on suppressing unwanted behaviors and teaching new skills [74,75]. Behavioral approaches have also been used for enuresis and encopresis. The "bell and pad treatment" for enuresis has been in use since its description in 1938 by Mowrer and Mowrer [76]. This technique is effective in 75–80% of cases but also has a relapse rate of about 40%. The dry-bed training technique of Azrin and colleagues incorporates several behavioral techniques, including positive practice, reinforcement, punishment, and the urine alarm and thus may be more effective than the urine alarm only [77]. Behavior therapy for functional encopresis uses positive conditioned reinforcement and/or regular checks toward full cleanliness. Laxatives or suppositories are often used as adjuncts.

Behavior Therapy Techniques Particularly Used for Internalizing Disorders Desensitization has been widely `used to reduce children's fears, as in the gradual exposure of a child to a conditioned stimulus such as separation, test-taking, or frightening animals [78]. An extension of this technique is *participant modeling,* in which a parent models a lack of fear of a particular animal, for example, and the child is then able to follow this behavior. In *systematic desensitization,* the child works with the therapist to establish a hierarchy of fears about anxiety-provoking stimuli; these stimuli are then provided during therapy from the least to the most anxiety producing. This may be done either in imagination or *in vivo,* as in taking a child to school who has school phobia. *Flooding* or *implosion therapy* involves having the child come into contact with the most feared item in the hierarchy. It has been found useful for children not responding favorably to gradual desensitization, but its general use is discouraged because it is often anxiety producing and may be used as a punishment technique.

Other behavioral therapies for anxiety or depression that stress a more cognitive approach include *cognitive behavior therapy* (CBT) and *interpersonal therapy.* As Petti has noted [79], in the former therapy, cognitive distortions or errors in reasoning such as those noted by Beck and colleagues [80] and Kovacs and Beck [81] include arbitrary inferences, selective abstraction (details taken out of context), personalization (being blamed for particular events), and dichotomous thinking (which does not allow for intermediate positions).

Therapists using such cognitive techniques explore the basis for faulty assumptions and teach alternate coping skills such as assigning measures of probability and reassigning attribution. In contrast, cognitive behavioral techniques help patients test their dysfunctional cognitions and change their behavior by using homework assignments or time structuring, increasing specific activities, or carrying out exercises related to specific situations. Some studies have described the successful use of cognitive therapy in adolescents with issues such as depression and distorted perceptions regarding appearance, sexuality, and competency [82,83].

Challenging assumptions may be difficult with children, and Leahy has suggested using a dichotomy such as "the bad thoughts monster" and "the smart thoughts man" [84].

A variant of the cognitive approach, which has been particularly used for depression, is interpersonal therapy, as described by Moreau and colleagues [85]. In contrast to the more cognitive style of therapy for depression, interpersonal psychotherapy emphasizes particular emotional and cognitive situations that exist between the patient and stressful circumstances or persons. By going through these areas, it is possible for the patient not only to recognize how certain situations may provoke depression but also to work on alternate strategies. Behavior therapy has been used for child and adolescent depression, dealing with poor self-esteem, social isolation, and hopelessness, and self-control training has demonstrated efficacy in treating depression in children and adolescents. As noted, it has also been shown to be effective in a recent study by March and colleagues of depression treated using the combination of fluoxetine and CBT, where again the combination was more effective than either individually, but the CBT had a more robust effect [86]. OCD has been shown by March and colleagues to be responsive to *exposure and response prevention* techniques [87]. This technique, combined with medication to offset the more severe forms of OCD, has been shown to be particularly effective and often utilizes manuals that lead to a more rational CBT approach.

In contrast to the above cognitive approaches, *rational emotive therapy* emphasizes an active dispute with the patient concerning fundamental dysfunctional thoughts and teaches the evaluation of actions [88]. Waters used rational emotive therapy for disturbed youth and focused on cognitions and the identification of sources causing specific problems [89]. Goals for young children are to identify emotions, distinguish thoughts from feelings, be alert to self-talk, connect self-talk and feelings, and develop rational coping statements. There is a possibility of confrontation in this technique, which may cause concern.

Interpersonal cognitive problem solving, which Shure and Spivack found effective with pupils in poor urban preschools, is conducted by teachers and stresses alternate solution thinking as well as means-end thinking, which in turn leads to better interpersonal adjustment and less psychopathology [90]. *Self-management skills* in cognitive therapy include self-regulation for some phobias and self-instructional training; the latter may be particularly useful for children with concrete thinking or learning problems and either low to average intelligence or retardation [91, 92].

In summary, the various behavior therapies presented have been found to be particularly useful for treating internalizing disorders.

Adlerian Psychotherapy

Although not generally described in many compendia of therapy, the Adlerian or NeoAdlerian approach described by Dinkmeyer and McKay is often extremely useful, especially with intelligent verbal children with oppositional defiant disorder whose parents are also intelligent and verbal [93]. The "goals of misbehavior" as defined in this form of therapy include: (i) requiring attention in which children only feel they belong when they are being noticed or served; (ii) power, in which children feel that they belong only when in control; and (iii) revenge, in which children feel that hurting others is necessary because they cannot be loved. Displays of inadequacy also convince others not to expect anything from the child. In contrast, the goals of positive behavior include involvement and contribution, feelings of power and autonomy, feelings of justice and fairness, and feeling the opportunity to withdraw from conflict (it is not necessary to fight all battles!).

These points are described in the manual on *Systematic Training for Effective Parenting* [93]. In contrast to behavior therapy, which emphasizes doing things to or with the child, Adlerian therapy aims to give the child as much power as possible, including allowing the child to make choices. These choices are often demarcated by the parent, as in "You have a choice – to stop hitting your brother or to go to your room," but are nonetheless choices. If the child cannot make a decision, then the parent has the option of taking over and making the decision for the child. The child is told, however, that the parent is willing to hand back the decision to the child as soon as the child is capable of doing this. The general phraseology is, "I see that you are unable to choose how to sort out your problem. I will take care of your problem, but then I will solve it my way. You may have your problem back at any time when you are able to solve it."

It is important for the parents to give directions as neutrally as possible, and for the therapist to reinforce this. Usually a prior group program of parent training is useful. A somewhat counterintuitive approach is that when a child is being aggressive or oppositional, parents should be free to remove themselves from the scene, on the basis that quarreling cannot occur in the absence, of one of the two parties.

Family and Group Therapies

Family therapy focuses on treating the family as the defined unit for therapy: problems evolve from the family structure and history, and although the child or adolescent may be the "identified patient," the basic problems rest within the family. This approach therefore stresses interactional components, although Sholevar has noted [94, 95] that earlier patterns of family therapy stressed psychoanalytic principles. Minuchin developed structural family therapy based on working with multiproblem families from low socioeconomic groups [96]. Earlier systemic approaches to family therapy were based on general systems theory, including the concept of cybernetics, which held that families tend to maintain equilibrium: a tension always exists between homeostasis and change, balancing stability and self-preservation with change and adaptation. Strategic and structural family therapy arose from this theory and focused on observable as well as reported family behavior. Structural family therapy requires that dysfunctional family structures are observed when the family is in action and allows for active suggestions for change. Strategic family therapy primarily emphasizes deciphering the family communication rules that underlie problems, leading to planned strategies for change and greater emphasis on cognition.

Other schools of family therapy include behavioral approaches such as the parent behavioral training model for family therapy described by Griest and Wells [97]. Another behavioral approach is functional family therapy, in which maladaptive behavior evolving from the family context becomes more interpersonally adaptive [98]. Further forms of family therapy include extended family therapy and object relations family therapy; the former obviously relates to extended family and social networks, and the latter returns to the psychoanalytic roots of family therapy, in which internal psychological development occurs in relation to significant caretakers.

There are a number of schools of family therapy, whose basic components are often associated with particular therapists who in turn tend to have their own disciples. The style of family therapy used is frequently overly dependent on the practitioner's schooling. Alternatively, family therapists may eschew labels for an "eclectic" approach; frequently, however, the therapist functions flexibly with patients but then has difficulty defining what he or she is doing.

Family diagnosis as such is not a major feature of family therapy, although a number of clinicians, including Epstein and colleagues [99], have advanced concepts for family therapy diagnosis. Other "diagnostic" models and typologies include the systems model of family competence and adaptability versus family interaction styles versus the Olson circumplex model, which measures dimensions of family behavior such as cohesion, adaptability, and communication [100]. Combrinck-Graham described families in a more developmental fashion, with the introduction of the family life cycle [101]. Family therapies can therefore evolve from more behavioral to intercommunicational and intrapsychic functioning, in line with the general sequential model of psychotherapy.

Group Therapy for Children and Adolescents

As described by Knauss [102], group therapy started with psychoeducational models and later group analytic models, as with that of Anthony [103], and then evolved to activity group therapy, focusing on observation of the child's behavioral and motoric communications in a particular group action. Most group therapists now use a mixture of developmental and group assignment frameworks, either with parents in parallel treatment with younger children or with groups of children who have common or at least interconnected problems. One of the technical difficulties is to focus on what represents a group. The group allows for a commonality in approach, but it may lead to a number of children or adolescents held to be similar for therapy purposes, but actually very different individually and clinically. The observation that other children have similar problems is nonetheless useful in reducing a child's anxiety and may lead to the evolution of shared coping skills.

A number of special populations therefore exist, including those for social skills, underachievement in school, divorce, abused children, and drug-using children, as well as parent/family groups stressing family evolution and parent training.

As discussed in the following section, groups can be used in an evolutionary fashion from behavioral to more communicational emphases. Group therapies are often attractive to a number of insurance companies, because they give the impression that more can be achieved for a greater number of children with less cost; the hard evidence for this is unclear, however. In one analysis, group therapy treatment was found to be more effective than individual treatment in 31% of the cases [104]. Some studies have discussed the effects of group therapy for particular diagnoses. Fine and colleagues, for example, found that depressed adolescents in a therapeutic support group showed a greater decrease in depressive symptoms and increased self-support than those not receiving group therapy [105].

In summary, group therapy is an important but somewhat understudied mode of therapy for children and adolescents. It is already undertaken with great enthusiasm in several settings but will benefit from more rigorous research.

Special Population Therapies

Because of the high prevalence of children and adolescents with problems not easily amenable to therapy, as in conduct disorders, there has been an increased interest in using multiple arenas for intervention. Some of the more dramatic forms, such as the use of "boot camps" have not been shown to work [106], but others such as the Multi- Systemic Therapy (MST) of Bourdin and colleagues have been tested satisfactorily, and show considerable promise [107].

Therapeutic Interventions: Models for Selection and Utilization of Different Forms of Child and Adolescent Psychotherapy

A General Model for Sequential Strategies in Child and Adolescent Psychotherapy

To simplify the complex array of possible psychotherapies, a general model will first be presented, focusing particularly on the strategies used or required to attain particular goals. In turn, the type of therapy used will be selected for its utility for stipulated goals at particular times during the course of the therapy. To this extent, the idea of adhering only to one particular form of psychotherapy – especially one with dedicated disciples – for all cases is nonsensical. It attempts to fit the patient into a Procrustean bed in conformity to the therapist's particular enthusiasms or limitations of training, rather than being responsive to the patient's needs. Good therapists can alter their approaches flexibly as need be, ideally with the knowledge and assent of the patient and/or parents, while still largely remaining within their preferred or initial psychotherapeutic métier. Implicit in this approach is that the therapist must be broadly and flexibly trained. This is why general strategies rather than labeled therapies are stressed in this section.

Psychotherapies with their attendant strategies can be conceptualized as existing in a spectrum between more goal-directed, behaviorally oriented modes and more nondirective analytic therapies [108]. Intermediate are those directed relationship therapies that use the therapist as a partial model for limited patterns of social interaction, as in assertiveness training techniques [109], or as a total model of an adult or parent figure (Table 6.1).

In addition, so as to include all the various models of individual, family, and group therapies as noted, the concept of "child (or adolescent) patient" is used synonymously with "patient unit" to stipulate that the therapy may be with the individual child, the parent(s), the parents plus child, the family, the group, the immediate society in general, or other units. Again, the "patient unit" may vary from time to time, but always within the context of evolving clinical realities. Put another way, the therapist should be able to define at any time why he or she is following a certain pattern of therapeutic intervention in a case – as in the rest of medicine!

The various psychotherapeutic strategies, viewed as a continuum or spectrum, can be classified from more directive to more nondirective, and also as more suppressive to more expressive. There is a general parallel between these two dimensions, although they are not necessarily synonymous. The model to be presented will also describe how a variety of interweaving therapies may be selected depending on the diagnosis of the child, family, or group, and also point out how the style of therapy may evolve over time, related in part to what occurs in therapy and to other events or clinical considerations. The model also indicates how both the therapeutic relationship and the therapy style are also dependent on diagnosis. Therapy often evolves from simpler to more complex phases, or sometimes vice versa, using a sequential approach that allows for interphase negotiations with the child and family about how to proceed throughout therapy. Such an approach is particularly suited to episodic and planned therapies with associated specified outcome goals; both apply to the realities of practice in the current clinical environment.

Table 6.1 Patterns in sequential child psychotherapy.

Therapy spectrum:	Directive			Nondirective
Therapy type	Custodial-supportive: "Do therapy to the patient"	Part-relationship: "Do therapy to or with the patient"	Complex relationship: "Do therapy with the patient"	Analytic relationship: "Be with the patient while he or she re-experiences or works through past issues"
Associated strategies	Supportive	Concrete reward system	Negotiated behavioral rehearsals	Verbal or play therapy; re-experiencing
	Suppressive	Induced partial modeling	Induced full modeling	Corrective experience with new skills; tension relief

The strategies associated with this sequence of directive to nondirective child therapies frequently evolve from behavioral methods to more dynamic approaches, especially with action-oriented and mistrustful children, as suggested by the left-right sequence in Table 6.1. Such an evolving sequence of strategies, however, has also been found useful in more internalizing children with subjective inner distress. In sequential psychotherapy, after a full initial clinical diagnosis, there follows a first stage of initial contract negotiation with different styles as required by the type of case (as described below), followed by a second stage of rehearsal of more simple interactional and affectual behaviors, and a possible third stage of exploration of more complex intrapsychic, intercommunicational, and intrafamilial issues. To illustrate these points, examples follow of the three-stage, sequential psychotherapy approaches to children with different diagnoses. However, this sequence is not invariant, and may vary with different children.

Stage 1: Initial Contract Negotiation and Formation, with Different Styles of Therapist–Patient Relationship

Several clinical variants of stage 1 occur, requiring different styles of approach by the therapist. Examples of three common styles follow. These are generally defined by the context of the relationship.

Style A: Therapist as Manipulated Helper: "What's in it For You to be in Therapy?"

In children with disruptive behavior disorders, interactions with authority figures are usually both unsatisfactory and punitive. Such children are often mistrustful, action-oriented, and desirous of escaping from the therapeutic situation. Therapists must formulate the initial contract in terms of "What's in it for you?" They stress the therapist's role as a helpful adult, pointing out how the child might, for example, be able to remain in school or avoid further punishment by the law if he or she conforms to certain rules. Therapists are not the law but merely members of that particular society. As manipulated helpers, and not the prime authority figure, they are able to avoid moralizing – but they do indicate the logical consequences involved in the child's antisocial actions.

Therapists should refrain from imposing their own values; a decision to avoid attacking other children to avert the response that follows from school authorities is sufficient motivation for therapy to proceed. Once this understanding has been reached, the child and therapist can move on to specific behavioral rehearsals in the second stage of sequential psychotherapy.

Style B: Therapist as Nonmanipulated Helper: "How Can I Help – or Take Good Enough Care of You?"

In a more trusting child the therapeutic relationship can become more personalized. In a suicidal child, for example, formation of the initial contract stressed that the child should be cared for in a structured and protective setting. This fulfilled the child's need for nurturance protection. This general point of "good enough" care is similar to Winnicott's concepts [110]. In another child with asthma and associated depression, the initial contract for "good enough" care involved assurance of adequate pediatric help while avoiding the overprotection and subsequent shame-rage reactions that had plagued the child in relationships with his own family.

The therapist in this situation is cast into a nurturing role with a child who can accept the usefulness of helping adults and has therefore achieved a degree of trust, or at least a suspension of mistrust. If this is not initially possible for the child, a brief period of more neutral contractual maneuvering in the "what's in it for you?" style may be required.

Style C: Therapist as Empathic Participant: "What's It Like Being You?"

The two former patterns in contract formation have stressed doing things with or for the child. In contrast, questions asked about "What's it like being you?" relate to the therapist's wish to understand the child and also achieve some notion of the child's own perceptions.

In all three styles the therapist's total understanding of the child must of necessity be limited; the child is still guarded, and the time available for obtaining information is short. But the therapist does signal his or her basic interest in the child as a person, and the contractual position of usefulness, helpfulness, and empathy reflects an honest transaction between one person and another.

During this initial contract formation, there may have been an unfolding elaboration of roles, from the therapist as a nonpersonalizing informer of consequences or routes of legal or social redress, to that of parenting caretaker in the second style, to that of an interested and empathic person in the third style. Many children and adolescents may progress through all three styles in contract formulation, but such a sequence is not invariable or even necessary for successful therapy. Such contractual groundwork provides a basis for the second stage in sequential psychotherapy.

Stage 2: From Instrumental to Interactional Patterns: "Doing Therapy To or With the Patient"

This stage initially employs an elaboration of simple to more complex behavior modification methods. Therapists may initially use such concrete reward systems and behavioral rehearsals, but then develop more complex interactional patterns by using themselves as models of interactions, while augmenting the child's capacity to observe himself or herself interacting more favorably and successfully. Similarly, the children progress in their perception of the therapist. Whereas initially they may regard the therapist as somebody to be manipulated for gain, they are secondarily involved with the therapist as a model toward whom they have ambivalent liking. Finally, they understand being with the therapist and share their excitement about increasing capacities. Following the formation of the initial contract, a number of possible therapies may therefore occur.

The next two case examples illustrate this approach with children with different diagnoses and attitudes towards the therapist.

The Child with Externalizing Disruptive Behavior Disorders

These children are best approached by directive therapies for agreed-on target behaviors such as high intensity aggression or other maladaptive social behaviors. Often such target behaviors are best approached by using rewards and time-outs for positive and negative behavior. This therapeutic interchange in the "What's in it for you?" relationship spells out to children the consequences of their actions but also avoids the intense and often exhortative personalizing that has often taken place with other adult figures.

In group interactions dominance-submission maneuvers with other children usually predominate, since such children have frequently not managed to achieve sharing or a capacity to delay gratification. As a result, basic socialization therapy with peers and adults can sometimes be employed. Often group approaches are used: group peer interactions may be broken down into such simple behavioral objectives as "spending more time with the group by avoiding fights and tantrums," with later sequential elaboration into more complex patterns of "doing something that somebody would like," and then into "doing something so that someone will try to please a third person."

In later individual or group therapy, verbal-limiting techniques may be used once a child has experience with more concrete reward systems. The primary therapist can also use direct modeling to channel the child into more effective modes of affectual assertion. Role-playing techniques of possible aggressive techniques may be employed, along with role reversals; here, the child can try out different patterns of verbal and physical behavior and demonstrate in a concrete way that such interactions are possible.

The Child with Internalizing and/or Psychophysiological Disorders

The sequential psychotherapy model is also relevant for children and adolescents with internalizing or psychophysiological disorders. In the suicidal child mentioned previously in the vignette in Style B, one of the key conflicts addressed in therapy related to his ineffective aggressive assertion. This in turn followed from his unmastered and murderous rages toward his mother, arising from a recently threatened separation from his father. Such murderous rages were immediately internalized because of the strict family conscience structure, leading to internalizing aggression and a resultant suicidal attempt. The key strategy area (after basic nurturance was achieved) was to encourage effective aggression. Accordingly, aggressive-assertive role playing was used, with role reversal to decrease the child's anxiety when necessary. With coaxing and support, he managed to express his anger first at the therapist in a role, and then in a real fashion – playing the person who would not allow him to return home for the weekend. He initially became more comfortable in therapy sessions, but as he expressed conscious anger during later sessions, he suddenly became aware of murderous rage impulses, followed immediately by a wish to kill himself and an absolute conviction of his own wickedness.

These emotions were dealt with directly by telling him about the nature of such early and primitive feelings, and by demonstrating that the therapist did not "drop dead" or attack him for his anger – even when the child said he "really meant it." The child then relaxed, although further working through was required as part of a continuing desensitization process.

In another example, an asthmatic child also had his aggression toward his mother identified, but initial attempts to have this well-socialized, charming child express and channel his anger were unsuccessful. In one session, however, a childcare worker to whom the patient related warmly as a mothering person role played his attacking and rejecting mother. The patient immediately became suffused with rage and attempted to attack her physically. Afterward, they were able to rehearse this sequence with good results.

In a further example, which exemplifies the good results of working directly with a pediatrician and psychologist, a little girl who did well with her father and other members of her family, as well as her teachers, had multiple rage episodes directed at her mother, exemplified particularly by strong impulses to push her mother down the stairs, resulting in possible damage to the mother, especially about the legs. The main feature was the mother asserted that she had a generally good relationship with the girl, but that the symptom was related in time to a preverbal period when she had been discovered to have congenital dislocation of the hips, and was placed immobilized into a hip spica for a prolonged period. The pediatrician who referred her confirmed the clinical history, and she was subsequently placed into play therapy. During this, it emerged that during the girl's first years of life her mother was absent from her care due to post-partum depression. The girl also felt her mother had avoided holding and playing with her because she was a damaged child.

In summary, the second stage of behavioral rehearsals focuses on a series of simple to more complex behavioral, interactional, and affectual rehearsal systems. Such intervention increases children's learned ability to perform social maneuvers, as well as their internalization and comfort in their own abilities, which is often associated with more positive self-esteem.

Renegotiation at the End of the Second Stage: "Do You Want To Go On, or Stop at This Stage?"

In sequential psychotherapy it is frequently possible to stop at the end of the second stage. In the case of the disruptive behavior-disordered child, the acquisition of more appropriate social behaviors usually leads to better acceptance by the family and society, although there may be technical difficulties. For example, counter-reactions by the family may follow the use of reward systems; parents may feel that a child should not be rewarded for fulfilling only normal expectations. Alternatively, guilty, self-punitive behaviors may emerge from the behavior-disordered child once more effective social maneuvers have been learned; this may arise from an internalizing of the anger that had previously been contained by the aggressive acting out. Again, the emphasis on behavioral reinforcers throughout the second stage might result in the parents and child still dealing with each other at the end of this stage of therapy as "good" or "bad," rather than as loving or loved persons. Hence the very use of social learning techniques might lead to the child's using adults in a more facile nature, but still with problems in affectual expression.

Many behavior-disordered children who have been brought up in an object-oriented or sensitization fashion may experience considerable difficulty with affect verbalization [111]. But both they and their parents are often capable of a general but strong warmth, which is released once more effective modes of expression and interaction are demonstrated. Once satisfactory behavioral interchanges have been elaborated, increased comfort between child and parent is often sufficient to allow the termination of therapy [112].

Many children and parents will accept the symptom change in social and affectual behavior accomplished during this second stage, and in the renegotiation phase will tell the therapist of their wish to stop therapy at this point. In other cases, the child or family will wish to explore more complex issues.

Stage 3: "Let's Go On": Exploration of More Complex Intrapsychic, Intercommunicational, and Intrafamilial Issues

In more verbal and subjectively oriented children, the behaviorally oriented techniques used in the second phase facilitate exploration during the third stage into more complex individual and familial psychodynamic material.

In the depressed suicidal child described earlier, the rehearsal of more effective aggressive-assertive patterns was initially paralleled by an increase in rage toward his mother. Further exploration in therapy revealed that he had always been angry at his mother for her threats of deserting the family. He also felt that his death by strangulation might cause his mother to feel guilty in this life, and also to be punished in the next life for her lack of attention to him. This led to an associated fantasy of their being linked together in life and death, since he would also be punished in Hell because of his suicide.

The ambivalent association between the child and his mother was also sustained by the family structure. The mother had formed a close alliance with the child, using him as a shield against the aggressive and sexual advances of her husband. Moreover, her basic ambivalence toward the boy was heightened because she became pregnant with him soon after she had adopted her first daughter, at a time when she felt – or had convinced her husband – that it was not possible for her to have a child. The child's perception of himself as unloved and unwanted was at the heart of his depression.

An interesting question asked by behavior therapy colleagues is whether knowledge of such dynamic material alters subsequent therapeutic strategies. In practice, such knowledge does seem to be useful. In the above case, knowledge of the genesis of the child's depression and anger, as well as the family's current and past dynamics, was addressed directly in family therapy, as was current nondominance of the father. Behavioral and insight approaches often coexist; the prime symptom of aggression in this patient was treated concomitantly by rehearsal of increasingly modulated aggressive behaviors. The child later observed that he was more comfortable in expressing anger toward his peers and his parents; as he did this, his suicidal wishes decreased and he was able to cry. His extremes of murderous rage had been modulated into more useful affects, which resulted in his being more spontaneously cheerful and less depressed. Therapeutic strategies therefore continued to come directly from previous stages of behavioral rehearsal, even though new treatment dealing with family relationships, sexual impulses, and other aspects then entered into therapy.

In the case of the child with asthma described above, the demonstration of increased capacity added to his general self-esteem and capacity to envision himself as exploring the world. Although he had previously avoided school, the child now planned successful re-entry. He began learning again and also started to play with other children; this replaced his previous behavior of sitting sadly with adults, endlessly reciting tales of the sports heroes he had observed in hours of passively looking at television.

The model of sequential psychotherapy presented therefore indicates a reasonable and rational approach for planning the initial moves and subsequent strategies to be used in therapy with many different types of children. The different stages are as follows:

(1) an initial diagnostic evaluation;
(2) a period of contractual negotiation;
(3) a stage of behavioral, interactional, and affectual rehearsal;
(4) a possible stage of further exploration into more involved intrapsychic, environmental, and intrafamilial issues.

Although the complexities of the case often suggest many complicated possibilities, initial therapeutic strategies are often couched in rather simple behavioral terms. Similarly, even though strategies become more complex as therapy progresses, they still maintain their inner consistency. As children achieve greater skills, they internalize increasing self-esteem and are therefore able to attack the more internalized and often frightening material that emerges in therapy. Even when such material emerges, behaviorally based approaches often provide the best inroads to these complex interactional and intrapsychic problems.

One final caveat might be made about either simple or complex accounts of the mechanisms of therapy. Despite the simple or elegant hypotheses that might be made, the focus or impetus for change might follow from basic and simple perceptions of the patient. Dr Stanley Greben, anoted Canadian analyst and colleague, wrote a book about an individual analysis, which contained complex descriptions of the analytic process. In contrast, the patient's remark at the end of the analysis was: "He was always there!"

Summary

In this chapter, the processes of diagnosis and psychopharmacological and other psychotherapeutic treatments in children and adolescents have been outlined. A sequential model is described that allows for a rational selection of therapies for the complex problems met by child and adolescent psychiatrists. Such an approach, which leads to the sequential descriptions of defined goals and objectives, is increasingly important in an era marked by growing impetus for accountability. Finally, the complex and rapidly adumbrating areas of "specific" forms of psychotherapy have been briefly discussed. Child psychiatrists and others training in this area need to have a broad training, probably with an emphasis in a particular area. But they should also be able to tailor their approaches to the varying clinical needs of the child, parent, or society. It is hoped that this brief summary will help child psychiatrists choose competently and selectively from among the often-bewildering mosaic of available therapies.

References

1. March JS, Szatmari P, Bukstein O, *et al.* AACAP 2005 Research Forum: speeding the adoption of evidence-based practice in pediatric psychiatry. *J Am Acad Child Adolesc Psychiat* 2007;**46**:1098–1110.
2. Steinhauer PD, Bradley SJ, Gauthier Y. Child and adult psychiatry: comparison and contrast. *Can J Psychiat* 1992;**37**:440–449.
3. Bernet W. Introduction: Tenth Anniversary of AACAP Practice Parameters. *J Am Acad Child Adolesc Psychiat* 2002;**41**:S1–S3.
4. Birmaher B, Brent D, Bernet W, *et al.* Practice parameter for the assessment and treatment of children and adolescents with depressive disorders. *J Am Acad Child Adolesc Psychiat* 2007;**46**:1503–1526.
5. McClellan J, Kowatch R, Findling RL. Practice parameter for the assessment and treatment of children and adolescents with bipolar disorder. *J Am Acad Child Adolesc Psychiat* 2007;**46**:107–125.
6. Findling RL. Evolution of the treatment of attention-deficit/hyperactivity disorder in children: a review. *Clin Ther* 2008;**30**:942–957.
7. Geller B. Obsessive-compulsive and spectrum disorders in children and adolescents. *Psychiatr Clin N Am* 2006; **29**:353–370.
8. Chang KD. The use of atypical antipsychotics in pediatric bipolar disorder. *J Clin Psychiatry* 2008;**69**(Suppl. 4):4–8.

9. Mabry-Hernandez IR, Koenig HC. Screening and treatment for major depressive disorder in children and adolescents. *Am Fam Physician* 2010;**82**:185–186.

10. Kazdin AE. Psychotherapy for children and adolescents. *Annu Rev Psychol* 2003;**54**:253–276.

11. Volkmar FR, Schwab-Stone M, First M. Classification in child and adolescent psychiatry: Principles and issues. In: Volkmar FR, Martin A (eds) *Lewis's Child and Adolescent Psychiatry: A Comprehensive Textbook*, 4th edn. Philadelphia: Lippincott Williams & Wilkins, 2007; pp. 302–309.

12. Donnelly CL. Childhood ADHD and comorbid ODD: diagnosis and contemporary treatments. *CNS Spectr* 2009;**14**:3–6.

13. American Psychiatric Association: *Diagnostic and Statistical Manual of Mental Disorders*, 4th edn, Text Revision. Washington, DC: American Psychiatric Association, 2000.

14. Sorensen MJ, Mors O, Thomsen PH. DSM-IV or ICD-10-DCR diagnoses in child and adolescent psychiatry: does it matter? *Eur Child Adolesc Psychiat* 2005;**14**:335–340.

15. First MB, Pincus HA. Classification in psychiatry: ICD-10 v. DSM-IV. A response. *Br J Psychiat* 1999;**175**:205–209.

16. Carrey N, Gregson J. A context for classification in child psychiatry. *J Can Acad Child Adolesc Psychiat* 2008;**17**:50–57.

17. Geller B, Williams M, Zimerman B, Frazier J. *Washington University in St. Louis Kiddie Schedule for Affective Disorders and Schizophrenia (WASH-U-KSADS)*. St Louis: Washington University, 1996.

18. Reich W. Diagnostic interview for children and adolescents (DICA). *J Am Acad Child Adolesc Psychiat* 2000;**39**:59–66.

19. Scahill L, Riddle MA, McSwiggin-Hardin M, *et al.* Children's Yale-Brown Obsessive Compulsive Scale: reliability and validity. *J Am Acad Child Adolesc Psychiat* 1997;**36**:844–852.

20. Poznanski EO, Cook SC, Carroll BJ. A depression rating scale for children. *Pediatrics* 1979;**64**:442–450.

21. Young RC, Biggs JT, Ziegler VE, Meyer DA. A rating scale for mania: reliability, validity and sensitivity. *Br J Psychiat* 1978;**133**:429–435.

22. Feighner J, Robbins E, Guze SB, Woodruff RA, Winokur G, Munoz R. Diagnostic criteria for use in psychiatric research. *Arch Gen Psychiat* 1972;**26**:57–63.

23. de Bildt A, Sytema S, Ketelaars C, *et al.* Interrelationship between Autism Diagnostic Observation Schedule-Generic (ADOS-G), Autism Diagnostic Interview-Revised (ADI-R), and the Diagnostic and Statistical Manual of Mental Disorders (DSM-IV-TR) classification in children and adolescents with mental retardation. *J Autism Dev Disord* 2004;**34**:129–137.

24. Achenbach TM, Edelbrock CS. The classification of child psychopathology: A review and analysis of empirical efforts. *Psychol Bull* 1978;**85**:1275–1301.

25. Szatmari P. More than counting: milestones in child and adolescent psychiatric epidemiology. *J Am Acad Child Adolesc Psychiat* 2009;**48**:353–355.

26. Kessler RC. Psychiatric epidemiology: challenges and opportunities. *Int Rev Psychiat* 2007;**19**:509–521.

27. Epstein NB, Bishop DS, Baldwin LM. McMaster model of family functioning: A view of the normal family. In: Walsh F (ed.) *Normal Family Processes*. New York: Guilford Press, 1982; pp. 115–141.

28. Freud A. *Normality and Pathology in Childhood*. New York: International University Press, 1965.

29. Nagera H. *The Developmental Approach in Childhood Psychopathology*. New York: Aronson, 1981.

30. PDM Task Force. *Psychodynamic Diagnostic Manual*. Silver Spring, MD: Alliance of Psychoanalytic Organizations, 2006.

31. Cantwell DP. DSM-III studies. In: Rutter M, Tuma H, Lann IS (eds) *Assessment and Diagnosis in Child Psychopathology*. New York: Guilford Press, 1985; pp. 3–36.

32. Rutter M. Isle of Wight revisited: Twenty-five years of child psychiatric epidemiology. *J Am Acad Child Adolesc Psychiat* 1989;**28**:633–653.

33. Vaughan Van Hecke A, Mundy PC, Acra CF, *et al.* Infant joint attention, temperament, and social competence in preschool children. *Child Dev* 2007;**78**:53–69.

34. Kanner L. Do behavior symptoms always indicate psychopathology? *J Child Psychol Psychiat* 1960;**1**:17–25.

35. Werner EE, Smith RS. Overcoming the odds: High-risk children from birth to adulthood. Ithaca, NY: Cornell University Press, 1992.

36. LaRoche C. Children of parents with major affective disorders: A review of the past 5 years. *Psychiatr Clin North Am* 1989;**12**:919–932.

37. Farrington DP. The Twelfth Jack Tizard Memorial Lecture. The development of offending and antisocial behavior from childhood: key findings from the Cambridge Study in Delinquent Development. *J Child Psychol Psychiat* 1995;**36**:929–964.

38. Kay J. The essentials of psychodynamic psychotherapy. *Focus* American Psychiatric Association 2006;**4**:167–172.

39. Cabaniss DL, Arbuckle MR, Douglas C. Beyond the supportive-expressive continuum: an integrated approach to psychodynamic psychotherapy in clinical practice. *Focus American Psychiatric Association* 2010;**8**:25–31.

40. Weerasekera P. Psychotherapy update for the practicing psychiatrist: promoting evidence-based practice. *Focus* American Psychiatric Association 2010;**8**:3–18.

41. Sanders KM. Mindfulness and psychotherapy. *Focus* American Psychiatric Association 2010;**8**:19–24.

42. Diamond GS, Wintersteen MB, Brown GK, *et al.* Attachment-based family therapy for adolescents with suicidal ideation: a randomized controlled trial. *J Am Acad Child Adolesc Psychiat* 2010;**49**:122–131.

43. Jensen PS, Arnold LE, Swanson JM, *et al.* 3-year follow-up of the NIMH MTA Study. *J Am Acad Child Adolesc Psychiat* 2007;**46**:989–1002.

44. March JS, Silva S, Benedetto V. The Treatment for Adolescents With Depression Study (TADS) methods and message at 12 weeks. *J Am Acad Child Adolesc Psychiat* 2006;**45**:1393–1403.

45. Rey JM, Martin A. Selective serotonin reuptake inhibitors and suicidality in juveniles: review of the evidence and implications for clinical practice. *Child Adolesc Psychiatr Clinic* 2006;**15**:221–237.

46. Rappaport N, Prince JB, Bostic JQ. Lost in the black box: juvenile depression, suicide, and the FDA's black box. *Pediatrics* 2005;**147**:719–720.

47. Kay J. Psychotherapy and medication. In: Gabbard G, Beck J, Holmes J (eds) *Oxford Textbook of Psychotherapy*. New York: Oxford University Press, 2005; pp. 463–476.

48. Green WH. *Child and Adolescent Clinical Psychopharmacology,* 4th edn. Baltimore: Williams & Wilkins, 2006.

49. Correll CU, Manu P, Olshanskiy V, Napolitano B, Kane JM, Malhotra AK. Cardiometabolic risk of second-generation antipsychotic medications during first-time use in children and adolescents. *JAMA* 2009;**302**:1765–1773.

50. Mehler-Wex C, Kölch M, Kirchheiner J, Antony G, Fegert JM, Gerlach M. Drug monitoring in child and adolescent psychiatry for improved efficacy and safety of psychopharmacotherapy. *Child Adolesc Psychiat Ment H* 2009;**3**:14.

51. de Leon J, Arranz MJ, Ruaño G. Pharmacogenetic testing in psychiatry: a review of features and clinical realities. *Clin Lab Med* 2008;**28**:599–617.

52. Ritvo RZ, Ritvo S. Intensive individual psychodynamic psychotherapy: The therapeutic relationship and the technique of interpretation. In: Lewis M (ed.) *Child and Adolescent Psychiatry: A Comprehensive Textbook,* 3rd edn. Baltimore: Lippincott Williams & Wilkins, 2002; pp. 974–983.

53. Delgado SV. Psychodynamic psychotherapy for children and adolescents: an old friend revisited. *Psychiatry* 2008;**5**:67–72.

54. Piaget J. *The Child's Conception of the World.* New York: Harcourt Brace, 1929.

55. Coppolillo HP. Use of play in psychodynamic psychotherapy. In: Lewis M (ed.) *Child and Adolescent Psychiatry: A Comprehensive Textbook,* 3rd edn. Baltimore: Lippincott Williams & Wilkins, 2002; pp. 992–997.

56. Freud A. *The Psycho-analytical Treatment of Children.* London: Imago, 1946.

57. Klein M. *The Psycho-Analysis of Children.* London. Hogarth, 1932.

58. Winnicott DW. *Therapeutic Consultations in Child Psychiatry.* New York: Basic Books, 1971.

59. O'Brien J. The psychotherapy of children with attention-deficit hyperactivity disorder and their parents. In O'Brien JD, Pilowsky D, Lewis O (eds) *Psychotherapies with Children and Adolescents.* Washington, DC: American Psychiatric Press, 1992; pp. 109–124.

60. Weiss B, Weisz JR. The impact of methodological factors on child therapy effectiveness. *J Am Acad Child Adolesc Psychiat* 1990;**31**:703–709.

61. Weisz JR, Weiss B, Donnenberg GR. The lab versus the clinic: Effects of child and adolescent psychotherapy. *Am Psychol* 1992;**47**:1578–1588.

62. Fonagy P, Target M. The efficacy of psycho-analysis for children with disruptive disorders. *J Am Acad Child Adolesc Psychiat* 1994;**33**:45–55.

63. Wolpe J, Plaud JJ. Pavlov's contributions to behavior therapy: The obvious and the not so obvious. *Am Psychol* 1997;**52**:966–972.

64. Pavlov IP. *Conditioned Reflexes: An Investigation of the Physiological Activity of the Cerebral Cortex.* London: Oxford University Press, 1927.

65. Watson JB, Ryanor R. Conditioned emotional reactions. *J Exp Psychol* 1920;**3**:1–14.

66. Skinner BF. *Science and Human Behavior.* New York: Free Press, 1953.

67. Grant P, Young PR, DeRubeis RJ. Cognitive and behavior therapies. In: Gabbard G, Beck J, Holmes J (eds) *Oxford Textbook of Psychotherapy.* New York: Oxford University Press, 2005; pp. 35–43.

68. Bandura A. *Social Learning Theory.* Englewood Cliffs, NJ: Prentice-Hall, 1986.

69. Lovaas OI, Koegel RL, Simmons JQ, Long JS. Some generalization and follow-up measures on autistic children in behavior therapy. *J Appl BehavAnal* 1973;**6**: 131–166.

70. Shaffer A, Kotchic BA, Dorsey S, Forehand R. The past present and future of behavioral parent training: interventions for child and adolescent problem behavior. *The Behavior Analyst Today* 2001;**2**:91–105.

71. Kazdin AE, Siegel T, Bass D. Cognitive problem-solving skills training and parent management training in the treatment of antisocial behavior in children. *J Consult Clin Psychol* 1992;**60**:733–747.

72. Horn WF. Additive effects of psychostimulants, parent training, and self-control therapy with ADHD children. *J Am Acad Child Adolesc Psychiat* 1991;**30**:233–240.

73. Molina B, Hinshaw SP, Swanson JM, *et al.* The MTA at 8 Years: prospective follow-up of children treated for combined-type ADHD in a multisite study. *J Am Acad Child Adolesc Psychiat* 2009;**48**:484–500.

74. Eason LJ, White MJ, Newsom C. Generalized reduction of self-stimulatory behavior: An effect of teaching appropriate play to autistic children. *Ann Intervent Dev Disabil* 1982;**2**:157–169.

75. Foxx RM, Azrin N. The elimination of autistic self-stimulatory behavior by overcorrection. *J Appl Behav Anal* 1973;**6**:1–14.

76. Mowrer OH, Mowrer WM. Enuresis: A method for its study and treatment. *Am J Orthopsychiatry* 1938;**8**: 436–459.

77. Azrin NH, Sneed TJ, Foxx RM. Dry-bed training: Rapid elimination of childhood enuresis. *Behav Res Ther* 1974;**12**:147–156.

78. Boettcher MA, Piacentini J. Cognitive and behavioral therapies. In:Volkmar FR, Martin A (eds) *Lewis's Child and Adolescent Psychiatry: A Comprehensive Textbook,* 4th edn. Philadelphia: Lippincott Williams & Wilkins, 2007; pp. 832–840.

79. Petti TA. Cognitive therapies. In: Lewis M (ed.) *Child and Adolescent Psychiatry: A Comprehensive Textbook,* 3rd edn. Baltimore: Williams & Wilkins, 2002; pp. 832–840.

80. Beck AT, Rush AJ, Shaw BF, *et al. Cognitive Therapy of Depression.* New York: Guilford Press, 1979.

81. Kovacs M, Beck AT. An empirical-clinical approach towards a definition of childhood depression. In: Schulterbrandt JG, Raskin A (eds) *Depression in Children: Diagnosis, Treatment and Conceptual Models.* New York: Raven Press, 1977; pp. 1–25.

82. Reinecke MA, Jacobs RH. Cognitive-behavioral therapy for depression. In: Dulcan MK (ed.) *Dulcan's Textbook of Child and Adolescent Psychiatry.* Washington, DC: American Psychiatric Publishing, 2010; pp. 907–914.

83. Friedberg RD, McClure JM. *Clinical Practice of Cognitive Therapy with Children and Adolescents.* New York: Guilford Press, 2002.

84. Leahy RL. Cognitive therapy of childhood depression: Developmental considerations. In: Shirk SR (ed.) *Cognitive Development and Child Psychotherapy.* New York: Plenum Publishing, 1988; pp. 187–204.

85. Moreau D, Mufson L, Weissman MM, Klerman GL. Interpersonal psychotherapy for adolescent depression: Description of modification and preliminary application. *J Am Acad Child Adolesc Psychiat* 1991;**30**:642–651.

86. March JS. Fluoxetine, cognitive-behavioral therapy, and their combination for adolescents with depression: Treatment for Adolescents with Depression Study (TADS) randomized controlled trial. *JAMA* 2004;**292**:807–820.

87. March JS, Franklin M, Nelson A, Foa E. Cognitive-behavioral psychotherapy for pediatric obsessive-compulsive disorder. *J Clin Child Psychol* 2001;**30**:8–18.

88. Ellis A. Early theories and practices of rational emotive behavior theory and how they have been augmented and revised during the last three decades. *J Rational-Emotive Cogn-Behav Ther* 2003;**21**:219–243.

89. Waters V. Rational emotive therapy. In: Reynolds CR, Gurkin TB (eds) *The Handbook of School Psychology*. New York: John Wiley & Sons, 1982; pp. 570–579.

90. Shure MB, Spivack G. Interpersonal cognitive problem solving. In: Price RH, Cowen EL, Lotion RP, Ramos-McKay J (eds) *Fourteen Ounces of Prevention: A Casebook for Practitioners*. Washington, DC: American Psychological Association, 1988; pp. 69–82.

91. Manassis K, Mendlowitz SL, Scapillato D, *et al.* Group and individual cognitive-behavioral therapy for childhood anxiety disorders: arandomized trial. *J Am Acad Child Adolesc Psychiat* 2002;**41**:1423–1430.

92. Whitman T, Burgio L, Johnson MB. Cognitive behavioral interventions with mentally retarded children. In: Meyers AW, Craighead WE (eds) *Cognitive Behavior Therapy with Children*. New York: Plenum Publishing, 1984; pp. 193–228.

93. Dinkmeyer D, McKay GD. *Parents' Handbook: Systematic Training for Effective Training for Effective Parenting*. Circle Pines, MN: American Guidance Service, 1976.

94. Sholevar GP. Family therapy. In: Volkmar FR, Martin A (eds) *Lewis's Child and Adolescent Psychiatry: A Comprehensive Textbook*, 4th edn. Philadelphia: Lippincott Williams & Wilkins, 2007; pp. 854–864.

95. Bloch S, Harari E. Family therapy. In: Gabbard G, Beck J, Holmes J (eds) *Oxford Textbook of Psychotherapy*. New York: Oxford University Press, 2005; pp. 57–66.

96. Minuchin S. *Families and Family Therapy*. Cambridge, MA: Harvard University Press, 1974.

97. Griest DL, Wells KC. Behavior family therapy for conduct disorders in children. *Behav Ther* 1983;**14**:37–53.

98. Sexton TL, Alexander JF. *Functional Family Therapy*. Bulletin. Office of Juvenile Justice and Delinquency Prevention, 2000.

99. Epstein NB, Schlesinger SE. Treatment of family problems. In: Reineeke M, Datrilio F, Freeman A (eds) *Treatment of Family Problems in Cognitive Therapy for Children and Adolescents*, 2nd edn. New York: Guilford Press, 2003; pp. 304–337.

100. Perosa L, Perosa S. Adolescent perceptions of cohesion, adaptability, and communication: revisiting the Circumplex Model. *The Family Journal* 2001;**9**:407–420.

101. Combrinck-Graham L. Developments in family systems theory and research. *J Am Acad Child Adolesc Psychiat* 1990;**29**:501–512.

102. Knauss W. Group psychotherapy. In: Gabbard G, Beck J, Holmes J (eds) *Oxford Textbook of Psychotherapy*. New York: Oxford University Press, 2005; pp. 35–43.

103. Anthony EJ. Group-analytic psychotherapy with children and adolescents. In: Foulkes SH, Anthony EJ (eds) *Group Psychotherapy*. Baltimore: Penguin Books, 1965; pp. 186–232.

104. Toseland RW, Siporin M. When to recommend group treatment: A review of the clinical and the research literature. *Int J Group Psychother* 1986;**36**:171–201.

105. Fine S, Forth A, Gilbert M, Haley G. Group therapy for adolescent depressive disorder: A comparison of social skills and therapeutic support. *J Am Acad Child Adolesc Psychiat* 1991;**30**:79–85.

106. Russell KC. A nation-wide survey of outdoor behavioral healthcare programs foradolescentswith problem behaviors. *J Experiential Education* 2003;**25**:322–331.

107. Henggeler SW, Clingempeel WG, Brondino MJ, Pickrel SG. Four year follow-up of multisystemic therapy with substance-abusing and substance-dependent juvenile offenders *J Am Acad Child Adolesc Psychiat* 2002;**41**:868–874.

108. McConville BJ. Opening moves and sequential strategies in child psychiatry. *Can Psychiatric Assoc J* 1976;**21**:295–301.

109. Bandura A, Walters RH. *Social Learning and Personality Development*. New York:Holt, Rinehart & Winston, 1963.

110. Winnicott DW. *The Maturational Processes and the Facilitating Environment*. New York: International Universities Press, 1965; pp. 145–146.

111. Singer RD, Singer A. *Psychological Development in Children*. Toronto: WB Saunders Co., 1969; pp. 274–297.

112. Rait D, Glick I. Reintegrating family therapy training in psychiatric residency programs: making the case. *Acad Psychiat* 2008;**32**:76–80.

7

Assessment of Infants and Toddlers

Martin J. Drell

In this chapter, I explain the basics of conducting a clinically based infant assessment. I do so by answering three questions:

(1) What are the fundamental aspects of an infant assessment?
(2) What models can be used to conceptualize infant assessments?
(3) How does one actually conduct an infant assessment?

As I address each of these questions, I suggest general modifications and accommodations to make when assessing very young children. Various articles address the specific content of infant assessments in more detail [1–5].

Fundamental Aspects of an Infant Assessment

The purpose of the assessment is to define the problem and elucidate its cause. An assessment is triggered by the perception that there is a problem. In the case of very young children, the perception is usually voiced by caregivers. (Due to the wide variation in caretaking situations, for this chapter I will use the more generic term "caregivers" rather than "parents.") These perceived problems generally center on aspects of normal daily activities such as eating, sleeping, bathroom functions, motor activities, and interactions. Based on their own experiences including those with other very young children, what they read, and what they are told by others, the caregivers have a general idea of what their child should be doing. When their child does not meet these expectations, they become concerned and try to figure out whether there is a problem and, if so, what to do about it. In most cases, this perception of something being wrong is not enough to lead to a formal assessment. Caregivers assume that the problem is transient, that it is within the range of normal behavior, or they deny that there is a problem. And indeed, due to the dynamic nature of very young

children, their relationships, and the unending march of development, the problems noted often change with time or even resolve. It is only when caregivers perceive that there is a significant problem and/or the problem endures despite their best efforts to solve or deny it that they seek an assessment.

The overall goal of an infant assessment is to collaborate with the caregivers to identify and clarify the problem, mutually agree on the factors that contribute to the problem, and design an appropriate treatment strategy. If any members of this "team" of caregivers and professionals disagree, this constitutes a separate therapeutic problem. Often, important clinical information can be ascertained while working from disagreement among the parties involved toward mutual agreement. Like any diagnostic assessment, such a process provides an absolutely unique entree into how the caregivers see the world, get along with people in this world, and solve problems.

CASE ONE

A couple brought in their 24-month-old son for an evaluation. The mother was upset that her child was hyperactive and unmanageable. The father felt that there was no problem, stating that "boys are just that way." He went on to denigrate his wife's parenting skills. The evaluation showed a child who was caught in the middle of his parents' marital problems. The child's behavior was a response to these difficulties. The behaviors ceased immediately after the parents were counseled on the impact of their difficulties on the child and sought marital therapy. They were astounded that a 2-year-old could pay attention to these issues. This is an example of how disagreements about what the problem is can be used in the treatment effort.

Clinical Child Psychiatry, Third Edition. Edited by William M. Klykylo and Jerald Kay.
© 2012 John Wiley & Sons, Ltd. Published 2012 by John Wiley & Sons, Ltd.

Most experts agree that it is helpful to gather data from many sources. As in the first case study, differences in perception often occur between the various persons involved. It is also vital to observe the infant and to judge the infant's interactions with the key persons in the infant's life, as well as with the assessor. The importance of these interactions is a key focus in infant work. Finally, most experts admit that no one specialty or person has a mastery of all the knowledge needed to assess infants and their caregivers. As a result, infant assessments often involve the expertise of numerous disciplines, including, but not limited to, child and adolescent psychiatry, pediatrics, clinical psychology, developmental psychology, speech and hearing physical therapy, genetics, and social work. Each of these disciplines has its own approaches, knowledge base, and formal assessment tools. When integrated, the information provided by these disciplines can be invaluable in defining problems and formulating what needs to be done to help moderate them.

Models of Infant Assessment

I utilize a systemically oriented, developmental, biopsychosocial model. Systemic refers to the belief that people are best understood when they are viewed as important interacting parts of a larger family system that is in turn part of still larger social systems such as peer groups, religious groups, organizations, and cultures. This model emphasizes the importance of the continuous interaction of all these systems and it assumes the continual evolution over time of problems and people. The systemic approach is dynamic and implies interest in the antecedents of the problem as well as its consequences.

A developmental perspective implies that children develop and mature over time. It stresses the need to examine the child against established norms for other children of his or her age. This perspective recognizes that development occurs in numerous areas of the child's life. Numerous standardized assessments are available to screen these areas of development (see Table 7.1) [5].

The areas focused on include:

Personal/socio-emotional. Does the child smile? Does the child respond to his or her caregivers in ways that indicate that they are special? Does the child respond differentially to strangers? Does the child indicate his or her needs? Does the child imitate other people? What are the child's emotional responses and the range of these responses?

Fine motor-adaptive. Does the child grasp a rattle? Does the child sit? Does the child have the ability to transfer an object from one hand to the other?
Language/communication. Does the child laugh? Does the child turn in response to another's voice? Does the child imitate speech sounds? Does the child have the ability to communicate its needs despite not having formal speech? Does the child speak? How complex is his or her speech?
Gross motor. Can the child roll over? Can the child sit? Can the child stand? Can the child walk? Can the child walk backward? Can the child walk upstairs? Can the child kick and throw a ball? Can the child balance on one foot?

All these skills have been tested on thousands of children to determine what are the normal ranges of behaviors in each category. A failure to develop appropriately in any of these areas may indicate a deviation. Certain types of developmental failure are indicative of specific types of problems and disorders. For example, children with early autistic disorder show a cluster of abnormalities in their ability to interact with people, in their ability to play, and perhaps in some of their motor skills. A fundamental component of assessing young children is appreciating what is normal and abnormal development for a particular age group. This is learned over time by seeing many young children.

A biopsychosocial approach implies that problems (and their solutions) evolve from the interaction of biologic, psychologic, and social phenomena. These phenomena should not be considered all negative and include protective factors and individual resilences. During assessments, one must identify and attend to these strengths and weaknesses and the possibility of problems in all these overarching categories. Unfortunately, when dealing with infants or toddlers and their caregivers, there has been a tendency to accept the first reasonable, yet perhaps oversimplified, theory. For example, in the 1950s it was thought that autistic disorder was caused by faulty caregiving, especially by the mother. The experts who believed this at the time were correct in their observation that the parents of autistic children acted differently than the parents of other children. They were incorrect, however, in attributing the cause of the disorder to the parenting. Subsequent research has shown that the abnormalities in parenting noted are within the normal, expectable responses of parents faced with a young child who is different and who therefore poses unique parenting challenges and responses. The cause of early infant autism is now believed to be neurodevelopmental (i.e., a disruption in early brain development). Numerous

Table 7.1 Selected measures of early childhood symptoms [5].

Measure	Ages (months)	Domains	Format	Number of items	Validity	Reliability	Special characteristics
Ages and Stages Questionnaires: Socio-Emotional (Squires *et al.* 2001)[26][a]	6–60	Self-regulation, compliance, communication, adaptive functioning, autonomy, affect, and interaction with people	3-point Likert scale Different forms for each age group (months): 6, 18, 24, 30, 36, 48, 60	22–36	Sensitivity in predicting a positive score on the CBCL and Vineland. Socio-Emotional Early Childhood Scales, or a known diagnosis: 71–85%; lower in younger groups Specificity: 90–98%	Test-retest reliability after 1–3 weeks is excellent ($r = 0.91$)	Screening measure; includes strength-based items; validity using broadly defined
Child Behavior Checklist $1\frac{1}{2}$–5 (Achenbach and Rescorla 2000)[24][a]	18–60	Internalizing, externalizing, and total problems	3-point Likert scale.	99	Clinically referred children have higher scores than non-clinically referred children (effect size = 0.3%); 77% referred sample vs 26%	1-week test-retest reliability: mean = 0.85 (parent report), 0.81 (teacher report)	Computer scoring system; validated teacher rating form
Infant-Toddler Social and Emotional Assessment (Briggs-Gowan 1998)[25][a]	12–26	Internalizing, externalizing, dysregulation, and competence	3-point Likert scale	166	Correlation with CBCL total problem scores: $r = 0.47$ (internalizing problems); $r = -0.67$ (externalizing problems) Correlation with observer ratings: $r = 0.20$–0.31	Mean 1-month test-retest reliability: $r = 0.82$–0.90 for domains	Includes strengths; BITSEA screener (a companion measure) available

BITSEA, Brief Infant-Toddler Social and Emotional Assessment; CBCL, Child Behavior Checklist.

[a]Purchasing information: www.brookespublishing.com/store/books/squires-asqse/index.htm.

[†]Purchasing information: www.aseba.com.

[‡]Purchasing information: http://pearsonassess.com.

[‡]Reproduced from Gleason and Zeanah, p. 11 [5], with permission.

prenatal, perinatal, and postnatal biological events are also known to cause the types of behaviors that lead to the diagnosis of autistic disorder. A short list of these includes maternal rubella, untreated phenylketonuria, tuberous sclerosis, anoxia during birth, encephalitis, infantile spasms, and fragile X syndrome. Neurodevelopmental problems also affect a young child's social skills, which in turn have consequences for the caretakers. A systems oriented developmental, biopsychosocial approach assumes that the behaviors of the caregivers, in turn, reciprocally affect the social skills of the child, which may in turn affect the biology and brain development of the child.

Development is a dynamic process that affects and is changed by interacting biologic, psychologic, and social events. Thankfully, for the assessor, these interactions usually have a predictable quality that facilitates diagnosis. As with the psychiatric disorders of older children and adults, there are key behaviors and interactions that can be used to differentiate the infant disorders from one another.

In 1989, Stern-Bruschweiler and Stern proposed a systemic model for conceptualizing the role of the mother or primary caregiver in mother-infant therapies [6]. I find this model helpful in my approach to infant and toddler assessments. The model consists of four interdependent elements in constant dynamic equilibrium (Figure 7.1) [6]. These elements are the following:

(1) The infant's overt interactive behavior.
(2) The mother's overt interactive behavior (1 and 2 together constitute "the interaction").
(3) The infant's representation of the interaction (i.e., how the infant understands what is happening in the

situation, including what's happening to him or her and others in the interactions).
(4) The mother's representation of the interaction.

All four elements together constitute "the relationship." In the assessment, this translates into the need to evaluate all four elements, as shown in Figure 7.1 and described below.

As the assessor gathers the history, occasionally there is such a clear hypothesis about the origins of the problem that a successful intervention can be mounted. In most cases, however, when things are not so clear, the clinician will want to assess the behaviors and interactions of the infant and the caregivers through interactional sessions.

(1) What the mother (and other key persons involved in the infant's caregiving system, including pediatricians) thinks is happening. This constitutes the R_M (mother's representation) part of the model.
(2) How the mother and the other involved caregivers behave and interact with the infant (and each other) as well as how the infant behaves and interacts with the mother and other caregivers. This constitutes the B_M (behaviors of the mother)/B_I (behaviors of the infant) part of the model, which defines "the interaction."
(3) What the infant thinks is happening. This coincides with the R_I, (infant's representation) part of the model. Knowledge concerning the representations of infants is sparse and remains speculative, since it is difficult for researchers to ascertain with certainty what goes on in an infant's mind [7].

An infant assessment, then, involves asking questions about what may have occurred to get things to

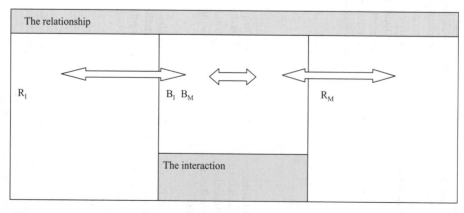

Figure 7.1 The Stern-Bruschweiler and Stern model [6].

their present state and then developing a coherent story concerning the relationship of these four elements.

Conducting an Infant Assessment

There are varying ways to accumulate the essential data for a comprehensive assessment. All the techniques are directed at clarifying the nature of the problem and constructing a formulation that will serve as the basis for a treatment plan. This section is organized around the three major categories of information set forth in the Stern-Bruschweiler and Stern model.

Assessing the Perceptions of the Mother and Other Caretakers

The first step of any evaluation is to identify those people involved with the infant. One then asks each of these individuals to define the problem. Consider speaking to the person who made the initial contact with you, since this person has probably been chosen as the spokesperson for the family. It is often best to start with the family's perceptions/representations and move from there. Often this means dealing with the fears, misperceptions, misunderstandings, and defenses of the family, all of which can interfere with an accurate accounting of what is happening. The same processes of inquiry, analysis, and understanding are critical to each step of the treatment.

People to be interviewed are those who can provide information on problem definition, who might have been involved in the creation of the problem, and who might be involved in solving the problem. This almost always includes the parents, and it can also include grandparents, siblings, and other caregivers such as foster parents, community agencies involved in the care of young children, pediatricians, professionals from other medical disciplines, and daycare providers.

Having identified these key people, the clinician must investigate their unique stories concerning the infant under assessment. One should cover the five Ws: when, where, why, what, and who. Make sure everyone is asked about their impression of the problem. It is important to collect data on antecedents, behaviors, and consequences (the "ABCs" in the terminology of behavior modification). Thus, the assessment will investigate events before the problem started, while the problem occurs, and what happens as a result of the problem. Are there times and situations when the problem doesn't occur or things that make the problem better

or worse? It is important to determine with whom the problem occurs, since the infant's behavior can be person specific. The clinician should understand that at all stages in the assessment, perceptions of key people vary. Problems are, of course, in the eye of the beholder. Often one caregiver may feel that there is no problem (e.g., "He's just a spirited boy" or "My parents told me I was just like that when I was that age, and I turned out OK"). When faced with differing perceptions, the assessor should ask questions about these differences. This line of questioning elicits people's differing perceptions of what is normal or not normal. It also allows the assessor to identify misconceptions or knowledge deficits about infants that can be remedied through education. These misconceptions often involve the over- or under-estimation of the capabilities of infants. Such differences of perception are often the first sign the assessor receives of problems between the caregivers that may be contributing to the infant's or toddler's behavior.

It is wise to ask questions about how and why the caregiver has arrived at his or her conception. "How did you come to that idea?"; "What does the infant do that leads you to believe that?"; "Who told you that?" If these initial questions are not productive, the answer often can productively be pursued by asking about the past history of the caregiver. This approach is reflective of the early infant work of Selma Fraiberg on what she called "ghosts in the nursery" [8]. In this pioneering work, Fraiberg hypothesized that many infant and toddler problems stem from unresolved caregiver conflicts that distort their interactions and behaviors with their children in the "here and now." To emphasize this point, I often tell caregivers: "You raise your kids exactly as you were raised or exactly the opposite, and both are wrong because you aren't your parents and your child isn't you!" This starts caregivers thinking about their pasts.

A more formal technique for getting at the "ghosts in the nursery" uses family of origin work, a type of treatment originated by Murray Bowen, wherein specific, detailed information is gathered about the caregivers' families [9]. In some cases this is done in separate sessions (one with each caregiver) to discuss how each caregiver's family functioned as they grew up. Caregivers are told that such information is valuable in learning about the forces that molded them into the people and the caregivers they are. Ghosts from the past can lead to inconsistent or nonexistent disciplinary habits and confusing interactions for infants and their caregivers. Frequently family of origin issues arise naturally during the assessment as caregivers associate to events, often stressful, in their past lives.

CASE TWO

A mother brought her 2-year-old in for an evaluation to see if he was hyperactive. The child was indeed more hyperactive than most children his age. In the interview, I was puzzled that the mother put extraordinary emphasis on the fact that she had read that hyperactive children had something wrong with their brains. After a successful behavioral intervention and parenting work, the child's behavior moderated. Rather than being pleased, the mother continued to worry about her son and the possibility of brain damage. She especially wanted to know if he would "get better." More careful family of origin work on my part unearthed a brother with profound mental retardation who had been sent to live in an institution at an early age. A discussion of the impact of this brother on the mother's family when she was growing up provided clues about the mother's concern over "damaged brains" that do not get better. Therapeutic work with the mother to differentiate her son's problems from those of her brother's relieved her fears and the impact of those fears on her relationship to her son.

The assessor should gather information concerning the infant's development and maturation, including gestation, birth, perinatal events, and developmental milestones. The assessor should also ask about medical problems, medical procedures, current medications, allergies, and hospitalizations. Information should be received from the pediatrician when indicated, especially if there is suspicion of a biological disorder. In cases in which the infant has not had routine pediatric care, this should be suggested as a means of providing preventive care.

CASE THREE

A mother was very concerned about her 12-month-old daughter who was not responding to her. She worried that her daughter might have autistic disorder. The assessment showed that the child was hearing impaired. Referral to speech and hearing specialists led to a dramatic improvement in the responses of her child and a shift in the mother's concerns that facilitated treatment.

The assessment should seek to elicit key events in the past history of the infant and his or her family that might perturb or influence the families' interactions. These events include deaths in the family, the subsequent reactions to these deaths by family members, separations, medical or emotional problems in other family members that might change the caregiver–infant interaction (e.g., postpartum depression or medical illness of a caregiver), accidents, fires, or persons being laid off from work.

CASE FOUR

The 22-month-old daughter of a single father whose wife had recently died in an auto accident was having temper tantrums daily and was kicking, refusing to go to sleep at the proper time, and being incredibly oppositional. The father was overwhelmed both with his grief and with his new duties as a single parent. The father was helped to appreciate that his daughter had equally strong feelings concerning the death of her mother. He was instructed to talk to his daughter about the death and to "open this area" for discussion. He was counseled on what to expect from his daughter and how to deal with her emotions. He was further supported in the process by the therapist, who helped the father with his own grief. As part of the process, the father and daughter put together a scrapbook of mementos and pictures of the mother. The oppositional symptoms lessened over several weeks.

In cases in which the assessor has specific questions concerning the child's development or lacks the knowledge base or expertise to properly assess his or her development, referral to a developmentally trained psychologist is suggested. These psychologists have access to and knowledge of specific developmental tests and instruments that usually yield a clear profile of the infant's strengths and weaknesses (Table 7.1) [5].

Assessing the Interaction

The interactional approach may include sessions with the evaluator and the infant as well as with the infant and family members. Sessions with the toddler help the assessor better to understand the infant outside the context of his or her caretaking environment. Sleep disorders, attention-deficit hyperactivity disorder, developmental disabilities, and anxiety disorders can prove important in the genesis of interactional problems. In short, if the evaluator is overwhelmed by the child, uncomfortable with the child, or cannot elicit normal interactions with the child, then this is important information. Likewise, it is equally important if the evaluator has no difficulty interacting with a child who appears normally behaved. It may indicate that the problem stems from something the caregivers are doing or not doing to which the infant is reacting with relationship- or situation-specific problematic behaviors. A differentiation between infants with "specific" problems with specific persons versus infants whose problems are pervasive and involve numerous persons across various settings is a key part of any assessment.

CASE FIVE

A 2-year-old with severe temper tantrums played beautifully with the evaluator. The same 2-year-old was then observed while she played with her mother. This play session was punctuated by numerous temper tantrums. The evaluator noted that these occurred when the mother intervened to finish play sequences that the 2-year-old wanted to do herself. The mother would repeatedly tell her child that she was "doing it wrong" and, in frustration, would take over the play. At this point, the child would complain. If the mother did not turn the play back over to the child, then the child would begin to tantrum.

Interactive sessions can provide information that cannot be gathered by caregiver interviews alone, as some problems are outside the awareness of the parents. Calling such patterns to the attention of the caregivers during the assessment can allow the caregivers to see their child's problems in a new light. Caregivers can be quite resistant to such insights, however. Because of this, the material elicited by the assessor must be handled with great therapeutic sensitivity. The evaluator must be empathic to the fear and guilt in many caregivers that they are responsible for their child's problems. In cases in which the interactions are too subtle, too complex, or too confusing to keep track of in real time, videotaping the sessions can be useful. Be sure to obtain appropriate consent for these procedures.

CASE SIX

A mother was concerned that her 3-month-old son was not breastfeeding properly. The history proved noncontributory, so the breastfeeding was videotaped. This showed that the son would interrupt his feeding at regular intervals to make eye contact with his mother. Whenever the mother did not reciprocate the eye contact, the baby would become upset and interrupt the feeding until eye contact was made. Once this pattern was identified, the mother was able to adjust her responsiveness, which caused the feedings to improve.

CASE SEVEN

A father complained that his 21-month-old was not obedient. In a videotaped play sequence, it was noted that the father would ask his young son to do something but would not give his son adequate time to respond. The fact that the son did not respond immediately frustrated the father, who would then re-ask his son in a louder voice. The son who wanted to respond but didn't have time also became frustrated and began to say "No." At this point, the father became angry and began to yell at his child, who he felt was being disrespectful. The evaluator showed the videotape sequence to the father, who was able to see how his son was really trying to please him. The father was given some developmental guidance on what a 21-month-old is capable of and was told to wait at least 3 seconds for a response. This allowed the son to respond to his father's requests. The father-son relationship improved measurably after this session.

It is not uncommon to tape interactions (usually between the person performing the assessment and the infant, and between the infant and his or her caregiver) and to repeatedly replay the tape, often in "slow motion," to catch all of these nuances. Often combinations of *unstructured time* (free play in which you ask the caregiver to be with the child as they normally would be at home) and *structured time* (in which you ask the caregiver to perform a specific interactive task such as

Table 7.2   Typical set of toys.

1. Doll house and family figures	12. Stuffed bear
2. Tea set	13. Fisher-Price hourglass
3. Trucks	14. Playskool school bus and seven passengers
4. Nesting cups	15. Playskool teddy bear shape sorter
5. Pop-it beads	16. Fisher-Price stacking rings
6. Playpath, with small balls in large ball	17. Fisher-Price ring stand
7. Wooden blocks	18. Plastic bowl and lid
8. Pounding bench and hammer	19. Pie plate
9. Dolls	20. Wooden spoon
10. Books	21. Gabriel busy driver
11. Play telephone (2)	22. Fisher-Price musical roller (push toy)

From Harmon (1986). [10]

feeding or playing a simple game with the infant) are more helpful and time conserving than videotaping a regular session. To facilitate interactions, the assessor is advised to equip his or her office with toys, games, furniture, and equipment developmentally suitable for very young children. Any combination of age-appropriate toys will do (Table 7.2) [10]. If the evaluator does not have toys, he or she can ask the caregivers to bring favored examples of the child's play equipment from home. This, however, does not allow the evaluator to see what play is like with new toys (a crude test of curiosity) or toys that might be too difficult for the child's developmental level (a crude test of frustration tolerance).

CASE EIGHT

A mother complained that her 6-month-old infant cried incessantly and seemed not to like her. The history proved unhelpful. During a subsequent observation session, the evaluator noted that the mother was grossly over-stimulating the child with her constant intrusive rocking and bouncing of the infant. It was further noted that the mother would become increasingly frustrated and increase her intrusive behaviors the more the child cried, thus further exacerbating the situation. The evaluator then videotaped the interaction and showed it to the mother, who was able to moderate her responses. Her infant's crying subsequently decreased. The mother was quite pleased by the change in her infant and admitted that she had been told that rocking and forceful bouncing were what one should do when babies begin to cry.

In several cases, I have suggested that the caregivers set up a video camera at home to record problematic behavior. This is especially helpful in those instances in which the infant, for whatever reason, does not display the problem behaviors during the assessment. Home videos can provide wonderful additional material and often can be a vindication for caregivers, who can be quite embarrassed and angry when their infant fails to "show" the problem to the evaluator.

Some clinicians have a routine for their evaluative sessions. Some have very structured and set assessments that include specific questions, tests, and tasks based on the type of problem noted, such as eating disorders, temper tantrums, and sleep disorders. The latter approach is especially useful for research and for gathering a personal database on the range of interactions noted in infant work [11–13].

While interacting with the infant, the assessor should conduct a mental status evaluation to provide a baseline snapshot of how the child looks, acts, and responds. Such baselines are extremely valuable to provide a historical account and to assist in monitoring subsequent behavioral changes. Assessors new to this population could profitably use the four developmental domains (personal/socio-emotional, fine motor, language/communication, and gross-motor) mentioned earlier to help them organize their remarks. A more comprehensive and fine-grained approach has been offered by researchers of infants and toddlers, who have formally attempted to define an appropriate mental status examination for this population [14]. Their attempts include the following categories:

Physical appearance, including dysmorphic features.
Motor functioning, tone, coordination, gross and fine tics, abnormal movements, seizure activity.
Reaction to new settings and people, adaptation during evaluation.

Self-regulation: state regulation, sensory regulation, activity level, attention span, frustration tolerance, unusual behaviors.

Speech and language, expressive and receptive language, speech production.

Thought: hallucinations, dissociative states, nightmares, fears.

Affect and mood: behavioral, nonverbal cues to affect, intensity, range, modes of expression.

Play: structure, content, symbolic functioning, expressions of and control of aggression.

Intellectual functioning.

Relatedness: to parent figures, other caregivers, examiner.

Assessing the Perceptions of the Infant

The third category of information in the Stern-Bruschweiler and Stern model is assessing the subjective experience of the infant. This often proves difficult because of the lack of knowledge about the mental processes of infants [7]. The younger the child is, the greater the challenge. We cannot easily ask infants to tell us their opinions of their problems. We can, however, make assumptions based on how infants interact with their caregivers and the evaluator. These assumptions are based on response patterns such as smiles, reaching for objects, putting objects in their mouth, periods of rapt attention, noting what is attended to, crying, pouting, insistent grunts, falling asleep, crawling away, and avoiding certain people or objects.

As infants grow older, they develop an increased ability to share their experiences. The most significant of these advances is the addition of babbling at 4 to 5 months, words at 12 months, and the ability to think symbolically at 16 to 18 months. The latter two abilities allow skilled assessors to engage the infant in play therapy-type assessments. The developmental achievements that occur at around 18 months, which include the ability to truly pretend play, to pretend with other people, to use one object to represent another, to use personal pronouns, and to realize the difference between self and others, distinguish infancy from toddlerhood. Just as an assessor uses different strategies for children in middle childhood versus adolescence because of their different developmental levels, an infant assessor needs different strategies for toddlers versus infants. Strategies for working with toddlers often include spending more individual time with the toddler than with an infant, with a corresponding emphasis on relationship building. Within this relationship, there is an increased use of words and play. Toddler assessments also take into consideration the fact that toddlers increasingly spend

time with people other than their caregivers. Thus, toddler assessments more often include information about daycare, siblings, and peer interactions.

Putting it all Together

Having conducted a thorough assessment in which you have assessed the perceptions of the key players involved in the presenting problem, viewed their interactions, assessed the infant's and caregivers' interactions with you, taken a past history and a developmental history, performed a mental status examination, and tried to assess what is going on in the child's mind, a reasonable formulation of the problem should be made. The assessor should be able to view the problem systemically and determine its developmentally influenced biopsychosocial causes. At this point, the assessor should share this formulation with the caregivers and gather their feedback concerning their reactions. Any discrepancies between the assessor's perception of the problem and those of the caregivers should be clearly addressed. These discrepancies can be due to simple straightforward misinterpretations and misunderstandings of the facts, but they may also be due to resistances. When resistances arise, the assessor should interrupt the process and try to empathically understand their causes. Such sensitive dealing with resistances ensures that the therapeutic relationship is maintained and that treatment can continue.

No effective treatment can occur unless the caregivers "buy into" the formulation. This is not the same, however, as saying that the formulation cannot change over time as new information is gained. My particular style is to share my formulations with the caregivers as the assessment unfolds. I talk out loud and share my best guess as to what is occurring at the moment and challenge the caregivers to tell me what is right or wrong with my guesses. This technique involves the caregivers and gives them a feel for the way I think, prioritize, and solve problems. It also allows for modeling and numerous mid-course corrections as the evaluation proceeds.

If the assessor has gathered the appropriate data and is unable to arrive at a formulation, some key element or point has probably been missed. Such a situation should prompt the evaluator to reanalyze the questions asked and the data gathered and to consider further assessment. This might include more structured assessment tools and/or taping of the interactions. If this, in turn, fails to clarify the situation, then a consultation is probably needed. A consultant can bring additional expertise and more objective "fresh eyes" to the situation. In some cases, especially nonurgent and/or com-

plex ones, the family and assessor need to take a "wait
and see" approach, in which time either clarifies missing
elements, solves the problem, or the problem evolves
into another more identifiable form.

Should the assessor wish to make a diagnosis, he or
she can do so using the *Diagnostic and Statistical Manual of Mental Disorders,* Fourth Edition, Text Revision
(DSM-IV-TR), which includes the standard diagnostic
nomenclature for the field [15]. Unfortunately, the
DSM-IV-TR was not developed with very young children as its main priority. It contains only a few infant
and toddler diagnoses (e.g., separation anxiety disorder,
reactive attachment disorder, early infant autism, and
pica) and does not capture the interactive realities of

most infant and toddler problems [16]. A group of infant
experts have attempted to address the weaknesses of the
DSM-IV-TR by designing a diagnostic classification
especially for children younger than 4 years of age. It
is entitled *Diagnostic Classification: Zero to Three-Revised* (Table 7.3) [17, 18]. Like the DSM-IV, the classification system consists of five axes, each of which focuses
on varying factors thought to be important to an infant's
or a toddler's problems. Owing to the differing developmental realities of this population, the axes are not all
similar to those of the DSM-IV-TR. The *Diagnostic
Classification: Zero to Three-Revised* has allowed a new
generation of infant/toddlers diagnosis and research
to occur [19–26].

Table 7.3   Diagnostic Classification: Zero to Three-R. Reprinted from Diagnostic Classification: Zero to Three-
Revised. Diagnostic Classification of Mental Health and Developmental Disorders of Infancy and Early Childhood:
Revised Edition. Arlington, VA: Zero to Three; 2005. With permission.

The diagnostic framework is multiaxial. It consists of five axes:

Axis I: Clinical disorders
Traumatic stress disorder
Disorders of affect
   Anxiety disorders of infancy and early childhood
   Mood disorder: Prolonged bereavement or grief reaction
   Mood disorder: Depression of infancy and early childhood
   Mixed disorder of emotional expressiveness
   Childhood gender identity disorder
   Reactive attachment deprivation or maltreatment disorder of infancy
Adjustment disorder
Regulatory disorders
   Type I – Hypersensitive
   Type II – Underreactive
   Type III – Motorically disorganized, impulsive
   Type IV – Other
Sleep behavior disorder
Eating behavior disorder
Disorders of relating and communicating
   Multisystemic developmental disorder

Axis II: Relationship classification
Over-involved relationship
Under-involved relationship
Anxious/tense relationship
Angry/hostile relationship
Verbally abusive
Physically abusive
Sexually abusive

Axis III: Medical and developmental disorders and conditions

Axis IV: Emotional and social functioning
Challenges to child's primary support group
   Challenges in the social environment
   Birth of a sibling
   Change in primary caregiver

Table 7.3 (*Continued*)

Child adopted
Child in foster care
Child in institutional care
Death of a parent
Death of other family member
Death of nonfamily significant other
Domestic violence
Emotional abuse
Marital discord
Medical illness of parent(s) (specify acute or chronic)
Medical illness of sibling(s) (specify acute or chronic)
Neglect
New adult in household (e.g., boyfriend)
New child (not by birth) in home (e.g., adoption, stepsibling, cousin)
Parental divorce or separation
Parental mental illness
Parental remarriage
Parental separation from child (e.g., out-of-town employment, hospitalization)
Parental separation (work)
Parental substance abuse
Physical abuse
Removal of child from home
Severe discord or violence with sibling
Sexual abuse
Sibling mental illness
Sibling substance abuse
Challenges in social environment
   Cultural conflicts
   Discrimination
   Inadequate social support for the family
   Single parenting
Educational/childcare challenges
   More than 9 hours/day in out-of-home care
   Multiple changes in childcare provider
   Parent without high school diploma
   Parent illiteracy or low literacy
   Poor quality early learning environment (e.g., health and safety concerns; high child/staff ratios and large groups: inadequate trained staff; lack of attention to social and emotional development)
Housing challenges
   Dislocation from home
   Homelessness
   Multiple moves
   Problems maintaining heat, electricity, water, and telephone
   Unsafe neighborhood
   Unsafe or overcrowded housing
Economic challenges
   Food insecurity
   Heavy indebtedness
   Poverty or near poverty
Occupational challenges
   Dangerous or stressful parental work conditions (civilian)

(*Continued*)

Table 7.3　(*Continued*)

Military deployment
Parental unemployment
Threat of parental job loss
Health-care access challenges
　Inadequate health services in area
　Lack of or inadequate health insurance
Health of child
　Hospitalization of child
　Medical illness in child (acute or chronic); child accident/injury (e.g., animal bite, passenger in vehicular accident)
　Medical procedure(s) performed on child (e.g., spinal tap)
Legal/criminal justice challenges
　Child Protective Services involvement
　Child victim of crime
　Custody dispute in the context of parental divorce
　Immigration status
Other
　Abduction (specify by family member or nonfamily member)
　Child witness to violence (in the home)
　Child witness to violence (out of the home)
　Epidemic (e.g., AIDS)
　Natural disaster (e.g., fire, hurricane)
　War/terrorism
　Other

From *Diagnostic Classification: Zero to Three-Revised* (2005) [17].

Conclusion

Although performing a clinically based psychiatric assessment of a very young child can be intimidating, it can be successfully achieved by keeping track of the fundamental aspects of any assessment and modifying them to the needs of infants and toddlers. The assessor must have a solid understanding of development in this age range, as in all other ages of children and adults.

References

1. Greenspan S, Wieder S. The Assessment and diagnosis of infant disorders: developmental level, individual differences, and relationship-based interactions. In: Osofsky J, Fitzgerald H (eds) *Early Intervention, Evaluation, and Assessment*, Vol. II. New York: John Wiley & Sons, 2000; pp. 207–237.
2. Meisels S, Atkins-Burnett S. The elements of early childhood assessment. In: Shonkoff J, Meisels S (eds) *Handbook of Early Childhood Intervention*, 2nd edn. Cambridge, UK: Cambridge University Press, 2000; pp. 231–257.
3. Seligman S. Clinical interviews with families of infants. In: Zeanah C (ed.) *Handbook of Infant Mental Health*, 2nd edn. New York: Guilford Press, 2000; pp. 211–221.
4. Gilliam W, Mayes L. Development assessment of infants and toddlers. In: Zeanah C (ed.) *Handbook of Infant Mental Health*, 2nd edn. New York: Guilford Press, 2000; pp. 236–248.
5. Gleason MM, Zeanah C. Assessing infants and toddlers: Table 1-3: Selected measures of early childhood symptoms. In: *Dulcan's Textbook of Child and Adolescent Psychiatry*. Washington, DC: American Psychiatric Publishing, 2010; p. 11.
6. Stern-Bruschweiler N, Stern D. A model for conceptualizing the role of the mother's representational world in various mother-infant therapies. *Infant Ment Health J* 1989;**10**:142–156.
7. Stern D. *Diary of Baby.* New York: Basic Books, 1990.
8. Fraiberg S, Adelson E, Shapiro V. Ghosts in the nursery: A psychoanalytic approach to the problems of impaired infant-mother relationship. In: Fraiberg S (ed.) *Clinical Studies in Infant Mental Health: The First Year of Life.* New York: Basic Books, 1980; pp. 164–166.
9. Bowen M. *Family Therapy in Clinical Practice.* New York: Jason Aronson, 1978.
10. Harmon R. How to do an infant psychiatry assessment: Fundamental knowledge for clinical work with infants and toddlers. Paper presented to the pre-meeting institute, American Academy of Child and Adolescent Psychiatry, Los Angeles, 1986.
11. Dickson A, Kronenberg A. The Importance of relationship-based evaluations for traumatized young children and their caregivers. In: Osofsky JD (ed.) *Clinical Work with Traumatized Young Children.* New York: Guilford Press, 2011; pp. 114–135.
12. Crowell JA, Feldman SS, Ginsberg N. Assessment of mother-child interaction in preschoolers with behavior problems. *J Am Acad Child Adolesc Psychiatr* 1988;**27**: 303–311.

13. Miron D, Lewis ML, Zeanah CH. Clinical use of observational procedures in early childhood relationship assessment. In: Zeanah CH (ed.) *Handbook of Infant Mental Health,* 3rd edn. New York: Guilford Press, 2009; pp. 252–265.

14. Benham A. The observation and assessment of young children including the infant-toddler mental status exam. In: Zeanah C (ed.) *Handbook of Infant Mental Health,* 2nd edn. New York: Guilford Press, 2000; pp. 249–265.

15. American Psychiatric Association. *Diagnostic and Statistical Manual of Mental Disorders,* 4th edn, Text Revision. Washington, DC: American Psychiatric Association, 2000.

16. Gadow K, Sprafkin J, Nolan E. DSM-IV symptoms in community and clinic preschool children. *J Am Acad Child Adolesc Psychiat* 2001;**40**:1383–1392.

17. *Diagnostic Classification: Zero to Three-R. Diagnostic Classification of Mental Health and Developmental Disorders of Infancy and Early Childhood,* Revised Edition. Arlington, VA: Zero to Three, 1994.

18. Wright C, Northcutt C. Brief clinical report: schematic decision trees for DC: 0–3. *Infant Ment Health J* 2004;**25**:171–174.

19. Scheeringa M, Zeanah C, Myers L, Putnam F. New findings on alternative criteria for PTSD in preschool children. *J Am Acad Child Adolesc Psychiatry* 2003;**42**: 561–570.

20. Luby J, Heffelfinger A, Mrakotsky C, *et al.* The clinical picture of depression in preschool children. *J Am Acad Child Adolesc Psychiatry* 2003;**42**:340–348.

21. Luby J, Heffelfinger A, Koenig-McNaught A, Brown K, Spitznagel E. The Preschool Feelings Checklist: a brief and sensitive screening measure for depression in young children. *J Am Acad Child Adolesc Psychiatry* 2004;**43**: 708–717.

22. Thomas J, Guskin K. Disruptive behavior in young children: what does it mean? *J Am Acad Child Adolesc Psychiatry* 2001;**40**:44–51.

23. Crowell JA. Assessment of attachment security in a clinical setting: observations of parents and children. *J Dev Behav Pediatr* 2003;**24**:199–204.

24. Achenbach T, Rescorla L. *Manual for the ASEBA Preschool Form.* Burlington: University of Vermont, 2000.

25. Briggs-Gowan M. Preliminary acceptability and psychometrics of the Infant-Toddler Social and Emotional Assessment (ITSEA): a new adult-report questionnaire. *Infant Ment Health J* 1998;**19**:422–445.

26. Squires J, Bricker D, Heo K, *et al.* Identification of social-emotional problems in young children using a parent-completed screening measure. *Early Child Res Q* 2001;**16**:405–429.

8

Play Therapy

Susan C. Mumford

Childhood ain't what it used to be, so say professionals and parents alike. The whirlwind of activities in which children have become involved often leaves families overscheduled, with woefully little time for spontaneous interactions. Concern about the accelerated pace of children's lives emerged in the mid-1980s. The "hurried child" was now reported to be missing crucial elements of childhood as he or she rushed from one activity to another. However, despite this call for simplification, there has been little change in the complexity of life for many children [1]. The dramatic surge in the identification of childhood mental health disorders in part reflects the mounting pressures on today's children. New treatment tools such as trauma focused-cognitive behavioral therapy and Theraplay® have emerged in response to this need. However, the onset of managed care has reduced care options for patients and treatment restrictions have discouraged some mental health experts from serving as participating providers. For the child patient in particular, receiving appropriate treatment has become especially challenging as the treatment balance tilts toward pharmacology rather than psychotherapy or a mixture of the two. Despite this trend, play therapy, the traditional therapeutic approach with children, remains a viable treatment option. The purpose of this chapter is to familiarize the reader with the basic principles of play therapy including its history, definition, and technique.

History

As early as 1905, Sigmund Freud's writings contained references to play [2]. Freud maintained that play facilitates instinctual discharge as well as mastery of traumatic or unpleasant events. It provides a safe medium through which the repetition compulsion functions to help the child patient gain control over otherwise unmanageable feelings or situations. Play allows for the process of catharsis and reflects both the child's wishes and wish fulfillment. Fantasy, and the break it offers from reality, facilitates the growth of the ego in children. In the fluid atmosphere of fantasy, the ego can reckon with both id and superego demands, enabling the child to experiment with novel solutions to conflict. Freud followed up these early discussions of play with the publication of "Little Hans," one of the first pieces about psychotherapy with a child. Melanie Klein and Anna Freud subsequently emerged as the major theorists of child development and one of its natural subsets, play. Both offered significant but different ways of treating the conflicts of children. Klein's theory of object relations, which placed great importance on the pre-oedipal period of human development, distinguished her from classical psychoanalysts. Her revolutionary work posited that children have a rich and complicated internal life that can be shown to the therapist through the use of toys. Klein used her knowledge of adult psychoanalysis as her technical template, especially the principles of free association, transference, and interpretation. She believed that the child patient free associated not only with words but also with their play activities and these associations could be interpreted. Moreover, Klein saw that the transference provided clues about the child's past and their unconscious world. She was attuned to the importance of selecting toys that were not function-specific but instead could be used by the child in a variety of ways. This concept has of course, stood the test of time and remains a technical underpinning of play therapy today [3].

While Anna Freud never published a monograph exclusively on the subject of play, many of her writings focused on the development of ego capacities and defenses that make play possible [4]. She postulated that the seeds of the ability to play are planted in the early interactions between a baby and his or her mother. Through play with their own bodies, and those of their mothers, babies learn the rudiments of self/other differentiation and by extension, reality and fantasy. Anna

Clinical Child Psychiatry, Third Edition. Edited by William M. Klykylo and Jerald Kay.
© 2012 John Wiley & Sons, Ltd. Published 2012 by John Wiley & Sons, Ltd.

Freud believed that play both facilitates and reflects the child's growth process, which ideally results in personal autonomy, a developed sense of self, and the ability to work. Play provides a way to explore and master internal and external conflicts and gives clues about the child's unconscious strivings. Anna Freud's particular interest in the development of the ego and its impact on id and superego functioning is well known. Moreover, her concept of developmental lines illustrates the cumulative nature of child development – how successes or problems in one phase affect growth in the next. This idea remains useful today as child therapists are responsible for identifying where a patient's development went off track and what is needed to return him or her to a normal developmental point.

In addition to both the Freuds and Klein, there were a number of early pioneers who made significant contributions to the theory of play. Robert Waelder [5] echoed Freud's idea about the usefulness of the repetition compulsion in his writings about trauma, how it can be worked through in play by turning passive into active. Waelder also conceptualized that play permits children to break down the whole untoward nature of a traumatic event into manageable pieces. Erik Erikson [6], known for his epigenetic view of development, pointed out that play allows children to prepare for adult life by experimenting with different roles and identities. In addition to his work with mothers and babies, D.W. Winnicott [7] also provided much to the understanding of the origins and purpose of play and its persistence through the life span. Winnicott conceptualized that the newborn initially makes no differentiation between him/herself and mother. Next, the infant makes minute movements away from mother, out of this unified position with her. A space is then created that is not mother, not baby, but something in between (Figure 8.1). Winnicott termed this important creation "potential space." He identified it as the cradle of creativity, the place that allows for the selection of a transitional object and the emergence of the capacity to play. Understanding of this concept is crucial for child therapists whose assessment of a patient

must, first, confirm the patient's ability to play and, second, assess its quality and range. [8]

Play and Play Therapy

Although many parents are familiar with the clinical term "play therapy," few understand the complexity of this simple-sounding treatment. It is therefore incumbent upon the professional to be well informed about the properties of play, how they are therapeutic, and to be able to share this information with parents in a clear and cogent manner. Despite this obligation, some professionals find themselves more comfortable doing play therapy rather than explaining what it actually is.

The Function of Play Therapy

Play is marked by a variety of characteristics that, when used in therapy, contribute to an improvement in the child's functioning. Fueling children's maturation is their innate developmental thrust forward, their built-in ability to progress. Child therapists are able to use this energy as an ally in psychotherapy. Moreover, the natural power of play has been harnessed for treatment by clinicians representing a number of theory bases including psychodynamic, cognitive behavioral, child-centered, Adlerian, and short-term play therapy [9]. Despite differences in orientation, there are some shared features including recognition of the value of a strong therapeutic alliance, the need to work with the child patient differently than with the adult patient, the importance of viewing children developmentally, and an appreciation for play as the language of the child [10]. An example of two different concepts of play therapy are as follows. Cognitive behavioral play therapy uses play to subtly communicate cognitive change. It introduces children to different, more adaptive responses to their difficulties, which are then modeled using developmentally appropriate materials. The therapist conveys through play possible solutions to problems that resemble those of the patient [11]. The psychodynamic play therapist relies on four main interventions. Confrontation and then clarification are used to facilitate the growth of the observing ego. The therapist helps the child to understand what is occurring internally and points out defenses before drives. Interpretation is used to help the patient see the history of a problem, the purpose of defenses, and to facilitate the working through process. Finally, the psychotherapeutic process itself loosens the child's defensive structure, enabling more adaptive defenses to emerge, as well as providing increased drive satisfaction in a healthier fashion [12,13].

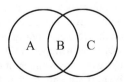

Figure 8.1 Schematic representation of Winnicott's concept of the "potential space" created during development of an infant. A, Mother; B, Potential Space; C, Infant.

The Characteristics of Play

The process of play therapy, made possible because of the relationship between the therapist and the patient, builds on the properties of play. Four properties of play are as follows.

First, *play is fun:* it provides not only pleasure for the child but also a sense of internal satisfaction. It is the external manifestation of a child's imagination and in this way, straddles the boundary between fantasy and reality. Creativity is both nurtured and expressed by play. It is a medium for self-definition and expression and valuable for the unfettered freedom it provides. Play is a process through which children acquire self-confidence and a sense of efficacy as they find solutions to problems in their own time and on their own terms. It provides an outlet for children's creativity. These features are implicit in the therapeutic process. While play certainly has elements of frivolity and excitement, it is also intense and serious. It is meaningful for the child and loaded with affect. It is often helpful for the therapist to follow the lead of a child in play, to include asking the child what he or she would have the therapist do or say.

CASE STUDY

Clinical Example: Child-Led Play

A child, aged nine, is being treated for adjustment difficulties stemming from a move to a new city. She has set up an elaborate scenario using the dolls and dolls' house, a game she informs the therapist that she often plays with her 8-year-old sister. The patient gives the therapist a doll. The therapist then asks if the patient wishes she had more friends to play with in her new neighborhood. However, in response the child suddenly shrieks "What are you saying? You don't know how to play!"

In this example, the therapist appears to have associated the patient's description of the game and subsequent invitation to play it with her as a possible indication of loneliness. The patient's sharp response clearly showed that the therapist had followed her own line of thinking instead of that of the child. It would have been more effective for the therapist to have instead remained silent, accepted the doll from the patient, and awaited what came next. In this way, the therapist would have followed the child's lead and allowed the play to unfold in a more natural fashion.

Second, *play is absorbing*. It can be so encompassing for children that they can appear to be oblivious to other activities around them and have difficulty stopping play before they are ready. The play activity can be complete in and of itself and it is not necessarily something a child does in order to accomplish something else. This qualifier does not mean that play cannot be goal-directed (e.g., build a fort, set up a doll house), but rather, that these goals are part of the larger play activity in general. The process of abreaction is also accomplished through play; the child relives painful situations and experiences the affect belonging to them.

CASE STUDY

Clinical Example: Absorption in Play

A child, aged eight, with significant concerns about his place in his family, has been working on a huge, multifaceted Lego® scene with his therapist for a number of sessions. The particular structure is a castle that houses the orphaned but determined child "hero" of the game. Great attention is given to the assembly of this structure and is accompanied by a rich narration of the hero's struggles. Aware of the child's absorption in his play, the therapist provides him with a 5-minute reminder of the session's end. He responds with dismay "but I just got here!"

The above example describes a clinical situation where the patient is intensely invested in his play. Attention to the aspects of "real life" such as the passage of time is therefore temporarily suspended. Being so immersed in the play scene, the patient is caught off guard by the session's approaching end. The therapist has anticipated this response and thus announces the time but the child is still surprised.

Third, *displacement is operative in child's play*. Due to children's ability to move freely between reality and fantasy without conflict, they can transfer their own affect and personal situation into the play arena. Children change passive into active; they can be the initiators of events rather than the recipients they may feel themselves to be in real life. Displacement permits distance from the original problem as well as from uncomfortable emotions that go along with it. It prevents children from becoming overwhelmed by their feelings or needing to overly inhibit them to keep them in check. Displacement also allows the child patient to talk or act in ways that are not possible without the protection the defense provides. Another important function of displacement is that it permits the child's ego to balance id and superego influences and to be employed in resolution of the difficulty.

CASE STUDY

Clinical Example: Displacement In Play

A 6-year-old boy is being seen by a child therapist following removal from his home due to child endangerment. While he has been quite laconic with the therapist about the events in his life, his play is very expressive. Using the dolls' house, the patient acts out scenes of parental violence. A mother doll is shown threatening a child doll whom the patient has hidden behind a piece of doll furniture. Suddenly, the patient moves the child doll out into the open and forcefully tells the mother to stop or he will put her in jail.

In this example, displacement allows the child to express himself in a way that is not possible in his day-to-day life. Feelings or fears that cannot be otherwise released can be shown through play, giving the child access to them in a safe, manageable way. Furthermore, displacement does not need to be interpreted in order for a child to progress. Clinical gains can be made with the defense left intact.

Fourth, *children's capacity for imaginative play dovetails with their cognitive growth*. Piaget [14] postulated that there are four periods of intellectual development: sensorimotor (birth–age 2 years), preoperational (2 years–7 years), concrete operational (7 years–11 years), and formal operational (11 years and beyond). According to Piaget, between the ages of 2 and 4 years, a child acquires the ability to form symbols. Through symbolism, mental representations are created of experiences, people, and objects and remain in the child's mind. Internalization frees the child from having to see an object to know it exists; a mental image or a word is sufficient. Through symbolic play, a child can bridge the gap between the concrete and abstract. Symbolism gives children's play its distinctly individualized flavor because the children can manipulate the play to reflect their own particular needs and wishes. Piaget's study of the cognitive development of older children (ages 4 through 11) included the use of language, communication, the meaning of rules, and moral judgments. [14] Again, cognitive maturation will be reflected in the increasingly complex play of older child patients.

CASE STUDY

Clinical Example: Symbolism In Play

A patient, age four, was recently adopted, having lived with his maternal grandmother for most of his life. His mother, a drug addict with occasional periods of abstinence, came and left the home unpredictably. During his first treatment session the child exhibited little interest in the toys, with the exception of several puppets, which he named "the monster catchers." He kept one puppet and gave the other to the therapist and pointed to the space under the couch. The patient declared that it was the hiding spot for the monster, a monster who came and went and repeatedly evaded our attempts, as monster catchers, to get him.

The Child Therapist

In psychotherapy with both adults and children, the therapist's warmth, sensitivity, and nonjudgmental attitude are the basis for the therapeutic alliance and critical to therapeutic success. However, due to the immaturity of the child's cognitive and psychic development, the therapist must possess a unique set of behavioral and emotional traits to effectively work with a child. Most importantly, the therapist must genuinely enjoy children, have the capacity to be authentic, and to be at ease in the child's presence [3]. It is beneficial for the therapist to have had a personal psychotherapy so that their own life experiences do not unduly influence interactions with the child patient. Accordingly, therapists should have easy access to their own imagination and be comfortable playing while simultaneously watching and reflecting upon the child's particular situation. To be able to enter the child's world through play yet also remain outside of it requires a great deal of mental elasticity, but without it, the therapist is likely to be more of an observer of rather than a participant in the therapy. Empathy, the capacity to feel what the patient feels, is of course vital to any sound therapeutic relationship. With child patients, it may be easier to feel sympathy for their situation rather than empathy with their feelings unless the therapist is able to tolerate and give veracity to his or her own childhood experiences and residual childlike emotions. Further, empathy enables the therapist to respect the reality of patients' struggles as well as their attempts, however imperfect, to deal with them [15].

Consistency in technique, acceptance of the patient, and flexibility are essential as the child patient can be very attuned to clinical variations or insincerities. The therapist should be patient, tolerant, and honest with the children, which will enhance the patients' ability to be that way with themselves; the therapist in this way serves as an ego ideal. Children most often have not requested psychotherapy and can therefore be suspicious, withdrawn, or concerned that the therapy is a punishment or a consequence of their behavior. Also, children may not necessarily feel troubled or believe they need help despite the worries of others. The therapist must be able to convey the helpful intent of the therapy to the patient and to develop a shared understanding of the problem to be addressed. The therapist needs to assure the child patient that their interactions will take place in a safe, confidential atmosphere. This particular issue can be challenging as the therapist must know how to inform the parents about the treatment but also protect the child's confidences. Most research about the role and characteristics of the therapist has been done by those who work with children; there has been minimal study about how children themselves view the therapist. Ethical considerations and difficulty obtaining a sufficient sample size obviously have hampered this type of research. However, the available data suggest that children most valued the therapist's kindness, helpfulness, and ability to understand and reflect back feelings [16].

Play Materials and the Play Space

Beginning therapists are often unsure about both the materials needed to equip the playroom as well as the rationale behind the selection. Toys or play, in and of themselves, are not therapeutic. Rather it is the way in which they are used in treatment that makes them effective. It is suggested that from the outset the therapist refers to the toys in the office as "play equipment" or "play materials." In this way, through both words and actions, the child starts to see that toys and play have different meanings and purposes than they do outside of the office. The toys chosen by the therapist should be interesting and intriguing; they should capture the child's attention and imagination. They need to be capable of being used symbolically as this is how the child communicates thoughts, fantasies, and wishes. In short, the toys used in therapy should facilitate the child's self-expression. These criteria contraindicate, for example, theme toys or toys of well-known television or movie characters, which might have a fixed identify rather than one created by the child. The toys should be in good repair and clean; a worn-out toy could leave the patient feeling devalued. A therapist may see a number of children in the same office so it can be helpful for the individual patient to have his or her own container in which to place special items or projects. This move contributes to the child's sense of place and belonging in the office as well as to a positive therapeutic atmosphere of safety, containment, and continuity.

Toys that are useful in therapy can be divided into three categories: toys that draw out real-life experiences; those that elicit or reflect anger or aggressive emotions; and those materials that facilitate creative expression [17]. Real-life toys include a doll house and a doll family, cars, airplanes, stuffed animals, zoo animals as well as a toy telephone, puppets, a doctor's/first aid kit, and a few soft baby dolls with bottles. These items naturally appeal, both consciously and unconsciously, to the child's experiences and relationships in daily life and provide a means for exploration and expression. This basic inventory of real-life toys is quite sufficient for most play therapies. However, if the patient has a particular situation that calls for the addition of specific toys, the therapist could provide them.

CASE STUDY

Clinical Example: Play Materials For A Specific Situation

A 7-year-old girl was seen due to anxiety after witnessing her mother being injured in an accident. The patient and her mother were riding bicycles when the mother accidentally rode off the sidewalk and suffered serious injuries. Mother was taken by ambulance to the hospital in the presence of the patient and remained in a coma for several days. Aware of this situation, the therapist added a doll-sized bicycle to her toy supply before meeting with the child. The patient used the doll bicycle during the first session in her play.

All children have aggressive feelings, including those who are referred for very different reasons. However, because they have a limited ability to fully express emotions with words, children can be helped by having aggressive toys with which to play out these feelings. Moreover, the child patient may feel safer engaging these feelings in a displaced way with the therapist than in other settings; this is true especially for inhibited children. Aggressive-type toys include army men and related equipment (e.g., tanks, fighter jets), wild animals – especially with mouths open, teeth exposed – angry-appearing puppets, and police cars. Some therapists provide punching bags or foam balls and bats for a physical release of aggression or energy. With these types of toys, a child's aggression can be easily visible to the therapist and can be interpreted with words. However, the expression of a particular affect is not dependent on having a corresponding toy in reality; anger can be expressed through other means than through, per se, army men or dinosaurs. Children will use materials in nonconventional ways to reveal themselves and therapists need to be alert to the wide variety of meanings a particular action or toy may have.

CASE STUDY

Clinical Example

A 4-year-old girl with an unstable, chaotic family history (i.e., exposure to continual parental arguments, mother often absent from home) presented for an evaluation due to noncompliance and aggressive behavior at preschool and home. During the second diagnostic session, the child used the doll family and doll house to play out a very angry scene between family members. Later in the hour, she took the marble game and very carefully arranged the marbles in an intricate pattern. Suddenly, while muttering "crash" and "bonk," the patient took another marble and obliterated the design. Upon observing the child's subsequent morose affect, the therapist commented, "You seem so sad that all the crashing and bonking has wrecked what you worked so hard on."

The above vignette raises several points. First, aggressive affect can be expressed through many mediums, not just with "aggressive"-looking objects. Here, it is expressed with the dolls and marbles. Second, more meaning can be attributed to the patient's sadness than just the destruction of her marble design. It is possible that the ruin of her arrangement is also a reference to the damage she experienced as a result of the constant fighting (crashing and bonking) at home or a reaction formation to minimize unconscious guilt she may have felt about her contribution to the parents' problems. These additional, possible interpretations demonstrate the need for therapists to remain attuned to more than the play scene's surface meaning.

The final category of toys refers to tactile and creative materials such as crayons, markers, colored pencils, tape and paper, and modeling clay or Play-Doh®. Some therapists use sand and water tables with child patients but this type of equipment clearly requires a large office space and the therapist's tolerance for potential spills. Additionally, blocks and Legos® of a wide variety of shapes and sizes can be useful in several ways. First, they offer the patient a chance to build, disassemble, and recreate new structures. Although concrete, the use of blocks can metaphorically mirror treatment, a process that builds, takes apart, and recreates new ways of thinking and being in the world. Second, they can easily be used in conjunction with many other toys; they are not function-specific. Third, they are appealing to a wide age group, from preschooler through elementary school-aged patients.

CASE STUDY

Clinical example

A 7-year-old boy, who was reported to be an excellent student and well-behaved child at school, was referred due to his explosive rages and out-of-control behavior at home. The patient was an avid race car fan and during an early session in the treatment, constructed an elaborate race track out of blocks. Special attention was given to reinforcing the walls with extra blocks in case of a car crash. The therapist noted how race car drivers who were concerned about spinning out of control and crashing might find these well-constructed walls both necessary and valuable.

While not undoing the displacement, the therapist responded to one of the likely meanings the patient had communicated with blocks.

The above listing of toy possibilities is not exhaustive; other materials such as books, bendable figures, board games, flashlights, and cards can be useful. Board games can be particularly useful when working with older children, latency-age and adolescents who are too old for "pretend" play. The elements of board games – turn taking, following rules, winning or losing – simulate aspects of real life. They also lend structure to the interaction between the therapist and patient. To conclude, individual therapists may find through their own experience and experimentation, additional toys that enrich therapy with children. It is how the toys are used and how the play is developed and understood by the child that is therapeutically valuable. The child patient uses the toys to express his or her inner world and to make sense of his or her experiences in the presence of the therapist; this combination is what is mutative.

Conducting Child Psychotherapy

Getting Started: The Evaluation Period

The Therapist's Relationship with Parents

While evaluation is an ongoing part of therapy, a thorough diagnostic assessment is vital for effective treatment planning. The first step in the assessment of a child is to meet with the parents. As previously noted, it is not often the child who has sought treatment, but rather the parents due to either their own concerns or those that have been brought to their attention by others, such as the school or neighbors. Moreover, the child is obviously having some developmental difficulty that is troubling to the parents even if it is ostensibly not bothersome to the child. It is therefore important for the therapist to remember the vulnerable position parents are in when they seek help and to respond to them in a nonjudgmental fashion. It is essential that from the initial contact forward, the parents view the therapist as accepting, helpful, and trustworthy; there can be no treatment of the child without ongoing support from the parents.

During the 1960s and 1970s, young patients were most frequently seen in hospital settings or child guidance clinics that were equipped to simultaneously work with the parents. While this model is not often practiced today, treatment of children is still indisputably more effective when the problems of the parents are addressed as well. [18] The treatment plan of a child patient should include provision for parental contact. Additionally, the therapist should be prepared to recommend additional services for the parents if needed to support the child's progress.

The therapist first meets with both parents to explain the diagnostic assessment procedure. Depending on the setting (e.g., clinic, private office), this process will take between one and four sessions. The first is generally with parents alone, the following one(s) with the child, and the final one with the parents to explain treatment recommendations. If the parents are divorced or separated, it is still highly preferable to have both parents present during the first session. Inclusion of both parents reduces the risk that the therapist becomes aligned primarily with one parent or hears only "one side of the story." Such a lopsided arrangement will certainly weaken the alliance with the more distant parent and potentially have a negative impact on the child as well. In some cases, regardless of marital status, one parent may refuse to participate or to support the treatment. The therapist should continue to invite that parent to meetings and most importantly, try to discuss the reasons for opposition to the treatment. This action is derived from Freud's original advice to address the negative transference in treatment while leaving intact the "unobjectionable positive transference" [2].

During the first session, the therapist should also obtain certain information about the child including:

(1) Both parents' perception of the (child's) presenting problem.
(2) Precipitant of/background to presenting problem.
(3) Basic developmental and medical history, including prior medications.
(4) Significant family history.
(5) Family history of mental illness, drug and/or alcohol or other addictions.
(6) History of school progress including peer relationships.
(7) Description of personality, fears, interests.
(8) Reason for seeking treatment at this time.
(9) Prior treatment/attempts to solve problem.
(10) Parents' perception of child's strengths and weaknesses.
(11) Parents' long-term hopes for and fears about the child.

Additionally, the basic administrative aspects of psychotherapy such as fees, cancellation policy, and confidentiality are reviewed in this initial meeting. The therapist also discusses ways to prepare the child for his or her first visit, something that parents are often uncertain how to do. It is not uncommon to have the child arrive for the appointment with no prior knowledge of where he or she was going or why. The parents need to simply inform the child that they have made an appointment with a special type of doctor, one who helps to figure out problems but who does not administer familiar types of medical care, such as giving shots. The parents indicate that it is their belief that the therapist can assist the child and them with the current difficulties. They can also state that this type of doctor uses toys and games as the treatment equipment and that the child will have a chance to investigate these during the appointment. While parents should answer if the child has additional questions, it is not necessary to inundate the child with a detailed description of the play therapy process. Such an explanation could both confuse the child and generate anxiety. More information about therapy can be furnished in a natural way as the sessions go along.

Meeting the Child Patient

Regardless of the child's age, upon meeting the child, the therapist should greet the child by name before the parents. This action makes it evident to both child and parent who the patient is and where the therapist's focus will be. Some children may be apprehensive about separating from the parent. It is not recommended that the child be "forced" to separate but rather, that the therapist acknowledge the child's concern, and if need be, suggest that the parent accompany the therapist and child to the office. In this way, the child is certain that the parent knows where he/she is and vice versa. If the child continues to be uncomfortable, the parent should be permitted to stay. Preschoolers may initially need the parent to remain for the entire session but the therapist must ensure that the attention is fixed on the child. Having a parent in the room may pose an extra challenge for some therapists (particularly new ones) as feelings of inhibition, self-consciousness and professional uncertainty may surface. It is helpful for the therapist to keep in mind that despite his or her discomfort, the parent is undoubtedly feeling more nervous and that the parental focus is probably on the child.

The First Session

How to proceed during the first session will depend to some degree on the therapist's theoretical orientation. Nondirective play therapy recommends following the child's thoughts and actions and refraining from doing more than reflecting back to the child. Brief psychodynamic therapy starts with the identification of general treatment goals [19]. However, the common denominator among all theory bases is the requirement for a therapeutic alliance, and the therapist's actions and comments should be made with this end point in mind. Acceptance and respect for the patient, essential components of the alliance, need to be conveyed to the patient early in the therapy. Like other aspects of psychotherapy, these features will be communicated to the child patient somewhat differently than to the adult. The question of acceptance, which may be raised in subtle ways by adults, is often more apparent with children and may call for a more direct response.

CASE STUDY

Clinical Example

A child, aged six, reluctantly entered the therapist's office having been referred for difficulties with anger. She had lived in multiple foster homes and had grown used to new settings and new rules; her outbursts seemed to have become worse with each change. She announced to the therapist that she was like a tornado. She added that tornadoes occurred outdoors, were very dangerous, and needed to be avoided. The therapist commented that the patient seemed to know a lot about tornadoes and it might be scary to feel like one. Perhaps the best idea would be to stay in the office where they could learn more about tornadoes and tornado-feelings together.

In this example, the patient clearly is concerned about the destructiveness of her anger and the potential impact it might have on the therapist. Respect for the patient and acceptance of her anger is communicated by the therapist in the following ways:

(1) The therapist does not undo the displacement. She stays with the child's language and talks about tornado-feelings, not her actual anger. She accepts the patient's need for the defense.
(2) The therapist's statement to remain in the office and work together obviously conveys acceptance of the patient and her feelings. It also suggests to her, perhaps unconsciously, that the therapist will be able to "weather her storms."
(3) The therapist's statement confirming the patient's knowledge of "tornadoes" shows awareness and respect for her experiences.

Many children will look for some direction from the therapist in the first several sessions as they might from the adults at home or school. It can therefore be helpful to familiarize the child with the office and any relevant limitations, such as the therapist's desk or file cabinet. When showing the toys, it is important to include a statement about the unique role they play in therapy. For instance, the therapist might say: "Here is where I keep the play materials. We will use them as we play and work together to help us better understand your feelings." This type of introduction makes the point to the child, right from the start, that toys are used differently in therapy than in other settings. It also identifies the therapist as a person who will work with the child, rather than instruct him or her. During the initial sessions, the therapist's task is to provide an atmosphere of safety and acceptance, as well as to note the emergence of play themes. The concerns and conflicts of most children can be expressed through play even when they are not or cannot be discussed verbally [17]. The therapist's remarks should be tailored to the child's developmental level. Without probing or pressing, the therapist's statements should correspond to the child's moves and comments.

CASE STUDY

Clinical Example

A 3 year 6-month-old boy was referred for an evaluation due to aggressive behavior. The therapist and the boy's mother agreed that the mother could remain in the office for the first several sessions, although the mother was advised to be as unobtrusive as possible. The patient quickly left mother's side and easily explored the office, looking under chairs and eyeing toys that were quite visible on the shelf. The therapist commented, "there are so many new things to look at in this place. You do not need mother right now; you can be an explorer on your own." The boy found a foam ball and threw it to the therapist, who returned the pitch stating: "We can play something together, now that you've found the ball!" The patient then went to the dolls' house and threw the baby doll out the window, and said that "the family did not need that baby anyway." The therapist, knowing about the recent birth of a sibling, added: "The family seemed fine the way it was before baby sister was born."

In this example, the therapist pulled out what appeared to be the main threads in the interaction between herself and the patient without overinterpreting or patronizing. First, the therapist noticed that the child is able to leave mother's side to investigate the new place. Such curiosity is both desirable and developmentally appropriate; the therapist's comment speaks to this achievement. Second, the therapist noted the patient's effort to initiate contact with her. Her subsequent action and comment demonstrated her willingness to reciprocate. Third, the therapist slightly extended and thereby perhaps clarified the child's comment. Fourth, the therapist did not make a link between the patient's action and his real-life sibling. To have made a direct connection between the patient's action and his home situation would have been premature for several reasons. This particular session was diagnostic, in which the purpose leans more toward observation and formulation than interpretation. Second, such a remark would have undone the displacement, potentially leaving the child inadequately defended. Third, the child might have been made anxious by the comment and inhibit his play as a result.

Continuing Therapy

One of the basic precepts of psychotherapy is to begin "where the patient is." Child patients will respond to the therapist with emotions and behaviors that reflect not only where their development has been derailed but also the defenses with which they have protected themselves. In the beginning period of treatment, child patients learn that the therapist is a person whom they can trust and who can accept their needs, wishes, and fears. A connection then forms between patient and therapist, which in turn, enables the child to invest in the therapy. During the middle phase of treatment, the therapist and child work together to achieve a sense of a more organized self. The patient has an idea of his or her conflicts and can safely explore them with the therapist. The final stage of treatment brings resolution to or a reduction of the child's difficulties and acceptance of the change that has occurred. It is not uncommon at this time to see the reappearance of original issues as the child deals with separating from the therapist, a person who has become very meaningful to the child.

Limit Setting

Psychotherapy with both adults and children involves the setting of limits. Indeed, from the outset, limits are demarcated by the therapist as he or she establishes the frame with the patient and details the conditions of therapy [20]. These requirements include at a minimum, the therapist's payment and cancellation policy, informed consent, and the limits of confidentiality. While most therapists are comfortable establishing limits, there is far more uncertainty when it comes to the testing or the enforcing of them. With child patients, whose behavior might result in damage to the office or therapist, limits are clearly necessary. There is agreement among most therapists that the office space, the therapist, and the patient cannot be hurt, and these rules must be clearly established and enforced. Otherwise, it is not necessary or even possible for the therapist to spell out every limit that might be required. It is more practical instead to limit the problematic behavior as it arises. Nonetheless, some therapists are uncomfortable with such ambiguity and it is beneficial to know at what point the child's behavior exceeds one's own limit of acceptable behavior. The following guidelines can be used to set limits [21].

- First, the therapist provides a verbal reflection to the child of his attitudes or wishes.

  Example: *I see that you want to take the puppets home with you and that is why you are trying to put them in your bag.*

- Second, the therapist verbally states the limit.

  Example: *I can tell that you want to take the puppets home very much, so much that you are trying to take them out of the office. But the play materials must stay here and you can use them when you are here.*

- Third, the therapist intervenes physically to control the child's behavior.

  Example: *While I know how much you want to take the puppets with you, they must stay here until next time [therapist removes them from the child].*

It can be very frightening to a child to feel that the adult is unable or unwilling to maintain adequate control. By defining and enforcing the limits of safe and acceptable behavior, the therapist assures the child that his or her impulses can be tolerated and contained.

Conclusion

Although methods of play therapy have both evolved and expanded over time, its value as a clinical intervention remains [22]. Play therapy provides a way for the child patient to define and understand personal struggles within a developmentally appropriate context.

References

1. Elkind D. *The Hurried Child*, 3rd edn. Perseus Books, 2001.
2. Freud S. *The Dynamics of Transference*, Standard Edition (12), 1912.
3. Axline V. *Play Therapy*. New York: Ballantine Books, 1947.
4. Marans S, Mayes L, Colonna A. Psychoanalytic views of children's play. In: Solnit AJ, Cohen DJ, Neubauer PB (eds) *The Many Meanings of Play*. New Haven, CN: Yale University Press, 1993; pp. 9–28.
5. Waelder R. The psychoanalytic theory of play. *Psychoanal Quart* 1933;**2**;208–224.
6. Erikson EH. *Childhood and Society*. New York: Norton, 1950.
7. Winnicott DW. *Playing and Reality*. London: Routledge, 1971.
8. Landreth G, Baggerly J, Tyndall-Lind A. Beyond adapting adult counseling skills for use with children: The paradigm shift to child-centered play therapy. *J Indiv Psychol* 1999;**55**:272–287.
9. Kottman T. Integrating the crucial Cs into Adlerian play therapy. *J Indiv Psychol* 1999;**55**:288–297.
10. Solnit AJ, Cohen DJ, Neubauer PB. *The Many Meanings of Play*. New Haven, CT: Yale University Press, 1993.
11. Knell S. Cognitive-behavioral play therapy. *J Clin Child Psychol* 1999;**27**:28–33.
12. Kottman T, Schaefer C. *Play Therapy in Action: A Casebook for Practitioners*. New Jersey: Jason Aronson, Inc.
13. Prat R. Imaginary Hide and Seek, A technique for opening psychic space in child psychotherapy. *J Child Psychother* 2001;**27**:2.
14. Ginsburg H, Opper S. *Piaget's Theory of Intellectual Development: An Introduction*. Englewood Cliffs, NJ: Prentice-Hall, 1969.
15. McWilliams N. *Psychoanalytic Psychotherapy*. New York: Guilford Press, 2004.
16. Caroll J. Play therapy: the children's views. *Child FamSoc Work* 2002;**7**:177–187.
17. Schaefer C. *The Therapeutic Powers of Play*. Jason Aronson, 1993.
18. Wilson K, Ryan V. Helping parents by working with their children in individual child therapy. *Child FamSoc Work* 2001;**6**:209–218.
19. Racusin R. Brief psychodynamic psychotherapy with young children. *J Am Acad Child AdolescPsychiat* 2000:**39**:791–793.
20. Luborsky L. *The Principles of Psychoanalytic Psychotherapy*. Basic Books, 1984.
21. Schaefer C. *The Therapeutic Use of Child's Play*. Jason Aronson, 1979.
22. LeBlanc M, Ritchie M. A meta-analysis of play therapy outcomes. *CounsPsychol Q* 2001;**14**:2.

9

Cognitive Behavioral Therapy

Christina C. Clark

Introduction

Today's mental health providers serving the needs of children, adolescents, and their families are strongly encouraged to implement treatment strategies that are evidence-based. For the purposes of this chapter, the term evidence-based practice (EBP) will be used to denote treatment that is formulated and delivered using evidence-based best practice recommendations and relies on current research [1]. Cognitive behavioral therapy (CBT) is increasingly recognized as an empirically supported method for psychosocial treatment with children and adolescents.

For this population, CBT has been shown to be an effective treatment for internalizing disorders [2], including anxiety [3–6], social phobia [7, 8], obsessive-compulsive disorder (OCD) [9], post-traumatic stress disorder (PTSD) [10], depression [11], anger/aggression [12, 13], disruptive behaviors disorders [14], including oppositional defiant disorder and conduct disorder (CD), substance abuse [15], and attention-deficit hyperactivity disorder (ADHD) [16]. Children with ADHD respond best to behavioral treatment that includes a parent training component [17].

As a result, various treatment approaches building on the research have been developed, then collected into clinically oriented volumes [18, 19] containing numerous CBT-oriented approaches for specific disorders/populations. Even more specifically, Ollendick and March [20] compiled a clinician-targeted volume of evidence-based psychosocial treatments for youth with anxiety and phobias. A special issue of *Child and Adolescent Psychiatric Clinics of North America* [21] devoted to CBT with youth included topics such as: flexible use of CBT in clinical practice; the history of CBT with youth; CBT for adolescent depression and suicide, anxiety disorders, obsessive-compulsive behavior, post-traumatic stress disorder, weight management/eating disorders, body dysmorphic disorder, tic disorders, chronic physical illness; CBT with younger (preschool/school-age) children; and core principles.

Given the mounting evidence for CBT to demonstrate such far-reaching utility [1, 21], practitioners would do children and adolescents a service by incorporating CBT into clinical settings. To do so, mental health practitioners need much more than a rudimentary knowledge of CBT or its techniques. CBT is not a one-size-fits-all approach nor is it merely a set of techniques or a "cookbook" approach. It is unlikely and impractical to believe that research protocols would or could be adopted in their entirety in clinical settings; on the other hand, too much variation from the original protocols has potential to dilute treatment effectiveness. Therefore, approaches that are flexible while adhering to CBT's fundamentals – "flexibility within fidelity" [22] – are recommended [23]. In order to equip clinicians to do this, dissemination of CBT has become a central focus.

This chapter is offered as part of the effort to disseminate knowledge and practice of CBT and, as such, may be used as a resource for clinicians interested in delivering CBT to children and adolescents. The overall approach of the chapter proposes the melding of basic principles of CBT with specifics from research: professionals in clinical settings need to keep up with current evidence-based findings. But how can this be done efficiently and effectively? Fortunately, modern technology (DVDs, podcasts, websites, webinars, online journals) has the potential to hasten and/or make this process more convenient for busy practitioners. More will be said about bridging the research-practice "gap" in the section discussing development as a CBT practitioner.

Before discussing CBT-specific information, a brief overview of important issues that should be considered regardless of theoretical approach is given. This is followed by specific CBT-oriented information, including a brief description of the CBT model and its principles. Following that, treatment will be discussed.

Clinical Child Psychiatry, Third Edition. Edited by William M. Klykylo and Jerald Kay.
© 2012 John Wiley & Sons, Ltd. Published 2012 by John Wiley & Sons, Ltd.

Finally, a set of guidelines that can help clinicians integrate theory and research into daily use with children and adolescents will be presented.

Special Issues

Children and adolescents constitute a "special population," and as such, require the clinician to pay particular attention to certain aspects of treatment. These considerations are not unique to CBT; however, as they are integral to clinical work with this population they will be briefly highlighted here. Included are ethical considerations, developmental factors, family involvement, and cultural factors. These issues are not discrete "entities," in other words, these considerations often interact or overlap.

Mental health professionals serving children, adolescents, and their families need to remain mindful of the complex nature of serving various family members and of the fact that children are still developing, i.e., they are vulnerable [24, 25]. Ethical considerations include, but are not limited to, issues related to referral, informed consent, and provision of effective treatment. Children and adolescents are typically brought to treatment by adults, usually parents [26, 27]. Although the child may be identified as the "patient," it is the adults who are typically stating what they would like treatment to address. Mental health providers consider the perspectives of all parties and attempt to determine what is likely to be in the best interest of the child [25] – which at times may be in direct opposition to what the parents are requesting, resulting in potential conflicts of interest [26]. However, the mental health provider who has followed ethical and legal guidelines regarding informed consent (e.g., encouraging participation and providing information in developmentally appropriate language [25]) has made it a habit to discuss expectations, responsibilities, risks/benefits, and outcome at the outset of treatment and as needed. Best practices for obtaining informed consent with children are briefly outlined by Fisher *et al.* [24].

Special attention to developmental factors, on the part of the clinician, is required throughout the therapy process. Doing so increases the likelihood that developmentally appropriate communication and assessment procedures occur, leading to developmentally titrated goals and selection of interventions. As a result, clinicians report that the child is often more engaged [28–31]. Furthermore, it would appear that the likelihood of progress is increased because, according to Holmbeck *et al.* [32], developmental sensitivity is thought to increase quality of treatment, though more developmentally oriented research is needed to determine whether this is true. In the meantime, Holmbeck and colleagues [32], in a

chapter discussing the relevance of developmental issues for therapists and researchers, have included a table of developmental milestones (Table 9.1) for child/adolescent therapists to integrate into treatment. Finally, it is useful to distinguish between "deficiency" and "distortion" [33–35] when working with children, and to recognize that either or both can occur. That is to say, the therapist needs to determine whether a child is engaging in inaccurate thinking or simply lacks skills/experience and aim interventions accordingly.

Generally speaking, the younger the child, the more likely it is that parents may become involved in treatment. This is because the child is still in the process of developing; therefore, they are dependent on parents for guidance and support. Furthermore, the younger the child, the more likely it is that problems are occurring within the family setting. Therefore, taking into account the interactions between the family and the child/adolescent will be an important part of understanding the child and delivering treatment. In most cases, the therapist should work to ensure that adults(s) involved have a good understanding of appropriate developmental expectations, as recommended by Holmbeck *et al.* [32]. In addition, the clinician facilitates parents' exploration of their own beliefs [36, 37] regarding developmental expectations and helps them to recognize when their own beliefs (thinking), feelings, and/or behavior may contribute to the child's problems.

The mention of parents elicits a parenthetical remark: Although many texts use the word "parent" to denote adults involved in the child's life, throughout this chapter the terms "parent" and "caregiver" will be used interchangeably to describe any adult who would live with and/or have major day-to-day responsibility for the child including biological and/or step-parents, grandparents, other biological relatives, foster-parents, adoptive parents, or other adults.

Other contextual areas that should be attended to by the clinician include school, peer group, religion, sexual orientation, social class, and ethnicity/culture [38]. To aid clinicians pay particular attention to these important areas, Friedberg and McClure [30] compiled a table of culturally sensitive questions (Table 9.2) and Fisher *et al.* [24]. briefly outline a set of best practices for culturally valid assessment and treatment.

Principles of Cognitive Behavioral Therapy

Cognitive therapists remain mindful of the basic principles regarding the process of cognitive therapy as they work with clients. These principles as outlined by Beck [39] include the idea that the process is collaborative, structured, active, time-limited, and goal-oriented.

Table 9.1 Developmental milestones and stages across childhood, adolescence, and emerging adulthood.

Infancy (0–2 years)	• Infants explore world via direct sensory–motor contact • Emergence of emotions • Object permanence and separation anxiety develop • Critical attachment period: secure parent–infant bond promotes trust and healthy growth of infant; insecure bonds create distrust and distress for infant • Initial use of sounds and words to communicate • Piaget's Sensorimotor stage
Toddler/preschool years (2–6 years)	• Use of multiple words and symbols to communicate • Learns self-care skills • Mainly characterized by egocentricity, but preschoolers appreciate differences in perspectives of others • Use of imagination, engagement in 'pretend' play • Increasing sense of autonomy and control of environment • Develop school readiness skills • Piaget's Preoperational stage
Middle childhood (6–10 years)	• Social, physical, and academic skills develop • Logical thinking and reasoning develops • Increased interaction with peers • Increasing self-control and emotion regulation • Piaget's Concrete Operational stage
Adolescence (10–18 years)	• Pubertal development; sexual development • Development of metacognition (i.e., use of higher-order strategizing in learning; thinking about one's own thinking) • Higher cognitive skills develop, including abstraction, consequential thinking, hypothetical reasoning, and perspective taking • Transformations in parent–child relationships; increase in family conflicts • Peer relationships increasingly important and intimate • Making transition from childhood to adulthood • Developing sense of identity and autonomous functioning • Piaget's Formal Operations stage
Emerging adulthood (18–25 years)	• Establishment of meaningful and enduring interpersonal relationships • Identity explorations in areas of love, work, and worldviews • Peak of certain risk behaviors • Obtaining education and training for long-term adult occupation

Reproduced from Holmbeck *et al.* [32], with permission.

The conceptualization of the client evolves continually as new information comes to light. Based on that conceptualization, numerous cognitive and/or behavioral techniques are suggested to aid the client in exploring and changing cognitions and/or behaviors. Typically, at the beginning the therapist takes on more of the responsibility for the content and direction of therapy; however, another principle holds that the ultimate goal is for the therapist to educate the client to become their own cognitive therapist.

Collaboration includes the notion of a positive therapeutic alliance with the client, and this is most likely achieved when the therapist demonstrates the well-known common factors including skills of "accurate empathy." This can be a particularly demanding and challenging task when working with children and adolescents, because it is not uncommon for caregivers to be involved in the treatment, in which case the therapist needs to consider how to work collaboratively with various members of the system without alienating or favoring anyone.

Sessions are structured (with mood-check, review of homework, agenda setting, addressing issues, feedback, and setting new homework) [39, 40]. While it may seem

Table 9.2 Sample questions addressing cultural context issues.

- What is the level of acculturation in the family?
- How does the level of acculturation shape symptom expression?
- What characterizes the child's ethnocultural identity?
- How does this identity influence symptom expression?
- What are the child and family thinking and feeling as a member of this culture?
- How do ethnocultural beliefs, values, and practices shape problem expression?
- How representative or typical is this family of the culture?
- What feelings and thoughts are proscribed as taboo?
- What feelings and thoughts are facilitated and promoted as a function of ethnocultural context?
- What ethnocultural specific socialization processes selectively reinforce some thoughts, feelings, and behaviors but not others?
- What types of prejudice and marginalization has the child/family encountered?
- How have these experiences shaped symptom expression?
- What beliefs about oneself, the world, and the future have developed as a result of these experiences?

Reproduced from Friedberg and McClure [30], with permission.

obvious, again, it is important to keep in mind what is developmentally appropriate with regard to structure. Therefore, as long as each of the session elements gets addressed during the therapy hour, younger children may require a greater amount of flexibility.

Content of the session (as well as "homework") needs to engage the child or adolescent. How is this done? We return to the theme of developmental "fit." In general, the younger the child, the more active and play-oriented treatment will be. Preschoolers may need toys, games, books, and/or a sandbox as, generally speaking, play is their "language." Relaxation skills can be delivered in a playful way, for example, using games like Simon Says or using soap bubbles to teach them to moderate their breathing. School-age children enjoy activities such as drawing, crafts, games, books, and age-appropriate workbooks, such as *Therapeutic Exercises for Children* [40]. Adolescents are frequently able to engage in talk therapy similar to that of adults but homework might involve journaling, poetry, or artwork. The therapist uses "guided discovery" to help the child, adolescent, and/or caregivers to increase understanding and to learn/practice new ways of thinking and behaving.

Setting goals is an opportunity for collaboration as well as for the therapist to gain additional understanding of beliefs and expectations of the child/adolescent, as well as the caregivers. Input from the child/adolescent should be solicited at the level judged to be developmentally appropriate.

In addition to helping the client with his/her current concerns, cognitive therapy takes an educative approach, that is, to prepare them to learn skills and general concepts that can be extended to their life after therapy. CBT attempts to help the client "become their own cognitive therapist" [39] by teaching the client skills to apply to current problems while simultaneously teaching them about the CBT model and learning to formulate a coherent "picture" (conceptualization) of themselves. Therefore, the therapist is not doing something to the client, but is teaching the client how to understand themselves and what to do to help themselves, both now and, hopefully, in the future. The therapist attempts to establish alliances with all participants and explains the conceptualization to individuals within the system at the level that is developmentally appropriate for each member.

The Model

Cognitive behavioral therapy (CBT) is based on a combination [5, 41] of behavioral principles such as classical and operant conditioning combined with concepts from social learning theory [30]. Cognitive therapy emphasizes the role of thinking (i.e., cognitive mediation), which mutually interacts with three other aspects of a person, namely, behavior, emotions, and physical reactions [42–44]. In turn, a person affects and is affected by, his/her environment [44]. Environment or context, which is particularly relevant for children and adolescents, includes peers, family, and teachers.

Given the emphasis on cognition as playing a major role in influencing emotions, behavior, and physical reactions, several points are relevant here. First, thinking is not a unitary concept: cognition is an information-processing system [28, 45]. This system comprises different levels of thinking, structures, and processes including automatic thoughts, intermediate beliefs (rules, attitudes, assumptions), schemas, and compensatory strategies [28, 39, 43]. Automatic thoughts are the most accessible level of thinking, which can be thought of as the running commentary that goes through your head during your daily activities. Intermediate beliefs are conditional and reveal assumptions or rules used by the patient to organize his/her experience. For example, a child who receives praise only when achieving may come to believe "If I work hard enough, I will be loved."

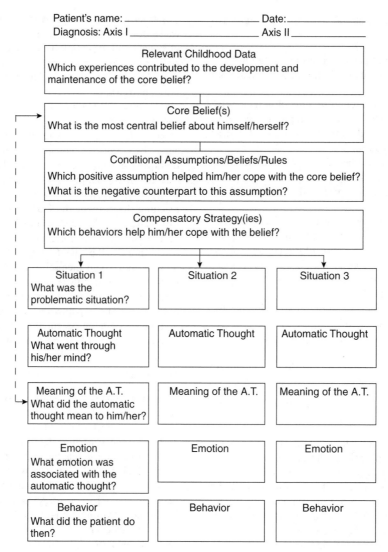

Figure 9.1 Cognitive Conceptualization Diagram.

Schemas or core beliefs are typically absolute, such as "I am unlovable" and are usually brought to light over time by the therapist. Compensatory strategies refer to the behaviors that help the patient deal with their beliefs [39]. Continuing with the example above, a compensatory strategy for a child with these beliefs would be for him/her to work to achieve what is expected by those whose love he/she wants. These levels of thinking are captured on the Cognitive Conceptualization Diagram [39], shown in Figure 9.1. Beck [39] provides detailed explanation of these structures and gives strategies for eliciting client cognitions as well as modifying them, although not geared specifically to children and adoles-

cents. Stallard [46] demonstrates the application of some of these concepts with children and adolescents.

Second, according to the content-specificity hypothesis proposed by Beck [45], cognitive content will reflect themes that correlate with specific disorders [43]. For example, anxiety disorders are characterized by cognitions related to themes of threat, whereas depression is characterized by themes of loss. A study including children and adolescents aged 7–16 demonstrated support for the content-specificity hypothesis, for both internalizing and externalizing disorders [47]. Finally, the distinction of "deficiency versus distortion" [27] is particularly relevant for the therapist working with children and adolescents because the distinction will influence intervention selection.

Adaptations

Although the cognitive behavioral model has produced evidence for positive treatment outcome, further investigation is needed to explore mediators and moderators of treatment [48] and to extend CBT's use to more diverse populations within children and adolescents. The process is underway. Attempts to adapt the CBT model to even younger children continue. For example, treatment of pediatric OCD has advanced within the last decade with results supporting the use of CBT as a viable treatment [49]. Since these investigations have not generally included children under the age of 7, recent work to extend the model to children aged 5–8 has been done [50]. To aid families and clinicians working with this population, recommendations for adaptations [51] and a workbook [52] for targeting treatment for OCD with this population have been developed.

Other extensions to young children include cognitive developmental therapy [31] (CDT) and cognitive behavioral play therapy [53, 54] (CBPT). Although CDT and CBPT have not been subjected to randomized controlled trial (RCT) studies, case studies are available to illustrate their principles. Both CDT and CBPT utilize play techniques. Although play has long been used as a technique in child-oriented therapy, there are few RCT studies to evaluate its effectiveness. Russ [55], apparently in an attempt to encourage the integration of play (in ways that are empirically supported), has compiled information that could be valuable to practitioners working with young children.

Developing the Conceptualization

Conceptualization is an essential cornerstone for effective delivery of CBT and refers to the process by which the therapist gathers and integrates information from several sources [30, 39, 56, 57] including: (i) knowledge of child/adolescent normal biopsychosocial development; [32] (ii) knowledge of child/adolescent psychopathology; (iii) knowledge of the cognitive behavioral model, including generic models of pathology and the content-specificity hypothesis; and (iv) specific presenting symptoms, including the background of the child/adolescent and his/her family. Once integrated, this information creates a "picture" of the client allowing the therapist to understand and make predictions (i.e., generate hypotheses) about the client and his/her family.

The rationale for developing a conceptualization is that, simply put, it leads to effective treatment [56].

Why? Because a cogent conceptualization that accounts for the client's problems and proposes to understand the underlying mechanisms will aid the therapist in delivering appropriate treatment, including selecting, timing, and tailoring interventions [56, 58]. Once the initial conceptualization is developed, the therapist uses the model to generate and test hypotheses regarding treatment approaches and specific interventions. As treatment progresses the therapist continues to collect information about the client while also deciding whether hypotheses are supported or disconfirmed. Therapists are not tied to their original ideas, because as scientist-practitioners, they revise the conceptualization in an iterative fashion [30, 39]. With each "successive approximation," however, the model should become clearer and more accurate, forming the basis for both within-session and extra-session [58] decisions about the client.

A second use for the conceptualization is to promote client self-awareness, leading to generalization of skills. This is accomplished by sharing the working model of the client with him/her. That being said, it is paramount that the therapist considers the capacity of the client to receive and process information. Expectations for the level of sophistication regarding the conceptualization would be based on the client's developmental level. For example, a young child may have the capacity to recognize and label feelings along with a recent situation whereas a school-age child may be able to begin to identify themes like "I always get mad when my Mom tells me no but not when my teacher tells me no." Adolescents, if motivated, may want to link their formative experiences with current patterns: "I was always worried that I would disappoint my Dad so I never tried new things to keep from failing at them." Clinicians could make use of the Cognitive Conceptualization Diagram [39] for adolescents and, with some adaptation/assistance from the therapist, may be able to have the teen complete it also. From the foundation of the well-developed conceptualization, the therapist begins to make use of it for treatment.

Treatment

A typical outline for an episode of CBT treatment is shown in Table 9.3 [59]. Generally speaking, while making initial treatment recommendations, I explain that frequently each family member may need to do their own changing to help the child or adolescent who has been brought in for treatment. In addition, I provide the rationale for my decisions to the client (titrated to their developmental level) and his/her parents as well as expectations for therapy. Whenever possible, I prefer

Table 9.3 Outline of standard course of cognitive behavioral therapy

1. Therapist elicits information regarding the development of specific symptoms, as well as situational determinants and temporal course. Objective and subjective data are collected (preferably from multiple informants) regarding the nature of the presenting problem.
2. A goal list is developed with the child and the parents or other caregiver. Cognitive behavioral formulation and treatment recommendations are shared with the child and his or her parents.
3. Underlying beliefs, attitudes, assumptions, expectations, attributions, goals, and selfstatements or automatic thoughts are identified. Patients learn to monitor negative or maladaptive thoughts and emotions. Attempts at selfmonitoring are rewarded.
4. Specific behavioral and interpersonal skills deficits are identified.
5. Medical, social, and environmental factors maintaining the symptoms are identified. The latter may include stressful life events (both major and minor, short-term and chronic) or the modeling and reinforcement of the symptoms by others in the child's life.
6. Cognitive and behavioral interventions are selected and introduced based upon the specific needs of the child.
7. Homework is assigned. The patient practices the cognitive or behavioral skills during the session. Attempts are made to ensure that the interventions are clearly understood, that the child is motivated to attempt the assignment, and that they expect the intervention to be helpful. Factors that may interfere with the successful completion of the homework assignment are identified and addressed.
8. Effectiveness of the intervention is evaluated through objective ratings, behavioral observations, and subjective reports.
9. Relapse prevention interventions are introduced. Follow-up or booster sessions are scheduled.

to hold this meeting with everyone involved; however, in cases where it appears it may be counter-therapeutic (e.g., the parent's actions cause the child to "shut down"), I meet individually with separate parties. Expectations include responsibilities of both parties and an overview of the anticipated treatment process. For example, families who have a child with symptoms of OCD should understand that exposure with response prevention (E/RP) will likely be a significant aspect of treatment. At the beginning of treatment, however, the

details of how E/RP will be carried out are not yet known for that particular child.

Treatment focuses simultaneously on two levels of intervention: addressing the specific here-and-now problems of the client, and secondly, teaching the client skills and concepts that would prevent relapse as well as deal with future problems [39].

Research on how best to involve parents in CBT treatment has been limited; what is meant by a parental or family component to treatment has not been well-defined in the research studies; and adding parents to the treatment can present challenges. However, based on the number of evidence-based treatments that include parents and appear to be effective, clinicians need to routinely consider inclusion of parents. There are several reasons for this. Involving parents in treatment can help support the child: the parents act as a "coach," reminding the child what they've learned and helping him/her to use it between sessions or after termination. A second advantage of involving parents in treatment is the opportunity for the clinician to assess and address, if necessary, the parent-child relationship and its impact on the child's symptoms, parental beliefs, and expectations.

Typically treatment will consist of interventions that combine both behavioral and cognitive techniques [60] that have been selected by the therapist to fit that specific individual [30], as well as taking into account the client's developmental capacity [31]. Independent of technique, however, it is paramount that the therapist ensures that the child or adolescent understands the CBT model, namely, the link between thinking and feelings. Friedberg and McClure [30] suggest that clinicians select techniques based on the stage of therapy. For example, it would be prudent to ensure that the client can identify/distinguish thoughts and feelings before the therapist implements more complex techniques.

Determining whether the treatment strategy is effective should be evaluated on an ongoing basis by having the client describe their understanding as well as determining what mood or behavioral changes are occurring. If the therapist sees that a particular intervention is not working, the therapist will attempt to determine the source of difficulty so as to modify some aspect of the current approach or to select a new intervention. All these decisions are made based upon the revised conceptualization.

Examples of Treatment

Let us turn to some examples to illustrate, in particular, adapting CBT interventions to children at different stages of development. Consider a male who has been brought to treatment by his mother, who reports he has been having behavioral problems at school (arguing and fighting with peers). During the first interview, the mother provides information that supports a diagnosis of oppositional defiant disorder (ODD). Furthermore, you have decided that the child may be depressed based on your observation of him and his responses to some questions. During a later session, while the therapist and the child's mother are discussing an incident that occurred at school (the child is present in the room), the child wants to speak with his mother. He tries getting her attention twice, then yells, picks up an object, preparing to throw it at her.

Preschool Age (age 4^1/$_2$ years)

Mother: (angrily) That is not nice! You could hurt someone doing that!

Child: But mommy...

Therapist: What made you get ready to throw that?

C: She wouldn't listen to me.

TH: And how did you feel when she didn't listen?

C: Huh?

TH: (changing strategies to labeling) I wonder if you felt mad?

C: No.

TH: Well I heard your voice get loud, like a tiger growling, and your face got red. I think that goes with being mad. You got mad when she kept on talking.

C: (nods)

TH: I wonder what else you could have done?

C: I dunno.

TH: Here, let me show you. Well, you could just "zip your lip" (making zipping gesture and funny face, child smiles) until Mommy stopped talking, or you could have tried staying still and raising your hand, or if it was real real important (like having to go to the restroom), you could even flap your hand around like a flag like this! And that would let us know you can't wait for us to stop talking. But that's only something you do once in a while. Understand?

C: (nods yes)

TH: OK, let's practice with Mommy right now.

School Age (age 9)

Mother: (angrily) That is not nice! You could hurt someone doing that!

Child: But...

Therapist: What made you get ready to throw that?

C: She wouldn't listen to me.

TH: And how did you feel when she didn't listen?

C: Mad.

TH: Yeah, I can see how mad you must feel because I heard your voice getting louder and louder.

C: Yep.

TH: I wonder what you said to yourself inside your head when she didn't listen.

C: She never listens to me. All she ever does is yell (Starts to cry and mother starts to comfort him).

TH: I wonder if there was anything else in your head about your mom....

C: Maybe she loves my sister more.

Adolescence (14 years)

Mother: (angrily) That is not nice! You could hurt someone doing that!

Child: But...I didn't throw it.

Therapist: What made you get ready to throw that?

C: She wouldn't listen to me.

TH: And how did you feel when she didn't listen?

C: Frustrated.

TH: And what was going through your mind?

C: Parents never listen to their kids because they think they know everything!

TH: How often do you get as mad as today?

C: Almost every time we talk about school, because all they ever do is get on my back!

CASE STUDY

Case One: Preschool Age

Danny, age 5 years 6 months, was brought to treatment by his mother who was concerned about his growing oppositional and defiant behaviors, which occurred primarily in the home setting but had also started to manifest in kindergarten. Initially, the therapist recommended that Mom use a behavioral chart with three daily tasks, two that were already occurring (so she could practice praise and positive reinforcement) and one challenging task that tended to elicit opposition. After two weeks of using the chart, an exasperated Mom said that the client's behavior had actually become more oppositional, not less. In the meantime, the therapist asked his mother to note any patterns related to opposition. The only pattern she could see was that when Danny cried, he became more oppositional. Further discussion of recent events revealed that when Danny was asked to do the difficult task, he would frequently cry, to which Mom responded by saying it wasn't so hard or that it wouldn't take very long. When asked if she talked with him about his crying or attempted to comfort him, she expressed concerns that this would make him into a cry baby and he would try to get out of doing things. Two interventions took place over time to address the interaction between Danny and his mother. First, the therapist explained that expressing understanding of children's feelings does not mean that the parent has to "cave" to whatever the child wants. To gain a more in-depth understanding of how to deal with Danny's negative feelings, his mother was asked to read a parenting book that explains the role of parent as "coach." [61] At the same time, the therapist gathered information from play with Danny, then modeled for his mother how to "coach" Danny through difficult feelings. Due to his age, a small sandbox with plastic animals (he chose horses) was used to facilitate the play. The following example shows how information was collected:

TH: So, this horse here (pointing to smaller horse). Is it a boy or girl horse?
D: A boy.
TH: I wonder how old he is...
D: Five and a half!
TH: And I see that the mommy horse just asked him to take his nap.
D: Yep, and he doesn't want to.
TH: How do you know?
D: Because he wants to play.
TH: So he wants to play – oh, and I think I hear him crying.
D: Yup (frown).
TH: Hmmm. I wonder what the mommy horse could do to help him?
D: Tell him he can play.
TH: Well, but mommy horse wants him to have his nap. I know, she can tell him he can take his favorite book to read while he goes to sleep and then he can play when he wakes up. Or...mommy horse can say, "It isn't that hard to take a nap."
D: No, it's better if she says it's OK for him to take a book into his room.
TH: OK, so he goes and finds his favorite book – do you think he is still crying?
D: No, I don't hear him crying but he still would like to play.
TH: I know.

Comment: Although all of the oppositional behavior did not disappear, through the combination of his mother reading and learning how to interact in a more positive fashion with Danny, about 8 weeks into treatment, she stated, "You know, after reading that book, I realize that I was a big part of the problem." Over time, Danny continued to reveal more of his feelings and thoughts to his mother, who learned to tolerate negative affect and "coach" him.

This example illustrates how a parent's beliefs about developmental expectations can interact with and influence a child's behavior. It also demonstrates that the child was most likely operating from "deficits" that were addressed when his mother learned how to respond to him. Finally, the "coaching" stance of the parent is a good example of a parent modeling emotional regulation and problem-solving for the child.

CASE STUDY

Case Two: Middle Childhood

Alonzo, a 9-year 4-month-old Latino male, was brought for treatment by his single mother, who explained that he was being treated for ADHD by a psychiatrist, who advised the mother to seek psychological services to help her manage her son's temper outbursts. His mother has been working with his teacher to track his daily in-school behaviors, including turning in assignments, paying attention, transitioning, and not interrupting. The daily goal was to obtain an OK in each area, thereby earning points that he could "cash in" at school for rewards. Furthermore, his mother based home privileges on his school behaviors, as reported by his teacher. As long as Alonzo's behavior was in the acceptable range, all was fine. When it wasn't, however, he would receive a "warning" from the teacher with the purpose of giving him feedback to help him get back on track. In most cases, after he received a warning, he became angry, upset, and uncooperative, leading to more difficulties for the rest of the day. At a session with Alonzo and his mother, I asked Alonzo to explain what he thought was making it so difficult for him to meet his goal, leading to the following dialogue:

A: Well, when I hear the "warning" I think that my teacher is just trying to make me fail and once I miss my goal for the day, I can't have any fun at home.
TH: Wow, that sounds like a lot of pressure and like you feel the grown-ups are out to get you.
A: Right! Like last week – Mom told me that if I could get a perfect week, then I could buy a new computer game.
TH: So you were probably trying your hardest because I know how much you like computer games.
A: Yeah, and then I get a warning on Thursday! And it wasn't even my fault but the teacher wouldn't listen.

TH: So, when you get a "warning" – what does that mean?

A: It means I'm probably not going to make my goal for the day OR the week.

TH: Sounds like you worry a lot about not meeting your goal.

A: Yeah, and I get mad thinking about how they don't want me to earn my points.

TH: I wonder what would happen if you think of your warnings as strikes, like in baseball – you know, three strikes and you're out. Only your teacher gives you two strikes.

A: You mean like chances?

TH: Yep. It seems like you've been thinking that a warning is an out.

A: I do and then I just feel like giving up because it's too hard.

At this point, the therapist spoke with Alonzo's mother privately to set up a way that he could earn some privileges even if his day wasn't "perfect." She expressed concern that "if you give him an inch, he will take a mile" but we worked out a "graduated" system that would allow her to give him basic privileges for 70% achievement, better privileges for 80% achievement, and "deluxe" privileges for 90% and above. Any day with achievement below 60% would result in a loss of all privileges at home for that day. We included Alonzo in the discussion by asking him to rate his favorite privilege as a '1' and so on. Mom agreed to remind Alonzo to think of warnings as chances and we implemented the graduated reward system, to discourage the all-or-nothing thinking of both the adults and Alonzo. As soon as these two interventions were put into place, the conflict level between Alonzo and his mother was greatly reduced, though not absent by any means.

Comment: In this case, it is clear that the parent's beliefs and expectations were influencing the child's feelings and beliefs. The intervention modified beliefs of the parent and child as well as teaching them the skill of collaborative problem-solving.

Guidelines for CBT-Oriented Treatment

Mental health providers may wish to consider the following guidelines for a CBT-oriented approach in their work with children, adolescents, and their families.

Using CBT Principles

Familiarize oneself with, and *utilize in each session*, the principles of the CBT model. Cognitive therapists are active and directive, while creating an atmosphere that conveys a sense of "teamwork" comprising the therapist, the client, and if applicable, family members. That team utilizes structure (e.g., agenda and homework) to work together cooperatively to explore existing beliefs and behaviors (collaborative empiricism), as well as to create new ones (skill-building and/or correcting distorted beliefs).

Assessment

Conduct an assessment that includes instruments that will lead to a conceptualization that is specifically CBT-oriented and/or that are conducive to evidence-based practice; for example, semi-structured interviews that have been used by researchers [62]. Semi-structured interviews, in comparison to unstructured interviews, generally produce more reliable and valid diagnoses, as well as sometimes collecting broad-based information for the case conceptualization, leading to decisions about treatment [62] including the choice and timing of specific techniques or interventions. Specifically, as information is collected related to presenting problems and symptoms, the mental health provider frames the information according to the CBT model of the person (thinking-feeling-behavior-body). Similar to other models, assessment will also include the mutual interaction between the person (child or adolescent) and the child's context, including family, school, culture, etc. Here, what distinguishes the CBT approach from other models is that the cognitive therapist listens for beliefs and observes behaviors (while connecting them to affect and physiological symptoms), so that the data can be organized into a CBT conceptualization. Thinking or cognition is further organized, to the degree that it is developmentally appropriate, into a system that reflects the way in which the client constructs his/her world. Common terms comprising this system include automatic thoughts, conditional beliefs/values/rules, and core beliefs/schemas.

A brief example may serve to clarify. Using three different scenarios that could occur, let's look at how different responses on the part of the caregiver may contribute to a difference in how interventions would be planned. Suppose a mother, Julie, brings her 7-year-old son, Danny, to see you because he has started to have nightmares within the past 3 months, around the same time she returned to full-time employment outside the home. The therapist, using collaboration, asks Julie if she has any ideas about what has triggered this episode and (to assess problem-solving ability) what she typically does to help him. Note that although this appears casual and conversational, the therapist is gathering information about the "world view" (cognitions, beliefs, values, rules) of the caregiver and the caregiver's coping strategies (behaviors, skills, problem-solving abilities). This information is key, as children and adolescents are affected by and influenced by the cognitions and behaviors of their caregivers.

Scenario One:

Julie: I think Danny is angry with me and spoiled. He always has to have things his way, I don't really think he wants me to work.
Therapist: And what do you do to help him when he wakes up?
J: I tell him to go back to bed and stop feeling sorry for himself. He's in first grade now and it's time to start growing up.

Scenario Two:

Julie: I feel so guilty because I can't be there for him to be a good mom.
Th: And what do you do to help him when he wakes up?
J: I hold him for a few minutes and comfort him. And then after I tuck him in I can't get back to sleep myself because I wonder if I'm permanently damaging him by sending him to daycare.

Scenario Three:

Julie: I'm not really sure. Maybe it is just a phase.
Th: And what do you do to help him when he wakes up?
Julie: I don't really do anything, I mean, I try to console him by telling him we all have bad dreams sometimes but he just cries. I don't know if anything can really help. Won't he just grow out of it?

Admittedly, before knowing additional details about this child and family, one would not make major treatment decisions. However, after just two questions posed by the therapist, we see three very diverse responses that exemplify the worldviews of the caregivers and give important clues (evidence) that will be used by the therapist to add to the case formulation, eventually leading to hypotheses. As information from caregivers is collected, the therapist fits it with what is known about the child (organizing it according to thinking-feeling-behavior-body domains) and imagines (hypothesizes) the dynamic interplay both intrapersonally and interpersonally.

Quite possibly, the same cognitive techniques would be used in eventually all three scenarios, though perhaps in a different sequence. For example, education about development, education about anxiety, helping the caregiver learn how to soothe the child, or intervening directly with the child. However, the starting point would depend on the conceptualization. In Scenario one, Julie is stressed and angry, while also not understanding how to be of comfort to Danny. She is likely to

be defensive if told that her stress and statements to him may be exacerbating the problem. Therefore, I would start with the child as the focus (since she sees him as the "problem"). I would explain to Mom that the child may benefit from learning how to help himself by learning relaxation exercises. For younger children, like Danny, I request that the caregiver learns the skills simultaneously so that they can support the child by helping him/her to remember homework assignments (practicing the skills) or in case the child "forgets" something about the procedure between sessions. While explaining the skill to them both, I routinely mention that adults get stressed too, so can benefit from learning relaxation techniques. Rarely have I had an instance where a parent resisted this approach. Instead, parents express relief that someone recognizes their stress and doesn't blame them for it, yet gently encourages them to address it. If this aspect of treatment goes smoothly, and a solid relationship between myself and the caregiver begins to blossom, I then consider addressing parent beliefs. Specifically, for caregivers who are angry and stressed, it should be a gradual approach (maybe just addressing one of their beliefs as part of a session focused on the child) and one that conveys empathy. As the relationship becomes more well established a more formal and direct focus on parent beliefs may be pursued.

Assessment procedures should be developmentally sensitive. As information is collected, the therapist organizes it within a CBT-oriented conceptualization. There are many assessment instruments available, and for young children, assessment will be done via interview and observation (probably during play or interacting with the caregiver). For school-age and younger adolescents, I prefer instruments that are particularly "CBT-friendly." For instance, the Beck Youth Inventories of Emotional and Social Impairment (BYI) [63], which were developed and normed for children ages 8 through 14, consists of five separate self-report inventories that measure levels of depression, anxiety, anger, disruptive behavior, and self-concept. A "combination" inventory is also available. Each 20-item inventory is written at the second-grade reading level, can be completed within 5–10 minutes, and scored easily by the therapist during the session, providing an opportunity for discussion of specific items and conveying information to the client and/or family members. I typically ask additional details about items, adding brief notes. A review [64] of the BYI notes their limitations, including insufficient evidence for their use by themselves to measure treatment effects. However, clinicians are well advised to consider assessment data, including results from self-report instruments, within the context of other information [65] about the child/adolescent and their functioning.

For assessing anger (ages 7–12), I have also used the Children's Anger Response Checklist (CARC) [66]. Features of the CARC that were particularly useful were the Likert-scale (operationalized using faces depicting different degrees of anger) and the fact that the scale uses 10 stories illustrating potentially frustrating situations. As the clinician and child explore the child's anger reaction to each situation, responses are organized according to the domains B, C, E, or P (behavioral, cognitive, emotional, or physiological). Although the 10 vignettes give a sense of the child's anger, in general, sometimes I wanted to gather information about events specific to a child. Therefore, using the general CARC format, I included vignettes based on issues that a particular child was grappling with. Personally, I found the scoring to be time-consuming, but clinically, the CARC yielded valuable qualitative information. For example, some children had absolutely no awareness of any physiological signs of anger (but their parents did!). Some children were eager to discuss their feelings, others became so upset during the CARC administration that we had to take a break and use coping skills before continuing.

As the therapist conducts the assessment, several questions (not necessarily mutually exclusive) the therapist wants to be able to answer fairly quickly (one to two visits) include:

- Are the child's presenting problems due to deficiency or distortion?
- What is this child's "system of thinking" (how has this child constructed his/her world and how well can the child articulate/understand information about feelings, thinking, behavior, and bodily symptoms?).
- Will it be helpful/necessary for the child's caregiver to be involved in treatment? If so, what will be their role?

The Working Model

Formulate your own "working model" of the client that reflects a CBT orientation. In other words, the information about a child (or adolescent and their family) can be organized such that the child's thinking, feelings, behavior, and physical functioning present an internally consistent "picture." Furthermore, to the degree that it is possible (depending on developmental level), the formulation should include various levels of cognition (automatic thoughts, beliefs, conditional assumptions, rules, schemas) that comprise the client's "system of thinking" about themselves, others (particularly significant people and events), and the future. For adolescents and some school-age children, the clinician can make use of Beck's Cognitive Conceptualization Diagram [39] to organize the material in a one-page format. Key

would be the child's ability to articulate automatic thoughts as well as the accompanying feelings, etc.

Clearly, the more cognitively developed a child is, the more ability he/she will have to articulate such information. When that is not the case, however, the therapist makes inferences through observation and attempts to examine the evidence for or against the inference. For example, the cardinal question of CBT, "What was *just now* going through your mind?" in the presence of heightened affect is not generally developmentally appropriate for a 5-year-old. Instead, information would be gathered during story-telling or a structured play that touches on areas of difficulty for the child.

In my own experience, I have discovered several benefits of a well-developed – yet dynamic – conceptualization. First, even as this CBT-oriented "picture" of the client continues to be refined, it provides a sense of continuity in my own thinking about the client, leading to an increased ability to recall details of the client's experiences as well as the ability to identify and explore recurrent themes. It can be quite comforting for clients (and their caregivers) to find that they "make sense" to someone else, even when they haven't yet been able to put the pieces together themselves. Second, the formulation allows for a quick guide to the timing and selection of intervention techniques, as well as how to tailor them to the individual. Finally, the conceptualization even guides the sharing of the conceptualization with the client (and/or caregiver). Why is this important? Because CBT is focused at two levels simultaneously: addressing current concerns while at the same time teaching skills that the client can utilize throughout the lifespan.

Blending Creative and Scientific Aspects

Integrate the creative and scientific aspects of treatment. The creative portion comes naturally to most practitioners in the caring professions and consists of the collaborative, warm, caring relationship that demonstrates to the client the humanity of the therapist. Without this foundation, even the most sophisticated, accurate, and brilliant CBT intervention is likely to have minimal impact.

The scientific aspect of treatment includes using outcome measures and incorporating research findings, protocols, or manuals and standard CBT techniques, as well as using a scientific approach to treatment. Some outcome measures have already been mentioned above, the results of which should be considered as data [65] in the context of the overall picture of the child/adolescent. Frequency of administration of outcome measures can be adjusted depending on the severity of the client's symptoms, the number of measures, and length of each, as well as time to score and interpret. Other factors that may influence the therapist's decision to have a client complete outcome measures over the course of treatment could be when there appears to be a significant change in symptom severity (increase or decrease), to help guide decisions regarding changes in frequency of sessions or when deciding to end treatment, and prior to reporting to a third party. For instance, when clients have been given medication by another provider, it can be helpful feedback to the prescriber to have specific information. For example, "When I saw this client at intake, the score they obtained on the Beck Depression Inventory for Youth [63] (BDI-Y) fell at the 88th percentile. Now, 2 months later, they have seen me for six sessions and because I knew they were coming to see you next Tuesday, I had them take the BDI-Y again, with a current score at the 67th percentile." On the other hand, the conversation could go like this: "When I saw this client at intake, the score they obtained on the BDI-Y fell at the 88th percentile. Their parent tells me they aren't due to see you again for another 6 weeks; however, today, when meeting with the family for the third session, the client completed the BDI-Y again and obtained a score at the 95th percentile."

Empirical literature should be regularly reviewed in order for the clinician to stay familiar with which treatments appear to be the most effective. Recent collections of evidence-based practices for children and adolescents [18–20] contain numerous CBT-oriented treatments, including information about specific disorders, age range treated, and parental involvement (whether and how much). Furthermore, specific and practical information about program protocols (delineated by sessions or steps) and manuals (for both therapist and clients) or assessment instruments are included. Treatment guidelines included in these resources address ADHD, anger for school age children, depression, disruptive behavior disorder, firesetting, OCD, ODD/CD, and anxiety, among others.

For example, the Coping Cat program developed at the Temple University Child and Adolescent Anxiety Disorders Clinic (CAADC) is designed for children aged 7 through 13 years who have been diagnosed with anxiety disorders, including social phobia, generalized anxiety disorder, and separation anxiety [67]. A total of 16 to 18 sessions (including two parent sessions) are divided into two phases. Phase one is oriented toward helping the client first acquire coping skills to deal with anxiety, then to practice the skills in phase two. Clients utilize the Coping Cat Workbook [68] in parallel with the treatment sessions. Therapists model the skills and assist with practice (exposure tasks).

Because a number of these treatment protocols were found to have effective treatment outcomes, therapists should use them. However, the manuals should be used in a flexible fashion. Doing so benefits both therapist and client, as the therapist retains the freedom to utilize clinical skills to "fit" the treatment to the client and his/her needs. This is best done based on the conceptualization of the client the therapist has developed. Furthermore, the client benefits as they get the "best of both worlds" – treatment that has been shown to be effective for other children with similar problems but tailored specifically for him/her by a person who cares about and understands their particular situation. Since many of the evidence-based treatments or manuals use techniques that would be considered part of the standard CBT repertoire, therapists should be familiar with these techniques, the rationale for using them, and the general procedure for implementing them.

No matter whether a therapist is using a strict treatment protocol, adapting a manual, or individualizing CBT techniques and methods in treatment, it goes (almost) without saying that the therapist will combine their interpersonal skills with analytic skills to make clinical decisions and to evaluate progress. The standard way in which this is done is to use the scientific method, which consists of the following feedback loop: data collection, development of hypothesis, testing of the hypothesis, then evaluating (i.e., data collection) leading to a revision of the hypothesis. This process occurs throughout each session as the clinician interacts with the client, makes choices about when and how to intervene, and then judges the outcome. An example will serve to illustrate how "second nature" this way of thinking becomes for the clinician.

CASE STUDY

Example

Janine is a 13-year-old female who presented due to weekly sleep problems and anxiety in several domains of her life: school, appearance, and her mother, who is having some medical issues but not serious ones. Until the past quarter, she had always been on the Honor Roll. Being so bright and motivated to feel better, she easily grasped the CBT model, and could identify her feelings and bodily symptoms, as well as articulate her automatic thoughts. By session 2, the therapist observes that Janine has many of the foundational abilities that are needed for her to learn about Thought Records, and thus plans to introduce them to her in session 3. For homework, the therapist suggests that Janine records anxious thoughts and rates how much they bother her, using a numeric rating from 1 to 10, 10 being the highest. When Janine returns to session 3, she reports that her sleep problems have worsened. At this point, the therapist wants to collect information so she can decide how best to proceed with the session.

Scenario One:

Therapist: So, was there anything upsetting that happened during the week?

Janine: Well, my mom told me she has to get another medical test – for high blood pressure.

Th: And that made you feel?

J: Basically terrified.

Th: And did you write something about this on your list of anxious thoughts?

J: Yes, "My mother might die."

Th: Well that sounds pretty upsetting. Do you think that had anything to do with you having more sleep problems this week?

J: Yeah, I guess I hadn't really thought about it.

Th: Did you get a chance to talk with your mom yet?

J: No, I'm afraid to bring it up, could you help me talk with her?

Th: Sure, let's ask her to come into the session.

Comment: In this case, the therapist has enough information to hypothesize that Janine's anxiety about her mother may have exacerbated the sleep problems. By having her mother come into the session, the therapist shows empathy, support, and caring yet simultaneously plans to model for Janine how to talk with her mother about her concerns. Furthermore, in a sense, the information that will be discussed will be a variation of the Thought Record, as the therapist plans on showing the client how to gather evidence that will dispute her anxious thoughts about her mother dying. After they've first discussed it all, the therapist can assist Janine to write it down in a way that makes sense to her and that she can access again in the future.

Scenario Two:

Therapist: So, was there anything upsetting that happened during the week?

Janine: Not really – just sort of the same.

Th: When did your sleep problems seem to get worse?

J: Well, maybe a couple days after I came here.

Th: What would be happening when you were sleeping?

J: Well, I was working on making that list of worries after I did my homework – like right before bed.

Th: Yes?

J: Well, then when I would wake up that was all that I kept thinking about.

Th: Your list? You mean, like "I better get up and add something to it?"

J: No, more like everything that was on the list kept coming back into my head. Kind of how it was before – only worse.

Th: I see. And then it was hard for you to get back to sleep?

J: Yes.

Th: OK, tell you what. Would it be alright with you if I keep your list because I know you worked hard on it but I have something else that I want us to do today and we'll come back to the list later.

J: Sure.

Comment: In this case, the therapist hypothesizes that the sleep problems were exacerbated due to the client focusing on anxious thoughts. Therefore, although the client appears to have excellent cognitive abilities to engage in Thought Records, the therapist is going to switch temporarily to behavioral techniques (relaxation techniques such as abdominal breathing, progressive muscle relaxation, and distraction – music, e.g.) to help the client cope. Within a session or two, the therapist believes they will return to Thought Records, but she will take one thought at a time off the list that the client has allowed her to keep in the file in the therapy office.

While the scientific method is not unique to CBT practitioners, the way in which the CBT practitioner collects (assessment instruments, the way in which questions are asked, etc.) and organizes information takes place within the context of a CBT framework.

Using Standard CBT Interventions

Familiarize yourself with standard CBT interventions while remembering to adapt them to the developmental level of the child or adolescent. Details of CBT interventions and techniques are described elsewhere; however, the CBT therapist would have in their "toolbox" a collection of both behavioral and cognitive techniques. Typical behavioral techniques include relaxation training, distraction, systematic desensitization, modeling, role-playing, pleasant activity scheduling, graduated exposure (imaginal and *in vivo*), behavioral experiments, and contingency management (including shaping, extinction, positive reinforcement, and punishment). Typical cognitive techniques include guided discovery using Socratic questioning, examining the evidence to address cognitive distortions, self-instruction, and problem-solving. Frequently, both cognitive and behavioral techniques may be combined in a single intervention, for example, into a "lesson" or module [69, 70]. In fact, clinicians are advised to consider collecting "empirically supported treatment modules." [33]

The therapist, then, instead of thinking of treatment as a string of interventions, considers the overall stages of components of treatment needed in order to address the child's problems. A good example of this is described by Kendall and colleagues [69] in working with anxious children. Although the Coping Cat program uses a treatment protocol with two phases, education and exposure, the overall strategy of treatment could be conceptualized in "modules" consisting of somatic education, relaxation, self-talk, exposure, self-reward, and consolidation. Each module may consist of several cognitive and/or behavioral interventions. For example, a goal of the self-talk "module" would be to help the child identify his/her anxious feelings and related anxious thought(s), but then to generate an alternative thought that would help reduce anxiety level. During the education phase of treatment, the child may be learning about his/her anxiety as well as how to potentially cope via self-talk. During the exposure phase, the skills are actually put into practice.

One of the most challenging tasks of the CBT practitioner is to adapt standard interventions to a child's developmental level, especially at younger ages. As previously mentioned, some work has recently been done in this area; however, there is less empirical information available for younger children; therefore, the practitioner needs to utilize a scientific approach, as previously described. In general, some rules of thumb to follow in this area include:

- the younger the child, the more often caregivers will be involved;
- the younger the child, the more often treatment will consist of behavioral interventions;
- the younger the child, the more often treatment will be activity or play-based;
- the younger the child, the more often treatment will address deficiencies (versus distortions);
- the younger the child, the more treatment will occur *in vivo* (caregiver would carry out homework assignments or support child to do so);
- the younger the child, the less often the conceptualization is shared (but may be shared with caregiver).

Adapting interventions to the child's or adolescent's developmental stage and individual interests appears to increase the effectiveness of the treatment, since it would be relevant and interesting, probably increasing motivation. Let us examine how a cognitive technique – Thought Records – might be developmentally adapted.

In general, adolescents can be treated more similarly to adults in terms of their ability to self-reflect and engage in analysis. Frequently, when I have presented the Thought Record to adolescents and asked them to complete between-session samples, they see it as another homework task. So, instead I find out about their interests – journaling, poetry, art, music – to make use of what they already do as a vehicle of discovery. Amanda, a 17-year-old female, who presented with anger (especially at home) and depression, had experienced a recent breakup. When she told me about the paintings and drawings she enjoyed doing, I asked her to bring some into the session. Seeing such work is a powerful communication to the therapist! As she described her work to me, I asked the cardinal CBT question, "What was going through your mind?" to obtain information while also assisting her to connect her thoughts and feelings, as well as to address her frequent belief "I'll never find another boyfriend."

For school-age children, having brief, engaging, and structured written work is quite similar to school tasks. Therefore, a workbook like *Therapeutic Exercises for Children* [40] (TEC) is ideal. TEC consists of 18 exercises designed for children aged 8–12 years who are struggling with anxiety or depression. Each exercise has a name, guidelines for the therapist, tips for children, and a sample. Specifically, the Thought Record has been developmentally adapted with the exercise Catching Feelings and Thoughts, making use of illustrations, coloring, and thought bubbles. Another workbook available online (electronic book available at www.netLibrary.com), *Think Good, Feel Good: A Comprehensive Behaviour Therapy Workbook for Children and Young People* [46], contains CBT-oriented exercises and worksheets.

I would be unlikely to attempt to adapt a Thought Record for a child under age 8 because a Thought Records assumes the presence of a "distortion" and has the goal of refuting it with a logical analysis by examining the evidence. At this age, treatment occurs more often in the here-and-now (*in vivo*). Therefore, I would typically use play, drawing, storytelling, puppets, or games with or without parent participation. Depending on the presenting issue, I would try to design the session so that it would bring to light issues that need to be addressed. For example, suppose a 6-year-old girl, Janie, tells you that nobody likes her or ever wants to play with her. You find from talking with her teacher that other children do keep a bit distant from her since she tends to be somewhat "bossy." Play in the sessions can be set up to help her learn turn-taking and/or problem-solving. This can be accomplished first by reading a book [71] about the difficulties of sharing and assessing the child's ability to recognize affect (her own and others') or by the therapist putting on a puppet show. Sharing skills could then be modeled by the puppets, then practiced by the client in the session.

Role of Psychoeducation

Use client and/or parent education to promote understanding of the CBT model and CBT techniques, *as well as their relevance* to the client in his/her life. This process actually starts with the initial contact and continues throughout treatment. An obvious way in which education occurs is with the CBT interventions themselves. Suppose the treatment of an anxious child, Dee, is going to involve relaxation and distraction techniques, cognitive restructuring, and exposure. Unless contraindicated, I prefer to have the parent and child together when I am explaining the general treatment approach (except in the case of very young children) and usually direct my conversation to the child at their level with the parent observing. Several benefits follow. The child receives treatment aimed at their capacity and the parent has the opportunity to observe how I will be interacting with their child. Furthermore, the parent becomes familiar with the content so they can understand and support their child's treatment.

A second way in which education occurs is whenever the conceptualization is explained. Again, depending on the circumstances, the way in which I share the conceptualization is individualized for each client. Generally speaking, when treatment goals are initially formulated and we decide to focus on particular skills or interventions, I provide the rationale framed in CBT terms. As treatment progresses, I have found that other parts of the conceptualization may come to light. At a later point in treatment, different parts of the conceptualization may be able to be linked together.

A third aspect of education concerns homework or between-session assignments to help the child practice the skills, whether behavioral or cognitive. The explanation I usually give for the assignments is that it will be hard to feel much better if the only time they practice new ways of thinking and feeling is in my office. Homework assignments, like interventions within sessions, are fitted to the developmental level of the child. For example, school-age children can use structured workbooks but adolescents may prefer to write poems or keep journals to explore their feelings and thoughts.

A final (last but definitely not least) way to utilize education is to assist parents in exploring general issues like development or to find additional information about the particular issues their child might be dealing with, such as anxiety or depression. Education is not particular to CBT providers; however, as a CBT-oriented provider, I prefer to recommend materials that are consistent with the model and that fit the interests and time constraints of the parents. Two general development books I frequently recommend are *Your Child*

[72] and *Your Adolescent* [73], both edited by a past president of the American Academy of Child and Adolescent Psychiatry. For knowledge about emotional development, the books by the Philadelphia Child Guidance Center (covering young children [74], childhood [75], and adolescence [76]) are beneficial. A good source for helping parents to understand how to handle their child's (unpleasant) emotions is *The Heart of Parenting* [77] audiotape with or without its companion book [61]. For parents who want to examine and alter beliefs about themselves and their children, I recommend *Why Can't I Be The Parent I Want to Be?* [78] Parents of anxious children may want to review *Helping Your Anxious Child* [79] or *Worried No More* [80]. For parents whose children struggle with OCD, *Freeing Your Child From Obsessive-Compulsive Disorder* [81] and *What To Do When your Child has Obsessive-Compulsive Disorder* [82] may be helpful. *More Than Moody* [83] describes and explains depression in adolescence, while *Helping Your Teen Beat Depression* [84] takes a problem-solving stance. For parents who want accessible information, internet sites such as the NYU Child Study Center's Giving Children Back Their Childhood (www.aboutourkids.org) are extremely useful, covering a wide array of topics.

Importance of Feedback

Seek feedback from the client and/or caregivers, both informally and formally. Some agencies have used a written feedback form that can be completed periodically, even after each therapy session. In addition, as part of the CBT session structure, feedback is given/asked for toward the end of the session. Feedback is likely to be part of any therapist's work, so what is different about this process for a CBT provider?

As a CBT therapist, I view feedback (especially negative) as absolutely vital! That is why I have learned to encourage it and welcome it. Numerous benefits occur when the client is encouraged in this direction. First, it adds to the sense of collaboration and to the therapeutic relationship. Second, since feedback is seen as a two-way exchange, it reduces (though probably does not eliminate) the power differential inherent in the therapist-client relationship. Third, the therapist can get a sense of client (or caregiver) beliefs, always adding this information to expand the conceptualization.

Although part of the CBT session structure is to solicit feedback, in my experience I have found that clients seemed to give me responses like "fine" or "Everything was good." Instead, I have developed several ways of making sure to give the client the message that the sessions are a safe place to give feedback (including negative) by doing the following.

During the session (usually session 2) when I socialize the client to the CBT model, I explain that we will be working together "like a team, to help you/your child with your problems. Therefore, it is really important and helpful if you tell me when something I say doesn't make sense or if you don't agree with it. Do you think you can do that?" Frequently, this begins to elicit client beliefs. For example, if the response is "But I don't want to hurt your feelings," then I might ask for an example of what would be "horrible enough" to hurt my feelings, and address their concerns. If the response is more like "But you are the expert and I should not be questioning you," I give them permission to do so, explaining that their concerns may not have anything to do with my expertise.

However, having such conversations only at the outset of treatment is not enough. Therefore, I have incorporated listening for feedback or asking for it once or twice (or at key points) during a session. That way it becomes second nature to the client and is part of our ongoing "dialogue." Key points have become fairly clear to me by attending to client affect, then asking the cardinal question: "What just went through your mind?" For example, when working with a mother of a 4-year-old female who was having trouble with transitions and complying with commands, I had spent several sessions modeling behavioral techniques like ignoring and redirection. As I "coached" the mother, preparing her to use these techniques for a few minutes at the next session, her affect shifted, getting "cloudy." As I asked "What was going through your mind?" she hesitantly responded by saying "You are asking me to do something before I am ready," related to her feeling irritable and anxious. With this information, I was able to find out more about how to support her and to address her concerns. This brief interaction strengthened our relationship but alerted me to her belief that she lacked a skill, a concern that could be addressed.

Finally, another method for obtaining feedback is via written forms. Some practitioners use brief client self-report measures that specifically assess the strength of the therapeutic relationship [85]. These would likely be most appropriate for adolescents or parents involved in treatment. In addition, Friedberg *et al.* [86] developed written feedback forms specifically for children aged 8–11 and 12–16 to measure engagement as well as what was helpful (or not) to the client.

Developing CBT Competency

Mental health professionals who choose to deliver CBT-oriented treatment need to possess a solid background in CBT, its history, theory, and classic techniques. Equally important is the ability to continually monitor and expand their own development, which frequently occurs within two interdependent domains: professional and personal. Following are suggestions for how to expand one's competence as a CBT provider.

Gain the professional foundations by reading the "classics" of CBT, including *Cognitive Therapy: Basics and Beyond* [39], especially the sections covering guidelines in treatment planning and problems encountered in therapy. For information specific to children and adolescents, two books that are loyal to basic CBT theory while including numerous practical suggestions for clinical application are *Clinical Practice of Cognitive Therapy with Children and Adolescents: The Nuts and Bolts* [30] and its companion volume with a modular treatment focus, *Cognitive Therapy Techniques for Children and Adolescents* [87]. Review and use practice guidelines such as those included in articles appearing in the special issue of the *Journal of Clinical Child and Adolescent Psychology* [48] update regarding evidence-based psychosocial treatments for children and adolescents.

Participate in organizations that support EBP and its dissemination, including the Association for Behavioral and Cognitive Therapies (ABCT) [88], the Anxiety Disorders Association of America (ADAA) [89], and the Society of Clinical Child and Adolescent Psychology (SCCAP) [90] – Division 53 of the APA (American Psychological Association). As part of the dissemination effort regarding EBP, the ABCT and SCCAP collaborated to educate clinicians and the public alike by providing extensive information on the ABCT website [91] about disorders affecting children and adolescents, as well as EBP treatments.

Utilize technology to access current EBP information conveniently and frequently. Extensive online resources are available at the websites for the ABCT and ADAA, including full pdf text articles, videos, and podcasts. At the time of writing, for example, the ADAA website offered several podcasts including "What Clinicians Need to Know About Treating Children with Anxiety Disorders" [92] presented by Dr Ronald Rapee. In addition to using podcasts for themselves, clinicians may choose to recommend such resources to caregivers. Embedded video clips for selected articles in the electronic version of the journal *Cognitive and Behavioral Practice* (an ABCT journal included with membership) was an innovation launched in 2009 [93] in order to illustrate treatment techniques. Subsequently, articles utilizing video segments to demonstrate parent training for young children with disruptive disorders [94] and to model examples of the flexibility of the Coping Cat Program for treating anxious youth [95, 96] have appeared.

DVDs provide opportunities to observe clinicians actually delivering CBT-based techniques. For anxious children in the 7 to 15-year-old range, see Kendall's 'The

Coping Cat Therapist: Session by Session Guide' [97]. DVDs featuring highly skilled therapists demonstrating cognitive behavioral methods (albeit with adults) facilitate the ability to witness "CBT in action." Specific topics covered include: cognitive therapy (Judith Beck) [98], cognitive behavioral therapy (Jacqueline Persons) [99], cognitive therapy over time (Keith Dobson) [100], cognitive behavioral therapy for clients with multiple problems (Gayle Iwamasa) [101], obsessive-compulsive disorder, perfectionism and behavior therapy (Martin Antony) [102–104], social phobia (Marie Albano) [105], generalized anxiety disorder (Michelle Craske) [106], panic disorder (David Clark) [107], and depression (Joan Davidson, Jacqueline Persons, and Michael Tompkins), which is actually a five-part series demonstrating cognitive fundamentals (case formulation [108], session structure [109], activity scheduling [110], thought record [111], and schema change [112]). Other technique-oriented DVDs include problem-solving (Christine Maguth Nezu, Arthur Nezu) [113] and Christine Padesky demonstrating guided discovery [114] and testing automatic thoughts [115].

Focus on simpler cases and/or specific disorders initially. Use a manualized treatment and CBT techniques with clients while seeking consultation or supervision from a well-trained cognitive behavioral therapist; see the Academy of Cognitive Therapists' website (www.academyofct.org) to locate someone in your area. Make use of the Cognitive Therapy Rating Scale (CTRS) [116]. The CTRS and its manual, both available online (www.academyofct.org), is a detailed tool that can be used to evaluate the strengths and weaknesses of a cognitive therapist.

Connect with CBT-oriented colleagues nationally and locally. Join organizations such as the Academy of Cognitive Therapy (ACT) and ABCT. The ABCT holds its annual convention in November, which offers presentations by leaders in CBT treatment. Even when attending non-ABCT workshops, make it a priority to attend workshops that are offered by well-known child and adolescent CBT-practitioners. Finally, add other CBT-oriented websites (www.beckinstitute.org and www.academyofct.org) to your Favorites list on your computer and review them regularly.

At the personal level, CBT practitioners can learn much from paying attention to their own automatic thoughts [54] during the therapy process concerning various issues or reactions concerning clients. In fact, completing Thought Records to examine one's own automatic thoughts and related emotions, as well as completing a self-conceptualization using the Cognitive Conceptualization Diagram [39] can be quite informative. As one gets in the habit of reflecting on the cardinal question "What just went through my mind?" there is an ever-increasing awareness of the connection between one's own thoughts and feelings, and this information can be used during sessions. In fact, at times it may be appropriate to self-disclose (for the benefit of the client) automatic thoughts or feelings. For example, Jake, a 14-year-old male, who presented for depression comes in for the sixth session and, once again, "forgot" to bring his homework. You notice you feel irritated but don't realize it shows until he tentatively asks "Are you mad at me?" At that point, you can deny it (and deprive him of his accurate perception) or you can acknowledge the truth, explaining, "Yeah, I noticed that I am kind of frustrated and what was going through my mind is that you must feel real overwhelmed and it's hard to do anything because the last time you were here we tried to make your homework as easy as possible. It is more that I want to see you start to feel better and be able to start to do things to help yourself." This very brief self-disclosure accomplishes a number of objectives: it builds rapport by being open to feedback from the client and showing one's own humanity; it models the ability to connect feeling and thought; and it demonstrates that the therapist both understands the depth of the client's distress without criticizing him and believes that the client will be able to help himself at some point in the future.

Concluding Remarks

The CBT model has continued to demonstrate that its techniques are a promising approach to ameliorate the psychological problems of children and adolescents. Applications of the model have recently been extended to include culturally diverse populations, younger age groups, and new issues. Efforts to educate clinicians and the public alike about CBT's effectiveness are advancing; at the same time, dissemination of quality CBT to the clinical world remains challenging for a variety of reasons. As others have noted [48, 117, 118], researchers need to discover how change occurs during treatment, under what conditions, and for what populations, and how to more easily translate research findings to clinical settings.

In the meantime, many children and adolescents are being helped with CBT-oriented psychosocial treatment. Practitioners currently working in the field can do a service to this population by using this chapter as a resource in their journey to provide quality CBT treatment.

References

1. March JS. The future of psychotherapy for mentally ill children and adolescents. *J Child Psychol Psychiat* 2009;**50**:170–179.

2. Compton SN, March JS, Brent D, Albano AM, Weersing R, Curry J. Cognitive-behavioral psychotherapy for anxiety and depressive disorders in children and adolescents: An evidence-based medicine review. *J Am Acad Child Adolesc Psychiat* 2004;**43**:930–959.

3. Christophersen ER, Mortweet SL. *Treatments that Work with Children: Empirically Supported Strategies for Managing Childhood Problems.* Washington, DC: American Psychological Association, 2001.

4. Hudson JL, Rapee RM, Deveney C, Schniering CA, Lyneham HJ, Bovopoulous N. Cognitive behavioral treatment versus an active control for children and adolescents with anxiety disorders: A randomized trial. *J Am Acad Child Adolesc Psychiat* 2009;**48**:533–544.

5. Kendall PC, Hudson JL, Gosch E, Flannery-Schroeder E, Suveg C. Cognitive-behavioral therapy for anxiety disordered youth: A randomized clinical trial evaluating child and family modalities. *J Consul Clin Psychol* 2008;**76**:282–297.

6. Silverman WK, Pina AA, Viswesvaran C. Evidence-based psychosocial treatments for phobic and anxiety disorders in children and adolescents. *J Clin Child Adolesc Psychol* 2008;**37**:105–130.

7. Garcia-Lopez LJ, Olivares J, Beidel D, Albano AM, Turner S, Rosa AI. Efficacy of three treatment protocols for adolescents with social anxiety disorder: a 5-year follow-up assessment. *J Anxiety Disord* 2008;**20**:175–191.

8. Velting ON, Setzer N, Albano AM. Update on and advances in assessment and cognitive-behavioral treatment of anxiety disorders in children and adolescents. *Prof Psychol Res Pract* 2004;**35**:42–54.

9. Barrett PM, Farrell L, Pina AA, Peris RS, Piacentini J. Evidence-based psychosocial treatments for child and adolescent obsessive-compulsive disorder. *J Clin Child Adolesc Psychol* 2008;**37**:131–155.

10. Silverman WK, Ortiz CD, Viswesvaran C, *et al.* Evidence-based psychosocial treatments for child and adolescent exposed to traumatic events: A review and meta-analysis. *J Clin Child Adolesc Psychol* 2008;**37**:156–183.

11. David-Ferdon C, Kaslow NJ. Evidence-based psychosocial treatments for child and adolescent depression. *J Clin Child Adolesc Psychol* 2008;**37**:62–104.

12. Lochman JE, Boxmeyer CL, Powell NP, Barry TD, Pardini DA. Anger control training for aggressive youth. In: Weisz JR, Kazdin AE (eds) *Evidence-Based Psychotherapies for Children and Adolescents*, 2nd edn. New York: Guilford Press, 2010; pp. 227–242.

13. Kazdin AE. Problem-solving skills training and parent management training for oppositional defiant disorder and conduct disorder. In: Weisz JR, Kazdin AE (eds) *Evidence-Based Psychotherapies for Children and Adolescents*, 2nd edn. New York: Guilford Press, 2010; pp. 211–226.

14. Eyberg SM, Nelson MM, Boggs SR. Evidence-based psychosocial treatments for child and adolescents with disruptive behavior. *J Clin Child Adolesc Psychol* 2008;**37**:215–237.

15. Waldron HB, Turner CW. Evidence-based psychosocial treatments for adolescent substance abuse. *J Clin Child Adolesc Psychol* 2008;**37**:238–261.

16. Pelham WE, Fabiano GA. Evidence-based psychosocial treatments for attention-deficit/hyperactivity disorder. *J Clin Child Adolesc Psychol* 2008;**37**:184–214.

17. Kaiser NM, Pfiffner LJ. Evidence-based psychosocial treatments for childhood ADHD. *Psychiat Ann* 2011;**41**:9–15.

18. Hibbs ED, Jensen PS (eds). *Psychosocial Treatments for Child and Adolescent Disorders: Empirically Based Strategies for Clinical Practice*, 2nd edn. Washington, DC: American Psychological Association, 2005.

19. Weisz JR, Kazdin AE (eds). *Evidence-Based Psychotherapies for Children and Adolescents*, 2nd edn. New York: Guilford Press, 2010.

20. Ollendick TH, March JS (eds). *Phobic and Anxiety Disorders in Children and Adolescents: A Clinician's Guide to Effective Psychosocial and Pharmacological Interventions.* New York: Oxford University Press, 2004.

21. *Child Adolesc Psychiat Clin N Am* 2011; **20**.

22. Kendall PC, Suveg CS, Kingery JN. Facilitating the dissemination and application of cognitive-behavioral therapy for anxiety in youth. *J Cognitive Psychother Int Q* 2006;**20**:243–245.

23. Kendall PC, Beidas RS. Smoothing the trail for dissemination of evidence-based practices for youth: Flexibility within fidelity. *Prof Psychol Res Pract* 2007;**38**:13–19.

24. Fisher CB, Hatashita-Wong M, Greene LI. Ethical and legal issues. In: Silverman WK, Ollendick TH (eds) *Developmental Issues in the Clinical Treatment of Children.* Boston: Allyn and Bacon,1999; pp. 470–486.

25. Rae WA, Fournier CJ. Ethical and legal issues in the treatment of children and families. In: Russ SW, Ollendick TH (eds) *Handbook of Psychotherapies with Children and Families.* New York: Plenum Publishers, 1999; pp. 67–83.

26. DeKraai MB, Sales BD, Hall SR. Informed consent, confidentiality, and duty to report laws in the conduct of child therapy. In: Morris RJ, Kratochwill TR (eds) *The Practice of Child Therapy,* 3rd edn. Boston: Allyn and Bacon, 1998; pp. 540–559.

27. Kendall PC. Guiding theory for therapy with children and adolescents. In: Kendall PC (ed.) *Child and Adolescent Therapy: Cognitive-Behavioral Procedures*, 3rd edn. New York: Guilford Press, 2006; pp. 3–32.

28. Kendall PC, Warman MJ. Emotional disorders in youth. In: Salkovskis PM (ed.) *Frontiers of Cognitive Therapy.* New York: Guilford Press, 1996, pp. 509–530.

29. Friedberg RD, Crosby LE, Friedberg BA, Rutter JG, Knight KR. Making cognitive behavioral therapy user-friendly to children. *Cognit Behav Pract* 1999;**6**:189–200.

30. Friedberg RD, McClure JM. *Clinical Practice of Cognitive Therapy with Children and Adolescents: The Nuts and Bolts.* New York: Guilford Press, 2002.

31. Ronen T. *Cognitive Developmental Therapy with Children.* New York: John Wiley & Sons, Ltd, 1997.

32. Holmbeck GN, Devine KA, Bruno EF. Developmental issues and considerations in research and practice. In: Weisz JR, Kazdin AE (eds) *Evidence-Based Psychotherapies for Children and Adolescents,* 2nd edn. New York: Guilford Press, 2010; pp. 28–39.

33. Kendall PC (ed.) *Child and Adolescent Therapy: Cognitive-Behavioral Procedures*, 3rd edn. New York: Guilford Press, 2006.

34. Kendall PC, MacDonald JP. Cognition in the psychopathology of youth and implications for treatment. In: Dobson KS, Kendall PC (eds) *Psychopathology and Cognition.* San Diego: Academic Press, 1993; pp. 387–427.

35. Kendall PC, Stark KD, Adam T. Cognitive deficit or cognitive distortion of childhood depression. *J Abnorm Child Psychol* 1990;**18**:255–270.

36. Shirk S. Development and cognitive therapy. *J Cognit Psychother* 2001;**15**:155–163.

37. Siqueland L, Diamond GS. Engaging parents in cognitive behavioral treatment for children with anxiety disorders. *Cognit BehavPrac* 1998;**5**:81–102.

38. Silverman WK, Ollendick TH (eds). *Developmental Issues in the Clinical Treatment of Children*. Boston: Allyn and Bacon, 1999.

39. Beck JS. *Cognitive Therapy: Basics and Beyond*. New York: Guilford Press, 1995.

40. Friedberg RD, Friedberg BA, Friedberg RJ. *Therapeutic Exercises for Children: Guided Discovery Using Cognitive-Behavioral Techniques*. Sarasota, FL: Professional Resource Press, 2001.

41. Krain AL, Kendall, PC. Cognitive-behavioral therapy. In: Russ SW, Ollendick TH (eds) *Handbook of Psychotherapies with Children and Families*. New York: Plenum Publishers, 1999; pp. 121–135.

42. Beck AT, Rush AJ, Shaw BF, Emery G. *Cognitive Therapy of Depression*. New York: Guilford Press, 1979.

43. Clark DA, Steer RA. Empirical status of the cognitive model of anxiety and depression. In: Salkovskis PM (ed.) *Frontiers of Cognitive Therapy*. New York: Guilford Press, 1996; pp. 75–96.

44. Greenberger D, Padesky CA. *Mind over Mood: A Cognitive Therapy Treatment Manual for Clients*. New York: Guilford Press, 1995.

45. Beck AT. *Cognitive Therapy and the Emotional Disorders*. New York: International Universities Press, 1976.

46. Stallard P. *Think Good, Feel Good: A Cognitive Behaviour Therapy Workbook for Children and Young People*. Chichester: John Wiley & Sons, Ltd, 2002 [electronic resource].

47. Schniering CA, Rapee RM. The relationship between automatic thoughts and negative emotions in children and adolescents: A test of cognitive content-specificity hypothesis. *J Abnorm Psychol* 2004;**113**:464–470.

48. Silverman WK, Hinshaw SP. The second special issue on evidence-based psychosocial treatments for children and adolescents: A 10-year update. *J Clin Child Adolesc Psychol* 2008;**37**:1–7.

49. Franklin MD, Freeman J, March JS. Treating pediatric obsessive-compulsive disorder using exposure-based cognitive-behavioral therapy. In: Weisz JR, Kazdin, AE (eds) *Evidence-Based Psychotherapies for Children and Adolescents*, 2nd edn. New York: Guilford Press, 2010; pp. 80–92.

50. Freeman JB, Garcia AM, Coyne L, *et al.* Early childhood OCD: Preliminary findings from a family-based cognitive-behavioral approach. *J Am Acad Child Adolesc Psychiatry* 2008;**47**:593–602.

51. Choate-Summers ML, Freeman JB, Garcia AM, Coyne L, Przeworski A, Leonard HL. Clinical considerations when tailoring cognitive behavioral treatment for young children with obsessive compulsive disorder. *Educ Treat Child* 2008;**31**:395–416.

52. Freeman JB, Garcia AM. *Family-Based Treatment for Young Children with OCD Workbook*. New York: Oxford University Press, 2008.

53. Knell SM. *Cognitive-Behavioral Play Therapy*. Northvale, New Jersey: Jason Aronson, Inc., 1993.

54. Knell SM. Cognitive-behavioral play therapy. In: Russ SW, Ollendick TH (eds) *Handbook of Psychotherapies with Children and Families*. New York: Plenum Publishers, 1999; pp. 385–404.

55. Russ SW. *Play in Child Development and Psychotherapy: Toward Empirically Supported Practice*. Mahwah, NJ: Lawrence Erlbaum Associates, 2004.

56. Needleman LD. *Cognitive Case Conceptualization: A Guidebook for Practitioners*. Mahwah, NJ: Lawrence Erlbaum, 1999.

57. Padesky CA. Developing cognitive therapist competency: Teaching and supervision models. In: Salkovskis PM (ed.) *Frontiers of Cognitive Therapy*. New York: Guilford Press, 1996; pp. 266–292.

58. Persons JB. *Cognitive Therapy in Practice: A Case Formulation Approach*. New York: Norton, 1989.

59. Reinecke MA, Dattilio FM, Freeman A. What makes for an effective treatment? In: Reinecke MA, Dattilio FM, Freeman A (eds) *Cognitive Therapy with Children and Adolescents: A Casebook for Clinical Practice*, 2nd edn. New York: Guilford Press, 2003; pp. 1–18.

60. Kendall PC, Panichelli-Mindel SM. Cognitive-behavioral treatments. *J Abnorm Child Psychol* 1995;**23**:107–124.

61. Gottman JM. *The Heart of Parenting: How to Raise an Emotionally Intelligent Child*. New York, NY: Simon & Schuster, 1997.

62. Silverman WK, Kurtines WM. Progress in developing an exposure-based transfer-of-control approach to treating internalizing disorders in youth. In: Hibbs ED, Jensen PS (eds) *Psychosocial Treatments for Child and Adolescent Disorders: Empirically Based Strategies for Clinical Practice*, 2nd edn. Washington, DC: American Psychological Association, 2005; pp. 445–476.

63. Beck JS, Beck AT, Jolly JB. *Beck Youth Inventories of Emotional & Social Impairment (BYI)*. San Antonio, TX: Psychological Corporation, 2001.

64. Bose-Deakins JE, Floyd RG. A review of the Beck youth inventories of emotional and social impairment. *J Sch Psychol* 2004;**42**:333–340.

65. Seligman LD, Ollendick TH, Langley AK, Baldacci HB. The utility of measures of child and adolescent anxiety. *J Clin Child Adolesc Psychol* 2004;**33**:557–565.

66. Feindler EL, Adler N, Brooks D, Bhumitra E. The children's anger response checklist: CARC. In: VandeCreek L (ed.) *Innovations in Clinical Practice: A Sourcebook*, Vol. 12. Sarasota, FL: Professional Resource Press, 1993; pp. 337–362.

67. Kendall PC, Furr JM, Podell JL. Child-focused treatment of anxiety. In: Weisz JR, Kazdin AE (eds) *Evidence-Based Psychotherapies for Children and Adolescents*, 2nd edn. New York: Guilford Press, 2010; pp. 45–60.

68. Kendall PC. *Coping Cat Workbook*. Ardmore, PA: Workbook Publishing, 1990.

69. Kendall PC, Chu B, Gifford A, Hayes C, Nauta M. Breathing life into a manual: Flexibility and creativity with manual-based treatments. *Cognit Behav Pract* 1998;**5**:177–198.

70. Curry JF, Reinecke MA. Modular therapy for adolescents with major depression. In: Reinecke MA, Dattilio FM, Freeman A (eds) *Cognitive Therapy with Children and Adolescents*, 2nd edn. New York: Guilford Press, 2003; pp. 95–127.

71. Ginns-Gruenberg D, Zacks A. Bibliotherapy: the use of children's literature as a therapeutic tool. In: Schaefer C (ed.) *Innovative Psychotherapy Techniques in Child and Adolescent Therapy*, 2nd edn. New York: John Wiley & Sons, Inc., 1999; pp. 454–490.

72. Pruitt DB (ed.) *Your Child: What Every Parent Needs to Know About Childhood Development from Birth to Preadolescence*. New York: HarperCollins Publishers, 1998.

73. Pruitt DB (ed.) *Your Adolescent: Emotional, Behavioral, and Cognitive Development from Early Adolescence*

Through the Teen Years. New York: HarperCollins Publishers, 1999.

74. Philadelphia Child Guidance Center, Maguire J. *Your Child's Emotional Health: The Early Years.* New York: Macmillan, 1994.

75. Philadelphia Child Guidance Center, Maguire J. *Your Child's Emotional Health: The Middle Years.* New York: Macmillan, 1994.

76. Philadelphia Child Guidance Center, Maguire J. *Your Child's Emotional Health: Adolescence.* New York: Macmillan; 1994.

77. Gottman J. The heart of parenting: raising an emotionally intelligent child. Los Angeles: Audio Renaissance Tapes, 1997.

78. Elliott CH, Smith LL. *Why Can't I Be the Parent I Want to Be?* Oakland, CA: New Harbinger, 1999.

79. Rapee RM, Spence SH, Cobham V, Wignall A. *Helping Your Anxious Child: A Step-by-step Guide for Parents.* Oakland, CA: New Harbinger Publications, Inc., 2000.

80. Wagner AP. *Worried No More: Help and Hope for Anxious Children.* Rochester, NY: Lighthouse Press, Inc., 2002.

81. Chansky TE. *Freeing Your Child from Obsessive-Compulsive Disorder.* New York: Crown Publishers, 2000.

82. Wagner AP. *What to do When Your Child has Obsessive-Compulsive Disorder: Strategies and Solutions.* Rochester, NY: Lighthouse Press, Inc., 2002.

83. Koplewicz HS. *More Than Moody: Recognizing and Treating Adolescent Depression.* New York: G.P. Putnam's Sons, 2002.

84. Manassis K, Levac AM. *Helping Your Teenager Beat Depression.* Bethesda, MD: Woodbine House, Inc., 2004.

85. Burns DD. *Therapist's Toolkit: Comprehensive Assessment and Treatment Tools for the Mental Health Professional.* Los Altos Hills, CA: David D. Burns, MD, 1995.

86. Friedberg RD, Miller R, Perymon A, Bottoms J, Aatre G. Using a session feedback form in cognitive therapy with children. *J Rational-Emotive Cogn Behav Ther* 2004;**22**:219–230.

87. Freidberg RD, McClure JM, Garcia JH. *Cognitive Therapy Techniques for Children and Adolescents.* New York: Guilford Press, 2009.

88. Association for Behavioral and Cognitive Therapies. http://www.abct.org/ (accessed 14 February 2011).

89. Anxiety Disorders Association of America. http://www.adaa.org/ (accessed 17 March 2011).

90. Society of Clinical Child and Adolescent Psychology. http://www.clinicalchildpsychology.org/ (accessed 17 March 2011).

91. http://www.abct.org/SCCAP/ (accessed 14 February 2011).

92. What Clinicians Need to Know About Treating Children With Anxiety Disorders. Podcast: http://www.adaa.org/resources-professionals/podcasts/what-clinicians-need-know-about-treating-children-with-anxiety-diso (accessed 31 March 2011).

93. Whittal ML. Looking to the future of cognitive and behavioral practice. *Cogn Behav Pract* 2009;**16**:367.

94. Borrego J Jr, Burrell TL. Using behavioral parent training to treat disruptive behavior disorders in young children: A how-to approach using video clips. *Cogn Behav Pract* 2009;**17**:25–34.

95. Podell JL, Mychailyszyn M, Edmunds J, Puleo CM, Kendall PC. The coping cat program for anxious youth: The FEAR plan comes to life. *Cogn Behav Pract* 2009;**17**:132–141.

96. Beidas RS, Benjamin CL, Puleo CM, Edmunds JM, Kendall PC. Flexible applications of the coping cat program for anxious youth. *Cogn Behav Pract* 2009;**17**:142–153.

97. The coping cat therapist: Session-by-session guide. Ardmore, PA: Workbook Publishing, 2006 [DVD].

98. Cognitive therapy. Washington, DC: American Psychological Association, 2005 [DVD].

99. Cognitive-behavioral therapy. Washington, DC: American Psychological Association, 2006 [DVD].

100. Cognitive therapy over time. Washington, DC: American Psychological Association, 2010 [DVD].

101. Cognitive-behavioral therapy for clients with multiple problems. Washington, DC: American Psychological Association, 2011 [DVD].

102. Obsessive-compulsive disorder. Washington, DC: American Psychological Association, 2007 [DVD].

103. Cognitive-behavioral therapy for perfectionism over time. Washington, DC: American Psychological Association, 2008 [DVD].

104. Behavioral therapy over time. Washington, DC: American Psychological Association, 2009 [DVD].

105. Shyness and social phobia. Washington, DC: American Psychological Association, 2006 [DVD].

106. Treating clients with generalized anxiety disorder. Washington, DC: American Psychological Association, 2008 [DVD].

107. Cognitive therapy for panic disorder. Washington, DC: American Psychological Association, 2006 [DVD].

108. Individualized case formulation and treatment planning. Washington, DC: American Psychological Association, 2007 [DVD].

109. Structure of the therapy session. Washington, DC: American Psychological Association, 2007 [DVD].

110. Activity scheduling. Washington, DC: American Psychological Association, 2006 [DVD].

111. Using the thought record. Washington, DC: American Psychological Association, 2007 [DVD].

112. Schema change methods. Washington, DC: American Psychological Association, 2006 [DVD].

113. Problem-solving therapy. Washington, DC: American Psychological Association, 2006 [DVD].

114. Guided discovery using Socratic dialogue. Richmond (CA): New Harbinger Publications, 1996 [DVD].

115. Testing automatic thoughts with thought records. Richmond (CA): New Harbinger Publications, 1996 [DVD].

116. Young J, Beck AT. Cognitive therapy scale: Rating manual. Unpublished manuscript. Philadelphia: University of Pennsylvania, 1980. Available at: http://www.academyofct.org/Upload/Documents/CTRS.pdf; http://www.academyofct.org/upload/documents/CTRS_Manual.pdf.

117. Weisz JR, Kazdin AE. The present and future of evidence-based psychotherapies for children and adolescents. In: Weisz JR, Kazdin, AE (eds) Evidence-Based Psychotherapies for Children and Adolescents, 2nd edn. New York: Guilford Press, 2010; pp. 557–572.

118. Norcross JC, Wampold BE. What works for whom: Tailoring psychotherapy to the person. *J Clin Psychol: In Session* 2011;**67**:127–132.

Section II
Common Child and Adolescent Psychiatric Disorders

10

Attention-Deficit Hyperactivity Disorder

David M. Rube, Tejal Kaur

Introduction

Attention-deficit hyperactivity disorder (ADHD) is one of the most common neuropsychiatric conditions of childhood and adolescence, and is also one of the best researched neurobiological conditions in medicine, with over 200 placebo-controlled medication trials displaying acute response [1]. The core symptoms of ADHD are manifest throughout the life cycle, from preschool through adult life; they interfere with a child's family and peer interactions, academic attainment, emotional development, self-esteem, and overall quality of life. Given the high prevalence, impairment, and societal cost of ADHD, treatment is not only essential, but also practical and efficacious.

History

In North America, children who survived the great encephalitis epidemics of 1917 and 1918 were noted to have many behavioral problems similar to those constituting what we call ADHD [2, 3]. The cases that were reported and others that have arisen due to birth trauma, head injury, exposure, or infections gave rise to the idea of a "brain-injured child syndrome." This concept evolved into that of minimal brain damage and eventually minimal brain dysfunction. Many challenges were raised to this label, however, because of the lack of evidence of brain injury in many of the children who exhibited the symptoms.

In the late 1950s and early 1960s, the "hyperactive child syndrome" was described by Burks and Chess [4, 5]. That syndrome was typified by daily movement that was greater than that of normal children of the same age. In the late 1960s, under the influence of the psychoanalytic movement, the second edition of the *Diagnostic and Statistical Manual of Mental Disorders* (DSM-II) [6] described all childhood disorders as "reactions," and the hyperactive child syndrome became the "hyperkinetic reaction of childhood." It was defined as a disorder of overactivity, restlessness, distractibility, and short attention span. It was asserted that the behavior usually diminishes in adolescence, leading to the ongoing myth that ADHD "disappears in adolescence."

In the revised edition of DSM-III (DSM-III-R) [7], the disorder was renamed ADHD (attention deficit hyperactivity disorder), with a single list of items incorporating all three symptoms and a single threshold for diagnosis. Since the publication of the DSM-III-R, researchers have found that the problems with hyperactivity and impulsivity were not separate but formed a single dimension of behavior. These conclusions led to the creation of two separate symptom lists when DSM-IV was published in 1994 [8]. The establishment of the inattention list once again permitted the diagnosis of a subtype of ADHD. The DSM-IV currently permits diagnosis of subtypes of attention-deficit hyperactivity disorder: inattentive type, hyperactive impulsive type, and, for children with problems from both lists, ADHD combined type.

Core Clinical Criteria

For a diagnosis of ADHD, DSM-IV requires an early age of onset (prior to age 7 years), the presence of impairment for 6 months or longer, and the presence of impairment in two or more settings (see Table 10.1). Inattention includes failing to give close attention to details, difficulty sustaining attention, not listening, not following through, difficulty organizing, losing things, becoming easily distracted, and forgetfulness. Hyperactivity includes fidgeting, being out of seat, running or climbing excessively, having difficulty playing quietly, being "on the go" or as if "driven by a motor," and talking excessively. The impulsivity symptom criteria include blurting out answers, having difficulty awaiting a turn, and often interrupting or intruding on others [8]. Core deficits include impairment in rule-governed

Clinical Child Psychiatry, Third Edition. Edited by William M. Klykylo and Jerald Kay.
© 2012 John Wiley & Sons, Ltd. Published 2012 by John Wiley & Sons, Ltd.

Table 10.1   Criteria for the diagnosis of attention-deficit hyperactivity disorder (ADHD).

The diagnosis requires evidence of inattention or hyperactivity and impulsivity or both

Inattention

Six or more of the following symptoms of inattention have persisted for at least six months to a degree that is maladaptive and inconsistent with developmental level:

Often fails to give close attention to details and makes careless mistakes

Often has difficulty sustaining attention

Often does not seem to listen

Often does not seem to follow through

Often has difficulty organizing tasks

Often avoids tasks that require sustained attention

Often loses things necessary for activities

Often is easily distracted

Often is forgetful

Hyperactivity and impulsivity

Six or more of the following symptoms of hyperactivity and impulsivity have persisted for at least six months to a degree that is maladaptive and inconsistent with developmental level:

Often fidgets

Often leaves seat

Often runs about or climbs excessively

Often has difficulty with quiet leisure activities

Often is 'on the go' or 'driven by a motor'

Often talks excessively

Often blurts out answers

Often has difficulty awaiting turn

Often interrupts or intrudes

Symptoms that cause impairment:

Are present before seven years of age

Are present in two or more settings (e.g., home, school, or work)

Do not occur exclusively during the course of a pervasive developmental disorder, schizophrenia, or another psychotic disorder

Are not better accounted for by another mental disorder (e.g., a mood disorder or an anxiety disorder)

The criteria are adapted from the *Diagnostic and Statistical Manual of Mental Disorders*, 4th edition, Text Revision.

behavior across a variety of settings and relative difficulty for age in inhibiting an impulsive response to internal wishes, needs, or external stimuli.

While the syndrome may manifest itself differently throughout the life cycle, school-age children are the most common presenting population to pediatricians, child psychiatrists, and psychologists. Weiss [9, 10] points out that these children typically present with:

- inappropriate or excessive activity, unrelated to the task at hand, which generally has an intrusive or annoying quality;
- poor sustained attention;
- difficulties in inhibiting impulses in social behavior and cognitive tasks;
- difficulties getting along with others;
- school underachievement;

- poor self-esteem secondary to difficulties getting along with others and school underachievement;
- other behavior disorders, learning disabilities, anxiety disorders, and depression.

Restlessness is measured by well-standardized rating scales and direct and indirect observation [11, 12]. Teachers and parents may not agree with one another, owing to the likelihood that children may act differently in different situations, particularly as the full range of ADHD symptoms are less likely to emerge in settings where a child likes a teacher or tries harder at home to please his or her parents. Consequently, a child being evaluated in a physician's office could sit perfectly still during the examination, and the clinician may use rating scales in settings where the child spends the majority of his time. Whalen and Henker [13] suggest that "each measure reflects a unique child × perceiver × setting example."

Bewildered parents will report their child's difficulties with attention. A common complaint is "he can play video games for hours but to do 20 minutes worth of homework requires 1 to 2 hours worth of screaming and temper tantrums." It seems that when a particular activity interests a child, he or she can pay attention for hours. However, these same children can have a poor attention span when attending to tasks they find boring, repetitive, or difficult and that give them no satisfaction.

Poor attention span should be carefully assessed, as it can also be very similar to the poor concentration seen in anxiety and mood disorders. Moreover, as many of the core symptoms of ADHD can appear cross-sectionally to mimic other Axis I psychiatric diagnoses, and vice versa, a thorough assessment should begin with a broad-based differential (see "Differential Diagnoses" and Table 10.2).

Difficulty Getting Along with Others

Peers often quickly reject children with ADHD because of their aggression, impulsivity, and noncompliance with rules [14]. Children with ADHD may be unpopular with their peers and may have difficulties with parents, siblings, and teachers [15]. These children may have few "best friends" and few enduring friendships, and this unpopularity and inability to establish and maintain friendships may be replaced in life by social isolation. In childhood, sometimes the only person willing to play with a hyperactive child is a younger child or a child with some other similar difficulty.

The negative effect of hyperactive children on others has been observed with respect to their teachers and ability to participate in both dyads and groups of children. Parents may also interact with a hyperactive child in a more negative and intrusive way. Furthermore, as ADHD often runs in families, one often discovers the likelihood that the parent may also have significant ADHD symptoms, which contribute to general disorganization in the household, which in turn often exacerbates ADHD and concomitant behavioral symptoms. Although working with parents to increase structure and behavioral modification strategies at home can prove beneficial, simultaneous addition of medication can lead to improved relationships with peers, teachers, and parents.

School Underachievement

Cantwell and Baker [16] showed that even when intelligence was controlled for, hyperactive children were behind normal children in their grade level in reading, spelling, and arithmetic. Even in the absence of comorbid learning disorder, the core symptoms of ADHD impair learning. ADHD children have poorer organizational skills, poor sequential memory, deficits in fine and gross motor skills affecting handwriting, and inefficient and unproductive cognitive styles. However, a recent longitudinal study beginning in kindergarten shows sustained improvement in academic performance in those with ADHD with ongoing medication treatment over 5 years compared to those without medication [17].

Low Self-Esteem

In general, when children receive praise and acceptance from parents, teachers, and students, their self-esteem and sense of self improves dramatically. However, children with ADHD have multiple difficulties in multiple areas of their lives. They are criticized and embarrassed. At times it is difficult for them to feel liked and successful. It is common for these children to feel "demoralized." With successful treatment, however, some of these symptoms may ameliorate.

Epidemiology of ADHD

Estimates of the prevalence of ADHD in school-age children range from 3% to 7% [18], with approximately half of those children ever having been treated with medication for ADHD (Centers for Disease Control and Prevention, 2005), and approximately 60–85% of children continuing to meet criteria for the disorder into adolescence [19, 20]. While determining the rates of persistent ADHD symptoms into adulthood is difficult methodologically, impairment tends to continue into adulthood, with potentially 90% of adults with childhood diagnoses of ADHD continuing to have at least five symptoms of ADHD and a Global Assessment of Functioning score below 60 [21]. In elementary school-age children, the ratio of boys to girls is typically 9:1 in a clinical setting, but approximates to 4:1 in community epidemiological surveys [22].

Teachers typically identify fewer girls than boys with ADHD symptoms. The male-to-female ratio ranges from 4:1 for the predominantly impulsive type, to 2:1 for the predominantly inattentive type. Even among children rated by teachers as meeting criteria for any subtype of ADHD, fewer girls than boys receive an ADHD diagnosis or stimulant treatment. Barkley [23] hypothesizes that these diagnostic criteria were set in a predominantly male distribution, which could create a higher threshold for the diagnosis for female subjects

Table 10.2 Mental health conditions that mimic or coexist with attention-deficit hyperactivity disorder (ADHD).

Disorder	Symptoms overlapping with ADHD	Features not characteristic of ADHD	Diagnostic problem
Learning disorders	Underachievement in school Disruptive behavior during academic activity Refusal to engage in academic tasks and use academic materials	Underachievement and disruptive behavior in academic work, rather than in multiple settings and activities	It can be difficult to determine which to evaluate first – a learning disorder or ADHD (follow the preponderance of symptoms)
Oppositional defiant disorder	Disruptive behavior, especially regarding rules Failure to follow directions	Defiance, rather than unsuccessful attempts to cooperate	Defiant behavior is often associated with a high level of activity It is difficult to determine the child's effort to comply in instances of a negative parent-child or teacher-child relationship
Conduct disorder	Disruptive behavior Encounters with law-enforcement and legal systems	Lack of remorse Intent to harm or do wrong Aggression and hostility Antisocial behavior	Fighting or running away may be reasonable reactions to adverse social circumstances
Anxiety, obsessive-compulsive disorder or post-traumatic stress disorder	Poor attention Fidgetiness Difficulty with transitions Physical reactivity to stimuli	Excessive worries Fearfulness Obsessions or compulsions Nightmares Re-experiences of trauma	Anxiety may be a source of high activity and inattention
Depression	Irritability Reactive impulsivity Demoralization	Pervasive and persistent feelings of irritability or sadness	It may be difficult to distinguish depression from a reaction to repeated failure, which is associated with ADHD
Bipolar disorder	Poor attention Hyperactivity Impulsivity Irritability	Expansive mood Grandiosity Manic quality	It is difficult to distinguish severe ADHD from early-onset bipolar disorder
Tic disorder	Poor attention Impulsive verbal or motor actions Disruptive activity	Repetitive vocal or motor movements	Tics may not be apparent to the patient, the family, or a casual observer
Adjustment disorder	Poor attention Hyperactivity Disruptive behavior Impulsivity Poor academic performance	Recent onset Precipitating event	Chronic stressors, such as having a sibling with mental illness, or attachment-and-loss issues may produce symptoms of anxiety and depression

relative to other female populations and for male subjects relative to other male populations. Anecdotally, a high percentage of females are not diagnosed with ADHD until they present in middle or late adolescence with a comorbid disorder such as depression, anxiety, or an eating disorder.

Etiology of ADHD

Recent evidence suggests genetics as a principal cause of ADHD, with estimated percentage of phenotypic variance accounted for by genetic factors being 76% expressed over multiple genes [24]; for a child of a parent with ADHD the risk of developing the disorder may be as high as 57% [25]. However, even nongenetic causes are neurobiological in nature, varying from severe early deprivation [26], maternal smoking during pregnancy [27], traumatic brain injury [28], fetal alcohol syndrome [29], and perinatal stress and low birthweight [30].

The presence of executive function deficits, particularly in domains of response inhibition, vigilance, working memory, and planning, has been shown in a recent meta-analysis of 83 studies including over 6000 subjects [31]. Yet, a subgroup of individuals with ADHD may not have executive deficits, and individuals tend to have varied symptom constellations, comorbidities, and severity, suggesting the presence of multiple pathways to ADHD [32–34].

While neuroimaging currently informs the neurobiological basis of ADHD, the research does not yet support its use in diagnosis or treatment. Similar to executive function deficits found on neuropsychological tests [31], studies suggest that patients with ADHD have functional differences in the caudate, frontal lobes, and anterior cingulate when performing executive function tasks [35]. Structural imaging studies suggest that children with ADHD have reduced cortical gray and white matter volume compared to controls, with volume deficits being more extensive in those who have never been treated compared to those treated with long-term stimulants [36, 37]. Individuals with ADHD, compared to controls, may also have reduced integrity and network homogeneity within the default mode network on functional imaging tests [38]. Stimulants seem to improve suppression of default-mode activity in the ventral anterior cingulate and posterior cingulate cortices, components of a circuit in which activity has been shown to correlate with the degree of mind-wandering during attentional tasks [39]. Future studies are needed to further elucidate what biomarkers may serve as endophenotypes of the illness and to elucidate treatment response and prognosis.

Environmental Toxins and Dietary Findings

In the 1970s, the "Feingold Diet," written by Dr Ben Feingold, claimed that half of all children with ADHD could be cured by a diet that eliminated all food additives. Evidence suggests that sugar content in diet does not seem to affect symptom assessment on multiple measures [40]. While another meta-analysis did find a small negative effect of food additives on ADHD symptoms [41], it is thought that the effects on ADHD may be mediated by genotype [42]. A recent study in the *Lancet* proposed that ADHD symptoms were largely attributed to diet; however, this study was fraught with many limitations, the most striking of which was that it was not blinded [43]. Further studies elucidating clinical correlates translating into treatment recommendations are not yet available.

Environmental toxins, such as lead exposure [44], particularly in inner city environments, and fetal alcohol syndrome [29] also tend to lead to higher rates of ADHD in exposed children.

Differential Diagnosis

As some parents are not aware what level of activity, concentration span, and compliance to commands can be expected from a normal child at different ages, particularly in boys, they may bring in children for evaluation when the level of hyperactivity may still be within developmental norms. Conversely, some parents will bring in the oldest sibling after the second child is between 3 to 5 years old, stating that they initially tolerated a child's hyperactivity because they felt that it was normal. When a child presents for evaluation, a thorough differential is necessary as a number of psychiatric disorders and family issues may resemble ADHD.

Learning-disabled children, even those without ADHD, are bored and discouraged at school because of their inability to learn at the same speed or keep up with the class. They may be restless and inattentive as a reaction to inappropriate school placement. A child with a speech and language impairment without ADHD may also be bored and restless and inattentive in the classroom. In these cases of isolated learning disorders without the presence of ADHD, inattention or hyperactivity would not be seen in varied settings. However, as learning disorders and ADHD are often comorbid, academic and behavioral symptoms consistent with a learning disorder may continue to be evident even after successful treatment of ADHD.

Conduct disorder and oppositional defiant disorder may also present with some degree of restlessness, inattention, and impulsivity. It is important in differentiating the two to obtain a symptom timeline, delineating which symptoms came first and which as a reaction to various problems that the child has at home and at school.

Adjustment disorders and anxiety disorders are also important diagnoses to differentiate from ADHD as overactivity can be a "common denominator" symptom of anxiety or post-traumatic stress disorder. Differentiating ADHD from anxiety would again be easier given a timeline of the various symptoms.

Similarly, understanding the timeline of symptoms can be helpful in differentiating affective disorders from ADHD as these conditions can produce hyperactivity and interfere with attention, but lead to episodic symptoms rather than being pervasive and consistent, which is seen in ADHD. While depressive symptoms may emerge as a process of demoralization from ADHD, usually depressive symptoms do not masquerade as ADHD. When full criteria for a major depressive episode are met, treatment is usually necessary for both the depressive disorder and the ADHD [45]. It is more complicated to tease apart whether bipolar disorder remains in the differential or as a comorbid condition, particularly given the complexities and competing views in diagnosing childhood onset bipolar disorder. Biederman and colleagues [46, 47] found that 16% of a sample of ADHD patients met the criteria for mania. However, when samples of young people with bipolar disorder are assessed, 90% of the preadolescents and 68% of the adolescents also meet criteria for ADHD [48, 49]. As diagnostic criteria for bipolar disorder in children are still being reassessed, currently it is most prudent to consider bipolar disorder in the differential of ADHD by making an educated clinical decision based on timeline of symptoms, chronicity versus episodicity, and assessing particular criteria such as grandiosity and euphoria, which seem more specific to bipolar disorder.

Assessing Comorbidity

Comorbidity tends to be the rule rather than the exception in children with ADHD. As many as two-thirds of elementary-school-age children with ADHD referred for a clinical evaluation have at least one other psychiatric disorder. As comorbidity predominates, it is essential that clinicians elicit developmental trajectories of symptom initiation and course, and identify comorbid conditions as well as differentiating when symptoms of a mood, anxiety, learning, or oppositional disorder may be mimicking ADHD (see Table 10.2).

Studies show that 54–84% of children and adolescents with ADHD also have oppositional defiant disorder,

and many of these kids will also develop conduct disorder [50–52]. Approximately 15–19% of youngsters with ADHD will develop a substance abuse disorder [53, 54], 25–35% will have a learning or language disorder [55], and up to one-third will have an anxiety disorder [52, 55–57]. Up to 33% may also have a depressive disorder [55], but elucidating the true comorbidity of bipolar disorder remains much more difficult given the overlapping symptom nature of ADHD and hypomania/mania [58]. It is therefore incumbent upon the evaluating clinician to assess a child with ADHD for the presence of other conditions [59] as the presence of a second or third comorbid disorder indicates a more serious problem with a worse prognosis [10]. When comorbid conditions exist, pharmacological treatment strategies are influenced by the condition that is currently the most impairing.

Diagnosis and Assessment

Diagnostic criteria for ADHD can be found in Table 10.1. The diagnosis of ADHD is a clinical diagnosis made on the basis of a clinical picture that begins early in life, is persistent over time and pervasive across different settings, and causes functional impairment at home, at school, or in leisure activity. While DSM-IV requires impairment in at least two settings (home, school, or job) to meet criteria for the disorder, the clinical consensus is that severe impairment in one setting warrants treatment [60].

The parent interview is the primary input in the assessment process. Interviewing the child alone can be helpful, and should be done particularly with kids of school age and above, but many children lack insight into their own difficulties and are unwilling or unable to report them [61]. Particular areas of focus include: age of onset of symptoms, settings in which impairment occurs, academic functioning and possibility of learning disorder, and teacher input either through rating scales or through old report cards or work samples if parents do not want to involve school [60]. As ADHD tends to run in families, family history and family functioning should be carefully assessed as not only can genetic risk contribute to a diagnosis of ADHD, but ongoing parental symptoms can contribute to a disorganized home setting, further exacerbating the child's symptoms [60].

As developmental and psychiatric disorders can either mimic or be comorbid with ADHD, besides assessing ADHD symptoms, clinicians should also ask parents about perinatal history, developmental milestones, medical history, and prior mental health history including treatment as delays in reaching developmental milestones or in social/language development suggest language disorders, mental retardation, or pervasive developmental disorders. Mental health history should include psychiatric symptoms in childhood, including symptoms of oppositional disorder, conduct disorder, depression, mania, anxiety, substance abuse, psychosis, and learning disability [60].

Rating scales may be helpful in gathering information from parents, teachers, other adults, and, in some cases, even the patient, during initial assessment and to document progress. Commonly used scales include the Conners Parent Rating Scale-Revised and Conners Teacher Rating Scale-Revised [62], which can be purchased from a publishing company, while the Swanson, Nolan and Pelham (SNAP-IV) [63] can be obtained free at http://adhd.net. Clinicians must be careful not to make a diagnosis on the basis of a score on a rating scale alone, but rather to take all information, including the interviews, into account. A classroom observation can also assess the teacher's style, as well as the child's social and academic environment [60].

Specialized tests, such as the Continuous Performance Test, the Wisconsin Card Sorting Test, the Matching Familiar Figures Test, and subtests of the Wechsler Intelligence Scale for Children-Fourth Edition (WISC-IV), should not be considered "diagnostic of ADHD." There is no specific diagnostic test for ADD, despite the frequent requests of parents and others for discrete psychological testing in which the conclusion is the diagnosis of ADHD. Psychological testing can elicit findings that are consistent with a child who has the diagnosis of ADHD, but the presence or absence of such findings should not dictate diagnosis or ongoing treatment.

A medical evaluation should include a complete medical history and a physical examination within the past 12 months. Any effects of medication and vision or hearing deficits should be ruled out. Unless there is strong supportive evidence in the medical history, neurological tests such as electroencephalography (EEG) or neuroimaging, or laboratory tests are not warranted. Speech and language evaluation may be required as suggested by clinical findings. Occupational therapy evaluation may also provide supplementary information regarding motor clumsiness or adaptive skills [60].

Treatment of ADHD

The evaluation and management of the treatments used for ADHD require cooperation from the patient, the parents, and the school. This makes the clinician's role as coordinator or case manager vital to the treatment. Once diagnosed, ADHD has an extended course requiring continuous treatment and treatment monitoring to deal with the ongoing challenges that these children and families face. The treatment plan should be individualized, targeting the symptoms that are presented (personal, family, and academic), and take into account the patient's, family's, and school's strengths and weaknesses.

Treatment planning should consist of medical treatment and management and psychosocial interventions, such as environmental modification, behavioral therapy, social skills intervention, and individual psychotherapy. The school and the teacher should be incorporated into the treatment plan, both as participants and as monitors of the treatment.

Psychoeducational treatment in ADHD is the provision of information to patients, parents, and teachers and is considered standard in both research protocols and clinical practice. It is also helpful to address the myths of ADHD and its treatment. For example, "Does ADHD vanish with puberty?" "Do stimulant medications act paradoxically, cause drug abuse, or stop working in puberty?" Information may be disseminated in a public group setting, through published books and newsletters, or by referral to support groups such as Children and Adults with Attention Deficit/Hyperactivity Disorder (CHADD; www.chadd.org) or the National Attention Deficit Disorder Association (www.add.org) (see Appendix 10.2).

Parent management training is also a part of the psychosocial interventions with ADHD. Parents may learn to use contingency management techniques in cooperation with schools, such as a school/home daily report card or a point token response-cost system (see "Multimodal Treatment" below).

This comprehensive treatment plan should be outlined in a clear methodic approach to the parents, the schools, and the patients (Table 10.3). Rating scales such as the Connors Parent Rating Scale-Revised and Conners Teacher Rating Scale-Revised [62], or the Swanson, Nolan and Pelham (SNAP-IV) [63], or custom-designed target symptom scales for daily behavioral report cards may be useful in monitoring progress.

Pharmacotherapy

Pharmacotherapy is often seen as a primary modality, particularly since the publication of the results of the Multimodal Treatment Study of Children with Attention-Deficit Hyperactivity Disorder (MTA) results, which pointed to the superiority of well-delivered medication treatment over psychosocial treatment and community standard care for ADHD symptoms [52]. Nevertheless, psychosocial treatments can be used successfully, either as a primary treatment or to augment

Table 10.3 Guidelines for the diagnosis and treatment of patients with attention-deficit hyperactivity disorder (ADHD).*

Diagnosis
   Comprehensive developmental, social, and family history
   Standardized checklists to assess behaviors
   Consideration of coexisting mental health disorders
   Physical examination, not to diagnose ADHD but to assess genetic and other conditions

Treatment
   Management of ADHD as a chronic health condition
   Establishment of treatment goals agreed on by the child, the family, and school personnel
   Medication with stimulants to manage symptoms (mono therapy)†
   Behavioral therapy for parent-child discord and persistent oppositional behavior

Desired outcomes of treatment
   Improved relationships with family, teachers, and peers
   Decreased frequency of disruptive behavior
   Improved quality of and efficiency in completing academic work, and increased quantity of work completed
   Increased independence in caring for self and carrying out age-appropriate activities
   Improved self-esteem
   Enhanced safety (e.g., care in crossing streets, staying with an adult in public places, and reduced risk-taking behavior)

*This information has been compiled from the guidelines of the American Academy of Child and Adolescent Psychiatry [60].
†Atomoxetine is recommended by the American Academy of Child and Adolescent Psychiatry as a possible alternative to stimulant medication [60].

medication treatment effects, and can be tailored to target symptoms of ADHD or comorbid disorders in school or at home. The therapeutic alliance between the clinician and the family is the most potent instrument for ensuring medication compliance. Faithful adherence to a prescribed regimen requires the cooperation of the parents, the patient, school personnel, and often additional caretakers. The child may have to take medication in a variety of settings, including in day care before school, in school, in after-school care, and at home in the evenings. Children and adolescents should not be responsible for administering their own medication, since they will often forget or refuse outright to take medication. However, as an adolescent approaches adulthood, assisting the patient in assuming responsibility for administering his or her own medication is important.

Psychostimulants

Although the precise mechanisms of action are not known, the therapeutic activity of the stimulants is often attributed to their blockade of the presynaptic dopamine transporter, which decreases reuptake and increases synaptic dopamine in the striatum and other brain regions. Stimulants also bind to the norepinephrine

transporter in the prefrontal cortex, enhancing both norepinephrine and dopamine as a result.

Psychostimulants have been the mainstay of treatment of ADHD, with effect sizes relative to placebo averaging around 1.0, which are considered quite high and one of the largest effects for most psychotropic medications [64]. At least 70% of children have a positive response to one of the major stimulants in a first trial. If a clinician conducts a trial of dextroamphetamine (dexamfetamine) or methylphenidate, the response rate to at least one of these is in the 85–90% range, depending on how response is defined [65].

Medical Work-Up   While there is no indication for routine cardiac evaluation prior to starting a psychostimulant in an otherwise healthy individual, in clinical practice it is not uncommon for an electrocardiogram to be ordered routinely. Practice guidelines, however, state that caution should be exercised in particular high-risk patients, who should be referred to cardiology for possible electrocardiography or echocardiography prior to starting stimulants, as well as followed by cardiology if stimulants are initiated and continued [60]. Indication of high risk include a history of severe palpitations, fainting, exercise intolerance not accounted for by obesity, structural cardiac abnormalities, or strong family history of sudden death [60].

Preparation and Dosage As either of the two stimulant types, methylphenidate or amphetamine, are equally efficacious in the treatment of ADHD, the physician may start with either. Practically, the choice of stimulant may also be determined by the delivery system: those that come in patches, or in beaded preparations that can be opened and sprinkled in food (such as yogurt, apple sauce, or pudding so that the medicine sticks to food and is not lost at the bottom of the container), can be good alternatives for kids who do not wish to swallow tablets (see Table 10.4).

In the past, physicians tended to begin with immediate release, ascertain dose, and then switch to longer-acting preparations. However, evidence suggests that the long-acting formulations are equally efficacious to the immediate-release forms [66], and can be started as initial treatment. Moreover, the long-acting preparations tend to be more practical because doses can be given before school, often eliminating the need for school-time dosing and maximizing the family's confidentiality. After selecting the starting dose, the physician may titrate up every 1–3 weeks until either maximal dose is reached, symptoms of ADHD remit, or side effects preclude further titration [60].

Immediate-acting formulations may be preferred for children under 16 kg for whom sufficiently low starting doses of long-acting preparations are not available, and in cases where long-acting preparations "wear off" during the day and "booster" short-acting formulations are required later in the day. While the behavior of children with ADHD tends to be worse later in the day compared to the morning, it is often more noticeable after morning stimulants are initiated as symptoms are largely improved for the first part of the day [67]. Often, small booster doses are given either at noon or early afternoon to help control symptoms at the end of the school day and when doing homework. Sometimes, a later dose may be given in an attempt to control hyperactivity around bedtime, which exacerbates insomnia. However, when dosing later in the day, the clinician should be particularly careful to adjust the time of dose so that the effects tend not to continue into the night leading to insomnia; the last dose of immediate-release medication is usually given no later than 5 hours before bedtime, and often even earlier.

Stimulant Use in Preschool Age Children The National Institute of Mental Health (NIMH)-funded Preschool ADHD Treatment Study (PATS) has validated the safety and efficacy of methylphenidate in preschoolers between 3 and 5.5 years old [68]. The study recruited a total of 303 children where children with less than 30% improvement in ADHD symptoms after parent training were eligible for an open-label followed by crossover double-blind placebo-controlled methylphenidate treatment phase. The mean best total daily dose of methylphenidate for the group was 14.2 ± 8.1 mg/day $(0.7 \pm 0.4$ mg/kg/day), significantly lower than the 30 mg/day reported for school-aged children in the Multimodal Treatment Study of Children with ADHD (MTA) [69]. Methylphenidate displayed efficacy in reducing ADHD symptoms with a graduated dose response [68] in comparison to placebo; however, effect sizes observed in preschoolers on methylphenidate (0.16–0.72) were smaller than those in school-aged children [70]. Furthermore, the PATS study showed that preschoolers metabolized methylphenidate (MPH) more slowly than did school-age children, suggesting that preschoolers may respond to lower and less frequent dosing [71].

While stimulants have been found effective in treating preschoolers [68], preschoolers, as opposed to school-age or adolescent patients, tended to show higher rates of irritability and crying [72], suggesting that doses should be titrated even more conservatively in this population, and particularly so in preschoolers with significant developmental delays, who are even more prone to such side effects [73].

Psychostimulant Treatment Guidelines The most recent and widely accepted algorithm for psychopharmacological treatment of ADHD is the Texas Children's Medication Algorithm Project (CMAP; www.dshs.state.tx.us/mhprograms/CMAP.shtm), which divides treatment into stages 0–6 with progression through stages if treatment response is insufficient [74].

Stage 0 – includes diagnostic assessment and family consultation.

Stage 1 – includes beginning with either an amphetamine or methylphenidate.

Stage 2 – includes switching to the group not used in stage 1 (methylphenidate vs amphetamine).

Stage 3 – includes use of atomoxetine, with an optional stage 3A of adding stimulant to atomoxetine.

Stage 4 – includes using either bupropion or tricyclic antidepressant (TCA).

Stage 5 – includes using either bupropion or TCA (whichever was not used in stage 4).

Stage 6 – includes use of an alpha-agonist, with subsequent clinical consultation if all stages lead to insufficient treatment response.

Table 10.4 Psychostimulant medications for treatment of attention-deficit hyperactivity disorder (ADHD).

Medication	Starting dose	MPH equivalent	Dose range	Duration	Comments
Immediate-release (IR)					
Methylphenidate (Ritalin)	5 mg t.i.d.		10–60 mg or 0.6–2.0 mg/kg	3–4 hours	Most studied and prescribed
Dexmethylphenidate (Focalin)	2.5 mg t.i.d.	5 mg t.i.d.	2.5–40 mg	4–5 hours	To convert from methylphenidate, start at 50% of current methylphenidate dose; may require t.i.d. dosing
Dextroamphetamine (Dexedrine)	2.5 mg b.i.d.	5 mg b.i.d.	5–60 mg or 0.3–1 mg/kg	3–5 hours	
Mixed amphetamine salts (Adderall)	2.5 mg b.i.d.	5 mg b.i.d.	10–40mg or 0.5–1.5 mg/kg	3–5 hours	
Extended-release (ER)					
Methylphenidate (Ritalin LA)	10 mg q.a.m.	5 mg b.i.d.	20–60 mg or 1.0 mg/kg	6–8 hours	Can be sprinkled onto food; released 50% as IR and 50% as ER
Methylphenidate (Metadate CD)	10 mg q.a.m.	3 mg q.a.m. and 7 mg q. noon	10–60 mg or 1.0 mg/kg	6–8 hours	Released 30% as IR and 70% as ER
MPH-OROS (Concerta)	18 mg q.a.m.	5 mg t.i.d.	18–72 mg	8–12 hours	OROS technology provides continuous release throughout day and limits potential for substance abuse
Methylphenidate transdermal (Daytrana)	10 mg q.a.m.	N/A	10–30 mg	8–12 hours	Patch provides continuous release throughout day and limits potential for substance abuse
Dexmethylphenidate (Focalin XR)	5–10 mg q.a.m.	5–10 mg b.i.d.	10–30 mg or 1 mg/kg	8–12 hours	To convert from methylphenidate, start at 50% of current methylphenidate dose; released 50% as IR and 50% as ER Can be sprinkled onto food
Mixed amphetamine salts (Adderall XR)	5–10 mg q.a.m.	5–10 mg b.i.d.	10–40 mg or 0.5–1.5 mg/kg	8–12 hours	May convert from IR to ER dose at total daily dose
Lisdexamfetamine (Vyvanse)	30 mg q.a.m.	10 mg b.i.d.	30–70 mg	8–12 hours	Prodrug conversion to dextroamfetamine limits potential for substance abuse Can be mixed into liquid

MPH, methylphenidate.

While combination psychopharmacological treatment of ADHD (not accounting for treatment of comorbidity) is not addressed in the CMAP algorithm, recent initial studies suggest that combination treatments such as adding alpha-agonists to stimulants [75] or adding stimulants to atomoxetine [76] can augment treatment response. Combination treatment may be considered in cases of residual symptoms, pharmacological synergism, improved tolerability, or psychiatric or medical comorbidity [76].

Side Effects of Stimulants Side effects of stimulant medication are similar for all the agents, tend to be brief in duration, and increase linearly with the dose (Table 10.5). In an individual patient, however, it is possible that if a patient has a side effect to one stimulant, he or she may not have any side effects with another. Mild appetite suppression is almost universal and may be managed by giving the medication after breakfast and lunch. It is very important when monitoring the patient to know the schedule of the patient's meals and give the medication accordingly. It is not uncommon for children who have a three-times-daily dosing regimen to have a late dinner or even "a midnight snack."

Sleep difficulties are common in these patients; however, difficulty falling asleep may be caused by direct stimulant effects, ADHD symptoms, oppositional behavior, separation anxiety, drug effect rebound, or a pre-existing sleep problem. The remedy should address the cause and may include behavior modification, giving clonidine or a small dose of stimulant before bedtime, decreasing the afternoon stimulant dose, or moving it to an earlier time. In a review of clonidine in sleep disturbances associated with ADHD, Prince *et al.* concluded that clonidine may be an effective agent for sleep disturbances associated with ADHD [77]. However, because of its short half-life, a percentage of children will develop early morning awakening. Melatonin has also been found to be helpful in promoting sleep onset in medicated and unmedicated children with ADHD, and is generally well tolerated [78–80]. If the sleep problems are direct symptoms of ADHD, a small dose of a stimulant may be helpful.

Another complaint sometimes associated with stimulant treatment is blunted affect. Patients may appear remote or less responsive than usual while on treatment. When affective blunting does occur, it is usually a dose-dependent adverse effect that can be successfully managed by dose reduction.

There has been some controversy about whether stimulant medication has been associated with decreased growth. It is important to balance the benefits of medication treatment with the risks of small reductions in height gain, which as yet have not been shown to be related to reductions in adult height [60, 81].

Some children have been noted to become more aggressive, emotionally labile, or even to experience psychotic symptoms on stimulants. When such side effects are noted, the physician should discontinue the current medication and restart another class of stimulant, or other medication [60, 82].

There has been a great deal of concern over cardiac risk and sudden death as rare, but important side effects. In 2005, the US Food and Drug Administration (FDA) reported 19 cases of sudden death in youth treated with stimulants for ADHD, with cardiac abnormalities found in two-thirds of the cases, leading to the FDA contraindicating stimulants in persons with known cardiac risks [83]. Gould *et al.* published the finding that there are higher rates of stimulant use (1.8%) in cases of sudden death compared with auto accidents, further suggesting that there may be a small, but statistically significant correlation between stimulant use and sudden death [84]. However, the incidence of sudden cardiac death is estimated at between 0.8 and 6.2 individuals per 100 000 persons in those less than 21 years old, and the increased risk of sudden death from athletic activity is estimated to be three times greater than the risk associated with stimulants [85]. Considering that it remains unclear whether cardiac risk on medications exceeds population risk in children, clinical screening is a standard of care and should be documented in medical records. The AACAP Practice Parameters recommend that cardiology referral is indicated if there is a personal history of syncope, family history of early sudden cardiac death, known cardiac abnormality, or abnormal cardiac exam. In the absence of such, while routine electrocardiogram (ECG) is reasonable, there is no evidence to suggest the practice of routine ECGs prior to starting treatment [60].

Atomoxetine

In January 2003, atomoxetine was released in the USA, becoming the first nonstimulant approved for the treatment of ADHD. It has an effect size of approximately 0.6 [64], which is much smaller than that of stimulant medications, which range around 1.0. However, it can be useful in cases of uncomplicated ADHD, refractory ADHD, or ADHD that is comorbid with either anxiety or depressive disorders or substance use disorders [74, 86].

Atomoxetine is a potent presynaptic, noradrenergic transport blocker with low affinity for any other receptors or transporters. Atomoxetine is labeled for once- or twice-daily use. It is administered in capsules that cannot be opened. Dosing follows a weight-based schedule because plasma levels vary considerably as a function of bodyweight (1.0–1.4 mg/kg). Although there is some immediate improvement, a longer period (approximately 4 weeks at the most effective tolerated dose) is required before the full effect of treatment is observed.

Table 10.5 Side effects, management, and contraindications of medications used to treat attention-deficit hyperactivity disorder (ADHD).

Medication	Side effects	Management for most common side effects	Considerations
Methylphenidate	Appetite suppression, stomach aches, headaches, irritability, weight loss, deceleration in rate of growth, exacerbation of psychosis, exacerbation of tics, mild increase in blood pressure and pulse	1. Mild **appetite suppression** is almost universal and may be managed by giving the medication after breakfast and lunch. Monitor patients' schedule of meals and give the medication accordingly 2. **Rebound effects** a. Increased structure after school b. Dose of medication in the afternoon that is smaller than the morning and midday doses c. Use of long-acting formulations d. Addition of clonidine or guanfacine to the regimen	Cardiovascular disease or hypertension, marked anxiety, agitation, glaucoma, use of monoamine oxidase inhibitors, seizures, tics, diversion of prescription for drug sales
Dextroamphetamine	As above	**Blunted affect** (may be complaint in all stimulants): a. Managed by dose reduction	As above
Atomoxetine	Appetite suppression, nausea, vomiting, fatigue, weight loss, deceleration in rate of growth, mild increase in blood pressure and pulse		Jaundice or other clinical or laboratory evidence of liver injury, use of monoamine oxidase inhibitors, narrow-angle glaucoma
Bupropion	Weight loss, insomnia, agitation, anxiety, dry mouth, seizures	**Insomnia** a. Address the cause, which may include behavior modification b. Giving clonidine or a small dose of stimulant before bedtime c. Decreasing the afternoon stimulant dose or moving it to an earlier time d. If sleep problems are direct symptoms of ADHD, a small dose of a stimulant may be helpful	Seizures, bulimia, anorexia nervosa, abrupt discontinuation of alcohol or benzodiazepines, use of monoamine oxidase inhibitors or other bupropion products such as Zyban
Alpha-agonists	Sedation, hypotension	**Sedation** a. Managed by dose reduction or termination	Cardiac disease, pre-existing hypotension, history of rebound hypertension

Adverse effects include sedation, nausea, and vomiting, decreased appetite, weight loss, and modest increase in pulse and blood pressure (comparable to stimulants). It is uncertain, but unlikely, whether atomoxetine affects growth, particularly after the initial effects of decreased appetite are accounted for, although effects appear to be small [87]. There have been reports of aggression, mania, and hypomania induction associated with atomoxetine [87]. Also, seizures and prolonged QTc interval with atomoxetine overdose have been reported [88].

In 2004, the FDA required a warning be added to atomoxetine because of reports that two patients (one adult and one child) had developed severe liver disease, from which both patients recovered. However, no evidence of hepatotoxicity was found in the clinical trials of 6000 patients. Current recommendations do not require routine monitoring of hepatic function, but patients who develop jaundice, dark urine, or other symptoms of hepatic disease should discontinue atomoxetine [60].

In 2005, the FDA issued an alert regarding suicidal ideation in children and adolescents taking atomoxetine. In 12 controlled trials with 1357 patients on atomoxetine and 851 control subjects, the average risk of suicidal ideation was 4/1000 in the atomoxetine group compared to none in the placebo group, but there were no completed suicides. Recommendations now include discussing this risk with families prior to starting atomoxetine and then monitoring closely after treatment initiation for emergence of suicidal ideation [60].

Adrenergic Agents

Clonidine and guanfacine are alpha-adrenergic agonists, both of which have long-acting forms that are FDA approved for treatment of ADHD (Kapvay and Intuniv, respectively). Intuniv is dosed at 0.05–0.12 mg/kg, with a starting dose of 1 mg in the morning and ranging from 1 to 4 mg daily. Kapvay has a starting dose of 0.1 mg at bedtime and ranges from 0.1 to 0.4 mg, which can be given daily or split b.i.d. Alpha-agonists have an effect size of approximately 0.6 in the treatment of ADHD [89], which is much lower than stimulant medications (range around 1.0), but can be useful in cases of uncomplicated ADHD, refractory ADHD, or ADHD with comorbidity such as oppositional defiant disorder, anxiety, or tics [74, 90]. Recent studies suggest that combination of alpha-agonists with stimulants may lead to improved response in partial responders, although these recent studies are not incorporated into current treatment algorithms [75].

Prior to starting treatment with these agents (see Table 10.4 for dosing information), the clinician should obtain a thorough cardiovascular history, vital signs, and the results of a recent physical or cardiac examination. History of syncope is a relative contraindication. The most common side effect is sedation, although this tends to decrease after several weeks. Dry mouth, nausea, and photophobia have also been reported. Glucose tolerance may decrease, especially in patients at risk for diabetes. Clonidine should be tapered instead of stopped suddenly to avoid a withdrawal syndrome consisting of motor restlessness, headache, agitation, increased blood pressure and pulse rate, and possible worsening of tics. Erratic compliance can increase the risk of cardiovascular events, and clonidine should not be prescribed unless it can be administered reliably.

Non-FDA-Approved Medication Treatments

Bupropion is a mixed catecholaminergic agonist that was a brought to market as an antidepressant, but may be useful as a second- or third-line agent in the treatment of ADHD, particularly in cases of ADHD comorbid with depression and/or substance abuse. It can be given in either immediate-release or long-acting form, but may not come in pill sizes small enough for children who weigh less than 25 kg. Bupropion may cause mild insomnia or loss of appetite. Extremely high single doses (> 400 mg) of bupropion may induce seizures even in patients without epilepsy [81].

There are controlled studies for tricyclic antidepressants in both children and adolescents that demonstrate their efficacy in the treatment of ADHD [92], leading to their use as second-line options for treatment of ADHD. However, reports in the 1990s of episodes of sudden death on tricyclic antidepressants have virtually eliminated them from consideration as a stimulant alternative [93, 94], especially considering the wider range of pharmacological alternatives available in recent years.

Multimodal Treatment

In the multimodal treatment study of children with ADHD (MTA), 579 children with ADHD combined type, aged 7 to 9.9 years, were assigned to 14 months of medication management (titration followed by monthly visits); intensive behavioral treatment (parent, school, and child components, with therapist involvement gradually reduced over time); the two combined; or standard community care (treatments by community providers) [95]. While all four treatment groups showed symptom reduction from baseline at 14 month follow-up, the two groups who received algorithmic medication management showed superior outcome compared to those who received either behavioral management alone or community care (of which two-thirds received medication, but had more limited physician follow-up and lower stimulant doses). Combined treatment did not prove superior to pharmacotherapy alone.

While the large MTA study displayed the efficacy of algorithmic stimulant treatment over psychosocial approaches, combined psychopharmacological and psychosocial intervention, and community treatment [52], the use of behavioral therapy is still widespread and indicated in cases when either ADHD symptoms are mild, comorbid conditions are present, parents reject psychopharmacological treatment, or when treating especially in low-income, minority populations, which have shown particular benefit with stimulant treatment with adjunctive behavioral treatments [60, 96–101].

Parent training has been suggested as a way to improve the social functioning of children with ADHD: teaching parents to recognize the importance of peer relationships, to use naturally occurring opportunities to teach social skills and self-evaluation, to take an active role in organizing the child's social life, and to facilitate consistency among adults in the child's environment.

During the training, parents are taught the following strategies: to give clear instructions, to positively reinforce good behavior, to ignore some behavior, and to use punishment effectively. One frequently used negative contingency is the time-out, which puts the child in an unstimulating situation in which naturally occurring positive reinforcement is not available. Since a high number of ADHD children have parents with ADHD, compliance with training programs and behavioral therapy is often difficult. Manual-based treatments for applying behavioral parent training to ADHD and ODD children are available [102, 103], which rely on principles such as parental psychoeducation, carefully assessing negative and positive behaviors, creating reward systems, using time-out effectively, and preparing for potential upcoming misbehavior.

Discontinuation of Treatment

If a child has been asymptomatic for at least one year, clinicians should assess whether psychopharmacological treatment continues to provide benefit; if not, they should consider a trial off medication, especially if the child has displayed lack of symptoms during missed doses or lack of need to increase medication during growth spurts. Optimal times for a trial off medication include vacation times, such as school breaks or summer, whereas particularly poor times would be at the start of a new school before the child's routine is established. If symptoms return, medication should be promptly restarted [60].

Long-Term Course into Adolescence and Young Adulthood

The 8-year follow-up arm of the MTA study [104] showed that there were no differences in 6- and 8-year outcomes based on randomized treatment during the 14-month MTA study, such that initial differences in groups disappeared once treatment was relaxed, due likely to medication discontinuation as well as less careful medication monitoring and dose adjustment in community settings. At 8 years, 62% had discontinued medication and only 32.5% received medication for more than half of the prior year. While treatment response during initial therapy was the best predictor of long-term outcome, best outcomes were associated with behavioral and socioeconomic advantage [104].

As children with ADHD are likely to continue to suffer from ongoing symptoms into adulthood (see "Epidemiology" above), they are at increased risk of ongoing psychosocial difficulties. Adults with a history of childhood ADHD have higher rates than controls of antisocial and criminal behavior [105], injuries and accidents [105], employment and marital difficulties, health problems, teen pregnancies [106] and children out of wedlock [107], and substance abuse [108]. They also report lower rates of employment, lower annual household income for those with a postgraduate degree, and lower educational attainment [109]. Although some worry that stimulants may increase the risk of substance use, a meta-analysis of open-label long-term studies of stimulant treatment in ADHD concluded that stimulant treatment does not increase the risk of substance abuse and may even have a protective effect [110, 111]. Although longitudinal studies of childhood ADHD with follow-up into adulthood are methodologically challenging to undertake, anecdotal clinical opinion is that sustained treatment beginning in childhood may generally ameliorate some of these negative outcomes into adulthood.

Summary and Conclusions

Despite being one of the best researched neurobiological conditions in medicine, and having pharmacological treatments with large effect sizes, ADHD is known to cause significant morbidity throughout the life course. Algorithms exist to guide clinicians in best practice, and appear particularly efficacious in cases of "straightforward" ADHD. However, considering the high proportion of cases of ADHD with other comorbidities, more studies are needed to ascertain best practice parameters when dealing with ADHD with comorbid psychiatric conditions, psychosocial adversity, and in cases of treatment refractory illness. As there is significant potential for poor outcomes, clinicians must engage in a thorough assessment and comprehensive treatment plan with the expectation that successful treatment may change the course of children's lives.

CASE ONE

Martin, a 6-year-old boy who was diagnosed with ADHD, came in for a clinical visit with his father one afternoon after baseball practice. The father stated that practice began at approximately 5.00 pm and that Martin's last dose of methylphenidate was at lunch at school. The father described Martin's performance at baseball practice as "awful." Martin saw no reason for his father's concern. The father stated that Martin would sit in the outfield and watch the birds, airplanes, and runners on a nearby track. He failed to pay attention when balls were thrown and hit. Adding an afternoon methylphenidate dose to Martin's regimen helped to improve his hitting, his batting average, and his status on the baseball team.

CASE TWO

Charles, a 7-year-old boy who developed severe side effects from methylphenidate, began a trial of dextroamphetamine, 5 mg twice a day and 2.5 mg at 4.00 pm. He has had persistent sleep problems, refusing to stay in his bed, wanting to sleep on the floor, and wanting his mother to lie with him. A dose of 1.25 mg dextroamphetamine at bedtime has completely resolved these problems. He now sleeps in his own bed all night. Pharmacologicl treatment of ADHD symptoms at bedtime in this case facilitated sleep without creating insomnia.

CASE THREE

Jose, a 10-year-old boy who was brought to the clinic for evaluation of treatment for his ADHD, was prescribed methylphenidate for his symptoms. Within 2 weeks the patient became increasingly irritable, complained that there were bugs around him that were trying to get him, and at times was afraid and had to hide under the furniture. He was using no other medication and there was no history of psychotic disorders in the family or previous psychotic episodes with the patient. The stimulants were discontinued and his symptoms persisted for 2 weeks, requiring approximately 5 days of low-dose thioridazine. Once the hallucinations ended, thioridazine was discontinued and the patient reported no further incidents of hallucinations. Hallucinosis is a rare but reported side effect of psychostimulants.

Appendix 10.1 Approach to Assessment and Treatment of ADHD

I. Initial Evaluation

A complete psychiatric assessment is indicated; see Practice Parameters for the Psychiatric Assessment of Children and Adolescents [60].

A. Interview with Parents

(1) Child's history
  (a) Developmental history.
  (b) DSM-IV symptoms of ADHD:
    i. presence or absence (may use symptom or criterion checklist);
    ii. development and context of symptoms and resulting impairment, including school (learning, academic productivity, and behavior), family, peers.
  (c) DSM-IV symptoms of possible alternate or comorbid psychiatric diagnoses.
  (d) History of psychiatric, psychological, pediatric, or neurological treatment for ADHD; details of medication trials.
  (e) Areas of relative strength (e.g., talents and abilities).

(f) Medical history:
  i. medical or neurological primary diagnosis (e.g., fetal alcohol syndrome, lead intoxication, thyroid disease, seizure disorder, migraine, head trauma, genetic or metabolic disorder, primary sleep disorder);
  ii. medications that could cause symptoms (e.g., phenobarbital, antihistamines, theophylline, sympathomimetics, steroids).
(3) Family history
  (a) ADHD, tic disorders, substance use disorders, conduct disorder, personality disorders, mood disorders, obsessive-compulsive disorder and other anxiety disorders, schizophrenia.
  (b) Developmental and learning disorders.
  (c) Family coping style, level of organization, and resources.
  (d) Past and present family stressors, crises, changes in family constellation.
  (e) Abuse or neglect.

B. Standardized Rating Scales Completed by Parents

C. School Information

From as many current and past teachers as possible:

(1) Standardized rating scales.
(2) Verbal reports of learning, academic productivity, and behavior.
(3) Testing reports (e.g., standardized group achievement tests; individual evaluations).
(4) Grade and attendance records.
(5) Individual educational plan, if applicable.
(6) Observations at school if feasible and if case is complex.

D. Child Diagnostic Interview

History and mental status examination:

(1) ADHD symptoms (note: may not be observable during interview and may be denied by child).
(2) Oppositional behavior.
(3) Aggressive behavior.
(4) Mood and affect.
(5) Anxiety.
(6) Obsessions or compulsions.
(7) Form, content, and logic of thinking and perception.
(8) Fine and gross motor coordination.
(9) Tics, stereotypes, or mannerisms.
(10) Speech and language abilities.
(11) Clinical estimate of intelligence.

E. Family Diagnostic Interview

(1) Patient's behavior with parents and siblings.
(2) Parental interventions and results.

F. Physical Evaluation

(1) Medical history and examination within 12 months or more recently if clinical condition has changed.
(2) Documentation of health history, immunizations, screening for lead level, etc.
(3) Measurement of lead level (if not done already) only if history suggests pica or environmental exposure.
(4) Documentation or evaluation of visual acuity.
(5) Documentation or evaluation of hearing acuity.
(6) Further medical or neurological evaluation as indicated.
(7) In preparation for pharmacotherapy:
  (a) baseline documentation of height, weight, vital signs, abnormal movements;
  (b) electrocardiogram and cardiology consult if risk factors pre-exist.

G. Referral for Additional Evaluations if Indicated

(1) Psychoeducational evaluation (individually administered):
  (a) intelligence quotient;
  (b) academic achievement;
  (c) learning disorders.
(2) Neuropsychological testing.
(3) Speech and language evaluation.
(4) Occupational therapy evaluation.
(5) Recreational therapy evaluation.

II. Psychiatric Differential Diagnosis

(A) Oppositional defiant disorder
(B) Conduct disorder
(C) Mood disorders – depression or mania
(D) Anxiety disorders
(E) Tic disorder (including Tourette's disorder)
(F) Pica
(G) Substance use disorder
(H) Learning disorder:
  (1) Pervasive developmental disorder
  (2) Mental retardation or borderline intellectual functioning.

III. Diagnosis

(A) Establish target symptoms and baseline impairment (rating scales may be useful).

(B) Consider treatment for comorbid conditions.
(C) Prioritize modalities to fit target symptoms and available resources:
    (1) Education about ADHD
    (2) Classroom placement and resources
    (3) Medication
    (4) Other modalities may assist with remaining target symptoms
(D) Monitor multiple domains of functioning:
    (1) Learning in key subjects (achievement tests, classroom tests, homework, classwork)
    (2) Academic productivity (homework, classwork)
    (3) Emotional functioning
    (4) Family interactions
    (5) Peer relationships
    (6) If on medication, appropriate monitoring of height, weight, vital signs, relevant laboratory parameters
(E) Re-evaluate efficacy and need for additional interventions
(F) Maintain long-term supportive contact with patient, family, and school:
    (1) Assure compliance with treatment
    (2) Address problems at new developmental stages or in response to family or environmental changes

Treatment

A. Education of parents, child, other significant adults

School interventions:

(1) Ensure appropriate class placement and availability of needed resources (e.g., tutoring)
(2) Consult or collaborate with teachers and other school personnel:
    (a) information about ADHD
    (b) educational techniques
    (c) behavior management
(3) Direct behavior modification program when possible, and if problems are severe in school setting

B. Medication

(1) Stimulants
(2) Atomoxetine
(3) Clonidine or guanfacine (primarily as an adjunct to a stimulant)
(4) Bupropion

C. Psychosocial interventions

(1) Parent behavior modification training
(2) Referral to parent support group, such as CHADD

(3) Family psychotherapy if family dysfunction is present
(4) Social skills group therapy for peer problems
(5) Individual therapy for comorbid problems, not core ADHD
(6) Summer day treatment

D. Ancillary treatments

(1) Speech and language therapy
(2) Occupational therapy
(3) Recreational therapy

E. Other treatments

These are outside the realm of the usual practice of child and adolescent psychiatry and are not recommended.

Children Aged 3 to 5 Years

Same protocol as above, except:

I. Evaluation

(A) Higher index of suspicion for neglect, abuse, or other environmental factors
(B) More likely to require lead level evaluation
(C) More likely to require evaluation of:
    (1) Speech and language disorders
    (2) Cognitive development

II. Treatment

(A) Increased emphasis on parent training
(B) Highly structured preschool
(C) Additive-free diet may occasionally be useful
(D) If medications are used, exercise more caution, use lower doses, and monitor more frequently

Adolescents

Same protocol as children aged 6 to 12 years, except:

  I. Higher index of suspicion for comorbidity with:
    (A) Conduct disorder
    (B) Substance use disorder
    (C) Suicidality
  II. Teacher reports less useful in middle and high school than in grammar school
 III. Patient must participate actively in treatment
 IV. Increased risk of medication abuse by patient or peers
  V. Greater need for vocational evaluation, counseling, or training
 VI. Evaluate patient's safe driving practices

Appendix 10.2 Readings for Parents, Patients, and Teachers

Books

Barkley RA. *Taking Charge of ADHD: The Complete, Authoritative Guide for Parents.* New York: Guilford Press, 1995.

Braswell I, Bloomquist M, Pederson S. *ADHD: A Guide to Understanding and Helping Children with Attention Deficit Hyperactivity Disorder in School Settings.* Minneapolis: University of Minnesota, 1991. [Department of Professional Development and Conference Services, Continuing Education and Extension, 315 Pillsbury Drive S.E., Minneapolis, MN 55455, 612-625-3504.]

Clark L. *The Time-Out Solutions: A Parent's Guide for Handling Everyday Behavior Problems.* Chicago: Contemporary Books, 1989. [Lots of detail on using time-out, but also other punishments and positive ways of increasing appropriate behavior. Includes examples, checklists, and tear-out reminder sheets.]

Fowler MC. *Maybe You Know My Kid: A Parent's Guide to Identifying, Understanding and Helping Your Child with Attention Deficit Hyperactive Disorder.* New York: Carol Publishing Group, 1990.

Garber SW, Garber MD, Spizman RE. *If Your Child is Hyperactive, Inattentive, Impulsive, Distractible ... Helping the ADD (Attention Deficit Disorder) Hyperactive Child.* New York: Villard Books, 1990. [A practical program for changing behavior with or without medication.]

Hallowell E, Ratey J. *Driven to Distraction: Recognizing and Coping with Attention Deficit Disorder from Childhood Through Adulthood.* New York: Pantheon Books, 1994. [Written by two psychiatrists who have ADHD themselves. Especially strong on the diagnosis and treatment of ADHD in adults.]

Hallowell EM, Ratey JI. *Answers to Distraction.* New York: Pantheon Books, 1994.

Ingersoll B. *Your Hyperactive Child: A Parent's Guide to Coping with Attention Deficit Disorder.* New York: Doubleday, 1988. [A comprehensive book with many examples. Includes brief guidelines for teachers and an appendix with behavioral management programs for classroom use.]

Ingersoll B, Goldstein S. *Attention Deficit Disorder and Learning Disabilities: Realities, Myths and Controversial Treatments.* New York: Doubleday Main Street Books, 1993. [An up-to-date review by two psychologists focusing on causes and treatment. Good coverage of common myths and unfounded claims.]

Kelly K, Ramundo P. *You Mean I'm Not Lazy, Stupid or Crazy?!* New York: Fireside Books, 1996.

Nadeau KG. *A Comprehensive Guide to Attention Deficit Disorder in Adults: Research, Diagnosis, and Treatment.* New York: Brunner/Mazel, 1995.

Nadeau K. *Survival Guide for College Students with ADD or LD.* New York: Magination Press, 1994. [A handy practical guide for the adolescent or young adult student with ADHD.]

Wender P. *Hyperactive Child, Adolescent and Adult.* New York: Oxford University Press, 1987.

Wender P. *Attention-Deficit Hyperactivity Disorder in Adults.* New York: Oxford University Press, 1995.

Websites

http://www.chadd.org (Children and Adults with Attention-Deficit/Hyperactivity Disorder).

http://www.nami.org (National Alliance on Mental Illness).

References

1. Prince JB. Pharmacotherapy of attention-deficit hyperactivity disorder in children and adolescents: update on new stimulant preparations, atomoxetine, and novel treatments. *Child Adolesc Psychiatr Clin N Am* 2006; **15**:13–50.
2. Ebaugh FG. Neuropsychiatric sequelae of acute epidemic encephalitis in children. 1923. *J Atten Disord* 2007;**11**: 336–338; discussion 339–340.
3. Holman L. Post-encephalitic behavior disorders in children. *Johns Hopkins Hosp Bull* 1922;**33**:372–375.
4. Chess S. Diagnosis and treatment of the hyperactive child. *NY State J Med* 1960;**60**:2379–2385.
5. Burks H. The hyperkinetic child. *Exceptional Children* 1960;**27**:18.
6. American Psychiatric Association. Committee on Nomenclature and Statistics. *Diagnostic and Statistical Manual of Mental Disorders* 2nd edn. Washington, DC: American Psychiatric Association, 1968.
7. American Psychiatric Association Work Group to Revise DSM-III. *Diagnostic and Statistical Manual of Mental Disorders,* 3rd edn, revised. Washington, DC: American Psychiatric Association. 1987.
8. American Psychiatric Association Task Force on DSM-IV. *Diagnostic and Statistical Manual of Mental Disorders,* 4th edn. Washington, DC: American Psychiatric Association, 1994; xxvii, 886 pp.
9. Weiss G. Attention deficit hyperactivity disorder. In: Lewis M (ed.) *Child and Adolescent Psychiatry, A Contemporary Approach,* 2nd edn. Baltimore: Williams & Wilkins, 1996; pp. 544–563.
10. Weiss G, Hechtman LT. *Hyperactive Children Grown Up: Empirical Findings and Theoretical Considerations,* 2nd edn. New York: Guilford Press, 1993.
11. Schachar R, Rutter M, Smith A. The characteristics of situationally and pervasively hyperactive children:

implications for syndrome definition. *J Child Psychol Psychiat* 1981;**22**:375–392.

12. Wolraich ML, Hannah JN, Pinnock TY, Baumgaertel A, Brown J. Comparison of diagnostic criteria for attention-deficit hyperactivity disorder in a county-wide sample. *J Am Acad Child Adolesc Psychiat* 1996;**35**:319–24.

13. Whalen CK, Henker B. Therapies for hyperactive children: comparisons, combinations, and compromises. *J Consult Clin Psychol* 1991;**59**:126–137.

14. Erhardt D, Hinshaw SP. Initial sociometric impressions of attention-deficit hyperactivity disorder and comparison boys: predictions from social behaviors and from nonbehavioral variables. *J Consult Clin Psychol* 1994;**62**:833–842.

15. Anderson CA, Hinshaw SP, Simmel C. Mother-child interactions in ADHD and comparison boys: relationships with overt and covert externalizing behavior. *J Abnorm Child Psychol* 1994;**22**:247–265.

16. Cantwell DP, Baker L. Issues in the classification of child and adolescent psychopathology. *J Am Acad Child Adolesc Psychiat* 1988;**27**:521–533.

17. Scheffler RM, Brown TT, Fulton BD, Hinshaw SP, Levine P, Stone S. Positive association between attention-deficit/hyperactivity disorder medication use and academic achievement during elementary school. *Pediatrics* 2009;**123**:1273–1279.

18. Goldman LS, Genel M, Bezman RJ, Slanetz PJ. Diagnosis and treatment of attention-deficit/hyperactivity disorder in children and adolescents. Council on Scientific Affairs, American Medical Association. *JAMA* 1998;**279**:1100–1107.

19. Barkley RA, Fischer M, Edelbrock CS, Smallish L. The adolescent outcome of hyperactive children diagnosed by research criteria: I. An 8-year prospective follow-up study. *J Am Acad Child Adolesc Psychiat* 1990;**29**:546–557.

20. Biederman J, Faraone S, Milberger S, *et al.* A prospective 4-year follow-up study of attention-deficit hyperactivity and related disorders. *Arch Gen Psychiat* 1996;**53**:437–446.

21. Biederman J, Mick E, Faraone SV. Age-dependent decline of symptoms of attention deficit hyperactivity disorder: impact of remission definition and symptom type. *Am J Psychiat* 2000;**157**:816–818.

22. Cohen P, Cohen J, Kasen S, *et al.* An epidemiological study of disorders in late childhood and adolescence – I. Age- and gender-specific prevalence. *J Child Psychol Psychiat* 1993;**34**:851–867.

23. Barkley R. Attention-deficit hyperactivity disorder. In: Mash RA (ed.) *Child Psychopathology*. New York: Guilford Press, 1996, pp. 63–112.

24. Faraone SV, Perlis RH, Doyle AE, *et al.* Molecular genetics of attention-deficit/hyperactivity disorder. *Biol Psychiat* 2005;**57**:1313–1323.

25. Biederman J, Faraone SV, Mick E, *et al.* High risk for attention deficit hyperactivity disorder among children of parents with childhood onset of the disorder: a pilot study. *Am J Psychiat* 1995;**152**:431–435.

26. Kreppner JM, O'Connor TG, Rutter M. Can inattention/overactivity be an institutional deprivation syndrome? *J Abnorm Child Psychol* 2001;**29**:513–528.

27. Mick E, Biederman J, Faraone SV, Sayer J, Kleinman S. Case-control study of attention-deficit hyperactivity disorder and maternal smoking, alcohol use, and drug use during pregnancy. *J Am Acad Child Adolesc Psychiat* 2002;**41**:378–385.

28. Max JE, Arndt S, Castillo CS, *et al.* Attention-deficit hyperactivity symptomatology after traumatic brain injury: a prospective study. *J Am Acad Child Adolesc Psychiat* 1998;**37**:841–847.

29. O'Malley KD, Nanson J. Clinical implications of a link between fetal alcohol spectrum disorder and attention-deficit hyperactivity disorder. *Can J Psychiat* 2002;**47**:349–354.

30. Mick E, Biederman J, Prince J, Fischer MJ, Faraone SV. Impact of low birth weight on attention-deficit hyperactivity disorder. *J Dev Behav Pediatr* 2002;**23**:16–22.

31. Willcutt EG, Doyle AE, Nigg JT, Faraone SV, Pennington BF. Validity of the executive function theory of attention-deficit/hyperactivity disorder: a meta-analytic review. *Biol Psychiat* 2005;**57**:1336–1346.

32. Nigg JT, Willcutt EG, Doyle AE, Sonuga-Barke EJ. Causal heterogeneity in attention-deficit/hyperactivity disorder: do we need neuropsychologically impaired subtypes? *Biol Psychiat* 2005;**57**:1224–1230.

33. Nigg JT. *What Causes ADHD? Understanding what goes Wrong and Why*. New York: Guilford Press, 2006.

34. Sonuga-Barke EJ, Halperin JM. Developmental phenotypes and causal pathways in attention deficit/hyperactivity disorder: potential targets for early intervention? *J Child Psychol Psychiat* 2010;**51**:368–389.

35. Bush G, Valera EM, Seidman LJ. Functional neuroimaging of attention-deficit/hyperactivity disorder: a review and suggested future directions. *Biol Psychiat* 2005;**57**:1273–1284.

36. Castellanos FX, Lee PP, Sharp W, *et al.* Developmental trajectories of brain volume abnormalities in children and adolescents with attention-deficit/hyperactivity disorder. *JAMA* 2002;**288**:1740–1748.

37. Sowell ER, Thompson PM, Welcome SE, Henkenius AL, Toga AW, Peterson BS. Cortical abnormalities in children and adolescents with attention-deficit hyperactivity disorder. *Lancet* 2003;**362**:1699–1707.

38. Uddin LQ, Kelly AM, Biswal BB, *et al.* Network homogeneity reveals decreased integrity of default-mode network in ADHD. *J Neurosci Methods* 2008;**169**:249–254.

39. Peterson BS, Potenza MM, Wang A, *et al.* An FMRI study of the effects of psychostimulants on default-mode processing during Stroop task performance in youths with ADHD. *Am J Psychiat* 2009;**166**:1286–1294.

40. Wolraich ML, Wilson DB, White JW. The effect of sugar on behavior or cognition in children. A meta-analysis. *JAMA* 1995;**274**:1617–1621.

41. Schab DW, Trinh NH. Do artificial food colors promote hyperactivity in children with hyperactive syndromes? A meta-analysis of double-blind placebo-controlled trials. *J Dev Behav Pediatr* 2004;**25**:423–434.

42. Stevenson J, Sonuga-Barke E, McCann D, *et al.* The role of histamine degradation gene polymorphisms in moderating the effects of food additives on children's ADHD symptoms. *Am J Psychiat* 2010;**167**:1108–1115.

43. Pelsser LM, Frankena K, Toorman J, *et al.* Effects of a restricted elimination diet on the behaviour of children with attention-deficit hyperactivity disorder (INCA study): a randomised controlled trial. *Lancet* 2011;**377**:494–503.

44. Lidsky TI, Schneider JS. Lead neurotoxicity in children: basic mechanisms and clinical correlates. *Brain* 2003; **126**:5–19.

45. Biederman J, Mick E, Faraone SV. Depression in attention deficit hyperactivity disorder (ADHD) children: 'true' depression or demoralization? *J Affect Disord* 1998;**47**:113–122.

46. Wozniak J, Biederman J, Kiely K, Ablon JS, Faraone SV, Mundy E, Mennin D. Mania-like symptoms suggestive of childhood-onset bipolar disorder in clinically referred children. *J Am Acad Child Adolesc Psychiatry* 1995;**34**:867–876.

47. Biederman J, Faraone S, Mick E, *et al.* Attention-deficit disorder and juvenile mania: an overlooked comorbidity? *J Am Acad Child Adolesc Psychiatry* (1996a);**35**(8): 997–1008.

48. Geller B, Williams M, Zimerman B, Frazier J, Beringer L, Warner KL. Prepubertal and early adolescent bipolarity differentiate from ADHD by manic symptoms, grandiose delusions, ultra-rapid or ultradian cycling. *J Affect Disord* 1998;**51**:81–91.

49. Geller B, Warner K, Williams M, Zimerman B. Prepubertal and young adolescent bipolarity versus ADHD: assessment and validity using the WASH-U-KSADS, CBCL and TRF. *J Affect Disord* 1998;**51**:93–100.

50. Barkley R. *Attention Deficit Hyperactivity Disorder: A Clinical Handbook,* 3rd edn. New York: Guilford Press, 2005.

51. Faraone SV, Biederman J, Jetton JG, Tsuang MT. Attention deficit disorder and conduct disorder: longitudinal evidence for a familial subtype. *Psychol Med* 1997;**27**: 291–300.

52. MTA-Cooperative-Group. Moderators and mediators of treatment response for children with attention-deficit/hyperactivity disorder: the Multimodal Treatment Study of children with Attention-deficit/hyperactivity disorder. *Arch Gen Psychiat* 1999;**56**:1088–1096.

53. Milberger S, Biederman J, Faraone SV, Chen L, Jones J. ADHD is associated with early initiation of cigarette smoking in children and adolescents. *J Am Acad Child Adolesc Psychiat* 1997;**36**:37–44.

54. Biederman J, Wilens T, Mick E, *et al.* Is ADHD a risk factor for psychoactive substance use disorders? Findings from a four-year prospective follow-up study. *J Am Acad Child Adolesc Psychiat* 1997;**36**:21–29.

55. Pliszka S, Carlson CL, Swanson JM. *ADHD with Comorbid Disorders: Clinical Assessment and Management.* New York: Guilford Press, 1999.

56. Biederman J, Newcorn J, SprichS. Comorbidity of attention deficit hyperactivity disorder with conduct, depressive, anxiety, and other disorders. *Am J Psychiat* 1991;**148**:564–577.

57. Tannock R. Attention deficit disorders with anxiety disorders. In: Brown T (ed.) *Attention Deficit Disorders and Comorbidities in Children, Adolescents and Adults.* New York: American Psychiatric Press, 2000; pp. 125–175.

58. Biederman J, Klein RG, Pine DS, Klein DF. Resolved: mania is mistaken for ADHD in prepubertal children. *J Am Acad Child Adolesc Psychiat* 1998;**37**:1091–1096; discussion 1096–1099.

59. Caron C, Rutter M. Comorbidity in child psychopathology: concepts, issues and research strategies. *J Child Psychol Psychiat* 1991;**32**:1063–1080.

60. Pliszka S. Practice parameter for the assessment and treatment of children and adolescents with attention-deficit/hyperactivity disorder. *J Am Acad Child Adolesc Psychiat* 2007;**46**:894–921.

61. Baker L, Cantwell DP, Mattison RE. Behavior problems in children with pure speech disorders and in children with combined speech and language disorders. *J Abnorm Child Psychol* 1980;**8**:245–256.

62. Conners CK, Wells K. *Conners Rating Scales-Revised.* Toronto: Multi-Health Systems, 1997.

63. Swanson J. *Swanson, Nolan, and Pelham (SNAP-IV).* 1992; available from: http://adhd.net.

64. Faraone SV, Spencer T, Aleardi M, Pagano C, Biederman J. Comparing the efficacy of medications used for ADHD using meta-analysis. Program and abstracts of the American Psychiatric Association 156th Annual Meeting; San Francisco, California, 2003.

65. Rapport MD, Stoner G, DuPaul DJ, Kelly KL, Tucker SB, Schoeler T. Attention deficit disorder and methylphenidate: a multilevel analysis of dose-response effects on children's impulsivity across settings. *J Am Acad Child Adolesc Psychiat* 1988;**27**:60–69.

66. Spencer TJ, Wilens TE, Biederman J, Weisler RH, Read SC, Pratt R. Efficacy and safety of mixed amphetamine salts extended release (Adderall XR) in the management of attention-deficit/hyperactivity disorder in adolescent patients: a 4-week, randomized, double-blind, placebo-controlled, parallel-group study. *Clin Ther* 2006;**28**: 266–279.

67. Swanson JM, Wigal S, Greenhil LL, *et al.* Analog classroom assessment of Adderall in children with ADHD. *J Am Acad Child Adolesc Psychiat* 1998;**37**:519–526.

68. Greenhill L, Kollins S, Abikoff H, *et al.* Efficacy and safety of immediate-release methylphenidate treatment for preschoolers with ADHD. *J Am Acad Child Adolesc Psychiat* 2006;**45**:1284–1293.

69. MTA-Cooperative-Group. Moderators and mediators of treatment response for children with attention-deficit/hyperactivity disorder: the Multimodal Treatment Study of Children with Attention-Deficit/Hyperactivity Disorder. *Arch Gen Psychiatry* 1999;**56**: 1088–1096.

70. Greenhill L, Kollins S, Abikoff H, *et al.* Efficacy and safety of immediate-release methylphenidate treatment for preschoolers with ADHD. *J Am Acad Child Adolesc Psychiatry* 2006;**45**:1284–1293.

71. Wigal SB, Gupta S, Greenhill L, *et al.* Pharmacokinetics of methylphenidate in preschoolers with attention-deficit/hyperactivity disorder. *J Child Adolesc Psychopharmacol* 2007;**17**:153–164.

72. Wigal T, Greenhill L, Chuang S, *et al.* Safety and tolerability of methylphenidate in preschool children with ADHD. *J Am Acad Child Adolesc Psychiat* 2006;**45**: 1294–1303.

73. Handen BL, Feldman HM, Lurier A, Murray PJ. Efficacy of methylphenidate among preschool children with developmental disabilities and ADHD. *J Am Acad Child Adolesc Psychiat* 1999;**38**:805–812.

74. Pliszka SR, Crismon ML, Hughes CW, *et al.* The Texas Children's Medication Algorithm Project: revision of the algorithm for pharmacotherapy of attention-deficit/hyperactivity disorder. *J Am Acad Child Adolesc Psychiat* 2006;**45**:642–657.

75. Wilens T. Combination of Guanfacine XR plus stimulants in the treatment of ADHD. Paper presented at Biological Psychiatry, New Orleans, 2010.

76. Wilens TE. Combined pharmacotherapy in pediatric psychopharmacology: friend or foe? *J Child Adolesc Psychopharmacol* 2009;**19**:483–484.

77. Prince JB, Wilens TE, Biederman J, Spencer TJ, Wozniak JR. Clonidine for sleep disturbances associated with attention-deficit hyperactivity disorder: a systematic chart review of 62 cases. *J Am Acad Child Adolesc Psychiat* 1996;**35**:599–605.

78. Weiss MD, Wasdell MB, Bomben MM, Rea KJ, Freeman RD. Sleep hygiene and melatonin treatment for children and adolescents with ADHD and initial insomnia. *J Am Acad Child Adolesc Psychiat* 2006;**45**:512–519.

79. Tjon Pian Gi CV, Broeren JP, Starreveld JS, Versteegh FG. Melatonin for treatment of sleeping disorders in children with attention deficit/hyperactivity disorder: a preliminary open label study. *Eur J Pediatr* 2003;**162**:554–555.

80. Van der Heijden KB, Smits MG, Van Someren EJ, Ridderinkhof KR, Gunning WB. Effect of melatonin on sleep, behavior, and cognition in ADHD and chronic sleep-onset insomnia. *J Am Acad Child Adolesc Psychiat* 2007;**46**:233–241.

81. Kramer JR, Loney J, Ponto LB, Roberts MA, Grossman S. Predictors of adult height and weight in boys treated with methylphenidate for childhood behavior problems. *J Am Acad Child Adolesc Psychiat* 2000;**39**:517–524.

82. Ross RG. Psychotic and manic-like symptoms during stimulant treatment of attention deficit hyperactivity disorder. *Am J Psychiat* 2006;**163**:1149–1152.

83. Nissen SE. ADHD drugs and cardiovascular risk. *N Engl J Med* 2006;**354**:1445–1448.

84. Gould MS, Walsh BT, Munfakh JL, et al. Sudden death and use of stimulant medications in youths. *Am J Psychiat* 2009;**166**:992–1001.

85. Denchev P, Kaltman JR, Schoenbaum M, Vitiello B. Modeled economic evaluation of alternative strategies to reduce sudden cardiac death among children treated for attention deficit/hyperactivity disorder. *Circulation* 2010;**121**:1329–1337.

86. Sumner C, Donnelly C, Lopez FA. Atomoxetine treatment for pediatric patients with ADHD and comorbid anxiety. Presented at Annual Meeting of American Psychiatric Association, 2005, Atlanta.

87. Wernicke JF, Kratochvil CJ. Safety profile of atomoxetine in the treatment of children and adolescents with ADHD. *J Clin Psychiat* 2002;**63**(Suppl. 12):50–55.

88. Wernicke JF, Faries D, Girod D, et al. Cardiovascular effects of atomoxetine in children, adolescents, and adults. *Drug Safety* 2003;**26**:729–740.

89. Connor DF, Fletcher KE, Swanson JM. A meta-analysis of clonidine for symptoms of attention-deficit hyperactivity disorder. *J Am Acad Child Adolesc Psychiat* 1999;**38**:1551–1559.

90. Spencer TJ, Greenbaum M, Ginsberg LD, Murphy WR. Safety and effectiveness of coadministration of guanfacine extended release and psychostimulants in children and adolescents with attention-deficit/hyperactivity disorder. *J Child Adolesc Psychopharmacol* 2009;**19**:501–510.

91. Conners CK, Casat CD, Gualtieri CT, et al. Bupropion hydrochloride in attention deficit disorder with hyperactivity. *J Am Acad Child Adolesc Psychiat* 1996;**35**:1314–1321.

92. Daly JM, Wilens T. The use of tricyclic antidepressants in children and adolescents. *Pediatr Clin North Am* 1998;**45**:1123–1135.

93. Riddle MA, Geller B, Ryan N. Another sudden death in a child treated with desipramine. *J Am Acad Child Adolesc Psychiat* 1993;**32**:792–797.

94. Riddle MA, Nelson JC, Kleinman CS, et al. Sudden death in children receiving Norpramin: a review of three reported cases and commentary. *J Am Acad Child Adolesc Psychiat* 1991;**30**:104–108.

95. [No authors] A 14-month randomized clinical trial of treatment strategies for attention-deficit/hyperactivity disorder. The MTA Cooperative Group. Multimodal Treatment Study of Children with ADHD. *Arch Gen Psychiat* 1999;**56**:1073–1086.

96. March JS, Swanson JM, Arnold LE, et al. Anxiety as a predictor and outcome variable in the multimodal treatment study of children with ADHD (MTA). *J Abnorm Child Psychol* 2000;**28**:527–541.

97. Sonuga-Barke EJ, Daley D, Thompson M, Laver-Bradbury C, Weeks A. Parent-based therapies for preschool attention-deficit/hyperactivity disorder: a randomized, controlled trial with a community sample. *J Am Acad Child Adolesc Psychiat* 2001;**40**:402–408.

98. Jensen PS, Hinshaw SP, Swanson JM, et al. Findings from the NIMH Multimodal Treatment Study of ADHD (MTA): implications and applications for primary care providers. *J Dev Behav Pediatr* 2001;**22**:60–73.

99. Arnold LE, Elliot M, Sachs L, et al. Effects of ethnicity on treatment attendance, stimulant response/dose, and 14-month outcome in ADHD. *J Consult Clin Psychol* 2003;**71**:713–727.

100. Moderators and mediators of treatment response for children with attention-deficit/hyperactivity disorder: the Multimodal Treatment Study of children with Attention-deficit/hyperactivity disorder. *Arch Gen Psychiat* 1999;**56**:1088–1096.

101. Hinshaw SP. Moderators and mediators of treatment outcome for youth with ADHD: understanding for whom and how interventions work. *J Pediatr Psychol* 2007;**32**:664–675.

102. Barkley RA. Defiant Children: A Clinician's Manual for Assessment and Parent Training, 2nd Vol. New York: Guilford, 1997.

103. Cunningham CE, Bremner R, Secord M. *COPE: The Community Parent Education Program. A School-Based Family Systems Oriented Workshop for Parents of Children with Disruptive Behavior Disorders*. Hamilton, ON: COPE Works, 1997.

104. Molina BS, Hinshaw SP, Swanson JM, et al. The MTA at 8 years: prospective follow-up of children treated for combined-type ADHD in a multisite study. *J Am Acad Child Adolesc Psychiat* 2009;**48**:484–500.

105. Barkley RA, Fischer M, Smallish L, Fletcher K. Young adult follow-up of hyperactive children: antisocial activities and drug use. *J Child Psychol Psychiatry* 2004;**45**:195–211.

106. Barkley RA, Fischer M, Smallish L, Fletcher K. Young adult outcome of hyperactive children: adaptive

functioning in major life activities. *J Am Acad Child Adolesc Psychiatry* 2006;**45**:192–202.

107. Johnston C. The impact of attention deficit hyperactivity disorder on social and vocational functioning in adults. In: Jensen PS, Cooper JR (eds) *Attention Deficit Hyperactivity Disorder: State of the Science, Best Practices*. Kingston, NJ: Civic Research Institute, 2002; pp. 6-2–6-21.

108. Wilens TE, Biederman J, Mick E, Faraone SV, Spencer T. Attention deficit hyperactivity disorder (ADHD) is associated with early onset substance use disorders. *J Nerv Ment Dis* 1997;**185**:475–482.

109. Biederman J, Faraone SV, Spencer TJ, Mick E, Monuteaux MC, Aleardi M. Functional impairments in adults with self-reports of diagnosed ADHD: A controlled study of 1001 adults in the community. *J Clin Psychiat* 2006;**67**:524–540.

110. Wilens TE, Faraone SV, Biederman J, Gunawardene S. Does stimulant therapy of attention-deficit/hyperactivity disorder beget later substance abuse? A meta-analytic review of the literature. *Pediatrics* 2003;**111**: 179–185.

111. Wilens TE, Adamson J, Monuteaux MC, *et al.* Effect of prior stimulant treatment for attention-deficit/hyperactivity disorder on subsequent risk for cigarette smoking and alcohol and drug use disorders in adolescents. *Arch Pediatr Adolesc Med* 2008;**162**:916–921.

11

Disruptive Behavior Disorders

Jennifer P. Edidin, Niranjan S. Karnik, Scott J. Hunter, Hans Steiner

Introduction

Disruptive behavior spectrum disorders (DBDs) constitute one of the most frequent presenting complaints to mental health professionals who provide care for children [1–3]. These behaviors, as a group, are often seen as signs and symptoms of other illness, but can in many instances be the primary manifestation of childhood psychopathology. The challenge for the treating clinician, then, is to differentiate normal from abnormal, as well as primary from secondary process. DBDs are challenging to treat and exact a high toll in terms of individual, familial, and societal loss. One of the hallmarks of these disorders, which include conduct disorder, oppositional defiant disorder (ODD), and disruptive behavior disorder not otherwise specified (DBD NOS), is that parents and others are usually more distressed by the behavior than is the child. As such, it is often hard to enlist the child's cooperation in the evaluation and treatment process.

This chapter presents the background on disruptive behavior spectrum disorders, with a focus on conduct disorder, as well as a method for evaluating and treating a child or adolescent presenting with a DBD. Beginning with a historical overview and definition of the disorder, it then considers epidemiology, etiology, diagnosis, course and natural history, treatment principles and guidelines, and finally prognosis and outcomes.

Definitions and Nosology

Conduct disorder first appeared in the second edition of the *Diagnostic and Statistical Manual of Mental Disorders* (DSM-II) in 1968 [4]. DSM-I included sociopathic personality, but this classification did not extend to children. Beginning with the DSM-II, disruptive behavior disorders comprised three categories: unsocialized aggressive reaction of childhood or adolescence, the runaway reaction of childhood, and the group delinquent reaction of childhood. DSM-III [5] expanded these subtypes and first introduced the term conduct disorder into the official nomenclature. Building on the DSM-II subtypes, DSM-III outlined four general variants of conduct disorder: socialized, undersocialized, aggressive, and nonaggressive. The 1987 revision, the DSM-III-R [6], further defined the category of conduct disorder by identifying the three most common variants of the previous classification: solitary aggressive, group type, and undifferentiated. A comparison of these definitions reveals the basic feature of conduct disorder: a pattern of behavior by an individual or group that violates age-appropriate and socially appropriate behavior.

The most recent editions of the DSM, the 1994 DSM-IV [7] and the 2000 DSM-IV-TR [8], ceased to differentiate by socialization and aggression, as validation has proved difficult. These versions instead emphasize aspects of the disorder that have been empirically validated. Two subtypes are defined: early or childhood onset and late or adolescent onset. There is also a coding for severity.

The essential feature of conduct disorder as defined by DSM-IV-TR is a "repetitive and persistent pattern of behavior in which the basic rights of others or major age-appropriate societal norms or rules are violated." These behaviors fall within four categories: (i) aggression to people and animals; (ii) destruction of property; (iii) deceitfulness or theft; and (iv) serious violation of rules (Table 11.1). Of the 15 types of behaviors within these categories, an individual must have shown three or more within the past 12 months and at least one within the past 6 months. Additionally, the behavior must cause clinically significant impairment in functioning.

The subtypes of conduct disorder (CD) provide useful diagnostic and prognostic information. Individuals with childhood or early-onset CD are more aggressive, show decreased socialization and regard for others, and have poor peer relationships. Their aggression usually shows a progression from oppositional defiant disorder (ODD)

Clinical Child Psychiatry, Third Edition. Edited by William M. Klykylo and Jerald Kay.
© 2012 John Wiley & Sons, Ltd. Published 2012 by John Wiley & Sons, Ltd.

Table 11.1   DSM-IV-TR criteria for conduct disorder. Reprinted with permission from the Diagnostic and Statistical Manual of Mental Disorders, Copyright 2000. American Psychiatric Association.

(A)   A repetitive and persistent pattern of behavior in which the basic rights of others or major age-appropriate societal norms or rules are violated, as manifested by the presence of three (or more) of the following criteria in the past 12 months, with at least one criterion present in the past 6 months:

Aggression to people and animals
(1)   often bullies, threatens, or intimidates others
(2)   often initiates physical fights
(3)   has used a weapon that can cause serious physical harm to others (e.g., a bat, brick, broken bottle, knife, gun)
(4)   has been physically cruel to people
(5)   has been physically cruel to animals
(6)   has stolen while confronting a victim (e.g., mugging, purse snatching, extortion, armed robbery)
(7)   has forced someone into sexual activity

Destruction of property
(8)   has deliberately engaged in fire setting with the intention of causing serious damage
(9)   has deliberately destroyed others' property (other than by fire setting)

Deceitfulness or theft
(10)   has broken into someone else's house, building, or car
(11)   often lies to obtain goods or favors or to avoid obligations (i.e., 'cons' others)
(12)   has stolen items of nontrivial value without confronting a victim (e.g., shoplifting, but without breaking and entering; forgery)

Serious violations of rules
(13)   often stays out at night despite parental prohibitions, beginning before age 13 years
(14)   has run away from home overnight at least twice while living in parental or parental surrogate home (or once without returning for a lengthy period)
(15)   is often truant from school, beginning before age 13 years
(B)   The disturbance in behavior causes clinically significant impairment in social, academic, or occupational functioning
(C)   If the individual is age 18 years or older, criteria are not met for antisocial personality disorder

Specify type based on age at onset:
Childhood-onset type – onset of at least one criterion characteristic of conduct disorder prior to age 10 years
Adolescent-onset type – absence of any criteria characteristic of conduct disorder prior to age 10 years

Specify severity:
Mild – few if any conduct problems in excess of those required to make the diagnosis and conduct problems cause only minor harm to others
Moderate – number of conduct problems and effect on others intermediate between 'mild' and 'severe'
Severe – many conduct problems in excess of those required to make the diagnosis or conduct problems cause considerable harm to others

---

during early childhood to a persistent course of conduct disorder during adolescence to antisocial personality disorder as adults. Individuals with adolescent or late-onset CD are typically less aggressive, show better peer socialization and relationships, and are more often female. Several additional alternative classifications have been proposed. As one example, Fergusson and colleagues have suggested a division based on overt (aggression, violence) and covert (theft, dishonesty) behaviors [9, 10]. Like the DSM-IV-TR subtypes, these two types show relatively distinct developmental patterns, comorbidities, and prognoses. Among the proposed changes to the current diagnosis of CD being considered for DSM-V is the inclusion of a specifier for individuals who present with the traits of callousness and an absence of emotion [11].

In contrast to conduct disorder, ODD is often viewed as a milder form or a precursor (Table 11.2). As with conduct disorder, the behaviors associated with ODD are typically more distressing to others than to the

Table 11.2 DSM-IV-TR criteria for oppositional defiant disorder. Reprinted with permission from the Diagnostic and Statistical Manual of Mental Disorders, Copyright 2000. American Psychiatric Association.

(A) A pattern of negativistic, hostile, and defiant behavior lasting at least six months, during which four (or more) of the following are present:

(1) often loses temper
(2) often argues with adults
(3) often actively defies or refuses to comply with adults' requests or rules
(4) often deliberately annoys people
(5) often blames others for his or her mistakes or misbehavior
(6) is often touchy or easily annoyed by others
(7) is often angry and resentful
(8) is often spiteful or vindictive

Note: Consider a criterion met only if the behavior occurs more frequently than is typically observed in individuals of comparable age and developmental level

(B) The disturbance in behavior causes clinically significant impairment in social, academic, or occupational functioning

(C) The behaviors do not occur exclusively during the course of a psychotic or mood disorder

(D) Criteria are not met for conduct disorder, and, if the individual is age 18 years or older, criteria are not met for antisocial personality disorder

---

individual exhibiting them and often contribute to a significant disruption in family, academic, and social functioning. Further, behaviors that are classified as ODD are also normal at certain developmental periods, particularly the toddler and adolescent years. Unlike conduct disorder, however, ODD behaviors usually do not involve serious violations of others' rights or delinquency.

ODD first appeared in the DSM-III as oppositional disorder. It defined a spectrum of behaviors characterized by hostility, usually toward an authority figure. The DSM-III-R added the term defiant to the disorder and broadened the range of behaviors encompassed by the diagnosis, including the use of obscene language or swearing. The DSM-IV dropped this last behavior but retained the term defiant. The key feature remains a "pattern of negativistic, hostile, and defiant behavior." Of the eight types of behavior

comprising ODD, an individual must demonstrate four or more over at least a 6-month period of time, and the behaviors must cause clinically significant impairment in functioning. In the upcoming version of the DSM, these criteria will likely remain the same; however, increased specificity about the frequency of behaviors, age of onset, and cultural factors influencing ODD may be included [12].

Given our increased knowledge base about the disruptive behavior disorders, it is believed quite likely that the DSM-V will include significant changes to the Disruptive Behavior Disorder category. Specifically, the broad diagnostic category may be renamed "Disruptive, Impulse Control, and Conduct Disorders." The broad diagnostic category also will consist of a wider range of disorders. In addition to diagnoses of conduct disorder and oppositional defiant disorder, pyromania, kleptomania, and intermittent explosive disorder, among other impulse control disorders, are being considered for inclusion. Moreover, in contrast to its current inclusion in the DBDs, Attention-Deficit/Hyperactivity Disorder (ADHD) will likely be moved into the broader category of neurodevelopmental disorders.

Pertinent to, and underlying the changes being proposed for DSM-V, recent developments in the etiology of disruptive behavior spectrum disorders have led to the understanding that there are two major forms of aggression in childhood. One is reactive aggression, which is characterized as being impulsive and generally triggered by anger or frustration on the part of the child. This type of aggression has a significant affective valence and is defensive in nature. As such, it is referred to as RADI (i.e., reactive, affective, defensive, impulsive) or "hot" aggression [13]. Individuals showing RADI aggression may feel remorse after committing an aggressive act and understand that it is maladaptive [13]. More disturbing in nature is the second form of aggression, referred to as PIP (i.e., proactive, instrumental, planned) or "cold" aggression [13], which is understood as proactive or instrumental. This form of aggression is planned and premeditated, and often is characterized by a lack of remorse or morality. Proactive aggression is highly correlated with future delinquency and psychopathy, whereas reactive aggression shows a lack of direct correlation, and appears to have significant connections to other causes of behavioral instability. Individuals who display the former type of aggression, RADI, may believe their behavior is adaptive, given that it often enables them to achieve goals and meet personal demands [13].

The neuroscience of aggression has begun to trace out the differences between these forms of aggression at a neuroanatomical level, and has begun to show that disruptions in underlying neural pathways may have functional behavioral impact [14–17]. Specifically, both the medial and orbitofrontal cortical pathways, which are part of the five major prefrontal pathways of the mind, have been implicated in potentially mediating aggression and violence and, as such, are a current focus of attention [16, 18–20]. Nevertheless, it is evident that these neurological risk factors are not deterministic and instead act in a dynamic relationship with the social world encompassing the child [21]. For a full summary of the neuroscience literature on maladaptive aggression in youth populations, please see the report from the American Academy of Child & Adolescent Psychiatry Workgroup on Juvenile Aggression and Impulsivity [13].

Epidemiology

Conduct disorder is generally recognized as the most common form of childhood psychopathology. It represents the most common reason for psychiatric consultation, accounting for 25–90% of consultations in some clinics [22]. The general population prevalence varies from 1.5% to 20%, depending on the method of data collection, time frame of study, and the particular site [22]. The male-to-female ratio varies from 3:1 to 5:1, depending on the age range studied; specifically, the gender difference decreases in mid-adolescence because of the increased rate observed among girls [23, 24]. Additionally, studies indicate that girls exhibit different types of violence and aggression than boys, and that these may contribute to lower rates of CD recorded among girls [24–26]. Girls tend to produce indirect, less overt aggressive violence and instead use social networks as a means of violence and aggression. That is to say they will shun or exclude people whom they wish to harm, and will do so in ways that utilize social and emotional, as well as environmental systems, rather than engaging aggressively using physical means. Further, due to the difficulty in diagnosing early onset, pervasive antisocial behavior in girls, our current estimates of prevalence in this population may be artificially low [27]. Still, the peak age of onset for all children is in late childhood and early adolescence, but ranges from preschool to late adolescence. The impact of conduct disorder extends beyond the above estimates. Because of costs at the familial, community, and state levels (i.e., the involvement of educational and legal systems), the actual impact is broader and more significant than that recorded on the individual level.

Etiology

As noted previously, the etiology of conduct disorder is multifactorial. The current model is that of premorbid genetic or neurological liability, which is worsened by psychosocial adversity and finally produced by high environmental risk. From this perspective, one can deduce that there are also protective factors that mediate the potential for DBDs and moderate resilience.

Early theories viewed the development of antisocial behavior in children from two perspectives: an internal deficit and an ecological adaptation. William Healy, who developed the first view, in 1915 described affected children as having a "psychic constitutional deficiency" [28]. He maintained that he had found both mental and physical defects in antisocial children, which supported his belief that the behavior was hereditary. Aichhorn, in 1935, proposed an opposing view that was rooted in the psychodynamic study of delinquency. He described the "neurotic delinquent," a youth who seeks to assuage neurotic guilt by seeking punishment through his or her delinquent deeds [29]. Today, both theories are encompassed within the broader model addressing the heterogeneous symptoms of conduct disorder, and multiple pathways need to be considered in their genesis.

Biological studies show abnormalities in the neurotransmitter systems of people with conduct disorders, including serotonin [30, 31], noradrenergic, and dopaminergic [32] activity. Among these different neurotransmitters, the best studied and supported pathway is serotonin dysregulation. Concurrent and extensive research has also supported the observation that autonomic arousal is predictive of conduct disorder; specifically, the autonomic nervous system shows low reactivity on a variety of parameters, including decreased heart rate and skin conductance, in youth with conduct disorder, with a slow resting heart rate being the most widely replicated finding [33, 34]. Finally, the neuroanatomy of aggression, as mentioned above, is becoming better understood and is helping to shape our understanding of the etiology of youth aggression [13–16].

Genetic studies suggest a possible heritable factor of conduct disorders. One study found concordance in monozygotic twins to be higher than in dizygotic twins [34, 35]; however, in a study that examined biological twins who were later adopted, both genetic and environmental factors were shown to be influential [36, 37]. Conduct disorder is perceived as the childhood precursor of antisocial personality disorder; therefore, estimates of heritability from adults with antisocial personality disorder could be useful to evaluate the genetic contribution to conduct disorder. Yet these studies are difficult to interpret, as most children with conduct disorder do not develop antisocial personality disorder in adulthood. Those who do may represent a subgroup with more severe pathology. Other longitudinal studies have found that there is greater genetic liability in early childhood-onset conduct disorder [38]. Early constitutional factors, such as temperament and restraint, may also be genetically mediated, and serve to influence the later development of DBDs. Clearly, genetic studies are presently incomplete. Nevertheless, it still seems likely that there is a heritable component that acts as a risk factor for the development of conduct disorder.

The high incidence of neurological abnormalities in children with conduct disorder provides further evidence that neurological factors may be significant. This high incidence, however, may actually represent an increased exposure to accidents, injuries, and illnesses that affect central nervous system (CNS) functioning. Among more seriously disordered youth, there does seem to be a significantly higher incidence of psychomotor seizures. In a small sample of incarcerated youths, Lewis and colleagues [39] found a 20-fold higher incidence of seizure disorder in those with conduct disorder over the general population. These youths also showed more subtle findings, including learning and communication disorders, impaired memory for behavior, executive dysfunction, and minor motor abnormalities. These findings have been replicated in subsequent studies [40, 41]. It has been posited that the neuropsychological deficits observed in youth with conduct disorder develop through both direct and indirect pathways, including problems with self-control and academic difficulties [40].

Other forms of psychiatric disability can act as risk factors. In particular, other disruptive behavior disorders (i.e., ADHD and ODD), as well as traits characteristic of disruptive behavior disorders (e.g., hyperactivity and impulsivity) have been found to represent a risk [42–45]. In addition, cognitive deficits and linguistic problems can act as predisposing factors, and chronic illness and disability have also been shown to be risk factors. Children who are chronically ill are significantly more likely to present with conduct problems compared to healthy peers [46]. Moreover, if the chronic condition affects the CNS, the risk can increase as much as five-fold [47]. Individual personality factors such as aggression and coping style may similarly predispose individuals to later conduct disorder and delinquency [48].

Several familial factors have been found to affect the incidence of conduct disorder. Poor family functioning, poor parenting, marital discord, and child abuse are proven risk factors. More specifically, drug and alcohol abuse [49–51], mood disorders [52, 53], psychotic disorders [54, 55], attention-deficit hyperactivity disorder (ADHD) and learning disorders [40, 49, 56–58], intrafamilial trauma [59, 60], and parental antisocial personality disorder [61, 62] also increase the risk. Although all of these factors are significant, the risk is highest for parenting practices that are abusive and injurious [62, 63].

Risk elements also exist at the community and social levels. Socioeconomic disadvantage, poor housing, crowding, and poverty exert negative influences; moreover, poor peer relations, limited role models and prosocial structures (e.g., schools and churches), and increased antisocial structures (e.g., organized violence and drug sales) represent another layer of risk [64]. These community risk factors are not limited to the development of conduct disorder and delinquency, however, as they can also increase the incidence of other forms of psychopathology, such as post-traumatic stress disorder (PTSD) [65–67].

Some attention should be given to protective factors. Increasingly, we find that there is evidence for a positive psychology that defines a set of factors that act to protect and even enhance the lives of young people who may traditionally be seen as at-risk [68, 69]. Within the individual domain, an easy temperament, intelligence, good rapport with others, good work habits at school, and areas of competence outside of school all offer protection and motivation to change [70, 71]. Within the family domain, a good relationship with at least one parent or another important adult affords a degree of protection; and in the community domain, prosocial peers and a school that promotes empowerment also emerge as protective factors [64].

Still, despite the presence of potential positive factors, it remains the case that after some point, for some individuals, protection is probably no longer possible, and the full display of the disorder arises, impacting and influencing ongoing adaptive functioning and development. Additionally, at a further point in time, the disorder becomes unresponsive to even the most concerted treatment effort. The challenge is to diagnose and intervene early, and as completely as possible, in order to stem the progression to an entrenched DBD, and improve outcomes.

Diagnosis

The clinical evaluation of a child for disruptive behavior spectrum disorders needs to take place across several dimensions, with multiple informants, employing diverse methods, and in different settings. Without this comprehensive approach, it becomes difficult not only to identify disordered behaviors but also to distinguish them from other potential etiologies.

The multidimensional category refers to evaluating individual, family, and community risk and protective factors. The assessment may begin with individual factors. This includes a thorough history and physical examination and appropriate laboratory and diagnostic studies. More than one informant should be consulted: both the child and his or her family should be interviewed, as well as teachers and other significant adults who have had the opportunity to observe the child. More than one method of assessment with each informant should be used: interviews, rating scales (e.g., Conners Scale, the Child Behavior Checklist, Response Evaluation Measure [72], and the child hostility inventory and child version of the Overt Aggression Scale), neuropsychological testing, and review of school records. Additionally, the child's behaviors may require assessment in more than one setting (e.g., office, home, and school). This gives the clinician a context in which to consider the behavior, as well as an indication of the chronicity and habituation of the behavior. One should assess the familial and community dimension similarly (Figure 11.1). After a complete assessment, one can begin to look at the number of disruptive behaviors present (severity), associated factors seen (comorbidity), and patterns of behavior displayed (subtypes). This allows one to generate a complete differential diagnosis and identify any comorbid conditions.

Comorbidity and Differential Diagnosis

As detailed earlier, conduct disorder is associated with many other psychiatric and nonpsychiatric disorders [58, 73–79]. The most common associated disorders are other disruptive behavior disorders. Up to 90% of children diagnosed with early-onset conduct disorder also meet criteria for ODD at an earlier age. In fact, because of the high degree of overlap between conduct disorder and ODD, many believe they are manifestations of the same illness at different levels of severity. Both conduct disorder and ODD are also associated with ADHD: Up to 45% of children with either conduct disorder or ODD also have ADHD. The concurrence of conduct disorder and ADHD is highest in the preteen years and decreases slightly in the teen years. There is a significant gender difference, however, as comorbid ADHD seems to predispose girls to the development of conduct disorder and to increase the intensity and chronicity of conduct disorder among boys. Alcohol and drug abuse represent two additional disorders that are significantly higher in individuals with conduct disorder [10, 78, 81–85].

Conduct disorder is associated with other psychiatric disorders. Mood disorders, particularly depressive and unipolar syndromes, occur in up to 50% of individuals

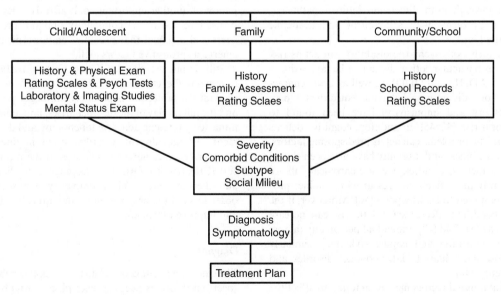

Figure 11.1 Diagnostic assessment.

with conduct disorder. Anxiety disorders also occur at a higher level for girls with conduct disorder. Learning disabilities, especially dyslexia, show a comorbidity of 20% with conduct disorder. Other developmental disabilities, such as intellectual disability and personality disorders (usually antisocial in boys and borderline in girls), occur frequently [86]. Head trauma, seizure disorders, and other neurological disorders are also comorbid conditions.

As a result of the frequent comorbidity, the differential diagnosis of conduct disorder is broad and raises the question of comorbid (i.e., simply coexisting) versus compound (i.e., complicating each other) psychopathologies. In addition to the comorbidities, the differential diagnosis includes psychotic disorders, intermittent explosive disorder, and other personality disorders apart from developing antisocial personality disorder. In essence, almost any condition with socially unacceptable behaviors can mimic conduct disorder. Most disorders other than conduct disorder, however, lack the critical determinant of persistently inappropriate behavior that violates the rules and rights of others. A careful family history, qualification of the frequency and severity of behaviors, and a thorough medical evaluation can help differentiate conduct disorder from other distinct and potentially more treatable conditions.

Course and Pattern

Among the disruptive behavior spectrum disorders, oppositional defiant disorder (ODD) is often seen as being the gateway diagnosis; however, not every child with ODD develops CD. Some studies suggest that the ODD-conduct disorder trajectory is more common for boys [38]. When compared to CD, ODD presents at earlier ages, and usually begins as a pattern of behavior that shows resistance to authority and parental control. To some extent, all children exhibit some qualities of this behavior, because this is the method through which children learn the rules of society. These behaviors enter the diagnostic realm when the pattern has become fixed or the behaviors are escalating, and thereby significantly impacting the child's (and family's) life.

In contrast, CD is a relatively stable diagnosis. In fact, untreated it may progress to severe behavioral disturbances and criminality. Conduct disorder with onset in childhood may predispose affected children to develop adult antisocial personality disorder; one study found that 30–50% of affected children showed this developmental course. As noted previously, different subtypes of conduct disorder have different trajectories [87]. Factors that predispose individuals to a more severe case

and poor outcome include (i) childhood onset and proactive type; (ii) comorbid conditions, especially ADHD; (iii) individual risk factors such as poor peer relations, labile temperament, and reduced intelligence; and (iv) familial risk factors such as family discord and disorganization.

Children with more chronic and severe conduct disorder show impairment across multiple areas: difficulties with social mechanics and the legal system, lower academic and vocation achievement, and severely hampered interpersonal development. They have a higher risk of suicidal or homicidal behavior and an increased rate of substance abuse. More extreme forms of the disorder may worsen associated comorbid conditions. It is when working with these more disturbed children that one really begins to appreciate the cost of this disease and the importance of skilled, expedient interventions and treatments.

Treatment

Disruptive behavior spectrum disorders should warrant conservative treatment during their early presentation. Particularly for the child who is diagnosed with ODD, family and individual therapy are the recommended interventions. Medications should not play a role at this stage unless there are comorbid conditions such as mood disorder that warrant pharmacological treatment. Should the illness begin to worsen despite these interventions, and the child begins to show early manifestations of conduct disorder, by attempting to harm themselves or others, or by exhibiting marked violence against property or animals, then the clinician can consider expanding the approach.

Because of the multitude of illnesses that can complicate conduct disorder, it is a complex illness to treat. In addition, since the behaviors are more distressing to others, it is difficult for a child or teen with conduct disorder to acknowledge the problem and comply with treatment. As with diagnosis and assessment, treatment should proceed from multiple perspectives on multiple levels and should use a variety of techniques.

The initial task is to decide on the treatment setting (Figure 11.2). This is usually determined by the affected child. Despite the fact that studies on criteria for hospitalization for those with CD are lacking, 88 if the behaviors are severe and pose a danger to either the child or others, the child should be treated as an inpatient. Initial intervention consists of providing a safe, secure environment and pharmacological treatment as needed. After the child has been stabilized, discharge is recommended as soon as possible. A transition to the outpatient setting allows patients more definitive, long-term treatment

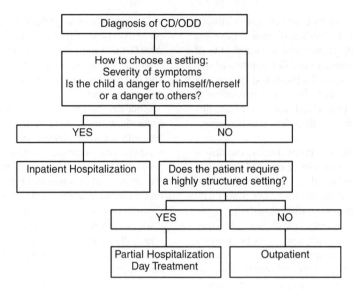

Figure 11.2   Treatment approach.

while they and their caretakers are still actively involved and committed [89].

With both inpatients and outpatients, it is important to consider the presence of comorbid conditions. If present, these conditions should be treated first, since this type of therapy often decreases the intensity and frequency of antisocial behavior. Usually a combined treatment approach is needed: individual psychotherapy, group psychotherapy, family psychotherapy, community interventions (i.e., educational support and restructuring) [90, 91], and medication all should be considered. The recommendations for medication follow traditional guidelines and target other complicating symptoms:

(1) psychostimulants, norepinepherine reuptake inhibitors, and clonidine for ADHD;
(2) selective serotonin reuptake inhibitors (SSRIs) for depression;
(3) diphenhydramine (Benadryl), benzodiazepines, SSRIs, and possibly buspirone (BuSpar) for anxiety [92, 93].

Rarely, if ever, is simple psychopharmacology sufficient for treatment; usually a comprehensive and extensive treatment package is needed.

Psychosocial approaches to conduct disorder include individual psychotherapy (behavioral, supportive, and insight oriented), group psychotherapy, and family psychotherapy. Behavioral and supportive variants of psychotherapy seem to have more success than insight-oriented psychotherapy, but there are ongoing investigations in the efficacy of psychoanalytic models [94–96].

Cognitive behavioral therapy can enhance the child's sense of self-control (internal locus of control) and begin to nurture healthy problem-solving skills [97–99]. Insight-oriented therapy, however, may still be useful: those who demonstrate greater distress and an interest about their behaviors, and those subtyped as reactive (responding to external stressors with rapid anger) may benefit from such a treatment approach. Group therapy may be helpful, since many youths are more comfortable discussing issues among peers than adults. Family therapy is also usually indicated, especially if the child is preadolescent or younger; often the behavior may be reinforced or suppressed by the reactions of family members. By providing a safe place to express these reactions, families may be able to identify ways to alter their reactions and avenues for meaningful family interactions, and family risk factors such as chronic discord, disorganization, and abuse can be addressed. Approaches focused on enhancing attachment to important caregivers have been found to decrease the rate of conduct disordered behaviors. Therapy for couples may also be appropriate if there is significant marital discord and conflicting or dysfunctional and injurious parenting styles.

Psychoeducational approaches to conduct disorder include social skills building and behavior modification for the affected youth, family, and community. Children can be taught more appropriate coping strategies and social skills, for which day treatment programs are particularly beneficial. If indicated, supplemental academic and vocational training can be provided. Parent-directed methods are also effective. For example, Parent-Child

Interaction Training (PCIT), during which the therapist observes interactions between the child and parent, and then provides in-the-moment feedback, has strong research support [62]. Parent management training (PMT) consists of positively reinforcing prosocial behavior and negatively reinforcing antisocial behavior. The latter refers to nonviolent punishments for previously defined behaviors. The key to this method is consistency, which requires parents to be patient and highly motivated; thus, like many of these treatment methods, it may not apply to every situation. The combination of child- and parent-directed methods is particularly effective in decreasing the incidence of aggressive and inappropriate behavior. Henggeler has described an intervention that acts at the community level called Multisystemic Treatment (MST). It combines child- and parent-directed interventions with community case management and family support services. This form of treatment utilizes specially trained therapists following small numbers of families and having a high degree of availability. Therapists work toward empowering the family and drawing in collateral support from other family members, friends, and community members over several months [100–104]. Borduin and colleagues [105], in their long-term follow-up study of 176 youths who were on average over 10 years out from the intervention, found substantially lower rates of recidivism, arrests, and days of confinement. The results are promising, especially for treatment-resistant populations such as violent juvenile delinquents.

Another intervention at the family level is Multidimensional Treatment Foster Care (MTFC), which uses an intensive model of foster care to rehabilitate young offenders. The program relies on foster parents following a very structured approach to monitoring and rewarding behaviors. Individual and family therapy are provided during the program, and there is also intensive case management. Foster parents receive additional support through group meetings and program support. The availability of these major modalities for treatment at the family level constitutes good empirically based arms of intervention at this level [106–110].

Although pharmacological interventions have had varying degrees of success, medication should still be considered as part of the comprehensive treatment plan. Divalproex sodium has been found to have good mood-stabilizing qualities in children and adolescents, and has expanded in use given its efficacy [92, 93]. Other mood stabilizers such as lithium and carbamazepine may help manage aggressive and impulsive behavior. Likewise, neuroleptics such as risperidone, olanzapine, and haloperidol may be used, and propranolol has been tried with some success. Stimulants like methylphenidate should be used with extreme caution

in this population as they can exacerbate behavioral swings and aggressive patterns. When using pharmacological treatment, one should first address any comorbid conditions and then define target symptoms and consider potential side effects [93]. All medications require careful consideration of risks and benefits, and increasingly good medical monitoring. Divalproex puts children at risk for major hepatic injury, and careful monitoring of blood levels as well as hepatic function is necessary. All atypical antipsychotics now carry a warning on the development of diabetes mellitus, and regular measurements of height, weight, and appropriate laboratory studies are now an expected part of care, based on recent recommendations by the American Diabetes Association and the American Psychiatric Association [111].

The future of psychopharmacological treatment in this population is likely found in recent approaches like that of Blader and colleagues [112], who conducted an augmentation trial for youth with ADHD and disruptive behaviors that did not respond to stimulant monotherapy. In this study divalproex was added to the regimen and the outcome of aggression examined. In addition to the finding of decreased aggression, the notable aspect to Blader's study was the incorporation of a sound psychosocial intervention for all participants. Future work needs to use this approach to research where combined interventions are utilized that better mirror the "real world" of clinical practice [113].

Prognosis

With appropriate treatment, much can be done to alter the course and outcome of patients with conduct disorder. Clearly, conduct disorders are developmental forms of psychopathology: risks accrue over many years and the combination of multiple risks ultimately produces the disorder. There is ample time, therefore, to intervene prior to the crystallization of a risk into a full-blown disorder. Interventions have a chance to work provided they are multifocal, use different methods, and are delivered consistently over extensive periods. Combined treatment approaches can significantly reduce the degree of disordered behaviors and the attendant rate of criminal activity and incarceration. True preventive methods, however, must take place fairly quickly after the onset of behaviors, probably in the first decade of life if not the first 5 years. Parents represent the first line of defense, followed by other important adults, teachers and the education system, peers, and the larger community. Although conduct disorders currently remain difficult to treat, much progress has been made; many research projects are exploring additional ways to decrease the cost to the individuals, family, and society.

Even with the best interventions, some individuals still fail and eventually enter criminal pathways and delinquency. Prevalence rates of disruptive behavior disorders among adjudicated youths range between 70% and 100% depending on the study [114–119]. This finding may reflect the fact that the criteria for conduct disorder mirror most of the social rules and laws that children are likely to break. Substance abuse seems to have a special role in this progression: once youngsters develop extensive substance abuse patterns, disorders, or even dependency, it becomes even more difficult to extricate them from a career of crime. Eighty percent of incarcerated juveniles report extensive experimentation, and 25% fulfill diagnostic criteria for dependency. Since drugs are expensive, youngsters are increasingly forced to resort to criminal activity to support their habits, with the resulting risk of arrest and criminal punishment. The clinician should always consider substance abuse and its treatment when dealing with an adjudicated youngster. Such treatment needs to be concomitant with the treatment of learning disabilities and psychosocial deficits.

Our approach to the youngster in the juvenile justice system deserves some special consideration. Many of our conduct-disordered patients ultimately end up in a system in which mental health becomes secondary to criminological management and considerations. Once a juvenile has been adjudicated, his or her life becomes more complex and difficult, as does access to mental health professionals. Nevertheless, clinicians have a vital role to fulfill, since they can more easily prescribe treatment and rehabilitation that were not previously available. We like to view periods of confinement as an opportunity to deal with the treatment needs of those who, for a variety of reasons, have failed to respond to previous interventions. There is evidence that youngsters in confinement have high rates of psychopathology, which interferes with rehabilitative programs and has a bearing on their future recidivism after release. The task before us when dealing with juveniles in prison is as follows:

(1) Establish diagnostic profiles and comorbidities, which dictate what interventions are most appropriate for certain youngsters; ADHD, affective disorders, and PTSD occur at very high rates and have immediate management implications.
(2) Assist the staff in making appropriate recommendations to the youthful offender parole board regarding dispositions within the system and after release.

(3) Assess crises that arise during confinement that have been triggered by events in prison or by contacts (or lack thereof) with families.
(4) Serve as a consultant to the system regarding the appropriate timing of release of the youngsters and their readiness to face the external world.

Future Directions

The future directions for care of children with disruptive disorders are manifold. Both the neuroscience and neuropsychology of aggression are producing new insights. One recent example is found in a report from Jean Decety and colleagues on the development of moral sensitivity in children [120]. Using a combination of neuropsychological assessment and functional neuroimaging, Decety and colleagues found that moral sensitivity changes as a function of age and that particular areas of the brain seem to differentially respond to moral stimuli in a developmental fashion [120]. This finding parallels long-established theories of moral development outlined by Kohlberg and others, but adds a fascinating layer of neurobiology to these understandings. The field is changing rapidly; as our understanding of the neuropsychology of aggression advances so will the options for interventions using a multiplicity of cognitive, behavioral, pharmacologic, and neurochemical techniques. Even as these choices expand, it is prudent for the treating clinician to be ever mindful of the social and family milieu of the child, and the potential interventions that can be made using the social resources around the child, including parents, schools, and peers. These options used in concert with judicious pharmacological options are likely to have the best and most lasting effects for the child.

References

1. Steiner H. Practice parameters for the assessment and treatment of children and adolescents with conduct disorder. *J Am Acad Child Adolesc Psychiat* 1997;**36**:122S–139S.
2. Steiner H, Dunne JE. Summary of the practice parameters for the assessment and treatment of children and adolescents with conduct disorder. *J Am Acad Child Adolesc Psychiat* 1997;**36**:1482–1485.
3. Merikangas KR, He J, Brody D, Fisher PW, Bourdon K, Kortez DS. Prevalence and treatment of mental disorders among US children in the 2001–2004 NHANES. *Pediatrics* 2010;**125**:75–81.
4. American Psychiatric Association. Committee on Nomenclature and Statistics. *Diagnostic and Statistical Manual of Mental Disorders*. Washington, DC: American Psychiatric Association, 1968.
5. American Psychiatric Association. Task Force on Nomenclature and Statistics. *Diagnostic and Statistical*

Manual of Mental Disorders. Washington, DC: American Psychiatric Association, 1978.

6. American Psychiatric Association. Work Group to Revise DSM-III. *Diagnostic and statistical Manual of Mental Disorders: DSM-III-R.* Washington, DC: American Psychiatric Association, 1987.

7. American Psychiatric Association. Task Force on DSM-IV. *Diagnostic and Statistical Manual of Mental Disorders: DSM-IV.* Washington, DC: American Psychiatric Association, 1994.

8. American Psychiatric Association. Task Force on DSM-IV. *Diagnostic and Statistical Manual of Mental Disorders: DSM-IV-TR.* Washington, DC: American Psychiatric Association, 2000.

9. Fergusson DM, Horwood LJ, Lynskey MT. Prevalence and comorbidity of DSM-III-R diagnoses in a birth cohort of 15 year olds. *J Am Acad Child Adolesc Psychiat* 1993;**32**:1127–1134.

10. Fergusson DM, Horwood LJ, Lynskey MT. Structure of DSM-III-R criteria for disruptive childhood behaviors: confirmatory factor models. *J Am Acad Child Adolesc Psychiat* 1994;**33**:1145–1155; discussion 155–157.

11. Moffitt TE, Arseneault L, Jaffee SR, *et al.* Research Review: DSM-V conduct disorder: research needs for an evidence base. *J Child Psychol Psychiat* 2008;**49**:3–33.

12. American Psychiatric Association. ADHD and Disruptive Behavior Disorders Work Group. Oppositional Defiant Disorder. 2010. Retrieved from: http://www.dsm5.org/ProposedRevision/Pages/proposedrevision.aspx?rid=106.

13. Blair RJR, Karnik NS, Coccaro EF, Steiner H. Taxonomy and neurobiology of aggression. In: Benedek EP, Ash P, Scott CL (eds) *Principles and Practice of Child and Adolescent Forensic Mental Health.* Arlington, VA: American Psychiatric Publishing, Inc., 2010; pp. 267–278.

14. Blair RJ. Neurocognitive models of aggression, the antisocial personality disorders, and psychopathy. *J Neurol Neurosurg Psychiat* 2001;**71**:727–731.

15. Blair RJ. Neurobiological basis of psychopathy. *Brit J Psychiat* 2003;**182**:5–7.

16. Blair RJ. The roles of orbital frontal cortex in the modulation of antisocial behavior. *Brain Cognition* 2004;**55**:198–208.

17. Richell RA, Mitchell DG, Newman C, Leonard A, Baron-Cohen S, Blair RJ. Theory of mind and psychopathy: can psychopathic individuals read the 'language of the eyes'? *Neuropsychologia* 2003;**41**:523–526.

18. Gansler DA, Lee AKW, Emerton BC, *et al.* Prefrontal regional correlates of self-control in male psychiatric patients: Impulsivity facets and aggression. *Psychiatr Res* 2011;**191**:16–23.

19. Herpertz SC, Huebner T, Marx I, *et al.* Emotional processing in male adolescents with childhood-onset conduct disorder. *J Child Psychol Psychiat* 2008;**49**:781–791.

20. Rubia K, Smith AB, Halari R, *et al.* Disorder-specific dissociation of orbitofrontal dysfunction in boys with pure conduct disorder during reward and ventrolateral prefrontal dysfunction in boys with pure ADHD during sustained attention. *Am J Psychiat* 2009;**166**:83–94.

21. Karnik NS. The social environment. In: Steiner H (ed.) *Handbook of Mental Health Interventions in Children and Adolescents: An Integrated Developmental Perspective.* San Francisco: Jossey-Bass, 2004; pp. 51–72.

22. Connor DF. *Aggression and Antisocial Behavior in Children and Adolescents: Research and Treatment.* New York: Guilford Press, 2002.

23. Cohen P, Cohen J, Kasen S, *et al.* An epidemiological study of disorders in late childhood and adolescence – I. Age- and gender-specific prevalence. *J Child Psychol Psychiat* 1993;**34**:851–867.

24. Maughan B, Rowe R, Messer J, Goodman R, Meltzer H. Conduct disorder and oppositional defiant disorder in a national sample: developmental epidemiology. *J Child Psychol Psychiat* 2004;**45**:609–621.

25. Card NA, Stucky BD, Sawalani GM, Little TD. Direct and indirect aggression during childhood and adolescence: a meta-analytic review of gender differences, intercorrelations, and relations to maladjustment. *Child Dev* 2008;**79**:1185–1229.

26. Hawkins S, Miller S, Steiner H. Aggression, psychopathology and delinquency: influences of gender and maturation. Where did the good girls go? In: Hayward C (ed.) *Gender Differences at Puberty.* London: Cambridge University Press, 2003; pp. 93–110.

27. Zoccolillo M, Tremblay R, Vitaro F. DSM-III-R and DSM-III criteria for conduct disorder in preadolescent girls: specific but insensitive. *J Am Acad Child Adolesc Psychiat* 1996;**35**:461–470.

28. Healy W. *The Individual Delinquent.* Boston: Little, Brown & Co., 1915.

29. Aichhorn A. *Wayward Youth.* New York: Viking Press, 1935.

30. Swann AC. Neuroreceptor mechanisms of aggression and its treatment. *J Clin Psychiat* 2003;**64**(Suppl 4):26–35.

31. Lee R, Coccaro E. The neuropsychopharmacology of criminality and aggression. *Can J Psychiat* 2001;**46**:35–44.

32. Pliszka SR, Rogeness GA, Renner P, Sherman J, Broussard T. Plasma neurochemistry in juvenile offenders. *J Am Acad Child Adolesc Psychiat* 1988;**27**:588–594.

33. Ortiz J, Raine A. Heart rate and antisocial behavior in children and adolescents: A meta-analysis. *J Am Acad Child Adolesc Psychiat* 2004;**43**:154–162.

34. Raine A. Biosocial studies of antisocial and violent behavior in children and adults: a review. *J Abnorm Child Psychol* 2002;**30**:311–326.

35. Raine A. *Biosocial Bases of Violence.* New York: Plenum Press, 1997.

36. Cadoret RJ, Cain CA, Crowe RR. Evidence for gene-environment interaction in the development of adolescent antisocial behavior. *Behav Genet* 1983;**13**:301–310.

37. Riggins-Caspers KM, Cadoret RJ, Knutson JF, Langbehn D. Biology-environment interaction and evocative biology-environment correlation: contributions of harsh discipline and parental psychopathology to problem adolescent behaviors. *Behav Genet* 2003;**33**:205–220.

38. Rowe R, Costello EJ, Angold A, Copeland WE, Maughan B. Developmental pathways in oppositional defiant disorder and conduct disorder. *J Abnorm Psychol* 2010;**119**:726–738.

39. Lewis DO, Pincus JH, Shanok SS, Glaser GH. Psychomotor epilepsy and violence in a group of incarcerated adolescent boys. *Am J Psychiat* 1982;**139**:882–887.

40. Närhi V, Lehto-Salo P, Ahonen T, Marttunen M. Neuropsychological subgroups of adolescents with conduct disorder. *Scand J Psychol* 2010;**51**:278–284.

41. Pajer K, Chung J, Leininger L, Wang W, Gardner W, Yeates K. Neuropsychological function in adolescent

girls with conduct disorder. *J Am Acad Child Adolesc Psychiat* 2008;**47**:416–425.

42. Hinshaw SP, Lee SS. Conduct and oppositional defiant disorders. In: Mash EJ, Barkley RA (eds) *Child Psychopathology*, 2nd edn. New York: Guillford Press, 2004; pp. 144–198.

43. Loeber R, Green SM, Keenan K, Lahey BB. Which boys will fare worse? Early predictors of the onset of conduct disorder in a six-year longitudinal study. *J Am Acad Child Adolesc Psychiat* 1995;**34**: 499–509.

44. Martel MM, Gremillion M, Eye AV, Nigg JT. The structure of childhood disruptive behaviors. *Psychol Assessment* 2010;**22**:816–826.

45. Offord DR, Boyle MH, Racine YA, *et al.* Outcome, prognosis, and risk in a longitudinal follow-up study. *J Am Acad Child Adolesc Psychiat* 1992;**31**:916–923.

46. Hysing M, Elgen I, Gillberg C, Lundervold AJ. Emotional and behavioural problems in subgroups of children with chronic illness: Results from a large-scale population study. *Child Care Hlth Dev* 2009;**35**:427–533.

47. Cadman D, Boyle MH, Offord DR, *et al.* Chronic illness and functional limitation in Ontario children: findings of the Ontario Child Health Study. *Can Med Assoc J* 1986;**135**:761–767.

48. Coon H, Carey G, Corley R, Fulker DW. Identifying children in the Colorado Adoption Project at risk for conduct disorder. *J Am Acad Child Adolesc Psychiat* 1992;**31**:503–511.

49. Disney ER, Elkins IJ, McGue M. Iacono WG. Effects of ADHD, conduct disorder, and gender on substance use and abuse in adolescence. *Am J Psychiat* 1999;**156**: 1515–1521.

50. Myers MG, Stewart DG, Brown SA. Progression from conduct disorder to antisocial personality disorder following treatment for adolescent substance abuse. *Am J Psychiat* 1998;**155**:479–485.

51. Fisckenscher A, Novins D. Gender differences and conduct disorder among American Indian adolescents in substance abuse treatment. *J Psychoactive Drugs* 2003;**35**:79–84.

52. Marmorstein NR, Iacono WG. Major depression and conduct disorder in a twin sample: gender, functioning, and risk for future psychopathology. *J Am Acad Child Adolesc Psychiat* 2003;**42**:225–233.

53. Knapp M, McCrone P, Fombonne E, Beecham J, Wostear G. The Maudsley long-term follow-up of child and adolescent depression: 3. Impact of comorbid conduct disorder on service use and costs in adulthood. *Brit J Psychiat* 2002;**180**:19–23.

54. Mueser KT, Drake RE, Ackerson, TH, Alterman AI, Miles KM, Noordsy DL. Antisocial personality disorder, conduct disorder, and substance abuse in schizophrenia. *J Abnorm Psychol* 1997;**106**:473–477.

55. Mueser KT, Rosenberg SD, Drake RE, *et al.* Conduct disorder, antisocial personality disorder and substance use disorders in schizophrenia and major affective disorders. *J Stud Alcohol* 1999;**60**:278–284.

56. Biederman J, Mick E, Faraone SV, Burback M. Patterns of remission and symptom decline in conduct disorder: a four-year prospective study of an ADHD sample. *J Am Acad Child Adolesc Psychiat* 2001;**40**:290–298.

57. Connor DF, Barkley RA, Davis HT. A pilot study of methylphenidate, clonidine, or the combination in ADHD comorbid with aggressive oppositional defiant or conduct disorder. *Clin Pediatr (Phila)* 2000;**39**: 15–25.

58. Rothenberger A, Banaschewski T, Heinrich H, Moll GH, Schmidt MH, Van't Klooster B. Comorbidity in ADHD-children: effects of coexisting conduct disorder or tic disorder on event-related brain potentials in an auditory selective-attention task. *Eur Arch Psychiat Clin Neurosci* 2000;**250**:101–110.

59. Plattner B, Silvermann MA, Redlich AD, *et al.* Pathways to dissociation: intrafamilial versus extrafamilial trauma in juvenile delinquents. *J Nerv Ment Dis* 2003;**191**: 781–788.

60. Steiner H, Carrion V, Plattner B, Koopman C. Dissociative symptoms in posttraumatic stress disorder: diagnosis and treatment. *Child Adolesc Psychiatr Clin N Am* 2003;**12**:231–249, viii.

61. Frick PJ, Lahey BB, Loeber R, Stouthamer-Loeber M, Christ MA, Hanson K. Familial risk factors to oppositional defiant disorder and conduct disorder: parental psychopathology and maternal parenting. *J Consult Clin Psychol* 1992;**60**:49–55.

62. Loeber R, Burke J, Pardini DA. Perspectives on oppositional defiant disorder, conduct disorder, and psychopathic features. *J Child Psychol Psychiat* 2009;**50**: 133–142.

63. Burke JD, Pardini DA, Loeber R. Reciprocal relationships between parenting behavior and disruptive psychopathology from childhood through adolescence. *J Abnorm Child Psychol* 2008;**26**:679–692.

64. Bassarath L. Conduct disorder: a biopsychosocial review. *Can J Psychiat* 2001;**46**:609–616.

65. Ruchkin VV, Schwab-Stone M, Koposov R, Vermeiren R, Steiner H. Violence exposure, posttraumatic stress, and personality in juvenile delinquents. *J Am Acad Child Adolesc Psychiat* 2002;**41**:322–329.

66. Steiner H, Garcia IG, Matthews Z. Posttraumatic stress disorder in incarcerated juvenile delinquents. *J Am Acad Child Adolesc Psychiat* 1997;**36**:357–365.

67. Cauffman E, Feldman SS, Waterman J, Steiner H. Posttraumatic stress disorder among female juvenile offenders. *J Am Acad Child Adolesc Psychiat* 1998;**37**:1209–1216.

68. Furstenberg FF. *Managing to Make It: Urban Families and Adolescent Success.* Chicago: University of Chicago Press, 1999.

69. Seligman ME, Csikszentmihalyi M. Positive psychology. An introduction. *Am Psychol* 2000;**55**:5–14.

70. Rae-Grant N, Thomas BH, Offord DR, Boyle MH. Risk, protective factors, and the prevalence of behavioral and emotional disorders in children and adolescents. *J Am Acad Child Adolesc Psychiat* 1989;**28**:262–268.

71. Salekin RT, Lee Z, Schrum Dillard CL, Kubak FA. Child psychopathy and protective factors: IQ and motivation to change. *Psychol Public Pol L* 2010;**16**:158–176.

72. Steiner H, Araujo KB, Koopman C. The response evaluation measure (REM-71): a new instrument for the measurement of defenses in adults and adolescents. *Am J Psychiat* 2001;**158**:467–473.

73. Fischer M, Barkley RA, Smallish L, Fletcher K. Young adult follow-up of hyperactive children: self-reported psychiatric disorders, comorbidity, and the role of childhood conduct problems and teen CD. *J Abnorm Child Psychol* 2002;**30**:463–475.

74. Goodwin RD, Hamilton SP. Lifetime comorbidity of antisocial personality disorder and anxiety disorders

among adults in the community. *Psychiatry Res* 2003;**117**:159–166.

75. Lahey BB, Loeber R, Burke J, Rathouz PJ, Mcburnett K. Waxing and waning in concert: dynamic comorbidity of conduct disorder with other disruptive and emotional problems over 7 years among clinic-referred boys. *J Abnorm Psychol* 2002;**111**:556–567.

76. Miller-Johnson S, Lochman JE, Coie JD, Terry R, Hyman C. Comorbidity of conduct and depressive problems at sixth grade: substance use outcomes across adolescence. *J Abnorm Child Psychol* 1998;**26**:221–232.

77. Newcorn JH, Halperin JM, Jensen PS, *et al.* Symptom profiles in children with ADHD: effects of comorbidity and gender. *J Am Acad Child Adolesc Psychiat* 2001;**40**:137–146.

78. Nock MK, Kazdin AE, Hiripi E, Kessler RC. Prevalence, subtypes, and correlates of DSM-IV conduct disorder in the National Comorbidity Survey replication. *Psychol Med* 2006;**36**:699–710.

79. Thapar A, Harrington R, McGuffin P. Examining the comorbidity of ADHD-related behaviours and conduct problems using a twin study design. *Brit J Psychiat* 2001;**179**:224–229.

80. Fergusson DM, Horwood LJ, Lynskey MT. The comorbidities of adolescent problem behaviors: a latent class model. *J Abnorm Child Psychol* 1994;**22**:339–354.

81. Fergusson DM, Horwood LJ, Lynskey MT. The stability of disruptive childhood behaviors. *J Abnorm Child Psychol* 1995;**23**:379–396.

82. Fergusson DM, Lynskey M, Horwood LJ. The adolescent outcomes of adoption: a 16-year longitudinal study. *J Child Psychol Psychiat* 1995;**36**:597–615.

83. Fergusson DM, Lynskey MT, Horwood LJ. Factors associated with continuity and changes in disruptive behavior patterns between childhood and adolescence. *J Abnorm Child Psychol* 1996;**24**:533–553.

84. Fergusson DM, Lynskey MT, Horwood LJ. Origins of comorbidity between conduct and affective disorders. *J Am Acad Child Adolesc Psychiat* 1996;**35**:451–460.

85. Neighbors B, Kempton T, Forehand R. Co-occurrence of substance abuse with conduct, anxiety, and depression disorders in juvenile delinquents. *Addict Behav,* 1992;**17**:379–386.

86. Eppright TD, Kashani JH, Robison BD, Reid JC. Comorbidity of conduct disorder and personality disorders in an incarcerated juvenile population. *Am J Psychiat* 1993;**150**:1233–1236.

87. Loeber R. Antisocial behavior: more enduring than changeable? *J Am Acad Child Adolesc Psychiat* 1991; **30**:393–397.

88. Lock J, Strauss GD. Psychiatric hospitalization of adolescents for conduct disorder. *Hosp Community Psych* 1994;**45**:925–928.

89. Kazdin AE, Whitley MK. Treatment of parental stress to enhance therapeutic change among children referred for aggressive and antisocial behavior. *J Consult Clin Psychol* 2003;**71**:504–515.

90. Kazdin AE. Treatments for aggressive and antisocial children. *Child Adolesc Psychiatr Clin N Am* 2000;**9**: 841–858.

91. Kazdin AE, Wassell G. Predictors of barriers to treatment and therapeutic change in outpatient therapy for antisocial children and their families. *Ment Health Serv Res* 2000;**2**:27–40.

92. Steiner H, Petersen ML, Saxena K, Ford S, Matthews Z. Divalproex sodium for the treatment of conduct disorder: a randomized controlled clinical trial. *J Clin Psychiat* 2003;**64**:1183–1191.

93. Steiner H, Saxena K, Chang K. Psychopharmacologic strategies for the treatment of aggression in juveniles. *CNS Spectr* 2003;**8**:298–308.

94. Fonagy P, Target M. The efficacy of psychoanalysis for children with disruptive disorders. *J Am Acad Child Adolesc Psychiat* 1994;**33**:45–55.

95. Fonagy P, Target M. Understanding the violent patient: the use of the body and the role of the father. *Int J Psychoanal* 1995;**76**:487–501.

96. Fonagy P, Target M. The place of psychodynamic theory in developmental psychopathology. *Dev Psychopathol* 2000;**12**:407–425.

97. Kazdin AE, Bass D, Siegel T, Thomas C. Cognitive-behavioral therapy and relationship therapy in the treatment of children referred for antisocial behavior. *J Consult Clin Psychol* 1989;**57**:522–535.

98. Kazdin AE, Siegel TC, Bass D. Cognitive problem-solving skills training and parent management training in the treatment of antisocial behavior in children. *J Consult Clin Psychol* 1992;**60**:733–747.

99. Rohde P, Clarke GN, Mace DE, Jorgensen JS, Seeley JR. An efficacy/effectiveness study of cognitive-behavioral treatment for adolescents with comorbid major depression and conduct disorder. *J Am Acad Child Adolesc Psychiat* 2004;**43**:660–668.

100. Borduin CM. Multisystemic treatment of criminality and violence in adolescents. *J Am Acad Child Adolesc Psychiat* 1999;**38**:242–249.

101. Curtis NM, Ronan KR, Borduin CM. Multisystemic treatment: A meta-analysis of outcome studies. *J Fam Psychol* 2004;**8**:411–419.

102. Henggeler SW, Melton GB, Smith LA. Family preservation using multisystemic therapy: an effective alternative to incarcerating serious juvenile offenders. *J Consult Clin Psychol* 1992;**60**:953–961.

103. Henggeler SW, Melton GB, Brondino MJ, Scherer DG, Hanley JH. Multisystemic therapy with violent and chronic juvenile offenders and their families: the role of treatment fidelity in successful dissemination. *J Consult Clin Psychol* 1997;**65**:821–833.

104. Schaeffer CM, Borduin CM. Long-term follow-up to a randomized clinical trial of multisystemic therapy with serious and violent juvenile offenders, *J Consult Clin Psychol* 2005;**73**:445–453.

105. Borduin CM, Mann BJ, Cone LT, *et al.* Multisystemic treatment of serious juvenile offenders: Long-term prevention of criminality and violence. *J Consult Clin Psych* 1995;**63**:569–578.

106. Chamberlain P, Reid JB. Comparison of two community alternatives to incarceration for chronic juvenile offenders. *J Consult Clin Psychol* 1998;**66**:624–633.

107. Chamberlain P, Weinrott M. Specialized foster care: Treating seriously emotionally disturbed children. *Child Today* 1990;**19**:24–27.

108. Eddy JM, Chamberlain P. Family management and deviant peer association as mediators of the impact of treatment condition on youth antisocial behavior. *J Consult Clin Psychol* 2000;**68**:857–863.

109. Leve LD, Chamberlain P, Reid JB. Intervention outcomes for girls referred from juvenile justice: Effects on

delinquency. *J Consult Clin Psychol* 2005;**73**: 1181–1185.

110. Liddle HA, Dakof GA, Parker K, Diamond GS, Barrett K, Tejeda M. Multidimensional family therapy for adolescent drug abuse: Results of a randomized clinical trial. *Am J Drug Alcohol Abuse* 2001; **27**:651–688.

111. American Diabetes Association and the American Psychiatric Association. Consensus development conference on antipsychotic drugs and obesity and diabetes. *Diabetes Care* 2004;**27**:596–601.

112. Blader JC, Schooler NR, Jensen PS, Pliszka SR, Kafantaris V. Adjunctive divalproex versus placebo for children with ADHD and aggression refractory to stimulant monotherapy. *Am J Psychiat* 2009;**166**:1392–1401.

113. Steiner H, Karnik NS. Integrated treatment of aggression in the context of ADHD in children refractory to stimulant monotherapy: a window into the future of child psychopharmacology. *Am J Psychiat* 2009;**166**:1315–1317.

114. Haapasalo J, Hamalainen T. Childhood family problems and current psychiatric problems among young violent and property offenders. *J Am Acad Child Adolesc Psychiat* 1996;**35**:1394–1401.

115. Pliszka SR, Sherman JO, Barrow MV, Irick S. Affective disorder in juvenile offenders: A preliminary study. *Am J Psychiat* 2000;**157**:130–132.

116. Ruchkin V, Koposov R, Vermeiren R, Schwab-Stone M. Psychopathology and age at onset of conduct problems in juvenile delinquents. *J Clin Psychiat* 2003;**64**: 913–920.

117. Ulzen TP, Hamilton H. The nature and characteristics of psychiatric comorbidity in incarcerated adolescents. *Can J Psychiat* 1998;**43**:57–63.

118. Vermeiren R, De Clippele A, Deboutte D. A descriptive survey of Flemish delinquent adolescents. *J Adolesc* 2000;**23**:277–285.

119. Vermeiren R, Schwab-Stone M, Ruchkin V, De Clippele A, Deboutte D. Predicting recidivism in delinquent adolescents from psychological and psychiatric assessment. *Compr Psychiatry* 2002;**43**:142–149.

120. Decety J, Michalska KJ, Kinzler KD. The contribution of emotion and cognition to moral sensitivity: a neurodevelopmental study. *Cereb Cortex* 2011; DOI:10.1093/cercor/bhr111.

12

Child and Adolescent Affective Disorders and their Treatment

Rick T. Bowers, Christina G. Weston, Julia Jackson

Introduction

The purpose of this chapter is to help the clinician understand how to diagnose and treat affective disorders in children and adolescents. While diagnosing mental health disorders in youth can be challenging, new research has yielded evidence-based treatments that can be offered to patients with more certainty of their effectiveness. It also is beginning to elucidate the developmental differences children have compared with adults when diagnosing affective disorders.

Depressive Disorders

Historical Perspectives

In the early twentieth century when modern psychiatry was established the psychoanalytic school of thought was dominant. At that time it was thought that children were unable to experience a major depressive episode similar to those experienced by adults. This was because depression was felt to be the result of an intrapsychic conflict between the ego and persecutory superego. Since young children weren't believed to develop a superego until late adolescence, they were thought not to have the capacity for intrapsychic conflict or depression. This view persisted despite descriptions at the time by Spitz of a depressive clinical syndrome in hospitalized infants termed anaclitic depression [1]. As time passed the age at which depression was felt to exist in youth gradually moved, from acceptance of its existence in teenagers to school-age children. Most recently Luby and colleagues have been examining depression in preschoolers and have found empirical data that have validated the existence of preschool depression [2]. Once experts began to accept the existence of depression in children of all ages,

parents began to seek treatment for the emotional pain they were appreciating in their children, and child psychiatric researchers began to investigate the etiology, diagnosis, and treatment of the disorder.

Clinical Description

The diagnostic criteria for depressive disorders in the *Diagnostic and Statistical Manual of Mental Disorders* (DSM-IV-TR [3] generally use the same criteria to diagnose mood disorders in children, adolescents, and adults. It is important to keep in mind that as children develop their ability to articulate their internal life and the way they express their depressive symptoms will change. A child's level of intellectual and emotional maturity affects the way they communicate their innermost feelings to others and also how those feelings are perceived by adults. When evaluating children for depression it is important to rely on multiple sources of information. Parents are necessary to help make a diagnosis in younger children but one must rely on the child as well as other sources of information to establish a diagnosis. Evaluations of parental versus self-reports demonstrate that parents are more effective at recognizing externalizing disorders such as oppositional defiant disorder (ODD) or attention-deficit hyperactivity disorder (ADHD) in their children but they are much less able to detect internalizing disorders such as depression or anxiety [4]. Specific depression symptoms in DSM-IV-TR have similar occurrence rates across the lifespan; however, some neurovegetative and cognitive impairments do seem to have different age-related rates of occurrence. Table 12.1 describes some of the developmental differences in the clinical presentation of depression across the lifespan [3, 5, 6].

Clinical Child Psychiatry, Third Edition. Edited by William M. Klykylo and Jerald Kay.
© 2012 John Wiley & Sons, Ltd. Published 2012 by John Wiley & Sons, Ltd.

Table 12.1 Developmental difference in clinical presentation of depression throughout the lifespan.

Age	Frequency	Sex ratio M:F	Symptoms of major depressive disorder (MDD)
3–6	0.3–0.5%	1:1	Diminished interest in play
			Self-destructive or worthlessness play themes
			Symptoms present but may not be persistent over 2 weeks
7–12	2–5%	1:1	More somatic complaints (e.g., "my head hurts")
			Unexplained irritability or outbursts of crying
			Complaints of boredom
12–18	5–10%	1:3	Poor school performance
			More irritability, impulsivity and reckless behavior
			Suicidal thoughts and attempts increase
19+	17–20%	1:2	DSM-IV-TR criteria 5 of 9 symptoms
			More decreased appetite and weight loss seen than in children
			More hypersomnia in young and middle-aged adults

Adapted from refs [5–7].

Major Depressive Disorders

The DSM-IV-TR characterizes major depression as the presence of a single major depressive episode, with five or more of the following symptoms present during the same 2-week period, and at least one of the symptoms being either depressed mood or loss of interest in pleasure. Symptoms include the following (DSM-IV-TR):

(1) Depressed mood for most of the day and nearly every day.
(2) Markedly diminished interest or pleasure in almost all activities nearly every day.
(3) Significant weight loss or gain due to decrease or increase in appetite resulting in a 5% change in bodyweight in a month.
(4) Insomnia or hypersomnia nearly every day.
(5) Psychomotor agitation or retardation nearly every day.
(6) Fatigue or loss of energy nearly every day.
(7) Feelings of excessive worthlessness or guilt.
(8) Diminished ability to think or concentrate.
(9) Current thoughts of death and/or suicidal ideation that may include a plan or an actual suicide attempt.

In addition to the above symptoms the DSM specifies that the symptoms must cause clinically significant distress or impairment in the child/adolescent's academic, social, or other important areas of functioning that reflect a change from their previous level of functioning. Symptoms must also not be attributable to abuse of substances, use of medications, other psychiatric illness, bereavement, or a medical illness. Many of the symptoms are more appropriate for adults; for example, since children are growing it would be rare for them to have a significant decrease in appetite that would cause a 5% change in bodyweight. This can make it difficult for children to meet the minimum number of five symptoms required to make a diagnosis of major depressive disorder in DSM-IV-TR.

Younger children and preschoolers often have not developed enough language skills and cognitive capacity to describe their mood states, which can make it difficult to utilize them as informants. Luby and colleagues have studied preschool depression and have proposed some developmental modifications. They found that although symptoms are present over a 2-week period they do not necessarily persist for the entire 2 weeks, but still represent a change in the previous level of functioning. Decreased interest is seen in decreased interest in play activities. Feelings of worthlessness and inappropriate guilt are seen in play themes. Suicidal or self-destructive themes are persistently evident in play only [5]. It had previously been believed that young children had "masked depression" or symptoms such as somatization and regression. When rates of typical and masked depressive symptoms in depressed preschoolers were compared it was found that typical depressive symptoms occurred at higher rates [2]. In this study somatic complaints occurred in 40% of depressed preschoolers. The typical symptoms of depression occurred at higher rates. Sadness/irritability occurred 98% of the time, while appetite, sleep, and concentration problems occurred over 80% of the time. As children enter school and develop increased cognitive capacities their clinical symptoms of depression can be seen in relation to their societal expectations of going to school and developing relationships with peers.

Signs and Symptoms of Depression in Children

The signs and symptoms of depression in children can be summarized as follows [7–9]:

(1) Complain of sadness or report a negative self-concept when it pertains to their behavior, intelligence, appearance, or acceptance by peers: "I'm stupid, I'm ugly," etc.
(2) Complain of frequent vague somatic complaints such as fatigue, stomachache or headache (to miss school) possibly as they are verbally unable to express their inner feelings.
(3) Disengagement from peers and social withdrawal typified by refusal to engage with friends or hobbies, or participate in extracurricular activities.
(4) Isolation – choose to stay in their rooms, sleep extensively, and are more irritable when interacting with family.
(5) More sensitive to perceived criticism or rejection with vocal outbursts or crying.
(6) May fail to make expected weight gains.
(7) Behavioral problems with temper tantrums.
(8) Thoughts of death or suicide may have nonverbal cues such as giving away a favorite possession (rare completions in children under 12).
(9) Can show more anxiety and auditory hallucinations than adolescents.

As children mature and become teenagers they develop metacognition and are more able to report their actual feeling states and neurovegetative disturbances. It can still be a clinical challenge to understand their clinical symptoms and how they relate to symptoms of depression. It is also important to distinguish depressive symptoms from the occasional transient periods of adolescent turmoil where emotional upheaval is not uncommon. As adolescents are developing more relationships outside their family their initial symptoms may be more evident to their friends and teachers than their parents. Collateral information provided by parents, friends, teachers, coaches, and others may be invaluable in making a proper diagnosis. Making the diagnosis and developing a treatment plan is crucial as teenagers may have more feelings of hopelessness, suicidal ideation, and engage more frequently in suicide attempts. Suicide is the third leading cause of death for teenagers and they have much higher rates of completed suicides than younger children [10].

Signs and Symptoms of Depression in Adolescents

In adolescents, the major signs and symptoms of depression are as follows [7, 11, 12]:

(1) Irritability, boredom, anxiety, or a feeling of hopelessness.
(2) Withdrawal from friends and previous activities and isolation from family when at home.
(3) May show their sadness by writing poetry or stories with morbid themes, be preoccupied with nihilistic music, or wear black clothes.
(4) Sleep disturbance manifested by staying awake all night watching TV or on the internet, difficulty getting up for school, and sleeping during the day.
(5) Poor motivation to attend school, frequently skipped classes, poor concentration leading to low grades.
(6) Rebellious behavior, alcohol or drug use, and promiscuous sexual activity.
(7) Preoccupation with death and dying. Suicide attempts can be more serious and lethal.

When identifying depression in youth it is important to get an understanding of the course of the illness. Children and adolescents can also have seasonal affective disorder. This occurs when there is a temporal relationship between the onset of a depression and the change of seasons and decrease in sunlight. This pattern must have been duplicated in three separate years. It is important to account for developmental issues as children start school in late summer and fall, which can be a significant stressor for some. Depressed mood can start in the winter quarter, after their first marking period is complete.

Dysthymia

This is a chronic low-grade depression in which the DSM-IV-TR criteria were altered for children and adolescents. The criteria allowed that for children and adolescents the mood can be primarily irritable (instead of sad) and have a duration of at least one year compared with a duration of 2 years in adults. This depressed or irritable mood must occur most days or more days than not, and the person must have never been without symptoms for more than 2 months at a time. Two of the following additional symptoms are required: changes in appetite, sleep difficulty, fatigue, low self-esteem, poor concentration or difficulty with making decisions, and feelings of hopelessness [3]. While the symptoms are very similar to major depression they are less severe and don't impair daily living as significantly as is seen in major depression. In one study 70% of dysthymic children and adolescents eventually developed major depression [13]. This highlights the importance of identifying these youths and intervening before they develop a more debilitating major depressive disorder.

Depressive Disorder Not Otherwise Specified

Depression not otherwise specified (NOS) is also referred to as "minor" or subsyndromal depression, and is diagnosed in the presence of depressed mood, irritability, or anhedonia and up to three symptoms of Major Depression [14]. Since many of the descriptive criteria in the DSM-IV-TR were derived from adult studies, often many children and adolescents are diagnosed with Depressive Disorder NOS since they do not have enough symptoms to meet MDD. In a study of youths with subthreshold depression the subjects were found to have elevated risks for depression later in life and had more suicidal behaviors [14]. Their risk of future adverse outcome was the same as those who had been diagnosed with MDD. This study shows that this type of mood disorder does result in significant distress and impairment and is sufficient to warrant a diagnosis and develop a treatment plan.

CASE STUDY

Case example: Depression

S.T. is a 14-year-old ninth grader whose adoptive parents sought treatment for ongoing bouts of irritability and anger. S.T.'s parents described her as typically a pleasant and compliant child at home but shy and reserved in social interaction outside of the home. Approximately 8 months ago S.T. began spending increasingly more time in her room. Her sleep became problematic, with S.T. lying awake until the early morning hours reading or journaling. After finally falling asleep she would "toss and turn" until morning. She began failing her classes at school, despite making the honor roll previously, and told her parents she no longer wanted to play volleyball. Teachers advised her parents that S.T. falls asleep in class and daydreams frequently. She lacked focus or motivation, and had become short and irritable, with peers and teachers alike. Her parents complained that S.T. is easily overwhelmed and is quick to engage in angry verbal outbursts, which often end with her slamming her bedroom door. On exam S.T. appeared sad, exhibiting downcast eyes and a restricted range of affect. She was dressed in oversized athletic clothes, did not wear makeup, and had her hair pulled back in an unkempt ponytail. She related that she hates her life and wishes she were with her real family. She lamented that she causes more problems than she's worth, and wishes she could just disappear. She denied having thoughts of ending her life, though her parents offered that on two separate occasions in the past week she screamed "I want to kill myself!" S.T. maintained that she was just frustrated and wasn't planning on ending her life. She admitted to making superficial cuts on her thighs in the past month, however, in an attempt to feel better emotionally. She expressed fear that she is going crazy because, approximately 2 weeks ago, she started hearing a mumbling, incoherent voice when she is alone. Her parents are concerned that she feels left out because her mother is often overwhelmed with parenting five children and her dad is frequently away on business trips. Her mother describes their home as "chaotic," with much yelling and fighting between S.T. and her adopted brothers and sisters. S.T.'s mother reports primarily yelling and removing privileges when disciplining her children. She shares that she has struggled with depression for most of her life, but never sought treatment. Due to S.T.'s ongoing angry outbursts, she's been grounded for some time, and feels there is no one to talk to, particularly now that she lost her phone and computer privileges. S.T. was referred for individual and family therapy. Individual therapy helped S.T. reframe her negative view of herself and the world and taught her positive coping strategies. Family therapy addressed the distant relationship between her parents and siblings and provided her parents with more effective parenting strategies. Her parents eventually began marital therapy, and S.T.'s mother sought treatment for her own depressive symptoms. S.T. was concurrently started on fluoxetine after discussing the risks, benefits, and side effects of antidepressant medication including the need for close monitoring for suicidality or activation symptoms. After approximately 4 months of treatment S.T. described feeling significantly better, and no longer experienced self-injurious behavior or thoughts of ending her life.

Epidemiology and Prevalence of Depressive Disorders

The prevalence of depression in children and adolescents varies depending on the population sampled and the methods used to diagnose depression. In the Great Smokey Mountain population study, the 3-month prevalence of psychiatric disorders in children aged 9–16 was examined. Depressive disorder rates were combined to include MDD, dysthymia, and depression NOS [15]. In this study rates of depression for children aged 9–12 years averaged 2.13%; in adolescents aged 13–16 years the rates of depression averaged 3%. Studies have found that the incidence of depression increases with age. A review of rates of depression in studies of preschool-aged children found a range from 0.3% to 1.4% [16]. The point prevalence of depression increases with age to range from 1% to 2% in prepubertal children, and 3% to 8% of adolescents, and increases to a lifetime prevalence of 20% by the completion of adolescence [17]. The National Comorbidity Survey Replication – Adolescent Supplement Study found that 11.7% of adolescents met criteria for MDD or dysthymia. Females were twice as likely as males to have depression. It also found that mood disorders increased uniformly with age, with a twofold increase from the 13–14-year-old group to the 17–18-year-old group [18].

In recent years there has been concern, in the popular press as well as in academic journals, about an "epidemic" of depression [19, 20]. Concern that this has been occurring has been raised by evidence of increased antidepressant prescriptions for children and adolescents; retrospective recall by successive birth cohort of adults with depression; rising adolescent suicide rates until 1990; and an increase in emotional problems seen in three cohorts of adolescents in Britain. [21, 22] This prompted Costello and colleagues to conduct a meta-analysis of all studies that used structured interviews to diagnose depression in populations under 18. They found 26 studies from 1965 to 1996, and the overall prevalence estimates of depression were: under 13 years old, 2.8%; 13–18-year-olds, 5.6%; and these had not increased over the past 30 years. The authors concluded that the perception of an "epidemic" may have arisen from heightened awareness of a disorder that had been previously underdiagnosed by clinicians [22]. It is likely that increased publicity and awareness of the existence of depression is contributing to this perception of an epidemic. Hopefully increased awareness will lead to a decrease in stigma and more families will seek help for their depressed children and adolescents.

Etiology and Pathogenesis

Although science has made significant progress in understanding the causes of depression in youth a complete understanding of the etiology often remains a mystery. As with most areas of psychiatry explanatory models have been adapted from studies of depressive disorders in adults. Currently no one model or combination of models can satisfactorily provide a causal mechanism to explain the production of depression in children. As each case is unique it is best to examine the biological, psychological, and environmental factors unique to each patient to provide the best explanation for the etiology of a child's depression.

Depression Risk Factors

Stressors in a youth's environment can be a contributing factor in the development of depression. In a 14-month longitudinal study of adolescents it was found that youth conflict with parents was significantly predictive of adolescents having depressive symptoms compared to peers [23]. When parents are stressed often that contributes to a child feeling stressed. One study found that early maternal stress was predictive of childhood depressive symptoms, while later maternal stress predicted depression in adolescents [24]. The same study also found that maternal depression also predicted childhood and adolescent depression. Another study of depressed children found that 30% had mothers with moderate to severe depression at baseline assessment. The mothers with more severe depression had more severe levels of depression in their children. Fortunately maternal depressive severity wasn't related to improvement in the child's depression over time [25]. In addition to family risk factors, youths who have other comorbid disorders such as anxiety, antisocial behavior, and attention difficulties also have a higher incidence of depression. One study found that 25–50% of depressed youths also have a comorbid anxiety disorder, while 10–15% of anxious youths have a depressive disorder [26]. Youths followed longitudinally who had high levels of antisocial behavior in first and second grades were found to have higher levels of depressive symptoms in eighth grade [23]. In a longitudinal study, Ashford and colleagues examined children at 2–3 and later 4–5 years and again at 11 years. They found that at 2–3 years of age children with low socioeconomic status and family stress were more likely to have internalizing problems at age 11. Furthermore, 4–5-year-olds with high levels of parenting stress were also more likely to have internalizing problems at age 11 [27]. The authors also found that the risk for internalizing problems increased from 15.5% when children had one risk factor to 48% when children had more than two risk factors. This suggests that the creation of effective prevention programs to decrease parenting stress in the families of preschoolers can lead to a decrease in future childhood depression.

Genetic Model of Depressive Disorders

In treating children and adolescents, it is very common to find other close family members who also suffer from an affective disturbance. Indeed, the available literature indicates that the genetic contribution to mood disorders is significantly greater when the symptoms first appear in childhood or adolescence.

Utilizing one of the best methods to study heredity via twin studies, Akiskal and Weller reported that the concordance rate for mood disorders in monozygotic twins is 76% declining to 19% in dizygotic twins [28]. Monozygotic twins reared apart in this study showed a concordance rate of 67%, indicating an environmental factor as well. Thus, it seems the rate of depression in adopted children is correlated with the rate of depression in their biological rather than their adoptive parents.

Family studie [29]. of depression in adults have shown that a positive family history for depression increases the likelihood of depression occurring in relatives. This genetic loading and predisposition seem to be increased even further for relatives of children and adolescents with major depression. The earlier the age of onset of depression in children, the greater the degree of genetic loading for the affective disorder; first-degree relatives of prepubertal children with depression have the greatest risk, and the first-degree relatives of adolescents with depression have a somewhat lesser risk [30, 31].

Conversely, a stud [32]. involving children and adolescents indicated that having a single parent with a unipolar or bipolar affective disorder imparts to the offspring a 25% risk of developing an affective disturbance, and having two parents affected imparts a 75% risk.

In summary, the overwhelming evidence suggests that early-onset major depression is associated with marked psychiatric and medical comorbidity, and a protracted course leading to significant functional impairment with a reduced life expectancy due to a higher rate of comorbid medical illnesses and suicide [33, 34].

Biological Factors

It is believed that affective disorders may result from or produce biological changes of a brief or lasting duration. Biological inquiry and tests have sought to elucidate these biological changes in the hopes of developing a laboratory test that could confirm or rule out an affective disorder as well as monitor response to treatment.

Biological markers are differentiated either as *state markers*, which are detectable only during the episode and eventually revert to normal, or *trait markers*, which are detectable prior to the onset of the illness in question.

A recent task forc [35]. reviewed evidence for the use of biological markers in depression. Ideally, a biological marker could be used to "describe a biological change associated with depression that could be used to indicate the presence and severity of the condition and predict drug or other treatments' response as well as the clinical prognosis."

In evaluating all of the numerous potential biological markers of depression including biochemical markers, serotonergic markers, neurotrophic factors, immunological markers, neuroimaging, neurophysiological, and neuropsychological markers the task force proposed that those listed below warrant the most attention:

- decreased platelet imipramine binding (5-HTT serotonin transporter);
- decreased 5-HT1A serotonin receptor expression;
- increase of soluble interleukin-2 receptor (SIL-2R) and interleukin-6 in serum;
- decreased brain-derived neurotrophic factor (BDNF) and fibroblast growth factor (FGF-1) in serum;
- hypocholesterolemia;
- low blood folate levels;
- impaired suppression of the dexamethasone suppression test; cortisol hypersecretion.

However, none of these markers has been shown to be adequately specific to contribute to the diagnosis of major depression and warrant inclusion as a diagnostic aid of major depression. Given the lack of conclusive data regarding these tests and their costs (often several hundred or several thousand dollars), these studies have limited use, especially in the present medical environment of cost constraints, as they have limited predictive or diagnostic value. In short, they may help to confirm a diagnosis of depression but not diagnose it. These current studies are likely to be increasingly relegated to patients in specific research protocols or studies. This research is promising for the discovery and development of future biological markers that will aid the clinician in diagnosing and directing effective treatments of patients.

Adding sometimes to the delay in accurately diagnosing and implementing appropriate treatment is the fact that numerous conditions are known to mimic depressive disorders. Unfortunately, there is no consensus as to what should constitute a routine screening battery of blood work and tests to rule out many of these potentially treatable disorders. A chemistry panel may indicate an electrolyte disturbance or alteration in calcium, which could affect one's mental state. A complete blood count (CBC) with differential may help to identify a central nervous system infection or anemia, which would prompt the physician to pursue a vitamin B12 or folate deficiency, as such disorders are well known to have psychiatric manifestations. A thyroid-stimulating hormone (TSH) and a free thyroid (T4 free) serum level will typically screen for most thyroid disorders. Testing for sexually transmitted diseases that affect the CNS, such as syphilis or AIDS, is increasingly relevant in an age when so many youths are sexually active or unfortunately sexually abused. An elevation of liver enzymes could signal alcohol abuse or mononucleosis. If accompanying mental or neurological symptoms are present these liver abnormalities may also indicate Wilson's disease or a porphyria, which can be further evaluated via a ceruloplasmin level or 24-hour quantitative urine screen for porphyrins, respectively. Other mental or neurological symptoms may indicate the need for an electroencephalogram (EEG) or brain imaging with computed axial tomography (CAT), magnetic resonance imaging (MRI), or positron emission tomography (PET). Lastly, as the knowledge base grows about the most prevalent type of metabolic disorders known as mitochondrial disease, which can theoretically contribute to such psychiatric conditions as developmental disorders, depression, bipolar disorder, and schizophrenia, clinicians will have to consider mitochondrial disorders in the differential of many psychiatric disorders.

Assessment

When examining a child with suspected depression it is important to complete a comprehensive assessment, which is described in Chapter 00. When evaluating depression specifically it is important to gather information from the child and parents, and collateral from teachers and other involved parties. It is often helpful to assess the severity of symptoms with standardized instruments with normative data, which identifies when symptoms are clinically significant. It is useful to keep in mind that most depression-rating scales have poor construct validity and tend to measure general distress rather than depression specifically. Depression instruments developed for use in youths and recommended for screening clinically referred youths are the Child Depression Inventory, and the Children's Depression Rating Scale-Revised (CDRS-R) [36]. The CDRS-R examines more of the physiological symptoms of depression while the CDI examines more of the cognitive symptoms. One of the drawbacks of these scales is that they have low specificity for diagnosing clinical depression and are not generally used alone to make the

diagnosis. They often are used to screen for depression and assess its severity, and shorter versions of the scale can be used to assess clinical improvement.

In the past structured and semi-structured interviews were considered the domain of research psychiatrists. These assessment tools are increasingly finding their way into clinical practice and are a means of making diagnosis more reliable and accurate. Initially it can feel to clinicians that they are putting an artificial element into the diagnostic process and that it is more time consuming. Once a provider becomes proficient with using the structured interview, it need not extend the diagnostic process. It offers more reliability and certainty that the diagnosis is correct and allows for more confidence in treatment planning. Many structured instruments are now available for use in children and adolescents. The Diagnostic Interview Schedule for Children verstion IV (DISC-IV) can be administered with a computer and headphones, which allows for information to be gathered before meeting with the psychiatrist, making their interview more focused and allowing for greater rapport building. Some instruments are respondent or "structured" interviews, which consist of a series of questions that are asked verbatim. Investigator-based or "semi-structured" interviews allow the more clinically trained interviewer to ask about specific behaviors and mood states with questions they deem appropriate.

Treatment

When a depressed youth and his or her family present for help a comprehensive diagnostic assessment and subsequent formulation serve as the foundation for the treatment plan. In the assessment the strengths and weaknesses of the patient and their family/environment should be identified as they pertain to the intrapsychic make-up, family, peers, school, and community. This can guide the selection of a treatment modality that can address the factors that precipitated the condition and the factors that are maintaining it. It is important to choose treatments that are a good fit for the patient and their families and have an evidence base that indicate that they are likely to be successful. One must be careful to avoid using a treatment approach primarily because it aligns with the therapist's theoretical orientation when other approaches may be more beneficial for the patient and family. It is also important to be mindful that youths are emotionally and financially dependent on their caregivers and that treatment must address family dynamics along with other environmental interventions. A nonjudgmental attitude that doesn't overemphasize blame and highlights the positive healthy functioning of the child and family are necessary. The therapist and treatment team must work to be seen by the patient and family as an advocate or resource for positive change.

Since the publication of the initial results of the Treatment for Adolescents with Depression Study (TADS) in 2004, which found that the combination of fluoxetine and cognitive behavioral therapy (CBT) was superior to either treatment alone, there has been renewed interest in using combination treatment for depressed youths [37]. In subsequent analysis of the study youths with combined treatment were found to have the largest number of adolescents without functional impairment 34.6% compared to only 20.2% with fluoxetine alone and 13.5% with CBT alone [38]. It was also found that depression response is fastest with combined treatment [39]. The TADS study only examined treatment of depression in adolescents and only used CBT as the psychotherapy type. It is important to be familiar with a variety of psychotherapies or psychosocial treatments when the treatment plan is developed so as to customize the treatment to meet the patient's and family's needs.

Psychosocial Treatments

In a recent review of evidence-based psychosocial treatments for child and adolescent depression, studies of treatment outcomes were reviewed using the Task Force on the Promotion and Dissemination of Psychological Procedures guidelines [40]. These guidelines deem an intervention to be *well-established* if there are two well-conducted experiments of between-group design that demonstrate efficacy either by showing its superiority to a pill or psychological placebo or to another treatment, or its equivalence to an already established treatment.

A treatment is deemed *probably efficacious* when two experiments demonstrate that the treatment is more effective than a no-treatment control group in improving functioning or the studies meet all of the criteria for a well-established treatment except that it is only shown by one research team. Treatments are characterized as *experimental* if they have shown treatment effects in only a limited evaluation and one randomized controlled trial. In their analysis the task force authors divided the available studies into childhood treatments and adolescent treatments.

In a recent meta-analysis of youth psychotherapy for depression, 75% of the studies used a cognitive change emphasis (through CBT or other cognitive approaches) [41]. The authors found that noncognitive treatments also had robust treatment findings; however, the effect size for all studies was only 0.34, which is a small to medium effect. This was much less than previous studies, which found significantly higher effect size [41]. Commonly used CBT techniques are described in Table 12.2. In a review of childhood treatment studies 10 rigorous studies were identified that used psychosocial treatment in depressed children [40]. CBT was deemed a well-established treatment in individual, group, and child group with parent formats. They also found the Penn Prevention Program and self-control therapy to be two *probably efficacious* treatments for children. The Penn Prevention Program was developed as a cognitive behavioral model designed to reduce depressive symptoms among at-risk 10–15-year-olds in school settings. It has a cognitive and a social problem-solving component [42]. The cognitive component teaches children to identify their negative

Table 12.2 Strategies commonly used in cognitive behavioral therapy (CBT) for children and adolescents.

Strategy	Description
Mood monitoring and psychoeducation	Youths and parents are given information about the symptoms and course of depression and how the CBT model can help. They are taught how to monitor their moods, behaviors, and thoughts to identify patterns
Pleasant activity scheduling and behavioral activation	Youths are asked to identify and plan to engage in enjoyable activities. They are taught to choose activities that are pleasurable and also allow for mastery of a skill or task. They are encouraged to create a rewarding, nonstressful, and mood-elevating environment in the long term
Cognitive restructuring	Youths are encouraged to identify their automatic thoughts and core schemes and assess the accuracy of these beliefs and how they affect their mood. Youths are taught to engage in "rational" thinking about themselves, the world, and their future possibilities
Skill-building techniques often used in CBT programs	Relaxation techniques are taught to cope with stressors; conflict resolution and general problem-solving skills are frequently taught

Adapted from Weesing and Brent (2006) [134].

beliefs and dispute them with more likely alternatives. The social problem-solving component focuses on setting goals, perspective taking, information gathering, finding action alternatives, and self-instruction. The children are taught how to handle family conflict and realization training, and encouraged to enhance their social support network. Self-Control Therapy is another school-based intervention developed by Stark and colleagues as a group intervention. It is based on a cognitive behavioral model and teaches self-management skills. It has been studied in a 12- and 24–26-session program and both were found to be superior to traditional counseling [43, 44].

Adolescents have had a greater number of depression treatment studies than children. A recent review of psychotherapy studies since 1998 found that 18 studies of treatment outcomes in depressed adolescents have been published [40]. Twelve of these included adolescents who met criteria for depression, and six were conducted with adolescents at risk for depression as they had elevated depressive symptoms. The majority of the interventions focused on CBT or interpersonal psychotherapy (IPT). In their review David-Ferdon and Kaslow felt that CBT individual and adolescent group interventions qualified as "well-established" treatments. Adolescent group CBT plus parent component and individual plus parent/family component from the TADS study were felt to be in the "probably efficacious" category. IPT also qualified as a "well-established" treatment. Family systems theory and several other therapies were categorized as "experimental." [40].

Interpersonal therapy for adolescents (IPT-A) was first developed by Mufson and colleagues [45]. Patients are taught how their depression and the quality of their interpersonal relationships affect each other. It differs from the adult version in that it has a shorter treatment duration (16–20 weeks), involves parents, allows therapists to liaison between schools and families, and re-conceptualizes the sick role to have a limited focus [46]. It has been adapted to adolescent development to focus on separation from parents, development of romantic interpersonal relationships, initial experience with grief, and dealing with peer pressures. It has been investigated in a hospital-based clinic and a school based clinic [47,48]. In the initial small study, by week 12 of the protocol 75% of the IPT-A-treated patients were recovered compared with 46% of those who received usual clinic management [47]. In the school-based study, adolescents with depression were given therapy at school-based primary care clinics by staff who had received a day of training and an hour of weekly group supervision. The youths who received IPT-A were compared to those who received treatment as usual. They were found to have greater symptom reduction, more rapid symptom improvement, and better functioning by week 8 [48]. This second study was important in that it showed that research-based psychotherapy treatments can be translated to real world settings and be effective [46]. When selecting a psychotherapy for adolescents it is important to also look at the patients' unique characteristics. In the TADS study it was found that adolescents with low levels of cognitive distortion did equally well when they received medication or combined medication and CBT, suggesting that they didn't receive any additional benefit from the therapy [49]. This highlights the importance of selecting psychotherapy or other treatment that best fits patients' unique needs. In addition to best fit it is important to be aware of what resources are available in the community and to refer patients appropriately when additional specialty care is needed. In some remote areas it can be a challenge to find any therapist, especially one with competence in newer evidence-based therapies.

Pharmacotherapy and other Somatic Treatments

Research [50, 51] has shown that, as in adults, depression in children and adolescents is treatable via medical and psychotherapies, with the combination being preferable.

Tricyclic antidepressants (TCAs) were the first compounds to be utilized on a large scale to treat depressive disturbances in children and adolescents. No TCA antidepressant has ever been approved by the US Food and Drug Administration (FDA) for use in depressed children, and in fact most double-blind placebo-controlled studies using imipramine in depressed children have shown the medication to be not significantly better than placebo. One notable sideline of these studies is that the placebo rate surpassed 50–70% in some of these studies and thus as with the more contemporary selective serotonin reuptake inhibitor (SSRI) trials with similarly high placebo rates, it hindered the ability of these clinical trials to demonstrate a positive response rate versus placebo. With the advent of the SSRI class of antidepressants and their ease of use, preferable side-effect profile, and safety, TCAs are seldom used now.

The introduction of the SSRI fluoxetine to the American market in 1987 quickly led to the SSRIs becoming the most widely prescribed antidepressants for adults and youths in short fashion even though initial FDA approval was for adults only. Fluoxetine was the first SSRI to receive FDA approval for treatment of children and adolescents with depression (major depressive disorder) from 7 to 17 years of age but that was not until 2006. This delay in pediatric FDA approval for fluoxetine and other SSRIs has in part been due to the high placebo rate in these SSRI studies.

There are now 17 randomized, placebo-controlled trials of various antidepressant agent classes, including citalopram, escitalopram, fluoxetine, mirtazapine, nefazodone, paroxetine, sertraline, and venlafaxine. The placebo-corrected effect sizes vary significantly and overall are less than expected when compared to adult studies. There do seem to be several factors that may account for the variance in these studies. Factors that seem to result in higher effect sizes include a placebo run-in period to minimize the placebo response rate, fewer trial sites per study, and non-industry studies such as those completed by the National Institute of Mental Health (NIMH), where there may be greater expertise in patient selection, treatment, and assessment reliability. The two non-industry federally sponsored fluoxetine trials with fewer and more experienced sites reported a very acceptable placebo response rate of 30–35% and resulted in a standardized moderate effect size estimate of 0.5. Even in the industry-sponsored trials where some of the mean placebo response rates were over 50% it is notable that more than 50% of youths treated also responded to antidepressant therapy. While not ideal such results may give clinicians confidence in using antidepressants in their own practice settings where they have control over patient selection and the treatment process. This becomes even more relevant when one considers outcome data from studies such as the TADS, which employed best practice treatment approaches utilizing medication (fluoxetine) plus CBT psychotherapy. Despite the combined therapy approach the TADS data indicate that only 23% of study participants reached remission at week 12, and still only 60% reached remission by week 36. Thus, there is much room for improvement in the treatment of adolescent depression given the high morbidity to the adolescent, the associated family burden [52]. the relapsing course, and the concern of mortality given that depression is strongly associated with suicidal events in as many as 50% of adolescents with the disorder [53].

The TADS data support several useful clinical guidelines (discussed later) for treating adolescents to promote optimal treatment outcomes given the significant limitations of currently available medical and psychotherapeutic modalities. While our knowledge of antidepressant treatments in youths has progressed significantly it is still comparatively limited compared to what is known about treating depression in adults (e.g., Star*D Trials). Basic clinical questions such as whether to switch or augment medical or psychotherapy interventions when treatment response is inadequate have yet to be answered conclusively. New

NIMH-funded research such as the Treatment of Resistant Depression in Adolescents (TORDIA) study [54]. will investigate how best to treat adolescents whose depression is resistant to the first SSRI medication they have tried, should help answer this important treatment question. Lastly, the NIMH is also supporting the Treatment of Adolescent Suicide Attempters (TASA) study [55]. which is investigating the treatment of adolescents who have attempted suicide; treatment options will include antidepressant medications, CBT, or both. See Figure 12.1 for a depression treatment algorithm.

Much is still to be learned about the specifics of prepubertal-onset MDD, which is more likely to become bipolar disorder in adulthood [56, 57], as distinguished from juvenile-onset MDD and from adult-onset MDD.

Juvenile-onset depression is heterogeneous, and pioneering studies such as the Dunedin Multidisciplinary Health and Development Stud [58]. helped to elucidate that specific early-childhood risk factors examined by the authors (i.e., perinatal insults, motor skills, psychopathological characteristics, instability in the family of origin, and behavioral and socioemotional problems) were associated with juvenile-onset MDD but not with adult-onset MDD. Such data influence one's treatment approach and could guide the implementation of specific and unique treatment interventions. Ongoing epidemiological and family study findings have helped clinicians to better understand the clinical course and treatment of juvenile-onset depression.

Future studies to clarify phenotypic versus genotypic variants as well as physiological markers through techniques such as gene mapping or neuroimaging will hopefully allow more selective treatments to be implemented and positive predictive responses to be realized [59].

Prognosis

It is helpful when working with depressed children and their families to be aware of the possible developmental trajectories of the illness. In a Dutch longitudinal study of over 2000 youths the trajectories of the subjects were examined by gender and six distinct developmental trajectories were identified [60]. Boys in the study were found to fit into one of six trajectories:

(1) Very low decreasing males.
(2) Low stable males.
(3) Moderate increasing males.
(4) High decreasing males.
(5) High childhood peak males.
(6) Increasing high males.

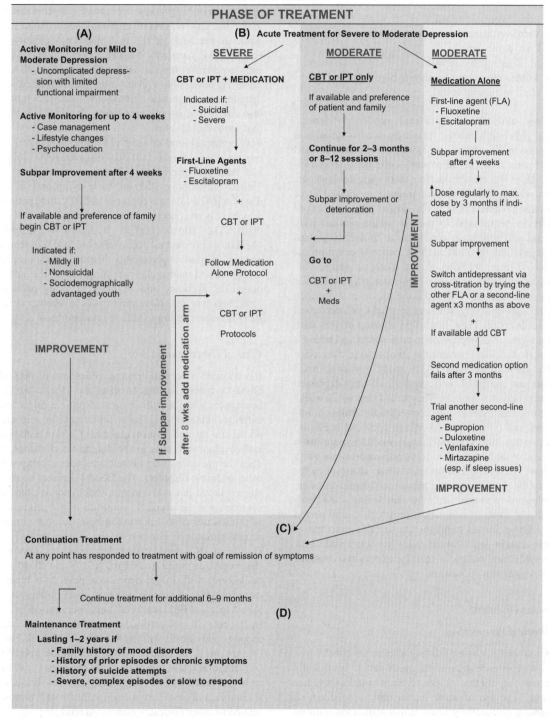

Figure 12.1 Treatment of pediatric major depressive disorder. CBT, cognitive behavioral therapy; IPT, interpersonal therapy.

Girls in the study were found to fit into six slightly different trajectories:

(1) Low decreasing females.
(2) Very low increasing females (increasing adolescence).
(3) Low stable females.
(4) Moderate stable females.
(5) Adolescence onset increasing high females.
(6) High increasing females.

This study found significant gender differences. Only girls had a chronic trajectory of early childhood depression. Two boys' trajectories were found that had decreasing levels of depression – one became asymptomatic in late childhood, the other in late adolescence. Boys with elevated depression trajectories showed lower educational attainment while similar girls were more likely to be referred to mental health services [60]. Mazza and colleagues conducted a similar study with a population of children with depressive symptoms followed in school from second to eighth grade. This study found five different depressive trajectories for males and females [61]. Like the previous study they found a group of boys whose depression levels decreased by adolescence. They didn't find a group of girls with high increases of depression in adolescence as Dekker's group found, likely because the group wasn't followed in later adolescence. The TADS study examined three treatment groups of moderately to severely depressed teenagers over 9 months. They found that by 24 weeks all three treatment groups converged in remission outcomes and 60% of youths overall achieved remission [62]. In this study youths who had residual symptoms at the end of the 12-week treatment phase were more likely to have not achieved remission at weeks 18 and 36 of the study. They also found that between 65% and 72% of the adolescents who achieved remission during acute treatment were able to maintain it during the study period [62]. These studies highlight the variable outcome of depression in youths: while many get better with time, some will have relapse of their symptoms and continue to struggle with depression.

Bipolar Disorders

Historical Perspectives

Similar to the debate regarding whether or not children could experience depression, much debate historically surrounded whether or not children could experience mania. The use of adult mania criteria to diagnose pediatric mania likely resulted in a significant number of pediatric mania cases going undetected. This presumed diagnostic deficit persisted despite reports from respected clinicians such as Kraepelin, who in 1921 published the finding that 4% of manic-depressive patients experienced prepubertal bipolar symptomatology [63]. Also, case reports of early childhood mania were made as far back as the mid-nineteenth century by Esquirol [64]. Currently it is well accepted that children can experience bipolar affective disorders (BAD); however, developing a clear consensus regarding age-appropriate diagnostic criteria for pediatric bipolar disorder (PBD) is only now being clarified. It is clear that one should always take into consideration the developmental level of the child in question. Over the past decade the diagnosis of PBD has risen 4000% [65]. It has been estimated that 1–2 million children in the United States have PBD or early symptoms of the disorder [66]. Prior to acceptance of PBD, these patients may have been conceptualized as having conduct disorder (CD), attention-deficit hyperactivity disorder (ADHD), oppositional defiant disorder (ODD), schizophrenia, borderline personality disorder, or poor socialization due to inadequate parenting. Given the lack of diagnostic accuracy and certainty in many pediatric cases, however, questions still exist as to whether or not PBD is being overdiagnosed or misdiagnosed.

Clinical Description

It is uncommon for children and adolescents to meet full DSM-IV criteria for bipolar disorder. More often one encounters a child with cyclical explosive anger and extremes of emotional lability. Differentiating expected adolescent turmoil ("sturm und drang") from pathological development adds to the diagnostic challenge, as does the presence of significant symptom overlap with other pediatric disorders. The DSM-IV makes no comparable developmental concessions for pediatric bipolar disorder, and the atypical symptoms of the prodromal state (absence of distinct mood episodes and chronic mixed symptoms) complicate the diagnostic picture. One must also consider that depression is commonly the presenting symptom of PBD [67]. Some 20–40% of adolescents with major depression developed bipolar disorder within 5 years of the first onset of depression [68]. Aspects of PBD that need diagnostic consensus are: (i) the necessity of cardinal symptoms such as elated mood or grandiosity; (ii) the role of irritability in PBD; (iii) the need for clearly demarcated mood episodes; (iv) temporal relationships of mood episodes; (v) symptoms that lack DSM-IV symptom or duration thresholds for mania; and (vi) differentiating mania from symptoms related to other disorders such as ADHD [69].

It is now understood that bipolar disorder presents differently in young children and adolescents compared to adults. Pavuluri *et al* [70]. cited empirical evidence supporting two variants of PBD: prepubertal and early-onset bipolar disorder (PEA-BD), which encompasses children under the age of 12 years; and adolescent-onset bipolar disorder (AO-BD), which encompasses postpubertal adolescents. Phenomenological studies indicate that each variant exhibits a unique presentation. PEA-BD children demonstrated more irritability, higher levels of emotional lability, rapid cycling (ultradian), minimal interepisode recovery, and high comorbidity with ADHD and ODD. They also tended to have higher symptom chronicity, and a seeming absence of distinct mood cycling. Thus, the "rapid cycling" (four or more episodes per year) variant of bipolar disorder appears to occur less commonly in PBD compared to adult bipolar disorder. One might conceptualize PBD as a disorder of rapidly changing affective states interspersed with chronic episodes with incomplete recoveries. Geller [71]. studied 60 bipolar patients aged 7–16 years by using specific definitions of cycling. Eighty-three percent were found to have rapid mood cycling. Among these, 8% exhibited "ultra-rapid" cycling (episodes lasting a few days to a few weeks), and 75% experienced "ultradian" cycling (mood variation occurring within the same 24-hour period). When mania occurred, 87% involved a mixed episode.

Bipolar children commonly display extreme moodiness, difficulty falling asleep, poor concentration, hyperactivity, impulsivity, declining grades, explosive anger or "rages" that may take an hour or two to de-escalate, dysphoric mood states, poor frustration tolerance, and disruptive behaviors. More classic symptoms of mania such as hypersexuality, racing thoughts, pressured speech, and flights of ideas may also be present. Occasionally, collateral information reports severe and targeted aggressive behavior. Hallucinations and delusional thinking may also be evident. Emily L. Fergu [72]. of the NIMH proposed that the presence of the following five symptoms predicts PBD in 91% of cases: grandiosity, suicidal gesture, irritability, decreased attention span, and racing thoughts. In a meta-analysis of seven PBD studies the most common symptoms of pediatric mania were increased energy (89%), distractibility (84%), pressured speech (82%), irritability (81%), grandiosity (78%), racing thoughts (74%), decreased need for sleep (72%), euphoria (70%), poor judgment (69%), flight of ideas (57%), and hypersexuality (38%) [73]. Significant variability existed for euphoria (14–89%) and irritability (22–92%), however, suggesting that these symptoms may have been assessed differently by the different research groups.

There is general clinical consensus that PBD may present with a dysphoric rather than euphoric mood state, a chronic rather than episodic course, and a predominantly mixed presentation encompassing symptoms of both mania and depression concurrently. This phenotype may include explosive tantrums involving rapid escalation and slow de-escalation, and general behavioral dyscontrol. With adolescence, classic cycling of manic and depressive states may occur more commonly. AO-BD children may demonstrate an increase in overt symptoms of mania such as elation, euphoria, and grandiosity. AO-BD is also correlated with high rates of anxiety, substance use, and episodic mood states in at least 25% of research subjects [95–97].

Distinguishing PBD from ADHD can be challenging, particularly in prepubertal children, who tend to exhibit more symptom overlap between the disorders. Gelle [71]. opined that high rates of ADHD comorbid with PBD are due to "phenocopy ADHD." In essence, prepubertal bipolar children will concurrently meet criteria for ADHD, though will not continue to meet these criteria as they age. In a prior study, Geller and Luby found that the prevalence of ADHD comorbid with PBD decreased from 100% during prepuberty to 70% during young adolescence to 30% among older adolescents [74]. In a separate study, Kutcher cited a 29–98% comorbidity between PBD and ADHD within the United States, but only 10% comorbidity between PBD and ADHD in studies completed outside of the United States [75]. It is clear that additional research and clarification in this area are needed, as a misdiagnosis of ADHD or depression and subsequent initiation of a stimulant or antidepressant medication in a PBD patient could lead to significant mood destabilization. Geller *et al.* suggested that euphoric mood, grandiosity, decreased need for sleep, racing thoughts, and hypersexuality are typically only seen in PBD and can assist with distinguishing between BPD and ADHD [76].

Depressive symptoms in children with BPD are not uncommon, but less research exists regarding this topic. In one study Martin *et al.* discovered that children aged 10–14 years were at highest risk for switch to mania following SSRI treatment after a diagnosis of depression [77]. This leads one to question whether prepubertal depression is a risk factor for subsequent development of PBD, though it is well known that a depressed child is more likely to have unipolar depression than bipolar depression.

Duration of mood episodes differs considerably between PBD and adult BPD. Geller *et al.* reported a mean mood episode duration of 3.6 years in BPD youths [78]. Similarly, a 4-year prospective longitudinal study of early adolescent BPD published in 2004 revealed a pediatric manic episode duration of 79.2 ± 66.7 weeks [79]. The chronic symptoms seen in this study were deemed representative of ultradian rapid cycling, psychosis, and mixed mania. Related to the above, some researchers hypothesize that bipolar youths have chronic manic symptoms encompassing several years of mixed symptomatology. In the Course and Outcome of Bipolar Illness in Youth (COBY) study of children aged over 2 years, subjects spent 37.9% of the time symptom free, 22.4% of the time in a DSM-IV qualified mood episode, 37.9% of the time in a subsyndromal episode, and 3.1% of the time experiencing psychosis. (Birmaher et al. 2006) Data regarding polarity shifts revealed that 30% of subjects changed polarity 20 + times yearly, 47% changed polarity 10 + times yearly, 61% changed polarity 5 times yearly, and only 19% of subjects changed polarity once per year or less [80]. BP-NOS diagnosis, lower SES, and lifetime psychosis groups appeared to have an increased risk for high polarity. BP-1 youths in the COBY study spent more time symptomatic, exhibited more mixed/cycling episodes, and experienced an increase in polarity switches compared to adult patients with BP-1. This research appears to support the idea that BPD youths are more often symptomatic and experience more overall psychopathology than adult BPD individuals.

Cyclothymia

Symptoms of cyclothymia resemble bipolar spectrum disorders, particularly PBD; however, mood states in cyclothymia tend to be less intense and are associated with less functional impairment. To meet diagnostic criteria for cyclothymia one must demonstrate numerous episodes of both hypomanic and depressed symptoms that last at least 1 year while concurrently experiencing no more than 2 months without symptoms.

Bipolar II Disorder

Criteria for Bipolar II Disorder are met when there is a history of at least one major depressive episode, at least one hypomanic episode, and no history of a full manic or mixed episode.

Bipolar Disorder Not Otherwise Specified (BP NOS)

This diagnosis describes the situation in which a clinician concludes that a bipolar spectrum disorder is present, yet symptoms do not meet criteria for a specific bipolar disorder. Presumably due to a lack of diagnostic consensus, BP NOS has become the most controversial diagnosis used in children who exhibit chronic, nonepisodic affect and behavior dysregulation, as well as

mood episodes that do not meet DSM-IV duration criteria [81]. It now appears that a large subset of this BP NOS group with chronic irritability likely represents a syndrome distinct from Bipolar Disorder and labeled Severe Mood Dysregulated in research settings such as the NIMH, as discussed below, or referred to as Temper Dysregulation Disorder with Dysphoria (TDD) by other research groups. Practice parameters of the American Association of Child and Adolescent Psychiatry (AACAP) recommend that a diagnosis of BP NOS be given to children with "chronic manic-like symptoms which constitute baseline functioning," and for children whose manic symptoms are between hours and 4 days in duration [82]. Children with mania of too short a duration to meet DSM criteria were diagnosed as BP NOS in the COBY study [80]. After 2 years 25% of this group progressed to BD-I or BD-II.

Leibenluft et al. classified a group of children in their clinic population with severe chronic and impairing irritability and anger as severe mood dysregulated (SMD) or "broad phenotype" BPD [83]. Their seemingly unremitting irritability resembles the baseline low mood seen in dysthymia. Children with SMD may also exhibit symptoms such as poor sleep, distractibility, racing thoughts, intrusiveness, and psychomotor agitation. Generally, symptoms in SMD children should last at least 1 year, start before the age of 12 years, and result in significant functional impairment. It does not appear, however, that SMD represents the same diagnostic entity as PBD. In the Great Smokey Mountain Study, for example, only 1% of youths meeting SMD criteria converted to BD-I or BD-II over an 8-year period [84]. In a separate study only 3% of SMD children evidenced a family history of BPD compared to 33% of BPD children [85]. Distinguishing between SMD and PBD carries substantial treatment implications, particularly if SMD children are treated with PBD medication inappropriately, and not treated with medication or psychosocial treatments more appropriate to their actual diagnosis [81].

An Indepth Look at the Proposed DSM-V Diagnosis of Severe Mood Dysregulated (SMD) or Temper Dysregulation Disorder with Dysphoria (TDD)

In the last decade there appeared to be a strong movement in the clinical research arena to accept an alternative view that within the condition of pediatric bipolar affective disorder (PBAD) there existed a pediatric variant presentation that was typified by chronic severe irritability but without clearly demarcated cyclic episodes of irritability or manic symptoms. This variation, however, was contradictory with the present DSM-IV criterion A, which stipulates a "distinct period" of abnormally elevated, expansive, or irritable mood. Ongoing longitudinal studies and family history now seem to indicate that this initial proposed reclassification is not accurate as a true bipolar variant. This new syndrome, for which various names have been proposed and more recently termed "severe mood dysregulation" (SMD) by the research group at the NIMH, is, however, a condition that is as debilitating/impairing for children as is classic bipolar affective disorder. At the time of writing there is much controversy regarding creating a new diagnostic classification and it remains undetermined at this point if this syndrome will be included in DSM-V as field trials are currently underway to determine validity and to clarify criteria. As the prevalence of this very debilitating syndrome is much higher than PBAD it appears that research into this condition would warrant priority consideration, but first a diagnosis must be agreed upon. As such a thorough discussion of what is known about SMD is included in this chapter as it will eventually need to be addressed as a new, unique affective disorder or variant of an existing disorder with a modifier.

Clinicians are frequently faced with children presenting with a constellation of symptoms that typically include chronic dysphoric affective instability, ADHD, and severe ODD. This condition is most commonly diagnosed as BAD and to a lesser degree ADHD or ODD. This in some fashion would seem to account for the marked increase in the diagnosis of pediatric BAD in the United States that has occurred in the last 15 years, with studies citing 5- to 15-fold increases in inpatient and outpatient diagnosis [86, 87].

Severe mood dysregulation is unfortunately not rare, with an initial estimated prevalence of 3.2%, which is much higher than the reported prevalence for PBAD of 0.1% or even the 1.9% prevalence for ADHD [88]. To compound this higher prevalence issue is the finding that in the NIMH samples the mean Children's Global Assessment Scale (CGAS) score for the 107 youths diagnosed with BAD was 46.5 while the CGAS score for the 146 youths diagnosed with SMD was 45.8. The comparable degree of severity of impairment between these two disorders indicates that while SMD is not BAD, as discussed later, it is nevertheless a disorder that warrants acute treatment on a level akin to that implemented with BAD. Indeed this constellation of symptoms is often the reason these children are placed in costly specialized school programs or require institutionalization. The high prevalence rates and typical negative outcomes are why many clinicians would argue the issue of explosive rage reactions is the most critical

issue facing child psychiatry at this time. This speaks to the need to have a diagnosis that accurately quantifies these symptoms so that NIMH grants can be funded to define appropriate treatment strategies. These treatments would likely include pharmacotherapy, and a diagnosis is needed for research to proceed that could lead to FDA-approved therapies.

Clinical Features

The longitudinal data, some for up to 20 years, collected from clinical and community samples involved in studies such as those done at the NIMH have brought a degree of clinical distinction between the SMD and BAD groups while providing insights into a possible pathophysiological continuum between BAD and major depressive disorder, discussed later.

In a large longitudinal epidemiological study, Brotman *et al.* looked at large community samples that had been monitored for as long as 20 years. In comparing youths who met post hoc proxy criteria for severe mood dysregulation at a mean age of 10.6 years it was found that the SMD group were seven times more likely to meet criteria for a unipolar MDD at a mean age of 18.3 years compared to youths who did not meet these criteria [84].

Longitudinal data from a NIMH clinical research sample assessed the rates of future mood episodes in 84 youths with severe mood dysregulation and 93 youths with DSM-IV BAD over a median of 28.4 months [89]. During this follow-up period only one patient (1.2%) with SMD but 58 (62.4%) of the BAD group displayed evidence of at least one new manic, hypomanic, or mixed episode. Thus, the conclusion of this study, albeit a clinical sample with only a roughly 2-year follow-up period, was that the "rates of prospectively observed manic episodes were 50 times higher in bipolar disorder than in severe mood dysregulation."

An additional longitudinal community sample study by Stringaris *et al.* (89) followed 631 subjects who as adolescents at a mean age of 13.8 years demonstrated chronic irritability into adulthood at a mean age of 33.2 years. The symptom of chronic irritability in adolescence predicted major depressive disorder (odds ratio (OR) = 1.33), generalized anxiety disorder (OR = 1.72), and dysthymia (OR = 1.81) but not BAD.

There seems to be a confluence of evidence from these studies that chronic irritability[1] does not predict BAD but has some predictive value for unipolar depressive affective disorders and generalized anxiety disorder. A possible continuum could be viewed between these affective disorders as shown in Figure 12.2.

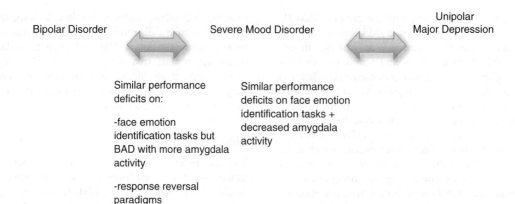

Figure 12.2 Possible continuum between bipolar disorder, severe mood disorder, and unipolar major depression. Face emotion identification tasks measure the ability to accurately process social cues, which is a core social-emotional function that supports both emotional regulation and social competence [57].

CASE STUDY

Case Example: Bipolar Disorder

B.A. is a 10-year-old boy whose single mother originally sought his treatment for a new onset of depressive symptoms in the context of parental divorce. He was initially diagnosed with an adjustment disorder with depressed mood, and was referred for individual and family therapy. Due to ongoing and worsening depressive symptoms, however, including the development of suicidal ideation with a plan to stab himself with a knife, B.A. was started on fluoxetine 10 mg daily and continued in individual therapy. B.A.'s depression improved over the first several months of treatment, but later recurred in the context of being bullied and teased after switching to a new school. B.A. complained that he was smaller than his classmates and therefore could no longer play football, a sport he previously loved playing with his now absent father. Fluoxetine was increased to 20 mg daily and he was maintained in individual therapy to address sadness relating to the loss of his father and poor self-esteem related to abandonment by his father and mistreatment from peers at school. After approximately 1 week of B.A. taking the higher dose of fluoxetine, B.A.'s mother called his psychiatrist in a frantic state, describing how B.A. had become increasingly irritable, angry, and destructive. He was suspended from school the day prior for engaging an older student in a fistfight, then threatening to kill him. At home he broke a chair when he was asked to pick up his dirty clothes, and kicked several holes in his walls after losing game privileges for cursing at his mother. He accused her of being incapable of running a household, and voiced that he was going to run away, find a better mom, and grow up to be rich with fourteen racecars. With additional questioning, B.A.'s mother shared that he is awake off and on throughout the night, and two nights ago was found at the kitchen computer naked, searching multiple women's lingerie sites. She expressed that "he's just not himself," and stated he purposefully trips the family dog then lies about it afterward. She described him as loud and noted that he jumps from topic to topic in conversation. She voiced worry about his new-found proclivity to steal candy when shopping with her. After telling him he could go to jail for such an offense he flippantly replied, "Nope, I'm too young for jail and juvie would just let me go." Most worrisome, and what ultimately prompted her phone call, was his resurgence of suicidal ideation and new development of homicidal ideation toward his estranged father. B.A. was hospitalized to ensure his safety and the safety of others. Fluoxetine was discontinued and he was started on a mood stabilizer for presumed PBD. During his hospitalization his mother discovered that B.A.'s paternal uncle and father are in treatment for bipolar disorder. She shared that she and two of her sisters suffer from anxiety and depression, and that B.A.'s paternal grandfather completed suicide years ago. B.A.'s mood stabilized while in hospital and he was discharged without further suicidal or homicidal ideation. He remained stable for several months with medication management and therapy. Due to uncertainty regarding whether or not his manic symptoms resulted from PBD or represented mania induced by fluoxetine, he was carefully tapered off his mood stabilizer. His agitation, aggression, irritability, and destructive behavior quickly recurred off medication, however, and B.A. was diagnosed with PBD. With ongoing mood stabilizer and psychotherapeutic treatment, as well as initiation of a modified school plan and family services, B.A. made significant treatment gains and was able to function more appropriately in both the home and school environment.

Epidemiology and Prevalence of Bipolar Disorders

The current lack of uniformity and diagnostic consensus among providers diagnosing PBD renders it difficult to determine an accurate prevalence rate. One epidemiological study reported a lifetime prevalence of adolescent BPD of approximately 1% [90]. A separate study completed several years later estimated a lifetime prevalence of 3.3% in children with SMD [84]. Retrospective studies of adults with BPD estimate that 60% experienced the onset of their disorder before the age of 20, and 10–20% experienced symptom onset before the age of 10 [91]. While PBD is less prevalent than pediatric depression in community samples, prevalence rates of PBD rise considerably in restricted samples such as inpatient populations. Base rates of PBD or manic symptoms varied from 0.6% in a high-school epidemiological study, to 6–8% in general outpatient clinics, to 30% on an inpatient service [92]. As such, available epidemiological data suggest that PBD is not an uncommon diagnosis, particularly in psychiatrically referred children. The author R.T.B. would argue that these markedly elevated rates of PBD in inpatient populations are partially due to an attempt by treating clinicians to substantiate the need for inpatient treatment in a group of often very aggressive and unstable youths who may not meet formal diagnostic criteria for PBD but need insurance coverage to approve their admissions.

Etiology and Pathogenesis of Bipolar Disorders

While significant progress has been achieved in the diagnosis and treatment of PBD, a comprehensive understanding of the etiology of this disorder is lacking. There are, however, a multitude of explanatory models, many of which address biopsychosocial factors as etiological agents. It has been shown that BPD aggregates in families [93, 94], which is presumed to be related to a combination of genetic factors (discussed later) and intrafamilial interactions.

Environmental Influences

Clinically it appears clear that intrafamilial and environmental interactions play a role in the onset and development of pediatric affective disturbance. It is not uncommon to encounter an affectively disturbed child who is under the care of an affectively disturbed parent. Parental psychopathology or substance misuse, child abuse, and poor parent-child relations are just a few factors commonly associated with pediatric mood disorders.

The complex interplay between frequently comorbid externalizing behaviors, and resultant environmental stressors, is also theorized to contribute to affective disturbance in children. PBD is increasingly associated as a risk factor for the development of substance use disorders [95]. Additionally, Pavuluri et al. estimated that 50–80% of PBD patients have comorbid ADHD and 20–60% have disruptive behavior disorders [96]. Rates of ODD comorbid with BPD are as high as 47–88% [78, 97]. Akiskal theorized that temperament excesses generate negative life events such as substance use, sleep disturbance, and volatile family relationships, which in turn contribute to the manifestation of affective disorders [98].

Inherent temperament may likewise contribute to the development of PBD. It has been hypothesized that temperamental dysregulation not only provides a framework for affective episodes to develop, but also may be genetically linked to bipolar illness [98]. Akiskal's hypothesis alludes to the concept of "bipolar spectrum" illness, encompassing temperamental dysregulation at one end and severe manic or mixed mood states at the other. As cited earlier, however, recent research highlighted apparent differences between SMD and PBD, which casts doubt on the concept of an overly broad bipolar spectrum illness. It appears important that diagnostic criteria for PBD do not expand to the extent they no longer can differentiate true bipolar illness from affective dysregulation resultant from inconsistent parenting, parental psychopathology, or other psychosocial disturbances.

Genetic Model of Bipolar Disorders

There is conclusive supporting evidence from twin, family, and adoption studies that bipolar disorder has a strong genetic component. Akiska [99]. states that genetic studies have shown that if one parent has bipolar disorder the risk to the offspring of developing BPD is 30–40%, and when both parents are diagnosed with bipolar disorder the risk is 50–70%. Twin studies show the concordance rate of mania in monozygotic twins to be 65%, versus 14% in dizygotic twins [100]. An adoption study by Mendlewicz and Raine [101]. found that 31% of the biological parents of adopted children who developed mania suffered from BPD, whereas only 2% of the adoptive parents did so. Klein and colleague [102]. found an association of cyclothymia among the adolescent offspring of bipolar adults. Among the children or siblings of bipolar adults, however, depressive spectrum disorders (major depression, dysthymia, and melancholic) were actually the most common finding.

Pedigree studie [103]. involving the chromosomal mapping of identified families with a high incidence of affective disorders including BPD (such as those found within the Amish community) initially led to the hope that a bipolar gene could be identified. Akiska [99]. reported that molecular genetic studies have focused on "hot spots" on chromosomes 18 and 22 as the most promising leads for bipolar-related genes. He indicates there is evidence that panic attacks associated with BPD have been strongly linked with genes on chromosome 18, and there is some genetic overlap with schizophrenia on both chromosomes 18 and 22. A collaborative analysis [104–106] of the three largest genome-wide association studies of bipolar disorder implicates two genes, coding for the proteins *ANK3* (ankyrin G) on chromosome 10q21 and *CACNA1C* (alpha 1C subunit of the L-type voltage-gated calcium channel) on chromosome 12p13, that either regulate or are subunits of sodium or calcium ion channels. Collateral evidence further supports the role of *ANK3* and subunits of the calcium channel in bipolar disorder as they are both downregulated in the mouse brain in response to lithium treatment [107]. These findings suggest that bipolar disorder might be, in part, an ion channelopathy, similar to epilepsy. Another interesting candidate gene for mania is the *CLOCK* gene involved in circadian periodicity [108]. A mouse *CLOCK* mutant was recently shown to exhibit features of mania.

It is clinically relevant that several medical conditions such as obsessive-compulsive disorder and migraine headaches appear to be associated with bipolar disorder as these conditions are comorbid at higher prevalence rates than one would predict based on their individual prevalence rates in the population. A large retrospective database study that utilized a US health insurer's managed care claims indicated that bipolar disorder is an independent risk factor lipid disorders. [109, 110]

Assessment and Formulation of Bipolar Disorders

As with many youth psychiatric disorders, assessment for PBD is a complex task. Diagnostic interviews should include an interview of the child and parents separately and together. Teacher or school counselor input is often a necessary diagnostic component when applicable, and can help differentiate between behaviors specific to only one environment versus more pervasive and global behaviors and alterations in mood states. One must also consider potential organic etiologies of affective disturbance such as lab abnormalities, genetic defects, or neurological disorders. Occasionally psychological or neuropsychological testing may be indicated to assist with diagnostic clarification. It is important additionally to consider socio-cultural factors, which may assist or complicate the diagnostic understanding of a particular child.

The age of the child will often dictate how data are collected. A heavier reliance on parental report is likely to ensue with younger or socially anxious children. Historically, dynamically oriented play therapy was used to further understand a child's intrapsychic conflicts; however, this often lengthy diagnostic style is limited by increasing demands from insurance companies for brief treatment, and heavy reliance on DSM-IV-TR criteria to justify diagnoses. In younger childhood, it will be necessary to modify questions about affective states, often relying on the use of several descriptive phrases or statements, to assist the child's understanding. By middle childhood, most children will be able to accurately describe their mood states. Mood diaries or mood charts may help when assessing PBD, and can be downloaded from the Child and Adolescent Bipolar Foundation (www.bpkids.org). One should also consider that children have been shown to more accurately identify internalizing disorders in comparison to their parents, whereas parents appear better at identifying externalizing behaviors than youths.

Although structured and semi-structured interviews were once used almost exclusively in research domains, their use in clinical settings is on the rise. In research settings the Washington University Kiddie Schedule for Affective Disorders and Schizophrenia (Wash-U-KSADS) is considered the "gold standard" for diagnosis of PBD; however, it requires several hours to administer, rendering it impractical in clinical settings. Wash-U-KSADS includes prepubertal-specific mania items,

Table 12.3 Structured or semi-structured interviews for assessing mood disorders in children and adolescents.

	K-SADS	DICA	DISC	CAPA	CAS	ISC
Type	Semi-structured	Structured	Structured	Semi-structured	Semi-structured	Semi-structured
Ages (years)	6–17	6–17	8–17	7–17	7–17	8–17
Period assessed	Present or lifetime	Lifetime	Past year	Present	Present	Present
Administrator	Clinician	Clinician	Lay	Clinician or trained lay (4–5 weeks of training)	Clinician	Clinician

assesses added items such as ultradian cycling, and includes developmentally appropriate descriptors for pediatric symptoms such as grandiosity [111]. Six structured and semi-structured interviews for assessment of youth mood disorders are listed in Table 12.3.

A few screening tools have been investigated to determine their usefulness in detecting PBD. The Child Behavior Checklist-Pediatric Bipolar Disorder profile (CBCL-PBD) appears to help differentiate between PBD and ADHD. A "deviant" profile suggesting aggressive, anxious-depressed, and elevated inattentive symptoms is likely to indicate BPD [112–114]. Similarly, in a longitudinal study of youth with ADHD, positive CBCL-PBD scores were associated with increased comorbidity of BPD, MDD, and CD, when studied for an average of 7.4 years. In a comparison of six common screening instruments, it was discovered that parent report is more likely than youth or teacher report to assist with accurately diagnosing BPD in youths aged 5–17 years [115].

It is important to note that screening tools are not diagnostic tools, but rather generate information that, when used in conjunction with a clinical interview, may assist with diagnostic understanding. As proficiency in using common screening instruments improves, the length of time to administer them should decrease, and one will benefit not only from an additional diagnostic tool, but also objective measures to follow throughout treatment.

Treatment of Bipolar Disorders

Psychosocial Therapies

Psychosocial interventions including psychotherapy and psychoeducation are essential components of an effective PBD treatment plan. Considering that 50% of adult patients with mood disorders were found to be noncompliant with their medication [116].it appears clear that medication alone is unlikely to ensure the best possible prognosis for youths with BPD. Ongoing education about the illness and acceptance of the same

may improve medication compliance. Additionally, family members often serve a valuable role in monitoring and reporting symptoms when properly educated. Sharing knowledge of known triggers for mood episodes, such as stress, insomnia, or substance use, promotes healthy lifestyle choices that promote mood stability.

Supportive interventions are vital, particularly during the acute phase of treatment. Listening, empathizing with the child and family, restoring hope, and affording case management are fundamental components of support [117]. The child and family should be educated on risks associated with various treatments, as well as the risks of not treating BPD.

Community involvement and support is often a necessary component of treatment. Given that PBD is typically a chronic and recurrent disorder, family members may benefit from practical information such as how to apply for Family Medical Leave when available, or how to find support resources in their local area or online. Simple knowledge that their child's extreme mood swings and misbehavior are due to PBD and chronic illness, and not to inadequate parenting, also provides family relief [118].

Evidence-based psychotherapeutic treatment modalities are emerging, and show promise in successfully managing aspects of PBD. Child-and-family-focused cognitive behavior therapy (CFF-CBT) incorporates treatment of both BPD youths aged 8–12 years and their families [119]. This approach integrates developmentally appropriate reward-based CBT with psychotherapy that emphasizes empathic validation. The additional intensive focus on parents' own treatment, as well as education about effective parenting techniques for a BPD child, is valuable. CFF-CBT consists of 12 sessions and follows the "Rainbow" mnemonic: R – routine, A – affect regulation, I – I can do it, N – no negative thoughts and live in the now, B – be a good friend, O – oh, how can we solve it, and W – ways to get support (120). A three-year follow-up study of children who received CCF-CBT with booster treatment showed maintenance of treatment gains [120].

Multi-family psychoeducation groups (MFPG) were developed as a group treatment for parents and school-aged children with bipolar and depression spectrum disorders [121]. This treatment approach emphasizes medication compliance and coping strategies. Children identify favorable creative, physical, social, and relaxing activities that are then used to ward off negative emotional states. In a trial evaluating the effectiveness of MFPG, 35 children and families showed improved family relations, enhanced ability to access services, increased perceived social support from parents, and expanded knowledge about the BPD disease process [122].

Family focused therapy (FFT-A), a manualized treatment for adolescent BPD, emphasizes coping skills, reduced expressed emotion from caregivers, and improving family communication and problem solving [123]. In FFT-A, psychoeducation, communication enhancement, and problem-solving skills training are delivered over 21 sessions, and involve the child, the parents, and available siblings. In a 2-year clinical trial, adolescents who received FFT-A demonstrated lower depression severity scores, and quicker recovery from depression [124].

While the aforementioned structured treatments for youth BPD show promise, ongoing studies are needed to validate their effectiveness. Preliminary data suggest that such modalities offer an opportunity for improved treatment engagement and quality of life for children and families affected by PBD.

Pharmacotherapy and Other Somatic Treatments

Antipsychotics Beginning in late 2009 several of the atypical antipsychotics have received FDA approval for the treatment of bipolar disorder in youths, including risperidone, aripiprazole, quetiapine, olanzapine, and lithium (Table 12.4).

Lithium was the first medication to be approved for pediatric bipolar disorder and risperidone the second. Although FDA approval was given to the four atypical antipsychotic listed in Table 12.4 mood stabilizers for the treatment of pediatric bipolar disorder, the FDA panel expressed concerns about side effects of these medications, especially the propensity for weight gain and metabolic issues such as diabetes or lipid disorders. One study found that teens are more prone than adults to weight gain when taking atypical antipsychotic drugs. Some have speculated that the higher density of histamine receptors in the pediatric versus the adult brain may account for this greater propensity for weight gain. The study found children and teens can gain nearly 9 kg (20 pounds) and become obese within just 11 weeks [125]. Reviewing the weight gain reported in the randomized controlled trials (RCTs) one could rank the weight gain from most to least as olanzapine > risperidone > quetiapine ≫ aripiprazole > ziprasidone = 0.

Ziprasidone was initially voted to be "acceptably safe" and effective for the treatment of bipolar disorder in teenagers and children by a FDA panel of outside medical experts that reviewed trial data for the FDA in 2009. However, there were comparatively more concerns about its efficacy compared to the other agents in the subgroups of younger patients aged 10 to 14 and patients weighing less than 45 kg, where ziprasidone did not achieve statistically significant differences versus placebo given the small numbers of patients in these subgroups precluded any meaningful conclusion. It is likely that safety record and poor clinical efficacy as well as concerns about data collection at certain study

Table 12.4 Medications having FDA approval for treating bipolar disorder in children and adolescents.

Agent	Indication	Dosage
Risperidone	Acute treatment of manic and mixed episodes associated with bipolar I disorder in children and adolescents (10–17 years of age)	0.5–6.0 mg/day
Aripiprazole	Acute and maintenance treatment of manic or mixed episodes associated with bipolar I disorder in children and adolescents (10–17 years of age), both as monotherapy and as an adjunct to lithium or divalproex	10–30 mg/day
Quetiapine	Acute treatment of manic episodes associated with bipolar I disorder in children and adolescents (10–17 years of age), both as monotherapy and as an adjunct to lithium or divalproex	400–600 mg/day
Olanzapine	Acute treatment of manic and mixed episodes associated with bipolar 1 disorder in adolescents (13–17 years of age)	2.5–20 mg/day
Lithium	Approved for the treatment of bipolar disorder in adolescents aged 12 years and above	Blood level 0.6–1.2

Note: Issues related to ziprasidone's lack of formal FDA approval are discussed in the text.

sites, ziprasidone's final formal FDA approval never materialized.

Now that clinicians have several FDA-approved medications for pediatric bipolar disorder, initiating treatment with one of these agents as first-line treatment seems appropriate. See Figure 12.3 for a suggested treatment algorithm. While the studies indicate some variance in the number needed to treat (NNT), which is the number of patients that need to be treated for one to benefit, values were predominantly in the 3 to 4 range, which indicates a clinically significant treatment effect. It is not always possible to accurately compare efficacy data across different studies and as such many clinicians are apt to select an initial medication based on its side-effect profile and how that relates to the patient. The patient variables considered could include body mass index (BMI), health history, family history, or target symptoms.

(1) Amongst the options, due to the above risks of weight gain and metabolic syndrome, one could consider first a trial with aripiprazole (or possibly ziprasidone in older adolescents) due to its preferable weight gain profile, especially if the patient is overweight or there is a family history of obesity, diabetes, or lipid disorders. Severe sleep onset issues may lead one to initiate treatment with quetiapine.

(2) If the initial atypical agent fails a second atypical may be tried.

(3) If these two agents fail one could next try risperidone or quetiapine while monitoring closely for weight gain.

(4) If the response to an antipsychotic mood stabilizer is judged to be marginal or absent, consider switching to an antiepileptic mood stabilizer (valproate, carbamazepine, lamotrigine) or lithium. A National Institute of Mental Health (NIMH)-funded study comparing lithium, divalproex, and placebo indicated a moderate effect size for these two agents versus placebo with a slight advantage to divalproex [126].

(5) If a partial response is appreciated by the clinician to an antipsychotic mood stabilizer consider augmentation with an antiepileptic mood stabilizer or lithium.

(6) For more treatment-resistant patients one must look at non-FDA-approved options. Numerous open-label trials in adults [127, 128] as well as in children and adolescents [129, 130] have demonstrated mood-stabilizing effects of clozapine in treatment-resistant bipolar disorder patients. Many believe that clozapine is a very efficacious mood-stabilizing agent as well as the most efficacious antipsychotic agent, but no FDA approval exists for its use for

bipolar disorder in adults or the pediatric population, largely due to its generic status and its side-effect profile, which inhibits the completion of large studies in the pediatric population. There are many case reports showing that selected agents such as thyroid agents (T3 or T4), calcium channel blockers (CCB), other antiepileptic mood stabilizers such as oxcarbazepine or topiramate, or even ECT may be beneficial for selected patients, but unfortunately little exists in the literature to direct patient selection for a specific medication.

Most of these algorithms address manic or mixed states, but depressive phases can be more prolonged, frequent, and problematic. Recent adult studies indicate no benefit overall with antidepressants in BAD depression [131]. but many clinicians continue to try this although a short-term trial may be preferable given the risk of affective switching to mania. The largest randomized placebo-controlled study to date was a 2006 study sponsored by the NIMH and Stanley Medical Research Institute, which found higher switch rates with venlafaxine compared to bupropion or sertraline [132]. Lamictal may be reasonable in this area as while there is no pediatric FDA approval for pediatric BAD there is a great deal of experience/safety data using lamotrigine in the pediatric population given its anti-seizure indications.

For children aged under 10 years requiring treatment for bipolar disorder there are very limited data to guide one. Biederman *et al.* evaluated short-term safety and efficacy in 31 preschoolers (4–6 years) in an open-label prospective study and found both risperidone (at 1 week) and olanzapine (at 2 weeks) resulted in a rapid reduction of symptoms of mania in children with BPD. However, there were substantial adverse effects and the benefit may not outweigh the risk in this population [133].

Medications in BPD frequently contribute to weight gain and obesity. Weight control measures may include augmenting with topiramate at 200–400 mg/day, metformin (1000–2000 mg/day in divided dosages), or possibly in combination with stimulants (if comorbid ADHD is present) to help avoid excessive weight gain.

Conclusion

Pediatric affective disorders, particularly pediatric bipolar disorder, are undoubtedly among the most challenging diagnoses to establish and treat in all medicine. Diagnostic uncertainty is due not only to the ubiquitous nature of primary pediatric mood symptoms, such as irritability and temper outbursts, but also to the relative paucity of evidence-based research compared to a

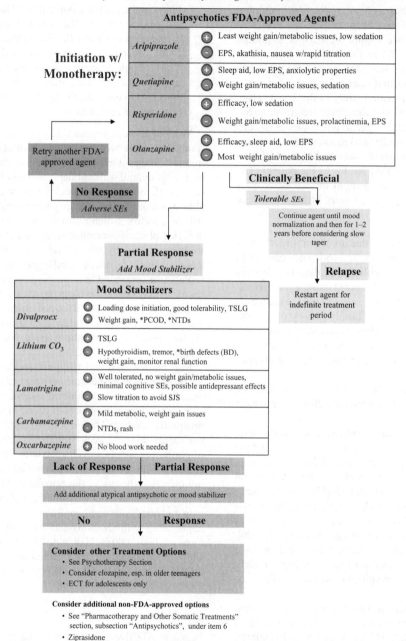

Figure 12.3 Treatment algorithm for pediatric bipolar disorder.

variety of other diagnoses in medicine. Fortunately, research and interest in pediatric affective disorders are on the rise, lending exciting hope for ever-expanding diagnostic and treatment clarity, in support of the ultimate goal of achieving accurate and effective treatment for our patients. The purpose of this chapter is to present the most up-to-date diagnostic and treatment recommendations at this time, such that success may be achieved to benefit our patients and providers alike. It is hoped that by reading this chapter you will have the framework and knowledge necessary to feel comfortable not only in diagnosing but also in treating these often devastating diagnoses, and that the lives of both patients and their families may be maximally benefited.

Notes

1   Irritability – the two defined components of irritability are: (i) temper outbursts that are developmentally inappropriate, frequent, and extreme; and (ii) negatively valenced mood (anger or sadness) between outbursts.

References

1. Spitz R. Anaclitic depression: an enquiry into the genesis of psychiatric conditions in early childhood. *Psychoanal Study Child* 1946;**1**:47–53.
2. Luby JL, Heffelinger A, Markotskky C, *et al*. The clinical picture of depression in preschool children. *J Am Acad Child Adolesc Psychiat* 2003;**42**:340–348.
3. American Psychiatric Association. *Diagnostic and Statistical Manual of Mental Disorders, 4th edn, Text Revision.* Washington, DC: American Psychiatric Association, 2000.
4. Cantwell DP, Lewinsohn PM, Rohde P, Seeley JR. Correspondence between adolescent report and parent report of psychiatric diagnostic criteria. *J Am Acad Child Adolesc Psychiat* 1997;**36**:610–619.
5. Luby JL, Heffelinger AK, Mratosky C, *et al*. Preschool major depressive disorder: preliminary validation for developmentally modified DSM-IV criteria. *J Am Acad Clin Adolesc Psychiat* 2002;**41**: 928–937.
6. American Academy of Child and Adolescent Psychiatry. Practice parameters for the assessment and treatment of children and adolescents with depressive disorders. *J Am Acad Clin Adolesc Psychiat* 2007;**46**: 1503–1526.
7. Birmaher B, Brent DA, Benson RS, for the American Academy of Child and Adolescent Psychiatry. Summary of the practice parameters for the assessment and treatment of children and adolescents with depressive disorders. *J Am Acad Clin Adolesc Psychiat* 1998;**37**: 1234–1238.
8. Dopheide JA. Recognizing and treating depression in children and adolescents. *Am J Health-Syst Pharm* 2006;**63**:233–243.
9. Weller EB, Weller RA, Danielyan AK. Mood disorders in prepubertal children. In: Wiener JM, Dulcan MK (eds) *Textbook of Child and Adolescent Psychiatry,* 3rd edn. Washington, DC: American Psychiatric Publishing, 2004; pp. 411–435.
10. Anderson RN. Deaths: leading causes for 2000. *Natl Vital Stat Rep* 2002;**51**:1–62.
11. Birmaher B, Williamson ED, Dahl RE, Axelson DA, *et al*. Clinical presentation and course of depression in youth: does onset in childhood differ from onset in adolescence? *J Am Acad Clin Adolesc Psychiat* 2004;**43**: 63–70.
12. Weller EB, Weller RA, Danielyan AK. Mood disorders in adolescents. In: Wiener JM, Dulcan MK (eds) *Textbook of Child and Adolescent Psychiatry,* 3rd, edn. Washington, DC: American Psychiatric Publishing, 2004; pp. 437–481.
13. Kovacs M, Akiskal HS, Gatsonis C, Parrone PL. Childhood-onset dysthymic disorder. Clinical features and prospective naturalistic outcome. *Arch Gen Psychiat* 1994;**51**:365–374.
14. Fergusson DM, Horwood LJ, Ridder ME, Beautrais AL. Subthreshold depression in adolescence and mental health outcomes in adulthood. *Arch Gen Psychiat* 2005;**62**:66–72.
15. Costello EJ, Mustillo S, Erkanli A, Keelor G, Angold A. Prevalence and development of psychiatric disorders in childhood and adolescence. *Arch Gen Psychiat* 2003;**60**: 837–844.
16. Stalets MM, Luby JL. Preschool depression. *Child Adolesc Psychiatr Clin N Am* 2006;**15**:899–917.
17. Zalsman G, Brent DA, Weersing VR. Depressive disorders in childhood and adolescence: an overview of epidemiology, clinical manifestation and risk factors. *Child Adolesc Psychiatr Clin N Am* 2006;**15**:827–841.
18. Merikangas KR, He J, Burstein M, Swanson SA, *et al*. Lifetime prevalence of mental disorders in U.S. adolescents: results from the national comorbidity survey replication adolescent supplement (NCS–A). *J Am Acad Clin Adolesc Psychiat* 2010;**49**:980–989.
19. Kessler R, Avenevoli S, Merikangas K. Mood disorders in children and adolescents: An epidemiologic perspective. *Biol Psychiat* 2001;**49**:1002–1014.
20. Healy B. Dying of depression. *US News and World Report* 2003;**135**:67.
21. Zito JM, Safer DJ, DosReis S, *et al*. Psychotropic practice patterns for youth: A 10-year perspective. *Arch Pediatr Adolesc Med* 2003;**157**:17–25.
22. Costello EJ, Erkanli A, Angold A. Is there an epidemic of child or adolescent depression? *J Child Psychol Psychiat* 2006;**47**:1263–1271.
23. Mazza JJ, Abbott RD, Fleming CB, *et al*. Early predictors of adolescent depression: A 7-year longitudinal study. *J Early Adolesc* 2009;**29**:664–692.
24. Duggal S, Carlson EA, Sroufe LA, Egeland B. Depressive symptomology in childhood and adolescence. *Dev Psychopathol* 2001;**13**:143–164.
25. Kennard BD, Hughes JL, Stewart SM, *et al*. Maternal depressive symptoms in pediatric major depressive disorder: Relationship to acute treatment outcomes. *J Am Acad Child Adolesc Psychiat* 2008;**47**:694–699.
26. Axelson DA, Birmaher B. Relations between anxiety and depressive disorders in childhood and adolescence. *Depression and Anxiety* 2001;**14**:67–78.

27. Ashford J, Smit F, Pol A, Cuijpers P, Koot JM. Early risk indicators of internalizing problems in late childhood: a 9 year longitudinal study. *J Child Psychol Psychiat* 2008;**49**:774–780.

28. Wender PH, Kety SS, Rosenthal D, *et al.* Psychiatric disorders in the biological and adoptive families of adoptive individuals with affective disorders. *Arch Gen Psychiat* 1986;**43**:923.

29. Weissman MM, Gershon ES, Kidd KK. Psychiatric disorders in the relatives of probands with affective disorders: The Yale-NIMH collaborative family study. *Arch Gen Psychiat* 1984;**41**:13.

30. Puig-Antich J, Goetz D, Davies M, *et al.* A controlled family history study of prepubertal major depressive disorder. *Arch Gen Psychiat* 1988;**46**:406–420.

31. Strober M, Carlson G, Ryan N, *et al.* Advances in the psychopharmacology of childhood and adolescent affective disorders. Paper presented at the Scientific Proceedings of the annual meeting of the American Academy of Child and Adolescent Psychiatry, Washington, DC, 1987.

32. Gershon ES, Hamovit J, Guroff JJ, *et al.* A family study of schizoaffective, bipolar I, bipolar II, unipolar, and normal control probands. *Arch Gen Psychiat* 1982;**39**:1157.

33. Harris EC, Barraclough B. Excess mortality of mental disorder. *Brit J Psychiat* 1998;**173**:11–53.

34. Harris EC, Barraclough B. Suicide as an outcome for mental disorders. A meta-analysis. *Brit J Psychiat* 1997;**170**:205–228.

35. Mössner R, Mikova O, Koutsilieri E, *et al.* Consensus paper of the WFSBP Task Force on Biological Markers: biological markers in depression. *World J Biol Psychiat* 2007;**8**:141–174.

36. Myers K, Winters NC. Ten-year review of rating scales. II: Scales for internalizing disorders. *J Am Acad Child Adolesc Psychiat* 2002;**41**:634–659.

37. TADS. Fluoxetine, cognitive-behavioral therapy and their combination for adolescents with depression: Treatment for Adolescents With Depression Study. *JAMA* 2004;**292**:807–820.

38. Vitiello B, Rohde P, Silva S, *et al.* Functioning and quality of life in the treatment for adolescents with depression study. *J Am Acad Clin Adolesc Psychiat* 2006;**45**:1414–1426.

39. Kratochvil C, Emslie G, Silva S, *et al.* Acute time to response in the Treatment for Adolescents with Depression Study (TADS). *J Am Acad Clin Adolesc Psychiat* 2006;**45**:1412–1418.

40. David-Ferdon C, Kaslow NJ. Evidence-based psychosocial treatments for child and adolescent depression. *J Clin Child Adolesc Psychol* 2008;**37**:62–104.

41. Weisz JR, McCarty CA, Valeri SM. Effects of psychotherapy for depression in children and adolescents: a meta-analysis. *Psychol Bull* 2006;**132**(1):132–149.

42. Gillham JR, Reivich KH, Freres DR, *et al.* School-based prevention of depression and anxiety symptoms in early adolescence: A pilot of a parent intervention component. *School Psychol Quart* 2006;**21**:323–351.

43. Stark KD, Rouse L, Livingston R. Treatment of depression during childhood and adolescence: Cognitive behavioral procedures for the individual and family. In: Kendall P (ed.) *Child and Adolescent Therapy*. New York: Guilford Press, 1991; pp. 165–206.

44. Stark KD, Reynolds WM, Kaslow NJ. A comparison of the relative efficacy of self-control therapy and behavior

problems-solving therapy for depression in children. *J Abnorm Child Psychol* 1987;**15**:91–113.

45. Mufson L, Moreau D, Weissman MM, *et al.* Modification of interpersonal psychotherapy with depressed adolescents (IPT-A): phase I and II studies. *J Am Acad Child Adolesc Psychiat* 1994;**33**:695–705.

46. Klomek AB, Mufson L. Interpersonal psychotherapy for depressed adolescents. *Child Adolesc Psychiatr Clin N Am* 2006;**15**:959–975.

47. Mufson L, Weissman MM, Moreau D, *et al.* Efficacy of interpersonal psychotherapy for depressed adolescents. *Arch Gen Psychiat* 1999;**56**:573–579.

48. Mufson L, Dorta KP, Wikramarante P, *et al.* A randomized effectiveness trial of interpersonal psychotherapy for depressed adolescents. *Arch Gen Psychiat* 2004;**61**: 577–584.

49. Curry J, Rohde P, Simons A, *et al.* Predictors and moderators of acute outcome in the Treatment for Adolescents with Depression Study (TADS). *J Am Acad Child Adolesc Psychiat* 2006;**45**:1427–1439.

50. Emslie GJ, Rush AJ, Weinberg WA, *et al.* A double-blind, randomized, placebo-controlled trial of fluoxetine in children and adolescents with depression. *Arch Gen Psychiat* 1997;**54**:1031–1037.

51. March J, Silva S, Petrycki S, *et al.,* Treatment for Adolescents With Depression Study (TADS) Team. Fluoxetine, cognitive-behavioral therapy, and their combination for adolescents with depression: Treatment for Adolescents with Depression Study (TADS) randomized controlled trial. *JAMA* 2004;**292**:807–820.

52. Angold A, Messer SC, Stangl D, Farmer EM, Costello EJ, Burns BJ. Perceived parental burden and service use for child and adolescent psychiatric disorders. *Am J Public Health* 1998;**88**:75–80.

53. Gould MS, King R, Greenwald S, *et al.* Psychopathology associated with suicidal ideation and attempts among children and adolescents. *J Am Acad Child Adolesc Psychiat* 1998;**37**:915–923.

54. Treatment of SSRI-Resistant Depression in Adolescents (TORDIA). See: http://clinicaltrials.gov/ct/show/ NCT0018902?amp;order-1.

55. Treatment of Adolescent Suicide Attempters (TASA). See: http://clinicaltrials.gov/ct/show/NCT00080158?amp;order-1.

56. Harrington R, Fudge H, Rutter M, Pickles A, Hill J. Adult outcomes of childhood and adolescent depression, 1: psychiatric status. Arch Gen Psychiat 1990;**47**:465–473.

57. Weissman MM, Wolk S, Wickramaratne P, *et al.* Children with prepubertal-onset major depressive disorder and anxiety grown up. *Arch Gen Psychiat* 1999;**56**:794–801.

58. Jaffee SR, Moffitt TE, Caspi A, Fombonne E, Poulton R, Martin J. Differences in early-childhood risk factors for juvenile-onset and adult-onset depression. *Arch Gen Psychiat* 2002;**59**:215–222.

59. Emslie G. Letters to the Editor – Le mieux est l'ennemi du bien. *J Am Acad Child Adolesc Psychiat* 2010;**49**:185–186.

60. Dekker MC, Ferdinant RF, Van Lang DJ, Bongers IL, Vander Ende J, Verhulst FC. Developmental trajectories of depressive symptoms from early childhood to late adolescence: gender differences and adult outcome. *J Child Psychol Psychiat* 2007;**48**:657–666.

61. Mazza JJ, Fleming CB, Abbott RD, Haggerty KP, Catalano RF. Identifying trajectories of adolescents' depressive phenomena: an examination of early risk factors. *J Youth Adolescence* 2010;**39**:579–593.

62. Kennard BD, Silva SG, Tonev S, *et al.* Remission and recovery in the Treatment for Adolescents with Depression Study (TADS): acute and long-term outcomes. *J Am Acad Child Adolesc Psychiat* 2009;**48**:186–195.

63. Kraepelin E. *Manic Depressive Insanity and Paranoia.* Edinburgh: Livingstone, 1921.

64. Esquirol E. *Mental Maladies* (Hunt EK, trans.). Philadelphia: Lea and Blanehard, 1845.

65. Moreno C, Laje G, Blanco C, Jiang H, Schmidt AB, Olfson M. National trends in the outpatient diagnosis and treatment of bipolar disorder in youth. *Arch Gen Psychiat* 2007;**64**:1032–1039.

66. Chang K. Challenges in the diagnosis and treatment of pediatric bipolar depression. Dialog Clin Neurosci 2009;**11**:73–80.

67. Lish JD, Dime-Meenan S, Whybrow PC, Price RA, Hirschfeld RM. The National Depressive and Manic-Depressive Association (DMDA) survey of bipolar members. *J Affect Disord* 1994;**31**:281–94.

68. Birmaher B, Ryan ND, Williamson DE, *et al.* Childhood and adolescent depression: A review of the past 10 years. Part I. *J Am Acad Child Adolesc Psychiat* 1996;**35**:1427–1439.

69. Birmaher B, Axelson D, Pavuluri M. In: Martin A, Volkmar F (eds) *Lewis's Child and Adolescent Psychiatry.* Philadelphia PA: Lippincott Williams & Wilkins, 2007; pp. 513–528.

70. Pavuluri M, Naylor M, Janicak P. Recognition and treatment of pediatric bipolar disorder. *Contemp Psychiat* 2002;April:1–9.

71. Geller B. Prepubertal and early adolescent bipolarity differentiate from ADHD by manic symptoms, grandiose delusions, ultra-rapid or ultradian cycling. *J Affect Disord* 1998;**51**:81–91.

72. Fergus E. How can we differentiate between ADHD, bipolar disorder in children? *Brown University Child and Adolescent Psychopharmacology Update* 1999;**1**(5):4–5.

73. Kowatch RA, Youngstrom EA, Danielyan A, Findling R. Review and meta-analysis of the phenomenology and clinical characteristics of mania in children and adolescents. *Bipolar Disord* 2005;**7**:483–496.

74. Geller B, Luby J. Child and adolescent bipolar disorder: A review of the past 10 years. *J Am Acad Child Adolesc Psychiat* 1997;**36**:1168–1176.

75. Kutcher S. Bipolar disorder in children and adolescents: Identification, diagnosis, and treatment. Presented at the World Assembly for Mental Health, Vancouver, Canada, 24 July 2001.

76. Geller B, Zimerman B, Williams M, *et al.* DSM-IV mania symptoms in a prepubertal and early adolescent bipolar disorder phenotype compared to attention-deficit hyperactivity and normal controls. *J Child Adolesc Psychopharmacol* 2002;**12**:11–25.

77. Martin A, Young C, Leckman JF, Mukonoweshuro C, Rosenheck R, Leslie D. Age effects on antidepressant-induced manic conversion. *Arch Pediatr Adolesc Med* 2004;**158**:773–780.

78. Geller B, Zimerman B, Williams M, *et al.* Diagnostic characteristics of 93 cases of prepubertal and early adolescent bipolar disorder phenotype by gender, puberty and co-morbid attention deficit hyperactivity disorder. *J Child Adolesc Psychopharmacol* 2000;**10**:157–164.

79. Geller B, Tillman R, Craney JL, Belhofner K. Four-year prospective outcome and natural history of mania in children with prebupertal and early adolescent bipolar disorder phenotype. *Arch Gen Psychiat* 2004;**61**:459–467.

80. Birmaher B, Axelson D, Strober M, *et al.* Clinical course of children and adolescents with bipolar spectrum disorders. *Arch Gen Psychiat* 2006;**63**:175–183.

81. Leibenluft E, Rich BA. Pediatric bipolar disorder. *Ann Rev Clin Psychol* 2008;**4**:163–187.

82. McClellan J, Kowatch R, Findling RL. Practice parameter for the assessment and treatment of children and adolescents with bipolar disorder. *J Am Acad Child Adolesc Psychiat* 2007;**46**:107–125.

83. Leibenluft E, Charney DS, Towbin KE, Bhangoo RK, Pine DS. Defining clinical phenotypes of juvenile mania. *Am J Psychiat* 2003;**160**:430–437.

84. Brotman MA, Schmuajuk M, Rich BA, *et al.* Prevalence, clinical correlates, and longitudinal course of severe mood dysregulation in children. *Biol Psychiat* 2006;**60**:991–997.

85. Brotman MA, Kassem L, Reising MM, *et al.* Parental diagnosis in youth with narrow phenotype bipolar disorder or severe mood dysregulation. *Am J Psychiat* 2007;**164**:1238–1241.

86. Blader JC, Carlson GA. Increased rates of bipolar disorder diagnoses among US child, adolescent, and adult inpatients, 1996–2004. *Biol Psychiat* 2007;**62**:107–114.

87. Moreno C, Laje G, Blanco C, Jiang H, Schmidt AB, Olfson M. National trends in the outpatient diagnosis and treatment of bipolar disorder in youth. *Arch Gen Psychiat* 2007;**64**:1032–1039.

88. Costello EJ, Foley DL, Angold A. 10-year research update review: the epidemiology of child and adolescent psychiatric disorders, II: developmental epidemiology. *J Am Acad Child Adolesc Psychiat* 2006;**45**:8–25.

89. Stringaris A, Baroni A, Haimm C, *et al.* Pediatric bipolar disorder versus severe mood dysregulation: risks for manic episodes on follow-up. *J Am Acad Child Adol Psychiat* 2010;**49**:397–405.

90. Lewinson PM, Klein DN, Seeley JR. Bipolar disorders in a community sample of older adolescents: prevalence, phenomenology, comorbidity and course. *J Am Acad Child Adolesc Psychiat* 1995;**34**:454–63.

91. Egeland et. Al. 2000; Lish, Dime–Meenan, Whybrow, Price & Hirschfeld; Loranger and Levine, 1978.

92. Youngstrom EA, Duax J. Evidence-based assessment of pediatric bipolar disorder, part I: base rate and family history. *J Am Acad Child Adolesc Psychiat* 2005;**44**:712–717.

93. Weussnan MM, Gershon ES, Kidd KK. Psychiatric disorders in the relatives of probands with affective disorders: The Yale-NIMH collaborative family study. *Arch Gen Psychiat* 1984;**41**:13.

94. Fergus EL. Offspring study of pediatric bipolar disorder. Poster presented at AACAP annual meeting, 1999.

95. Joshi G, Wilens T. Comorbidity in pediatric bipolar disorder. *Child Adolesc Psychiatr Clin N Am* 2009;**18**:291–319.

96. Pavuluri MN, Birmaher B, Naylor M. Pediatric bipolar disorder: Ten year review. *J Am Acad Child Adolesc Psychiat* 2005;**44**:846–871.

97. Findling RL, Gracious BL, McNamara NK, *et al.* Rapid continuous cycling and psychiatric co-morbidity in pediatric bipolar I disorder. *Bipolar Disord* 2001;**3**:202–210.

98. Akiskal HS. Development pathways to bipolarity: Are juvenile-onset depressions pre-bipolar? *J Am Acad Child Adolesc Psychiat* 1995;**34**:754–763.

99. Akiskal H. Recent progress in genetic studies of bipolar disorder. Presented at the World Assembly for Mental Health, Vancouver, Canada, 24 July 2001.

100. Nurnberger JI, Gershon E. Genetics. In: Paykel ES (ed.) *Handbook of Affective Disorders*. Edinburgh: Churchill-Livingstone, 1982.

101. Mendlewicz J, Rainer JD. Adoption study supporting genetic transmission in manic depressive illness. *Nature* 1977;**265**:327–329.

102. Klein DN, Depue RA, Slater JF. Cyclothymia in the adolescent offspring of parents with bipolar affective disorder. *J Abnorm Psychol* 1985;**94**:115–127.

103. Egeland J, Sussex J. Suicide and family loading for affective disorders. *JAMA* 1985;**254**:915.

104. Baum AE, Akula N, Cabanero M, *et al.* A genome-wide association study implicates diacylglycerol kinase eta (DGKH) and several other genes in the etiology of bipolar disorder. *Mol Psychiat* 2008;**13**:197–207.

105. Wellcome Trust Case Control Consortium. Genome-wide association study of 14,000 cases of seven common diseases and 3,000 shared controls. *Nature* 2007;**447**:661–678.

106. Sklar P, Smoller JW, Fan J, *et al.* Whole-genome association study of bipolar disorder. *Mol Psychiat* 2008;**13**:558–569.

107. McQuillin A, Rizig M, Gurling HM. *Pharmacogenet Genomics* 2007;**17**:605–617.

108. Post RM, Speer AM, Hough CJ, Xing G. Neurobiology of bipolar illness: implications for future study and therapeutics. *Ann Clin Psychiat* 2003;**15**:85–94.

109. McNamara D. Elevated risk for lipid disorders seen in bipolar. *Clinical Psychiatry News* 2009, September.

110. Poster at a meeting of the New Clinical Drug Evaluation Unit sponsored by the National Institute of Mental Health, Hollywood, FLA.

111. Geller B. Prepubertal and early adolescent bipolarity differentiate from ADHD by manic symptoms, grandiose delusions, ultra-rapid or ultradian cycling. *J Affect Disord* 1998;**51**:81–91.

112. Hudziak JJ, Although RR, Rettew DC, Faraone SV, Boomsma DI. The prevalence and genetic architecture of CBCL-juvenile bipolar disorder. *Biol Psychiat* 2005;**58**:562–568.

113. Mick E, Biederman J, Pandina G, Faraone SV. A preliminary meta-analysis of the Child Behavior Checklist in pediatric bipolar disorder. *Biol Psychiat* 2003;**53**: 1021–1027.

114. Biederman J, Petty CR, Monuteaux MC, *et al.* The Child Behavior Checklist-Pediatric Bipolar Disorder Profile predicts a subsequent diagnosis of bipolar disorder and associate impairments in ADHD youth growing up: a longitudinal analysis. *J Clin Psychiat* 2009;**70**:732–740.

115. Youngstrom EA, Findling RL, Calabrese JR, *et al.* Comparing the diagnostic accuracy of six potential screening instruments for bipolar disorder in youths aged 5 to 17 years. *J Am Acad Child Adolesc Psychiat* 2004;**43**: 847–858.

116. Basco MR, Rush AJ. Compliance with pharmacotherapy in mood disorders. *Psych Ann* 1995;**25**:78–82.

117. Colom F, Vieta E. A perspective on the use of psycho education, cognitive behavioral therapy and interpersonal therapy for bipolar patients. *Bipolar Disord* 2004;**6**:480–486.

118. Birmaher B, Axelson D, Pavuluri M. In: Martin A, Volkmar F (eds) *Lewis's Child and Adolescent Psychiatry*. Philadelphia, PA: Lippincott Williams & Wilkins, 2007; pp. 513–528.

119. Pavuluri MN, Graczyk PA, Henry DB, Carbray JA, Heidenreich J, Miklowitz DJ. Child and family-focused cognitive-behavioral therapy for pediatric bipolar disorder: development and preliminary results. *J Am Acad Child Adolesc Psychiat* 2004;**43**:528–537.

120. West AE, Pavuluri MN. Maintenance model of integrated psychosocial treatment in pediatric bipolar disorder. *J Am Acad Child Adolesc Psychiat* 2007;**46**: 205–212.

121. Fristad M, Goldberg-Arnold J, Gavazzi S. Multifamily psycho education groups (MFPG) for parents of children with bipolar disorder. *Bipolar Disord* 2002;**4**: 254–262.

122. Fristad M, Gavazzi S, Mackinaw-Koons B. Family psycho education: an adjunctive intervention for children with bipolar disorder. *Biol Psychiat* 2003;**53**:100–108.

123. Miklowitz DJ, George EL, Axelson DA, *et al.* Family-focused treatment for adolescents with bipolar disorder. *J Affect Disord* 2004;**82**(Suppl. 1):113–128.

124. Miklowitz DJ, Axelson DA, Birmaher B, et al. Family-focused treatment for adolescents with bipolar disorder: results of a 2-year randomized trial. *Arch Gen Psychiat* 2008;**65**:1052–1061.

125. Correll CU, Manu P, Olshanskiy V, *et al.* Cardiometabolic risk of second-generation antipsychotic medications during first-time use in children and adolescents. *JAMA* 2009;**302**:1765–1773.

126. Kowatch R, Findling R, Scheffer R, *et al.* Placebo controlled trial of divalproex versus lithium for bipolar disorder. Paper presented at Annual Meeting of the American Academy of Child and Adolescent Psychiatry, 23–28 October 2007, Boston, MA.

127. Suppes T, McElroy S, Gilbert J, Dessain E, Cole J. Clozapine in the treatment of dysphoric mania. *Biol Psychiat* 1992;**32**:270–280.

128. Suppes T, Phillips K, Judd C. Clozapine treatment of nonpsychotic rapid cycling bipolar disorder: a report of three cases. *Biol Psychiat* 1994;**36**:338–340.

129. Kowatch RA, Suppes T, Gilfillan SK, Fuentes RM, Grannemann BD, Emslie GJ. Clozapine treatment for children and adolescents with schizophrenia and bipolar disorder: a clinical case series. *J Child Adolesc Psychopharmacol* 1995;**5**:241–253.

130. Masi G, Mucci M, Millepiedi S. Clozapine in adolescent inpatients with acute mania. *J Child Adolesc Psychopharmacol* 2002;**12**:93–99.

131. Sachs GS, Nierenberg AA, Calabrese JR, *et al.* Effectiveness of adjunctive antidepressant treatment for bipolar depression. *N Engl J Med* 2007;**356**:1711–1722.

132. Leverich GS, Altshuler LL, Frye MA, *et al.* Risk of switch in mood polarity to hypomania or mania in patients with bipolar depression during acute and continuation trials of venlafaxine, sertraline, and bupropion as adjuncts to mood stabilizers. *Am J Psychiat* 2006;**163**: 232–239.

133. Biederman J, Mick E, Hammerness P, *et al.* Open-label, 8 week trial of olanzapine and risperidone for the treatment of bipolar disorder in preschool-age children. *Biol Psychiat* 2005;**58**:589–594.

134. Weersing VR, Brent DA. Cognitive behavioral therapy for depression in youth. *Child Adolesc Psychiatr Clin N Am* 2006;**15**:939–957.

13

Anxiety Disorders in Childhood and Adolescence

Craig L. Donnelly, Jesse C. Rhoads

Introduction

Fear and anxiety are common experiences across childhood and adolescence. It is in the adaptive management and development of coping strategies for these affective states that the processes of mastery, autonomy, skill acquisition, and cognitive maturation unfold. The clinician evaluating childhood anxiety disorders faces the task of differentiating the normal, protective, transient, and developmentally appropriate expressions of anxiety from pathological anxiety. Expertise in the early identification of pathological anxiety is important given the fact that less than one-third of youths with anxiety disorders actually receive treatment services [1].

Anxiety disorders are characterized as "internalizing" disorders, along with depression and dysthymia, and stand in distinction to the "externalizing" disorders of childhood such as oppositional defiant disorder (ODD), conduct disorder (CD), and attention-deficit hyperactivity disorder (ADHD). Anxiety disorders are among the most common psychiatric disorders in children and adolescents, affecting 31.9% of children under the age of 18 at some point in their lives, with 8.3% having a severely impairing disorder [2]. The latest version of the *Diagnostic and Statistical Manual of Mental Disorders, Fourth Edition, Text Revision* (DSM-IV-TR) [3] has refined the diagnostic nomenclature of childhood anxiety disorders to attain greater consistency with the adult anxiety disorders. In using the criteria to reach a diagnostic threshold, the clinician is expected to exercise clinical judgment in terms of the severity, degree of distress, and relative dysfunction manifested by the individual child.

The developmental course of anxiety, its appropriateness, and boundaries with other psychiatric disorders are areas of intense research interest in child psychiatry, and yet surprisingly few empirical data exist in these areas. To effectively engage the assessment process a wide and thorough clinical perspective is necessary.

First, clinicians need to maintain a high level of suspicion for anxiety disorders when evaluating children. Anxiety disorders are not rare and often mimic or are comorbid with other childhood disorders. Symptoms such as school refusal, tantrums, or irritability may be less reflective of oppositional behavior than an underlying social phobia or generalized anxiety disorder. Second, children need to be evaluated within a biopsychosocial framework. Genetic vulnerability, biological etiologies, life experience, social and family contexts, and developmental phase are interwoven to a greater or lesser extent in the expression of pathological anxiety, and their roles need to be clarified. The clinician must understand the inner experiential context and the external behavioral contingencies in which the anxious child is operating. Third, given the uniqueness of each child and the complex interplay among the internal and external variables that drive anxiety, a multimodal approach to diagnosis and treatment is warranted.

This chapter will provide the basics for evaluating and treating each of the recognized childhood anxiety disorders. In using this chapter, the clinician should bear in mind that the assessment and treatment of childhood anxiety is often quite complex and time consuming. The clinician undertaking this task should not hesitate to consult an expert in childhood anxiety if time constraints, lack of experience, or the intricacies of a particular child's presentation prove problematic.

Separation Anxiety

Definition

Separation anxiety disorder (SAD) is the sole anxiety disorder classified in DSM-IV-TR as one of the

Clinical Child Psychiatry, Third Edition. Edited by William M. Klykylo and Jerald Kay.
© 2012 John Wiley & Sons, Ltd. Published 2012 by John Wiley & Sons, Ltd.

"Disorders Usually Diagnosed in Infancy, Childhood or Adolescence." Its cardinal feature is excessive anxiety engendered by separation from major attachment figures or the home environment. Four weeks' duration and clinically significant or subjectively distressful impairment in social, academic, or occupational functioning are necessary to make this diagnosis.

Sometime past their first birthday, normal children begin to exhibit signs of distress when confronted with possible separation from their caretakers. This adaptive anxiety response, called separation protest, peaks at about 15 months of age, after which it continues on a course of resolution. This is qualitatively different from the experience of children with SAD, who, at a later age, exhibit excessive distress and abnormal reactivity at the thought of, or at the time of actual, separation from a parent. Children with SAD may be burdened with unrelenting worries about losing or possible harm befalling a parent or loved one. Getting lost or kidnapped are frequent fears. They may be reluctant to attend school, go to bed at night, or be alone in the house without their major attachment figure present. These children often suffer nightmares with themes of separation, and will complain of multiple somatic symptoms, such as headaches, stomach aches, or nausea. They are often fretful and whiny, and pester their parents with reassurance seeking. Children with separation anxiety are typically unable to do sleepovers at friends' houses or endure overnight summer camps. Commonly, children and their parents seek treatment in the context of school refusal or excessive somatic complaints.

Incidence and Prevalence

The estimated prevalence of SAD has been noted to be 4–5% [4]; however, results from the National Comorbidity Survey Replication-Adolescent Supplement (NCS-A) show a higher lifetime prevalence of 7.6% [2], making it one of the most common childhood psychiatric disorders. About half of all anxious children seeking psychiatric assessment have separation anxiety [5]. Most studies report a higher rate of SAD for girls than boys; [6] however, the symptom presentation does not differ between the sexes [6]. SAD can be diagnosed until age 18, but it is primarily a disorder of prepubertal children, with an average age of onset of 7.5 years [7], making SAD one of the earliest anxiety disorders to be diagnosed in children. Two age-related trends are worth noting: Younger children report more symptoms and experience more distress than older children; and, as children age, prevalence rates go down [8]. Interestingly, while most children with anxiety disorders come from the middle to upper-middle classes, children with SAD

more frequently come from lower socioeconomic homes [4], which may relate to an interaction between an otherwise "hidden" biological propensity that is more likely to be expressed owing to the cumulative stress burden, which is likely to be higher among children in impoverished settings.

Etiology and Natural History

Attempts have been made to attribute the onset of separation anxiety to an inadequately resolved separation/individuation conflict [9], vulnerability determined by temperament [10], security of attachment [11], or behavioral contingencies. Genetic and familial/environmental factors have also been advanced as causes. Decisive empirical or epidemiological proof supporting any of these theories is lacking. Multiple and interactive etiologies appear most likely.

The fact that SAD is a risk factor for panic disorder (PD) has led some investigators to posit a developmental link between them [12, 13]. Evidence in support of a specific SAD-PD link is mixed, given that SAD is a risk factor for other anxiety disorders as well. A more recent formulation is that SAD may persist into adulthood as part of the same "panic diathesis," or panic spectrum; [14, 15] however, Aschenbrand et al. found that having SAD did not increase the risk of developing panic 7 years later. However, this study looked only at children who were treated for anxiety, and it remains unclear if untreated SAD leads to panic disorder [16]. The SAD-PD link is still controversial and some studies support a link [16–19].

Separation anxiety is typically a disorder of middle childhood (ages 7–9), although it has also been described in adolescents. If the disorder develops acutely, a precipitating stressor can often be identified. Common precipitating factors include a move, change of school, loss of a loved one, illness in the family, or prolonged absence from school. Sometimes the symptoms develop more insidiously, worsening over 3–6 months before a clinical referral is necessitated. Separation anxiety waxes and wanes, with exacerbations in times of stress. While some children recover fully after a single episode, others may experience a more protracted and chronic course. Later age of onset, comorbidities, familial pathology, and missing more than 1 year of school seem to be associated with a greater risk of chronicity [20].

Comorbidities with separation anxiety are common. As many as 60% of the children diagnosed with separation anxiety have at least one comorbid anxiety disorder, and 30% have two [21], the most likely being generalized anxiety disorder and specific phobias. Separation anxiety is also closely associated with depression; one-third of children diagnosed with SAD have comorbid major depression [7]. Conversely, SAD is the most commonly diagnosed anxiety disorder for prepubertal children with depression [22]. Typically, separation anxiety precedes depression, raising the question of whether the mood disorder is a consequence of enduring functional impairment. When SAD is comorbid with panic disorder, there is greater functional impairment [23]. Finally, there has been an association between SAD and the development of future psychopathology. One study found that 75% of children in a cohort with SAD developed a major depressive episode in young adulthood [24].

Diagnosis

Children suffering from SAD often come to the clinician's attention when problems with school attendance develop. Presentation may range from great reluctance to refusal and temper tantrums if parents insist on taking the child to school (Table 13.1). Separation from loved ones is often an issue around sleep time, and the separation-anxious child often winds up in the parents' bed. Increasing anxiety interferes with spending the night at a friend's house or going to camp. Once separation takes place, these children may worry incessantly about the misfortunes that might befall their loved ones. Nightmares with prominent themes of separation are sometimes reported. Fears of being lost and never reunited with their families often beset these children. Typically the "storm" is resolved once the child is returned to home. Somatic complaints such as morning stomach aches, headaches, nausea, and vomiting are more often seen in younger children, while older ones may also complain of palpitations and feeling faint.

Table 13.1 Separation anxiety disorder: diagnostic features and associated disorders.

Discriminating features	Associated disorders
Middle childhood (7–10)	Phobia
Fears specific to separation from primary attachment figure	Generalized anxiety disorder
Frequent reassurance seeking	
Bedtime anxiety, cannot do overnights at friends	
Crying/whining, irritable and fretful in anticipation of separation	
Frequently described as clingy	

A detailed history is the most helpful diagnostic resource. As is true for most of the internalizing disorders, accounts from the child are usually more telling than parent and teacher reports. Descriptions of the events preceding the separation, response to parents' departure, ensuing behavior (usually in school) and the consequences of separation are helpful in understanding the pattern of distress and precipitants. Gathering a comprehensive family history of psychiatric disorders is important, given the notable family patterns involving SAD. Clinicians should be sensitive to hearing the family's expressed and unexpressed feelings about the child as well as separation from the child, as these may be precipitating and maintaining factors. For example, as is typical with many childhood anxiety disorders, parents initial and well-intended attempts to reassure the child may be inadvertently supporting the child's anxiety and/or reinforcing escape/avoidance responses. Cooperation with a pediatrician is valuable, especially when somatic complaints are prominent.

Anxiety rating scales such as the Screen for Child Anxiety Related Emotional Disorders (SCARED) [25], the Multidimensional Anxiety Scale for Children (MASC) [26], or the Separation Anxiety Scale for Children (SASC) [27], may be used diagnostically and as measures of treatment outcome. General psychiatric symptom rating scales, such as the Connors Parent and Teacher Questionnaires [28], may assist in the diagnosis of comorbid disorders, which are common in these children. Routinely available laboratory studies do not increase the accuracy of the diagnosis.

Differential Diagnosis

The clinician must differentiate separation anxiety from developmentally appropriate fears accompanying separation from loved ones. These developmentally normal separation fears occur earlier in childhood, have milder presentations, and tend to be transient and self-limiting. Functional impairment is not a typical feature of fears accompanying normal development (see Table 13.2 for a list of normal developmental fears).

Delineation of SAD from other disorders sharing "school refusal" as a symptom is sometimes a challenging task. After conduct disorder and oppositional defiant disorder (i.e., truancy) have been ruled out, one should carefully evaluate evidence for other anxiety disorders. School refusal may be based in a specific phobia (e.g., test taking and/or fear of humiliation), in situationally bound panic disorder, or in social phobia as well as SAD.

Generalized anxiety disorder (GAD) has a more varied presentation and the fears involved tend to

Table 13.2 Normal development fears.

Age	Source of fear
Birth to 6 months	Loud noises, loss of physical support, rapid position changes, rapidly approaching unfamiliar objects
7–12 months	Strangers, looming objects, sudden confrontation by unexpected objects or unfamiliar people
1–5 years	Strangers, storms, animals, the dark, separation from parents, objects, machines, loud noises, the toilet, monsters, ghosts, insects, bodily harm
6–12 years	Supernatural beings, bodily injury, disease (AIDS, cancer), burglars, staying alone, failure, criticism, punishment
12–18 years	Tests and exams in school, school performance, bodily injury, appearance, peer scrutiny, athletic performance, social embarrassment

stem from matters other than separation. Although children with separation anxiety can experience panic attacks, in panic disorder attacks will occur in other unrelated situations. Relative comfort in social settings will differentiate separation anxiety from social phobia. Specific phobias are characterized by well-defined and usually singular phobic objects; distress can occur even in the presence of an attachment figure. Pervasiveness of a mood disorder, especially if it precedes the onset of separation anxiety, demands a separate diagnosis. Teasing apart major depression from separation anxiety is not always easy as they often occur together, but both diagnoses should be given, when appropriate, as treatment interventions differ for the two disorders.

Psychotic disorders, post-traumatic stress disorder, pervasive developmental disorders, and learning disorders should also be addressed. Familial dysfunction, substance abuse, medical problems (especially ones causing abdominal distress), and iatrogenically caused syndromes (e.g., neuroleptic-induced anxieties) need to be ruled out.

Several additional points bear emphasizing. First, children with SAD commonly have parents with an anxiety or depressive disorder. Careful assessment and, if necessary, treatment of the parent may be called for. This may entail simple psychoeducation of the parents regarding their inadvertent support of the child's anxiety versus frank treatment for an anxiety disorder in the parent. Second, a complete evaluation is important as over half of children with SAD have a second comorbid anxiety diagnosis, which can unnecessarily complicate treatment if it is missed.

Treatment

If the child presents with school refusal, this needs addressing. Treatment of school refusal is discussed in

a subsequent section. For separation difficulties that do not involve school, use of psychoeducational, behavioral, and cognitive techniques is recommended.

Psychoeducational interventions targeting the family members should focus on explaining the diagnoses given to the child, how these relate to the child's current maladaptive behaviors, and how behavioral, cognitive, and emotional changes made by members of the family may help the child. Educating parents about age-appropriate developmental tasks, informing them how they might encourage and support their child's attainment of these, and instructions on how to deal with negative family dynamics should also be undertaken where required. The essential and core feature of this approach is to assist parents in helping their child confront the separation experience and avoid the typical escape/avoidance response that reinforces the anxiety. Gradual mastery of minor separations, with parents modeling coping and nondistress and reinforcing the child's successes, supports children in facing and overcoming separation fears. Note that for mild cases of separation anxiety, this may be sufficient treatment.

Behavioral techniques have been demonstrated to be successful in SAD-related behaviors. Shaping the desired behavior through contingency management by positively reinforcing nonfearful behavior and withdrawing rewards for anxious behaviors may yield results. Modeling and exposure-based treatments have also been reported as effective. In these, children are rewarded for practicing "being brave" and are taught new skills for managing old anxious behaviors. Success in this endeavor depends upon identification of manageable target behaviors, practicing new behaviors, and appropriate reinforcement strategies.

Cognitive interventions focusing on the maladaptiveness of "catastrophic" thoughts and their replacement with more adaptive cognitions, in combination with self-instruction and teaching realistic appraisal of fear-producing circumstances, can be fruitful. Generally referred to as CBT (cognitive behavioral therapy), this type of treatment is now widely used with children, and some manualized protocols are becoming available [29].

Some somatic complaints can be countered by instruction in deep muscle relaxation or tension-relaxation exercises that can serve as anxiety counter-responses. Group and family therapies can be valuable adjunct treatments and may be more efficient means for skill teaching, modeling, and generalization.

Psychopharmacologic approaches may be useful in selected cases, especially when combined with psychosocial interventions. The reader is referred to recent summaries of the psychopharmacologic literature for comprehensive assessment of current options [30–32]. Psychotropic agents should be reserved for more refractory and complicated cases, or when anxiety is so severe that it limits therapy-based exposure practice [33]. Although there is no currently approved medication for the treatment of SAD, standard of care consensus suggests that the selective serotonin reuptake inhibitors (SSRIs) are first-line pharmacotherapy. Adjunctive medications may include clonazepam, particularly while awaiting benefit of the SSRI, although this strategy might best be reserved for older children. Tricyclic antidepressants (e.g., clomipramine, imipramine) have been used successfully in the past, although use of these agents is currently limited due to their side-effect profile and potential for cardiac toxicity. It should be borne in mind that CBT is likely to be the most powerful and enduring treatment. Studies of combined CBT and medication therapies have shown that combined treatment leads to a better response rate [34].

School Refusal

Definition

School refusal is not an anxiety disorder diagnosis per se, but it bears mentioning as it often presents in relation to other psychiatric diagnoses. School refusal is defined as difficulty attending school, associated with emotional distress, especially anxiety and depression [35]. It should be differentiated from other forms of school absenteeism [36]. It is distinguished from truancy and conduct disorder because the child is home from school with the parent's knowledge, and the child does not have any associated antisocial behaviors, such as lying, stealing, or destructiveness. As noted, school refusal is not a separate diagnostic entity, but rather a symptom of other diagnoses. It is most commonly thought to be a behavioral manifestation of separation anxiety disorder (SAD); however, accumulating evidence supports significant heterogeneity in its presentation. Not all children with separation anxiety become school refusers, and not all children who refuse to go to school meet criteria for separation anxiety [20].

Incidence and Prevalence

Some 1–2% of all school-aged children and 5% of all clinic-referred children become school refusers. Boys and girls are equally affected. There is an unequal distribution of cases of school refusers across the age span, with certain ages and school grades showing a greater vulnerability to the behavior. Peak expression of school refusal tends to come at ages 5–6, 10–11 and 13–15 [37]. These ages represent the times that children typically face transition entry into elementary, middle, and high school, respectively.

Etiology and Natural History

There is a wide variation in the presentation of school refusal, suggesting multiple etiologies. Some children go to school, but spend much of their day in distress in the nurse's office, making multiple phone contacts with parents. Others refuse to leave home. Some make partial progress toward school, but become anxious while en route. Some miss weeks and months of school, others manage to attend school on an intermittent basis. When school refusers are confronted with going to school, they manifest true physiological distress with increased muscle tension and breathing irregularities [38]. Many complain of feeling ill, most frequently complaining of headaches or stomach distress. When fear is involved, it is directed differentially, depending on the age of the child. Younger children fear separation from their parent(s), older children fear their teachers or other children. Social-evaluative fears dominate the presentation of adolescents.

School refusers meet criteria for other psychiatric disorders more often than not. Kearney and Albano examined 143 youths with school refusal and found that 22.4% had separation anxiety disorder, 22.4% had generalized anxiety disorder, 8.4% had oppositional defiant disorder, and 4.9% had depression. Interestingly, nearly one-third of their sample had no psychiatric diagnosis [39]. Some family patterns are identifiable; school refusers with separation anxiety disorder have an increased likelihood of having a parent with panic disorder, with or without agoraphobia. School refusers diagnosed with specific phobias have an increased likelihood of having a parent who also has specific phobias or social phobia. Several types of problematic family function have been identified, such as the enmeshed family, the conflictive family, the isolated family, and the detached family [40]. However, many school-refusing children have healthy families [40]. Single-parent families are overrepresented in this group of children [41].

Diagnosis

Because of the variability in the clinical presentations of school refusal, evaluations prior to treatment should engage multiple informants. The child and the family should undergo clinical interviews. Members of the school, daycare staff, and the family doctor are all potentially important sources of collateral information. Patterns of family dynamics need to be explored for potential weaknesses, for example, inadequate parental oversight or conflicting parental tactics. Psychoeducational reports and discussion with teachers should be requested from the school, if these are available. It is important to understand if school violence or victimization (bullying) is contributing to school refusal [36]. Developmental patterns need to be reviewed, especially language and academic and social skills. A thorough medical exam should be undertaken to rule out any organic cause for the child's somatic complaints, if these are part of the presentation. Once the primary diagnosis is made, search should continue for associated comorbid disorders as they are common [42].

Differential Diagnosis

Because school refusal is not a diagnostic entity, the goal of a clinical evaluation will be to identify the primary disorder, of which the school refusal is a symptom (Table 13.3). Consideration needs to be given to separation anxiety disorder, generalized anxiety disorder, specific phobias, including school and social phobia, and depression. Other anxiety disorders, such as post-traumatic stress disorder and panic disorder, need to be considered. Competing explanations for school attendance failure are uncomplicated truancy versus truancy as part of conduct disorder. Both are distinguished from school refusal because truant and/or conduct disordered children do not suffer significant emotional distress as part of their attempts to attend school. Additionally, unlike parents of school refusers, parents of truant children are typically not aware of their children's failure to be in school. The potential for learning disabilities or developmental disabilities needs to be ruled out, and a more straightforward fear of failure needs to be identified, when present.

Treatment

In uncomplicated cases where school refusal has not lasted more than 2 weeks, treatment is fairly straightforward. After informing the parents about the nature of

Table 13.3 Differential diagnosis of school refusal.

Diagnosis	Features
Separation Anxiety Disorder	Fears separation from parent or attachment figure. Spends out of school time in presence of parent
Generalized Anxiety Disorder	Anxiety in multiple domains, not limited to school setting, fretful, overly conscientious/fearful
Specific Phobia	Exhibits anxiety toward teacher, other student, activity, test taking or other specific object or circumstance
Social Phobia	Social setting per se is the primary fear. May fear scrutiny in test taking, being observed in bathroom, etc.
Panic Disorder	May have situationally bound or predisposed panic attacks. Some panic attacks have occurred out of school or unexpectedly, anticipatory anxiety, agoraphobia
Post-Traumatic Stress Disorder	Multiple symptoms in addition to school refusal: irritability, depression, re-experiencing, all related to a specified trauma
Obsessive-Compulsive Disorder	Presence of obsessive thoughts/compulsive rituals that may be a source of embarrassment or result in phobic avoidance
Conduct/Oppositional Defiant Disorder (Truancy)	Multiple oppositional/disruptive behavior symptoms in addition to school refusal, "hangs out" with friends when not in school, often complicated by substance abuse or antisocial behavior

the disorder and eliciting their cooperation as well as that of school authorities, the child is encouraged to return to school as soon as possible. Parents are instructed to show empathy and understanding for the child's distress but to insist in a firm and consistent manner on regular school attendance. The child is supported and provided with skills to master the fears and worries incumbent in the separation. This may involve the parent being present in the classroom for a brief period and then fading out their presence. Reward and praise should accompany desired behavior.

If school refusal has become entrenched, especially in older adolescents, therapy is much more difficult. Under these circumstances, CBT is considered first-line treatment for school refusal. King and Bernstein [35] recommend the use of the School Refusal Assessment Scale (SRAS) [40, 43] as an aid to identification of the negative and positive reinforcers that maintain the school refusal behavior. Associated with the SRAS are manuals that prescribe treatments for each of the functional conditions identified [44], and involving the school as well as family. Whether or not this or other protocols are used, success will likely depend upon successful identification of the positive reinforcers at home and the negative reinforcers at school, and some combination of relaxation therapy, systematic desensitization, modeling, shaping, and contingency management [44] involving the school as well as family. A gradual return to school is the typical goal. Identifying the common negative perceptions, such as "the kids think I'm stupid," and replacing them with more positive and realistic perceptions is frequently part of the plan. Teaching self-monitoring skills and counter-anxiety responses is common. Extended treatment to involve the family and the teacher helps to make the behavioral plan consistent throughout the course of the child's day. The best treatments span the home and school domains.

Several reports of successful CBT treatments of school refusal are in the literature [35]. Interestingly, there is also one report [45] of a successful "placebo" treatment group, which underwent "educational therapy" to be compared with an experimental CBT-based therapy. Educational therapy consisted of a combination of educational presentations, supportive psychotherapy, and a daily diary for the recording of thoughts and fears. No treatment for modifying thoughts or encouragement for confronting fears was given. On all measures, the "educational therapy" matched the CBT for success. While it is not clear what elements of the educational therapy made it successful, and perhaps a common element of exposure was at work

in both groups, the possibility is open for alternative types of therapy as potential remedial tools.

The use of medications has been addressed in several studies. While most reports involve the use of tricyclic antidepressants (with or without CBT), the general feeling of clinicians is that these medications should not be considered first line, given new reports of the effectiveness of the safer SSRIs, such as fluoxetine in treating anxiety disorders in children [46]. Additionally, it is the general clinical opinion that medication should not be added to treatment until a trial of CBT-based therapy has been undertaken, extremely severe or debilitating cases [37].

Finally, the prognosis of school refusal behaviors is better for younger children and for children with a higher baseline of school attendance prior to the initiation of treatment. Older children, and those with longer periods of failed school attendance, fare worse [38].

Generalized Anxiety Disorder

Definition

In 1994 with the publication of DSM-IV, the American Psychiatric Association replaced the diagnostic category "Overanxious Disorder" (OAD) with "Generalized Anxiety Disorder" (GAD) for use with the pediatric population. Diagnostic modification of the criteria for adult GAD included the reduction in the number of physical/somatic complaints required, from three to one (of six alternatives), as well as a replacement of the former descriptor "unrealistic worries," with "excessive anxiety and worry that is difficult to control." To be diagnosed with GAD, the child or adolescent must additionally experience excessive worry that impairs daily function and continues for at least 6 months.

Several challenges complicate the diagnosis of GAD in this population. Due to the significant overlap of anxiety with depressive symptoms in children – such as concentrating, irritability, and sleep disturbance – clinicians face the task of differentiating GAD from depressive disorders. This is complicated by the high comorbidity of GAD with depressive disorders that is found in children and adolescents [42, 47] as well as adults [48]. In order to better discriminate between the disorders, work is continuing to identify those symptoms of GAD that are most common in pediatric populations. In their report of 58 children, Masi et al [47]. reported that the most common symptoms of GAD are tension, apprehension, need for reassurance, irritability, negative self-image, and physical complaints. Less common symptoms were psychomotor agitation, fear of sleeping alone, and fear of being alone. GAD is also frequently comorbid with other anxiety disorders and at times the clinical picture will overlap with other anxiety disorders. It is important to understand that childhood GAD needs to be evaluated within a developmental context [49].

Additionally, some amount of anxiety is typical of normal development [50]. Fears, worries, and scary dreams are experienced by the majority of children at one time or another. This leaves the distinction between pathological and developmentally appropriate anxiety to be made by the clinician (see Table 13.2). Pathological worries of children with GAD tend to encompass more domains of concerns (such as health of family members, school performance, social relationships), be associated with greater distress, cause stronger daily interference, are more difficult to control [50, 51], and, to a lesser extent, occur more frequently [52] than those of healthy children.

Incidence and Prevalence

Current understanding of the epidemiology of GAD in children and adolescents continues to rely heavily on data collected using the older diagnostic entity "Overanxious Disorder" (OAD) [47]. Using the older criteria, youth prevalence rates for GAD are estimated to be from 2.2% to 5.7%; [2, 53, 54] prevalence rates increase with age [55]. The mean age of onset of GAD/OAD is reported to be 8.8 years [56]. Younger females and males are equally likely to receive the diagnosis, although this changes in adolescence when it becomes more common in girls [57]. Muris and colleagues reported that 3.8% of boys and 9.0% of girls met diagnostic criteria in their sample of 8–13-year-olds [50]. Comorbidities with GAD are high; Masi et al. [58] reported that 87% of their 7–13-year-old group had comorbid diagnoses, most frequently a depressive disorder (62%). SAD was a common comorbidity for younger children (42%). Studies of anxious youth found that 36% of the sample are comorbid for GAD, Social Phobia and SAD [18].

Etiology and Natural History

Freud postulated that anxiety is a byproduct of suppression of unacceptable libidinous or aggressive drives. In a later revision of this theory, he postulated "signal anxiety" as a warning to the approach of highly conflictual and potentially devastating repressed material [59].

Behavioral theories conceptualize anxiety as an arousal response inadvertently rewarded and perpetuated. Recent cognitive theories tend to view maladaptive cognitions associated with arousal as precipitants, which are subsequently reinforced through escape or avoidance. Familial factors, such as high levels of parental expectation and an emphasis on achievement, or

conversely, excessive permissiveness, may facilitate the development of anxiety.

Data indicate that behavioral inhibition (BI), a temperamental profile described as a stable tendency to be avoidant, quiet, and behaviorally restrained in unfamiliar situations, seen in about 20% of Caucasian children, may constitute a substantial risk for the development of GAD (OAD) [60]. Increasing evidence supports BI as a distinct physiological profile [61], with a substantial heritability index, as documented in twin studies [62].

Van Oort et al. tracked the developmental trajectory of anxiety disorders and found that in GAD, anxiety symptoms initially decreased during early adolescence and increased from middle to late adolescence [63]. Neurobiological theories suggest disturbance in the hypothalamic-pituitary-adrenal axis, and in regulation of thyroid and growth hormone secretion as possible causes of anxiety. Gamma-amino butyric acid (GABA), noradrenaline, serotonin, and adenosine dysfunction have all been implicated as contributing to anxiety [64]. Not surprisingly, offspring of parents with anxiety disorders are more likely to be anxious themselves compared to nonpsychiatric controls (odds ratio 3.91) [65].

De Bellis and colleagues identified structural differences in both the amygdala and the superior temporal gyrus (STG) associated with pediatric GAD. In two separate reports, they initially described significantly larger right and total amygdala volumes [66], and later identified STG increases in both total and white matter volume, which were more pronounced on the right side [67]. Further, their index of this asymmetry correlated with child reports on the SCARED (Screen for Child Anxiety Related Emotional Disorders) scale. Although a theoretical accounting of these findings would be premature, the data are intriguing in that they link regions of the brain known to be involved with fear responses (amygdala) and social intelligence (STG) to GAD in a clinically meaningful way. Additionally, the right > left structural asymmetry fits nicely with demonstrations of right-sided prefrontal activation in behaviorally inhibited children as well as increased responses to angry faces and novel situations that have been reported [61]. In the future, we may be able to use functional magnetic resonance imaging (fMRI) of the amygdala to gauge potential response to somatic or psychotherapeutic interventions [68].

Diagnosis

The differential diagnosis of GAD can be complicated, as it frequently involves symptom overlap with other

Table 13.4 Generalized anxiety disorder: diagnostic features and associated disorders.

Discriminating features	Associated disorders
Anxiety in multiple settings	Separation anxiety disorder
Common anxiety disorder in 12–19-year-olds	Specific phobia
Often overlooked/ underdiagnosed	
Fretful, reassurance seeking	
Shifting sources of worry	
"Achey-painy"/somatic/ stomach pain	
Worries about inconsequential items/"what if" concerns	

anxiety disorders (Table 13.4). Children and adolescents with GAD tend to worry excessively about their performance and competence, even in the absence of external scrutiny. Ruminating about past mistakes and worrying about future adversities (i.e., "what if" concerns) may cause a decline in academic function and precipitate a referral. Parents will often report children's apprehension about "adult issues:" illness, old age, death, financial matters, wars, and natural disasters. Children with GAD are often seen as perfectionist and self-cautious, frequently seeking reassurance. Because they "cannot stop worrying" these youths often appear deconcentrated, restless, fragile, tense, and irritable. Where there is a discrepancy between their high expectations and the level of achievement, depression often ensues, especially in teenagers. Comorbid phobias, panic attacks, or panic disorder are not uncommon [58, 69]. Younger children sometimes have concomitant symptoms of separation anxiety and attention-deficit hyperactivity disorder [70]. Somatic complaints are common in youths with GAD, with the most common symptoms being restlessness, stomach aches, and palpitations [71]. The frequency of somatic symptoms increases as comorbidity increases.

An extensive and detailed history, including family history of psychiatric disorders, is important in establishing a correct diagnosis and differentiating GAD from other anxiety disorders. Multiple sources of information are preferable. Formal or informal reports from teachers, daycare providers, and past or present mental health providers can be invaluable. Assessment of family dynamics can reveal stressors to the child, which are not easy for the patient or family members to share without encouragement. As with all childhood anxiety disorders, gathering history from both child and parents is essential. Cooperation with the family doctor or

pediatrician and school authorities assures better evaluation and more effective treatment.

Several anxiety scales are available for use. These include: the Revised Children's Manifest Anxiety Scale (RCMAS) [72], the Multidimensional Anxiety Scale for Children (MASC) [26], the Child Behavior Checklist (CBCL) [73], and the Pediatric Anxiety Rating Scale (PARS) [74]. These scales have potential value both in identifying anxiety disorders and in monitoring treatment progress. Detailed descriptions of useful psychometric instruments are available [75, 76].

Differential Diagnosis

GAD can be differentiated from separation anxiety by its pervasive nature and presence across different contexts (e.g., school, home, and peer relations). Panic disorder is more "phasic" in comparison to the more "tonic" GAD. The content of anxiety in panic disorder is usually focused on future panic attacks. In specific phobia, fears center on the phobic object. Obsessive thoughts can be distinguished from GAD by their intrusive nature and concomitant compulsive rituals used to alleviate anxiety. In post-traumatic stress disorder (PTSD), anxiety is usually related to a past traumatic event or re-experiencing of the event. Prevalence of depressed mood, anhedonia, and vegetative signs set depressive episodes apart from GAD, in spite of significant symptom overlap.

Finally, medical conditions often present with symptoms that may mimic GAD. Caution is warranted so as not to overlook hyperthyroidism, diabetes mellitus, and the more rare syndromes such as pheochromocytoma or systemic lupus erythematosus. Excessive stimulant use, alcohol withdrawal, or drug dependence can also mimic GAD. The recreational use of steroids, primarily by adolescent boys, warrants monitoring as this practice has been associated with anxiety [77].

Treatment

Traditionally, psychodynamic therapy focused on the expanding awareness of the defensive and maladaptive nature of the anxiety. Empirical validation is lacking for this approach in the treatment of children. Neither does empirical support exist for the use of play therapy or supportive psychotherapy for pediatric GAD.

In contrast, CBT has received the most empirical support for the treatment of anxiety disorders in youths. This form of therapy is supported in recent practice parameters [78]. Common treatment components include desensitization, prolonged exposure, modeling, contingency management, and self-management/

cognitivestrategies [79]. Relaxation, visual imagery, self-affirmative statements, self-instruction, identifying faulty cognitions, and replacing them with adaptive thoughts have been combined in various ways in different cognitive behavioral approaches.

There is some evidence that CBT with a family therapy component improves treatment outcome [80], although this benefit may disappear with time [81]. If a child has at least one parent with anxiety, parental anxiety management combined with child-focused CBT is superior to the CBT component alone [82].

Several reports have been made of the successful use of The Coping Cat, a manualized treatment protocol developed by Kendall [83]. In two separate studies, 50% [84] and 64% [85] of participating children no longer met criteria for OAD after undergoing this manualized treatment approach. Long-term maintenance of improvement was documented in each of these randomized trials. More recently, comparisons have been made of the efficacy of The Coping Cat protocol when presented in individual versus group formats. Significant improvement was reported with both formats, with nonsignificant differences between them [86]. Psychiatric comorbidity and severity of pretreatment anxiety predict a worse outcome [87]. Due to the paucity of mental health care providers in the US, CBT may not be able to be delivered in all communities. Preliminary studies have shown that CBT delivered over the internet without a clinician can have a large effect size [88].

Increasingly, practitioners are turning to psychopharmacologic therapy for treatment of pediatric GAD. Many now consider SSRIs as first-line agents for pediatric GAD. The RUPP (Research Unit on Pediatric Psychopharmacology) Anxiety Subgroup has presented compelling evidence that these medications – specifically fluvoxamine (Luvox) – are both effective for anxiety disorders (including GAD) and tolerated well [89]. Other controlled studies support the efficacy and tolerability of sertraline [34], fluoxetine [90], citalopram [91], and extended-release venlafaxine [92] for pediatric GAD.

Limited information exists concerning the efficacy of benzodiazepine use in pediatric GAD. An early study of alprazolam failed to demonstrate significant improvement over placebo [93]. Concerns for previously demonstrated behavioral disinhibition [94], as well as theoretical concerns for dependence and abuse, are limiting clinical use of benzodiazepines in this context. Short-term use for highly anxious children, especially while awaiting onset of the action of an SSRI, remains a potential treatment choice.

Specific Phobia

Definition

A specific phobia is a marked and persistent fear of a specific object or situation whose exposure invariably provokes intense anxiety, much like a situationally bound or predisposed panic attack. Children with specific phobias will avoid the object or situation; if they cannot, they react with distress, often crying, exhibiting tantrums, freezing, or clinging. Although their fearful responses are excessive or unreasonable for the event, children may not recognize them as such. The DSM-IV-TR currently recognizes five types of phobias: animal, natural environment, blood-injection-injury, situational, and other types. To meet DSM-IV-TR criteria for specific phobia, the child must be in significant distress or suffer clinical impairment for at least 6 months.

Incidence and Prevalence

Specific phobia is a relatively common anxiety disorder for children. Prevalence is estimated to be 3–4% in some studies and is somewhat higher for girls than for boys [95]. A recent epidemiological survey showed a lifetime prevalence of 19.3%, with 0.8% having severe impairment [2]. It peaks in prevalence between 10 and 13 years of age [96, 97]. Some fears are common to normal development: preschoolers are often afraid of strangers, the dark, animals, and imaginary creatures; elementary children may fear animals, the dark, threats to safety, and thunder/lightning; adolescents may be agoraphobic or have fears with sexual or failure themes [98]. Normally, these fears decrease with age [99, 100]. Normal fears are distinguished from true phobias by their intensity and degree of impairment. Specific phobias may parallel age-related fears for content, or they may be unique.

Etiology and Natural History

Psychoanalytical theory viewed phobias as attempts to master anxiety and fear stemming from repressed conflictual libidinal and aggressive urges. Thus, fear disconnected from repressed material is displaced onto a phobic object, allowing the child a degree of control through the act of phobic avoidance.

Current theories emphasize the role of learned experiences in the generation and maintenance of phobias. Strong empirical evidence supports each of the three mechanisms touted in the three-pathway theory: [101] aversive classical conditioning, modeling, and negative information transmission [102]. Stated differently, children may learn phobias by having one (or more) frightening experiences with an object/situation (e.g., developing a phobia of dogs after having been bitten by one), by witnessing the behavior of somebody who has an established phobia (e.g., seeing an older sibling respond fearfully to dogs), or by direct instruction (e.g., hearing from a parent, "Don't go near dogs, they are dangerous and can hurt you"). Once developed, phobic fears are maintained by the positive consequences of avoidance.

There are some fears, shared by many children, which have been described as occurring spontaneously, without identifiable experiences of prior learning (e.g., fear of water, thunder). This has led to the intriguing notion of evolutionary-dependent, or "intrinsic," fears that are hard-wired, and that become phobias either because the child's experiences fail to habituate them properly, or due to some flaw in the child's internal "danger detection" system [96]. While acceptance of this non-associative theory of fear is mixed, evidence does suggest that genetic factors play a substantial role in propagating specific phobias [103].

Phobic symptoms tend to vacillate over time, and in the majority of children they will gradually subside without treatment. However, clinicians are cautioned against hasty dismissal of a child's fears. A portion of children will not get over their phobias, which may eventually hamper their normal development and functioning. Specific phobias have been reported to be highly comorbid with social phobia and separation anxiety disorder [104]. It has also been shown that children with natural environment type fears have more comorbid anxiety, more depressive symptoms, and less life satisfaction than children with animal phobias [105].

Diagnosis

Children usually present with excessive fear related to some well-circumscribed situation or object (Table 13.5). Often parents will complain that the child is preoccupied with the object, causing the fear or attempts to avoid it to interfere with family life. The child's play, relationship with peers and family members, as well as school per-

Table 13.5 Specific phobia: diagnostic features.

Discriminating features
Specific phobic object or circumstance
Anticipatory anxiety
Common fears are of: needles, animals, doctor's office
Restricted anxiety
Clearcut avoidance

formance can be negatively influenced by avoidance of a feared situation or even by incapacitating anticipatory anxiety.

Exposure to the phobic object elicits a response that has cognitive, emotional, behavioral, motoric, and physiological components. Each of these components presents the clinician with the opportunity for assessment by observation and clinical history, increasing diagnostic accuracy.

The path to correct diagnosis lies in a detailed history containing an accurate description of the sequence of events, fear-producing situation, consequences, and the intensity of fear. The behavioral component is usually measured indirectly by distance from the phobic object at which the subject experiences distress. Heart rate is a quantifiable correlate of physiological response. A comprehensive description of psychometric instruments may be found in King et al [106].

Differential Diagnosis

The initial task is to differentiate developmentally appropriate fears from a specific phobia. Specific phobia is not diagnosed if the child's anxiety is better accounted for by another disorder. In social phobia, fears are confined to social situations, especially if one's performance is subject to scrutiny. Fears in panic disorder are related to anticipation of re-experience of an attack. Anxiety peaks during separation from loved ones in separation anxiety disorder. In generalized anxiety disorder, fears and worries tend not to be confined to a specific object or situation. Post-traumatic stress disorder is characterized by fear and avoidance of memories related to past traumatic experiences. In anorexia nervosa, obsessions with food and its avoidance can be suggestive of a phobia although the eating disorder symptoms are pervasive and dominate the clinical picture. Bizarre fears are often a part of a psychotic disorder, but here the presence of a thought disorder is an obvious differentiating feature.

Treatment

Both exclusively behavioral as well as cognitive behavioral therapies are widely used to treat children with specific phobias. In their comprehensive review, Ollendick and King [107] identify participant modeling and contingency management techniques as the most efficacious. Thus, a combination of exposure, reinforced practice with shaping, positive reinforcement, and extinction techniques best predisposes to symptom control. They identify other therapeutic techniques, including variants of systematic desensitization, live or filmed modeling, and CBT as good choices for treatment. A recent study showed that even one session of exposure treatment may have lasting therapeutic benefit [108]. It has also been shown that this one session of treatment geared toward a specific phobia can lead to a reduction in comorbid anxiety and comorbid phobias [109]. Thus, the beneficial effects of the treatment of a specific phobia may generalize to other disorders. Self-control strategies (which use the cognitive tools of self-evaluation and self-reward) used in combination with contingency management and *in vivo* exposure (a variant of systematic desensitization) have been touted as a successful treatment combination [110].

Flooding, or implosive therapy, is not a recommended modality for the treatment of children. Psychodynamic therapy, described in numerous case studies, has had scarce empirical support.

Family therapy is a useful adjunct. It can be fruitful in dealing with disturbed family relationships, especially where they cause the child's phobia or serve to support it. Psychoeducation of parents about the basics of anxiety reinforcement and extinction is a necessary feature of treatment. Often, providing them with a "rule of thumb" that avoidance increases anxiety and exposure decreases it, can be helpful.

Anecdotal reports of benzodiazepine or antidepressant use for treatment of phobias should not encourage the clinician to pursue medication intervention. Psychosocial treatments are efficacious and are the standard of care.

Social Phobia (Social Anxiety Disorder)

Definition

Sociability is the preference for companionship and affiliation with others, and shyness is a form of social withdrawal accompanied by distress and inhibited behaviors. Both are enduring personality features, detectable at an early age and stable across development [111]. Children who indicate a desire for affiliation with other children but who experience significant distress in social settings may meet criteria for social phobia.

Social phobia (SP) and social anxiety disorder are interchangeable terms, with a trend toward preferred use of the latter in the adult literature. SP is characterized by a marked and persistent fear of one or more social or performance situations in which the individual is exposed to unfamiliar people or possible scrutiny. In children, there must be the capacity for age-appropriate social relationships and the anxiety must occur in peer settings, not just in adult interactions. Youngsters may express the anxiety in the form of crying, tantrums, freezing, or avoidance or may exhibit a full-blown panic attack. Children may not recognize that their fears are excessive, although adolescents typically do.

Incidence and Prevalence

Social phobia has the distinction of being the most common adult anxiety disorder, and is the third most common psychiatric disorder overall, with a lifetime prevalence of nearly 15%. Only depression and alcohol abuse occur more frequently. In children and adolescents, prior prevalence was frequently cited to be 1%, with the caveat that it is generally under-diagnosed in childhood and adolescence. A recent epidemiological survey showed a lifetime prevalence of 9.1% (in adolescents), with 1.3% having severe impairment [2]. Reasons for under-diagnosis include widespread failure of both parents and school personnel to identify the disorder, partly because they may not understand it to be anything other than "shyness," [112] and partly because these children, in their efforts to reduce their anxiety, do not draw attention to themselves and can be "invisible" to inattentive or misinformed adults.

Etiology and Natural History

Symptoms of SP begin to appear in adolescence, with diagnosis around age 15. Its typical course is chronic and unremitting, with lifelong symptoms that can lead to multiple, significant social impairments. Adults with SP are less likely to be married, more likely to be under-employed, and less likely to attain a high educational level [113]. Some 70–80% of adults with SP have at least one other psychiatric disorder, most frequently panic with agoraphobia, GAD, or simple phobia. In adults, the illness is now recognized for its pervasive and severely disabling nature.

Much less is known about pediatric SP. It has been diagnosed in children as young as 8 years of age, but is more commonly identified in early- to mid- adolescence. Its presentation varies with age. Younger children may cry, cling to their parents, or have temper tantrums when faced with a feared social situation. School-aged children may become oppositional and resist going to school. When in school, they may avoid class presentations, discussions, and physical education classes. Adolescents have an increased risk of alcohol abuse, school drop-out, suicide ideation, and suicide attempts. Conduct problems may appear [110]. Like adults with SP, children and adolescents are thought to have impaired social skills, although it has been suggested that it is less the absence of social skills and more the presence of anxiety that limits their use. Across all ages, somatic symptoms of distress, such as racing heart, sweating, tremulousness, lightheadedness, and gastrointestinal discomfort, are common [114].

Both concordance data [103] and proband studies [115] suggest a genetic predisposition to SP. Behavioral inhibition (BI), the predisposition to withdraw from novel circumstances, may be developmentally linked to SP [116]. High levels of parental criticism and over-control may be predisposing experiences [117], as may peer rejection and victimization experiences [118]. Once manifested, SP is maintained by negative perceptions and affect, social skill deficits, and the positive reinforcement of avoidance [119].

Diagnosis

Children with SP typically do not spontaneously report nor seek treatment for their disorder. Symptoms such as school refusal, test anxiety, shyness, poor peer relationships, difficulty using public restrooms, problems using the telephone, eating in front of others, and shrinking from social settings should alert the clinician to the need for a more systematic evaluation for social phobia. A thorough clinical evaluation should include interviews with both the child and the parents or primary caretakers, with a focus on physical symptoms, specific worries, and distressful situations characteristic of social phobia. Clinicians will often have to "pin down" the specific fears and situations with the child, as children are less adept at articulating their symptoms and will often report complaints in vague terms, for example, stomach aches, hating school, and "not liking" situations.

To date, there are no laboratory tests or physiological probes that have been demonstrated to be pathognomonic for SP. The Social Phobia and Anxiety Inventory for Children (SPAI-C) and the Social Phobia and Anxiety Inventory (SPAI) are empirically derived inventories meant to be used with children aged 8–14 years and over 14 years of age, respectively [120], for diagnostic assessment and clinical monitoring of treatment.

Differential Diagnosis

Panic disorder with agoraphobia, separation anxiety disorder, generalized anxiety disorder, and specific phobia are chief considerations in the differential diagnosis of SP.

Classically, SP is characterized by the avoidance of social situations in the absence of panic attacks (Table 13.6). Although social avoidance may occur in panic disorder with agoraphobia, it is the specific

Table 13.6 Social phobia: diagnostic features and associated disorders.

Discriminating features	Associated disorders
Relatively common, typically mid-teen onset	School refusal
Fear of social or performance settings	Panic attacks
Shyness	
General shy demeanor over time	
Somatic complaints to avoid social interactions	
Avoidance of peers	

fear of having a panic attack or being seen while having a panic attack that discriminates the two disorders. Fears in individuals with agoraphobia may or may not include the fear of scrutiny by others. Also, unlike SP, agoraphobic individuals may be reassured in social situations by the presence of a companion.

In separation anxiety disorder, the primary fear is one of separation from the primary caretaker. These individuals are usually comfortable in social settings in the home, whereas socially phobic individuals are distressed in social situations, even in the home.

In children with generalized anxiety disorder and specific phobia, fear of embarrassment or humiliation in social settings may occur but it is not the main focus of their anxiety. These individuals experience fear and anxiety apart from social contexts.

Social anxiety and avoidance are common in many disorders, for example, major depressive disorder, general medical disorders, and personality disorders, and the diagnosis of SP should not be made if another disorder better accounts for the social anxiety or if its occurrence is limited to the occurrence of the other disorder.

Finally, school refusal is a descriptive term for behavior that may indicate the presence of a specific phobia, separation anxiety, truancy, or SP, among other causes, but does not imply a specific psychiatric diagnosis.

Treatment

Rigorous treatment outcome data for children with SP are limited. While published support for the efficacy of cognitive behavioral therapies (CBT) are available, most studies do not focus on children with SP, but instead include them in the larger category of children with anxiety disorders [121]. Using the larger category of children with anxiety disorders, evidence does support the fact that CBT is more effective than nonspecific therapies [122]. Nonetheless, some SP-specific data are slowly becoming available. Beidel and colleagues [123] report considerable success with preadolescent children with SP symptoms, using a multifaceted behavioral treatment that combines social skills training with individual and group exposure sessions (but does not include cognitive restructuring), which Beidel calls Social Effectiveness Therapy for Children (SET-C). SET-C has been compared with fluoxetine and both treatments were superior to placebo, with the SET-C group showing greater improvement in social skills [124]. Albano and colleagues [125] have treated adolescents with a version of Cognitive-Behavioral Group Therapy for Adolescents (CBGT-A) adapted for SP, consisting of psychoeducation, cognitive restructuring, exposure, and skills building. Both short- and long-term control of symptoms were evidenced. Other reports have demonstrated the additional benefit of including parents in CBT-based treatment [126], and the potential for school-based CBT for adolescents [127]. Individual CBT is a more cost-effective treatment than family-oriented CBT [128]. The reports of successful interventions with CBT all share four treatment components: psychoeducation, exposure, skills building (relaxation training, cognitive restructuring, social skills, problem-solving skills), and homework [110]. Loneliness appears to be an important mediator of improvement in social anxiety, with one study showing that improvement in social anxiety and overall functioning are predicted by decreases in loneliness [129].

Following the lead of investigators of adult SP, preliminary reports on the utility of pharmacotherapy for children and adolescents with the disorder are beginning to appear. Both fluoxetine [130] and fluvoxamine [107] have been described as effective and well tolerated by children with anxiety disorders, including SP. Venlafaxine ER has also been shown to be effective and well tolerated in youths with social phobia [131]. A recent meta-analysis supports the efficacy of SSRIs for social anxiety in children [132].

Cognitive- and behavior-based strategies are the preferred treatment approaches for social phobia in children and adolescents. Where medications are indicated, despite the absence of FDA label indication in childhood, SSRIs are considered the pharmacologic treatment of choice. Empirical evidence and downward extrapolation from adult studies support the use of medication in treating social phobia.

Panic Disorder

Definition

Panic attacks are discrete, intense periods of fear and discomfort with cognitive and somatic symptoms that escalate in a crescendo fashion. Attacks may last minutes to, rarely, several hours. The attacks may be unexpected or "out of the blue," or they may be situationally predisposed (more likely but not always occurring in a specific context), or situationally bound (almost always occurring in a specific situation). Panic attacks, but not necessarily the disorder itself, may occur in association with specific phobias, PTSD, or SP, but by definition in panic disorder at least some of the panic attacks are unexpected.

Panic disorder (PD) is diagnosed when the attacks are recurrent, and at least one of the attacks is followed by a month or more period of worried anticipation for additional attacks and/or concern for negative consequences of an attack, to the point where it may change behavior. Agoraphobia (fear and avoidance of situations in which a panic attack may occur or in which escape may be difficult) may or may not complicate the disorder.

Incidence and Prevalence

Studies of adolescents in community samples report that between 2% and 18% of adolescents have experienced at least one four-symptom panic attack, when these are identified via a structured psychiatric interview. Higher prevalence reports of 43% to 60% are found with adolescent self-report questionnaires. Prevalence of PD is reported to be between 0.5% and 5%, with greater representation in pediatric psychiatric clinic populations, for example, up to 10% of referrals [133]. Females are more frequently afflicted than males [134]. Reliable epidemiological data are not available for preadolescents.

An earlier and well-accepted model of PD [135] posited that panic attacks were the result of "catastrophic misinterpretation" of ongoing somatic sensations. Because young children are considered lacking in the cognitive skills necessary to make these cognitive evaluations, it was long believed that children could not be diagnosed with PD [136]. Subsequent reports of clear panic attacks in children have challenged this theory, although it has remained useful for treatment.

Etiology and Natural History

Panic disorder may have a bimodal onset, the first peak occurring between the ages of 15 to 19 years, and the second, smaller peak in the mid-30s. Development of

PD in early childhood or after the mid-40s, although possible, is considered a rarity. Panic attacks, as well as PD, are more likely in older children and adolescents than in younger children [137]. In adolescence, boys and girls are equally likely to experience panic attacks, but a diagnosis of PD is made more frequently with girls [138].

Following a lively debate in the literature, which eventually acknowledged the existence of prepubertal panic attacks, some investigators still maintain that preadolescent "panic" is not a genuine disorder, but rather an associated feature of another disorder, such as SP [95]. A more common position is that SP is linked to PD, via genetics, experience, or in some other indirect way, such as a shared relation to major depressive disorder (MDD). While this issue remains open, there is evidence disputing a direct developmental link [16, 133].

The symptoms most frequently reported by children and adolescents during panic attacks change with age [139]. For the youngest children, the most common somatic complaints are palpitations, shortness of breath, sweating, fainting, and weakness. In adolescence, new somatic symptoms emerge, including chest pain, flushing, trembling, headache, and vertigo. Cognitive symptoms are a delayed manifestation, relative to somatic symptoms, with the earliest reports of children and early adolescents being typically limited to fear of dying. Fear of going crazy and depersonalization-derealization tend to follow.

Risk factors for PD include female sex, MDD, high anxiety sensitivity (an increased tendency to respond fearfully to anxiety symptoms), negative affectivity (a temperamental tendency toward fear, sadness, self-dissatisfaction, hostility, and worry in the face of negative stimuli), and a family history of MDD and PD [133, 138]. Up to 90% of children and adolescents with PD have comorbidities, most frequently MDD and other anxiety disorders (GAD, SAD, social phobia, agoraphobia). Up to 50% report somatoform disorders, substance use disorders, conduct disorder, oppositional defiant disorder, attention-deficit hyperactivity disorder, and bipolar disorder [133].

Diagnosis

A somewhat intricate relationship between PD, other anxiety disorders, and depression calls for a thorough clinical assessment (Table 13.7). A detailed history should be obtained from the patient, family members, teachers, and other professionals acquainted with the child. Discerning whether the child can predict the onset of the attack is important for differential diagnosis (e.g., a specific phobia vs situationally bound vs "out of the blue" panic attack). Pediatric and neurological exams

Table 13.7 Panic disorder: diagnostic features and associated disorders.

Discriminating features	Associated disorders
Rare in children, more common in teens	Agoraphobia
Unexpected anxiety attacks	Panic attacks
Sudden/crescendo anxiety, "fear of fear"	
Somatic anxiety, feelings of loss of control/disaster/ impending doom	
Somatic symptoms (tachypnea, chest tightness, tachycardia),	
Discrete episodes of extreme anxiety	

can be helpful in some instances to elucidate the origin of somatic complaints or unusual sensations. Anxiety symptom scales may provide useful diagnostic information and later assist in evaluating treatment progress.

Differential Diagnosis

It is essential to differentiate PD from medical conditions such as hyperthyroidism, hyperparathyroidism, pheochromocytoma, diabetes, asthma, seizures, vestibular dysfunction, or cardiac problems. Intoxication with stimulants or withdrawal from sedatives can produce symptoms that mimic panic attacks.

Differentiating PD from other anxiety disorders can be challenging. Fear and panic occurring only when a child is separated from an attachment figure points to separation anxiety rather than panic disorder. If the discomfort is experienced only in situations when one is subjected to scrutiny, social phobia is a more likely diagnosis. In specific phobia, fear and anxiety are an expected response to confrontation of the phobic object. Recollection of past trauma usually precedes emotional and autonomic distress in post-traumatic stress sufferers. Obsessions and compulsive rituals will help differentiate panic disorder from obsessive-compulsive disorder. The generic descriptor "school phobia" needs to be precisely defined symptomatically and operationally in order to differentiate its etiology as anxiety related (panic, phobic, or separation) or due to another cause (e.g., truancy).

The absence of panic-like symptoms will distinguish PD from dissociative disorders manifested by depersonalization/derealization. Although some psychotic disorders may have panic as an associated feature, PD patients do not have thought disorders.

Treatment

Behavioral, cognitive, and pharmacologic treatments of panic disorder in children have for the most part been extrapolated from the adult literature, with some necessary modifications. Ollendick [140] and Hoffman and Mattis [141] report success using modified CBT programs with adolescents diagnosed with PD. Diler [133] recommends that such therapies focus on modifying the patient's interpretation of their bodily processes, as well as changing the behaviors that maintain their previous "catastrophic" interpretations.

While no controlled trials to evaluate the efficacy of behavioral and cognitive approaches in children have been undertaken, anecdotal data suggest that systematic desensitization may be helpful in the treatment of agoraphobia. Exposure techniques may be particularly helpful in situationally bound and predisposed panic attacks.

Masi and colleagues [142] reported considerable success in their open-label treatment of adolescent PD with paroxetine. Diler [133] reviews small-scale studies describing success with imipramine, alprazolam, clonazepam, and other SSRIs. More systematic studies are necessary before a recommendation regarding pharmacotherapy can be made. However, clinical wisdom is leaning heavily in favor of the use of SSRIs when there is significant debility.

Obsessive-Compulsive Disorder

Definition

The essential features of obsessive-compulsive disorder (OCD) include the recurrence of obsessions and/or compulsions severe enough to be time consuming (i.e., more than 1 hour per day), and causing marked impairment or significant distress. Obsessions are recurrent and persistent thoughts, urges, impulses, or images that are experienced as intrusive and inappropriate and that cause anxiety or distress. Compulsions are repetitive behaviors (e.g., hand-washing, ordering, checking) or mental acts (e.g., praying, counting, repeating words silently) that the person feels driven to perform in response to an obsession. The behaviors or mental acts are aimed at preventing some dreaded event or situation, or in order to get something "just so." Children may or may not recognize that the obsessions or compulsions are unreasonable or excessive, and this criterion is not necessary in order to make a pediatric diagnosis.

Incidence and Prevalence

Obsessive-compulsive disorder is more common in children and adolescents than was once thought. Prevalence estimates, which have been widely discrepant in the past due to varied collection and diagnostic techniques [95], are now reported to be around 2% [143]. Cases of clinically significant OCD need to be distinguished from the subclinical obsessions and compulsions experienced by large numbers of children and adolescents in the course of normal development [100, 144].

Etiology and Natural History

Like adults, children with OCD tend to present with both obsessions and compulsions, although independent presentations of compulsions and (less likely) obsessions are possible. Young children in particular may present with ritualistic behaviors unassociated with compulsions and may not experience anxiety or feel distressed while performing them [145]. Symptoms tend to follow adult patterns: at some time during the course of the illness, washing rituals affect more than 85% of children with OCD, repeating rituals 51%, and checking rituals 46% [146]. Ordering, arranging, counting, collecting, ensuring symmetry, and a preoccupation with having said or done the right thing are all common.

The mean age of onset is 10.3 years, with males outnumbering females by a 3:2 ratio [143]. Surprisingly, symptoms are present for 5 to 8 years before they come to clinical attention [144]. The disproportionate representation of male relative to female cases in childhood OCD is different from the adult disorder (where males and females are equally affected) and likely due to the earlier age of onset for boys [147]. Early-onset OCD has been posited as a special subtype of OCD, perhaps genetically related to tic disorders, which are more prevalent for males [148].

OCD is characterized by a waxing and waning course, with symptoms often worsened by stress, although this is not invariant. Males are more likely than females to have a chronic rather than episodic course [149, 150]. In the vast majority of patients, specific symptoms are numerous, appear and disappear, vary in intensity, and change in content over the course of the illness.

Childhood-onset OCD is a chronic and debilitating illness. It is complicated by high comorbidity rates with other disorders, including mood disorders (8–73%), other anxiety disorders (13–70%), disruptive behavior disorders (3–57%), tic disorders/Tourette's syndrome (13–26%), speech/developmental disorders (13–27%), enuresis (7–37%), and pervasive developmental disorders (3–7%) [143]. Studies indicate that the majority of children with OCD will require long-term medication treatment and that although as many as 80% will experience improvement, a significant proportion (43–68%) will continue to meet diagnostic criteria for OCD [146].

Since the presentation of and initial support for the serotonin hypothesis [151], much new information has come to light with respect to the pathogenesis of OCD. While support for the major role played by serotonin has continued, other neurotransmitters, such as dopamine and glutamate, have been suggested as important mediators of the disorder. The cortico-striato-thalamo-cortical (CSTC) circuit has been identified, with dysfunction in this circuit tied to OCD symptoms in ways consistent with our understanding of mediating neurotransmitters [152]. Structural and functional imaging studies of children and adolescents with OCD are currently being undertaken; although they lag behind information obtained with adult patients, so far they support the accumulating data and developing theory of functional deficits in the CSTC circuit [153, 154].

Current clinical research focuses on the heterogeneity of OCD. Several factor analytic studies have consistently identified at least four stable dimensions: contamination/washing, aggressive/checking, hoarding, and asymmetry/ordering, each posited to represent a potential subtype, with different presumed genetic features, comorbidities, and responses to treatment. How these subtypes converge upon shared cortical and subcortical circuitry remains to be illuminated, although presumably it will involve a model of different phenotypes, different or overlapping etiologies, but a shared common pathway of expression.

Diagnosis

Accurate diagnosis of pediatric OCD is complicated by comorbid disorders, a waxing and waning course, changes in favored obsessions and compulsions, and potential confusion with developmentally appropriate expression of fearful preoccupations and rituals (Table 13.8). Additionally, many children feel shameful

Table 13.8 Obsessive-compulsive disorder: diagnostic features and associated disorders.

Discriminating features	Associated disorders
Ruminations and rituals	Second anxiety disorder
Washing, repeating, checking	Tics, Tourette's syndrome
"Just so" concerns	Attention-deficit
Counting, getting stuck	hyperactivity disorder
Rigid routines	
Need to confess	

about their obsessions and compulsions, making disclosure difficult. Consequently, careful history taking from the parents or primary caregiver and the use of semi-structured interview scales are useful in making the diagnosis. Input from siblings, teachers, and daycare providers can be helpful.

The primary instrument for assessing OCD in children and adolescents is the Children's version of the Yale-Brown Obsessive Compulsive Scale (CY-BOCS), which can be useful to rate the severity of the disorder as well as to monitor its treatment progress [155]. A companion instrument, the CY-BOCS Symptom Checklist, is an extremely useful paper-and-pencil checklist for parents and children to identify current and past obsessions and compulsions. It is a time-efficient way to survey a vast array of symptoms and is helpful in mapping treatment target symptoms. The Leyton Obsessional Inventory-Child Version (LOI-CV) [156] is an acceptable self-report assessment instrument. A shorter version of the LOI-CV is available, purporting to have similar psychometric soundness [157].

Differential Diagnosis

Because of the comorbidity of OCD and Tourette syndrome, a disorder of chronic motor and vocal tics, it is necessary to distinguish complex motor tics from a true ritual. Tics are usually not heralded by a preceding thought or obsession.

The stereotypies and repetitive movements seen in mental retardation and pervasive developmental disorder tend to be more fixed than the broader symptom picture of OCD.

Obsessive ruminations in depressed or dysthymic individuals can often mimic OCD symptoms, although in the former case mood symptoms predominate. Similarly, although obsessions or compulsions can occur in psychotic disorders, there is by definition no disorder in reality testing in OCD. The individual with OCD is often aware of the ridiculous or unreasonable nature of the cognition or behavior, although in younger children this is not a required feature of the diagnosis.

OCD symptoms associated with PANDAS (pediatric autoimmune neuropsychiatric disorders associated with streptococcal infections) have a temporal relationship with group A beta-hemolytic streptococcal infections and are sometimes associated with choreiform movements [158].

The eating rituals of anorexic or bulimic patients and the rigid personality traits characteristic of obsessive-compulsive personality disorder (OCPD) need to be considered in the differential diagnosis of OCD. OCPD is present in a minority of cases and often improves with successful treatment of OCD. Curiously, individuals with OCPD may not find their "symptoms" debilitating and may in fact believe their rigidity and obsessiveness are means to success.

Treatment

The American Academy of Child and Adolescent Psychiatry has established practice parameters for the treatment of OCD in pediatric patients [159]. Here, recommendation is made that CBT, with or without medication, be considered the first-line treatment. Graduated exposure and response prevention (E/RP) has been demonstrated to have a respectable success rate with durability of effect [160]. In this technique, identification of all obsessions and compulsions is followed by assignment of a stimulus hierarchy, ranked by "subjective units of discomfort" (SUDS). Exposure tasks are then undertaken with concurrent prevention of the usual obsessive or compulsive behavior. Repeated presentation of the anxiety-invoking stimulus ensues, based on least to greatest SUDS, in the absence of the avoidance response, until they evoke minimal anxiety. This treatment approach is based on the principle that anxiety responses will habituate and eventually extinguish in the presence of repeated presentations of the anxiety stimulus, in the absence of an escape or avoidance response (i.e., performing the compulsive ritual). The specifics of the treatment have been described elsewhere and a manualized treatment program of E/RP is available [161]. Mild cases of OCD are likely best treated initially with behavioral techniques exclusively, with adjunctive pharmacologic treatment reserved for moderate-to-severe cases.

The greatest number of pharmacologic studies of childhood anxiety disorders to date have examined the use of SSRIs in pediatric OCD [162]. Pharmacotherapy with serotonergic agents such as clomipramine (at 3–5 mg/kg/day) [163] and various SSRIs (fluoxetine: up to 60 mg/day; sertraline: up to 200 mg/day; fluvoxamine: up to 200 mg/day) has demonstrated effectiveness in the treatment of children with OCD [164–166]. Three SSRIs, fluvoxamine (Luvox), sertraline (Zoloft), and fluoxetine (Prozac), have FDA label indications for the treatment of OCD in childhood and adolescence. Because side effects with the SSRIs tend to be fewer, these agents are typically preferred, with a 12-week trial of an adequate dose recommended before the trial is considered a failure. Following failure of a second SRI, a course of clomipramine should be considered. Augmentation with a neuroleptic, such as risperidone [167], is an alternative strategy for those with a limited response to SRIs. In general, published studies reveal that 40–50%

of patients will experience a 25–40% reduction in symptoms with their first trial of medication. Medication treatment may be particularly indicated in cases of OCD where primary obsessional OCD is present (e.g., primary obsessional slowness) and target compulsions amenable to CBT are lacking. Treatment reports of PANDAS-related OCD with immunoglobulin and plasmapheresis therapies have been primarily limited to specialty or research settings [158].

Selective Mutism

Definition

The term elective mutism was coined by Tramer in 1934 to describe a population of children who speak only in certain situations or to certain people. Historically, a variety of etiologies for this disorder have been presented, with support for a particular etiology frequently limited to a single case study. In this manner, the disorder has variously been attributed to early psychological trauma [168], dysfunctional family dynamics involving mother-child enmeshment [169], a learned behavior reinforced by the child's environment [170], a manifestation of unresolved conflict [171], or the defiant refusal to speak [172]. The heterogeneous nature of these proposed etiologies has been cited as one justification for the disorder's current classification as a Disorder Usually First Diagnosed in Infancy [173].

In 1994, DSM-IV renamed the disorder *selective mutism*. Consistent with that change has since come theoretical consideration of selective mutism as a symptom of an anxiety disorder, or a variant of a specific anxiety disorder, such as social phobia, which would address the "selective" nature of the mutism [174].

Selective mutism is characterized by the consistent failure to speak in specific social situations in which there is the expectancy for speech, despite speaking in other situations, such as the home. The failure to speak is not due to a lack of knowledge or comfort with social communication or a specific language (such as might occur for immigrants), and is debilitating to the individual. It is not diagnosed when better accounted for by embarrassment related to speech or language abilities, or by another psychiatric disorder.

Incidence/Prevalence

Prevalence estimates of selective mutism range from 0.03% to 2% [110]. While it has widely been assumed to be rare, some investigators are now calling this into question [175], as estimates are increasing with accumulating data. Most cases do not come to medical attention and resolve with age.

Etiology and Natural History

The mean age of onset ranges from 2.7 to 4.1 years [176]. Seventy percent of referrals occur during kindergarten years, with boys being referred an average of 2.3 years earlier than girls. The disorder is more common in girls than boys, with a ratio of about 3:1. Symptoms may be present several years before a referral is made, which typically occurs through the school in the early school-age years [177]. This time lag between onset of symptoms and diagnosis is likely due to symptoms not being present in the home.

A wide variety of psychiatric symptoms have been reported to be associated with selective mutism. Premorbid speech and language difficulties [178], developmental disorders [179], and Asperger's disorder [180] have all been reported to occur at elevated rates for this group. Higher rates of enuresis, encopresis, depression, and separation anxiety have been suggested [181], although demonstrations of these are not consistent [182].

Remarkably consistent are associations between selective mutism and anxiety disorders. Black and Uhde described a population of children with selective mutism, nearly all of whom (97%) also met criteria for social phobia or avoidant behavior, and most of whom (70%) had a parent who met the same criteria [182]. Dummit and colleagues [183] reported 100% of their sample of 50 to be comorbid for either social anxiety or avoidant disorder, and 48% of them had additional anxiety disorders. Kristensen [179] found selective mutism to have 74% comorbidity with anxiety disorders. In general, there is increasing evidence for a high association of selective mutism with anxiety disorders.

The majority of children with selective mutism appear to outgrow their disorder although it is not uncommon for the disorder to persist for several years in elementary school. There is some evidence to indicate that children who do not improve by the age of 10 years have an intractable form of the disorder [178].

Diagnosis

Diagnosis is based on clinical history (Table 13.9). Children with selective mutism should receive a complete medical history and physical examination. Neurological examination and developmental history should focus on motor, cognitive, language, and social milestones. Quality of temperament and social interactions, and the precise contexts in which speech occurs should be assessed. Formal hearing, speech, and language

Table 13.9 Selective mutism: diagnostic features and associated disorders.

Discriminating features	Associated disorders
Refusal to speak in school/ socially despite ability	Social phobia
Early childhood onset (3–6 years)	
Shyness, reticence with peers	
Tendency to isolate	

assessment (sometimes utilizing the child's audio-recorded speech) may be necessary.

Differential Diagnosis

Shyness, unfamiliarity with the language, or the presence of a communication disorder may be mistaken for selective mutism. Children with disorders such as schizophrenia, mental retardation, or Pervasive Developmental Disorder (PDD) may be unable to speak in social situations. However, selective mutism should only be diagnosed in a child with an established capacity to speak in some social situations, such as at home. The presence of a comorbid anxiety (e.g., social phobia), communication (e.g., stuttering), or other disorder should be diagnosed when present. It is worth noting that the presence of selective mutism *does not* imply that a child has been abused. Finally, rare cases of mutism can occur following operations on the posterior fossa, usually to remove large tumors, or on the corpus callosum, usually to improve intractable epilepsy [184].

Treatment

Historically, treatments for selective mutism have included a range of individual, family, behavioral, and psychodynamic modalities. Evidence-based treatment literature is limited. Psychodynamic treatments, in isolation, have generally fared poorly, although they may provide a supportive role, and facilitate social interactions and understanding of family issues unique to the child.

A multimodal approach with or without pharmacotherapy is the treatment of choice. The child should not be removed from the classroom for initiation of treatment. Cognitive behavioral therapy is the primary intervention aimed at reducing the child's anxiety inhibiting speech and positively reinforcing the child for speaking. An attitude of expectation for normal speech and reinforcement for efforts to speak are important. Behavioral treatments are time consuming, requiring persistence and the cooperation of parents, teachers, and other professionals. The child should not be removed from the classroom setting during treatment.

Psychosocial interventions utilizing modeling and peer pressure may be used to reinforce incremental or successive approximations of speech (e.g., hand raising, whispering) in the context of small groups of adults or peers. Family therapy may provide a powerful context for support, for understanding the dynamics of the mutism, and an opportunity for application of cognitive and behavioral interventions.

Pharmacotherapy for selective mutism includes the use of SSRIs, such as fluoxetine and sertraline [182, 185], and the monoamine oxidase inhibitor phenelzine (at doses up to 2 mg/kg/day) [186]. Evidence is preliminary at best, but a trial of an SSRI, or failing that phenelzine, should be considered when the symptoms of selective mutism are debilitating, of long duration, or refractory to other interventions.

Summary

Anxiety symptoms are ubiquitous in youth. In addition to being a burden on children and families, anxiety disorders in children are a great burden on society. A recent study showed that the average family of an anxious child costs society 21 times more money than the typical family [187]. Clinicians need to be familiar with the normal developmental course of anxieties in youth and their consequent mastery by children in order to differentiate normative versus pathological anxiety. Anxiety symptoms do not necessarily constitute an anxiety disorder. Adept assessment and management of anxiety symptoms through reassurance, anticipatory guidance, and psychoeducation of parents may forestall the development of full-blown anxiety syndromes.

Owing to anxiety disorders being among the most common psychiatric disorders in youth, clinicians need to maintain a high index of suspicion for them. A biopsychosocial approach to assessment utilizing multiple informants as well as paper-and-pencil assessment instruments will assist in the accurate screening and diagnosis of these disorders. The hallmark of all anxiety disorders is debility in life functioning attributable to fear or distress that is inappropriate in its intensity, frequency, or context.

Empirically driven theories and treatment strategies, often in manualized form, are emerging for children and adolescents with anxiety disorders. Data are beginning to emerge regarding the effectiveness of pharmacologic strategies for treating childhood anxiety, especially in regard to the SSRIs. Despite the current controversy regarding potential suicidal ideation in youth related to these agents, SSRIs can be used safely and effectively with judicious selection and appropriate symptom monitoring by clinicians. The most successful treatments are typically multimodal, involving interventions that are educational and skills based, with a focus on exposure and mastery, and that involve both the child and the important adults in the child's environment. The two case vignettes at the end of the chapter illustrate some of the complexities involved in assessment and treatment of rather typical anxiety disorder presentations in youth.

The field of child and adolescent anxiety disorder research is rapidly evolving, offering new insights into the etiology, developmental course, and outcome of childhood anxiety disorders as well as the promise for more effective treatment interventions.

Vignette 1: Anxiety Comorbid with ADHD in an Adolescent Female

History and Chief Complaint

Sheila, a 13-year-old eighth grader, presented for evaluation of depression on referral from her school guidance counselor. Sheila's history was significant for shyness noted in kindergarten and elementary school. She struggled academically throughout her early school years to attain average grades despite special education accommodations in the classroom. Her elementary school teachers described Sheila as being "spacey and disconnected." Psychoeducational testing revealed that Sheila had a full-scale IQ of 102 (Verbal = 104, Performance = 98) and did not meet criteria for a specific learning disability.

Sheila's parents described her as a shy and immature girl who was somewhat over-dependent, disorganized, and unsure of herself. Socially she had few friends and tended to avoid group activities or sports. At home, Sheila exhibited a low tolerance for frustration and was known to be "prickly" and bossy, often becoming irritable and frequently whining when her needs were not immediately met. She also engaged in frequent reassurance seeking from her parents and tended to have multiple somatic complaints including stomach aches, which contributed to her frequent absences from school.

The eighth grade represented a transition to a new school for Sheila. She started out the year without apparent problems but over the course of the first quarter, her academic performance began to decline. She had increasing trouble completing her homework without hours of prompting and assistance from her parents. She had frequent absences and tended to withdraw and isolate herself from peers while in school. Sensing that Sheila was depressed her guidance counselor advised Sheila's parents to pursue an evaluation for possible depression.

Psychiatric Evaluation

Sheila presented as a thin, quiet, early adolescent female who was appropriately, if plainly, dressed and groomed. She had difficulty maintaining eye contact, spoke in a quiet voice, and gave only brief answers to interviewer questions. There was no evidence of psychosis, suicidal ideation, or suicidal intent. Sheila's mood was self-described as "OK," but she appeared mildly dysphoric. Sheila denied frank depressed mood. She did, however, endorse multiple symptoms of anxiety as well as anxious cognitions. Sheila stated that she had great difficulty keeping focused on her teacher's lectures in the classroom setting and was often easily distracted by sounds in or outside the classroom as well as getting lost in her own thoughts. She reported that she was always anxious that she would be called on in class and that she would say something stupid and be laughed at by her peers. She was highly anxious of both peer criticism and performance situations such as test taking and in-class oral presentations. In these situations her heart would pound, her palms and underarms would sweat, her mouth would become dry, and she would feel short of breath. In several oral classroom presentations, Sheila reported that she became so paralyzed by her anxiety symptoms that she froze and subsequently fled the classroom. She reported that she had begun to anticipate these highly distressing anxiety episodes and that she feared entering the school building in the morning. Sheila's difficulties were compounded by a social scene that had intimidating cliques of seemingly confident and outgoing girls who were more physically mature than Sheila.

Family history was positive for a presumptive history of ADHD in Sheila's father. Sheila's mother had been treated as a late adolescent for depression.

Psychiatric Assessment

Assessment revealed that Sheila met DSM-IV diagnostic criteria for Attention-Deficit Hyperactivity, Inattentive Subtype as well as for Generalized Anxiety Disorder. In addition, although Sheila did not meet criteria for Panic Disorder, she did experience isolated situationally bound panic attacks in performance situations.

Treatment

Sheila was referred for cognitive behavioral therapy to target her anxiety symptoms with a focus on skills-based training. Special emphasis was given to targeting performance-based situations in which Sheila could practice exposure and response prevention as well as anxiety management training skills. Pharmacotherapy trials resulted in several medications being evaluated before arriving at a successful combination of a long-acting stimulant plus a selective serotonin reuptake inhibitor.

Discussion

Sheila's case highlights several important features of anxiety disorder presentations in adolescence. First, anxiety can often mimic other psychiatric disorders. Sheila's counselor mistakenly attributed her isolation, withdrawal, school absences, and academic struggles as signs of depression rather than the consequences of anxiety and ADHD. Second, anxiety disorders frequently occur comorbidly with other diagnoses. In this case Sheila's comorbid condition was ADHD, Inattentive Type, a diagnosis frequently overlooked in girls who present without disruptive behavioral problems. Comorbid psychiatric conditions can often display a complex array of symptoms that, taken together, may mimic other psychiatric disorders such as depression. In Sheila's case, a thorough and detailed psychiatric evaluation was able to pinpoint the presence of attention and concentration problems along with significant anxiety symptoms. The two disorders acted synergistically to exacerbate one another leading to a progressive downward spiral of performance across all important domains of Sheila's functioning. Finally, Sheila's treatment involved a multiple modality approach with combination CBT and pharmacotherapy. Because the combination of ADHD and anxiety can be difficult to treat pharmacologically, several medication trials were necessary before arriving at a successful combination.

Vignette 2: ADHD with Comorbid Anxiety in a School-Age Boy

History and Chief Complaint

Tommy, a 6-year-old first grader, was referred for psychiatric evaluation for attention-deficit hyperactivity disorder. Tommy's mother reported that he had been anxious and a "worry wort" since the age of two. Tommy's parents had divorced when he was 3 years old and he currently lived with his mother. Mother noted that Tommy had become increasingly irritable and clingy over the past year, subsequent to the death of his grandmother, to whom he was particularly close. Tommy had experienced academic and behavioral difficulties since kindergarten. Always an active and rambunctious youngster, Tommy was seen as disruptive and somewhat aggressive toward his peers in kindergarten. He would often throw temper tantrums in the morning and refuse to allow his mother to leave him in the kindergarten classroom. In first grade, Tommy's teacher noted that he appeared deconcentrated, had difficulty settling down to complete his work, and was often oppositional, argumentative, and disruptive with peers in class. Reading was difficult owing to Tommy's impatience and he was seen as a highly impulsive youngster with low frustration tolerance. Transitions were particularly difficult.

At home Mother reported that Tommy was a high-need youngster who was very busy. He demanded constant attention and could not engage in independent activities, even for short periods of time. Mother noted that she could not be in the bathroom by herself and that Tommy insisted on being there with her, although he would turn away from her in order to "give her privacy." Bedtime was difficult. Typically, it would take several hours for Tommy to get to sleep. He would cry out, leave his room for the company of his Mother, and make repeated demands for a drink, a story, or trips to the bathroom. At the time of psychiatric evaluation, Tommy's mother reported that she was exhausted and despite the seemingly endless time commitment to Tommy, the situation was worsening.

Psychiatric Evaluation

Tommy presented as a healthy appearing 6-year-old male who was noted to be fidgety and who continually interrupted his mother during the psychiatric interview. Tommy was seen as a highly distractible youngster who had difficulty sustaining his focus in either play activities or in direct conversation with the examiner. His mood was noted to be mildly irritable but he denied frank sadness, tearfulness, or depression. There was no evidence of psychosis, or hypomanic or manic symptoms. Tommy endorsed multiple fears and worries. Since the death of his grand-

mother, Tommy had been having nightmares that his mother was killed in an automobile accident. He had intrusive thoughts during the day that his mother would become ill or would die, and that he would be left alone in the world. He reported that these fears were especially strong in the morning, when his mother would drop him off at school, and in the evening prior to bedtime.

History was negative for abuse or trauma exposure. Family history was significant for probable ADHD, anger problems, and substance abuse in Tommy's father.

The Child Behavior Checklist, filled out by Tommy's mother and teacher, indicated that Tommy had clinically significant scores on both internalizing and externalizing symptom domains. His Connors ADHD rating scale, which his mother and teacher completed, indicated highly significant core symptoms of ADHD including concentration problems, impulsivity, and hyperactivity.

Assessment

Tommy was diagnosed with Attention-Deficit Hyperactivity Disorder, Combined Type; Oppositional Defiant Disorder; Separation Anxiety Disorder; and Generalized Anxiety Disorder.

Treatment

Treatment was initiated involving parent-guided behavioral management training to target Tommy's oppositional and defiant symptoms, along with individual skills-based CBT to give Tommy tactics that he could use to identify and combat his anxious thoughts. Tommy and his mother "rehearsed being brave" in progressively longer and longer separations, after which Tommy was reinforced with access to his Game Boy. Pharmacotherapy was initiated with a long-acting stimulant medication in the morning supplemented by clonidine at bedtime for sleep initiation. However, Tommy exhibited an increase in daytime anxiety symptoms and irritability in response to stimulant medication. Ultimately, Tommy was switched to a nonstimulant ADHD treatment and his stimulant and clonidine were tapered to discontinuation. Improvement was noted in core ADHD symptoms as well as anxiety. Tommy was able to separate from his mother without undue distress and sleep latency was less than 30 minutes.

Discussion

Owing to the disruptive nature of Tommy's behaviors, Tommy's teacher failed to see the significant anxiety component in Tommy's symptom picture. Much of Tommy's seemingly disruptive, oppositional, and hyperactive behaviors were in fact being driven, or at least exacerbated, by the significant anxiety that Tommy was experiencing. Treatment involved multiple modalities. Pharmacotherapy targeted Tommy's core ADHD and anxiety symptoms; CBT provided Tommy with anxiety management skills; and parent behavioral management training provided his mother with skills for dealing with Tommy's anxious and oppositional behaviors.

References

1. Merikangas KR, He JP, Burstein M, *et al.* Service utilization for lifetime mental disorders in U.S. adolescents: results of the National Comorbidity Survey-Adolescent Supplement (NCS-A). *J Am Acad Child Adolesc Psychiat* 2011;**50**:32–45.

2. Merikangas KR, He JP, Burstein M, *et al.* Lifetime prevalence of mental disorders in U.S. adolescents: results from the National Comorbidity Survey Replication-Adolescent Supplement (NCS-A). *J Am Acad Child Adolesc Psychiat* 2010;**49**:980–989.

3. American Psychiatric Association, American Psychiatric Association. Task Force on DSM-IV. *Diagnostic and Statistical Manual of Mental Disorders,* 4th edn, text revision (*DSM-IV-TR*). Washington, DC: American Psychiatric Association, 2000.

4. Masi G, Mucci M, Millepiedi S. Separation anxiety disorder in children and adolescents: epidemiology, diagnosis and management. *CNS Drugs* 2001;**15**:93–104.

5. Bell-Dolan D, Brazeal TJ. Separation anxiety disorder, overanxious disorder and school refusal. *Child Adolesc Psychiatr Clin N Am* 1993;**2**:563–580.

6. Compton SN, Nelson AH, March JS. Social phobia and separation anxiety symptoms in community and clinical samples of children and adolescents. *J Am Acad Child Adolesc Psychiat* 2000;**39**:1040–1046.

7. Last CG, Hersen M, Kazdin AE, Finkelstein R, Strauss CC. Comparison of DSM-III separation anxiety and overanxious disorders: demographic characteristics and patterns of comorbidity. *J Am Acad Child Adolesc Psychiat* 1987;**26**:527–531.

8. Francis G, Last CG, Strauss CC. Expression of separation anxiety disorder: the roles of age and gender. *Child Psychiatry Hum Dev* 1987;**18**:82–89.

9. Mahler MS, Pine F, Bergman A. *The Psychological Birth of the Human Infant: Symbiosis and Individuation.* New York: Basic Books, 1975.

10. Kagan J, Snidman N, Arcus D. Childhood derivatives of high and low reactivity in infancy. *Child Dev* 1998;**69**:1483–1493.

11. Dallaire DH, Weinraub M. Predicting children's separation anxiety at age 6: the contributions of infant-mother attachment security, maternal sensitivity, and maternal separation anxiety. *Attach Hum Dev* 2005;**7**:393–408.

12. Silove D, Manicavasagar V. Adults who feared school: is early separation anxiety specific to the pathogenesis of panic disorder? *Acta Psychiatr Scand* 1993;**88**:385–390.

13. Silove D, Harris M, Morgan A, *et al.* Is early separation anxiety a specific precursor of panic disorder-agoraphobia? A community study. *Psychol Med* 1995;**25**:405–411.

14. Fagiolini A, Shear MK, Cassano GB, Frank E. Is lifetime separation anxiety a manifestation of panic spectrum? *CNS Spectrums* 1998;**3**:63–73.

15. Manicavasagar V, Silove D. Is there an adult form of separation anxiety disorder? A brief clinical report. *Aust N Z J Psychiatry* 1997;**31**:299–303.

16. Aschenbrand SG, Kendall PC, Webb A, Safford SM, Flannery-Schroeder E. Is childhood separation anxiety disorder a predictor of adult panic disorder and agoraphobia? A seven-year longitudinal study. *J Am Acad Child Adolesc Psychiat* 2003;**42**:1478–1485.

17. Biederman J, Petty CR, Faraone SV, *et al.* Antecedents to panic disorder in nonreferred adults. *J Clin Psychiatry* 2006;**67**:1179–1186.

18. Biederman J, Petty CR, Hirshfeld-Becker DR, *et al.* Developmental trajectories of anxiety disorders in offspring at high risk for panic disorder and major depression. *Psychiatry Res* 2007;**153**:245–252.

19. Biederman J, Petty C, Faraone SV, *et al.* Childhood antecedents to panic disorder in referred and nonreferred adults. *J Child Adolesc Psychopharmacol* 2005;**15**:549–561.

20. March JS. *Anxiety Disorders in Children and Adolescents.* New York: Guilford Press, 1995.

21. Kashani JH, Orvaschel H. A community study of anxiety in children and adolescents. *Am J Psychiatry* 1990;**147**:313–318.

22. Keller MB, Lavori PW, Wunder J, Beardslee WR, Schwartz CE, Roth J. Chronic course of anxiety disorders in children and adolescents. *J Am Acad Child Adolesc Psychiat* 1992;**31**:595–599.

23. Doerfler LA, Toscano PF Jr, Connor DF. Separation anxiety and panic disorder in clinically referred youth. *J Anxiety Disord* 2008;**22**:602–611.

24. Lewinsohn PM, Holm-Denoma JM, Small JW, Seeley JR, Joiner TE Jr. Separation anxiety disorder in childhood as a risk factor for future mental illness. *J Am Acad Child Adolesc Psychiat* 2008;**47**:548–555.

25. Birmaher B, Brent DA, Chiappetta L, Bridge J, Monga S, Baugher M. Psychometric properties of the Screen for Child Anxiety Related Emotional Disorders (SCARED): a replication study. *J Am Acad Child Adolesc Psychiat* 1999;**38**:1230–1236.

26. March JS, Parker JD, Sullivan K, Stallings P, Conners CK. The Multidimensional Anxiety Scale for Children (MASC): factor structure, reliability, and validity. *J Am Acad Child Adolesc Psychiat* 1997;**36**:554–565.

27. Mendez X, Espada JP, Orgiles M, Hidalgo MD, Garcia-Fernandez JM. Psychometric properties and diagnostic ability of the separation anxiety scale for children (SASC). *Eur Child Adolesc Psychiatry* 2008;**17**:365–372.

28. Connors CK. *Connors Rating Scales-Revised Technical Manual.* North Tonawanda, NY: Multi-Health Systems, 1997.

29. Barrett PM, Lowrey-Webster D, Turner SM. *Effects of Cognitive and Behavioral Interventions in School* Brisbane, Australia: Academic Press, 2000.

30. Kratochvil CJ, Harrington MJ, Burke WJ, March JS. Pharmacotherapy of childhood anxiety disorders. *Curr Psychiatry Rep* 2002;**4**:264–269.

31. Murphy TK, Bengtson MA, Tan JY, Carbonell E, Levin GM. Selective serotonin reuptake inhibitors in the treat-

ment of paediatric anxiety disorders: a review. *Int Clin Psychopharmacol* 2000;**15**(Suppl. 2):S47–63.

32. Velosa JF, Riddle MA. Pharmacologic treatment of anxiety disorders in children and adolescents. *Child Adolesc Psychiatr Clin N Am* 2000;**9**:119–133.

33. Bernstein GA, Shaw K. Practice parameters for the assessment and treatment of children and adolescents with anxiety disorders. American Academy of Child and Adolescent Psychiatry. *J Am Acad Child Adolesc Psychiat* 1997;**36**(10 Suppl.):69S–84S.

34. Walkup JT, Albano AM, Piacentini J, *et al.* Cognitive behavioral therapy, sertraline, or a combination in childhood anxiety. *N Engl J Med* 2008;**359**:2753–2766.

35. King NJ, Bernstein GA. School refusal in children and adolescents: a review of the past 10 years. *J Am Acad Child Adolesc Psychiat* 2001;**40**:197–205.

36. Kearney CA. School absenteeism and school refusal behavior in youth: a contemporary review. *Clin Psychol Rev* 2008;**28**:451–471.

37. Heyne D, King NJ, Tonge BJ, Cooper H. School refusal: epidemiology and management. *Paediatr Drugs* 2001;**3**:719–732.

38. King NJ, Ollendick TH, Tonge BJ. *School Refusal: Assessment and Treatment.* Boston: Allyn & Bacon, 1995.

39. Kearney CA, Albano AM. The functional profiles of school refusal behavior. Diagnostic aspects. *Behav Modif* 2004;**28**:147–161.

40. Kearney CA, Silverman WK. Family environment of youngsters with school refusal behavior: A synopsis with implications for assessment and treatment. *Am J Fam Ther* 1995;**23**:59–72.

41. Bernstein GA, Borchardt CM. School refusal: Family constellation and family functioning. *J Anxiety Disord* 1996;**10**:1–19.

42. Kendall PC, Brady EU, Verduin TL. Comorbidity in childhood anxiety disorders and treatment outcome. *J Am Acad Child Adolesc Psychiat* 2001;**40**:787–794.

43. Kearney CA, Silverman WK. A preliminary analysis of a functional model of assessment and treatment for school refusal behavior. *Behav Modif* 1990;**14**:340–366.

44. Kearney CA. *School Refusal Behavior in Youth: a Functional Approach to Assessment and Treatment.* Washington, DC: American Psychological Association, 2001.

45. Last CG, Hansen C, Franco N. Cognitive-behavioral treatment of school phobia. *J Am Acad Child Adolesc Psychiat* 1998;**37**:404–411.

46. Labellarte MJ, Ginsburg GS, Walkup JT, Riddle MA. The treatment of anxiety disorders in children and adolescents. *Biol Psychiatry* 1999;**46**:1567–1578.

47. Masi G, Millepiedi S, Mucci M, Poli P, Bertini N, Milantoni L. Generalized anxiety disorder in referred children and adolescents. *J Am Acad Child Adolesc Psychiat* 2004;**43**:752–760.

48. Judd LL, Kessler RC, Paulus MP, Zeller PV, Wittchen HU, Kunovac JL. Comorbidity as a fundamental feature of generalized anxiety disorders: results from the National Comorbidity Study (NCS). *Acta Psychiatr Scand Suppl* 1998;**393**:6–11.

49. Kendall PC, Compton SN, Walkup JT, *et al.* Clinical characteristics of anxiety disordered youth. *J Anxiety Disord* 2010;**24**:360–365.

50. Muris P, Meesters C, Merckelbach H, Sermon A, Zwakhalen S. Worry in normal children. *J Am Acad Child Adolesc Psychiat* 1998;**37**:703–710.

51. Weems CF, Silverman WK, La Greca AM. What do youth referred for anxiety problems worry about? Worry and its relation to anxiety and anxiety disorders in children and adolescents. *J Abnorm Child Psychol* 2000;**28**:63–72.

52. Perrin S, Last CG. Worrisome thoughts in children clinically referred for anxiety disorder. *J Clin Child Psychol* 1997;**26**:181–189.

53. Costello EJ. Developments in child psychiatric epidemiology. *J Am Acad Child Adolesc Psychiat* 1989;**28**:836–841.

54. Shaffer D, Fisher P, Dulcan MK, *et al.* The NIMH Diagnostic Interview Schedule for Children Version 2.3 (DISC-2.3): description, acceptability, prevalence rates, and performance in the MECA Study. Methods for the Epidemiology of Child and Adolescent Mental Disorders Study. *J Am Acad Child Adolesc Psychiat* 1996;**35**:865–877.

55. McGee R, Feehan M, Williams S, Partridge F, Silva PA, Kelly J. DSM-III disorders in a large sample of adolescents. *J Am Acad Child Adolesc Psychiat* 1990;**29**:611–619.

56. Last CG, Perrin S, Hersen M, Kazdin AE. DSM-III-R anxiety disorders in children: sociodemographic and clinical characteristics. *J Am Acad Child Adolesc Psychiat* 1992;**31**:1070–1076.

57. Werry JS. Overanxious disorder: a review of its taxonomic properties. *J Am Acad Child Adolesc Psychiat* 1991;**30**:533–544.

58. Masi G, Mucci M, Favilla L, Romano R, Poli P. Symptomatology and comorbidity of generalized anxiety disorder in children and adolescents. *Compr Psychiatry* 1999;**40**:210–215.

59. Freud S. *Inhibitions, Symptoms and Anxiety* (revised edn). New York: Norton, 1977, 1959.

60. Biederman J, Rosenbaum JF, Bolduc-Murphy EA, *et al.* A 3-year follow-up of children with and without behavioral inhibition. *J Am Acad Child Adolesc Psychiat* 1993;**32**:814–821.

61. Kagan J, Snidman N. Early childhood predictors of adult anxiety disorders. *Biol Psychiatry* 1999;**46**:1536–1541.

62. Carey G, DiLalla DL. Personality and psychopathology: genetic perspectives. *J Abnorm Psychol* 1994;**103**:32–43.

63. Van Oort FV, Greaves-Lord K, Verhulst FC, Ormel J, Huizink AC. The developmental course of anxiety symptoms during adolescence: the TRAILS study. *J Child Psychol Psychiatry* 2009;**50**:1209–1217.

64. Millan MJ. The neurobiology and control of anxious states. *Prog Neurobiol* 2003;**70**:83–244.

65. Micco JA, Henin A, Mick E, *et al.* Anxiety and depressive disorders in offspring at high risk for anxiety: a meta-analysis. *J Anxiety Disord* 2009;**23**:1158–1164.

66. De Bellis MD, Casey BJ, Dahl RE, *et al.* A pilot study of amygdala volumes in pediatric generalized anxiety disorder. *Biol Psychiatry* 2000;**48**:51–57.

67. De Bellis MD, Keshavan MS, Shifflett H, *et al.* Superior temporal gyrus volumes in pediatric generalized anxiety disorder. *Biol Psychiatry* 2002;**51**:553–562.

68. McClure EB, Adler A, Monk CS, *et al.* fMRI predictors of treatment outcome in pediatric anxiety disorders. *Psychopharmacology* (Berl) 2007;**191**:97–105.

69. Verduin TL, Kendall PC. Differential occurrence of comorbidity within childhood anxiety disorders. *J Clin Child Adolesc Psychol* 2003;**32**:290–295.

70. Wilens TE, Biederman J, Brown S, *et al.* Psychiatric comorbidity and functioning in clinically referred preschool children and school-age youths with ADHD. *J Am Acad Child Adolesc Psychiat* 2002;**41**:262–268.

71. Ginsburg GS, Riddle MA, Davies M. Somatic symptoms in children and adolescents with anxiety disorders. *J Am Acad Child Adolesc Psychiat* 2006;**45**:1179–1187.

72. Reynolds CR, Richmond BO. What I think and feel: a revised measure of children's manifest anxiety. *J Abnorm Child Psychol* 1978;**6**:271–280.

73. Achenbach TM, Rescorla LA. *Manual for the ASEBA School Age Forms and Profiles.* Burlington, VT: University of Vermont Research Center for Children, Youth and Families, 2001.

74. The Pediatric Anxiety Rating Scale (PARS): development and psychometric properties. *J Am Acad Child Adolesc Psychiat* 2002;**41**:1061–1069.

75. Myers K, Winters NC. Ten-year review of rating scales. II: Scales for internalizing disorders. *J Am Acad Child Adolesc Psychiat* 2002;**41**:634–659.

76. Brooks SJ, Kutcher S. Diagnosis and measurement of anxiety disorder in adolescents: a review of commonly used instruments. *J Child Adolesc Psychopharmacol* 2003;**13**:351–400.

77. Clark AS, Henderson LP. Behavioral and physiological responses to anabolic-androgenic steroids. *Neurosci Biobehav Rev* 2003;**27**:413–436.

78. Connolly SD, Bernstein GA, Work Group on Quality Issues. Practice parameter for the assessment and treatment of children and adolescents with anxiety disorders. *J Am Acad Child Adolesc Psychiat* 2007;**46**:267–283.

79. Compton SN, March JS, Brent D, Albano AM, Weersing R, Curry J. Cognitive-behavioral psychotherapy for anxiety and depressive disorders in children and adolescents: an evidence-based medicine review. *J Am Acad Child Adolesc Psychiat* 2004;**43**:930–959.

80. Mendlowitz SL, Manassis K, Bradley S, Scapillato D, Miezitis S, Shaw BF. Cognitive-behavioral group treatments in childhood anxiety disorders: the role of parental involvement. *J Am Acad Child Adolesc Psychiat* 1999;**38**:1223–1229.

81. Barrett PM, Duffy AL, Dadds MR, Rapee RM. Cognitive-behavioral treatment of anxiety disorders in children: long-term (6-year) follow-up. *J Consult Clin Psychol* 2001;**69**:135–141.

82. Cobham VE, Dadds MR, Spence SH. The role of parental anxiety in the treatment of childhood anxiety. *J Consult Clin Psychol* 1998;**66**:893–905.

83. Kendall PC. *Coping Cat Workbook.* Ardmore, PA: Workbook Publishing, 1990.

84. Kendall PC, Southam-Gerow MA. Long-term follow-up of a cognitive-behavioral therapy for anxiety-disordered youth. *J Consult Clin Psychol* 1996;**64**:724–730.

85. Kendall PC. Treating anxiety disorders in children: results of a randomized clinical trial. *J Consult Clin Psychol* 1994;**62**:100–110.

86. Flannery-Schroeder E, Choudhury MS, Kendall PC. Group and individual cognitive-behavioral treatments for youth with anxiety disorders: 1-year follow-up. *Cognitive Ther Res* 2005;**29**:253–259.

87. Liber JM, van Widenfelt BM, van der Leeden AJ, Goedhart AW, Utens EM, Treffers PD. The relation of severity and comorbidity to treatment outcome with Cognitive Behavioral Therapy for childhood anxiety disorders. *J Abnorm Child Psychol* 2010;**38**:683–694.

88. Robinson E, Titov N, Andrews G, McIntyre K, Schwencke G, Solley K. Internet treatment for generalized anxiety disorder: a randomized controlled trial comparing clinician vs. technician assistance. *PLoS One* 2010;**5**:e10942.

89. Walkup J, Labellarte M, Riddle MA, *et al.* Treatment of pediatric anxiety disorders: An open-label extension of the Research Units on Pediatric Psychopharmacology Anxiety Study. *J Child Adolesc Psychopharmacol* 2002;**12**:175–188.

90. Birmaher B, Axelson DA, Monk K, *et al.* Fluoxetine for the treatment of childhood anxiety disorders. *J Am Acad Child Adolesc Psychiat* 2003;**42**:415–423.

91. Baumgartner JL, Emslie GJ, Crismon ML. Citalopram in children and adolescents with depression or anxiety. *Ann Pharmacother* 2002;**36**:1692–1697.

92. Rynn MA, Riddle MA, Yeung PP, Kunz NR. Efficacy and safety of extended-release venlafaxine in the treatment of generalized anxiety disorder in children and adolescents: two placebo-controlled trials. *Am J Psychiatry* 2007;**164**:290–300.

93. Simeon JG, Ferguson HB, Knott V, *et al.* Clinical, cognitive, and neurophysiological effects of alprazolam in children and adolescents with overanxious and avoidant disorders. *J Am Acad Child Adolesc Psychiat* 1992;**31**:29–33.

94. Graae F, Milner J, Rizzotto L, Klein RG. Clonazepam in childhood anxiety disorders. *J Am Acad Child Adolesc Psychiat* 1994;**33**:372–376.

95. Lewis M. *Child and Adolescent Psychiatry: A Comprehensive Textbook*, 3rd edn. Philadelphia: Lippincott Williams & Wilkins, 2002.

96. Fyer AJ. Current approaches to etiology and pathophysiology of specific phobia. *Biol Psychiatry* 1998;**44**:1295–1304.

97. Essau CA, Conradt J, Petermann F. Frequency, comorbidity, and psychosocial impairment of specific phobia in adolescents. *J Clin Child Psychol* 2000;**29**:221–231.

98. Marks IM. *Fears, Phobias, and Rituals: Panic, Anxiety, and their Disorders.* New York: Oxford University Press, 1987.

99. Gullone E. The development of normal fear: a century of research. *Clin Psychol Rev* 2000;**20**:429–451.

100. Evans DW, Leckman JF, Carter A, *et al.* Ritual, habit, and perfectionism: the prevalence and development of compulsive-like behavior in normal young children. *Child Dev* 1997;**68**:58–68.

101. Rachman S. The conditioning theory of fear-acquisition: a critical examination. *Behav Res Ther* 1977;**15**:375–387.

102. Muris P, Merckelbach H, de Jong P, Ollendick TH. The etiology of specific fears and phobias in children: a critique of the non-associative account. *Behav Res Ther* 2002;**40**:185–195.

103. Kendler KS, Neale MC, Kessler RC, Heath AC, Eaves LJ. The genetic epidemiology of phobias in women. The interrelationship of agoraphobia, social phobia, situational phobia, and simple phobia. *Arch Gen Psychiatry* 1992;**49**:273–281.

104. Lewinsohn PM, Zinbarg R, Seeley JR, Lewinsohn M, Sack WH. Lifetime comorbidity among anxiety disorders and between anxiety disorders and other mental disorders in adolescents. *J Anxiety Disord* 1997;**11**:377–394.

105. Ollendick TH, Raishevich N, Davis TE 3rd, Sirbu C, Ost LG. Specific phobia in youth: phenomenology and psychological characteristics. *Behav Ther* 2010;**41**:133–141.

106. King NJ, Ollendick TH, Murphy GC. Assessment of childhood phobias. *Clin Psychol Rev* 1997;**17**:667–687.

107. Ollendick TH, King NJ. Empirically supported treatments for children with phobic and anxiety disorders: current status. *J Clin Child Psychol* 1998;**27**:156–167.

108. Ollendick TH, Ost LG, Reuterskiold L, *et al.* One-session treatment of specific phobias in youth: a randomized clinical trial in the United States and Sweden. *J Consult Clin Psychol* 2009;**77**:504–516.

109. Ollendick TH, Ost LG, Reuterskiold L, Costa N. Comorbidity in youth with specific phobias: Impact of comorbidity on treatment outcome and the impact of treatment on comorbid disorders. *Behav Res Ther* 2010;**48**:827–831.

110. Wiener JM, Dulcan MK. *Textbook of Child and Adolescent Psychiatry*, 3rd edn. Washington, DC: American Psychiatric Publishing, 2004.

111. Thomas A, Chess S. *Temperament and Development*. New York: Brunner/Mazel, 1977.

112. Mash EJ, Barkley RA. *Child Psychopathology*. New York: Guilford Press, 1996.

113. Keller MB. The lifelong course of social anxiety disorder: a clinical perspective. *Acta Psychiatr Scand Suppl* 2003; (417):85–94.

114. Beidel DC, Turner SM, Morris TL. Psychopathology of childhood social phobia. *J Am Acad Child Adolesc Psychiat* 1999;**38**:643–650.

115. Stein MB, Chartier MJ, Kozak MV, King N, Kennedy JL. Genetic linkage to the serotonin transporter protein and 5HT2A receptor genes excluded in generalized social phobia. *Psychiatry Res* 1998;**81**:283–291.

116. Schwartz CE, Snidman N, Kagan J. Adolescent social anxiety as an outcome of inhibited temperament in childhood. *J Am Acad Child Adolesc Psychiat* 1999;**38**: 1008–1015.

117. Whaley SE, Pinto A, Sigman M. Characterizing interactions between anxious mothers and their children. *J Consult Clin Psychol* 1999;**67**:826–836.

118. La Greca AM, Lopez N. Social anxiety among adolescents: linkages with peer relations and friendships. *J Abnorm Child Psychol* 1998;**26**:83–94.

119. Kashdan TB, Herbert JD. Social anxiety disorder in childhood and adolescence: current status and future directions. *Clin Child Fam Psychol Rev* 2001;**4**:37–61.

120. Storch EA, Masia-Warner C, Dent HC, Roberti JW, Fisher PH. Psychometric evaluation of the Social Anxiety Scale for Adolescents and the Social Phobia and Anxiety Inventory for Children: construct validity and normative data. *J Anxiety Disord* 2004;**18**:665–679.

121. Zaider TI, Heimberg RG. Non-pharmacologic treatments for social anxiety disorder. *Acta Psychiatr Scand Suppl* 2003;(417):72–84.

122. Hudson JL, Rapee RM, Deveney C, Schniering CA, Lyneham HJ, Bovopoulos N. Cognitive-behavioral treatment versus an active control for children and adolescents with anxiety disorders: a randomized trial. *J Am Acad Child Adolesc Psychiat* 2009;**48**:533–544.

123. Beidel DC, Turner SM, Morris TL. Behavioral treatment of childhood social phobia. *J Consult Clin Psychol* 2000;**68**:1072–1080.

124. Beidel DC, Turner SM, Sallee FR, Ammerman RT, Crosby LA, Pathak S. SET-C versus fluoxetine in the treatment of childhood social phobia. *J Am Acad Child Adolesc Psychiat* 2007;**46**:1622–1632.

125. Albano AM, Marten PA, Holt CS, Heimberg RG, Barlow DH. Cognitive-behavioral group treatment for social phobia in adolescents. A preliminary study. *J Nerv Ment Dis* 1995;**183**:649–656.

126. Spence SH, Donovan C, Brechman-Toussaint M. The treatment of childhood social phobia: the effectiveness of a social skills training-based, cognitive-behavioural intervention, with and without parental involvement. *J Child Psychol Psychiat* 2000;**41**:713–726.

127. Masia CL, Klein RG, Storch EA, Corda B. School-based behavioral treatment for social anxiety disorder in adolescents: results of a pilot study. *J Am Acad Child Adolesc Psychiat* 2001;**40**:780–786.

128. Bodden DH, Dirksen CD, Bogels SM, *et al.* Costs and cost-effectiveness of family CBT versus individual CBT in clinically anxious children. *Clin Child Psychol Psychiatry* 2008;**13**:543–564.

129. Alfano CA, Pina AA, Villalta IK, Beidel DC, Ammerman RT, Crosby LE. Mediators and moderators of outcome in the behavioral treatment of childhood social phobia. *J Am Acad Child Adolesc Psychiat* 2009;**48**:945–953.

130. Birmaher B, Waterman GS, Ryan N, *et al.* Fluoxetine for childhood anxiety disorders. *J Am Acad Child Adolesc Psychiat* 1994;**33**:993–999.

131. March JS, Entusah AR, Rynn M, Albano AM, Tourian KA. A randomized controlled trial of venlafaxine ER versus placebo in pediatric social anxiety disorder. *Biol Psychiatry* 2007;**62**:1149–1154.

132. Segool NK, Carlson JS. Efficacy of cognitive-behavioral and pharmacological treatments for children with social anxiety. *Depress Anxiety* 2008;**25**:620–631.

133. Diler RS. Panic disorder in children and adolescents. *Yonsei Med J* 2003;**44**:174–179.

134. Whitaker A, Johnson J, Shaffer D, *et al.* Uncommon troubles in young people: prevalence estimates of selected psychiatric disorders in a nonreferred adolescent population. *Arch Gen Psychiatry* 1990;**47**:487–496.

135. Clark DM. A cognitive approach to panic. *Behav Res Ther* 1986;**24**:461–470.

136. Nelles WB, Barlow DH. Do children panic? *Clin Psychol Rev* 1988;**8**:359–372.

137. Hayward C, Killen JD, Hammer LD, *et al.* Pubertal stage and panic attack history in sixth- and seventh-grade girls. *Am J Psychiatry* 1992;**149**:1239–1243.

138. Hayward C, Killen JD, Kraemer HC, Taylor CB. Predictors of panic attacks in adolescents. *J Am Acad Child Adolesc Psychiat* 2000;**39**:207–214.

139. Masi G, Favilla L, Mucci M, Millepiedi S. Panic disorder in clinically referred children and adolescents. *Child Psychiatry Hum Dev* 2000;**31**:139–151.

140. Ollendick TH. Cognitive behavioral treatment of panic disorder with agoraphobia in adolescents: A multiple baseline design analysis. *Behav Ther* 1995;**26**:517–531.

141. Hoffman EC, Mattis SG. A developmental adaptation of panic control treatment for panic disorder in adolescence. *Cogn Behav Pract* 2000;**7**:253–261.

142. Masi G, Toni C, Mucci M, Millepiedi S, Mata B, Perugi G. Paroxetine in child and adolescent outpatients with panic disorder. *J Child Adolesc Psychopharmacol* 2001;**11**:151–157.

143. Martin A. *Pediatric Psychopharmacology: Principles and Practice.* Oxford, New York: Oxford University Press, 2003.

144. Zohar AH, Bruno R. Normative and pathological obsessive-compulsive behavior and ideation in childhood: a question of timing. *J Child Psychol Psychiatry* 1997;**38**:993–999.

145. Geller D, Biederman J, Jones J, *et al.* Is juvenile obsessive-compulsive disorder a developmental subtype of the disorder? A review of the pediatric literature. *J Am Acad Child Adolesc Psychiatry* 1998;**37**:420–427.

146. Leonard HL, Swedo SE, Lenane MC, *et al.* A 2- to 7-year follow-up study of 54 obsessive-compulsive children and adolescents. *Arch Gen Psychiatry* 1993;**50**:429–439.

147. Eichstedt JA, Arnold SL. Childhood-onset obsessive-compulsive disorder: a tic-related subtype of OCD? *Clin Psychol Rev* 2001;**21**:137–157.

148. Lochner C, Stein DJ. Heterogeneity of obsessive-compulsive disorder: a literature review. *Harv Rev Psychiatry* 2003;**11**:113–132.

149. Rettew DC, Swedo SE, Leonard HL, Lenane MC, Rapoport JL. Obsessions and compulsions across time in 79 children and adolescents with obsessive-compulsive disorder. *J Am Acad Child Adolesc Psychiat* 1992;**31**:1050–1056.

150. Lensi P, Cassano GB, Correddu G, Ravagli S, Kunovac JL, Akiskal HS. Obsessive-compulsive disorder. Familial-developmental history, symptomatology, comorbidity and course with special reference to gender-related differences. *Br J Psychiatry* 1996;**169**:101–107.

151. Thoren P, Asberg M, Bertilsson L, Mellstrom B, Sjoqvist F, Traskman L. Clomipramine treatment of obsessive-compulsive disorder. II. Biochemical aspects. *Arch Gen Psychiatry* 1980;**37**:1289–1294.

152. Charney DS, Nestler EJ, Bunney BS. *Neurobiology of Mental Illness.* New York: Oxford University Press, 1999.

153. Fitzgerald KD, Moore GJ, Paulson LA, Stewart CM, Rosenberg DR. Proton spectroscopic imaging of the thalamus in treatment-naive pediatric obsessive-compulsive disorder. *Biol Psychiatry* 2000;**47**:174–182.

154. Rosenberg DR, MacMaster FP, Keshavan MS, Fitzgerald KD, Stewart CM, Moore GJ. Decrease in caudate glutamatergic concentrations in pediatric obsessive-compulsive disorder patients taking paroxetine. *J Am Acad Child Adolesc Psychiat* 2000;**39**:1096–1103.

155. Scahill L, Riddle MA, McSwiggin-Hardin M, *et al.* Children's Yale-Brown Obsessive Compulsive Scale: reliability and validity. *J Am Acad Child Adolesc Psychiat* 1997;**36**:844–852.

156. Berg CJ, Rapoport JL, Flament M. The Leyton Obsessional Inventory-Child Version. *J Am Acad Child Psychiatry* 1986;**25**:84–91.

157. Bamber D, Tamplin A, Park RJ, Kyte ZA, Goodyer IM. Development of a short Leyton Obsessional Inventory for children and adolescents. *J Am Acad Child Adolesc Psychiat* 2002;**41**:1246–1252.

158. Swedo SE, Leonard HL, Garvey M, *et al.* Pediatric autoimmune neuropsychiatric disorders associated with streptococcal infections: clinical description of the first 50 cases. *Am J Psychiatry* 1998;**155**:264–271.

159. King RA, Leonard H, March JS. Summary of the practice parameters for the assessment and treatment of children with obsessive-compulsive disorder. *J Am Acad Child Adolesc Psychiat* 1998;**37**(10 Suppl):27s–45s.

160. March JS, Mulle K, Herbel B. Behavioral psychotherapy for children and adolescents with obsessive-compulsive disorder: an open trial of a new protocol-driven treatment package. *J Am Acad Child Adolesc Psychiat* 1994;**33**:333–341.

161. March JS, Mulle K. *OCD in Children and Adolescents: A Cognitive-Behavioral Treatment Manual.* New York: Guilford Press, 1998.

162. Ipser JC, Stein DJ, Hawkridge S, Hoppe L. Pharmacotherapy for anxiety disorders in children and adolescents. *Cochrane Database Syst Rev* 2009;(3)(3):CD005170. DOI: 10.1002/14651858.CD001206.pub2

163. DeVeaugh-Geiss J, Moroz G, Biederman J, *et al.* Clomipramine hydrochloride in childhood and adolescent obsessive-compulsive disorder – a multicenter trial. *J Am Acad Child Adolesc Psychiat* 1992;**31**:45–49.

164. March JS, Biederman J, Wolkow R, *et al.* Sertraline in children and adolescents with obsessive-compulsive disorder: a multicenter randomized controlled trial. *JAMA* 1998;**280**:1752–1756.

165. Riddle MA, Reeve EA, Yaryura-Tobias JA, *et al.* Fluvoxamine for children and adolescents with obsessive-compulsive disorder: a randomized, controlled, multicenter trial. *J Am Acad Child Adolesc Psychiat* 2001;**40**:222–229.

166. Geller DA, Hoog SL, Heiligenstein JH, *et al.* Fluoxetine treatment for obsessive-compulsive disorder in children and adolescents: a placebo-controlled clinical trial. *J Am Acad Child Adolesc Psychiat* 2001;**40**:773–779.

167. Fitzgerald KD, Stewart CM, Tawile V, Rosenberg DR. Risperidone augmentation of serotonin reuptake inhibitor treatment of pediatric obsessive compulsive disorder. *J Child Adolesc Psychopharmacol* 1999;**9**:115–123.

168. Hayden TL. Classification of elective mutism. *J Am Acad Child Psychiatry* 1980;**19**:118–133.

169. Meyers SV. Elective mutism in children: A family systems approach. *Am J Fam Therap* 1984;**12**:39–45.

170. Porjes MD. Intervention with the selectively mute child. *Psychol Schools* 1992;**29**:367–376.

171. Valner J, Nemiroff M. Silent eulogy. Elective mutism in a six-year-old Hispanic girl. *Psychoanal Study Child* 1995;**50**:327–340.

172. Hoffman S, Laub B. Paradoxical intervention using a polarization model of cotherapy in the treatment of elective mutism: A case study. *Contemp Fam Ther* 1986;**8**:136–143.

173. Anstendig KD. Is selective mutism an anxiety disorder? Rethinking its DSM-IV classification. *J Anxiety Disord* 1999;**13**:417–434.

174. Dow SP, Sonies BC, Scheib D, Moss SE, Leonard HL. Practical guidelines for the assessment and treatment of selective mutism. *J Am Acad Child Adolesc Psychiat* 1995;**34**:836–846.

175. Bergman RL, Piacentini J, McCracken JT. Prevalence and description of selective mutism in a school-based sample. *J Am Acad Child Adolesc Psychiat* 2002;**41**:938–946.

176. Viana AG, Beidel DC, Rabian B. Selective mutism: a review and integration of the last 15 years. *Clin Psychol Rev* 2009;**29**:57–67.

177. Kumpulainen K. Phenomenology and treatment of selective mutism. *CNS Drugs* 2002;**16**:175–180.

178. Kolvin I, Fundudis T. Elective mute children: psychological development and background factors. *J Child Psychol Psychiatry* 1981;**22**:219–232.

179. Kristensen H. Selective mutism and comorbidity with developmental disorder/delay, anxiety disorder, and elimination disorder. *J Am Acad Child Adolesc Psychiat* 2000;**39**:249–256.

180. Gillberg C. *Clinical Child Neuropsychiatry*. Cambridge, New York: Cambridge University Press, 1995.

181. Lahey BB, Kazdin AE (eds). *Advances in Clinical Child Psychology*. New York: Plenum Press, 1992.

182. Black B, Uhde TW. Treatment of elective mutism with fluoxetine: a double-blind, placebo-controlled study. *J Am Acad Child Adolesc Psychiat* 1994;**33**: 1000–1006.

183. Dummit ES 3rd, Klein RG, Tancer NK, Asche B, Martin J, Fairbanks JA. Systematic assessment of 50 children with selective mutism. *J Am Acad Child Adolesc Psychiat* 1997;**36**:653–660.

184. Gordon N. Mutism: elective or selective, and acquired. *Brain Dev* 2001;**23**:83–87.

185. Carlson JS, Kratochwill TR, Johnston HF. Sertraline treatment of 5 children diagnosed with selective mutism: a single-case research trial. *J Child Adolesc Psychopharmacol* 1999;**9**:293–306.

186. Golwyn DH, Sevlie CP. Phenelzine treatment of selective mutism in four prepubertal children. *J Child Adolesc Psychopharmacol* 1999;**9**:109–113.

187. Bodden DH, Dirksen CD, Bogels SM. Societal burden of clinically anxious youth referred for treatment: a cost-of-illness study. *J Abnorm Child Psychol* 2008;**36**:487–497.

14

Substance Use in Adolescents

Jacqueline Countryman

Introduction

Despite some evidence indicating that adolescent substance use is a normal part of development it is one of the strongest predictors of later adult substance abuse disorders [1]. Over 90% of adult addicts started substance use in adolescence [2]. Substance use among the adolescent population is increasing and is responsible for multiple problems including an increase in mortality among this age group [3]. The three leading causes of death in young people between the ages of 15 and 24 in the United States are, in descending order: accidents, homicides, and suicide. Alcohol and other drugs have contributed to each of these causes [4].

Most adolescents have not obtained a mature level of cognitive, emotional, social, or physical growth and will experiment with a range of attitudes and behaviors. This experimentation also includes use of substances. Typically adolescents start experimenting with "gateway" drugs including tobacco and alcohol. The use of substances in the preteen population has not been researched as well as the adolescent population, and therefore this chapter concentrates on the use of substances in adolescents.

Epidemiology

The most recent update on the National Institute on Drug Abuse Monitoring the Future Study looks at trends in 8th, 10th and 12th graders. The 2010 results show:

(1) Lifetime use of any illicit drug is 48%.
(2) Lifetime use of any illicit drug other than marijuana is 25%.
(3) Marijuana use continued to rise among teens. This is in contrast to the long gradual decline that had been occurring over the preceding decade.
(4) After a decline of several years in perceived risk for ecstasy, its use is increasing.

(5) Alcohol use including binge drinking (five or more drinks in a row on at least one occasion in the 2 weeks prior to the survey) has continued to decline.
(6) Eighth and tenth graders showed evidence of an increase in smoking.
(7) Vicodin use decreased among 12th graders to 8%. However, it continues to be one of the most widely used illicit drugs.
(8) LSD use is at historically low levels.
(9) Cocaine and crack use declined over the last decade.

The data indicate that while the use of individual drugs may fluctuate widely, the proportion of the population using any of them is much more stable [5].

Risk Factors

Family/Parent Factors

Parents and siblings are role models for adolescents. Their attitudes toward drinking and their drinking habits correlate with adolescents' drinking patterns [6]. The influence of siblings has been a stronger correlate on adolescent drug-taking behaviors than parents' influence. The gender of the parent also has been shown to be an influence on substance use. Mothers' drinking habits have been shown to be more relevant for adolescents' drinking than those of the fathers [7]. Family bonding has been shown to decrease the risk of alcohol and other drug use among adolescents [8].

Family environmental risk factors that stem from substance use include: excessively high family conflict, low parent-child attachment, poor parenting skills, lax or excessive punishment, physical or sexual abuse, ineffective communication, lack of sharing of prosocial family values, little time spent supervising and monitoring children's activities and friends, and no sharing of positive leisure time activities and ways to reduce stress [9]. The discipline style of the parent

Clinical Child Psychiatry, Third Edition. Edited by William M. Klykylo and Jerald Kay.
© 2012 John Wiley & Sons, Ltd. Published 2012 by John Wiley & Sons, Ltd.

influences substance use. Inconsistent and unpredictable parental discipline and parental permissiveness have been shown to increase the risk of substance use in adolescents [10].

Family protective factors include supportive parent-child relationships, positive discipline methods, monitoring and supervision, family advocacy for their children, and seeking information and support for the benefit of children [11].

Open communication with parents and feeling supported by parents are protective factors. Even when parents use substances there can be protective factors. Seeing the ramifications of substance use in their parents can deter adolescents from using [12]. Anti-drug parental attitudes are reasons why adolescents do not use drugs and alcohol [13]. Parental attitudes concerning drug use play a greater role for girls than boys. In contrast the community and neighborhood environment has a greater influence on boys than girls [14].

Peer Factors

Peer tolerance or approval of drug use, and whether friends have asked, encouraged, or pressured an adolescent all influence an adolescent's drug usage [15]. Parental norms have been found to be more important for early adolescents (mean age 13) and peer norms more important for middle adolescents (mean age 15). During mid-adolescence peer influence may peak as children spend more time with their peers than with family.[16] The single strongest predictor of adolescent substance use is having friends who use drugs; 88% of substance users stated that they had friends who also use [13].

Community Factors

Social environmental norms, role models, social support, and opportunities for nonuse of drugs have been shown to be related to adolescent drug use [17]. Other factors that have shown an influence include low socioeconomic status, high population density, physical deterioration of the neighborhood, and high crime [18]. With children an important component is the school environment. Those adolescents who feel connected to the school are at a lower risk for using and abusing substances [19]. Adolescents expected to have high academic achievement by their parents are also at lower risk [20]. Adolescents with poor academic achievement and low commitment to education are more likely to engage in substance use [12]. Work is also included in community factors, and those adolescents who work more than 20 hours per week are at a greater risk for use and abuse [21].

Genetic Factors

The role of genetics in alcoholism has been studied with adoption and twin studies. Studies done in the 1930s and 1940s in Denmark showed an association between alcoholic biological fathers and male adoptees developing alcoholism [21]. More recent research has implicated the A1 allele of the dopamine D2 receptor being associated with alcoholism [22]. Sons of alcoholics have a higher tolerance to the effects of alcohol and therefore may not notice the effects that alcohol can have until they drink larger quantities [23].

Cloninger has concluded that risk factors for alcoholism are mediated in large part by inborn, heritable differences in temperament and learning styles [24]. Cloninger type 2 alcoholics demonstrate interpersonal risk factors that lead to continued use. These risk factors are a high level of novelty seeking, a low level of harm avoidance, and a low level of reward dependence. They also show other risk factors including: early onset of spontaneous alcohol-seeking behavior; diagnosis during adolescence; rapid course of onset; possible genetic precursors that put them at risk for substance use; and severe symptoms of deviant behavior, including fighting and arrests while drinking.

Individual Factors

Traits that are associated with substance use are aggression, depression, impulsivity, sensation-seeking behavior, and positive attitudes toward substance use [13]. Gender and age are also risk factors. Males have higher rates of alcoholism than females. The age of greatest risk to initiate alcohol and marijuana use is between ages 16 and 18 [25]. Use of substances before age 15 increases the risk of future substance use/abuse. Table 14.1 lists risk factors associated with drug use.

Comorbidity

Studies of treatment-seeking adolescents with substance use disorders have documented that 50–90% also have non-substance-use comorbid psychiatric disorders [26]. Although a high prevalence of %. Some researchers have felt that methodological considerations, including the length of abstinence required before the diagnosis is made, the population studied, and the perspective of the examiner, affect prevalence rates for psychiatric disorders in persons who abuse substances and account for the variability. They see the prevalence rates artificially elevated by the tendency to make a diagnosis before abatement of some of the psychiatric symptomatology secondary to substance use [27].

Table 14.1 Risk factors associated with drug use.

I. Family/parent factors
Family conflict
Low parent-child attachment
Poor parenting
Lax/excessive punishment
Physical/sexual abuse
Ineffective communication
Little time supervising/monitoring children's
activities
Parental drug attitudes

II. Peer factors
Peer tolerance/approval of drug use
Peer rejection

III. Community factors
Low socioeconomic status
High population density
Physical deterioration of neighborhood
High crime
Availability of drugs in community

IV. School factors
No connection with school
Poor academic achievement

V. Genetic factors
Inherited susceptibility to drug abuse

VI. Individual factors
Age
-Gender
Aggression, especially early onset
Depression
Impulsivity
Sensation-seeking behavior
Positive attitudes towards substance use

Depression

Depression is thought to be the primary component of substance dependence in women [28]. The question of which came first is an ongoing one with depressive disorders. One study of inpatient adolescent substance abusers with major depression showed that 60% had a secondary depression and 16% had a primary diagnosis [29]. Another study showed that 53% of inpatients with substance use disorders had dysthymia prior to the substance problems [30].

Bipolar Disorder

In teenagers, the diagnosis of bipolar disorder is a difficult diagnosis to make and even more difficult when there is possible substance abuse. Studies have shown an increased risk of substance use disorders in adolescents diagnosed with bipolar disorder. Children who are treated at a younger age for bipolar disorder have a decreased risk of substance use. It is important to make the diagnosis of bipolar disorder during a period of abstinence from substance use because there is an overlap of manic symptoms with substance intoxication [31].

Anxiety Disorders

Anxiety disorders are among the most common psychiatric conditions in adolescents and often can be missed if there is a coexisting substance abuse disorder. Many patients first use substances to help reduce or relieve anxiety. In all countries the findings show that the onset of anxiety disorders is more likely to precede than to follow a substance use disorder [32]. Adolescents with anxiety often do not come to the attention of teachers and clinicians because they don't usually exhibit behavioral problems. The combination of shyness and aggressiveness has been shown to be a valid predictor of future cocaine use in boys [33]. Adolescents who have experienced trauma may use substances to help relieve symptoms of post-traumatic stress disorder [34]. General anxiety in middle adolescence places adolescents at risk for concurrent and subsequent substance use. Social phobia in middle adolescence may protect from substance use [35].

Schizophrenia

The onset of schizophrenia typically is in the late teenage years. The use of substances may precipitate an incipient psychosis [28]. Young persons with schizophrenia may abuse substances in an attempt to manage or deny their symptoms. Their use of substances often interferes with treatment for their psychotic disorder [36].

Recent reports have attributed a role to cannabis use in the development of schizophrenia. Several prospective studies have reported a greater prevalence of psychotic symptoms in cannabis users than in control groups. Studies have also shown that cannabis use is associated with a higher risk of development of schizophrenia [37, 38].

Attention-Deficit Hyperactivity Disorder

Attention-deficit hyperactivity disorder (ADHD) is a common comorbid diagnosis with adolescents who have substance abuse problems. There has been debate about whether ADHD is directly connected with the increased risk for substance abuse or if the presence of conduct disorder in addition to the ADHD is the true risk factor.

Children with ADHD with conduct disorder have a much greater risk for substance abuse than do children with ADHD alone [39]. Childhood ADHD has been associated with alcohol use disorder by young adulthood and with nicotine use by middle adolescence [40].

Studies have shown that individuals with ADHD begin drug use at an earlier age, experience more severe substance abuse, and have a more negative self-image before drug use [41]. Another reason for the high coincidence of ADHD and addictive illnesses is individuals trying to self-medicate their symptoms. Clinical findings indicate that affected patients report improvement in ADHD-specific symptoms when applying self-medication in the form of cannabis and cocaine [42].

The issue of whether medicating adolescents with psychostimulants increases their risk of substance abuse has been studied. Studies have been consistent in showing that successful treatment of adolescents with stimulants actually lowers their probability of developing a substance use disorder [37]. In fact one study showed that if an adolescent has ADHD and is treated, the risk for a substance use disorder is reduced by 85% [43]. Childhood ADHD has been associated with alcohol use disorder by young adulthood and with nicotine use by middle adolescence.

Conduct Disorder

Conduct disorder is one of the most common comorbid diagnoses with substance abuse, especially in boys [44]. Reebye *et al.* found that 52% of the preadolescents and adolescents they studied with conduct disorder also met criteria for a substance use disorder [45]. In the younger age group the probability of comorbidity was greater. The prognosis of adolescents who develop conduct disorder prior to a substance abuse disorder is poorer than for those who develop conduct disorder during the substance abuse disorder [46].

Eating Disorders

One-fourth of patients with an eating disorder have a history of substance abuse or are currently abusing substances [47]. Persons with eating disorders may abuse amphetamines to lose weight. The use of substances is more prevalent in bulimia nervosa than in anorexia nervosa.

Suicidality

In a study done by Shafii *et al.* postmortem analysis of adolescents who committed suicide demonstrated that 70% were drug and alcohol users [48].

Assessment

The first part of assessment should be a clinical interview with the patient and collateral sources. Part of substance abuse is deception and denial, and thus collateral sources are extremely important. Areas to explore include: substance use behaviors; psychiatric and behavior problems; school functioning; family functioning; peer relationships; and leisure activities. In the area of substance use behavior it is important to ask about the quantity, frequency, onset, type of substance used, negative consequences, context of use, and control of use. These questions need to be asked with each substance identified. As part of the clinical interview risk factors should be evaluated. Of particular importance is the parent's own history of substance use, attitudes about drug use, the type and level of discipline used within the home, and the level of attachment between the child and parent.

Laboratory measures are often used to detect use. Urinalysis is the most widely used test but is limited to the short and variable detection period for substances. Stimulants are detected up to 1–2 days after use. Cocaine is detected for several days after use. Sedative hypnotic drugs are variable ranging from 1 day to 1 week or more for the long-acting benzodiazepines, to about 2 weeks for long-acting barbiturates. Opiates are detected for up to 2 days. Cannabis can be detected for up to 30 days, especially with chronic use. A positive drug screening test does not confirm a diagnosis of abuse or dependence but does confirm use.

Self-report instruments can be used as an adjunct to the clinical interview but should not be relied upon as the only source to make a diagnosis. Table 14.2 lists several examples of self-report screening and diagnostic instruments that can be used with adolescents. Most can be self or clinician administered and take a short time to take and score.

The diagnosis of Substance Abuse and Substance Dependence are defined by the *Diagnostic and Statistical Manual, Fourth Edition, Text Revision* (DSM-IV-TR) as a maladaptive pattern of substance abuse leading to clinically significant impairment. Other criteria that distinguish between the two are listed in Table 14.3.

Medical Concerns

Alcohol and Other Central Nervous System Depressants

Clinicians who work with adolescents should be familiar with the presentation of alcohol intoxication, alcohol withdrawal, and symptoms of abuse and dependence,

Table 14.2 Self-help and diagnostic instruments.

Measure	Type
Adolescent Drug Abuse Diagnosis (ADAD; Friedman and Utada, 1989)[1]	Structured interview, comprehensive assessment drug/alcohol use
Adolescent Diagnostic Interview (ADI; Winters and Henly, 1993)[2]	Structured interview, diagnostic assessment
Diagnostic Interview Schedule for Children (DISC; Shaffer *et al.*, 1996)[3]	Structured interview; diagnostic assessment
Minnesota Multiphasic Personality Inventory-Adolescent (MMPI-A; Wood *et al.*, 1994)[4]	Self-administered screen, identifies and describes drug/alcohol-related problems
Personal Experience Inventory (PEI; Winters and Henly, 1989)[5]	Self-administered, comprehensive assessment; identifies drug/alcohol use patterns
Personal Experience Screening Questionnaire (PESQ; Winters, 1993)[6]	Self-administered screen; identifies drug/alcohol use
Problem Oriented Screening Instrument for Teenagers (POSIT; Rahden, 1991)[7]	Self-administered screen; identifies potential drug/alcohol use
Substance Abuse Subtle Screening Inventory (SASSI, Miller, 1990)[8]	Self-administered screen; identifies drug/alcohol use and tendency to deny use
Teen Addiction Severity Index (TASI; Kaminer *et al.*, 1991)[9]	Structured interview; comprehensive assessment

[1] Friedman A and Utada A. A method for diagnosing and planning the treatment of adolescent drug abusers. The Adolescent Drug Abuse Diagnosis Instrument. Journal of Drug Education. 1989, 19(4) 285-312.

[2] Winters K. and Henley G. Adolescent Diagnostic Interview (ADI) Manuel, Los Angeles, CA: Western Psychological Services, 1993.

[3] Shaffer D. et al. Diagnostic Interview Schedule for Children (IV) New York: Columbia University, 2003.

[4] Butcher J. et al. MMPI –A Manuel for administration, scoring, and interpretation. Minneapolis: University of Minnesota Press. 1992.

[5] Winters K. and Henley G. Personal Experience Inventory. Los Angeles: Western Psychological Services, 1989.

[6] Winters K. Personal Experience Screening Questionnaire. Los Angeles: Western Psychological Services, 1993.

[7] Rahdert E. The Adolescent Assessment/Referral System Manual. Rockville MD: US Department of Health and Human Services, ADAMHA, National Institute on Drug Abuse. DHHS Publ No (ADM) 91-1735.

[8] Miller G. Substance Abuse Subtle Screening Inventory. Springville IN: SASSI Institute 1985.

[9] Kaminer Y. et al. The Teen- Addiction Severity Index. Rationale and reliability. International Journal of the Addictions, 1991, 26(2) 219-226.

especially in the emergency room setting. The CAGE questionnaire can be used as a screening tool though it is used more in adults than in adolescents [49]. The CAGE consists of four questions with two or more positive answers suggestive of alcoholism:

(1) Have you ever felt the need to **C**ut down on your drinking?
(2) Have you ever felt **A**nnoyed that others criticized your drinking?
(3) Have you ever felt bad or **G**uilty about your drinking?
(4) Have you ever felt the need for an **E**ye-Opener first thing in the morning?

A more developmentally appropriate questionnaire is the CRAFFT [50]. It consists of six questions with two or more "yes" answers suggestive of a significant problem:

(1) Have you ever ridden in a **C**ar driven by someone (including yourself) who was "high" or had been using alcohol or drugs?
(2) Do you ever use alcohol or drugs to **R**elax, feel better about yourself, or fit in?
(3) Have you ever used alcohol or drugs while you are **A**lone?
(4) Do any of your **F**amily or **F**riends ever tell you that you should cut down on your drinking or drug use?
(5) Do you ever **F**orget things you did while using alcohol or drugs?
(6) Have you gotten in **T**rouble while you were using alcohol or drugs?

Alcohol intoxication in adolescents is identical to that in adults. This can be broken down into three stages. The initial stage consists of low levels of blood alcohol concentration (BAC) leading to an increase in

Table 14.3 DSM-IV-TR diagnoses of Substance Abuse and Substance Dependence.

Substance Abuse
  A. A maladaptive pattern of substance use leading to clinically significant impairment or distress, as manifested by
     one (or more) of the following, occurring within a 12-month period:
     (1) recurrent substance use resulting in a failure to fulfill major role obligations at work, school, or home
     (2) recurrent substance use in situations in which it is physically hazardous
     (3) recurrent substance-related legal problems
     (4) continued substance use despite having persistent or recurrent social or interpersonal problems caused or
         exacerbated by the effects of the substance.
  B. The symptoms have never met the criteria for Substance Dependence for this class of substance.

Substance Dependence
A maladaptive pattern of substance use, leading to clinically significant impairment or distress, as manifested by three
  (or more) of the following, occurring at any time in the same 12-month period:
     (1) Tolerance, as defined by either of the following:
         (a) a need for markedly increased amounts of the substance to achieve intoxication or desired effect;
         (b) markedly diminished effect with continued use of the same amount of the substance.
     (2) Withdrawal, as manifested by either of the following:
         (a) the characteristic withdrawal syndrome for the substance;
         (b) the same substance is taken to relieve or avoid withdrawal symptoms.
     (3) The substance is often taken in larger amounts or over a longer period than was intended.
     (4) There is a persistent desire or unsuccessful efforts to cut down or control substance use.
     (5) A great deal of time is spent in activities necessary to obtain the substance, use the substance, or recover from its
         effects.
     (6) Important social, occupational, or recreational activities are given up or reduced because of substance use.
     (7) The substance use is continued despite knowledge of having a persistent or recurrent physical or psychological
         problem that is likely to have been caused or exacerbated by the substance.

[10] Reproduced from: American Psychiatric Association. *Diagnostic and Statistical Manual, Fourth Edition, Text Revision* (DSM-IV-TR). Washington, DC: American Psychiatric Press, 2000.

disinhibition, increased feelings of self-confidence, impaired judgment, and a loss of fine motor tasks. The next stage, the excitement stage, begins with a BAC of 100 mg/dL and leads to impaired memory, increased distractibility, and impaired concentration. Above a BAC of 200 mg/dL persons exhibit confusion, disorientation, dizziness, ataxia, diplopia, and slurred speech.

Alcohol withdrawal for adolescents is usually not as severe as it is with adults possibly due to adolescents being in better health and using substances for less time than adults. The symptoms of alcohol withdrawal generally begin 24 hours after cessation of use and will resolve within several days. The treatment of uncomplicated alcohol withdrawal is generally the same in adolescents as in adults though the literature is sparse on this topic. Long-acting benzodiazepines are typically used and administered on a fixed or symptom-triggered schedule. Alcohol withdrawal seizures are typically seen 24–48 hours after last use. Delirium tremens is a medical emergency and is seen 48–120 hours after last use. Symptoms are autonomic instability, severe tremors, and mental status changes. It is rare in adolescents but requires ICU monitoring if seen.

Studies have shown that heavy chronic alcohol use persisting from adolescence to young adulthood may produce cognitive disadvantages, primarily in visuospatial and memory abilities. Youths who chronically use heavy quantities of alcohol and experience drug withdrawal symptoms may be particularly at risk for cognitive deterioration by young adulthood [51].

Marijuana

Intoxication symptoms include impaired motor coordination, anxiety, impaired judgment, conjunctival injection, increased appetite, dry mouth, and tachycardia. Withdrawal with marijuana is a controversial subject. The DSM-IV does not recognize cannabis withdrawal though it has been described in the literature [52]. Its symptoms are insomnia, irritability, restlessness, drug craving, depression, and nervousness. Pharmacological treatment for intoxication and withdrawal is rarely indicated.

Adolescents have been shown to be more vulnerable than adults to neurocognitive abnormalities associated with chronic heavy marijuana use. Adolescents demonstrate persisting deficits related to heavy use following discontinuation, particularly in the domains of learning, memory, and working memory [53].

Cocaine

During cocaine intoxication agitation and anxiety may occur. A person may also present with psychotic symptoms including formication. Other symptoms include hypertension, arrhythmias, or seizures. Withdrawal symptoms include mild depression, anxiety, and fatigue. Treatment for intoxication and withdrawal is typically supportive. Complications can arise from the method of use, including nasal perforation, HIV infection, hepatitis C infection, and infections at the injection site.

Opiates

Intoxication symptoms include initial euphoria followed by apathy, dysphoria, psychomotor agitation or retardation, impaired judgment, or impaired social or occupational functioning. Physical symptoms include pupillary constriction, drowsiness, slurred speech, and impaired attention. Naloxone use causes opiate withdrawal and can be life-saving. Withdrawal symptoms include dysphoric mood, nausea, muscle aches, lacrimation, piloerection, diarrhea, and yawning. Methadone or clonidine have been used for treatment [54].

Phencyclidine (PCP)

Intoxication symptoms include nystagmus, hypertension, numbness, ataxia, dysarthria, and seizures. Agitation and psychotic symptoms can result. Treatment is typically supportive. Severe intoxication may require medical or psychiatric monitoring. The DSM-IV does not recognize PCP withdrawal though in animal models symptoms include tremor, lethargy, piloerection, and seizures [55].

Ecstasy

Intoxication consists of disorientation, increased sociability, increased mental clarity, a feeling of closeness to others, and a general sense of well-being. Other physical symptoms noted with intoxication include hyperthermia, tachycardia, hypertension, agitation, and confusion. A "hangover" feeling is often noted 24–48 hours after last use consisting of confusion, depression, restlessness, insomnia, and paranoia. Treatment is supportive [56].

Ketamine

Ketamine is a noncompetitive NMDA (N-methyl-D-aspartate) receptor antagonist and is considered a psychotomimetic or schizophrenomimetic drug. In large doses it produces reactions similar to PCP. At lower doses it results in impaired attention and memory. At higher doses it can result in delirium, amnesia, hypertension, or depression [57]. Treatment is supportive [58].

Gamma-hydroxybutyrate (GHB)

GHB is a naturally occurring inhibitory neurotransmitter. It is used for its intoxicating, sedating, and euphoria-producing effects or for its growth hormone-releasing effects. Withdrawal from GHB has been described and looks similar to alcohol withdrawal [59].

Treatment

The primary goal of treatment for substance use disorders in adolescents is achieving and maintaining abstinence from substance use. This goal is difficult to achieve and practitioners need to keep in mind that because of the chronicity of the problem in some adolescents, and the self-limiting nature of substance use in other adolescents, a reduction of harm may be a more achievable goal.

Many adolescents with substance use disorders have comorbid psychiatric diagnosis or have social/family/educational problems that should also be addressed in the treatment plan.

Characteristics of treatment that have been shown to be related to improved abstinence and lower relapse rates are: [60, 61]

- Treatment that is intensive and of sufficient duration to achieve change. The intensity and duration should depend on the level of substance involvement, level of motivation of the adolescent and the family, the quality of social supports, the presence of a comorbid psychiatric diagnosis, and the existence of deficits in other psychosocial areas.
- Treatment should be comprehensive and target all areas that are noted to be dysfunctional in the adolescent's life.
- Treatment should encourage family involvement. Working with the parents to provide appropriate and effective limits should be a focus. Also any addiction noted in the parents should be addressed.
- Treatment should address the development of a drug-free lifestyle by the adolescent and his or her family.
- Treatment should include self-help groups for both the adolescent and the family.
- Treatment should be sensitive to the culture and socioeconomic limitations of the family.
- Treatment programs should work with social service agencies, juvenile justice, and the school system.
- Treatment should include an after-care component.

- Treatment should be multimodal to achieve the above goals.

Treatment Settings

As with any care rendered to patients the least restrictive setting that is safe and effective should be sought for adolescents with substance use disorders. The treatment settings that are available include: inpatient, residential, partial hospitalization, and outpatient treatment with or without community treatment (self-help groups). Factors that providers should examine to determine the appropriate level of care include:

- motivation and willingness to cooperate;
- need for structure and limit-setting;
- need for a safe environment;
- adolescent's ability to care for him/herself;
- comorbid conditions;
- availability of treatment settings;
- adolescent's/family's preference for treatment;
- past treatment failure in a less restrictive setting.

Listed in Table 14.4 are each treatment setting and when to utilize the setting for a specific patient.

Treatment Modalities

Cognitive Behavioral Therapy

Cognitive behavioral therapy (CBT) is used to identify negative thinking patterns and cognitive distortions and

Table 14.4 Treatment settings for patients with substance use disorders.

Setting	Appropriate disorders
Inpatient	Severe psychiatric disorders, treatment failure in less restrictive setting, patients with withdrawal risk/history
Residential	Severe personality disorders, inadequate psychosocial supports, history of treatment failure after inpatient care
Partial hospitalization	24-hour supervision not necessary, step-down from inpatient; stable social supports
Outpatient	Highly motivated, stable social supports, limited comorbid psychopathology, following successful treatment in higher level of care

then modify these to reduce negative feelings and behavior. Adolescents in a CBT program have demonstrated a reduction in the severity of substance use [62, 63].

Behavioral Therapy

Inpatient, residential, and partial hospitalization programs often use the operant conditioning methods that are part of behavioral therapy. This includes rewarding and punishing the adolescent for appropriate and inappropriate behaviors. Parent management training is also included in behavioral therapy. Behavioral contingency contracting pairs a specific behavior to a positive reinforcer after a certain goal is obtained. Parents are then trained on how to continue this method when the adolescent returns home.

Dynamic and Interpersonal Therapy

These methods are used often in clinical practice with adolescents with substance use disorders. However, there are no controlled studies in this population.

Self-Help Groups

Participation in self-help groups is a part of many treatment programs. Adolescents receive support from other recovering peers. Role models for recovery and abstinence are available. The 12-step approach (Table 14.5) is the most widely used to treat adolescents with substance use disorders. The philosophy of the 12-step approach is that recovery from addiction is possible only if the person recognizes his/her problem with drugs/alcohol and admits that he/she is unable to use substances in moderation without significant consequences. Spiritual growth is seen as critical to this process. There has been little published research on the use of 12-step approaches with adolescents. Studies that have been done show a lower substance use rate in those who attend Alcoholics Anonymous (AA) or Narcotics Anonymous (NA) groups than those who do not [64].

Family Therapy

Family approaches have been found to be critical for good outcomes in adolescent substance use. This makes sense when looking at the number of risk factors for substance use that involve the family or parents. A combined child-parent intervention showed substantial and significant effects on heavy weekly drinking as opposed to child- or parent-only interventions [65]. Goals of family therapy include psychoeducation, assisting the family in getting the adolescent into treatment, assisting the family in establishing structure with

Table 14.5 The 12 Steps of Alcoholics Anonymous and Narcotics Anonymous.

---

(1) We admitted we were powerless over alcohol (our addiction) – that our lives had become unmanageable.

(2) We came to believe that a Power greater than ourselves could restore us to sanity.

(3) We made a decision to turn our will and our lives over to the care of God, as we understood Him.

(4) We made a searching and fearless moral inventory of ourselves.

(5) We admitted to God, to ourselves, and to another human being the exact nature of our wrongs.

(6) We were entirely ready to have God remove all these defects of character.

(7) We humbly asked Him to remove our shortcomings.

(8) We made a list of persons we had harmed and became willing to make amends to them all.

(9) We made direct amends to such people wherever possible, except when to do so would injure them or others.

(10) We continued to take a personal inventory and when we were wrong promptly admitted it.

(11) We sought through prayer and medication to improve our conscious contact with God, as we understood Him, praying only for knowledge of His will for us and the power to carry that out.

(12) Having had a spiritual awakening as the result of these steps, we tried to carry this message to alcoholics (addicts) and to practice these principles in all our affairs.

---

consistent limit-setting and monitoring, and improving communication within the family. There are many approaches to family therapy. Cognitive-behavioral family-focused programs show the most evidence of effectiveness, the largest effect size, and the most lasting effects [66, 67]. In contrast, parent education programs have not been found to be effective. Structural-strategic family therapy has been shown to improve the parent-adolescent relationship and in turn reduce the adolescent's drug use [68]. Structural-strategic family therapy involves the whole family and focuses on the dysfunctional family structure and interactional patterns.

Community-Based Interventions

Multisystemic therapy (MST) has been shown to be an effective model for community-based alternatives for violent chronic juvenile offenders with substance use disorders. MST targets individual, family, peer, school, and community factors. Studies have shown that it reduces substance use and deviant behaviors in subjects [69, 70].

Motivational Enhancement Therapy (MET)

This is a brief therapy of two to four sessions that seeks to aid the patient to identify their goals for change, develop a plan for change, increase their motivation to achieve change, and make a commitment for change. The foundational belief of MET is that the patient's behaviors are at least partially under the patient's control and can be changed with the right motivation and plan of action. Adolescents who received motivational therapy had lower rates of alcohol and marijuana use [71]. A combination of MET and CBT exhibited greater reductions in substance use frequency, substance use problems, and illegal behaviors 12 months after treatment than with MET or CBT alone [72].

Medication Management

Few clinical trials have been conducted on pharmacotherapuetic agents for treating adolescent substance use disorders. Data from adult studies should be extrapolated to adolescents with caution. Treatment of withdrawal symptoms in adolescents is rare [73], but should proceed as would the treatment of withdrawal in adults. The use of pharmacological agents to decrease the subjective reinforcing effects of a substance is limited to case reports in the literature. The use of such agents should be reserved for treatment after other proven methods have been utilized. The use of aversive agents, such as disulfiram, should also be limited in use in adolescents due to concerns with safety and compliance.

The treatment of comorbid psychiatric disorders with psychopharmacological agents is critical in the overall treatment plan. A period of abstinence is recommended so that a definitive assessment can be made. Few studies have been done in this population. A placebo-controlled study has examined lithium use in children and adolescents with comorbid bipolar disorder and substance use disorders. Twenty-six subjects aged 7–18 years old were treated with lithium or placebo for 6 weeks. Positive urine toxicology screens decreased significantly, and global assessment of functioning improved in 46% of those receiving lithium versus 8% of those receiving placebo [74].

An assessment of the risk of abuse of a therapeutic agent by the adolescent or family should be done. All medications should be monitored under adult supervision. Also the choice of agent should be considered, with agents having lower abuse potential being chosen first.

Prevention

Clinicians need to be aware of the risk factors for substance use disorders in youths. These risk factors need to be targeted and appropriate interventions made.

School-based interventions are the mainstay of prevention research. Research by Botvin et al. showed significant reductions in drug use with long-term positive results after implementation of a classroom-based intervention [75]. Interactive as opposed to didactic programs have been shown to have greater effect [76]. Another preventive target is parent training. Parents who include consistent limit-setting and discipline combined with love, warmth, and involvement raise children who are engaged in fewer high-risk behaviors [77]. It has been shown that higher alcohol consumption in late adolescence continues into adulthood and is associated with alcohol problems including dependence [78]. Studies have also shown that cognitions regarding alcohol use in middle-school-aged adolescents predict subsequent heavy drinking during their high-school years [79]. Targeting these age groups with prevention programs could impact these associations.

Conclusion

Substance abuse and dependence is a major problem facing the adolescent population today. Research on this topic has made many advances over the past 10 years but much still needs to be discovered. We know a great deal about the risk and preventive factors involved in substance use disorders. We know that in treatment the involvement of the family is critical, and we know what treatments are the most effective. Further studies on the cause and on definitive treatments are needed to continue to help this population with this widespread problem.

References

1. Shedler J, Block J. Adolescent drug use and psychological health. *Am Psychol* 1990;**45**:612–630.
2. Sheehan M, Oppenheimer E, Taylor C. Who comes for treatment: drug misusers at three London agencies. *Br J Addict* 1988;**83**:311–320.
3. Johnston L, Bachman JG, O'Malley PM. *National Trends in Drug Use and Related Factors Among American High School Students and Young Adults, 1975–1987.* National Institute on Drug Abuse Publ. no. ADM-87-1587. Washington, DC: US Department of Health and Human Services, 1987.
4. Kaplan HI, Sadock BJ. *Synopsis of Psychiatry*, 8th edn. Baltimore: Williams & Wilkins, 1998.
5. Johnston L, O'Malley P, Bachman J. Monitoring the Future. National Results on Adolescent Drug Use: Overview of Key Findings 2010. Bethesda, MD: National Institute on Drug Abuse, 2010.
6. D'Amico EJ, Fromme K. Health risk behaviors of adolescent and young adult siblings. *Health Psychol* 1997;**16**:426–432.
7. White HR, Johnson V, Buyske S. Parental modeling and parenting behavior effects on offspring alcohol and cigarette use. A growth curve analysis. *J Subst Abuse* 2000;**12**:287–310.
8. Bahr SJ, Marcos AC, Maughan SL. Family, educational and peer influences on the alcohol use of female and male adolescents. *J Stud Alcohol* 1995;**56**:457–469.
9. Kumpfer KL. Special populations: etiology and prevention of vulnerability to chemical dependency in children of substance abusers. In: Brown BS, Mills AR (eds) *Youth at High Risk for Substance Abuse.* Rockville, MD: NIDA Monograph, 1987; pp. 1–71.
10. Dielman TE, Butchart AT, Shope JT, Miller M. Environmental correlates of adolescent substance use and misuse: implications for prevention programs. *Int J Addict* 1990–1991;**25**:855–880.
11. Bry BH, Catalano RF, Kumpfer KL, Lochman JE, Szapocznik J. Scientific findings from family prevention intervention research. In: Ashery RS, Robertson E, Kumpfer KL (eds) *Family Focused Prevention of Drug Abuse: Research and Interventions.* NIDA Research Monograph. Washington, DC: Superintendent of Documents, US Government Printing Office, 1998; pp. 103–129.
12. Patton LH. Adolescent substance abuse: risk factors and protective factors. *Pediatr Clin N Am* 1995;**42**:283–293.
13. Dembo R, Wothke W, Shemwell M, *et al.* A structural model of the influence of family problems and child abuse factors on serious delinquency among youths processed at a juvenile assessment center. *J Child Adolesc Subst Abuse* 2000;**10**:17–31.
14. Center for Substance Abuse Prevention. *Preventing Substance Abuse Among Children and Adolescents: Family-Centered Approaches. Prevention Enhancement Protocols System.* DHHS Publication No. 3223-FY'98. 1998; Washington DC: Superintendent of Documents, US Government Printing Office.
15. Graham JW, Marks G, Hansen WB. Social influence processes affecting adolescent substance use. *J Appl Psychol* 1991;**76**:291–298.
16. Biddle BJ, Bank BJ, Marlin MM. Parental and peer influences on adolescence. *Social Forces* 1980;**58**: 1057–1080.
17. Roski J, Perry CL, McGovern PG, Williams CL, Farbakhsh K, Veblen-Mortenson S. School and community influences on adolescent alcohol and drug use. *Health Educ Res* 1997;**12**:255–266.
18. Brook JS, Whiteman M, Gordon AS, Brook DW. The psychosocial etiology of adolescent drug use: A family interactional approach. *Gen Social Psychol Monographs* 1990;**116**.
19. Resnick MD, Harris LJ, Blum RW. The impact of caring and connectedness on adolescent health and well-being. *J Paediatr Child Health* 1993;**29**(Suppl 1):3–9.
20. Resnick MD, Bearman PS, Blum RW, *et al.* Protecting adolescents from harm: findings from the national longitudinal study on adolescent health. *JAMA* 1997;**278**: 823–832.
21. Goodwin DW, SChulsinger F, Hermansen L, *et al.* Alcohol problems in adoptees raised apart from alcoholic biological parents. *Arch Gen Psychiatry* 1973;**28(2)**: 238–243.

22. Blum K, Noble EP, Sheridan PJ, *et al.* Allelic association of human dopamine D2 receptor gene in alcoholism. *JAMA* 1990;**263**:2055–2060.

23. Schukit MA. A 10 year study of sons of alcoholics: preliminary results. *Alcohol Alcohol* 1999(Suppl (1): 147–149.

24. Cloninger CR. Neurogenetic adoptive mechanisms in alcoholism. *Science* 1987;**236**:410–416.

25. Beman DS. Risk factors leading to adolescent substance abuse. *Adolescence* 1995;**30**:201–208.

26. Clark DB, Bukstein OG. Psychopathology in adolescent alcohol abuse and dependence. *Alcohol Health Res World* 1998;**22**:117–126.

27. Miller NS, Fine J. Current epidemiology of comorbidity of psychiatric and addictive disorders. *Psychiatr Clin N Am* 1993;**16**:1–10.

28. Whitmore EA, Milulick SK, Thompson LL, *et al.* Influences on adolescent substance dependence, conduct disorders, depression, attention deficit hyperactivity disorder, and gender. *Drug Alcohol Depend* 1997;**47**:87–97.

29. Bukstein OG, Glancy LJ, Kaminer Y. Patterns of affective comorbidity in a clinical population of dually diagnosed adolescent substance abusers. *J Am Acad Child Adolesc Psychiatry* 1992;**31**:1041–1045.

30. Hovens JG, Cantwell DP, Kiriakos R. Psychiatric comorbidity in hospitalized adolescent substance abusers. *J Am Acad Child Adolesc Psychiatry* 1994;**33**:476–483.

31. Wilens TE, Biederman J, Millstein RB, *et al.* Risk for substance use disorders in youths with child and adolescent-onset bipolar disorder. *J Am Acad Child Adolesc Psychiatry* 1999;**38**:680–685.

32. Merikangas KR, Mehta RL, Molnar BE, *et al.* Comorbidity of substance use disorders with mood and anxiety disorders: Results of international consortium in psychiatric epidemiology. *Addict Behav* 1998; **23**:893–907.

33. Swan N. Early childhood behavior and temperament predict later substance abuse. *National Institute on Drug Abuse Notes* 1995;**10**:1–6.

34. Clark DB, Lesnick L, Hegedus AM. Traumas and other adverse life events in adolescents with alcohol use and dependence. *J Am Acad Child Adolesc Psychiatry* 1997;**36**:1744–1751.

35. Frojd S, Ranta K, Kaltiala-Heino R, Martunen M. Associations of social phobia and general anxiety with alcohol and drug use in a community sample of adolescents. *Alcohol Alcoholism* 2011;**46**:192–199.

36. Buckley PF. Substance abuse in schizophrenia; a review. *J Clin Psychiatry* 1999;**59**(Suppl 3):26–30.

37. Fergusson D, Horwood L, Swain-Campbell N. Cannabis dependence and psychotic symptoms in young people. *Psychol Med* 2003;**33**:15–21.

38. Arseneault L, Cannon M, Poulton R, Murray R, Caspi A, Moffitt TE. Cannabis use in adolescence and risk for adult psychosis: longitudinal prospective study. *Brit Med J* 2002;**325**:1212–1213.

39. Wilens TE, Biederman J, Spencer TJ. Attention deficit hyperactivity disorder and psychoactive substance use disorders. *Child Adolesc Psychiatr Clin N Am* 1996; **5**:73–91.

40. Charach A, Yeung E, Climans T, Lillie E. Childhood attention-deficit/hyperactivity disorder and future substance use disorders: comparative meta-analyses. *J Am Acad Child Adolesc Psychiatry* 2011;**50**:9–21.

41. Horner B, Scheibe K. Prevalence and implications of attention-deficit hyperactivity disorder among adolescents in treatment for substance abuse. *J Am Acad Child Adolesc Psychiatry* 1997;**36**:30–36.

42. Biederman J, Wilens T, Mick E, *et al.* Psychoactive substance use disorders in adults with attention deficit hyperactivity disorder (ADHD): Effects of ADHD and psychiatric comorbidity. *Am J Psychiatry* 1995;**152**: 1652–1658.

43. Biederman J, Wilens T, Mick E, *et al.* Pharmacotherapy of ADHD reduces risk of substance use disorder. *Pediatrics* 1999;**104**:e20.

44. American Academy of Child and Adolescent Psychiatry. Practice Parameters for the assessment and treatment of children and adolescents with substance abuse disorders. *J Am Acad Child Adolesc Psychiatry* 1998; **37**:122–126.

45. Reebye P, Moretti M, Lessard J. Conduct disorder and substance use disorders: comorbidity in a clinical sample of preadolescents and adolescents. *Can J Psychiatry* 1995; **40**:313–319.

46. Myers MG, Stewart DG, Brown SA. Progression of conduct disorder to antisocial personality disorder following treatment for adolescent substance abuse. *Am J Psychiatry* 1998;**155**:479–485.

47. Katz JL. Eating disorders: a primer for the substance abuse specialist. I: Clinical features. *J Subst Abuse Treat* 1990; **7**:143–149.

48. Shafii M, Stelz-Linarsky J, Derrick AM, *et al.* Comorbidity of mental disorders in the post mortem diagnosis of completed suicides in children and adolescents. *J Affect Disord* 1998;**15**:227–233.

49. Issacson JH, Schorling JB. Screening for alcohol problems in primary care. *Med Clin N Am* 1999;**83**:1547–1563.

50. Knight JR, Shrier LA, Bravender TD, *et al.* A new brief screen for adolescent substance abuse. *Arch Pediatr Adolesc Med* 1999;**153**:591–596.

51. Hanson KL, Medina KL, Padula CB, Tapert SF, Brown SA. Impact of adolescent alcohol and drug use on neuropsychological functioning in young adulthood: 10-year outcomes. *J Child Adolesc Subst Abuse* 2011; **20**:135–154.

52. Duffy A, Millin R. Case study: withdrawal syndrome in adolescent chronic cannabis users. *J Am Acad Child Adolesc Psychiatry* 1996;**35**:1618–1621.

53. Schweinsburg AD, Brown SA, Tapert SF. The influence of marijuana use on neurocognitive functioning in adolescents. *Curr Drug Abuse Rev* 2008;**1**:99–111.

54. Jaffe SL, Estroff TW. Use of medications with substance-abusing adolescents. In: Estroff TW (ed.) *Manual of Adolescent Substance Abuse Treatment.* Washington, DC: American Psychiatric Publishing, 2001; pp. 187–203.

55. Baldridge EB, Besson HA. Phencyclidine. *Emerg Med Clin N Am* 1990;**8**:541–550.

56. Schwartz RH, Miller NS. MDMA (ecstasy) and the rave: a review. *Pediatrics* 1997;**100**:705–708.

57. Krystat JH, Karper LP, Siebyl JP, *et al.* Subanesthetic effects of the noncompetitive NMDA antagonist, ketamine, in humans: psychotomimetic, perceptual, cognitive, and neuroendocrine responses. *Arch Gen Psychiatry* 1994;**51**:199–214.

58. Koesters SC, Rogers PD, Rajasingham CR. MDMA (ecstasy) and other club drugs: the new epidemic. *Pediatr Clin N Am* 2002;**49**:415–433.

59. Galloway GP, Frederick SL, Staggers FE, et al. Gamma-hydroxybutyrate: an emerging drug of abuse that causes physical dependence. Addiction 1997;92:89–96.

60. Friedman AS, Beschner GM (eds). Treatment Services for Adolescent Substance Abusers. DHSS Pub No. (ADM) 85-1342. Washington, DC: US Government Printing Office, 1985.

61. Fleisch B. Approaches in the Treatment of Adolescents with Emotional and Substance Abuse Problems. DHSS Pub. No. (ADM) 91-1744. Washington, DC: US Government Printing Office, 1991.

62. Kaminer Y. Alcohol and drug abuse: Adolescent substance abuse treatment: Where do we go from here? Psychiatr Serv 2001;52:147–149.

63. Kaminer Y, Burleson JA. Psychotherapies for adolescent substance abusers: 15 month follow-up of a pilot study. Am J Addict 1999;8:114–119.

64. Alford GS, Koehler RA, Leonard J. Alcoholics Anonymous-Narcotics Anonymous model inpatient treatment of chemically dependent adolescents: A 2-year outcome study. J Studies Alcohol 1991;52:118–126.

65. Koning IM, van den Eijnden RJ, Verdurmen JE, Engles RC, Vollebergh WA. Long-term effects of a parent and student intervention on alcohol use in adolescents: a cluster randomized controlled trial. Am J Prev Med 2011;36: 75–78.

66. Taylor TK, Biglan A. Behavioral family interventions for improving child-rearing: a review for clinicians and policy makers. Clin Child Fam Psychol Rev 1998;1:41–60.

67. Webster-Stratton C, Taylor T. Nipping early risk factors in the bud: Preventing substance abuse, delinquency, and violence in adolescence through interventions targeted at young children–8 years. Prev Sci 2000;2:165–192.

68. Joanning H, Quinn TF, Mullen R. Treating adolescent drug abuse: a comparison of family systems therapy, group therapy, and family drug education. J Marital Fam Ther 1992;18:345–356.

69. Henggeler SW, Melton GB, Smith LA, et al. Family preservation using multi-systemic treatment: Long term follow-up to a clinical trial with serious juvenile offenders. J Child Fam Studies 1993;2:283–293.

70. Henggeler SW, Schoenwald SK, Pickrel SG, et al. Treatment Manual for Family Preservation Using Multisystemic Therapy. Charleston: Medical University of South Carolina,1994.

71. Stein LA, Lebeau R, Colby SM, et al. Motivational interviewing for incarcerated adolescents: effects of depressive symptoms on reducing alcohol and marijuana use after release. J Stud Alcohol Drugs 2011;72:497–506.

72. Ramchand R, Griffin BA, Suttorp M, et al. Using a cross-study design to assess the efficacy of Motivational Enhancement Therapy-Cognitive Behavioral Therapy 5 (MET/CBT5) in treating adolescents with cannabis-related disorders. J Stud Alcohol Drugs 2011;72: 380–389.

73. Martin CS, Kaczynski NA, Maiston SA, et al. Patterns of alcohol abuse and dependence symptoms in adolescent drinkers. J Studies Alcohol 1995;56:672–680.

74. Geller B, Cooper TB, Watts HE, et al. Early findings from a pharmacokinetically designed double-blind and placebo-controlled study of lithium for adolescents co-morbid with bipolar and substance dependency disorders. Prog Neuropsychopharmacol Biol Psychiat 1992; 16:281–299.

75. Botvin GJ, Baker E, Dusenbury L, et al. Long-term follow-up results of a randomized drug abuse prevention trial in a white middle-class population. JAMA 1995; 273:1106–1112.

76. Tobler NS, Stratton HS. Effectiveness of school-based drug prevention programs: a meta-analysis of the research. J Prim Prevent 1997;18:71–128.

77. Brook JS, Brook DW, Gordon AS, et al. The psychological etiology of adolescent drug use: a family interactional approach. Gen Soc Gen Psychol Monographs 1990; 116:111–267.

78. McCambridge J, McAlaney J, Rowe R. Adult consequences of late adolescent alcohol consumption: a systematic review of cohort studies. PLoS Med 2011;8(2): e1000413.

79. Andrews JA, Hampson S, Peterson M. Early adolescent cognitions as predictors of heavy alcohol use in high school. Addict Behav 2011;36:448–455.

15

Childhood Trauma

Julia Huemer, Sidney Edsall, and Niranjan S. Karnik, Hans Steiner

Introduction

Childhood trauma is a common presenting issue for the practicing clinician. The range of phenomena that bring about these issues can range from pediatric acute and chronic illness, to sexual abuse, and even entail mass trauma as the events surrounding the destruction of the World Trade Center in New York City highlight. Clinicians working with these varied populations of children need to be cognizant of current advances in the neurobiological underpinnings of trauma and post-traumatic stress, and its implications on treatment, as well as being sensitive to the social and family milieu that can help form the basis of good therapeutic interventions.

History of Trauma-Related Diagnosis

The diagnosis and treatment of psychological sequelae associated with traumatic events have changed greatly over the years and have only recently expanded to include children. Initially, the definition of traumatic events and the research that ensued were limited to war duty. The experiences of soldiers in World Wars I and II led to terms such as shell shock and combat fatigue and established a relationship between traumatic events and the resulting behavior and affect. It was not until the Vietnam War and the 1970s that the diagnosis of post-traumatic stress disorder (PTSD) was formally introduced into the mental health nomenclature. Although the early conceptualizations of the effects of trauma were significant in shaping our current understanding, the research in this area was largely based on adult men. Only in the last 20 years has the conceptualization of trauma and the incidents that induce trauma-related psychopathology been broadened to include the experiences of the general population, women, specific ethnic groups, and most recently, those of children [1–3]. Recent publications suggest an adaptation and revision of the diagnostic criteria of pediatric PTSD [4].

The association between the range of traumatic events and the resulting psychological and biological effects continues to challenge researchers and clinicians in the mental health community.

Traumatic events can be described as impacting children on at least one of the following three levels: the self, the community, and the environment (Figure 15.1). Depending on their developmental stage, children may be particularly susceptible to the adverse effects of trauma because of their dependency on adults for care and safety, their limited ability to influence the events and surroundings in which they live, and their cognitive and emotional level of development. Over the past decade, there has been a considerable amount of research examining the impact of trauma on children. Studies to date suggest the psychiatric consequences of trauma are influenced by several variables, such as the level of exposure and duration of trauma, [5, 6] preexisting psychopathology prior to trauma exposure [7–9], the impact of trauma on a child's social structure [10], and biological factors contributing to a child's predisposition to trauma-related pathology as well as resilience in the development of pathology [11]. In addition, a child's subjective experience of potential harm during trauma has been found to be associated with trauma-related symptoms as opposed to more objective accounts of traumatic events [12–14]. It is also apparent that different types of trauma impact children to varying degrees. For example, exposure to natural disasters results in a lower rate of PTSD development compared to more chronic, war-related traumas [15]. Interpersonal-related traumas, such as physical or sexual abuse, seem to be associated with the highest rates of PTSD [15–18].

Studies assessing the psychological sequelae of physical and sexual abuse in children have revealed the presence of significant trauma-related pathology [19–22]. The duration of abuse, the closeness of the perpetrator, and the use of violence all influence the severity of

Clinical Child Psychiatry, Third Edition. Edited by William M. Klykylo and Jerald Kay.
© 2012 John Wiley & Sons, Ltd. Published 2012 by John Wiley & Sons, Ltd.

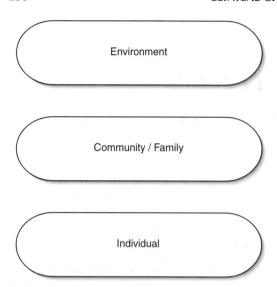

Figure 15.1 Levels of trauma experience.

psychological symptoms that present during and following abuse [21]. Sexual abuse in children is associated with the development of depression, anxiety, behavioral problems, sexualized behaviors, and PTSD [20, 22]. Victims of sexual abuse as children are at higher risk for having psychiatric problems in adulthood as well, including substance use disorders, social anxiety, and depression, and are at higher risk for attempting suicide [23, 24]. Children who experience significant accidents, such as those involving motor vehicles and fires, or who suffer life-threatening illness and invasive medical procedures, are at risk for developing psychological symptoms [25–27]. Additionally, children who are victims of violent crimes such as robbery, assault, and attempted murder are at high risk for developing PTSD, anxiety, and depressive disorders [28], and may demonstrate increased rates of internalizing and externalizing behavioral problems [29].

Children who witness violence in their immediate environment may develop trauma-related pathology. Violence within the family, such as abuse between parents or abuse between a parent and sibling, can create an environment of fear resulting in psychological distress and symptomatology [30–32]. Children who witness the assault or murder of a parent exhibit trauma-related symptoms such as anxiety, hypervigilance, and decreased concentration [33].

Trauma within the community can cause psychiatric disturbance in children, as reflected by research of violence in US inner cities [13, 28, 34–36]. US inner city environments can parallel the environments of combat zones, as violence and aggression create an atmosphere of potential danger and fear for personal safety and security. Ninety-two percent of 90 female adolescents living within a US urban environment and presenting for routine medical care endorsed at least one trauma, including witnessing community violence (86%) and hearing about a homicide (68%) [37]. Other community-based studies have reported that more than 80% of inner-city adolescents have seen someone physically assaulted, 40% have seen someone shot or stabbed, and almost 25% have witnessed a homicide [35, 38, 39]. Mazza et al., in 1999, reported a significant relationship between violence exposure and PTSD symptomatology, suicidal ideation, and depression in 94 young adolescents from an inner-city school within the United States [40].

Terrorism-induced trauma imposes a unique stress on the community and the individual. Due to its unpredictability and devastating effects, terrorism can create an environment of fear and intimidation within society persisting for prolonged periods of time. Few studies have been conducted to determine the effects on children in the aftermath of terrorist events such as the 11 September 2001 terrorist attacks, the 1995 bombing of the Alfred P. Murrah Building in Oklahoma City, the Scud missile attacks in Israel, state terrorism attacks in Guatemala between 1981 and 1983, and terrorist activity in Northern Ireland [41]. The rates of PTSD in children exposed to terrorism activity range from 28% to 50% [42–44]. Other psychiatric problems have been associated with terrorism, such as depression, anxiety, separation problems, mood changes, sleep difficulties, behavioral problems, and regressive symptoms [41, 42, 44].

The terrorist attacks of 11 September 2001 have increased concerns for personal safety and security in both adults and children. Schuster et al., in 2001, surveyed 560 adults throughout the United States 3–5 days after 11 September. Thirty-five percent of adults surveyed noted their children were experiencing one or more stress symptoms. Parents experiencing stress reactions were more likely to report symptoms in their children [45]. Pfefferbaum et al. examined the impact of peri-traumatic responses in over 2000 middle-school children 7 weeks after the 1995 Oklahoma City bombing, finding that peri-traumatic responses such as nervousness, fear, or fear that a family member or friend would be hurt, were the strongest predictors of PTSD reactions [12].

Research addressing the effects of war on children in Cambodia [46, 47], South Africa [48], Kuwait [49], Rwanda [50], and the Israeli-Palestinian conflict [51] have documented the psychological sequelae resulting from wartime experiences. As expected, traumatic events and development of pathology vary between populations due to multiple psychosocial factors. Of note, 3000 Rwandan children, interviewed 13 months after the genocide in April 1994, described exposure to extreme levels of violence in the form of witnessing the deaths of close family members and others in massacres. The majority of these children (90%) had believed they would die and 61% had severe levels of PTSD symptoms, predominantly presenting as avoidance and intrusive thoughts [50]. Eighty-seven percent of Palestinian children living in areas of bombardment were found to have moderate to severe levels of PTSD [51].

War also creates significant numbers of child refugees, who are uniquely at risk for developing trauma-related pathology due to the multiple and compounding stressors experienced before escape from their country of origin, during their flight from home, and during resettlement [52]. An estimated 300 000 children under 18 have fought in armed conflicts, and there are approximately 10 million refugee children in the world [53]. In addition, traumatic events often occur during detainment in refugee camps. For example, among Cuban refugees detained in a refugee camp prior to arrival in the United States, 80% witnessed acts of violence, 37% saw someone attempt or commit suicide, and 19% were separated from family members [54]. Yet refugee children have also been reported to have significant levels of resiliency. Ideological commitment to issues of war, peace, patriotism, and the political enemy were found to be associated with less anxiety, insecurity, and depression in Israeli Jewish young adolescents faced with low levels of war exposure [55]. Social support, parental well-being, and maintaining connections to one's culture of origin have also been found to be protective in refugee children [56, 57].

Indirect exposure to violence, such as television viewing of traumatic events, has been shown to increase children's risk for trauma-related symptoms, in particular PTSD-related symptoms [12, 49, 58, 59]. For example, PTSD symptoms in Kuwaiti children following the Gulf War were found to be positively correlated with television coverage exposure of combat-related events [49]. Terr et al. studied children's reactions to the Challenger space shuttle explosion. They described the children's experience as "distant trauma," insofar as they had witnessed the disaster at the time of its occurrence, but indirectly via television and from a safe distance from the disaster. The children's symptom patterns were similar to PTSD, in addition to trauma-specific fear, fear of being alone, clinging to others, and event-specific fears [58]. Following the 11 September terrorist attacks, the number of hours of television

viewing by children was correlated with the number of reported stress symptoms [60]. Also, children who have experienced direct loss are more likely to watch television coverage of a traumatic event [43, 59], thereby exacerbating their trauma-related symptoms.

Natural disasters such as flash floods, hurricanes, and earthquakes have all been found to produce trauma-related pathology in children [61–64]. Anxiety, depression, PTSD symptoms and diagnosis, as well as behavior problems such as aggression and enuresis, have been found in children who survive these types of trauma. The perceived severity of the disaster, level of injury, and level of pre-disaster functioning are all moderating factors that can contribute to the extent of psychological distress [62, 64, 65]. Physical proximity to a trauma has also been associated with increased PTSD symptomatology [6, 66]. Vernberg et al. described how children's level of exposure to Hurricane Andrew, including their perceived life threat, was highly predictive of later development of PTSD symptoms [64].

Displacement and relocation may have varying effects on children. Children whose families are displaced because of political violence have higher levels of psychiatric symptoms compared to families who are not displaced [67]. Relocation due to nonwar situations, as may occur during natural disasters, has been shown to have comparatively fewer negative psychological effects on children [68].

It is also important to recognize that children's responses to traumatic events can be influenced by their parents' response. Positive correlations have been found between children's and parents' symptomatology following trauma [51, 56, 69, 70]. In addition, having a parent who models appropriate coping mechanisms, as well as having a stable and secure emotional relationship with at least one parent, has been shown to increase resiliency in children experiencing trauma-related stress [56, 70, 71]. Other psychosocial factors that have been associated with children's resiliency during and after traumatic events include social support and community educational, political, and religious support [56, 72]. It is apparent that further understanding of resilient factors will help to better identify children's optimal coping strategies, and differentiate these strategies from those of their parents.

Epidemiology

The pattern in which trauma-related pathology occurs in the general population is an issue of ongoing study. Studies involving children are scarce, due in part to difficulties in reporting traumatic events and in the diagnostic process, both of which will be discussed later.

Although literature is lacking in this area, several studies have generated a fairly complete picture.

One of the most important studies in this field describes that more than two-thirds of children report at least one traumatic event by 16 years of age. Among them, 13.4% develop some PTS symptoms. Few PTS symptoms or psychiatric disorders are observed for individuals who are affected by their first event. Fewer than 0.5% of children in this epidemiological assessment fulfill the criteria for full-blown DSM-IV PTSD. Violent or sexual trauma is related to the highest rates of symptoms. The post-traumatic stress symptoms were predicted by previous multiple traumas, anxiety disorders, and family adversity. Lifetime co-occurrence of other psychiatric disorders with traumatic events and PTSD symptoms happened most frequently with anxiety and depressive disorders [73].

A person in the general population has an approximately 69% chance of experiencing an extraordinary event during his or her lifetime [74]. Of the individuals that do experience such an event, about 20% become traumatized. Tragic deaths are the most frequent form of trauma experienced, and sexual assault yields the highest rates of trauma-related pathology. Motor vehicle crashes present the most adverse combination of frequency and impact but low socioeconomic status also puts individuals at risk [75, 76]. Approximately one-fifth of all psychiatric outpatients show symptoms of PTSD [74].

In an urban population study, Breslau and colleagues [8, 77] reported that over one-third of a sample of young adults experienced some type of trauma in their lifetime, as defined in the *Diagnostic and Statistical Manual of Mental Disorders, Third Edition, Revised* (DSM-III-R). Approximately 24% of these individuals (9% of the total sample) also exhibited symptoms consistent with a diagnosis of PTSD. A separate assessment of the general adolescent population reported that 40% of the adolescents evaluated experienced some type of traumatic event during their teen years [9, 78]. Of those adolescents, approximately 14% (6% of the sample population) later developed PTSD. No differences across gender were identified for the occurrence of trauma, but females were six times more likely than males to develop PTSD. A study of urban school-age children found that 57% of the students sampled had been the victim of a violent act or knew someone who had been a victim [34]. More recently, Cuffe and colleagues found that 3% of females and 1% of males in a community sample of older adolescents met DSM-IV criteria for PTSD [79].

Rates of trauma-related symptoms are often higher in those populations whose risk of exposure to traumatic events is greater than that of the general population.

Incarcerated delinquent males, for example, present with high rates of active PTSD and dissociative symptoms [80, 81]. Approximately 32% of these males meet the full criteria for a trauma-related diagnosis, and 15% fulfill partial criteria. Many of these youths come from communities in which they are exposed to community violence, which thus places them at greater risk for trauma-related pathology. In addition, many of these individuals are traumatized by the circumstances and events of their crime.

Among the children who experience specific traumas, the rates of PTSD vary depending on the methods used for data collection and the criteria used. For example, the rate of PTSD has been reported to be as high as 44% in cases of sexual abuse and 20% in cases of physical abuse, with an even larger percentage for partial criteria [19, 82–84]. The variability reported is due in part to differences in abuse circumstances. The closeness of the relationship between the child and the perpetrator (i.e., parent vs stranger), the duration of the abuse, and the level of violence all contribute to the presence of a PTSD diagnosis. Females and young children appear to be more susceptible to the disorder [21]. Methodological design and length of time post trauma vary among the studies and likely account for some differences in rates; few studies use longitudinal designs with adequate follow-up time.

As many as 38% of children exposed to violence in the community show symptoms of PTSD. A study conducted by Fitzpatrick and Boldizar found that 27% of African American youths between the ages of 7 and 18 years exhibited PTSD symptoms as a result of community violence [28]. Studies of the effects of natural disasters vary greatly in their method of reporting PTSD, owing to the length of time post trauma at which the children are evaluated and to the type of disaster. Rates of PTSD and PTSD symptoms range from as high as 54% immediately following a disaster such as an earthquake, to 37% 2 years following a flood, to 7% 6 months following a hurricane [63, 66, 85–87]. The more intense a child's experience during and following a disaster, the more likely the child is to develop PTSD symptoms. Factors influencing the development of symptoms include the severity of the disaster, the extent of injury, the degree of material and personal loss, and the level of trait anxiety [61, 62].

The picture that emerges is incomplete but useful. Only a fraction of people going through extraordinary situations become ill, and this varies depending on the intensity of the experience and nature of the trauma. Although a substantial amount of information is known about the factors that contribute to the presence of trauma-related symptoms for specific types of trauma, less is known about what factors protect children from developing symptoms or, conversely, place them at risk. Research discussed later in this chapter suggests that personality and coping styles play a part in a child's response to events [80, 88, 89]. Further information is needed on the clinical profiles and prevalence of PTSD and trauma-related symptoms in the clinical child and adolescent population. Future studies should also obtain profiles of the general population and examine the influence of protective factors that insulate those who do not develop psychopathology [90].

Developmental Traumatology

The field of developmental traumatology is a relatively new focus of child psychiatric study. It is defined as a systematic investigation of biological, psychological, and sociological impacts on children who have experienced maltreatment and/or trauma, in an attempt to identify varying biopsychosocial effects throughout the developmental stages of a child into adulthood [1]. This area of study attempts to clarify the interactions between biological and environmental variables in the developing child, such as genetic constitution, psychosocial stressors, and identification of critical periods of vulnerability and resilience for traumatic experiences. Information regarding psychosocial stressors, such as low socioeconomic status, parental mental illnesses, and poor social support, can be integrated with research from developmental psychopathology, developmental neuroscience, and stress and trauma research. Developmental traumatology is the study of these complex interactions, as stressful life experiences can affect biological systems leading to a variety of psychiatric and psychological consequences [91].

Recent advances in neuroimaging and neurochemical research have shed considerable light onto the biological effects of trauma in children. These effects can have significant and ongoing developmental impact on children. Neurobiological systems provide the structural framework not only for physical and cognitive development, but also for emotional and behavioral development. Acute and chronic stress causes significant alterations in these neurobiological pathways [11, 92]. Stress also impacts the regulation and expression of genes, which in effect impacts the development of the brain and its processes [93, 94].

Neurobiological Processes Involved in the Stress Response

Research regarding the neurobiological aspects of PTSD and its development from single and/or multiple

traumatic event(s) in childhood is limited to date. Initial findings appear to show that PTSD in childhood is a different developmental process compared to PTSD in adults. These differences may be reflected in the finding that children appear to be less resilient to trauma than adults. Results of a meta-analysis demonstrated children and adolescents who have experienced trauma are approximately 1.5 times more likely to be diagnosed with PTSD compared to adults [95].

Traumatic stress activates the catecholamine system, that is, the sympathetic nervous system, leading to increases in heart rate, blood pressure, metabolic rate, and alertness. In addition, during a stress response, corticotropin-releasing hormone (CRH) is released from the hypothalamus, thereby activating the hypothalamic-pituitary-adrenal (HPA) axis by stimulating secretion of adrenocorticotropin (ACTH) from the pituitary. Cortisol is then released from the adrenal glands, further stimulating the sympathetic nervous system during stress. These biological processes are consistent with the "fight-or-flight" response evolutionarily adapted to protect the individual from danger and potential harm, but which in chronic experience may become counterproductive. HPA regulation eventually leads to restoration of basal cortisol levels via negative feedback inhibition. It is hypothesized that dysregulation of the catecholamine system and HPA axis in response to stress and trauma may significantly contribute to the negative symptoms of PTSD.

It has generally been hypothesized that early stress on brain development could exert only deleterious effects on neural development. An alternative hypothesis has been proposed, suggesting that early stressors can create new developmental pathways, allowing the brain to adapt itself for continued survival and reproduction, despite existence in a stressful environment [92, 94]. Nonetheless, elevated levels of catecholamines and dysregulation of the HPA axis associated with stress and trauma appear to lead to adverse neuronal development through a variety of mechanisms. There is evidence of accelerated loss of neurons [96–98], delays in myelination [99], decreased number and length of dendritic processes [100], disruptions in neural pruning [101], inhibition of neurogenesis [102, 103], and decreases in brain-derived neurotrophic factor expression [104]. Early stressful experiences have also been shown to have neurobiological structural consequences, such as reduced corpus callosum size, attenuated development of the left neocortex, hippocampus, and amygdala, enhanced electrical irritability in limbic structures, and reduced functional activity of the cerebellar vermis [92]. Loss of the corpus callosum volume can lead to reduced communication between the hemispheres, and has been shown to produce lateralization that can lead to catecholamine dysregulation. The brain regions affected during stressful experiences appear to have one or more of the following features: (i) a prolonged postnatal development; (ii) a high density of glucocorticoid receptors; and (iii) some degree of postnatal neurogenesis [92]. While the picture at this point is still preliminary, there appears to be increasing evidence that collectively damage to these areas of the brain can lead to difficulties in social integration, attachment, and bonding, as well as mood and anxiety disorders. These features suggest there are potential ongoing developmental consequences of traumatic stress. In order to better understand the neurobiological and psychological sequelae of trauma, it is worthwhile to review neurobiological findings in children at varying developmental stages into adulthood.

The Catecholamine System and Trauma

There has been significant evidence to suggest that maltreated children and adolescents with mood and anxiety symptoms have altered catecholamine levels. Maltreated children with PTSD have been shown to have elevated concentrations of urinary norepinephrine and dopamine over 24 hours compared to nontraumatized children diagnosed with over-anxious disorder and healthy controls, with a significant positive correlation between urinary catecholamine levels and duration of trauma and severity of PTSD symptoms [105]. Increased 24-hour urinary norepinephrine concentrations in neglected depressed male children have been reported [106], as well as greater 24-hour urinary catecholamine and catecholamine metabolite concentrations in dysthymic, sexually abused girls [107]. This is a consistent finding in adult populations, as adult patients with chronic PTSD have been shown to have increased circulating levels of norepinephrine [108] and increased reactivity of α_2-adrenergic receptors [109].

The Hypothalamic-Pituitary-Adrenal Axis and Trauma

The HPA axis has also been implicated in the pathophysiology of PTSD, although current PTSD research reflects conflicting theories regarding the regulation of the HPA axis in PTSD, both in child and adult populations. Still, it appears some trends in HPA axis research have been identified. For example, most studies of traumatized pediatric populations have found increased basal levels of cortisol, whereas cortisol levels in adult populations with PTSD are generally decreased.

The theory that adults with PTSD have low basal cortisol levels is supported by evidence of lower plasma cortisol levels in adult combat veteran populations

with PTSD compared to controls without PTSD [110], and findings of low urinary cortisol excretion in adult holocaust survivors with PTSD compared to holocaust survivors without PTSD [111]. It is hypothesized that cortisol levels in adults with chronic PTSD are decreased compared to nontraumatized control subjects due to a downregulation of anterior pituitary CRH receptors secondary to chronic elevations in CRH levels, and also to an enhanced negative feedback inhibition of cortisol at the level of the pituitary [112]. This downregulation may be an adaptive response, as chronically elevated cortisol levels are potentially neurotoxic. This theory is supported by studies by Yehuda et al. demonstrating that combat veterans with PTSD have an exaggerated cortisol suppression following the administration of low-dose dexamethasone (an analog of cortisol) and an exaggerated decline of cytosolic lymphocyte glucocorticoid receptors compared to those without PTSD [113]. Also compatible with this hypothesis are the findings that individuals with PTSD have high levels of corticotropin-releasing factor (CRF) in their cerebrospinal fluid (CSF) [114], a blunted adrenocorticotropin hormone (ACTH) response to CRH [115], and an enhanced ACTH response to doses of metyrapone suppressing cortisol production [116].

Other studies have not been compatible with the above-mentioned theory regarding PTSD in adults. Specifically, three studies reported elevated 24-hour urinary cortisol excretion in adult patients with PTSD [117–119]. In addition, a greater ACTH response to CRF in PTSD compared to control subjects has been reported [120], as well as greater ACTH responses to current psychosocial stress among women with histories of childhood physical and sexual abuse compared to women with no such histories [121]. These studies postulate an alternative theory explaining baseline low cortisol levels, namely a chronically low adrenal output of cortisol, or rather, adrenal insufficiency [122]. These discrepant findings may be associated with the confounding effects of assay methodology as well as potential current life stressors influencing the regulation of the HPA axis.

Studies of the HPA axis and its regulation following trauma in children have generally demonstrated elevated cortisol levels, suggesting different biological consequences of traumatic stress compared to adult populations. De Bellis et al. reported that maltreated prepubertal children diagnosed with PTSD have increased 24-hour urinary cortisol levels compared to matched control subjects [105]. Carrion et al. demonstrated significantly elevated salivary cortisol levels in children with trauma exposure histories and PTSD symptoms when compared with control groups [123]. Gunnar *et al.* demonstrated elevated salivary cortisol levels in 6–12-year-old children raised in Romanian orphanages for 8 months of their lives compared with early adopted and Canadian-born children tested at 6.5 years after adoption [124] (Table 15.1). In a relatively large study, Hart *et al.* demonstrated that depressed maltreated children had elevated afternoon salivary cortisol levels compared to depressed nonmaltreated children [125].

In contrast, Goenjian *et al.* studied adolescents 5 years after the 1988 Armenian earthquake and reported reduced levels of cortisol in children in closest proximity to the disaster [126]. Also King *et al.* found that girls with a history of sexual abuse within the last 2 months had lower cortisol in comparison to control subjects [127]. Comparing and interpreting the results of these studies in children, as well as in adult PTSD studies, is limited by varying methodological approaches and differing population samples. While there is no absolute consensus on whether cortisol levels in children with PTSD are elevated or decreased, most studies show an elevation in cortisol levels in children diagnosed with PTSD.

It is possible that some variations in study results could also be explained by examining the developmental stage when trauma occurred as well as the duration of time elapsed since exposure to trauma in children as well as adults. One could postulate that CRH and cortisol levels are elevated acutely after a trauma. Long-term, or rather, developmental effects of trauma could eventually lead to decreased levels of cortisol due to chronic elevations in CRH and the enhanced negative feedback on the HPA axis. This hypothesis is supported by a study comparing pituitary volume differences using magnetic resonance imaging (MRI) in children of varying ages with PTSD and nontraumatized healthy comparison subjects [128]. Although there were no differences seen in pituitary volumes between PTSD and control subjects, there was a significant age-by-group effect for PTSD subjects showing greater differences in pituitary volume with age compared to control subjects. Post hoc analyses revealed pituitary volumes were significantly larger in pubertal and postpubertal maltreated subjects with PTSD compared to control subjects, but were similar in prepubertal maltreated subjects with PTSD and control subjects. Pituitary volume changes in response to stress and dysregulation of the HPA axis have already been demonstrated in various research models. Chronically administering CRH to rats produces an increase in the number and size of pituitary corticotroph cells [129, 130]. Also, suicide victims have been shown to have larger pituitary corticotroph cells [131].

Clearly, neurobiological research regarding PTSD in children is only beginning to elucidate the biological effects of trauma. While preliminary data and developing theory regarding HPA regulation in children with PTSD are provocative, the evidence is incomplete to date. Further research is needed to clarify HPA regulation in PTSD in children at varying developmental stages.

In this context, recent studies on PTSD in children and adolescents expand the view beyond neuroendocrinology by combining different methodological approaches. One study, for instance, revealed a significantly negative association between left ventral prefrontal cortex gray matter and prebedtime cortisol levels [132].

Neuroanatomical Findings Associated with Traumatic Stress

A growing body of evidence is reflecting significant involvement of glucocorticoids (cortisol) and their impact on the hippocampus in a stress response [133]. There is significant evidence for hippocampal atrophy in adult populations with PTSD [134–137], Cushing syndrome (characterized by a pathological oversecretion of glucocorticoids) [138, 139], and recurrent major depressive disorder [140, 141] (also frequently associated with oversecretion of glucocorticoids). There is also significant evidence that glucocorticoid toxicity may, in part, be mediated by prolonged elevations in excitatory amino acids such as glutamate [142].

With the use of high-resolution magnetic resonance imaging (MRI), significant hippocampal atrophy, compared to control subjects, has been demonstrated in adult combat veterans with the diagnosis of PTSD [134, 135]. In addition, studies have reported significant left hippocampal volume reduction in adult populations with histories of childhood trauma and a current diagnosis of PTSD [136, 137].

In contrast, studies of children with PTSD have not demonstrated any significant differences in hippocampal volumes compared to normal controls. Carrion *et al.* did not observe any significant differences in hippocampal volumes between abused children with the diagnosis of PTSD and subthreshold diagnosis of PTSD compared to normal control subjects [143]. De Bellis *et al.*, in 1999 and in a subsequent study in 2002, studied hippocampal volumes using MRI in maltreated children with PTSD and healthy controls, and found no significant differences in volume [144, 145]. Rather, it was reported that subjects with PTSD had smaller intracranial, cerebral, and prefrontal cortex, prefrontal cortical white matter, right temporal lobe volumes, and smaller areas

Table 15.1 HPA studies of PTSD and trauma in children.

Study	N	Location	Population	DSM diagnosis	Findings
Goenjian et al. 1996	37 Trauma exposed from 1988 Armenia earthquake (five years after event)	Armenia	Adolescents	PTSD symptoms	Lower morning salivary cortisol, and greater suppression with dexmethasone challenge
De Bellis et al. 1999	18 PTSD Overanxious disorder (OAD) 24 Control	USA	Ages 8–12 mixed gender	PTSD diagnosis	Urine catecholamines PTSD > OAD = Control
Gunnar et al. 2001	18 Romanian orphans (adopted at eight months) 15 Early adopted (prior to four months) 27 Canadian born	Canada/Romania	Ages 6–12	None	Salivary cortisol greater in eight-month institutionalized infants
King et al. 2001	10 girls with sexual abuse histories 10 Control	USA	Ages 5–7 girls	None	Lower basal cortisol levels than controls
Carrion et al. 2002	51 PTSD symptoms 31 Control	USA	Ages 7–14 mixed gender	PTSD symptoms	Salivary cortisol elevated in PTSD > control

of the corpus callosum. Teicher *et al.* found a marked reduction in the middle portions of the corpus callosum in child psychiatric inpatients with a substantiated history of abuse or neglect versus control subjects [146]. De Bellis *et al.* (1999) also reported reduced corpus callosum size in children with a history of abuse and PTSD, with more notable volume changes in males than females. This neurobiological finding may be associated with decreased communication between the cortical hemispheres, which may be related to memory difficulties and dissociative disorders, both of which are often found to be comorbid with PTSD.

There are several possible explanations for the differences in neuroanatomical findings between adult and child populations with diagnoses of PTSD. One possibility may be associated with the fact that many adults with PTSD have comorbid substance use disorders, and reduced hippocampal volumes may be associated with such alcohol and/or drug use. De Bellis *et al.* has demonstrated a decrease in hippocampal volumes in adolescent-onset alcohol abuse [147]. Yet neuroimaging studies described in adults have continued to reflect significant hippocampal volume changes even after matching controls for years of substance use [135, 136] or adjusting volume changes for cumulative alcohol exposure [134, 137].

Another possible cause of these discrepancies could be that neurobiological findings may take time to present, suggesting the stress response is gradual and progressive in nature. The hippocampus, as well as other brain structures, is known to have continued neurogenesis postnatally. In addition, the hippocampus has been shown to have an overproduction of axonal and dendritic arborization, as well as synapses and receptors, which are not pruned and eliminated until the postpubertal period [148–150]. Animal models suggest that psychological and physical stress produce measurable changes in brain-derived neurotrophic factor (BDNF), which has effects on neurogenesis and prevention of apoptosis [151]. Cumulatively, these findings suggest that the effects of childhood trauma could have ongoing developmental implications for brain structure and function. Traumatic injury could therefore be partially dependent on the individual's stage of postnatal neural development.

A third possibility may be that the neurobiological finding of a smaller hippocampal volume is actually not a result of chronic stress, but rather is a predisposition for the development of PTSD. This is supported by a study comparing monozygotic twin veterans and normal control subjects. It was found that combat veterans with PTSD, as well as their identical twins without exposure to trauma, both had smaller hippocampi com-

pared to normal, nontraumatized controls. In addition, veterans with PTSD had significantly smaller hippocampal volumes compared to their nontraumatized twins [152]. This may suggest that smaller hippocampal volumes may be a both predisposition to the development of PTSD as well as an effect of trauma in adults.

The majority of research involving metabolic activity of the brain in PTSD has been conducted in adult populations although there are a few recent studies in children as well. Positron-emission tomography and functional magnetic resonance imaging have shown increased reactivity in the amygdala and anterior paralimbic region [153, 154] and decreased reactivity in the anterior cingulate and orbitofrontal areas in adults with a history of childhood sexual abuse who are asked to read trauma-related scripts [155]. Preliminary studies in child populations with PTSD have reported some similar changes in metabolic activity, implicating specific brain areas as being metabolically affected in PTSD. Using proton magnetic resonance spectroscopy, De Bellis *et al.* found a decreased ratio of *N*-acetylaspartate to creatine in the anterior cingulate in 11 maltreated children and adolescents with PTSD compared to control subjects, suggesting the anterior cingulate's metabolism is altered in childhood PTSD [156]. Of note, these brain areas described have been implicated in the fear response.

One caveat to these studies must be noted. Functional imaging studies are labor intensive to produce, and although they have yielded interesting preliminary data, the sample sizes so far are generally small, numbering less than 20 in the best studies. The data emerging must therefore be interpreted with caution, and clinicians are strongly discouraged at this point from using imaging techniques as the sole or primary basis for diagnosis. Expense, expertise, and the need to interpret images very carefully are cautionary flags for the practicing clinician. In contrast, these cautions need not extend to the endocrine literature, which is much better established and represents a long history of research with some degree of clinical correlation. But here again, the diagnostic value of this information remains in doubt and only further studies will shed light on these complex pathways and their utility in practice.

Research on the neurobiological and neuroanatomical effects of PTSD from single and/or multiple traumatic event(s) in childhood is limited to date. Initial findings may appear to demonstrate that PTSD in childhood is a different developmental process compared to PTSD in adults, with potentially evolving neurobiological consequences during the course of an individual's early life. It is important to consider the likelihood of prolonged effects from childhood trauma, not only impacting the development of coping strategies, impact on interpersonal relationships and academic performance, but also the neurobiological effects in children and adolescent populations. These neurobiological effects may indeed demonstrate significant impact on behavior and cognition, and may in part be influenced by the neurobiological developmental stages in children and adolescents. Further research is needed to clarify these complexities in PTSD development in childhood through adolescence and into young adulthood.

The Workup

The Interview

When making a trauma-related diagnosis in children, the clinician should recognize that the necessary information is often not forthcoming. Since most of the symptoms of PTSD and acute stress disorder (ASD) [157] are of an internalizing kind, the younger the child, the worse he or she is as a self-observer and reporter. Much information about internal states is provided by the parents of young children and is displayed by the children in play. As children reach school age, they develop some psychological structures to report complex internal states; these reports can nevertheless involve fairly simple reports and misunderstanding.

Children, in particular young children, often do not associate the emotional repercussions with the traumatic events that caused them; as a result, they are not likely to volunteer information regarding events that may seem far in the past. Children who are sexually abused are often sworn to secrecy by the abuser and are therefore less likely to reveal the occurrence of the trauma. Parents often bring their children to treatment with recognition of problematic behavior but without specific knowledge of the trauma from which it originated. The situation is further complicated in adolescence. Although most adolescents have the capacity to self-observe, many do not have the motivation to collaborate in their own treatment. Adolescents as well as children often presume personal responsibility and guilt and may experience threats from the perpetrator, all of which decrease the likelihood of reporting.

When assessing for traumatic events (Figure 15.2), it is crucial that the clinician administers interviews with the child, as well as with the parents or primary caregiver, to establish as accurate a history as possible. This is especially important because many trauma victims deny or minimize the factors surrounding the event, depending on the stage of trauma recovery. In addition, contact with teachers, school counselors, and

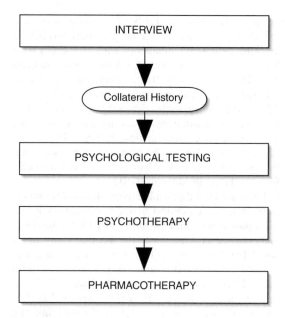

Figure 15.2 Evaluation of trauma in children.

school psychologists should be made to form a more objective assessment of the child's behavior in structured settings. The absence of a thorough assessment from different parties can lead to misdiagnosis, ineffective treatment, and a continuation of symptoms as well as the appearance of new symptoms.

Trauma can often be the hidden cause of psychopathology in the absence of significant reported life events. This does not mean, however, that one should assume trauma as a fallback diagnosis. Rather, when a child presents with difficulties in attention and concentration or mood changes, the clinician should explore possible experiences with traumatic events and the reactions that ensued. In the absence of an explained cause of behavior difficulties, traumatic events should be investigated but not assumed. It is becoming increasingly apparent that memory is a complex experience, and that the mind is capable of repressing trauma [158, 159]. Nevertheless, care must be taken when interviewing children if the clinical data are to be used for judicial or investigative purposes. Children and adolescents are suggestible, and thus leading questions (e.g., the type of questions that are usually part of a structured interview), although never a good strategy in clinical practice, are especially problematic in this context. Combining structured techniques with skilled clinical exploration is likely the best method for conducting interviews where trauma is suspected. We advocate that clinicians prepare an unstructured format for the child and family or guardinans to allow open-ended exploration of leads that may arise, and then proceed in a more structured and thorough way to obtain details of the history. While we believe this combination approach represents a good set of practices, there may be circumstances where alternative approaches are needed and therefore clinical judgment is always necessary.

The differentiation of false from true traumatic memories is complex and inconsistent. Williams, in her study of victims of sexual abuse 17 years after the event, found that younger age at the time of abuse and closeness of relationship with the abuser correlated with the inability to recall the event [160]. A functional MRI study by John Gabrieli and colleagues demonstrated that prefrontal cortical and right hippocampal regions of the brain exhibit higher degrees of activation in individuals who repressed unwanted memories [161]. Their study, while limited to adults in nontraumatic situations, sheds light on the ways that the brain may produce traumatic forgetting and also leads to the realization that memories might indeed emerge at a later time in the event that these pathways normalize at a neurochemical level.

It is clear that memories are reconstructed and not simply laid down, and thus not simply recalled as a photographic image or 100% accurate event. Memories are narrated and constantly being reconstructed, and individuals can therefore be induced to believe that certain events happened when in fact they did not; however, it is not yet clear whether complex events typically reported by trauma victims can also be implanted. In clinical practice, we have helped several patients with this kind of problem and were impressed with several features of the emergence of long-forgotten material:

(1) The emergence occurred in the context of a long-established and trusted therapeutic relationship after many months of treatment for other related problems.
(2) The emergence was triggered by a current event in the patient's life that in some form was reminiscent of the original event.
(3) The traumatic event did not come as a total surprise, since the patient usually assessed the victimizer to be a problematic person in his or her life.
(4) The memories were disjointed and fragmented at first and were accompanied by appropriate emotions such as anxiety and rage, but there was a general hesitancy to draw the appropriate inferences.
(5) Nightmares at times re-emerged that had been present a long time ago.
(6) Our own clinical conduct during the time of the emergence of these traumatic events was at all times receptive and facilitative but never pressuring and prescriptive.

As further research is conducted to help deal with these complex issues, clinicians can be helpful to patients but still not "muddy the waters."

Assessment

Psychological and neuropsychological testing can be beneficial in assessing a trauma-related diagnosis, particularly when there is a question of differential diagnosis or comorbidity or when children are reluctant or unable to discuss the trauma or their feelings [162]. In addition to the standard psychological assessment measures, more specific measures have been designed to assess problematic behavior of children who have been sexually abused [163, 164]. The presence of commonly occurring traumas that often lead to psychopathology can also be investigated with specific measures such as the Impact of Event Scale and the Response Evaluation Measure (REM-71) [165, 166]. Other measures, such as the Child Behavior Checklist and the Schedule for Affective Disorders and Schizophrenia, can help assess the presence of certain target symptoms such as depression, anxiety, and dissociation. Further measures for the assessment of PTSD are subsumed in a recent publication [167] as well as online [168].

Treatment

PTSD and trauma-related psychopathology have been treated for many decades. Numerous studies have reported many different kinds of interventions, for example, eye roll movements, hypnosis, psychoanalysis, cognitive therapy, and psychopharmacology.

Only a handful of studies, however, were conducted to allow the formation of firm conclusions about treatment efficacy, and none of those studies involved children and adolescents. The present literature concludes (after much extrapolation from adult studies – which is itself problematic as demonstrated in the depression literature) that psychopharmacology and various forms of psychotherapy are all moderately effective, that many interventions show promise (none of them being superior to others *a priori*), and that most interventions have not been rigorously tested in children and adolescents. It also appears that various treatments target different aspects of the syndrome. Medications seem to reduce intrusion and "startle response" problems, as do behavioral treatments. Psychodynamic treatments seem to work better on avoidance symptoms, although this result is variable across studies and has not been adequately studied in children. There are likely to be differences across ages, given the different nature of child PTSD.

Factors that Influence Treatment

As in the treatment of any disorder, the culture of the patient should be considered. The race, ethnicity, and religion of a patient can influence his or her willingness to present symptoms that may be considered taboo or embarrassing. In cases of sexual abuse, patients may be embarrassed about what took place and attribute blame to themselves. Family and communities may also blame, ostracize, and distance themselves from the victim. If a family member has perpetrated the abuse, some cultures may dictate that the perpetrator be taken care of within the family (e.g., moved to another location) and resent the interference of "outsiders." Behaviors such as hitting or alienating a child for unacceptable behavior may be the standard form of punishment in certain countries and cultures. Although this behavior should be understood within its cultural framework, it should not be sanctioned as acceptable in the USA. Behaviors that occur because of cultural differences and a lack of knowledge regarding the laws in the USA can often be resolved in family therapy.

The limits of confidentiality can significantly affect therapy with trauma victims. Although the specific laws vary slightly among federal states, clinicians are legally and ethically obligated to report suspected abuse, and in most cases are legally protected in making reports that turn out to be without merit. Parents, children, and adolescents should all be informed about the limits of confidentiality. In cases in which abuse is the presenting problem, the issue of confidentiality can be addressed at the beginning of therapy in relation to the trauma; patients should be made aware, however, that these limits also apply to other instances of abuse that might be revealed during the course of therapy. This is an important point to stress, since traumatized or abused patients have often experienced more than one significant trauma.

Clearly defining the limits of confidentiality does not preclude difficulties from arising later in therapy, should confidentiality be broken. Reporting information revealed during therapy to the police and to child protection agencies can bring up issues of trust, security, and betrayal for patients, particularly if they are not in agreement with the reporting. One-fourth of families drop out of therapy after a report is made. The integrity of the therapeutic relationship is influenced by the manner in which the need to report is presented, the identity and relationship of the perpetrator to the patient, and the ability of the patient to cope with the effect of such reporting on his or her relationships, both in and out of therapy.

Psychotherapy

Individual treatment is the mainstay of intervention. In our clinic, we usually prescribe a mixture of behavioral interventions that are delivered in the context of a psychodynamic treatment package. The psychodynamic elements are intended to help develop a treatment alliance with children, help the clinician manage the therapeutic relationship, and possibly target memories in order to uncover important details of the original trauma. The typical course progresses in three stages. Phase one is exploratory (two to five sessions); the nature and extent of the traumatic event is established while a solid working alliance is built. This phase is completed when the patient and clinician agree on a scenario of the events that traumatized the patient and on a course of exposure or desensitization (depending on the comorbidity), the familial resources, and the patient's ego strengths and defense profile. More resilient patients with many resources usually receive some form of exposure, in which the traumatic event is reworked and the patient rapidly works up to flooding therapy. These patients, however, are still cognizant of some of the severe side effects this method may produce. More complicated cases should be approached gradually, with a model based on the prevention of relapse.

In phase two (6 to 15 sessions), the behavioral program is carried out and is supplemented by further exploratory sessions as needed to work through patient resistance. In the first two phases, ongoing treatment is provided every week. After these phases, regular clinic contact is terminated. In the third phase of treatment (up to 2 to 3 years as necessary, with very intermittent contacts), the patient is encouraged to practice on his or her own and to return when progress stops or symptoms recur. Such relapses are then handled in the course of one to three sessions. Play therapy and drawings are productive with younger children, and more traditional forms of therapy benefit older adolescents. At all phases of treatment, the patient's need for psychopharmacology is assessed.

Cognitive behavioral therapy (CBT) has shown effectiveness in treating children who are victims of sexual abuse [169]. Judith Cohen and colleagues have shown specific benefit to children experiencing PTSD as a result of sexual abuse by using trauma-focused cognitive behavioral therapy (TF-CBT) over a child-centered therapeutic approach for both children and their parents [22]. TF-CBT develops skills in expressing feelings, coping, and developing a sense of the connections between emotion, behavior, and feeling. It also includes some exposure by using narrative, processing, parenting skills, and psychoeducation. Along a similar line, Barry Nurcombe and colleagues, in a review of the limited published studies for the treatment of sexual abuse, likewise found benefit from CBT, as well as from group therapy and play therapy [170]. Ramchandani and Jones in their review of the literature on treatment of sexually abused children, likewise concluded that in randomized clinical trials CBT has garnered the most evidence for its efficaciousness [171].

Additional Forms of Therapy

Psychoeducation can be extremely beneficial for parents of children who have experienced a trauma. Often parents are scared, confused, and uncertain about the origins of their child's behavior and the prevalence of symptoms. They often need to learn new strategies and parenting skills to deal with problematic behavior such as anger outbursts and flashbacks. In addition, children and especially adolescents can gain security in knowing that their symptoms are valid and within the normal range of experiences for individuals affected by a traumatic event.

Group therapy often helps children and adolescents understand that their symptoms are experienced by others, and allows them to learn coping strategies from those who have been through similar circumstances. Group therapy should begin following an initial assessment of the trauma and related symptoms. It is not recommended as the initial form of therapy in the case of severe trauma, since children are likely to experience symptoms during the initial telling of their traumas that may be better managed in initial individual sessions. An initial assessment should differentiate between those patients who can present their experience in a group and withstand the exposure to others' traumas and those who require individual work prior to sharing with others. For the latter patients, once individual therapy has started, group therapy can be used as a means of continued support.

Particularly in the instance of abuse, family therapy can be beneficial for the patient as well as the individual family members. These approaches have been manualized and tested in community settings [170]. When one member of a family experiences a trauma, everyone in the family is affected. Feelings of insecurity, fear, guilt, and shame can all be present in family members as a result of the trauma. These feelings along with changes in the family routine because of care for the identified patient can upset the previously held dynamics of the family. When the perpetrator of abuse is within the family, family therapy is essential for assessing family structure and relationships within the family, as well as the development of new roles within the family. Decisions about whether to include the perpetrator in therapy should be decided on a case-by-case basis and should take into consideration the stage of recovery of the victim, the perpetrator's understanding of the abuse and his or her involvement in treatment, and reunification issues.

Psychopharmacology

If the evidence for the efficacy of drugs is not strong in adults, it is quite weak for the treatment of children and adolescents with PTSD. Studies on psychopharmacological treatment options are summarized in a recent review [172].

At present, one can only extrapolate from studies of adults, which is of course problematic. Psychotherapeutic interventions should be tried first; only if patients fail to progress or if symptoms are so overwhelming as to incapacitate the patient should the clinician consider medications. A trial of medicine should be started if symptoms do not begin to recede after about 4 weeks of adequate intervention or when symptoms are so incapacitating as to make management impossible and there is pronounced interference with developmental tasks.

What are the appropriate targets for treatment? Based on what can be gleaned from the adult literature, predominantly the intrusion and hyperactivity-related symptoms of PTSD respond to intervention. Post and colleagues propose a kindling model for the development of PTSD [173, 174]. Three general stages can be discerned. First, there are the traumatic events that serve to prime the system and can result in acute stress disorder. Second, there is the development of PTSD with the presence of flashbacks, nightmares, hyperarousal, avoidance, and numbing. In the third phase, chronic PTSD develops whereby explosiveness, irritability, panics, generalized anxiety, depression, social phobia, and somatization can occur. Pharmacologically, these stages can be approached with different sets of medications but will likely require multiple interventions including psychotherapy and family therapy. The kindling theory of PTSD holds that prompt intervention to address core symptoms is necessary in order to prevent further progression of the disease, and medications may play one significant role in this process.

Selective serotonin reuptake inhibitors (SSRIs) have been the mainstay of PTSD treatment. The evidence for their utility in children is supported by limited studies, and most practitioners draw from the adult literature on this point. Seedat and colleagues studied eight adolescents with a 20 mg fixed dose of citalopram and found improvements in arousal level and startle response [175]. The use of SSRIs in children has become a point of controversy in recent years, and all drugs in this class now have a block box warning for the possible development of suicidal ideation with the initiation of SSRI therapy. Clinicians need to monitor all children for this potential effect, and caution should be exercised when starting any new medication.

Limited data are available on the use of mood stabilizers like divalproex sodium for populations with high levels of PTSD and comorbid conduct disorder [176]. Studies by our group have shown that divalproex sodium can significantly reduce intrusion, avoidance, and arousal in children with PTSD [177]. The efficacy of mood stabilizers seems consistent with Post's kindling theory of PTSD, in that this medication can reduce arousal, irritability, and explosiveness, and thereby theoretically blunt the transition from PTSD to chronic PTSD.

Should SSRIs and mood stabilizers fail, then consideration can be given to using beta-blockers [178], alpha-blockers [179], and atypicals. Each of these classes of medications has had some limited success in treating PTSD symptoms in children. Minor tranquilizers are apparently not useful on an ongoing basis, changing little of the core pathology of PTSD, but can be used for brief symptomatic relief. One has to be mindful of the potential abuse of these drugs, especially in teenagers or in chaotic families in which parents might avail themselves of medications prescribed for their children.

Drugs should never be considered the primary mode of treating PTSD in this age group, and all patients, given the current state of knowledge, should receive a carefully reviewed and comprehensive psychotherapy package.

Conclusion

It is evident that knowledge about childhood trauma is rapidly changing. The field of developmental traumatology is newly emerging and evolving, and the results will likely change our understanding of the mind and the effects of early trauma. In addition, as the neuroscience underlying childhood trauma becomes clearer, the resulting changes in interventions from pharmacological, psychotherapeutic, and sociotherapeutic perspectives [180] will have to alter and progress. It is incumbent on practitioners to be vigilant about these coming changes in order to provide the highest level of care for this population of children.

References

1. Ohmi H, Kojima S, Awai Y, *et al.* Post-traumatic stress disorder in pre-school aged children after a gas explosion. *Eur J Pediatr* 2002;**161**:643–648.
2. Scheeringa MS, Zeanah CH, Drell MJ, Larrieu JA. Two approaches to the diagnosis of posttraumatic stress disorder in infancy and early childhood. *J Am Acad Child Adolesc Psychiatry* 1995;**34**:191–200.
3. Shaw JA, Applegate B, Schorr C. Twenty-one-month follow-up study of school-age children exposed to Hurricane Andrew. *J Am Acad Child Adolesc Psychiatry* 1996;**35**:359–364.
4. American Psychiatric Associaton. Posttraumatic Stress Disorder. 2011. Available from: http://www.dsm5.org/ProposedRevisions/Pages/proposedrevision.aspx?rid=165.
5. Allwood MA, Bell-Dolan D, Husain SA. Children's trauma and adjustment reactions to violent and nonviolent war experiences. *J Am Acad Child Adolesc Psychiatry* 2002;**41**:450–457.
6. March JS, Amaya-Jackson L, Terry R, Costanzo P. Posttraumatic symptomatology in children and adolescents after an industrial fire. *J Am Acad Child Adolesc Psychiatry* 1997;**36**:1080–1088.
7. Breslau N, Chilcoat HD, Kessler RC, Davis GC. Previous exposure to trauma and PTSD effects of subsequent trauma: results from the Detroit Area Survey of Trauma. *Am J Psychiatry* 1999;**156**:902–907.
8. Breslau N, Davis GC. Posttraumatic stress disorder in an urban population of young adults: risk factors for chronicity. *Am J Psychiatry* 1992;**149**:671–675.
9. Giaconia RM, Reinherz HZ, Silverman AB, Pakiz B, Frost AK, Cohen E. Traumas and posttraumatic stress disorder in a community population of older adolescents. *J Am Acad Child Adolesc Psychiatry* 1995;**34**:1369–1380.
10. Pine DS, Cohen JA. Trauma in children and adolescents: risk and treatment of psychiatric sequelae. *Biol Psychiatry* 2002;**51**:519–531.
11. De Bellis MD. Developmental traumatology: The psychobiological development of maltreated children and its implications for research, treatment and policy. *Dev Psychopathol* 2001;**13**:539–564.
12. Pfefferbaum B, Doughty DE, Reddy C, *et al.* Exposure and peritraumatic response as predictors of posttraumatic stress in children following the 1995 Oklahoma City bombing. *J Urban Health* 2002;**79**:354–363.
13. Schwarz ED, Kowalski JM. Malignant memories: PTSD in children and adults after a school shooting. *J Am Acad Child Adolesc Psychiatry* 1991;**30**:936–944.
14. Aaron J, Zaglul H, Emery RE. Posttraumatic stress in children following acute physical injury. *J Pediatr Psychol* 1999;**24**:335–343.
15. Yehuda R. Post-traumatic stress disorder. *N Engl J Med* 2002;**346**:108–114.
16. Fergusson DM, Lynskey MT, Horwood LJ. Childhood sexual abuse and psychiatric disorder in young adulthood: I. Prevalence of sexual abuse and factors associated with sexual abuse. *J Am Acad Child Adolesc Psychiatry* 1996;**35**:1355–1364.

17. Brown J, Cohen P, Johnson JG, Smailes EM. Childhood abuse and neglect: specificity of effects on adolescent and young adult depression and suicidality. *J Am Acad Child Adolesc Psychiatry* 1999;**38**:1490–1496.

18. Fergusson DM, Horwood LJ, Lynskey MT. Childhood sexual abuse and psychiatric disorder in young adulthood: II. Psychiatric outcomes of childhood sexual abuse. *J Am Acad Child Adolesc Psychiatry* 1996;**35**:1365–1374.

19. Adam BS, Everett BL, O'Neal E. PTSD in physically and sexually abused psychiatrically hospitalized children. *Child Psychiatry Hum Dev* 1992;**23**:3–8.

20. Saywitz KJ, Mannarino AP, Berliner L, Cohen JA. Treatment for sexually abused children and adolescents. *Am Psychol* 2000;**55**:1040–1049.

21. Wolfe DA, Sas L, Wekerle C. Factors associated with the development of posttraumatic stress disorder among child victims of sexual abuse. *Child Abuse Negl* 1994;**18**:37–50.

22. Cohen JA, Deblinger E, Mannarino AP, Steer RA. A multisite, randomized controlled trial for children with sexual abuse-related PTSD symptoms. *J Am Acad Child Adolesc Psychiatry* 2004;**43**:393–402.

23. Nelson EC, Heath AC, Madden PA, *et al.* Association between self-reported childhood sexual abuse and adverse psychosocial outcomes: results from a twin study. *Arch Gen Psychiatry* 2002;**59**:139–145.

24. Brent DA, Oquendo M, Birmaher B, *et al.* Familial pathways to early-onset suicide attempt: risk for suicidal behavior in offspring of mood-disordered suicide attempters. *Arch Gen Psychiatry* 2002;**59**:801–807.

25. Jaworowski S. Traffic accident injuries of children: the need for prospective studies of psychiatric sequelae. *Isr J Psychiatry Relat Sci* 1992;**29**:174–184.

26. Jones RW, Peterson LW. Post-traumatic stress disorder in a child following an automobile accident. *J Fam Pract* 1993;**36**:223–225.

27. Stoddard FJ, Norman DK, Murphy JM, Beardslee WR. Psychiatric outcome of burned children and adolescents. *J Am Acad Child Adolesc Psychiatry* 1989;**28**:589–595.

28. Fitzpatrick KM, Boldizar JP. The prevalence and consequences of exposure to violence among African-American youth. *J Am Acad Child Adolesc Psychiatry* 1993;**32**:424–430.

29. Youngstrom E, Weist MD, Albus KE. Exploring violence exposure, stress, protective factors and behavioral problems among inner-city youth. *Am J Community Psychol* 2003;**32**:115–129.

30. Silva RR, Alpert M, Munoz DM, Singh S, Matzner F, Dummit S. Stress and vulnerability to posttraumatic stress disorder in children and adolescents. *Am J Psychiatry* 2000;**157**:1229–1235.

31. Wolfe DA, Jaffe P, Wilson SK, Zak L. Children of battered women: the relation of child behavior to family violence and maternal stress. *J Consult Clin Psychol* 1985;**53**:657–665.

32. Eth S, Pynoos RS. Children who witness the homicide of a parent. *Psychiatry* 1994;**57**:287–306.

33. Burman S, Allen-Meares P. Neglected victims of murder: children's witness to parental homicide. *Soc Work* 1994;**39**:28–34.

34. Freeman LN, Mokros H, Poznanski EO. Violent events reported by normal urban school-aged children: characteristics and depression correlates. *J Am Acad Child Adolesc Psychiatry* 1993;**32**:419–423.

35. Schwab-Stone ME, Ayers TS, Kasprow W, *et al.* No safe haven: a study of violence exposure in an urban community. *J Am Acad Child Adolesc Psychiatry* 1995;**34**:1343–1352.

36. Pynoos RS, Frederick C, Nader K, *et al.* Life threat and posttraumatic stress in school-age children. *Arch Gen Psychiatry* 1987;**44**:1057–1063.

37. Lipschitz DS, Rasmusson AM, Anyan W, Cromwell P, Southwick SM. Clinical and functional correlates of posttraumatic stress disorder in urban adolescent girls at a primary care clinic. *J Am Acad Child Adolesc Psychiatry* 2000;**39**:1104–1111.

38. Bell CC, Jenkins EJ. Community violence and children on Chicago's southside. *Psychiatry* 1993;**56**:46–54.

39. Schubiner H, Scott R, Tzelepis A. Exposure to violence among inner-city youth. *J Adolesc Health* 1993;**14**:214–219.

40. Mazza JJ, Reynolds WM. Exposure to violence in young inner-city adolescents: relationships with suicidal ideation, depression, and PTSD symptomatology. *J Abnorm Child Psychol* 1999;**27**:203–213.

41. Fremont WP. Childhood reactions to terrorism-induced trauma: a review of the past 10 years. *J Am Acad Child Adolesc Psychiatry* 2004;**43**:381–392.

42. Laor N, Wolmer L, Mayes LC, *et al.* Israeli preschoolers under Scud missile attacks. A developmental perspective on risk-modifying factors. *Arch Gen Psychiatry* 1996;**53**:416–423.

43. Pfefferbaum B, Nixon SJ, Tucker PM, *et al.* Posttraumatic stress responses in bereaved children after the Oklahoma City bombing. *J Am Acad Child Adolesc Psychiatry* 1999;**38**:1372–1379.

44. Koplewicz HS, Vogel JM, Solanto MV, *et al.* Child and parent response to the 1993 World Trade Center bombing. *J Trauma Stress* 2002;**15**:77–85.

45. Schuster MA, Stein BD, Jaycox L, *et al.* A national survey of stress reactions after the September 11, 2001, terrorist attacks. *N Engl J Med* 2001;**345**:1507–1512.

46. Sack WH, Clarke G, Him C, *et al.* A 6-year follow-up study of Cambodian refugee adolescents traumatized as children. *J Am Acad Child Adolesc Psychiatry* 1993;**32**:431–437.

47. Sack WH, Clarke GN, Seeley J. Posttraumatic stress disorder across two generations of Cambodian refugees. *J Am Acad Child Adolesc Psychiatry* 1995;**34**:1160–1166.

48. Magwaza AS, Killian BJ, Petersen I, Pillay Y. The effects of chronic violence on preschool children living in South African townships. *Child Abuse Negl* 1993;**17**:795–803.

49. Nader KO, Pynoos RS, Fairbanks LA, al-Ajeel M, al-Asfour A. A preliminary study of PTSD and grief among the children of Kuwait following the Gulf crisis. *Br J Clin Psychol* 1993;**32**:407–416.

50. Dyregrov A, Gupta L, Gjestad R, Mukanoheli E. Trauma exposure and psychological reactions to genocide among Rwandan children. *J Trauma Stress* 2000;**13**:3–21.

51. Qouta S, Punamaki RL, El Sarraj E. Prevalence and determinants of PTSD among Palestinian children exposed to military violence. *Eur Child Adolesc Psychiatry* 2003;**12**:265–272.

52. Lustig SL, Kia-Keating M, Knight WG, *et al.* Review of child and adolescent refugee mental health. *J Am Acad Child Adolesc Psychiatry* 2004;**43**:24–36.

53. Westermeyer J. Psychiatric services for refugee children: an overview. In: Westermeyer J (ed.) *Refugee Mental*

Health in Resettlement Countries: The Series in Clinical and Community Psychology. Washington, DC: Hemisphere Publishing, 1991; pp. 235–245.

54. Rothe EM, Lewis J, Castillo-Matos H, Martinez O, Busquets R, Martinez I. Posttraumatic stress disorder among Cuban children and adolescents after release from a refugee camp. *Psychiatr Serv* 2002;**53**:970–976.

55. Punamaki RL. Can ideological commitment protect children's psychological well-being in situations of political violence? *Child Dev* 1996;**67**:55–69.

56. Smith P, Perrin S, Yule W, Rabe-Hesketh S. War exposure and maternal reactions in the psychological adjustment of children from Bosnia-Hercegovina. *J Child Psychol Psychiatry* 2001;**42**:395–404.

57. Servan-Schreiber D, Le Lin B, Birmaher B. Prevalence of posttraumatic stress disorder and major depressive disorder in Tibetan refugee children. *J Am Acad Child Adolesc Psychiatry* 1998;**37**:874–879.

58. Terr LC, Bloch DA, Michel BA, Shi H, Reinhardt JA, Metayer S. Children's symptoms in the wake of Challenger: a field study of distant-traumatic effects and an outline of related conditions. *Am J Psychiatry* 1999;**156**:1536–1544.

59. Pfefferbaum B, Nixon SJ, Tivis RD, *et al.* Television exposure in children after a terrorist incident. *Psychiatry* 2001;**64**:202–211.

60. Schlenger WE, Caddell JM, Ebert L, *et al.* Psychological reactions to terrorist attacks: findings from the National Study of Americans' Reactions to September 11. *JAMA* 2002;**288**:581–588.

61. Shannon MP, Lonigan CJ, Finch AJ Jr, Taylor CM. Children exposed to disaster: I. Epidemiology of posttraumatic symptoms and symptom profiles. *J Am Acad Child Adolesc Psychiatry* 1994;**33**:80–93.

62. Lonigan CJ, Shannon MP, Taylor CM, Finch AJ Jr, Sallee FR. Children exposed to disaster: II. Risk factors for the development of post-traumatic symptomatology. *J Am Acad Child Adolesc Psychiatry* 1994;**33**:94–105.

63. Garrison CZ, Bryant ES, Addy CL, Spurrier PG, Freedy JR, Kilpatrick DG. Posttraumatic stress disorder in adolescents after Hurricane Andrew. *J Am Acad Child Adolesc Psychiatry* 1995;**34**:1193–1201.

64. Vernberg EM, Silverman WK, La Greca AM, Prinstein MJ. Prediction of posttraumatic stress symptoms in children after hurricane Andrew. *J Abnorm Psychol* 1996;**105**:237–248.

65. La Greca AM, Silverman WK, Wasserstein SB. Children's predisaster functioning as a predictor of posttraumatic stress following Hurricane Andrew. *J Consult Clin Psychol* 1998;**66**:883–892.

66. Goenjian AK, Pynoos RS, Steinberg AM, *et al.* Psychiatric comorbidity in children after the 1988 earthquake in Armenia. *J Am Acad Child Adolesc Psychiatry* 1995;**34**:1174–1184.

67. Goldstein RD, Wampler NS, Wise PH. War experiences and distress symptoms of Bosnian children. *Pediatrics* 1997;**100**:873–878.

68. Najarian LM, Goenjian AK, Pelcovitz D, Mandel F, Najarian B. Relocation after a disaster: posttraumatic stress disorder in Armenia after the earthquake. *J Am Acad Child Adolesc Psychiatry* 1996;**35**:374–383.

69. Laor N, Wolmer L, Cohen DJ. Mothers' functioning and children's symptoms 5 years after a SCUD missile attack. *Am J Psychiatry* 2001;**158**:1020–1026.

70. Bryce JW, Walker N, Ghorayeb F, Kanj M. Life experiences, response styles and mental health among mothers and children in Beirut, Lebanon. *Soc Sci Med* 1989;**28**:685–695.

71. Breton JJ, Valla JP, Lambert J. Industrial disaster and mental health of children and their parents. *J Am Acad Child Adolesc Psychiatry* 1993;**32**:438–445.

72. Garbarino J, Kostelny K. Child maltreatment as a community problem. *Child Abuse Negl* 1992;**16**:455–464.

73. Copeland WE, Keeler G, Angold A, Costello EJ. Traumatic events and posttraumatic stress in childhood. *Arch Gen Psychiatry* 2007;**64**:577–584.

74. Brom D, Kleber RJ, Witztum E. The prevalence of posttraumatic psychopathology in the general and the clinical population. *Isr J Psychiatry Relat Sci* 1992;**28**:53–63.

75. Norris FH. Epidemiology of trauma: frequency and impact of different potentially traumatic events on different demographic groups. *J Consult Clin Psychol* 1992;**60**:409–418.

76. Norris FH, Murphy AD, Baker CK, Perilla JL, Rodriguez FG, Rodriguez Jde J. Epidemiology of trauma and posttraumatic stress disorder in Mexico. *J Abnorm Psychol* 2003;**112**:646–656.

77. Breslau N, Davis GC, Andreski P, Peterson E. Traumatic events and posttraumatic stress disorder in an urban population of young adults. *Arch Gen Psychiatry* 1991;**48**:216–222.

78. Silverman AB, Reinherz HZ, Giaconia RM. The long-term sequelae of child and adolescent abuse: a longitudinal community study. *Child Abuse Negl* 1996;**20**:709–723.

79. Cuffe SP, Addy CL, Garrison CZ, *et al.* Prevalence of PTSD in a community sample of older adolescents. *J Am Acad Child Adolesc Psychiatry* 1998;**37**:147–154.

80. Steiner H, Garcia IG, Matthews Z. Posttraumatic stress disorder in incarcerated juvenile delinquents. *J Am Acad Child Adolesc Psychiatry* 1997;**36**:357–365.

81. Steiner H, Carrion V, Plattner B, Koopman C. Dissociative symptoms in posttraumatic stress disorder: diagnosis and treatment. *Child Adolesc Psychiatr Clin N Am* 2003;**12**:231–249, viii.

82. McLeer SV, Deblinger E, Henry D, Orvaschel H. Sexually abused children at high risk for post-traumatic stress disorder. *J Am Acad Child Adolesc Psychiatry* 1992;**31**:875–879.

83. Deblinger E, McLeer SV, Atkins MS, Ralphe D, Foa E. Post-traumatic stress in sexually abused, physically abused, and nonabused children. *Child Abuse Negl* 1989;**13**:403–408.

84. McLeer SV, Deblinger E, Atkins MS, Foa EB, Ralphe DL. Post-traumatic stress disorder in sexually abused children. *J Am Acad Child Adolesc Psychiatry* 1988;**27**:650–654.

85. Green BL, Korol M, Grace MC, *et al.* Children and disaster: age, gender, and parental effects on PTSD symptoms. *J Am Acad Child Adolesc Psychiatry* 1991;**30**:945–951.

86. Green BL, Lindy JD, Grace MC, *et al.* Buffalo Creek survivors in the second decade: stability of stress symptoms. *Am J Orthopsychiatry* 1990;**60**:43–54.

87. Pynoos RS, Goenjian A, Tashjian M, *et al.* Post-traumatic stress reactions in children after the 1988 Armenian earthquake. *Br J Psychiatry* 1993;**163**:239–247.

88. Yehuda R, McFarlane AC. Conflict between current knowledge about posttraumatic stress disorder and its original conceptual basis. *Am J Psychiatry* 1995; **152**:1705–1713.

89. Yehud R, Hallig SL, Grossman R. Childhood trauma and risk for PTSD: relationship to intergenerational effects of trauma, parental PTSD, and cortisol excretion. *Dev Psychopathol* 2001;**13**:733–753.

90. Seligman ME, Csikszentmihalyi M. Positive psychology. An introduction. *Am Psychol* 2000;**55**:5–14.

91. De Bellis MD, Hooper SR, Woolley DP, Shenk CE. Demographic, maltreatment, and neurobiological correlates of PTSD symptoms in children and adolescents. *J Pediatr Psychol* 2010;**35**:570–577.

92. Teicher MH, Andersen SL, Polcari A, Anderson CM, Navalta CP, Kim DM. The neurobiological consequences of early stress and childhood maltreatment. *Neurosci Biobehav Rev* 2003;**27**:33–44.

93. Sapolsky RM, Romero LM, Munck AU. How do glucocorticoids influence stress responses? Integrating permissive, suppressive, stimulatory, and preparative actions. *Endocr Rev* 2000;**21**:55–89.

94. Sapolsky RM. Stress and plasticity in the limbic system. *Neurochem Res* 2003;**28**:1735–1742.

95. Traumatic Stress and Psychopathology Victor G Carrion, Sarah J Erickson, Mary E Bancroft, Julia Huemer and Belinda Plattner; Hans Steiner (ed.); in: Handbook of Developmental Psychiatry, 2011, World Scientific). New York: Guilford Publications, 1996.

96. Edwards E, Harkins K, Wright G, Henn F. Effects of bilateral adrenalectomy on the induction of learned helplessness behavior. *Neuropsychopharmacology* 1990; **3**:109–114.

97. Sapolsky RM, Uno H, Rebert CS, Finch CE. Hippocampal damage associated with prolonged glucocorticoid exposure in primates. *J Neurosci* 1990;**10**:2897–2902.

98. Simantov R, Blinder E, Ratovitski T, Tauber M, Gabbay M, Porat S. Dopamine-induced apoptosis in human neuronal cells: inhibition by nucleic acids antisense to the dopamine transporter. *Neuroscience* 1996;**74**:39–50.

99. Dunlop SA, Archer MA, Quinlivan JA, Beazley LD, Newnham JP. Repeated prenatal corticosteroids delay myelination in the ovine central nervous system. *J Matern Fetal Med* 1997;**6**:309–313.

100. Sapolsky RM. Stress, glucocorticoids, and damage to the nervous system: the current state of confusion. *Stress* 1996;**1**:1–19.

101. Todd RD. Neural development is regulated by classical neurotransmitters: dopamine D2 receptor stimulation enhances neurite outgrowth. *Biol Psychiatry* 1992; **31**:794–807.

102. Gould E, Tanapat P, Cameron HA. Adrenal steroids suppress granule cell death in the developing dentate gyrus through an NMDA receptor-dependent mechanism. *Brain Res Dev Brain Res* 1997;**103**:91–93.

103. Gould E, Tanapat P, McEwen BS, Flugge G, Fuchs E. Proliferation of granule cell precursors in the dentate gyrus of adult monkeys is diminished by stress. *Proc Natl Acad Sci U S A* 1998;**95**:3168–3171.

104. Smith MA, Makino S, Kvetnansky R, Post RM. Effects of stress on neurotrophic factor expression in the rat brain. *Ann N Y Acad Sci* 1995;**771**:234–239.

105. De Bellis MD, Baum AS, Birmaher B, *et al.* A.E. Bennett Research Award. Developmental traumatology. Part I:

Biological stress systems. *Biol Psychiatry* 1999; **45**:1259–1270.

106. Queiroz EA, Lombardi AB, Furtado CR, *et al.* Biochemical correlate of depression in children. *Arq Neuropsiquiatr* 1991;**49**:418–425.

107. De Bellis MD, Chrousos GP, Dorn LD, *et al.* Hypothalamic-pituitary-adrenal axis dysregulation in sexually abused girls. *J Clin Endocrinol Metab* 1994; **78**:249–255.

108. Yehuda R, Siever LJ, Teicher MH, *et al.* Plasma norepinephrine and 3-methoxy-4-hydroxyphenylglycol concentrations and severity of depression in combat posttraumatic stress disorder and major depressive disorder. *Biol Psychiatry* 1998;**44**:56–63.

109. Southwick SM, Krystal JH, Morgan CA, *et al.* Abnormal noradrenergic function in posttraumatic stress disorder. *Arch Gen Psychiatry* 1993;**50**:266–274.

110. Boscarino JA. Posttraumatic stress disorder, exposure to combat, and lower plasma cortisol among Vietnam veterans: findings and clinical implications. *J Consult Clin Psychol* 1996;**64**:191–201.

111. Yehuda R, Kahana B, Binder-Brynes K, Southwick SM, Mason JW, Giller EL. Low urinary cortisol excretion in Holocaust survivors with posttraumatic stress disorder. *Am J Psychiatry* 1995;**152**:982–986.

112. Yehuda R, Golier JA, Halligan SL, Meaney M, Bierer LM. The ACTH response to dexamethasone in PTSD. *Am J Psychiatry* 2004;**161**:1397–1403.

113. Yehuda R, Boisoneau D, Lowy MT, Giller EL Jr. Dose-response changes in plasma cortisol and lymphocyte glucocorticoid receptors following dexamethasone administration in combat veterans with and without posttraumatic stress disorder. *Arch Gen Psychiatry.* 1995;**52**:583–593.

114. Bremner JD, Licinio J, Darnell A, *et al.* Elevated CSF corticotropin-releasing factor concentrations in posttraumatic stress disorder. *Am J Psychiatry* 1997;**154**:624–629.

115. Smith MA, Davidson J, Ritchie JC, *et al.* The corticotropin-releasing hormone test in patients with posttraumatic stress disorder. *Biol Psychiatry* 1989;**26**:349–355.

116. Yehuda R, Teicher MH, Trestman RL, Levengood RA, Siever LJ. Cortisol regulation in posttraumatic stress disorder and major depression: a chronobiological analysis. *Biol Psychiatry* 1996;**40**:79–88.

117. Lemieux AM, Coe CL. Abuse-related posttraumatic stress disorder: evidence for chronic neuroendocrine activation in women. *Psychosom Med* 1995;**57**:105–115.

118. Maes M, Lin A, Bonaccorso S, *et al.* Increased 24-hour urinary cortisol excretion in patients with post-traumatic stress disorder and patients with major depression, but not in patients with fibromyalgia. *Acta Psychiatr Scand* 1998;**98**:328–335.

119. Pitman RK, Orr SP. Twenty-four hour urinary cortisol and catecholamine excretion in combat-related posttraumatic stress disorder. *Biol Psychiatry* 1990;**27**:245–247.

120. Rasmusson A, Lipschitz DS, Wang S, *et al.* Increased pituitary and adrenal reactivity in premenopausal women with posttraumatic stress disorder. *Biol Psychiatry* 2001;**50**:965–977.

121. Heim C, Newport DJ, Heit S, *et al.* Pituitary-adrenal and autonomic responses to stress in women after sexual and physical abuse in childhood. *JAMA* 2000; **284**:592–597.

122. Kanter ED, Wilkinson CW, Radant AD, et al. Gluco-corticoid feedback sensitivity and adrenocortical responsiveness in posttraumatic stress disorder. *Biol Psychiatry* 2001;**50**:238–245.

123. Carrion VG, Weems CF, Ray RD, Glaser B, Hessl D. Reiss AL. Diurnal salivary cortisol in pediatric posttraumatic stress disorder. *Biol Psychiatry* 2002;**51**:575–582.

124. Gunnar MR, Morison SJ, Chisholm K, Schuder M. Salivary cortisol levels in children adopted from Romanian orphanages. *Dev Psychopathol* 2001;**13**:611–628.

125. Hart J, Gunnar M, Cichetti D. Altered neuroendocrine activity in maltreated children related to symptoms of depression. *Dev Psychopathol* 1996;**8**:201–214.

126. Goenjian AK, Yehuda R, Pynoos RS, et al. Basal cortisol, dexamethasone suppression of cortisol, and MHPG in adolescents after the 1988 earthquake in Armenia. *Am J Psychiatry* 1996;**153**:929–934.

127. King JA, Mandansky D, King S, Fletcher KE, Brewer J. Early sexual abuse and low cortisol. *Psychiatry Clin Neurosci* 2001;**55**:71–74.

128. Thomas LA, De Bellis MD. Pituitary volumes in pediatric maltreatment-related posttraumatic stress disorder. *Biol Psychiatry* 2004;**55**:752–758.

129. Gertz BJ, Contreras LN, McComb DJ, Kovacs K, Tyrrell JB, Dallman MF. Chronic administration of corticotropin-releasing factor increases pituitary corticotroph number. *Endocrinology* 1987;**120**:381–388.

130. Westlund KN, Aguilera G, Childs GV. Quantification of morphological changes in pituitary corticotropes produced by in vivo corticotropin-releasing factor stimulation and adrenalectomy. *Endocrinology* 1985;**116**:439–445.

131. Lopez JF, Palkovits M, Arato M, Mansour A, Akil H, Watson SJ. Localization and quantification of pro-opiomelanocortin mRNA and glucocorticoid receptor mRNA in pituitaries of suicide victims. *Neuroendocrinology* 1992;**56**:491–501.

132. Carrion VG, Weems CF, Richert K, Hoffman BC, Reiss AL. Decreased prefrontal cortical volume associated with increased bedtime cortisol in traumatized youth. *Biol Psychiatry* 2010;**68**:491–493.

133. Sapolsky RM. Glucocorticoids and hippocampal atrophy in neuropsychiatric disorders. *Arch Gen Psychiatry* 2000;**57**:925–935.

134. Gurvits TV, Shenton ME, Hokama H, et al. Magnetic resonance imaging study of hippocampal volume in chronic, combat-related posttraumatic stress disorder. *Biol Psychiatry* 1996;**40**:1091–1099.

135. Bremner JD, Randall P, Scott TM, et al. MRI-based measurement of hippocampal volume in patients with combat-related posttraumatic stress disorder. *Am J Psychiatry* 1995;**152**:973–981.

136. Bremner JD, Randall P, Vermetten E, et al. Magnetic resonance imaging-based measurement of hippocampal volume in posttraumatic stress disorder related to childhood physical and sexual abuse – a preliminary report. *Biol Psychiatry* 1997;**41**:23–32.

137. Stein MB, Koverola C, Hanna C, Torchia MG, McClarty B. Hippocampal volume in women victimized by childhood sexual abuse. *Psychol Med* 1997;**27**:951–959.

138. Starkman MN, Gebarski SS, Berent S, Schteingart DE. Hippocampal formation volume, memory dysfunction, and cortisol levels in patients with Cushing's syndrome. *Biol Psychiatry* 1992;**32**:756–765.

139. Starkman MN, Giordani B, Gebarski SS, Berent S, Schork MA, Schteingart DE. Decrease in cortisol reverses human hippocampal atrophy following treatment of Cushing's disease. *Biol Psychiatry* 1999;**46**:1595–1602.

140. Bremner JD, Narayan M, Anderson ER, Staib LH, Miller HL, Charney DS. Hippocampal volume reduction in major depression. *Am J Psychiatry* 2000;**157**:115–118.

141. Sheline YI, Wang PW, Gado MH, Csernansky JG, Vannier MW. Hippocampal atrophy in recurrent major depression. *Proc Natl Acad Sci U S A* 1996;**93**:3908–3913.

142. Moghaddam B, Bolinao ML, Stein-Behrens B, Sapolsky R. Glucocorticoids mediate the stress-induced extracellular accumulation of glutamate. *Brain Res* 1994;**655**:251–254.

143. Carrion VG, Weems CF, Eliez S, et al. Attenuation of frontal asymmetry in pediatric posttraumatic stress disorder. *Biol Psychiatry* 2001;**50**:943–951.

144. De Bellis MD, Keshavan MS, Clark DB, et al. A.E. Bennett Research Award. Developmental traumatology. Part II: Brain development. *Biol Psychiatry* 1999;**45**:1271–1284.

145. De Bellis MD, Keshavan MS, Shifflett H, et al. Brain structures in pediatric maltreatment-related posttraumatic stress disorder: a sociodemographically matched study. *Biol Psychiatry* 2002;**52**:1066–1078.

146. Teicher MH, Ito Y, Glod CA, Andersen SL, Dumont N, Ackerman E. Preliminary evidence for abnormal cortical development in physically and sexually abused children using EEG coherence and MRI. *Ann N Y Acad Sci* 1997;**821**:160–175.

147. De Bellis MD, Clark DB, Beers SR, et al. Hippocampal volume in adolescent-onset alcohol use disorders. *Am J Psychiatry* 2000;**157**:737–744.

148. Purves D, Lichtman JW. Elimination of synapses in the developing nervous system. *Science* 1980;**210**:153–157.

149. Rakic P, Bourgeois JP, Eckenhoff MF, Zecevic N, Goldman-Rakic PS. Concurrent overproduction of synapses in diverse regions of the primate cerebral cortex. *Science* 1986;**232**:232–235.

150. Cowan WM, Fawcett JW, O'Leary DD, Stanfield BB. Regressive events in neurogenesis. *Science* 1984;**225**:1258–1265.

151. Rasmusson AM, Shi L, Duman R. Downregulation of BDNF mRNA in the hippocampal dentate gyrus after re-exposure to cues previously associated with footshock. *Neuropsychopharmacology* 2002;**27**:133–142.

152. Gilbertson MW, Shenton ME, Ciszewski A, et al. Smaller hippocampal volume predicts pathologic vulnerability to psychological trauma. *Nat Neurosci* 2002;**5**:1242–1247.

153. Rauch SL, Whalen PJ, Shin LM, et al. Exaggerated amygdala response to masked facial stimuli in posttraumatic stress disorder: a functional MRI study. *Biol Psychiatry* 2000;**47**:769–776.

154. Lieberzon I, Taylor SF, Amdur R. et al. Brain activation in PTSD in response to trauma-related stimuli. *Biol Psychiatry* 1999;**45**:817–826.

155. Shin LM, McNally RJ, Kosslyn SM, et al. Regional cerebral blood flow during script-driven imagery in childhood sexual abuse-related PTSD: A PET investigation. *Am J Psychiatry* 1999;**156**:575–584.

156. De Bellis MD, Keshavan MS, Spencer S, Hall J. N-Acetylaspartate concentration in the anterior cingulate of maltreated children and adolescents with PTSD. *Am J Psychiatry* 2000;**157**:1175–1177.

157. Shaw RJ, Robinson TE, Steiner H. Acute stress disorder following ventilation. *Psychosomatics* 2002;**43**:74–76.
158. DePrince AP, Freyd JJ. Forgetting trauma stimuli. *Psychol Sci* 2004;**15**:488–492.
159. Freyd JJ. Blind to betrayal: new perspectives on memory for trauma. *Harv Ment Health Lett* 1999;**15**:4–6.
160. Williams LM. Recall of childhood trauma: a prospective study of women's memories of child sexual abuse. *J Consult Clin Psychol* 1994;**62**:1167–1176.
161. Anderson MC, Ochsner KN, Kuhl B, *et al.* Neural systems underlying the suppression of unwanted memories. *Science* 2004;**303**:232–235.
162. Carrion VG, Steiner H. Trauma and dissociation in delinquent adolescents. *J Am Acad Child Adolesc Psychiatry* 2000;**39**:353–359.
163. Friedrich WN, Fisher JL, Dittner CA, *et al.* Child Sexual Behavior Inventory: normative, psychiatric, and sexual abuse comparisons. *Child Maltreat* 2001;**6**:37–49.
164. Briere J, American Professional Society on the Abuse of Children. *The APSAC Handbook on Child Maltreatment.* Thousand Oaks: Sage Publications, 1996.
165. Steiner H, Araujo KB, Koopman C. The response evaluation measure (REM-71): a new instrument for the measurement of defenses in adults and adolescents. *Am J Psychiatry* 2001;**158**:467–473.
166. Horowitz M, Wilner N, Alvarez W. Impact of Event Scale: a measure of subjective stress. *Psychosom Med* 1979;**41**:209–218.
167. Hawkins SS, Radcliffe J. Current measures of PTSD for children and adolescents. *J Pediatr Psychol* 2006; **31**:420–430.
168. National Child Traumatic Stress Network. Measures Review Database. Available from: http://www.nctsnet. org/resources/online-research/measures-review.
169. Deblinger E, McLeer SV, Henry D. Cognitive behavioral treatment for sexually abused children suffering posttraumatic stress: preliminary findings. *J Am Acad Child Adolesc Psychiatry* 1990;**29**:747–752.
170. Nurcombe B, Wooding S, Marrington P, Bickman L, Roberts G. Child sexual abuse II: treatment. *Aust N Z J Psychiatry* 2000;**34**:92–97.
171. Ramchandani P, Jones DP. Treating psychological symptoms in sexually abused children: from research findings to service provision. *Br J Psychiatry* 2003; **183**:484–490.
172. Huemer J, Erhart F, Steiner H. Posttraumatic stress disorder in children and adolescents: a review of psychopharmacological treatment. *Child Psychiatry Hum Dev* 2010;**41**:624–640.
173. Post RM, Weiss SR, Li H, *et al.* Neural plasticity and emotional memory. *Biol Psychiatry* 1998;**10**: 829–855.
174. Post RM, Weiss SRB. Sensitization and kindling phenomena in mood, anxiety, and obsessive-compulsive disoders: the role of serotonergic mechanisms in illness progression. *Biol Psychiatry* 1998;**44**:193–206.
175. Seedat S, Lockhat R, Kaminer D, Zungu-Dirwayi N, Stein DJ. An open trial of citalopram in adolescents with post-traumatic stress disorder. *Int Clin Psychopharmacol* 2001;**16**:21–25.
176. Steiner H, Petersen ML, Saxena K, Ford S, Matthews Z. Divalproex sodium for the treatment of conduct disorder: a randomized controlled clinical trial. *J Clin Psychiatry* 2003;**64**:1183–1191.
177. Steiner H, Saxena KS, Carrion V, Khanzode LA, Silverman M, Chang K. Divalproex sodium for the treatment of PTSD and conduct disordered youth: a pilot randomized controlled clinical trial. *Child Psychiatry Hum Dev.* 2007 Oct;**38**(3):183–93. Epub 2007 Jun 15.
178. Famularo R, Kinscherff R, Fenton T. Propranolol treatment for childhood posttraumatic stress disorder, acute type. A pilot study. *Am J Dis Child* 1988; **142**:1244–1247.
179. Harmon RJ, Riggs PD. Clonidine for posttraumatic stress disorder in preschool children. *J Am Acad Child Adolesc Psychiatry* 1996;**35**:1247–1249.
180. Steiner H. *Handbook of Mental Health Interventions in Children and Adolescents: An Integrated Developmental Approach,* 1st edn. San Francisco, CA: Jossey-Bass Publishers, 2004.

16

Attachment and its Disorders

Jerald Kay

Evidence is accumulating that human beings of all ages are happiest and able to deploy their talents to best advantage when they are confident that, standing behind them, there are one or more trusted persons who will come to their aid should difficulties arise…an attachment figure.

Bowlby (1969) [1]

It has been more than half a century since John Bowlby developed the concept of attachment. Attachment is the affectional connection that a baby develops with its primary caregiver, most often the mothering person, which becomes increasingly discriminating and enduring. It is the availability and responsiveness of the mother or other caretaker that is ultimately the most influential in determining the strength and safety of the attachment system. Bowlby's attachment theory has been integrated into other psychological theories and has experienced an extraordinary growth in its scientific base. His concepts have proved to be persistent and increasingly relevant to a broader and more sophisticated scientific understanding of the centrality of early experience in human development. In addition to the introduction of rigorous methods of assessing attachment, neurobiological studies of humans, primates, and nonprimates have provided strong support for attachment theory concepts. Moreover, psychiatry and psychology have continually demonstrated the impact of attachment and its disruption on childhood, adolescent, and adult stages of life. It is because of it exceptional power to exert influence on the entire lifespan and subsequent interpersonal relationships in so many dynamically interactive sectors of an individual's life that it especially behooves the child and adolescent mental health professional to become knowledgeable about attachment theory and its helpful role in understanding the etiology, prevention, and treatment of psychopathology.

The History of Attachment Theory

Like August Aichhorn [2] and others, John Bowlby's work started with experience involving juvenile delinquency. His retrospective study of 44 such subjects suggested to him that a distinguishing characteristic of these children appeared to lie in a history of disruptive early experiences with mothering [3]. Although Bowlby was a psychoanalyst, his work was greeted initially with strong contempt by the psychoanalytic community [4]. Moreover, his work, even at present, is viewed suspiciously by child and adult psychoanalysts. Criticisms have centered on Bowlby's simplistic and reductionistic model for understanding behavior, which was considered by many to have evolved more from the field of ethology than classical psychoanalysis. This included his jettisoning of the dual drive theory, dismissal of the centrality of the oedipal conflict, underappreciation for the emotional internalized world, exclusive focus on one domain of the parent-infant relationship, and minimization of the specific characteristics the baby contributes to attachment. In essence, his model retained little of analytic metapsychology although Bowlby constantly sought to maintain a relationship with the analytic community in Britain. It is ironic therefore that his contributions instigated the most intense scientific study of any psychoanalytic model and it has produced the strongest research base. As a result, there is now more interest in Bowlby's ideas and newer findings from attachment studies among analysts and child and adolescent psychiatrists than at any time in the past [4–8].

Core Concepts of Attachment Theory

The infant's attachment behavior is an attempt to bring stability, predictability, and consistency to his or her world through drawing the mother closer. These behaviors include crying, vocalizing, and smiling. Other manifestations

Clinical Child Psychiatry, Third Edition. Edited by William M. Klykylo and Jerald Kay.
© 2012 John Wiley & Sons, Ltd. Published 2012 by John Wiley & Sons, Ltd.

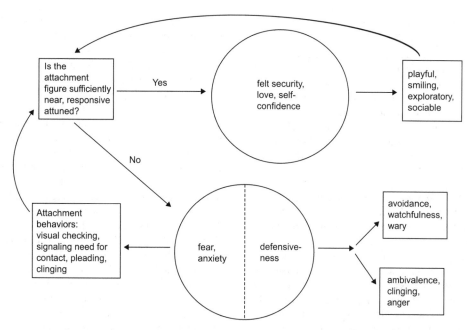

Figure 16.1 The attachment behavioral system. Reprinted from From: Holmes J. *John Bowlby and Attachment Theory*. London: Routledge, 1993; p. 76. With permission.

are greeting responses, crying when mother leaves, lifting of arms (often expressing the wish to be picked up), following the mother and clinging to her, and later, the rapid return to closeness with mother after the child's exploring activities. As will be addressed later, attachment is critical to acquisition of the infant's ability to regulate affect. This process begins with the experience of distress or fear leading to the activation of attachment through proximity-seeking resulting in the downregulation of emotions. Without sound attachment, the infant is ultimately left without a capacity to self-soothe. Figure 16.1 illustrates the attachment behavioral system.

Bowlby [1, 9, 10] classified attachment in a biologically driven (innate) epigenetic model consisting of four stages, including:

- Birth through 2 months – phase of *limited discrimination* and social responsiveness.
- 2–7 months – phase of *limited preference* toward discriminating familiar figures.
- 7–24 months – phase of *focused attachment* and secure base achievement with initiative in seeking proximity and contact.
- 24–36 months – phase of *goal-corrected partnership* with child's attempt to shape mother's ways of relating to accommodate the child's wishes.

Bowlby' tripartite attachment theory consists of: (i) an attachment behavioral system (that attempts to en-

sure closeness); (ii) development of internal models of self and others (internal representation); and (iii) the creation of a homeostatic system (to help the child deal with emotional, environmental, and physiological stress). He focused on the impact of levels of deprivation resulting from an infant's broken bond or failure to achieve a secure connection with the mother. The former attachment disorganization was referred to as partial deprivation and the latter was termed complete deprivation, both of which conditions may confer significant and enduring psychological, and in some cases, physical vulnerabilities leading to mental disorders later in life.

Clinicians are most familiar with Bowlby's description of what occurs when the child is separated from the mother for prolonged periods. He spoke of this process as consisting of three phases experienced by the separated or abandoned child: protest, despair, and detachment. These phases are demonstrated powerfully in the Robertsons' movies of children in naturalistic settings who experienced painful separation [11]. Each phase was marked by the child's readily observable behaviors, as illustrated in Table 16.1. However, it is important to note that separation comprises two distinct processes. The first is the physical act of disruption of the mother-child relationship, but undoubtedly more important is the child's appraisal or assessment of the separation experience. In other words, it is the meaning attributed to the phenomenon that is so powerful.

Table 16.1 Separation behaviors.

Phase	Responses
Protest	Resentment, crying, and attempts to find mother
Despair	Sadness, aggressive behavior toward others, social withdrawal
Detachment	Reaching out to other adults, social reintegration, negative/ambivalent reactions to reunification with mother

Solomon and George [12] noted that Bowlby's contributions provided a reconceptualization of numerous psychological responses to separation, threat of separation, and loss. For example, some symptoms heretofore attributed to anxiety, phobia, depression, aggression, incomplete mourning, and the failure to establish and maintain healthy interpersonal relationships, could be viewed in an overarching theory more reasonably explaining psychological vulnerability in terms of very early disorganizing and at times traumatizing caretaker-infant experiences.

The Developmental Significance of Attachment

There is an extensive literature on and theories about what occurs in the mental life of infants and children during the attachment process. At the risk of oversimplifying, the most intriguing and clinically useful of these theories focuses on the process of internalization. Internalization is the mechanism for building psychological structure. More specifically, it is an attempt to describe how children achieve an increasingly stable and sophisticated view of themselves and the world around them. The acquisition of internal representations of infants and those who care for them are the building blocks of identity formation and individuation. The former includes the capacity for relatedness and cohesiveness of self and the latter refers to the establishment of autonomy or separateness.

Studies have demonstrated how early internal representations are the result of emotional and physical reciprocity between infant and mother [13, 14]. That is, primitive representations are products of co-regulation of synchronies and asynchronies in communication patterns (vocalization, gestures, and facial expressions) within the mother-infant dyad. How the mother responds to unintended empathic failures or disengagements is also an important contributor to the representational process. Providing misattunement and separation are not traumatic, they are equally as potent in promoting healthy psychological development.

It is important to note that mirroring the child's affective state does not imply simple reflection [15]. Rather, an attuned mother exaggerates or distorts her responses, which allow the infant to begin to recognize his or her own emotional response as being separate from that of the mother's. Fonagy's [4] concept of mentalization is predicated on the mother's ability to promote both relatedness and separateness in the infant through her marked affective responses. Mentalization is the capacity of the infant to ascertain the mental states of the self and of others. It describes a process of the infant's recognition that someone else has a different mind from his or her own. It is acquired through repeated experiences in judging facial expression, tone of voice, and other nonverbal communications [4]. These experiences are encoded in implicit (nondeclarative) memory and in parallel with explicit (declarative) memory that has a temporal dimension. This is a critical accomplishment in that it establishes the basis for secure attachment. Conversely, the failure to mirror the child's affective state results in disorganized attachment through problematic internalization and therefore less than optimal identity formation and individuation. Above all, the mother's ability to mirror her infant's internal state is responsible for acquisition of affect regulation.

Recent research has suggested how the attachment process may contribute to the development of empathy. There are a set of motor neurons in the premotor cortex that encode in procedural memory the actions of others whether they are performed or merely observed passively. Initial research has focused on grasping and reaching movements, but Leslie et al [16]. have shown that subjects imitate not only hand movements but also facial expressions as measured by functional magnetic resonance imaging (fMRI). They found evidence for a common cortical imitation circuit involving, but not limited to, Broca's area, bilateral dorsal and ventral premotor areas, and the superior temporal gyrus. This neuronal circuit facilitates an unconscious recognition of goal detection in another person through shared representations of the observer and the observed, and may be a neural substrate for empathy.

Attachment Theory Research

Bowlby's ideas have prompted many different avenues of inquiry. While there has been reinterpretation of some of the findings and explanations of Ainsworth's [17] important studies of attachment types, Ainsworth nevertheless moved attachment theory forward through the application of rigorous observation. Her most substantial contributions are associated with the development of the Strange Situation test, which permitted observation, and analysis of clear differentiation between the characteristics of children's attachment patterns or styles. The Strange Situation provides an examination of the response of 1–2-year-old children to being left for two very brief periods. To summarize a large body of data, Ainsworth and colleagues concluded there are distinct ways in which children deal with separation, reflecting attachment styles she identified as secure, anxious/ resistant (avoidant), or anxious/avoidant. Securely attached infants and toddlers actively seek out their mothers and demonstrate observable relief at reunification. These children are confident that the parent will be available in times of need. A smaller number of children, however, demonstrate some level of indifference to the separation-reunion experience and appear uncertain whether the parent will be available and helpful. Ainsworth characterized this group as having anxious/ resistant (ambivalent) attachment and associated this style with unpredictable or inconsistent mothering. A third group of children display attempts to reconnect with their mothers but their capacity to be soothed upon reunion is impaired. This appears to reflect a lack of confidence in mother. Ainsworth termed this group anxious/avoidant.

More recent research identified a fourth type of child, who attempts to seek proximity through unusual means like hiding or simply denying the presence of the mother. Main and Soloman [18] identified this attachment style as disorganized/disoriented. In addition, these children demonstrate conflicted behaviors upon reunion with their mother including, but not limited to, hitting, freezing, unusual posturing, and non-goal-directed activity. A number of clinician-researchers have attributed the disorganized style of the child to experiencing the mother (who is

likely to have experienced a major loss, trauma, or significant psychopathology in her life) as either frightened (insecure in her caretaking) or frightening (unreliable comforting and soothing in times of need because of her significant misattunement with the child). This critical body of thought focuses on disorganization of children's behavior after separation and not on resistance or avoidance as patterns of attachment. Interestingly, it has been the disorganized/disoriented attachment type that has proven more reliable [19] and perhaps a better predictor of future psychopathology [20–22].

Attachment research with infants and adults now focuses on two dimensions. The first is the organized-disorganized vertical axis reflecting the soundness of psychological integrity and dealing with affect. The second, horizontal dimension, dismissing/deactivating and preoccupied/hyperactivating, portrays a person's ability through a specific set of defenses to handle negative affect. Those with dismissing style will minimize affect and those with a preoccupied style will respond intensely in their attempts to establish closeness and intimacy [23].

Since the development of the Strange Situation test, numerous new measures of attachment in early and later life have been developed. Table 16.2 summarizes many, but not all of these refinements.

Neurobiological Aspects of Animal Attachment

As noted previously, early in his career Bowlby's work was criticized by many in the psychoanalytic community as being too reliant on ethology. It is ironic; therefore, that some of the most evocative and exciting neurobio-

Table 16.2 Some measures of attachment.

Measure	Features
Separation Anxiety Test	Pictures of attachment scenes prompt children's responses based on their attachment styles
Attachment Interview for Childhood and Adolescence	Focuses on here and now relationships with parents in preteens and teens
Adult Attachment Interview	Most reliable measure of adult attachment styles as elicited through the narrative construction of significant childhood experiences (parental responses correlate highly with precise attachment style in their child within the Strange Situation)
Inventory of Parent and Peer Attachment	Self-report measures in adolescents of childhood attachment and in close current relationships
Attachment History Questionnaire	Assesses adults' memories of attachment-related experiences in childhood focusing, for example, on separation from parents, discipline, quality of attachment and supportive relationships, with emphasis on assessing pathological disruptions and distortions
Attachment Style Questionnaire	Evaluates romantic attachment in adulthood
Relationship Questionnaire	Delineates model of self and model of others as they reflect on four basic childhood attachment styles

logical research on attachment and stress in the last decade has involved primates and rodents. This is a very rich and rapidly expanding field that has consistently supported the long-term effects of stressful maternal separation and attachment difficulties in offspring. Because a complete review of this work is beyond the scope of this chapter, discussion will focus on a representative sample of studies.

Monkeys share with humans many characteristics of social development. When these primates experience early life separations, they have revealed lifelong detrimental neuroendocrine consequences. In one of many studies using rhesus monkeys, Suomi [24] was able to demonstrate that while surrogate mothering and socialization by normally reared peers was helpful in socially integrating monkeys separated from their mothers early after birth, there were nevertheless enduring responses to stress that clearly distinguished the separated monkeys. Most importantly, separated monkeys when exposed to environmental challenges such as separation later in life, responded with more extreme behavioral and physiological reactions, including higher levels of cortisol production, which has been linked repeatedly with such effects as impaired hippocampal neurogenesis [25–27]. Similarly, using the variable foraging model, which produces inconsistency and unpredictability in mother feeding [28], anxious mothers disrupt the attachment of their offspring, which results in a marked inability to deal with emotions and stress when the offspring reaches adolescence. Kraemer and Clarke [29] noted that peer-reared monkeys with inconsistent attachment figures not only demonstrated exaggerated fear responses but also had high levels of cortisol throughout adulthood.

A recent review of the impact of altering the early social experience of monkeys supported the findings of subsequent emotional and neurophysiological disturbances [30]. Moreover, it is apparent that animals with high-risk genotypes such as having two short alleles for the serotonin transporter gene (5-HTTLPR) or low monoamine oxidase A (MAO-A) transcription activity interact with experience to produce less resilience in affective stability and in levels of aggression [31, 32]. Either of these genetic patterns can also affect the competency of the mother's attachment since child rearing is ultimately a reciprocal experience.

With respect to rodent research, perinatal separation, even for very short periods, and abuse or neglect coupled with genetic variability appear to be associated with enduring changes in many areas of later life functioning, including:

- emotional and behavioral regulation;
- cognitive function;

- coping style;
- neuroendocrine response to stress;
- brain morphology [33, 34].

As an example, an elegant design, although unreplicated, was developed by the Emory University group to study the impact of early maternal separation and neglect in rats and its role in depression [35, 36]. From days 2 to 14 after birth, rat pups were separated for 3 hours each day. The offspring developed anhedonia, and decreased eating, sleeping, and reproductive behavior. They also displayed increased restless activity and withdrawal. Of perhaps even greater significance, the separated rat pups, as opposed to their nonseparated littermates, were treated differently by their mothers. Moreover, at 90 days, the pups were exposed to a stressor consisting of a puff of air into the eye, and responded with increased adrenocorticotropin (ACTH) and double the normal of corticotropin-releasing factor (CRF) in their amygdalae.

Early maternal separation in rats has been shown to be associated with both decreased brain-derived neurotrophic factor (BDNF) and NMDA (N-methyl-D-aspartate) receptors [37], as well as increased cell death in the brain [38]. BDNF plays a vital role not only in neurogenesis but also in the maintenance of neurons and synapses.

Insel [39] has studied another important neurobiological basis for attachment through investigation of the neuropeptides oxytocin and vasopressin in voles and rats. While it would be an oversimplification to attribute the basis for attachment in these animals and humans to these peptides only, this line of inquiry nevertheless has raised some poignant issues, not the least of which is their potential role in understanding the pathophysiology of abnormal social attachment in such conditions as infantile autism.

Insel studied prairie voles and montane voles, which display the following characteristics:

- Prairie voles:
  social;
  monogamous/protective of female;
  extended mothering;
  male parenting of offspring.
- Montane voles:
  asocial;
  no partner preference;
  females abandon young between 8 and 14 days;
  minimal parenting of offspring.

When the male prairie vole is given a vasopressin antagonist, both the partner preference and aggressivity toward other voles disappeared. After mating, the female prairie vole releases oxytocin, which is vital to establishing the pair bond. However, when the female is given an oxytocin antagonist, she behaves more like the female montane vole. Moreover, upon separation from the mother, the 5-day-old prairie vole demonstrates signs of distress through vocalization and corticosterone production. Insel found that prairie and montane voles also have different oxytocin and vasopressin receptor distribution in the brain, and that after giving birth the female montane vole, at least for a short time, possesses an oxytocin receptor configuration similar to that of the maternal prairie vole. Last, in Insel's studies of rats, females showed little maternal interest when not pregnant. This behavior changes immediately prior to birthing. Insel demonstrated that if oxytocin release is prevented through either lesioning or through the use of antagonist, the onset of maternal care behavior is inhibited. These findings raise provocative questions about a role for oxytocin in human maternal behavior and attachment styles, and have spawned a number of studies in humans utilizing the administration of intranasal oxytocin and its relationship to prosocial effects including anxiety, impaired social functioning, facial recognition, and mentalization, to name but a few [40].

The effect of exogenous oxytocin on trust and cooperation in those with borderline personality disorder (BPD) was measured during a social dilemma game. Oxytocin increased trust and cooperation in control subjects but increased maladaptive aggressive responses in those diagnosed with BPD. The effect of oxytocin seems to be mediated by attachment style, and in high-anxiety/high-avoidance subjects cooperation was decreased. However, in subjects with high-anxiety/low-avoidance styles, cooperation increased [41]. Bartz et al. also studied the effect of intranasal oxytocin on memory of maternal care and closeness in 24 male healthy adults. They found that less anxiously attached subjects recalled their mothers more positively after administration of the oxytocin, but that those who were more anxiously attached experienced less caring and closeness.

There is an additional area of research that has examined the possible reinforcing role of opioid receptors in attachment [42]. Knockout mice, which lack the mu-opioid receptor gene, appear dramatically inhibited in their attachment behavior. For example, when separated briefly from mothers, these offspring showed diminished vocalization but not when exposed to male mice odors or cold. Moreover, these pups also had difficulty in discriminating the smell of their own nests from that of nests belonging to other mothers. This study raises the possibility of another molecular consequence and basis for attachment disorders. Parenthetically, research has demonstrated that there is increased mu-opioid receptor availability (decreased endogenous uploading) within the limbic system and prefrontal cortex areas in those with borderline personality disorder, which may account for why teenagers and adults utilize self-injurious behaviors like cutting, which release endogenous opioids [43].

Animal studies have focused on gene–environment interaction and the impact on subsequent behavioral and emotional changes. This work has examined the role of specific polymorphisms in serotonin transporter genes in conjunction with maternal separation, abuse, and neglect. [44, 45] Specifically, the serotonin transporter gene (5-HTT) has variations in the length of its promoter region, which is expressed in either short, intermediate, or long allelic forms. The short (ss) allele, compared with the long allele (ll), appears to result in decreased serotonin function, a deficiency that may negatively impact on attachment. The hypothesis is supported by the link between the treatment of anxiety and mood disorders with serotonin reuptake inhibitors and genetic variation in serotonin transporters in humans. A serotonin knockout mouse with impaired serotonin uptake ability [46] has both exaggerated stress responses as measured by increased hypothalamic-pituitary axis (HPA) activity and anxiety-like behaviors. These inquiries support earlier work demonstrating persistent behavioral and social difficulties as a result of separation and other early adverse experiences.

Neurobiological Aspects of Human Attachment

Within the last decade, human studies too have explored the role of gene–environment interaction in the adaptation of children. Caspi et al [47]. have elucidated a representative gene–environment consequence of an abnormally low level of monoamine oxidase A (MAO-A) and childhood maltreatment. Low levels of MAO-A have been associated with rodents that display increased aggression. Caspi and colleagues [47] studied more than 1000 children in Dunedin who were assessed every 2 years from ages 3 to 15 years, and then again at ages 18 and 21 years. This birth cohort was evenly distributed among boys and girls. Moreover, the sample remained intact (96%) even by the age of 26. The findings of this study are as follows:

- 64%, 28%, and 8% experienced no, probable, and severe maltreatment respectively;
- males with normal MAO-A levels and maltreatment experienced no increase in antisocial behavior;
- 85% of males with low MAO-A levels and maltreatment demonstrated significantly more antisocial behavior including:
  increase in conduct disorders;
  conviction for violent crimes (rape, robbery, assault).

The overarching finding of this study is that neither environmental trauma alone nor low activity of genes by itself is sufficient to cause antisocial behavior. Once again this study emphasizes the role of functional genetic polymorphism and early adverse experience. This finding has been replicated in the United States as well [48].

Other studies have explored the relationship between attachment problems and developmental issues. Essex *et al.* [49] examined the effect of maternal stress on subsequent childhood pathology. Salivary cortisol levels were measured in 282 $4^1/_2$-year-old children and more than 150 of their sibs. Measurements of maternal stress were gathered when the children were 1, 4, 12, and 54 months. Mental health symptoms of the children were assessed when they were in first grade. Children who experienced chronic maternal depression in their infancy were more likely to have elevated cortisol levels and more mental health symptoms in the first grade. Children who were experiencing only concurrent levels of high stress, but not stress during infancy, did not share these symptoms. As is the case with many studies of early stressful experiences, children become sensitized to subsequent stress and demonstrate abnormal glucocorticoid responses. Studies have demonstrated also that exposure to postnatal maternal depression produces abnormally high levels of cortisol that persist into adolescence [50].

Recently, the role of the serotonin transporter system in human attachment has been described with increasing specificity. Maternal sensitivity or responsiveness only increases attachment security in infants who possess the *ss* allele [51]. There is a genetic predisposition for adolescents to react impulsively when they perceive their autonomy is threatened. Attachment security moderates this response in those teenagers with the *ss* allele, permitting a response that is less self-defeating characterized by more socially appropriate assertiveness. Moreover, adolescents who were securely attached with the *ss* configuration had greater agreeable autonomy in parental interactions compared to insecurely attached peers, who reacted with more hostility [52]. Unresolved attachment in adults is more common in those with the short allele of the serotonin transporter gene as measured by the Adult Attachment Interview [53]. This implies that the emotional regulatory system is weakened, perhaps by less robust connections between the limbic system and prefrontal cortex.

In passing, it is important to note the enduring controversy regarding the explanatory power of gene–environment interaction [54]. Concern has been expressed over the publication bias in novel studies and their subsequent replications. The small sample size of many of these studies has also been criticized. However, Brzustowicz and Freedman have cautioned that in the case of the serotonin transporter studies, their clinical relevance is impressive and may precede the current understanding of the causes of psychopathology [56].

Adrenocorticoid activity among attachment styles has been a fruitful area of study. Since the HPA axis is an integral part of the response to stress and novelty, Spangler and Grossman [57] studied whether disorganized infants respond differently than securely attached infants. Disorganized infants were examined 30 minutes after the Strange Situation and were found to have significantly elevated cortisol levels. Those with insecure attachment had more moderate increases in cortisol, and securely attached infants showed no increase in HPA activity. Higher levels of cortisol appear to reflect that disorganized children have the least success in developing effective coping responses to novelty and stress.

There have been two thrusts in neurobiological research on attachment. Many researchers have examined the behavioral and social responses among attachment styles while others have focused more on brain structure and function as they related to maturation. As noted previously, repeated interaction between a mother and her infant provides the neural template for the baby's knowledge of him or herself and his or her evolving world. These attachment experiences constitute important implicit or procedural memory, which shapes brain structure and function. In essence, "neurons that fire together, wire together." That is, repeated affect-laden interaction between mother and infant provide neuronal organization to the evolving brain through synaptogenesis and pruning. There is a growing body of research addressing the impact of dysfunctional attachment on right-left cortical maturation and functioning [58]. The right brain has been noted to develop earlier than the left, and plays an important role in the developing capacity to modulate affect, aggression, and stress, all of which are necessary for the acquisition of social skills. It may be that early negative experiences not only disproportionately increase synaptic pruning but leave the infant in a persistent state of vulnerability to stress, as has been demonstrated in animal studies. The studies of child maltreatment and its impact on the corpus callosum also provide support for detrimental effects on brain maturation. The corpus callosum functions as the bridge between the right and left brain. Infants who have been abused or neglected have smaller callosal structures, leaving them at a disadvantage regarding the integration of feelings and the developing cognitive capacity of the left brain.

Attachment Disorganization and Psychopathology

For the clinician, perhaps the most clinically relevant research has been that of assessing the impact of attachment problems on the psychological development of children and the likelihood of ensuing psychopathology. This line of inquiry has resulted in some support for the detrimental effects of disorganized attachment on subsequent relationships and adaptive capacity, especially among high-risk children. In general, the following family risk factors have been shown to be associated with disorganized attachment:

- alcohol and substance abuse;
- bipolar disorder;
- chronic major depression;
- child maltreatment;
- parental history of abuse or significant loss.

The children of mothers with psychosocial problems have been shown to have higher levels of aggression [21] and more externalizing behavioral problems. Internalizing symptoms appear to be correlated more with avoidant attachment and not disorganized attachment style. The additive component of risk factors is illustrated in a study of disorganized children who also had difficult temperament styles as rated by mothers. These children were noted as exceptionally aggressive by teachers [20]. It seems that disorganized attachment style leads not only to aggression but also to controlling behavior in middle childhood, with parents frequently feeling helpless and intimidated by the child. The aggressive and controlling child also is less likely to be involved in productive peer relationships. It often appears to the clinician that the disorganized child is more likely to be seen as having poor social skills, less likely to modulate affect and arousal, and have less adaptability and resilience.

Unresolved parental loss appears to be a critical component in the development of attachment disorganization in children [59]. Mothers who have experienced unresolved trauma and/or significant loss in their lives relate to their infants in a frightening or hostile manner. Other mothers with unresolved loss and/or trauma are often frightened and experience helplessness about caring for their child. Both of these scenarios, despite maternal sensitivity to the child, may result in the mother's inability to control emotions and memories stemming from the loss and/or trauma. Frequently, the demands of caring for an infant prompt maternal behaviors that are perceived as threatening to the infant. The infant, in turn, is in an unresolvable situation because of the need to seek comfort from the mother who also becomes a source of danger. Main and Hesse

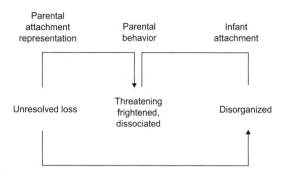

Figure 16.2 Theory of Main and Hess linking unresolved loss and infant disorganization. From Schuengel *et al.*, p. 73 [92].

argue that it is this repeated dyadic interaction that engenders the disorganized attachment. Figure 16.2 illustrates the role of unresolved loss and disorganized attachment. This work complements that of Blatt and Blass [60], who conceptualize attachment as a dialectic between two developmental pressures: the need to acquire the capacity to relate to others while at the same time acquiring a sense of identity. If acquiring the ability for relatedness did not go smoothly, later in life the clinician sees patients with dependency and the exaggerated wish for admiration and affirmation.

With respect to explaining disorganized attachment in both clinical studies and treatment, one of the most helpful theories is the relational diathesis model [5]. It posits that disorganized attachment can be viewed as a product of both the level of safety experienced by the infant as well as the magnitude of his or her psychological trauma. Moreover, it explains how unresolved loss and trauma often leads to successive traumatic experiences. Figure 16.3 presents this model in schematic form.

There is a growing literature about the effect of disorganized attachment on child and adult psychopathology, but two caveats are in order. First, although studies have supported Bowlby's notions that individual differences in attachment security can be continuous throughout life, they can also change from experience. Second, the most probable explanation of the contribution of disorganized attachment on psychopathology should include an interaction with other risk factors such as difficult child temperament, medical illness in the child and family members, family history of mental illness, marital conflict, social and financial adversity, and caretakers with poor parenting skills [61].

Problematic attachment has been correlated with dysfunctional behavior/disorders during infancy and childhood, and the *Diagnostic and Statistical Manual*

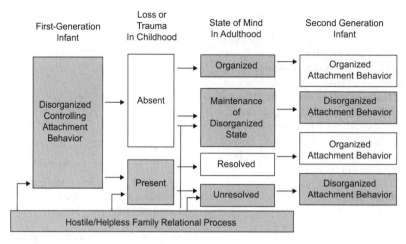

Figure 16.3   Proposed contributions of a relational diathesis. From Lyons-Ruth *et al.*, p. 44 [5].

of Mental Disorders, Fourth Edition, Text Revision (DSM-IV-TR) diagnostic category of Reactive Attachment Disorder (RAD) recognizes this as being characterized by the following characteristics:

- Before the age of 5, markedly disturbed and developmentally inappropriate social relatedness in the majority of contexts through either:
  - persistent failure to initiate or respond in a developmentally appropriate manner to most social interactions as manifest by highly excessively inhibited, hypervigilant, or highly ambivalent and contradictory responses such as responding to caregivers with a mixture of approach, avoidance, resistance to comforting, or frozen watchfulness (inhibited type);
  - or diffuse attachments with indiscriminate sociability and marked inability to exhibit appropriate selective attachments such as excessive familiarity with strangers or a lack of selectivity in attachment figures (disinhibited type).
- Disturbances are not accounted for by developmental delay (either as in mental retardation or pervasive developmental delay).

- Pathogenic care as evidenced by either persistent disregard of the child's basic emotional/physical needs or repeated changes of primary caregivers that prevent stable attachment [62].

A number of clinicians and researchers have criticized the DSM criteria for RAD [63]. Criticism has focused on the requirements of persistent disregard of the child's emotional and physical needs, which are not supported by research. As has been discussed at length, disorganized attachment is not always the result of willful maltreatment. While disorganized children have insecure attachment, the assumption that insecurely attached children are disorganized is incorrect and fails to acknowledge anxious resistant and anxious avoidant attachment styles. Other clinicians find the Diagnostic Classification of Mental Health and Developmental Disorders of Infancy and Early Childhood (DC:0–3) more comprehensive [64]. In this system, there are primary diagnostic categories for traumatic stress, and mood, anxiety, and regulatory disorders. Table 16.3 summarizes this approach in highlighting the centrality of early affective experiences.

Table 16.3   Basic functional emotional developmental capacities that depend on critical affective interactions.

Level/expected emotional function	Typical age range
Level 1: Shared attention and regulation	Birth to 3 months
Level 2: Engagement and relating	2 to 6 months
Level 3: Two-way purposeful interaction	4 to 9 months
Level 4: Shared social problem-solving	9 to 18 months
Level 5: Creating symbols and ideas	18 to 30 months
Level 6: Building logical bridges between ideas: logical thinking	30 to 48 months

Adapted from Greenspan and Wieder, p. 687 [54].

Research findings on the association between attachment styles and adaptation later in life are somewhat contradictory. However, there have been a number of studies demonstrating that problematic attachment styles do predict emotional and behavioral disorders in some populations. For example, anxiety symptoms and disorders in adolescence were predicted by an anxious resistant attachment style [65]. In this study, infants were administered the Strange Situation test at 1 year of age, and 172 of these children were assessed by structured clinical interview (Schedule for Affective Disorders and Schizophrenia for School-Aged Children) at 17.5 years. A birth cohort study of over 1000 subjects in New Zealand tested children at age 8 years and then followed them over the course of 21 years [66]. Subjects were assessed in middle childhood for anxious/withdrawn behavior and again at ages 16–18 and 18–21 for anxiety disorders. Increasing anxious/withdrawn behavior at age 8 was associated with higher risk in adolescence and young adulthood for panic disorder with agoraphobia, social and specific phobias, and major depression. Weinfeld *et al.* [67] conducted a 19-year prospective study of 12–18-month-old children using the Strange Situation, with follow-up in 125 subjects in young adulthood using the Adult Attachment Interview. Disorganized attachment in infants was significantly more likely to be insecure or unresolved in late adolescence, and this also predicted unresolved abuse scores for those who experienced childhood abuse.

A prospective study of high-risk children found that avoidant and disorganized attachment styles were associated with dissociative symptoms measured at four points in time over 19 years [68]. Carlson [22] also reported that disorganized attachment was associated with dissociation in young adulthood and also with behavioral problems in preschool, primary school, and high school. A study by Lyons-Ruth *et al.* [69] of 62 low-income families assessed attachment in infants at 18 months and at age 5 through preschool teacher ratings. The most potent predictor of hostile behavior toward classmates was earlier disorganized attachment style, with 71% of aggressive children having been designated as having disorganized attachment earlier in life.

There have been a number of studies of adoptive children with or without deprivation. O'Conner and Rutter [70] conducted a longitudinal examination of 152 Romanian children who experienced significant early hardship, and compared them to 52 adoptees from the UK. They found that duration of deprivation correlated highly with severity of attachment disorders. In addition, the attachment disorder behaviors were also associated with conduct and attentional problems. In a study by Roy and Pickles [71], hyperactivity and attentional problems were found to be higher in 19 children from group homes as opposed to a control group of the same number of children from foster care. Another study of these Romanian children [72] demonstrated that secure attachment was highest among the children who spent shorter times in the orphanage. In yet another Romanian study by Smyke *et al.*, [73] of 32 toddlers living in a typical unit within a large institution it was found that they were more likely to demonstrate emotional withdrawal and indiscriminate social attachment patterns compared to 33 toddlers living at home and to 29 children living on a unit designed to provide greater consistency by reducing the number of caretakers. A Greek study of 86 infants reared in residential care from birth and a control group of 41 infants raised with their two biological parents found that 62% of infants from the residential care setting demonstrated disorganized attachment as opposed to 25% of the latter group.

Treatment Implications of Disorganized Attachment

Perhaps the most straightforward way to approach this rich topic is by addressing three groups of intervention: prevention, treatment of children, and treatment of parents and other adult patients. In the case of poorly adjusted infants and children, it is assumed that treatment is not limited to the identified patient but frequently may include treatment of families and parents or other caretakers. For example, over 35 years ago Selma Fraiberg and colleagues [74] emphasized the importance of recognizing the contribution of unresolved parental childhood conflicts in poor adjustment of their infants. She called these unresolved problems "ghosts in the nursery," and described treatment as helping the parents attain insight through examination of their own childhood experiences and how they affected their ability to care for their infant.

Children with behavior problems and many psychiatric disorders undoubtedly constitute the majority of patients treated by child and adolescent psychiatrists. This book has emphasized the challenges in assessing infants, children, and adolescents, as well as treatment approaches to the most common child psychiatric disorders. It also addresses the centrality of those characteristics of the doctor-patient relationship that underlie every treatment situation with children, their parents, and their families. These include, but are not limited to, the engagement of patients and their families through establishing a nonjudgmental rapport, an empathic stance, a therapeutic alliance, and attention to a broad range of biological, social, and psychological considerations.

In this concluding section, it seems fitting to return to Bowlby's first interest, criminal and antisocial behavior that frequently is associated with disorganized attachment. A representative example of prevention of these problems is found in the work of Olds and colleagues [75]. They enrolled 400 young (less than 19 years old), unmarried, or of low socioeconomic status high-risk pregnant women with no previous live births. This randomized controlled trial (RCT) assigned mothers to standard well-child care in a clinic or to a nurse who made regularly scheduled home visits throughout pregnancy, up to the child's second birthday. The latter group of mothers received on average nine home visits during pregnancy and 23 visits after delivery. In their visits, nurses focused on maternal functioning within three dimensions. These included maternal personal development, health-related behaviors, and competent care of their children. A follow-up of 15-year-old teenagers of mothers receiving the intervention, compared to the former group in the standard well-child care clinic, showed:

- less running away;
- fewer arrests;
- fewer convictions;
- fewer sentences to youth corrections;
- less initiation of sexual intercourse;
- fewer sexual partners;
- less illicit substance abuse; and
- fewer school suspensions and teacher reports of disruptive behavior.

This study convincingly demonstrated that prenatal and early childhood intervention can dramatically decrease the likelihood of antisocial behavior among adolescents born into high-risk families. Of equal importance, this study substantiates the benefits of psychotherapy for parents, both to them and their children. The findings of this RCT complement those of the previously discussed Dunedin study, which examined the interaction between low MAO-A and adverse childhood experiences [47]. Both studies therefore demonstrate the inextricability of environment and genes in the pathogenesis of antisocial behavior. Other attachment-based studies offer promise in the prevention of the effects of maternal depression and other mental disorders on infants [76–78].

For psychiatrists and other mental health professionals who view psychotherapy, particularly psychodynamic psychotherapy, as a necessary component in the treatment of the many child, adolescent, and adult disorders, attachment theory has provided support for this treatment and highlighted the importance of a patient's attachment to the therapist [79]. It has deepened understanding of the psychological birth of the infant and has reaffirmed important underlying principles about the power of early experience in shaping a person's enduring view of themselves, the world around them, the intergenerational transmission of strengths and vulnerabilities, and, in some cases, the pathogenesis of mental disorders. Attachment theory has added considerable support to the study of personality development within a social context as expressed through earlier work of British object relationists (Winnicott and Fairbairn), neo-Freudians (Erikson), and self psychologists (Kohut). It has also played an important role in substantiating the effects of psychological trauma on both the mother and her child.

Among other contributions, attachment theory has brought a deeper understanding to the treatment of personality disorders. This is exemplified in some difficult-to-treat patients, very often with significant trauma history, who have an inadequate capacity for mentalization and self-reflection that interferes with the ability to understand mental functioning in themselves as well as the therapist [80]. Not infrequently, there are challenging countertransference issues in treating such patients, who may re-enact traumatic situations, which define the therapist as unhelpful and persecuting. An understanding of the impact of disorganized attachment and trauma on the ability to reflect provides the child psychiatrist with a nonpunitive and thereby more empathic view of symptoms. From this vantage point, the therapist can conceptualize the patient not in terms of deficits or manipulation, but rather of ultimately unsuccessful adaptation through the attempt to ward off pain from early loss and trauma and insecure attachment [81].

A specific treatment based on enhancing mentalization was developed by Fonagy and colleagues [82]. This evidence-based dynamic psychotherapy was initially created as a treatment for borderline personality disorder. However, throughout the last decade, mentalization-based therapy (MBT) has been widely adapted and integrated into many psychotherapies. MBT has four goals:

- To teach the difference between mentalizing and nonmentalizing narratives.
- To provide a method to reflect on nonmentalizing experiences.
- To promote an interest about the mental states of others.
- To acquire the ability to label explicit and feeling states that are outside of awareness.

In the psychotherapy of children and adolescents, attachment theory assists clinicians to focus on fear and not aggression. Slade [23] notes that the privileging of fear is based on Bowlby's concept that children, regardless of their unempathic experiences, must remain attached to the caregiver, even if this adult is the source of fear. Survival demands this adaptation. Despite the continued unhealthy relationship with the caregiver and/or subsequent persons, the child seeks the safety of the known. What is helpful in the therapeutic relationship, to state the obvious, is the creation of warm, nonjudgmental, empathic environment that does not constitute a threat to the patient's sense of safety. It permits the patient, through the establishment of a secure base, the opportunity to risk feeling and thinking what has previously been disavowed or dissociated. This in turn increases narrative competence and the patient's ability to develop a less distorted story of his or her life. The therapist then is able to tolerate strong affect and name what the patient is experiencing. The inability or the unwillingness of the patient to acknowledge the "unknown" or disavowed dooms the patient to re-enact unhelpful attachment patterns.

There have been some important RCTs of psychotherapy with mothers and preschoolers that have demonstrated significant efficacy. Lieberman *et al* [83]. conducted weekly child-parent psychotherapy with children exposed to marital violence. This treatment focuses on the mother-child relationship as the mechanism of change through increasing the mother's competence in responding to her child. Children in this treatment demonstrated decreased behavioral problems, traumatic stress symptoms, and diagnostic status. Mothers similarly showed decreased symptoms. Other RCTs utilizing mother-child psychotherapy have been efficacious with anxiously attached children [84], toddlers of depressed mothers [85], and neglected and maltreated preschoolers [86].

Does the attachment style of the therapist and patient influence psychotherapy? The short answer to this question is yes. Those teens and adults with a dismissing/deactivating type of attachment (analogous to the avoidant infant classification) favor defenses that minimize affect. For these patients, a goal of the psychotherapy is developing the capacity to tolerate and express emotions. For the preoccupied/hyperactivating attachment style (resistant infant style), the treatment goal is to contain and regulate that which remains overwhelming and or traumatizing [87]. Every patient has the capacity to evoke the therapist's attachment style [23].

Attachment theory has advanced the understanding of medical treatment and compliance. Using the Bartholomew and Horowitz [88] classification of secure, dismissing (avoidant), preoccupied (resistant), and fearful attachment styles, Ciechanowski and colleagues [89] studied 367 adult patients with type 1 or 2 diabetes within a primary care setting. Patients with dismissing attachment styles tend to undervalue close relationships and present in the doctor-patient relationship as overly self-reliant and minimizing symptoms and the need for other people. Those diabetics with dismissing attachment compared to secure attachment had poorer doctor-patient communication and glucose control, both of which were associated with elevated glycosylated hemoglobin (HbA 1c) levels. (An elevation of HbA 1c of 1% has been shown to be associated over a 10-year period with an approximate 60% increase in developing diabetic retinopathy.) In addition, those prescribed oral hypoglycemic agents were less likely to take these medications and monitor their blood glucose. This study supports research that has found dismissing attachment style to be associated with greater rejection of health providers, worse use of treatment, less self-disclosure in the treatment context, and fewer visits to health professionals [90, 91].

Attachment theory has also contributed to a richer understanding of cognitive development through its focus on the acquisition of models for internalization and perception. Finally, it has prompted important neurobiological research in animals and humans, which has substantiated the wisdom of dispensing with an artificially dichotomous view of nature and nurture and mind and brain.

Conclusion

Despite vehement initial rejection by psychoanalysis, attachment theory has proven to be an increasingly thoughtful contribution to the understanding of human development and psychopathology. Bowlby's theory described the intense innate need of the infant to affectionally connect with the primary caregiver. This connection provides the foundation for biological survival and psychological development and is a powerful motivator in the organization of the infant's mental life and his or her behavior. Moreover, it has a profound effect on all future interpersonal relationships through the establishment of a person's identity and world view. Last, attachment theory has elucidated the contributions to, and the enduring complications of, dysfunctional attachment and deepened the ability of psychiatrists to help their patients resolve these experiences.

References

1. Bowlby J. *Attachment and Loss,* Vol. 1: *Attachment.* London: Hogarth Press and the Institute of Psycho-Analysis, 1969.
2. Aichhorn A. *Wayward Youth.* London: Imago Publishing Company, 1951.

3. Bowlby J. Forty-four juvenile thieves: their characters and home life. *Int J Psychoanal* 1944;25:19–52

4. Fonagy P. *Attachment Theory and Psychoanalysis.* New York: Other Press, 2001.

5. Lyons-Ruth K, Bronfman E, Atwood G. A relational diathesis model of hostile-helpless states of mind: expressions in mother-infant interaction. In: Solomon J, George C (eds) *AttachmentDisorganization.* New York: Guilford Press, 1999; p. 44.

6. Slade A. Attachment theory and research: implications for the theory and practice of individual psychotherapy with adults. In: Cassidy J, Shaver PR (eds) *Handbook of Attachment: Theory, Research and Clinical Applications.* New York: Guilford Press, 1999; pp. 575–594.

7. Mitchell SA. *Relationality: from Attachment to Intersubjectivity.* Hillsdale, NJ: The Analytic Press, 2000; pp. 79–102.

8. Diamond D. Attachment disorganization: The reunion of attachment theory and psychoanalysis. *Psychoanal Psychol* 2004;21:276–299.

9. Bowlby J. *Attachment and Loss*, Vol. 2: *Separation: Anxiety and Anger.* London: Hogarth Press and Institute of Psycho-Analysis, 1973.

10. Bowlby J. *Attachment and Loss*, Vol. 3: *Loss: Sadness and Depression.* London: Hogarth Press and Institute of Psycho-Analysis, 1980.

11. Robertson J, Robertson J. *John, aged 17 months* [film]. London: Tavistock Institute of Human Relations, 1969.

12. Solomon J, George C. *Attachment Disorganization.* New York: Guilford Press, 1999.

13. Beebe B, Lachmann F, Jaffe J. Mother-infant interaction structures and presymbolic self and object representations. *Psychoanal Dialogues* 1977;7:113–182

14. Stern DN. *The Interpersonal World of the Infant: A View from Psychoanalysis and Developmental Psychology.* New York: Basic Books, 1985.

15. Fonagy P, Target M, Gergely G. Attachment and borderline personality disorder. A theory and some evidence. *Psychiatr Clin North Am* 2000;23:103–22, vii–viii.

16. Leslie KR, Johnson-Frey SH, Grafton ST. Functional imaging of face and hand imitation: towards a motor theory of empathy. *Neuroimage* 2004;21:601–607.

17. Ainsworth MDS, Blechar MC, Waters E, Wall S. *Patterns of Attachment: A Psychological Study of the Strange Situation.* Hillside, NJ: Erlbaum, 1978.

18. Main M, Solomon J. Procedures for identifying infants as disorganized/disoriented during the Ainsworth Strange Situation. In: Greenberg M, Ciccetti D, Cummings EM (eds) *Attachment During the Preschool Years: Theory, Research, and Intervention.* Chicago: University of Chicago Press, 1990; pp. 121–160.

19. Lyons-Ruth K, Repacholi B, McLeod S, Silver E. Disorganized attachment behavior in infancy: short-term stability, maternal and infant correlates, and risk-related subtypes. *Dev Psychopathol* 1991;3:377–396

20. Shaw DS, Owens EB, Vondra JI, Keenan K, Winslow EB. Early risk factors and pathways in the development of early disruptive behavior problems. *Dev Psychopathol* 1996;8:679–699.

21. Lyons-Ruth K. Attachment relationships among children with aggressive behavior problems: the role of disorganized early attachment problems. *J Consult Clin Psychol* 1996;64:64–73.

22. Carlson EA. A prospective longitudinal study of attachment disorganization/disorientation. *Child Dev* 1998;69: 1107–1128.

23. Slade A. The implications of attachment theory and research for adult psychotherapy. In: Cassidy J, Shaver PR (eds) *Handbook of Attachment: Theory, Research and Clinical Applications,* 2nd edn. New York: Guilford Press, 2008; pp. 762–782.

24. Suomi SJ. Attachment in rhesus monkeys. In: In: Cassidy J, Shaver PR (eds) *Handbook of Attachment: Theory, Research and Clinical Applications.* New York: Guilford Press, 1999; pp. 181–197.

25. Sapolsky RE, *et al.* Hippocampal damage associated with prolonged glucocorticoid exposure in primates. *J Neurosci* 1990:181–197.

26. Sapolsky RM: Glucocorticoids and hippocampal atrophy in neuropsychiatric disorders. *Arch Gen Psychiatry* 2000; 57(10):925–935.

27. Heim C, Plotsky PM, Nemeroff C: Importance of studying the contributions of early adverse experience to neurobiological findings in depression. Neuropsychopharmacology 2004;29(4):641–648.

28. Rosenblum LA, Coplan JD, Friedman S, Bassoff T, Gorman JM, Andrews MW. Adverse early experiences affect noradrenergic and serotonergic functioning in adult primates. *Biological Psychiatry* 1994;35:221–227.

29. Kraemer GW, Clarke AS. Social attachment, brain function and aggression. *Ann NY Acad Sci* 1996;794:121–135.

30. Stevens HE, Leckman JF, Coplan JD, Suomi SJ. Risk and resilience: early manipulation of Macaque social experience and persistent behavioral and neurophysiological outcomes. *J Am Acad Child Adolesc Psychiatry* 2009;48:114–127.

31. Champoux M, Bennet A, Shannon C, *et al.* Serotonin transporter gene polymorphism, differential early rearing, and behavior in rhesus monkeys. *Mol Psychiatry* 2002;7:1058–1063.

32. Barr CS, Newman TK, Becker ML, *et al.* The utility of the non-human primate model for studying gene by environment interactions in behavioral research. *Genes Brain Behav* 2003;2:336–340.

33. Sanchez MM, Ladd CO, Plotsky PM. Early adverse experience as a developmental risk factor for later psychopathology: evidence from rodent and primate models. *Dev Psychopathol* 2001;13:419–449.

34. Kalinichev M, Easterling KW, Plotsky PM, Holtzman SG. Long-lasting changes in stress-induced corticosterone response and anxiety-like behaviors as a consequence of neonatal maternal separation in Long-Evans rats. *Pharmacol Biochem Behav* 2002;73:131–140.

35. Nemeroff C. The corticotropin-releasing factor (CRF) hypothesis of depression: New findings and new directions. *Mol Psychiatry* 1996;1:336–342.

36. Nemeroff C: The neurobiology of depression. *Sci Am* 1998;278(6):42–49.

37. Roceri M, Hendriks W, Racagni G, Ellenbroek BA, Riva MA. Early maternal deprivation reduces the expression of BDNF and NMDA receptor subunits in rat hippocampus. *Mol Psychiatry* 2002;7:609–616

38. Zhang LX, Levine S, Dent G, *et al.* Maternal deprivation increases cell death in the infant rat brain. *Brain Res Dev Brain Res* 2002;133:1–11.

39. Insel TR. A neurobiological basis of social attachment. *Am J Psychiatry* 1997;154:726–735.

40. MacDonald K, MacDonald TM. The peptide that binds: a systematic review of oxytocin and its prosocial effects in humans. *Harv Rev Psychiatry* 2010;**18**:1–21.

41. Bartz J, Simeon D, Hamilton H, *et al.* Oxytocin can hinder trust and cooperation in borderline personality disorder. *Soc Cogn Affect Neurosci* 2010; 29 Nov [epub ahead of print].

42. Moles A, Kieffer BL, D'Amato FR. Deficit in attachment behavior in mice lacking the mu-opioid receptor gene. *Science* 2004;**304**:1983–1986.

43. Prossin AR, Love TM, Koeppe RA, Zubieta JK, Silk KR. Dysregulation of regional endogenous opioid function in borderline personality disorder. *Am J Psychiatry* 2010;**167**:925–933.

44. Suomi SJ. Gene-environment interactions and the neurobiology of social conflict. *Ann NY Acad Sci* 2003;**1008**:132–139.

45. Barr CS, Newman TK, Shannon C, *et al.* Rearing condition and rh5-HTTLPR interact to influence limbic-hypothalamic-pituitary-adrenal axis response to stress in infant macques. *Biol Psychiatry* 2004;**55**:733–738.

46. Holmes A, Murphy DL, Crawley JN. Abnormal behavioral phenotypes of serotonin transporter knockout mice: parallels with human anxiety and depression. *Biol Psychiatry* 2003;**54**:953–959.

47. Caspi A, McClay J, Moffitt TE, *et al.* Role of genotype in the cycle of violence in maltreated children. *Science* 2002;**297**:851–854.

48. Foley DL, Eaves LJ, Wormley B, *et al.* Childhood adversity, monoamine oxidase a genotype, and risk for conduct disorder. *Arch Gen Psychiatry* 2004;**61**:738–744.

49. Essex MJ, Klein MH, Cho E, Kalin NH. Maternal stress beginning in infancy may sensitize children to later stress exposure: effects on cortisol and behavior. *Biol Psychiatry* 2002;**52**:776–784.

50. Halligan SL, Herbert J, Goodyer IM, Murray L. Exposure to postnatal depression predicts elevated cortisol in adolescent offspring. *Biol Psychiatry* 2004;**55**:376–381.

51. Barry KA, Kochanska G, Phillibert RA. G x E interaction in the organization of attachment: mothers' responsiveness as a moderator of children's genotypes. *J Child Psychol Psychiatry* 2008;**49**:1313–1320.

52. Zimmerman P, Mohr C, Spangler G. Genetic and attachment influences on adolescents' regulation of autonomy and aggressiveness. *J Child Psychol Psychiatry* 2009;**50**:1339–1347.

53. Caspers KM, Paradiso S, Yucuis R, Troutman B, Arndt S, Philibert R. Association between the serotonin transporter promoter polymorphism (5-HTTLPR) and adult unresolved attachment. *Dev Psychol* 2009;**45**:64–76.

54. Caspi A, Hariri AR, Holmes A, Uher R, Moffitt TE. Genetic sensitivity to the environment: the case of the serotonin transporter gene and its implications for studying complex diseases and traits. *Am J Psychiatry* 2010;**167**:509–527.

55. Duncan LE, Keller MC. A critical review of the first 10 years of candidate gene-by-environment interaction research in psychiatry. *Am J Psychiatry* 2011 168:10;1041-1049.

56. Brzustowicz L, Freedman R. Digging more deeply for genetic effects in psychiatric illness. *Am J Psychiatry* 2011;**168**:1017–1020.

57. Spangler G, Grossmann KE. Biobehavioral organization in securely and insecurely attached infants. *Child Dev* 1993;**64**:1439–1450.

58. Shore AN. Early organization of the nonlinear right brain and development of a predisposition to psychiatric disorders. *Dev Psychopathol* 1997;**9**:595–631.

59. Main M, Hesse E. Parents' unresolved traumatic experiences are related to infant disorganized attachment status: Is frightened and/or frightening parental behavior the linking mechanism? In: Greenberg M, Ciccetti D, Cummings EM (eds) *Attachment in the Preschool Years: Theory Research and Intervention.* Chicago: University of Chicago Press, 1990; pp. 161–182.

60. Blatt SJ, Blass R. Relatedness and self definition: a dialectic model of personality development. In: Noam GG, Fischer KW (eds) *Development and Vulnerabilities in Close Relationships.* New York: Erlbaum, 1996; pp. 309–338.

61. Rutter ML. Psychosocial adversity and child psychopathology. *Brit J Psychiatry* 1999;**174**:480–493.

62. American Psychiatric Association. *Diagnostic and Statistical Manual of Mental Disorders, Fourth Edition, Text Revision.* Washington, DC: American Psychiatric Association, 2000; 130 pp.

63. Boris NW, Zeanah CH, Larrieu JA, Sheeringa MS, Heller SS. Attachment disorders in infancy and early childhood: a preliminary investigation of diagnostic criteria. *Am J Psychiatry* 1998;**155**:295–297.

64. Greenspan SI, Wieder S. Diagnostic classification in infancy and early childhood. In: Tasman A, Kay J, Lieberman JA, First MB, Maj M (eds) *Psychiatry,* 3rd edn. Chichester: John Wiley & Sons, Ltd, 2008; pp. 679–688.

65. Warren SL, Huston L, Egeland B, Sroufe LA. Child and adolescent disorders and early attachment. *J. Am Acad Child Adolesc Psychiatry* 1997;**36**:637–644.

66. Goodwin RD, Fergusson DM, Horwood LJ. Early anxious/withdrawn behaviours predict later internalizing disorders. *J Child Psychiatry* 2004;**45**:874–883.

67. Weinfeld NS, Whaley GJ, Egeland B. Continuity, discontinuity, and coherence in attachment from infancy to late adolescence: sequelae of organization and disorganization. *Attach Hum Dev* 2004;**6**:73–97.

68. Ogawa JR, Sroufe LA, Weinfield NS, Carlson EA, Egeland B. Development and the fragmented self: longitudinal study of dissociative symptomatology in a nonclinical sample. *Dev Psychopathol* 1997;**9**:855–879.

69. Lyons-Ruth K, Alpern L, Repacholi B. Disorganized infant attachment classification and maternal psychosocial problems as predictors of hostile-aggressive behavior in the preschool classroom. *Child Dev* 1993;**64**:572–585.

70. O'Conner TG, Rutter M. Attachment disorder behavior following early severe deprivation: extension and longitudinal follow-up. English and Romanian Adoptees Study Team. *J Am Acad Child Adolesc Psychiatry* 2000;**39**:703–712.

71. Roy PR, Pickles A. Institutional care: risk from family background or pattern of rearing? *J Child Psychol Psychiatry* 2000;**41**:139–149.

72. Marvin RS, Britner PA: Normative development: The ontogeny of attachment. In: Cassidy J, Shaver PR, eds. Handbook of Attachment: Theory, Research and Clinical Application. New York: Guilford Press, 1999:44–67.

73. Smyke AT, Dumitrescu A, Zeanah CH. Attachment disturbances in young children. I: The continuum of caretaking casualty. *J Am Acad Child Adolesc Psychiatry* 2002;**41**:972–982.

74. Fraiberg SH, Adelson E, Shapiro V. Ghosts in the nursery: a psychoanalytic approach to the problem of impaired

infant-mother relationships. *J Am Acad Child Psychiatry* 1975;**14**:387–422.

75. Olds D, Henderson CR, Cole R, *et al.* Long-term effects of nurse home visitation on children's criminal and antisocial behavior:15-year follow-up of a randomized controlled trial. *JAMA* 1998;**280**:1238–1244.

76. Bosquet M, Egeland B. Associations among maternal depressive symptomatology, state of mind and parent and child behaviors: implications for attachment-based interventions. *Attach Hum Dev* 2001;**3**:173–199.

77. McMahon C, Barnett B, Kowalenko N, Tennant C, Don N. Postnatal depression, anxiety and unsettled infant behaviour. *Aust N Z J Psychiatry* 2001;**35**:581–588.

78. Bifulco A, Figueiredo B, Guedeney N, *et al.* Maternal attachment style and depression associated with childbirth: preliminary results from a European and US cross-cultural study. *Br J Psychiatry Suppl* 2004;**46**:s31–37.

79. Parish M, Eagle MN. Attachment to the therapist. *Psychoanal Psychol* 2003;**20**:271–286.

80. Fonagy P. An attachment theory approach to treatment of the difficult patient. *Bull Menniger Clin* 1998;**62**:147–169.

81. Fonagy P, Target M, Steele M, Steele H, Leigh T, Levinson A, Kennedy R. Morality, disruptive behavior, borderline personality disorder, crime and their relationships to security of attachment. In: Atkinson L, Zucker KJ (eds) *Attachment and Psychopathology*. New York: Guilford, 1997; pp. 223–274.

82. Allen JG, Fonagy P (eds). *Handbook of Mentalization Based Treatment*. Chichester, UK: John Wiley & Sons, Ltd, 2006.

83. Lieberman AF, Van Horn P, Ippen CG. Toward evidence-based treatment: child-parent psychotherapy with preschoolers exposed to marital violence. *Am Acad Child Adolesc Psychiatry* 2005;**44**:1241–1248.

84. Lieberman AF, Weston DR, Pawl JH. Preventive intervention and outcome with anxiously attached dyads. *Child Dev* 1991;**62**:199–209.

85. Toth SL, Rogosch FA, Manly JT, Ciccheti D. The efficacy of toddler-parent psychotherapy to reorganize attachment in the young offspring of mothers with depressive disorder: a randomized preventive trial. *J Consult Clin Psychol* 2006;**74**:1006–1016.

86. Toth SL, Maughan A, Manly JT, Spagnola M, Cicchetti D. The relative efficacy of two interventions in altering maltreated preschool children's representational models: implications for attachment theory. *Dev Psychopathol* 2002;**14**:877–908.

87. Holmes J. *The Search for the Secure Base: Attachment Theory and Psychotherapy*. London: Taylor & Francis, 2001.

88. Bartholomew K, Horowitz LM. Attachment styles among young adults: a test of a four-category model. *J Pers Soc Psychol* 1991;**61**:226–244.

89. Ciechanowski PS, Katon WJ, Russo JE, Walker EA. The patient-provider relationship: Attachment theory and adherence to treatment in diabetes. *Am J Psychiatry* 2001;**158**:29–35.

90. Feeney J, Ryan S. Attachment style and affect regulation: relationships with health behavior and family experiences in illness in a student sample. *Health Psychol* 1994;**13**:334–345.

91. Dozier M. Attachment organization and treatment use for adults with serious psychopathological disorders. *Dev Psychopathol* 1990;**2**:47–60.

92. Schuengel C, Bakermans-Kranenburg M, van IJzendoorn, MDH, Blom M. Unresolved loss and infant disorganization: links to frightening maternal behavior. In: Solomon J, George C (eds) *Attachment Disorganization*. New York, NY: Guilford Press, 1999.

17

The Eating Disorders

Randy A. Sansone, Lori A. Sansone

Introduction

It is not known when the first cases of eating disorders initially emerged in human history. However, it is evident that these disorders have firmly asserted their clinical presence in modern times. In this chapter, we review the epidemiology, etiology, diagnosis, treatment, and outcome of these complex disorders. In synthesizing this material, we note that the eating disorders truly underscore the relevance of a biopsychosocial perspective in the evaluation and treatment of psychiatric disorders.

Epidemiology

Prevalence Rates

Over the past 50 years, the prevalence of eating disorders has dramatically increased. In a review of the literature, Hoek and van Hoeken [1] concluded that the average prevalence rate for anorexia nervosa (AN) and bulimia nervosa (BN) in young women is around 0.3% and 1%, respectively. Other researchers indicate that prevalence rates for AN vary between 0.5% and 1%, with subclinical cases accounting for up to 3.7% [2, 3], while prevalence rates for BN are between 1.1% and 4.2% [4]. Eating disorders appear to be more prevalent in industrialized and/or affluent countries, therefore rates vary dramatically across the globe.

Age of Onset

Most individuals begin to experience eating disorder symptoms between the ages of 12 and 35 years. For AN, the mean age of onset is 17 years, with infrequent inception after the age of 40. In our experience, late-onset cases of AN *can* occur and are oftentimes accompanied by paralleling psychosocial delays in development (i.e., the developmental position of the individual essentially conforms with the onset of adolescence, but not with their chronological age). Likewise, BN typically begins in either late adolescence or early adulthood [5].

Gender Distribution

Eating disorders occur more frequently in women than in men. Male-to-female ratios vary between 1 : 6 and 1 : 10. While there appear to be no distinct differences in the diagnostic approach of clinicians to males versus females [6], in our experience, males with eating disorders invariably suffer from obsessive-compulsive personality features, premorbid overweight/obesity, weight pressures related to lean body sports, and/or gender identity issues. BN in males may be under-recognized due to both gender patterns of mental health care utilization as well as social stigma.

Racial Distribution

Caucasian women have historically been over-represented among individuals with eating disorders and this trend appears to be continuing [7]. However, non-Caucasian women are also affected by these disorders [8], with some data suggesting that ethnic minorities may experience greater difficulties in accessing treatment [9].

Socioeconomic Profiles

The traditional perspective – that eating disordered individuals tend to come from middle to upper socioeconomic classes – is controversial. Some studies confirm this impression [10], while others do not [11, 12]. It may be that those who present for treatment have the requisite financial resources, in effect influencing the conclusions of these types of studies.

Clinical Child Psychiatry, Third Edition. Edited by William M. Klykylo and Jerald Kay.
© 2012 John Wiley & Sons, Ltd. Published 2012 by John Wiley & Sons, Ltd.

Sports and Professional Influences

Eating disorders appear to be more frequent among elite performers in specific types of sports and professions (e.g., gymnasts, ballet dancers). This same relationship exists among non-elite performers as well, particularly in fields that emphasize thinness or muscularity [13]. Eating disorders also occur at higher rates among occupations or professions that require a specific weight status for initial or continued employment (e.g., historically, flight attendants, the military, dancers).

Association with Medical Disorders

Eating disorders may be more prevalent in particular medical disorders, such as diabetes mellitus. For example, the prevalence of eating disorders among individuals with type 1 diabetes is twice that of their nondiabetic peers [14]. This particular comorbidity is associated with an increased risk of diabetic retinopathy [14], which suggests that the medical management of diabetes in individuals with eating disorders may be extremely challenging.

Etiology

Rather than a specific cause, eating disorders appear to be *multi-determined* and probably result from the complex intersection of a variety of contributory variables. In our experience, these biopsychosocial variables vary from case to case.

Genetic Factors

Genetics appear to influence the development of eating disorders, and several studies clearly indicate that eating pathology is more prevalent in the family members of probands (e.g., the first-degree relatives of individuals with either AN [3, 15] or BN [16] have higher rates of eating disorders). In addition, monozygotic twins demonstrate a higher concordance rate for eating disorders compared with dizygotic twins (approximately 50% vs 14%) [17, 18]. Overall, the empirically determined heritability of these disorders may be as high as 80% [19, 20].

What exactly is being genetically transmitted through generational lines remains unclear. It is likely that particular temperaments or personality traits (e.g., perfectionism) confer a nonspecific susceptibility. It also appears that specific types of psychiatric disorders (i.e., affective disorders, substance abuse [15, 21, 22]) as well as obsessive-compulsive spectrum disorders [23] and perfectionistic personality traits [24] are more common among the family members of those with eating disorders, suggesting genetic associations.

Neurohormonal Factors

While a variety of neurohormonal abnormalities have been confirmed among those with eating disorders, these generally appear to be secondary to the effects of nutritional deficits or starvation, rather than genuinely causal or etiological in nature. Examples of these secondary abnormalities include changes in luteinizing hormone, follicle-stimulating hormone, cortisol, and peptides as well as abnormal opioid and catecholamine metabolism. These biological changes typically normalize with weight restoration.

One causal neurohormonal possibility may be brain-derived neurotrophic factor (BDNF). Alterations in this neural factor appear to confer a susceptibility to restricting AN [25]. Specifically, researchers [25] have determined an association between restricting AN and the Met allele of the Val66Met BDNF.

The Self-Perpetuating Starvation State

The starvation state itself may initiate or perpetuate some of the symptoms found in eating disordered individuals. As examples, experimental starvation of normal volunteers resulted in food preoccupation, dysphoria, food hoarding, abnormal taste preferences, binge eating, and compulsive behaviors [26]. These findings suggest that starvation may be the impetus for several notable eating disorder symptoms. In addition, we have encountered several cases where initial unintentional weight loss due to medical illness or surgery precipitated eating pathology.

Family Factors

A variety of family factors have been associated with the development of eating disorders. In a study of infants, those with feeding problems tended to have mothers with eating disorders; these mothers demonstrated mealtime disorganization as well as strong controlling behaviors [27]. A parental marital status other than married may also confer risk [28]. Parent-child enmeshment (i.e., overinvolvement to the point where it is difficult to distinguish between the needs of the parent versus the wishes of the child) may ultimately set the stage for identity struggles, wherein the eating disorder functions as the vehicle for differentiation/individuation.

Other family factors may include impaired or poor communication within the family, conflict avoidance, strongly negative emotions within the family, boundary violations manifesting as physical or sexual abuse, and/or the excessive use of food as a soother or mood manager. Family preoccupation with food, body, and weight issues as well as dieting, exercise, and "health" preoccupation may also create an environment of risk in addition to having a parent with an eating disorder. However, according to a position paper by the Academy for Eating Disorders, "...[while] family factors can play a role in the genesis and maintenance of eating disorders, current knowledge refutes the idea that they are either the exclusive or even the primary mechanisms that underlie risk [29]."

Psychological Factors

Both obsessive-compulsive personality traits and perfectionism have long been associated with the development of eating disorders [30, 31]. In addition, Gowers and Shore [32] underscore the importance of poor impulse control and fears of losing control. To coalesce both perspectives, Favaro and Santonastaso [33] describe the coexistence of both impulsivity and compulsivity in individuals with eating disorders. Depression may be a mediating factor in the evolution of an eating disorder, particularly in terms of a susceptibility to media and peer influences [34].

Psychodynamic Factors

The psychodynamic value of an eating disorder, or the adaptive context, presumes that symptoms result in some potential benefit to the individual. These psychological benefits vary from individual to individual. As examples, severe weight loss may function to disable the individual to the point of a developmental arrest, thereby containing underlying fears about meeting the demands of an adult role, which may be perceived as overwhelming. Weight loss may also be seen as a means of securing popularity or social acceptability (i.e., thinner is better), resolving one's imperfections, engaging a significant other, refocusing parents from marital or other family problems to the afflicted individual, and/or achieving a sense of empowerment or control in situations or with life stressors that leave the individual feeling impotent. Sadly, at times, severe weight loss may also function to make one less sexually attractive to a sexual perpetrator.

Among those with comorbid borderline personality disorder, eating disorder symptoms may be viewed as functioning in two general ways: (i) to resolve food/body/weight issues, and (ii) to self-injure (i.e., a self-injury equivalent) in the same manner as other self-destructive behaviors. The functions of self-injury in these cases may include the regulation of overwhelming affects, consolidation of a self-destructive identity, engagement of others, displacement of anger from others to self, and/or a means to reorganize oneself from a transient psychotic episode [35]. According to Linehan [36], the primary function of such behavior is affect regulation or control.

Sociocultural Factors

As the bodyweights of citizens increase, thinness becomes increasingly rare and valued within a society. At least this appears to be the case in westernized societies. In westernized cultures, the influences connecting thinness with success are routinely reflected in the fashion and beauty industry as well as in the media. The cultural message for success appears to be less on personal development and education, and more on external body appearance. Given the inexperience and naïveté of adolescents, these cultural messages may be very profoundly and concretely incorporated. Interestingly, one group of investigators determined that while BN is a culture-bound syndrome, AN is not [37]; in keeping with these data, compared with AN, heritability estimates for BN show greater variability across cultures.

Negative Life Events

Whether negative life events actually cause an eating disorder, or act as a psychological trigger for pre-established factors, is unknown. However, the McKnight investigators [38] found that an increase in negative life events predicted the onset of eating disorders in a large sample of adolescent girls in grades 6 through 9. Negative life events may include appearance-based teasing [39]; trauma akin to that encountered in post-traumatic stress disorder [40], including sexual abuse; [41] and maladaptive paternal behavior [42]. The permutations of negative life events are probably endless.

Summary of Etiological Possibilities

To summarize, the risk for (or protection against) the development of eating disorders resides in several domains – biological, psychological, and social [43]. These variables seem to aggregate in specific developmental phases and likely interact with each other to ultimately result in symptoms. Eating disorders truly appear to be multi-determined disorders, with antecedent risk factors varying from case to case.

Diagnosis

Anorexia Nervosa

According to the *Diagnostic and Statistical Manual of Mental Disorders, Fourth Edition, Text Revision* (DSM-IV-TR) [5], the criteria for the diagnosis of AN include all of the following:

(1) refusal to maintain a minimally normal bodyweight for age and height (i.e., a bodyweight less than 85% of that expected);
(2) an intense fear of gaining weight or becoming fat despite subnormal weight status;
(3) disturbances in the perception or meaning of one's bodyweight or shape (e.g., excessive self-evaluation based upon weight or shape, denial of the seriousness of the current subnormal weight); and
(4) amenorrhea for at least 3 months.

Anorexia nervosa is subclassified into two types:

(1) restricting type, which is characterized by predominantly restrictive eating behavior (i.e., no binging or purging); or
(2) binge-eating/purging type, which is characterized by routine binge-eating episodes followed by purging behavior.

Adjunctive symptoms are noted in Table 17.1. In formulating the diagnosis of AN, significant weight loss, a consistent epidemiological context, and historical evidence of dieting behavior are essential.

Axis I Comorbidity

The starvation state encountered in AN tends to mimic many of the signs and symptoms of depression (e.g., insomnia, irritability, fatigue, dysphoria, psychomotor slowing, social withdrawal). Many of these ameliorate or resolve with weight restoration. Therefore, an accurate assessment for depression is probably most feasible when the patient is within 10% of a normal weight for height.

Starvation can also tend to intensify obsessive thinking and compulsive behavior. Weight restoration tends to improve these symptoms as well, although genuine obsessive-compulsive disorder may be present.

As for other types of symptoms, when Milos and colleagues [44] examined the Axis I and II diagnoses in a mixed sample of women with eating disorders, they found that about 50% suffered from anxiety disorders and affective disorders. Only 17% had no psychiatric comorbidity. In addition to the preceding comorbidities, substance use disorders are not uncommon, particularly among patients with binge-eating/purging behavior [45].

Axis II Comorbidity

Through a review of the literature, we determined that the most frequent personality disorder among individuals with restricting type AN is obsessive-compulsive personality disorder (about 22%). This is followed by avoidant personality disorder (about 19%), borderline or dependent personality disorders (around 10%), and Cluster A (i.e., the odd cluster) personality disorders (approximately 5%) [46]. Overall, Cluster C personality disorders (i.e., the anxious cluster) appear most predominant among this diagnostic group. The relationship between restrictive AN and obsessive-compulsive personality appears intuitive, given the high levels of restraint and control required to systematically starve oneself.

In those patients suffering from AN, binge-eating/purging type, the most frequent Axis II disorder is borderline personality disorder (25%), followed by avoidant or dependent personality disorders (about 15%), and histrionic personality disorder (10%) [46]. Thus,

Table 17.1 Adjunctive symptoms and behaviors in anorexia nervosa.

Intense drive for thinness	Relentless body preoccupation
Frequent weighings	Mirror gazing to scrutinize shape
Drive to attain smaller clothing sizes	Anxiety with food ingestion
Fears of becoming fat	Intense scrutiny of "fat" body areas
Preoccupation with food	Recurrent dreams about food
Cooking for others	Food hoarding
Food-centered conversation	Attempts to conceal weight loss
Denial of weight loss	Slow eating at meals
Rituals with eating	Body size mis-estimation
Irritability	Insomnia
Worry and obsessive thinking	Anxiety
Sexual disinterest	Depression
Light-headedness	Constipation
Amenorrhea	Thin, dry, brittle hair
Low body temperature	Dry skin
Increased body hair (lanugo)	

among anorexic individuals with binge-eating/purging symptoms, both Cluster B (i.e., the dramatic impulsive cluster) and Cluster C personality disorders appear predominant, with borderline personality clearly being the most common personality disorder. The relationship between binge-eating and purging echoes the self-regulation difficulties and impulsive behaviors encountered in borderline personality disorder.

Bulimia Nervosa

According to DSM-IV-TR [5], the criteria for BN are:

(1) recurrent episodes of binge eating (i.e., the consumption, within a discrete time period of usually less than 2 hours, of a large amount of food in a fashion that is perceived as out of control);
(2) recurrent compensatory behaviors (e.g., self-induced vomiting; the use of laxatives, diuretics, enemas, medication, fasting, and/or excessive exercise) to prevent weight gain;
(3) episode frequency of twice per week for at least 3 months; and
(4) self-evaluation that is unduly influenced by body shape or weight.

The eating pathology cannot occur exclusively during times of AN (otherwise, the diagnosis would be AN, binge-eating/purging type).

Bulimia nervosa is classified as:

(1) purging type (calorie eradication by vomiting, laxatives, diuretics, and/or enemas); or
(2) non-purging type (prevention of weight gain via fasting or excessive exercise).

Surprisingly, the exact parameters of a binge are yet to be defined, making the differentiation between overeating and binge eating somewhat clinically challenging. We assign binge status based upon the ingestion, in a single sitting, of $2^1/_2$ times the normal amount of food (i.e., about 2500 calories).

Adjunctive symptoms and behaviors in BN may relate to either the collection of voluminous amounts of food (e.g., high expenditures for food at the grocery store, excessive use of dormitory food cards, food hoarding), the need for social isolation to undertake a binge (e.g., calculated prompt departures after meals with others), and/or the remnants of purging (e.g., evidence of vomiting in the bathroom). Additional behaviors may include the excessive ingestion of high-calorie foods in a single sitting, the bagging and storage of vomitus, stealing of food from others, shoplifting food, and discarding remnants of associated weight-loss products (e.g., over-the-counter diet pills, laxatives, metabolic boosters) in

trash cans. In addition, according to one study, slightly over one-third of adolescents with eating disorders use herbal products; [47] not surprisingly, about one-third of these herbal users choose products to either decrease their appetites or induce vomiting.

Axis I Comorbidity

Common Axis I disorders in individuals with BN include mood (e.g., major depression, dysthymia), anxiety, and substance use disorders [48–50]. In turn, females with substance abuse appear to have relatively high rates of eating disorders (up to 25%) [51], with the majority suffering from BN (nearly two-thirds).

Axis II Comorbidity

In comparison with other types of eating disorders, including binge eating disorder, BN is the most studied with regard to Axis II comorbidity. According to our review of the literature [46], borderline personality disorder is the most frequent Axis II disorder (28%), followed by dependent and histrionic personality disorders (20%) [46]. Thus, the Cluster profile for BN in studies is predominantly Cluster B followed, to a lesser degree, by Cluster C.

Eating Disorder, Not Otherwise Specified

Individuals who have eating pathology but do not meet the criteria for AN or BN are diagnosed as eating disorder not otherwise specified. Examples might include variations of AN or BN (e.g., weight loss of more than 15%, but amenorrhea of less than 3 months duration; binge-purge frequencies of less than twice per week in a normal-weight individual). These oftentimes represent partial or subthreshold disorders that may either progress to full-syndrome disorders or recede spontaneously following brief intervention.

In addition to variations of AN and BN, this category presently includes binge eating disorder (see this topic later in the chapter), as well as other types of eating disorders, including night eating syndrome and purging disorder (i.e., purging without binging behavior in a normal-weight individual [52]) [53]. How this category will fare with the unfolding of DSM-V is currently unknown, but many of these disorders are as severe as the classic AN and BN [53].

The Eating Disorder Assessment

Adjunctive Assessment Measures

A number of tools are available for the assessment of eating disorders, and samples are shown in Table 17.2

Table 17.2 Assessment tools in eating disorders.

Assessment tool	First author	Description
Anorexia Nervosa Stages of Change Questionnaire	Rieger	20 items, self-report, Likert-style response options; measures readiness to change
Binge Eating Scale	Gormally	16 items, self-report, Likert-style response options; measures binge eating/purging
BULIT-R (Bulimia Test-Revised)	Thelen	39 items, self-report, Likert-style response options; measures binge eating/purging
Child Version of the Eating Disorder Examination	Bryant-Waugh	Semi-structured interview; child-adapted version of the Eating Disorders Examination
Disordered Eating Attitude Scale	Alvarenga	25 items, self-report, Likert-style response options; measures disordered eating attitudes
EAT-26 (Eating Attitudes Test-26)	Garner	26 items, self-report, Likert-style response options; measures general eating pathology
Eating Disorder Diagnostic Scale	Stice	22 items, self-report, various response formats; measures general eating pathology
Eating Disorder Examination	Fairburn	Semi-structured interview, graded responses (0–6); measures eating pathology over the past 28 days
Eating Disorders Inventory-2	Garner	91 items, self-report, Likert-style response options; measures general eating pathology
Eating Disorder Symptom Severity Scale	Henderson	Clinician-administered, 16 items; measures eating disorder behaviors, cognitions and anxiety, and treatment progress
McKnight Risk Factors Survey	Shisslak	103 items, self-report, various response formats; measures eating pathology, depression, perfectionism, risk/protection factors
Revised Restraint Scale	Herman	10 items, self-report, various response formats; measures restrained eating/dieting behavior
SCOFF Questionnaire	Morgan	5 items, self-report, yes/no responses; screening tool for eating disorders
The Binge Scale	Hawkins	19 items, self-report, Likert-style response options; measures binge eating/purging
The Change in Eating Disorder Symptoms Scale	Spangler	35-items, self-report, Likert-style response options; measures body preoccupation, body dissatisfaction, body checking, binge eating, restrictive eating, eating/food preoccupation, vomiting
Yale-Brown-Cornell Eating Disorder Scale	Mazure	82 items, semi-structured interview; measures general eating pathology and rituals

These instruments may be utilized as adjunctive tools to the DSM diagnostic criteria.

Laboratory Studies

As for laboratory studies, electrolytes, blood urea nitrogen (BUN), creatinine, thyroid assessment, and urinalysis should be considered in all patients [54]. For severely symptomatic or malnourished patients, additional laboratory studies might include calcium, magnesium, and phosphorus levels as well as liver function tests and an electrocardiogram [54]. In surreptitious cases of BN, the ratio of urine sodium to urine chloride is a reasonably good predictor, with ratios greater than 1:16 identifying 52% of cases [55]. Finally, an assessment for osteopenia using dual-energy X-ray absorptiometry (DEXA) should be considered in very-low-weight patients who have been symptomatic for 6–12 months or longer [54].

Medical Complications

The medical complications encountered in individuals with eating disorders typically relate to either starvation effects or the methods of purgation. These are summarized in Table 17.3 [56] In addition, Figure 17.1 illustrates lanugo, a fine downy body hair that emerges with

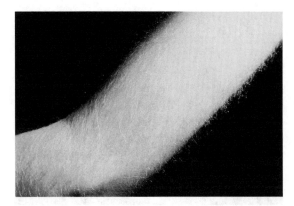

Figure 17.1 Lanugo in a patient with anorexia nervosa.

starvation. Figure 17.2 illustrates dental erosion (peri-mylolysis). In this figure, note that the upper front teeth show marked erosion due to their exposure to gastric acid during vomiting, while the lower teeth remain protected by the tongue. Figure 17.3 illustrates parotid gland enlargement, which occurs in some, but not all patients. The enlargement is typically bilateral, occurs with daily and multiple bouts of vomiting, and recedes with the cessation of vomiting. Although not invariably present in all patients who vomit, when present, this finding indicates that vomiting is usually occurring several times per day. Finally, Figure 17.4 illustrates Russell's sign, which is the roughened and calloused skin on the dorsal aspect of the hand due to its repeated impact on the front teeth during gag induction.

Table 17.3 Potential medical complications in eating disorders according to eating-disorder pathology.

Starvation	Self-induced vomiting	Laxative abuse	Diuretic abuse
Emaciation	Hoarseness Dental erosion	Acute-use discomfort:	Dehydration
Muscular wasting	↑ parotid/submandibular glands	abdominal pain	Light-headedness
Anemia	Aspiration	nausea	Tachycardia
Leukopenia	Pharyngeal/esophageal irritation	vomiting	Delirium
Thrombocytopenia	Esophageal/gastric tears	diarrhea	Seizures
↓ erythrocyte sedimentation rate	Hypokalemia	cramping	Cardiac arrhythmias
Impaired cell immunity	Hypochloremia	distention	Renal failure
Hypercholesterolemia		bloating	
Hypocalcemia		Laxative dependence	
Hypophosphatemia		Steatorrhea	
Hypokalemia		Protein-losing enteropathy	
Hypercortisolemia		Cathartic colon	
Hypoglycemia		Fixed drug eruptions (phenolphthalein)	
↑ growth hormone		Melanosis coli (senna, cascara)	
↓ estrogen			
↓ basal luteinizing hormone			
↓ basal follicle-stimulating hormone			
↑ liver enzymes			
↑ amylase			
Bradycardia			
Orthostatic hypotension			
Mitral valve motion abnormalities			
↓ cardiac index			
↓ left ventricular chamber size			
Systolic dysfunction			

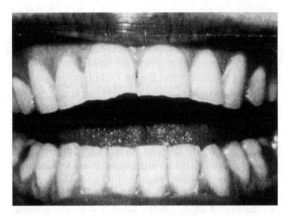

Figure 17.2   Dental erosion (perimylolysis) – a potential complication of self-induced vomiting. Stege P, Visco-Dangler, Rye L: Anorexia nervosa: Review including oral and dental manifestations. *JADA* 1982; **104** (**5**):648–652. © 1982 American Dental Association. All rights reserved. Reproduced by permission.

Several additional aspects of medical complications are worth noting. First, with multiple methods of purgation (e.g., vomiting, laxative abuse, diuretics), serum potassium losses may intensify. Acute potassium losses may cause seizures and cardiac arrhythmias whereas longstanding hypokalemia may result in kidney damage (i.e., hypokalemic nephropathy).

Second, prolonged amenorrhea due to malnutrition and starvation may result in osteoporosis in adulthood. Even with full weight recovery, bone mineral density among former anorexic individuals appears to be reduced relative to peers [57]. Treatment may entail consultation with a specialist, such as a pediatric endocrinologist or rheumatologist.

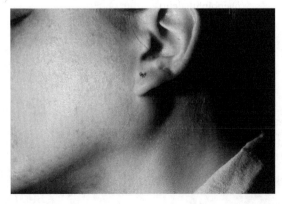

Figure 17.3   Parotid gland enlargement secondary to self-induced vomiting.

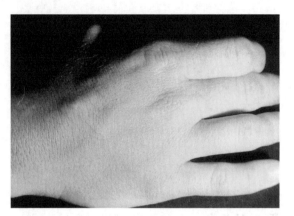

Figure 17.4   Roughened, calloused area on the dorsum of the gag-induction hand (Russell's sign).

Finally, compared with other psychiatric disorders, eating disorders carry a relatively high mortality rate [58]. In AN, mortality is related to the subsequent wasting of the myocardium and cardiac dysfunction. The crude mortality rate is approximately 6% [59]. The mortality rate for bulimia nervosa appears to be considerably less at 0.3% [60], and may be related to electrolyte disturbances (e.g., acute hypokalemia).

Treatment

Anorexia Nervosa

Treatment Engagement

At the outset of treatment, it can be very difficult to emotionally engage patients with AN. These patients seem to have genuine difficulty in recognizing or acknowledging their plight because of the intense denial associated with this disorder, the inability to recognize the extent of weight loss (i.e., body-image distortion), and on occasion parents who may be reticent to acknowledge that their "perfect" child has a psychiatric problem. In our experience, the best approach to building a therapeutic alliance is to initially validate the patient's physical symptoms. For example, the clinician may empathically acknowledge that the patient may feel dysphoric, cold, isolated, anxious, fearful, exhausted, and overwhelmed. This type of validation helps to establish some level of interpersonal connection with the patient, and is oftentimes an important foundation upon which to build rapport and a deeper alliance with the patient.

For the patient, the initial treatment encounter is invariably very threatening. From the patient's perspective, the clinician is, in a very pragmatic way, attempting to undermine their arduous efforts at weight loss. So, the clinician can anticipate a high degree of patient resistance. Validating this reality (e.g., "it must seem like we, the treatment team, are trying to undermine the very goal that you have worked so hard at") can demystify this genuine dilemma on a verbal level with the patient.

Determination of the Treatment Environment

During the evaluation, the determination of the initial treatment environment is of the utmost importance. This determination is based upon several factors, including the amount of weight lost, the rapidity of the weight loss, how the weight loss was achieved, the age of the patient, physical symptoms or laboratory abnormalities, and, frankly, local treatment resources. In addition to height and weight measurements, initial laboratory studies should be completed to reveal any existing metabolic imbalances. The primary care physician may already have completed laboratory studies and an electrocardiogram, and these should be obtained, if possible, prior to the evaluation. Initial and ongoing weight data are essential, and all clinicians should have immediate access to a scale in their office settings.

For eating disorder disposition alone, the determination of the treatment environment is primarily based upon the percent of weight lost. For those individuals who are 75% or less of expected weight for height, inpatient treatment is indicated, and we strongly recommend a milieu-based eating disorder treatment program. For patients with moderate or minimal weight loss, outpatient intervention is recommended.

Medical hospitalization is indicated for patients with significant electrolyte disturbances and/or cardiac arrhythmias (e.g., severe bradycardia, junctional rhythm). In these general hospital settings, the primary care physician or specialist (e.g., cardiologist) typically manages the patient.

In designing an overall treatment strategy, comorbid psychiatric conditions (e.g., substance abuse) will need to be considered as well. Initial disposition may relate to the comorbidity rather than the eating disorder (e.g., suicidal ideation and psychiatric hospitalization).

Behavior Modification for Inpatient Weight Restoration

At some point, most clinicians will face the task of inpatient weight restoration in patients with AN. While various forms of behavior modification are used, we have had consistent success with the following general approach.

After inpatient admission, we collect daily weights (in the morning, after voiding and just before breakfast; standard garb) for 3 days and then average these weights to determine a "starting weight" on a weight graph.

From this starting weight, we draw a line on graph paper (i.e., the weight graph) that designates one-quarter pound (113 g) of weight gain per day. Beginning at 1200 calories per day (5 MJ) in six divided feedings, we then titrate the patient's daily calorie levels in 300-calorie (1.26-MJ) increments to maintain his/her weight on the anticipated weight-gain schedule according to the weight-gain line. This enables the treatment team to monitor the patient's momentum around weight gain as well as observe for excessive or rapid refeeding. (Rapid refeeding may result in *refeeding syndrome*, which is characterized by severe hypokalemia, hypophosphatemia, and possibly death.) During weight restoration, the decisions around food choices, liquid supplements versus solid food, and the number of feedings per day are all negotiated individually. Patient progress is reinforced with increasing activity levels. At times, to maintain momentum, patients may be given the choice of a 300-calorie increase or a decrease in activity level. In conjunction with behavioral modification for weight restoration, we prescribe a multiple vitamin as well as calcium supplements that contain vitamin D.

With some minor modifications, this same approach can be used for outpatients as well. Examples of modifications might be weekly weighings at sessions rather than daily weighings as in the inpatient setting, less robust expectations around weight gain, and more flexibility around the menu plan. Liquid supplements or prepackaged puddings (i.e., precise calorie management) may be successfully utilized in the outpatient setting, particularly at the outset of treatment, when control and trust issues are high.

Psychotherapy Treatment

As for the integration of psychotherapy treatment, we observe three phases. During the first phase of treatment, when the patient is in an acute starvation state, the ability to abstract well and relate to others is compromised. Because the initial focus of treatment is weight restoration, we recommend cognitive and educational approaches, validation, and rapport building as well as contracting and negotiating around eating, weight gain, and activity levels.

As weight increases, the next phase of psychotherapy treatment often centers on exploring the various contributory factors that resulted in the eating disorder. During this phase, the psychotherapy focus is somewhat more psychodynamic in nature, with the examination of personal, home, and peer factors. This phase may also entail body-image work, further nutritional education, family work, and continuing cognitive restructuring.

In the final phase of treatment, the psychotherapy focus is more relational – that is, facilitating reconnection with others. This phase entails developing and practicing skills in social relationships. The patient may require specific interventions such as assertiveness training, dealing with the opposite sex, expressing emotional needs with others, resolving boundary issues, and sorting out compliance versus autonomy in relationships with others.

Because of the multi-determined nature of eating disorders, additional therapies may be chosen, based upon individual need. For example, all patients should receive educational intervention around nutritional issues, and almost all young adolescents will benefit from family therapy. When integrated into treatment, family members and significant others benefit from understanding their reactions to the disorder as well as rethinking their responses. In particular cases, specific skills training may be necessary such as relaxation and mindfulness training. Victims of abuse may benefit from trauma work. Because many patients with AN are young adolescents, developmental issues (i.e., separation/individuation, dating, peer relationships) as well as academic issues will need to be addressed in the treatment. For married patients, couples therapy may be indicated to address underlying marital conflicts.

Psychotropic Medications

During the acute phase of refeeding, psychotropic medications are not routinely recommended because they appear to have limited efficacy in low-weight states. Other concerns include the patient's greater susceptibility to side effects because of low bodyweight, the possible resolution of some mood and anxiety symptoms with weight restoration alone (e.g., depressive symptoms, obsessive thinking), and the patient's fear that the medication is intended as a weight-gain ploy by the treatment team.

Some studies have shown enhanced weight gain during weight restoration with particular medications for which weight gain is an anticipated side effect, such as olanzapine (Zyprexa). We have intentionally avoided these medications because of their inability to resolve the underlying psychological issues and the inability to effectively strategize an acceptable weight outcome. In other words, while these medications stimulate weight gain, it is not possible to predict how much weight will eventually be gained. In addition, there is currently insufficient evidence to confirm that atypical antipsychotics enhance weight gain in these circumstances [61].

Given the preceding advice about medication in low-weight patients with AN, we offer possible exceptions.

Some patients with severe obsessive-compulsive disorder are probably not disadvantaged by early intervention with a selective serotonin reuptake inhibitor (SSRI). The potential side-effect risks of this class of antidepressants are low and the potential benefits are high. Severe obsessive-compulsive symptoms that directly relate to food and weight issues (e.g., touching food is perceived as contamination) may so drastically impede a treatment that early intervention with medication is reasonable. There are also other clinical exceptions where early medication intervention is indicated (e.g., psychosis).

With regard to any medication intervention in low-weight patients, we strongly recommend small initial doses of medication with slow titration, as well as a credible discussion with the patient about the known weight effects of a prescribed medication. Among psychiatric patients in general, it is well known that many psychotropic medications cause weight gain, and such suspicions by the patient are well founded.

Following weight restoration to within 10% of a normal or previous body weight, we routinely consider medication intervention if adjunctive psychiatric symptoms persist (e.g., anxiety, depression). At the outset, we recommend SSRIs. This class of antidepressants has broad clinical efficacy (i.e., they are effective for various syndromes including depression, anxiety, panic, rumination, worry, obsessive-compulsive symptoms, posttraumatic stress disorder, impulsivity), which is particularly helpful in cases with complex psychiatric comorbidity. SSRIs also have tolerable side effects and reasonable safety in overdose with the possible exception of citalopram (Celexa), which may cause QT prolongation in overdose. In our experience, venlafaxine extended release (Effexor-XR) has also been useful, but has a more limited range of efficacy with regard to polysymptomatic patients. We avoid tricyclic antidepressants (TCAs) due to their cardiovascular effects, the risk of unpredictable weight gain, and potential lethality in overdose. Bupropion (Wellbutrin) is contraindicated in the treatment of eating disorders because of the heightened risk of seizures. Although there has been emerging concern about the risk of suicidal ideation in adolescents who are exposed to antidepressants and other types of psychotropic medications, we have infrequently encountered this dilemma in our work with patients with eating disorders.

Bulimia Nervosa

Compared with sufferers of AN, those with BN tend to establish an initial and easy rapport with the clinician. This observation may be related to these patients' later age at clinical presentation (i.e., greater developmental maturity), the type of eating disorder and associated personality features, higher levels of insight, and/or other related factors. So, typically at the initial evaluation, there is less resistance by the patient to dialoguing and participating in a treatment plan.

General Treatment Goals

While weight restoration is the initial focus in the treatment of AN, the normalization of eating patterns and the interruption of the binge/purge cycle are the initial goals in the treatment of BN. Given that the definition of "normalized eating patterns" is speculative, we recommend working towards 1800–2200 calories (7.5–9.2 MJ) per day, in four feedings (e.g., breakfast, lunch, dinner, snack).

When comorbid substance abuse is present, we generally recommend initial substance abuse treatment [62]. For patients with comorbid borderline personality disorder, we suggest initially focusing on self-regulation and self-harm behavior, and secondarily focusing on eating disorder issues [63].

Behavioral Strategies

A decisive majority of patients with BN can be managed in the outpatient setting. We initially have the patient keep a 1-week food record, then roughly estimate the daily calorie levels and establish an initial menu plan. We gradually advance the daily calorie levels by 300-calorie (1.26-MJ) increments to goal levels and simultaneously monitor weight status, either formally or informally (patient self-report). We strongly believe that a functional calorie deficit is a major contributory factor to binge eating.

With regard to further interrupting binge/purge behavior, we contract for reductions, explore and encourage alternative coping strategies, process behavior chains (i.e., explore thoughts, feelings, and behaviors before, during, and after each event), and examine the interpersonal costs of such behavior.

Psychotherapy Treatment

Various psychotherapy treatment strategies have been successfully used in BN. In this regard, Richards and colleagues [64] reviewed available treatment studies and concluded that there are substantially more studies in BN compared with AN. This seemingly adds some confidence to the empirical findings of treatment interventions in BN. However, the authors caution that the treatments in these studies may well be the result of *treatment default* (i.e., using only techniques confirmed by limited studies) rather than an inherent superiority of such treatments over other types of treatments.

Given the preceding caveat, it is evident that cognitive behavioral therapy is the most studied and empirically supported treatment approach for BN [64], particularly a recently enhanced version [65]. Interpersonal psychotherapy has also demonstrated efficacy in the treatment of BN. As in the treatment of AN, other types of therapies may be integrated into treatment, depending on individual needs. Psychodynamic psychotherapy may be incorporated into treatment, particularly in an effort to understand how earlier developmental issues are manifesting in adulthood. Acute problem-solving approaches are helpful for emergent issues. Family therapy may be useful in helping members to understand their reactions to the patient's symptoms as well as how to intervene in less stressful ways. Family issues may include dealing with blame and guilt, tightening family boundaries, developing healthier responses to patient behaviors, and adjusting the expectations of parents and/or significant others. For some older adolescents with highly dysfunctional families, therapeutic emancipation may be in order. Couples therapy or marital therapy may be extremely helpful, if only to develop ways for the couple to communicate neutrally about symptomatic behaviors, actively dialogue home and outside stressors, and work towards healthier ways to deal with negative emotions and feelings. In addition, partners can function as ongoing, full-time home coaches for patients, when feasible.

These preceding interventions may be undertaken in individual or group settings, including interpersonal psychotherapy [66]. Group treatments offer an efficient and economical means of delivering information and treatment strategies to a number of patients, although many patients benefit from the psychological intimacy of an individual treatment.

In addition, support groups are available in many areas and are typically open to new participants. Many have group facilitators who are either patients in partial or full recovery, or treatment professionals. These groups vary in philosophy, structure, clinical themes, and their individual screening processes. Rice and Faulkner outline the benefits and risks of such groups [67].

Novel interventions are also emerging for the treatment of eating disorders. These include motivational enhancement therapy, which was developed in the context of addictive disorders; dialectical behavior therapy, which was developed for the treatment of self-harm behavior in borderline personality; and manualized family therapy [68]. Like all newer treatments, their efficacy and patient-selection criteria are not explicitly known.

Technology is also augmenting our therapeutic armamentarium. For example, in small practices or practices with few eating disorder patients, the clinician may link patients together into a "support group" via the internet [69]. In addition, laptop computers may be effective as "therapy extension devices." [70] Finally, Taylor and colleagues [71] discuss the role of web-based prevention programs as well as psychoeducation and online treatment and support groups for patients with eating disorders.

Psychotropic Medications

Antidepressant medications appear to consistently reduce the frequency of binging and purging, regardless of the presence or not of depression. In our experience, antidepressant therapy initially results in a 50% or better reduction in eating disorder symptomatology, but complete amelioration of symptoms is rare in the clinical setting. Various types of antidepressants have been used including SSRIs, TCAs, monoamine oxidase inhibitors, and serotonin-norepinephrine reuptake inhibitors. As in AN, SSRIs are typically an initial starting place because of their mild side-effect profiles, positive safety records, and unique effects on rumination, worry, and impulsivity. In BN, higher-than-standard doses may be considered. Fluoxetine (Prozac) is the only antidepressant officially indicated by the US Food and Drug Administration (FDA) for the treatment of BN, although all of the SSRIs are effective.

As in AN, we avoid TCAs in individuals with BN. These antidepressants have significant side effects including weight gain and cardiovascular effects. The latter potential side effects are particularly problematic in patients with dehydration due to vomiting, laxatives, or diuretics. As noted earlier, TCAs are relatively lethal in overdose.

Monoamine oxidase inhibitors are risky interventions in patients with BN because of their potential to interact with various foods and drugs, causing acute hypertension and possibly cerebrovascular accidents. This risk is particularly heightened in the indiscriminant binge eater or the patient with borderline personality characteristics who engages in self-harm behavior through exposure to contraband food and drugs. For both AN and BN, the only contraindicated antidepressant is bupropion (Wellbutrin) because of the heightened risk of seizures.

Other types of medications have been helpful in the treatment of BN, including anticonvulsants and psychostimulants. However, these drugs have less empirical support, may be more complicated to use (e.g., laboratory studies and serum levels with anticonvulsants), and may be potentially hazardous in those patients prone to substance abuse (e.g., the abuse of psychostimulants).

In cases of psychiatric comorbidity, the corresponding psychotropic medication would be indicated (e.g., antipsychotics, lithium). However, the weight effects of individual drugs may pose more problems for those with eating disorders than the general psychiatric patient.

Outcome

Complexities of Outcome Assessment

It is genuinely difficult to draw conclusions about the treatment outcome of patients with eating disorders. As expected, outcomes markedly differ because the available studies vary in population types and methodologies (e.g., different ages of participants, levels of care, treatment settings, levels of psychiatric comorbidity and medical debility, treatment interventions). In addition, there is controversy regarding what constitutes remission versus recovery, and how to measure it.

Four general approaches for assessing treatment outcome have been proposed by Anderson and Williamson: [72] (i) structured interviews; (ii) self-report inventories; (iii) body mass indices or weights; and (iv) the use of test meals to assess comfort with eating. In pragmatic terms, the possibilities for outcome variables seem endless and may include the weight and nutritional status of the patient, level of eating difficulties, preoccupation with bodyweight, persistence of eating disorder symptoms, overall growth and physical development, menstrual functioning, mental state, psychosexual adjustment, psychosocial functioning, and mortality [73].

In an effort to promote a consistent approach to outcome measurement, researchers have developed a brief, self-report inventory, the Multifactorial Assessment of Eating Disorder Symptoms (MAEDS) [74]. The MAEDS assesses six symptom clusters: depression, binge eating, purging behavior, fears of fatness, restrictive eating, and the avoidance of forbidden foods. Only broader use will determine the viability and acceptability among clinicians and patients of this outcome measure, and other measures (e.g., the Eating Disorder Symptom Severity Scale).

Outcome of Eating Disorder Symptoms

One statistic that seems to echo throughout the outcome literature is that about one-third of eating-disorder patients experience a poor outcome. In support of this impression, Herzog and colleagues [75] found that at 90 months of follow-up, nearly one-third of patients relapsed. Keel [76] reported that 10–15 years after presentation for treatment, around 29% of those with BN still retained an eating disorder diagnosis. Herpertz-Dahlmann and colleagues [77] examined the 10-year outcome of adolescents with AN and determined that 31% had not fully recovered; there was a significant association between poor outcome and psychiatric co-morbidity. Steinhausen and colleagues [78] reported that after more than 6 years of follow-up, 30% of patients were unrecovered. In a 5-year outcome study, Ben-Tovim and colleagues [79] found that 32% of a mixed sample of patients still had a diagnosable eating disorder. Nakai and colleagues [80] found that in 4- to 10-year follow-up, 26–30% of patients either did not recover or died. Steinhausen and Weber examined 79 studies and found that 23% of participants had a chronic and contracted course [81]. Finally, Keel and Brown examined 26 recent outcome studies and concluded that 30% of individuals with BN remain ill up to 20 years following presentation [82]. Again, the recurring statistic appears to be that about one-third of eating disorder patients experience poor long-term outcomes. Conversely, these data indicate that nearly two-thirds of eating-disorder patients achieve partial or full remission, given time.

Whether poor outcome relates to Axis I or II comorbidity, severity of initial symptoms, history of abuse, age-of-onset, and/or other variables is unknown. However, males may fare better than females [83], borderline personality may predict diminished global functioning in follow-up [84], and severity of alcohol use may predict mortality in AN [85].

Fertility and Pregnancy Outcome

Another aspect of outcome is fertility among women with active eating disorders. Crow and colleagues [86] found that although menstrual irregularities were common among women with BN, there was little impact on patients' ability to achieve a pregnancy. Franko and colleagues [87] examined pregnancy complications and neonatal outcomes. While the majority of women had normal pregnancies, 6% had babies with birth defects. In this prospective study, over one-third of the women experienced postpartum depression, and there was also a higher frequency of cesarean section at delivery. On a side note, Carter and colleagues [88] found that pregnancy did not result in increased eating disorder symptomatology, which is relevant given the dramatic and acute increase in a patient's body size. Protecting the child from the ravages of an eating disorder may be a protective factor for the mother, as well.

Mortality

The crude mortality rates for AN and BN were noted earlier in this chapter. However, rates vary depending on the approach to analysis. For example, Crow and colleagues determined crude mortality rates for AN and BN at 4.0% and 3.9%, respectively [89]. It is important to be aware that, in addition to succumbing to the physical devastation of eating disorders, a number of individuals surrender to the emotional devastation through suicide. In support of this, AN is empirically associated with a heightened risk of suicide [90]. Again, the variables that contribute to this risk are unknown.

Binge Eating Disorder

Before closing this chapter, we would like to briefly review Binge Eating Disorder (BED), a provisional eating disorder in the DSM-IV-TR identified for additional study. Bunnell [91] and Walsh et al [92]. provide excellent overviews of this disorder, which we now summarize.

Binge eating disorder is characterized by a recurrent pattern of binge eating that occurs at least twice a week for a minimum period of 6 months. Unlike BN, there is no compensatory behavior (i.e., vomiting, fasting, exercise) to counter these episodes of massive calorie ingestion. Therefore, many BED patients are overweight although weight status, per se, is not a diagnostic criterion. The clinical characteristics of the binge eating behavior are like those encountered in BN; however, women with BED may eat at a normal rate.

The prevalence rate for BED in the community is up to 5%, in weight loss clinics up to 30%, and in those with body mass indices ≥40 up to 50%. These prevalence data indicate that BED is the most common eating disorder. Unlike the preceding eating disorders, a substantial number of males are affected, with the female-to-male ratio being 3:2. The age of onset is typically during the late teens to early 20s, the ethnicity of the patient population is quite diverse, and the age of presentation for treatment (i.e., 30 to 40 years) is later than that encountered in AN or BN. Comorbid diabetes occurs in up to 25% of patients with BED.

As in BN, many different types of treatment have been used including cognitive behavioral therapy, interpersonal psychotherapy, weight loss programs, and self-help treatments. Various medications are also being explored including SSRIs, anti-obesity drugs, and topiramate (Topamax). Surprisingly, the elimination of binging does not necessarily result in weight loss.

This diagnostic category remains under investigation, but may attain an independent status in the upcoming DSM edition.

Conclusions

Eating disorders are the epitome of the biopsychosocial model of assessment and intervention. They are multi-determined disorders with both psychological and medical sequelae, and they require creative and diverse therapeutic interventions. These disorders continue to be challenging for clinicians, with nearly one-third of patients being refractory to treatment. Only additional research, clinician perseverance, and supportive funding will enable the professional community to better understand these complex and intriguing patients.

References

1. Hoek HW, van Hoeken D. Review of the prevalence and incidence of eating disorders. *Int J Eat Disord* 2003;**34**:383–396.
2. Garfinkel PE, Lin E, Goering P, *et al*. Should amenorrhoea be necessary for the diagnosis of anorexia nervosa? Evidence from a Canadian community sample. *Br J Psychiatry* 1996;**168**:500–506.
3. Walters EE, Kendler KS. Anorexia nervosa and anorexic-like syndromes in a population-based female twin sample. *Am J Psychiatry* 1995;**152**:64–71.
4. Garfinkel RE, Lin E, Goering P, *et al*. Bulimia nervosa in a Canadian community sample: Prevalence and comparison in subgroups. *Am J Psychiatry* 1995;**152**:1052–1058.
5. American Psychiatric Association. *Diagnostic and Statistical Manual of Mental Disorders*, 4th edn, Text Revision. Washington, DC: APA, 2000.
6. Grace GF. Contrasting anorexia nervosa in males cross-nationally in the United States, Canada, and Great Britain. *Diss Abstr Int, Section B* 2003;**64**:2387.
7. Striegel-Moore RH, Dohm FA, Kraemer HC, *et al*. Eating disorders in White and Black women. *Am J Psychiatry* 2003;**160**:1326–1331.
8. Crago M, Shisslak CM, Estes LS. Eating disturbances among American minority groups: A review. *Int J Eat Disord* 1996;**19**:239–248.
9. Becker AE, Franko DL, Speck A, Herzog DB. Ethnicity and differential access to care for eating disorder symptoms. *Int J Eat Disord* 2003;**33**:205–212.
10. Gowers S, McMahon JB. Social class and prognosis in anorexia nervosa. *Int J Eat Disord* 1989;**8**:105–109.
11. Favaro A, Ferrara S, Santonastaso P. The spectrum of eating disorders in young women: A prevalence study in a general population sample. *Psychosom Med* 2003;**65**:701–708.
12. Gard MCE, Freeman CP. Dismantling of a myth: A review of eating disorders and socio-economic status. *Int J Eat Disord* 1996;**20**:1–12.
13. Ravaldi C, Vannacci A, Zucchi T, *et al*. Eating disorders and body image disturbances among ballet dancers, gymnasium users and body builders. *Psychopathology* 2003;**36**:247–254.
14. Rodin G, Olmsted MP, Rydall AC, *et al*. Eating disorders in young women with type 1 diabetes mellitus. *J Psychosom Res* 2002;**53**:943–949.
15. Strober M, Lampert C, Morrell W, Burroughs J, Jacobs C. A controlled family study of anorexia nervosa: Evidence of familial aggregation and lack of shared transmission with affective disorders. *Int J Eat Disord* 1990;**9**:239–253.
16. Stein D, Lilenfeld LR, Plotnicov K, *et al*. Familial aggregation of eating disorders: Results from a controlled family study of bulimia nervosa. *Int J Eating Disord* 1999;**26**:211–215.
17. Kendler KS, Maclean C, Neale M, Kessler R, Heath A, Eaves L. The genetic epidemiology of bulimia nervosa. *Am J Psychiatry* 1991;**148**:1627–1637.
18. Crisp AH, Hall A, Holland AJ. Nature and nurture in anorexia nervosa: A study of 34 pairs of twins, one pair of triplets and an adoptive family. *Int J Eat Disord* 1985;**4**:5–29.
19. Lamberg L. Advances in eating disorders offer food for thought. *JAMA* 2003;**290**:1437–1442.
20. Wade TD, Bulik CM, Neale M, Kendler KS. Anorexia nervosa and major depression: Shared genetic and environment risk factors. *Am J Psychiatry* 2000;**157**:469–471.
21. Lilenfeld LR, Kaye WH, Greeno CG, *et al*. Psychiatric disorders in women with bulimia nervosa and their first-degree relatives: Effects of comorbid substance dependence. *Int J Eat Disord* 1997;**22**:253–264.
22. Pyle RL, Mitchell JE, Eckert ED. Bulimia: A report of 34 cases. *J Clin Psychiatry* 1981;**42**:60–64.
23. Bellodi L, Cavallini MC, Bertelli S, Chiapparino D, Riboldi C, Smeraldi E. Morbidity risk for obsessive-compulsive spectrum disorders in first-degree relatives of patients with eating disorders. *Am J Psychiatry* 2001;**158**:563–569.
24. Lilenfeld LRR, Stein D, Bulik CM, *et al*. Personality traits among current eating disordered, recovered and never ill first-degree female relatives of bulimic and control women. *Psychol Med* 2000;**30**:1399–1410.
25. Ribases M, Gratacos M, Armengol L, *et al*. Met66 in the brain-derived neurotrophic factor (BDNF) precursor is associated with anorexia nervosa restrictive type. *Mol Psychiatry* 2003;**8**:745–751.
26. Keys A, Brozek J, Henschel A, Mickelsen O, Taylor HL (eds). *The Biology of Human Starvation*. Minneapolis: University of Minnesota Press, 1950; pp. 819–853.
27. Cooper PJ, Whelan E, Woolgar M, Morrell J, Murray L. Association between childhood feeding problems and maternal eating disorder: Role of the family environment. *Br J Psychiatry* 2004;**184**:210–215.
28. Martinez-Gonzalez MA, Gual P, Lahortiga F, Alonso Y, de Irala-Estevez J, Cervera S. Parental factors, mass media influences, and the onset of eating disorders in a prospective population-based cohort. *Pediatrics* 2003;**111**:315–320.
29. Le Grange D, Lock J, Loeb K, Nicholls D. Academy for Eating Disorders position paper: Role of the family in eating disorders. *Int J Eat Disord* 2010;**43**:1–5.
30. Bulik CM, Tozzi F, Anderson C, Mazzeo SE, Aggen S, Sullivan PF. The relation between eating disorders and components of perfectionism. *Am J Psychiatry* 2003;**160**:366–368.
31. Anderluch MB, Tchanturia K, Rabe-Hesketh S, Treasure J. Childhood obsessive-compulsive personality traits in adult women with eating disorders: Defining a broader eating disorder phenotype. *Am J Psychiatry* 2003;**160**:242–247.
32. Gowers SG, Shore A. Development of weight and shape concerns in the aetiology of eating disorders. *Br J Psychiatry* 2001;**179**:236–242.

33. Favaro A, Santonastaso P. The spectrum of self-injurious behavior in eating disorders. *Eat Disord* 2002;**1**:215–225.

34. Rodgers RF, Paxton SJ, Chabrol H. Depression as a moderator of sociocultural influences on eating disorder symptoms in adolescent females and males. *J Youth Adolesc* 2010;**39**:393–402.

35. Gunderson JG. *Borderline Personality Disorder*. Washington, DC: American Psychiatric Press, 1984.

36. Linehan MM. *Cognitive Behavioral Treatment of Borderline Personality*. New York: Guilford, 1993.

37. Keel PK, Klump KL. Are eating disorders culture-bound syndromes: Implications for conceptualizing their etiology. *Psychol Bull* 2003;**129**:747–769.

38. The McKnight Investigators. Risk factors for the onset of eating disorders in adolescent girls: Results of the McKnight Longitudinal Risk Factor Study. *Am J Psychiatry* 2003;**160**:248–254.

39. Menzel JE, Schaefer LM, Burke NL, Mayhew LL, Brannick MT, Thompson JK. Appearance-related teasing, body dissatisfaction, and disordered eating: A meta-analysis. *Body Image* 2010;**7**:261–270.

40. Tagay S, Schlegl S, Senf W. Traumatic events, posttraumatic stress symptomatology and somatoform symptoms in eating disorder patients. *Eur Eat Disord Rev* 2010;**18**:124–132.

41. Chen LP, Murad MH, Paras ML, *et al.* Sexual abuse and lifetime diagnosis of psychiatric disorders: Systematic review and meta-analysis. *Mayo Clin Proc* 2010;**85**:618–629.

42. Johnson JG, Cohen P, Kasen S, Brook JS. Childhood adversities associated with risk for eating disorders or weight problems during adolescence or early adulthood. *Am J Psychiatry* 2002;**159**:394–400.

43. Steiner N, Kwan W, Shaffer TG, *et al.* Risk and protective factors for juvenile eating disorders. *Eur Child Adolesc Psychiatry* 2003;**12**:138–146.

44. Milos GF, Spindler AM, Buddeberg C, Crameri A. Axes I and II comorbidity and treatment experiences in eating disorder subjects. *Psychother Psychosom* 2003;**72**:276–285.

45. Root TL, Pinheiro AP, Thornton L, *et al.* Substance use disorders in women with anorexia nervosa. *Int J Eat Disord* 2010;**43**:14–21.

46. Sansone RA, Levitt JL, Sansone LA. The prevalence of personality disorders among those with eating disorders. *Eat Disord* 2005;**13**:7–21.

47. Trigazis L, Tennankore D, Vohra S, Katzman DK. The use of herbal remedies by adolescents with eating disorders. *Int J Eat Disord* 2004;**35**:223–228.

48. Zaider TI, Johnson JG, Cockell SJ. Psychiatric comorbidity associated with eating disorder symptomatology among adolescents in the community. *Int J Eat Disord* 2000;**28**:58–67.

49. Grilo CM, Levy KN, Becker DF, Edell WS, McGlashan TH. Comorbidity of DSM-III-R axis I and II disorders among female inpatients with eating disorders. *Psychiatr Serv* 1996;**47**:426–429.

50. Braun DL, Sunday SR, Halmi KA. Psychiatric comorbidity in patients with eating disorders. *Psychol Med* 1994;**24**:859–867.

51. Matsumoto T, Kosaka K, Yamaguchi A, *et al.* Eating disorders in female substance use disorders: A preliminary research on the relationship of substances and eating behaviors. *Clin Psychiatry* 2003;**45**:119–127.

52. Keel PK, Striegel-Moore RH. The validity and clinical utility of purging disorder. *Int J Eat Disord* 2009;**42**:706–719.

53. Mitka M. DSM panel considers ways to clarify diagnostic criteria for eating disorders. *JAMA* 2010;**303**:2235–2237.

54. Work Group on Eating Disorders. Practice guideline for the treatment of patients with eating disorders (revision). *Am J Psychiatry* 2000;**157**:S1–39.

55. Crow SJ, Rosenberg ME, Mitchell JE, Thuras P. Urine electrolytes as markers of bulimia nervosa. *Int J Eat Disord* 2001;**30**:279–287.

56. Sansone RA, Correll TL. Eating disorders. *Hosp Physician* 2001;**5**:1–12.

57. Hartman D, Crisp A, Rooney B, Rackow C, Atkinson R, Patel S. Bone density of women who have recovered from anorexia nervosa. *Int J Eat Disord* 2000;**28**:107–112.

58. Neumaerker K-J. Mortality rates and causes of death. *Eur Eat Disord Rev* 2000;**8**:181–187.

59. Sansone RA, Sansone LA, Wiederman MW. Eating disorders: Diagnosis and management in the primary care setting. *Prim Care Rep* 1998;**4**:43–50.

60. Keel PK, Mitchell JE. Outcome in bulimia nervosa. *Am J Psychiatry* 1997;**154**:313–321.

61. McKnight RF, Park RJ. Atypical antipsychotics and anorexia nervosa: A review. *Eur Eat Disord Rev* 2010;**18**:10–21.

62. Sansone RA, Dennis AB. The treatment of eating disorder patients with substance abuse and borderline personality disorder. *Eat Disord* 1996;**4**:180–186.

63. Sansone RA, Johnson CL. Treating the eating disorder patient with borderline personality: Theory and technique. In: Barber J, Crits-Christoph P (eds) *Dynamic Therapies for Psychiatric Disorders (Axis I)*. New York: Basic Books, 1995; pp. 230–266.

64. Richards SP, Baldwin BM, Frost HA, Clark-Sly JB, Berrett ME, Hardman RK. What works for treating eating disorders? Conclusions of 28 outcome reviews. *Eat Disord* 2000;**8**:189–206.

65. Murphy R, Straebler S, Cooper Z, Fairburn CG. Cognitive behavioral therapy for eating disorders. *Psychiatr Clin North Am* 2010;**33**:611–627.

66. Wilfley DE, Frank MA, Welch R, Spurrell EB, Rounsaville BJ. Adapting interpersonal psychotherapy to a group format (IPT-G) for binge eating disorder: Toward a model for adapting empirically supported treatments. *Psychother Res* 1998;**8**:379–391.

67. Rice C, Faulkner J. Support and self-help groups. In: Harper-Guiffre H, MacKenzie KR (eds) *Group Psychotherapy for Eating Disorders*. Washington, DC: American Psychiatric Association, 1992; pp. 247–260.

68. Kotler LA, Boudreau GS, Devlin MJ. Emerging psychotherapies for eating disorders. *J Psychiatr Pract* 2003;**9**:431–441.

69. Sansone RA. Patient-to-patient e-mail support for clinical practices. *Eat Disord* 2001;**9**:373–375.

70. Norton M, Wonderlich SA, Myers T, Michell JE, Crosby RD. The use of palmtop computers in the treatment of bulimia nervosa. *Eur Eat Disord Rev* 2003;**11**:231–242.

71. Taylor CB, Jobson KO, Winzelberg A, Abascal L. The use of the Internet to provide evidence-based integrated treatment programs for mental health. *Psychiatr Ann* 2002;**32**:671–677.

72. Anderson DA, Williamson DA. Outcome measurement in eating disorders. In: IsHak WW, Tal B, Sederer LI (eds)

Outcome Measurement in Psychiatry: A Critical Review. Washington, DC: American Psychiatric Publishing, 2002; pp. 289–302.

73. Neiderman M. Prognosis and outcome. In: Lask B, Bryant-Waugh R (eds) *Anorexia Nervosa and Related Eating Disorders in Childhood and Adolescence,* 2nd edn. Hove, UK: Taylor & Francis, 2000; pp. 81–102.

74. Anderson DA, Williamson DA, Duchmann EG, Gleaves DH, Barbin JM. Development and validation of a multifactorial treatment outcome measure for eating disorders. *Assessment* 1999;**6**:7–20.

75. Herzog DB, Dorer DJ, Keel P, *et al.* Recovery and relapse in anorexia and bulimia nervosa: A 7.5-year follow-up study. *J Am Acad Child Adolesc Psychiatry* 1999;**38**: 829–837.

76. Keel PK. Long-term outcome of bulimia nervosa. *Diss Abstr Int, Section B* 1998;**58**:6812.

77. Herpertz-Dahlmann B, Muller B, Herpertz S, Heussen N, Hebebrand J, Remschmidt H. Prospective 10-year follow-up in adolescent anorexia nervosa: Course, outcome, psychiatric comorbidity, and psychosocial adaptation. *J Child Psychol Psychiatry* 2001;**42**:603–612.

78. Steinhausen H-C, Boyadjieva S, Griogoroiu-Serbanescu M, Neumaerker K-J. The outcome of adolescent eating disorders: Findings from an international collaborative study. *Eur Child Adolesc Psychiatry* 2003;**12**:191–198.

79. Ben-Tovim B, Walker K, Gilchrist P, Freeman R, Kalucy R, Esterman A. Outcome in patients with eating disorders: A 5-year study. *Lancet* 2001;**357**:1254–1257.

80. Nakai Y, Hamagaki S, Ishizaka Y, Takagi R, Takagi S, Ishikawa T. Predictors of outcome in eating disorders. *Clin Psychiatry* 2002;**44**:1305–1309.

81. Steinhausen HC, Weber S. The outcome of bulimia nervosa: Findings from one-quarter century of research. *Am J Psychiatry* 2009;**166**:1331–1341.

82. Keel PK, Brown TA. Update on course and outcome in eating disorders. *Int J Eat Disord* 2010;**43**:195–204.

83. Stoving RK, Andries A, Brixen K, Bilenberg N, Horder K. Gender differences in outcome of eating disorders: A retrospective cohort study. *Psychiatry Res* 2011;**186**: 362–366.

84. Rowe S, Jordan J, McIntosh V, *et al.* Dimensional measures of personality as a predictor of outcome at 5-year follow-up in women with bulimia nervosa. *Psychiatry Res* 2011;**185**:414–420.

85. Keel PK, Dorer DJ, Eddy KT, Franko D, Charatan DL, Herzog DB. Predictors of mortality in eating disorders. *Arch Gen Psychiatry* 2003;**60**:179–183.

86. Crow SJ, Thuras P, Keel PK, Mitchell JE. Long-term menstrual and reproductive function in patients with bulimia nervosa. *Am J Psychiatry* 2002;**159**:1048–1050.

87. Franko DL, Blais MA, Becker AE, *et al.* Pregnancy complications and neonatal outcomes in women with eating disorders. *Am J Psychiatry* 2001;**158**:1461–1466.

88. Carter FA, McIntosh VVW, Joyce PR, Frampton CM, Bulik CM. Bulimia nervosa, childbirth and psychopathology. *J Psychosom Res* 2003;**55**:357–361.

89. Crow SJ, Peterson CB, Swanson SA, *et al.* Increased mortality in bulimia nervosa and other eating disorders. *Am J Psychiatry* 2009;**166**:1342–1346.

90. Herzog DB, Greenwood DN, Dorer DJ, *et al.* Mortality in eating disorders: A descriptive study. *Int J Eating Disord* 2000;**28**:20–26.

91. Bunnell D. The "new" eating disorder. *Perspective* 2004; pp. 1, 4–6.

92. Walsh BT, Wilfley DE, Hudson JI. *Binge Eating Disorder: Progress in Understanding and Treatment.* Educational monograph. West Wayne, NJ: Health Learning Systems, 2003; pp. 1–14.

18

Elimination Disorders: Enuresis and Encopresis

Ryan C. Mast, Andrew B. Smith

Introduction

During the toddler phase (age 18 months to 3 years), a child's interest and attention turns toward the mastery of elimination. By the time they reach age 4, most children have achieved bowel and bladder continence. Bowel continence is typically mastered first. Acquiring continence generally proceeds in the following stages: (i) nighttime bowel control; (ii) daytime bowel control; (iii) daytime bladder control; and finally (iv) nighttime bladder control.

Piaget emphasized that it is the physical maturation of the child that enables continence to be achieved [1]. As a result of the normal maturation of the elimination system (coupled with effective potty training techniques), one-third of children in the United States are completely toilet-trained by age 24 months [2]. Potty training efforts prior to this physical maturation will be largely unsuccessful, and premature potty training may cause significant distress in the child and frustration for the parents, who might regard themselves as failures. A generally accepted tenet is to begin potty training when the child signals her or his readiness.

In general, females achieve continence earlier than males, and it is the more rapid physical maturation of females that is purportedly the cause. Therefore, males struggle with bedwetting longer than their female counterparts. However, an important caveat to this general trend is that females later have more difficulties with daytime bladder continence.

While most children (both boys and girls) are continent by the end of toddlerhood, some continue to struggle into adolescence. One percent of adults meet criteria for nocturnal enuresis according to the *Diagnostic and Statistical Manual of Mental Disorders, Fourth Edition, Text Revision* (DSM-IV-TR) [3, 4].

The achievement of continence does not occur in one day or one week. Parents should be made aware that progress often occurs in a step-wise series of successes and failures. You would not expect a child to start walking and never fall again. Falls are a normal part of learning to walk, and accidents are a normal part of potty training. As successful children learn to control elimination, they gain a sense of mastery. The sense of control gained here continues their march toward autonomy.

While the toddler is struggling to gain control of newfound physical capabilities, parents are also demonstrating growing interest in the child's mastery of elimination. This increased parental interest in the child's production of both urine and feces does not go unnoticed by the child. However, when a parent's potty training efforts become heavy-handed, the control of the child's body becomes a battlefield. Children may begin to resent the parent who attempts to control their internal body sensations through toilet training. This attack on their autonomy can have enduring consequences.

Erikson (in his Epigenetic Model) stated that the years from 1 to 3 are highlighted by the crisis of "Autonomy versus Shame and Doubt." [5] Bienenfeld notes that during this time, the developing nervous system allows the child to walk, retain feces, control urination, and exert other forms of self-control. If parents encourage self-sufficiency, then the child can develop a sense of autonomy. Children who sense their ability to handle their own problems have achieved an important milestone.

However, when parents demand too much too soon, don't allow toddlers to perform tasks for which they are ready, or ridicule children's inability to gain bladder/bowel control, then the children may develop shame and doubt about their ability to handle problems. The child

Clinical Child Psychiatry, Third Edition. Edited by William M. Klykylo and Jerald Kay.
© 2012 John Wiley & Sons, Ltd. Published 2012 by John Wiley & Sons, Ltd.

at the end of toddlerhood is able to say either: "I can exert myself and successfully accomplish tasks" or "I am incompetent and unsuccessful." Unless the latter is resolved, there can be severe consequences in adult life.

In addition to Piaget and Erikson, others have also noted the importance of this time in a child's development. Freud termed this phase of childhood the Anal and Urethral Phase of Development. Regarding this phase, Brenner noted, "Pleasurable and unpleasurable sensations are associated both with the retention of feces and with their expulsion, and these bodily processes, as well as feces themselves and fecal odors, are the objects of the child's most intense interest." [6] Gemelli noted that toddlers begin to "engage in a great variety of derivative play behaviors that resemble urination (e.g. playing with faucets, watering hoses and cans, and squirting devices)." [1] Later, during toddlerhood, children are not only fascinated by their own urination/feces, but also that of others (peers and family). During this time, children may get aggressive gratification out of withholding and depositing feces. During the Phallic Phase, urination is sometimes seen as an aggressive outlet.

Some have proposed that certain character styles might arise from failures during the Toddler Years. The anal retentive personality is described as the product of overly strict toilet training. Punishments and/or shaming may cause the child to retaliate by holding feces at all costs. When these children become adults, they may be stubborn, rigid, orderly, and compulsively neat. Some have postulated that obsessive-compulsive personality disorder might have some of its origins here.

The anal expulsive (or anal aggressive) personality is thought to be the product of overly subservient parents during toilet training. These parents reward desired behavior and suffer transparently during the child's failures. The children may become adults whose character style is described as sloppy and disorganized. They may be either overly generous or cruel.

The possible implications of elimination disorders on long-term mental health can therefore be significant. While the spontaneous remission rate of enuresis is reported to be 15% per year, a significant percentage of children remain affected by elimination disorders [3]. [7], Withholding treatment can have troubling consequences (including adult anxieties). Macdonald in his 1963 article "The Threat to Kill" proposed that the triad of: persistent bedwetting beyond the age of 5, obsession with firestarting, and cruelty to animals could lead to criminality [8]. While more than a few serial killers have had this triad in childhood, other investigators have examined this Triad of Sociopathy (also known as the MacDonald Triad) to determine if there is indeed a link

to homicidal behavior. This further research has put into question whether bedwetting should be included in the triad. The dyad of firestarting and cruelty to animals often does appear to be a dire prognostic sign. However, research indicates that bedwetting does not seem to have a direct link with sociopathic criminal/antisocial behavior.

While there does not appear to be a direct link between bedwetting and future criminal behavior, there may be an indirect link. The theoretical link is as follows: bedwetting that causes the child to be humiliated/abused by the guardian may lead the child to set fires and hurt animals in order to gain some sense of control (since they are unable to overpower the adult aggressor), and this can lead to sociopathic behavior. Therefore, the possible link between criminal behavior and bedwetting is not related to bedwetting itself, but to the child's and caregivers' responses to the bedwetting.

While some children with nocturnal enuresis may later engage in criminal behavior, most do not. In fact, even when bedwetting persists into the teenage years, many persevere and flourish. Many famous actors (including Michael Landon), star athletes, lawyers, medical professionals, and others in prominent positions have battled nocturnal enuresis in childhood. Some of these individuals have spoken candidly regarding their experiences. A few have revealed their caregivers' mishandling of their bedwetting. This mishandling has ranged from intentionally hanging sheets outside (as a form of shaming), to leaving the child in wet clothes as a punishment, to rubbing the child's face in the wet clothing, to overt physical abuse. Others have spoken of their caregivers' appropriate responses and interventions (as well as effective treatments).

Actress Suzanne Somers published her childhood struggles with nocturnal enuresis in her autobiography *Keeping Secrets* [9]. She detailed worries about wetting the bed at slumber parties. She also described how she was able to overcome nocturnal enuresis with the help of a wetness alarm.

While treatment modalities have evolved, nocturnal enuresis and (to a lesser extent) encopresis remain significantly problematic. Treatments for bedwetting include: education, watchful waiting, nonpharmacological interventions (e.g. bell and pad), and pharmacological interventions. There are times when "watchful waiting" is appropriate. As noted above, studies indicate that the yearly spontaneous remission rate for bedwetting is roughly 15%. However, high levels of distress caused by nocturnal enuresis can lead to anxiety. Therefore, when appropriate, some form of intervention is often indicated.

Although parents may report significant frustration with a child's continued bedwetting, a lack of bladder control before the age of 5 is generally considered a normal variant (unless there is an organic etiology). A lack of bowel control before age 4 is also typically considered a normal variant. Once these age barriers are crossed, clinicians should intervene (if this process has not already begun). Sometimes the intervention is simply education about the causes, incidence, treatments, and prognosis of elimination disorders.

Children with elimination disorders frequently present to primary care clinics. However, some parents do not raise the issue of continence until arriving at a psychiatric intake for the child's symptoms of anxiety, attention-deficit hyperactivity disorder (ADHD), acting-out behaviors, etc. While many seek treatment, some children are never evaluated for elimination disorders for a variety of reasons. Sometimes this silence is the result of watchful waiting, parental embarrassment, parental lack of understanding that there are treatments, or parental indifference. The toddler years can be a tumultuous time.

Enuresis

Enuresis has long plagued children, families, and clinicians. In Glicklich's 1951 article "An Historical Account of Enuresis," she reported that in 1550 BC the Papyrus Ebers recommended juniper berries, cypress, and beer in the treatment of enuresis [10].

Pliny the Elder in the first century suggested that "the incontinence of urine in infants is checked by giving boiled mice in their food." The consumption of an animal's bladder for the treatment of bladder problems ("organ therapy") gained popularity for a time. From antiquity to modern time, treatment modalities for enuresis have ranged from humane to horrific. These have included mechanical devices, cautery, and surgical interventions.

Gill outlined the following eras in the treatment of enuresis: the homeopathic or humor era of medieval medicine, the mechanical or primitive era of Victorian medicine, the pharmacological era from the late nineteenth century to today, the urological era from 1950 to 1980 (now largely obsolete), and the era of behavioral modification from the fifteenth century to today [11].

The difficulty in diagnosing and treating enuresis is therefore neither new nor straightforward. The number of treatments available today only underscores the reality that many etiologies of enuresis exist. Today, medications (e.g., desmopressin) and behavioral interventions (e.g., the bell and pad) are mainstays of treatment. As many have come to realize, behavioral modification works best when reward (instead of punishment) is utilized. Threats, ridicule, and physical punishment often increase anxiety and make enuretic symptoms worse.

While most children have mastered urinary continence by the time they turn 4 years old, many have not. As mentioned earlier, enuresis is not generally considered pathological unless it persists into the fifth year of life. By the time their child is age 5, parents may have tried a variety of methods in search of a cure. Significant anxiety, tension, frustration, and embarrassment are likely to exist by the time they present to the clinician. Parents may have a sense of inadequacy. A family's shame about enuresis can lead to secrecy and silence. Children and parents may feel anger about both the situation and toward one another. Parents may blame the child for being too lazy or irresponsible. Sentiments such as these may cause a worsening of symptoms as bedwetting becomes a battleground.

Definitions

Enuresis comes from the Greek word "enourein" (meaning to void urine). The DSM-IV-TR definition of enuresis is: the repeated voiding of urine into the bed or clothes at least twice per week for at least 3 consecutive months in a child who is at least 5 years old [12].

The timing of symptoms is a critical component in the diagnostic process. Wetting the bed only once is therefore not considered nocturnal enuresis. While the terms "bedwetting" and "nocturnal enuresis" are similar, they are not always synonymous.

Enuresis is often described as either *nocturnal* (voiding while asleep), *diurnal* (voiding while awake), or both. The etiology and treatment of diurnal enuresis are often very different from those of nocturnal enuresis. There is also no rule that a child will only have one cause of their enuresis (the etiology may be multifactorial).

Further classifications of enuresis include: primary or secondary. *Primary enuresis* describes when the child never accomplished continence through the night. *Secondary enuresis* is when the child achieved continence for at least 6 consecutive months, but then began wetting again.

Primary enuresis is usually due to maturational and/or physiological delays. Secondary enuresis is usually caused by either psychological factors or an underlying medical condition (e.g. urinary tract infection, diabetes). When the cause of secondary enuresis is psychological stress, it is sometimes termed *regressive enuresis* because it occurs in response to a perceived threat to the child's security. This regression stems from stressful circumstances (e.g., a move, the birth of a sibling, parental divorce, introduction of a new parent/caregiver, abuse, hospitalization, and/or school stressors/bullying).

Further classifications of enuresis exist. Some prefer to categorize nocturnal enuresis as either mono- or polysymptomatic. *Monosymptomatic nocturnal enuresis* is defined as nighttime wetting in children who are dry during the day (and who have no difficulties with urination while awake). *Polysymptomatic nocturnal enuresis* is defined as nighttime wetting along with daytime indicators of bladder dysfunction (e.g., urgency, frequency, and occasional accidental daytime voiding). While such cases may have some daytime symptoms, they do not meet full criteria for *both* nocturnal and diurnal enuresis.

Functional enuresis is wetting occurring in the absence of an identifiable organic cause. Examples of functional enuresis include: hormonal/biological rhythms and psychological stressors/mental retardation.

Nonfunctional enuresis is due to an identifiable organic etiology (e.g., due to a general medical condition). Strictly speaking, the diagnosis of *enuresis* (according to the DSM-IV-TR) cannot be made if wetting is due to a general medical condition. The inclusion of the term "nonfunctional enuresis" is included here because the concept is an important one. In the work-up of the patient with persistent bedwetting, one must first rule out a general medical condition. While urinary incontinence is not a new condition, the terminology used to describe the associated disorders continues to evolve.

Revenge enuresis is a method of retention typically in response to harsh training practices and/or a strict parent. *Enuresis due to a fancied injury* occurs after a child has had a physically traumatic experience that leaves the child to view him- or herself as damaged or injured (and therefore no longer in control of his or her urine flow).

Enuresis due to a lack of training occurs when families have decided not to potty train the child. This usually occurs in families that have had several members with enuresis. The family might have a sense that they can do nothing to help.

Detrusor-dependent enuresis is caused by spontaneous bladder contractions. *Volume-dependent enuresis* is caused by nocturnal polyuria.

Prevalence

Approximately one-third of US children achieve continence by age 2. The majority of children are toilet-trained by the end of the toddler phase. According to DSM-IV-TR, the diagnosis of nocturnal enuresis cannot be made before the age of 5.

While only 5–10% of 5-year-olds meet DSM-IV-TR criteria for nocturnal enuresis, it is important to note that as many as 20% of 5-year-olds have some bedwetting difficulties. Among enuretic 5-year-olds, there is a 4:1 male:female ratio. This ratio declines with age [2].

Without any formal treatment, approximately 15% of enuretic children will have a spontaneous resolution of symptoms each year. Criteria for nocturnal enuresis are met by 2–3% of 12-year-olds. By age 18, approximately 1% of the population still has enuretic symptoms. Many of these individuals will continue to have symptoms well into adulthood.

Overall, it has been estimated that between 5 and 7 million US children have primary nocturnal enuresis. Studies suggest that bedwetting is more common in African Americans and Asian immigrants to the United States compared to other populations. Primary enuresis remains twice as common as secondary enuresis. Nocturnal incontinence is more common than diurnal (daytime) incontinence.

Enuresis is not solely a problem of the United States and other industrialized nations. Most countries where data are available have similar incidence, prevalence, and spontaneous remission rates [13]. [14], Where variations in data do exist, it is sometimes related to a higher incidence of co-sleeping with parents (and other family members). In these cases, the parent may act as a *de facto* bell-and-pad alarm (awakening the child as soon as the parent feels the child wetting).

Diagnostic Criteria

DSM-IV-TR criteria for 307.6 Enuresis (Not Due to a General Medical Condition) include: repeated voiding of urine into bed or clothes (whether involuntary or intentional). The behavior is clinically significant as manifested by either a frequency of twice a week for at least 3 consecutive months or the presence of clinically significant distress or impairment in social, academic (occupational), or other important areas of functioning. Chronological age is at least 5 years (or equivalent developmental level). The behavior is not due exclusively to the direct physiological effect of a substance (e.g., a diuretic) or a general medical condition (e.g., diabetes, spina bifida, a seizure disorder). Three types are specified: Nocturnal Only, the most common subtype, defined as passage of urine only during nighttime sleep; Diurnal Only, defined as the passage of urine only during waking hours; and Nocturnal and Diurnal, defined as a combination of the two subtypes above.

Since publication of the DSM-IV-TR, some have argued for a revision of the criteria for enuresis. These criteria are continually being refined. Currently, several modifications are being given serious consideration for inclusion in the DSM-V [15]. These proposed revisions include:

- Criterion B currently requires either a minimum frequency or subjective distress. This is not reasonable – an isolated instance of incontinence might well cause more distress than frequent enuresis for which tolerance or habituation has occurred. Conversely, it makes no sense to require distress in the presence of very frequent incontinence, when such habituation might have taken place.
- The proposed Criterion D revision is: "The behavior is not due exclusively to the direct physiological effect of a substance (e.g., a diuretic, antipsychotic, or SSRI antidepressant) or to incontinence incurred as a result of polyuria or during loss of consciousness."

Etiology and Differential Diagnosis

Enuresis is typically thought of as either a storage or a voiding problem. In order to understand the pathology behind enuresis, one must first examine the normal progression of urinary continence. Urinary continence is achieved in three sequential steps. First, enlargement of bladder capacity occurs, followed by voluntary control of sphincter muscles (which normally occurs by age 3). Finally, voluntary control of the micturition reflex is attained. The neurological wiring and development required to master urination is complex and beyond the scope of this book. Suffice it to say that failure to achieve urinary continence can occur by a variety of methods.

Both nature and nurture play prominent roles in enuresis. When both parents have had enuresis, there is a 77% incidence of enuresis in their children. If one parent has had enuresis, the incidence is 44%. This compares with only a 15% incidence of enuresis in children without enuretic parents [3]. Twin studies show 68% concordance with monozygotes (identical twins) and 36% with dizygotes (fraternal twins).

Chromosomal linkages with nocturnal enuresis include: chromosome 13q (ENUR1), 12q (ENUR2), 4, 8, and 22. Chromosome 5 may also be implicated. Modes of transmission include autosomal dominant, autosomal recessive, and sporadic [16–19].

Determining the underlying cause of a child's enuresis can be complex. Nocturnal enuresis and diurnal enuresis typically have very different etiologies. Primary and secondary nocturnal enuresis often have very different underlying causes as well. Primary nocturnal enuresis is usually the result of developmental/maturational delays. Secondary nocturnal enuresis is often due to an organic or psychological cause. Diagnosis and treat-

ment are further complicated in those cases where the etiology of enuresis is multifactorial.

During the evaluation process, it is valuable to remember that most bedwetting is the result of a maturational delay (and not due to a general medical condition or due to psychological reasons). Approximately only 5–10% of cases are due to an underlying medical issue.

According to the DSM-IV-TR, the diagnosis of enuresis requires that the behavior is not due exclusively to the direct physiological effect of a substance (e.g., a diuretic) or a general medical condition. However, here we will include a discussion of incontinence caused by medications and general medical conditions because these factors are an important part of the history-taking and diagnostic process.

The typical causes of childhood urinary incontinence can be arranged according to the following categories: maturational, anatomical abnormalities, endocrine, urinary tract disease, neurological, medication-induced, and psychological (see Table 18.1).

Maturational

The most common cause of primary nocturnal enuresis is when the child fails to gain control of the typical neurological urinary mechanisms. Often these children also have speech and other motor delays. Conversely, if a child presents to the office due to speech or motor delays, it is important to also inquire about incontinence/bedwetting [20].

Anatomical Abnormalities

Examples of anatomical abnormalities include: bladder wall abnormalities (weak bladder and supporting musculature, detrusor overactivity, detrusor areflexia), low bladder pressure threshold causing early emptying, posterior urethral valves in males, ectopic ureter in females, tonsillar hypertrophy, and constipation. Surgery may be indicated in a small percentage of cases. Females with an ectopic ureter sometimes present with the complaint of frequent dribbling. Some cases of nocturnal enuresis may be related to obstructive sleep apnea (OSA). Proposed mechanisms are that OSA increases blood pressure, leading to increased release of atrial natriuretic peptide (ANP) from the atria and brain natriuretic peptide (BNP) from the ventricles of the heart [21]. As their names suggest, these peptides (ANP and BNP) can have natriuretic effects. ANP is involved in the homeostatic control of body water, sodium, potassium, and fat. It acts to reduce the water, sodium, and adipose loads on the circulatory system in an effort to reduce blood pressure and workload on the heart. It does so by inhibiting the renin-angiotensin-aldosterone axis (RAA

Table 18.1 Causes of childhood urinary incontinence.

Maturational
Failure of child to master control of urinary mechanisms
Anatomical abnormalities
Bladder wall abnormalities
Low bladder pressure threshold
Posterior urethral valve (males)
Ectopic ureter (females)
Tonsillar hypertrophy
Constipation
Obstructive sleep apnea
Post-void incontinence
Stress incontinence
Giggle incontinence
Endocrine
Diabetes mellitus
Diabetes insipidus
Abnormal release of vasopressin
Hyperthyroidism
Urinary tract disease
Urinary tract infection
Urinary outflow obstruction
Neurological
Loss of consciousness
Seizure disorder
Spinal cord disease/trauma
Spina bifida
Cerebral palsy
Mental retardation
Sleepwalking
Attention-deficit hyperactivity disorder (ADHD)
Medications
Lithium
Diuretics
Valproic acid
Clozapine and other antipsychotics
Selective serotonin reuptake inhibitors (SSRIs)
Theophylline and caffeine
Psychological
Stress (many different possibilities)
Reactive attachment disorder (RAD)
Volitional causes

axis). This action does reduce blood pressure, but it does so (in part) by increasing urinary output (which can lead to episodes of nocturnal enuresis) (Figure 18.1). OSA may also cause sleep fragmentation, and this has been proposed as a mechanism of nocturnal enuresis as well. In some cases, a tonsillectomy and adenoidectomy is warranted [22].

Other anatomical abnormalities leading to enuresis are postvoid, stress, and giggle incontinence. *Postvoid incontinence* is typically vaginal reflux of urine due to an improper voiding posture (typically in obese females who hold their legs together during urination). *Stress incontinence* occurs during running, coughing, or heavy lifting. *Giggle incontinence* (as the name suggests) occurs during periods of laughter. It has a typical onset in early to mid-pubescent females. Giggle incontinence probably represents a developmental defect, and long-term outcome is mostly unknown. Methylphenidate is the only treatment modality with any reported success for giggle incontinence.

Pressure placed on the bladder by constipation and large stools can also cause bladder incontinence. Fifteen percent of children with enuresis also have encopresis. Treating the encopresis sometimes causes a resolution of enuretic symptoms.

Endocrine

Diabetes mellitus, diabetes insipidus, abnormal nighttime release of vasopressin, and hyperthyroidism may all cause bedwetting. Due to circadian rhythms, the normal production of urine in the night is half of daytime urine production. Decreased urine production at night helps to keep the sleeper asleep by keeping them dry. This decrease in urine production is largely related to the increased secretion of vasopressin at night. There is a burst of vasopressin around sunset that causes the kidneys to reduce urine production. This hormone cycle is not present at birth, but most individuals develop it between the ages of 2 and 6 years old. However, in some cases, it may not develop until puberty (or not at all).

Urinary Tract Disease

Urinary tract infections (UTIs) and urinary outflow obstruction may cause bedwetting in a small percentage of children. However, the treatment of an existing UTI

OSA → ↑ BP → ↑ ANP release → ↑ Diuresis → ↓ BP → ↓ load on the heart.

Figure 18.1 Proposed mechanism by which obstructive sleep apnea (OSA) may cause nocturnal enuresis. ANP, atrial natriuretic peptide; BP, blood pressure.

rarely cures bedwetting. Therefore, in most cases, a UTI may be the result of bedwetting (and not the cause).

Neurological

There are numerous neurological deficits that can lead to enuresis. Examples include: loss of consciousness, seizure disorder, spinal cord disease/trauma (including tethered cord syndrome), spina bifida, cerebral palsy, mental retardation, other cognitive disorders, and sleepwalking (because children may think that they are in the bathroom when they are not). Kids with ADHD are 2.7 times more likely to have bedwetting issues. Children who are "deep sleepers" or who have other sleep disorders may wet the bed. Importantly, it has been reported that nocturnal enuresis occurs during all stages of sleep in proportion to the amount of time spent in each stage of sleep. Some have noted that bedwetting often occurs most frequently between 30 minutes and 3 hours after sleep onset. There have been mixed reports about whether children with nocturnal enuresis are more difficult to awaken. Parents have long reported this, and recent evidence suggests that this may be correct [23]. [24]. Simply stated, some children may be less prone to awaken themselves in response to sensations of a full bladder.

Medication-Induced

Lithium, diuretics, valproic acid, clozapine, other antipsychotics, selective serotonin reuptake inhibitors (SSRIs), theophylline, caffeine, and alcohol can all cause or increase bedwetting. SSRIs have been shown to improve enuresis in some cases and worsen/cause it in others [25]. Lithium (much like sodium) is a salt that is renally excreted. Alcohol acts as an antagonist to vasopressin in the kidney's collecting ducts (thereby preventing water reabsorption through aquaporin channels). It should be noted here that dandelions (which children sometimes eat) can have a potent diuretic effect.

Psychological

Stress (divorce, death, new sibling, hospitalization, abuse, school stress, or simply a change in sleeping arrangements/patterns), reactive attachment disorder (RAD), and volitional causes constitute some of the psychologically related causes of enuresis. Thirty percent of children with selective mutism also meet criteria for nocturnal enuresis. There is also a high comorbidity between nocturnal enuresis and depression/anxiety/ADHD. Enuresis treatment often improves depression and anxiety. The opposite (anxiety treatment curing enuresis) does not happen as often, but it does occur.

Regressive enuresis (enuresis in response to a psychological stressor) is sometimes described psychodynamically as the product of an unconscious desire for increased attention/care. A perceived threat to the child's security (a new sibling, death of a parent, etc.) may incite this desire in children. Understanding and treating the specific stressor causing regressive enuresis is paramount. It should be noted that there is a neurochemical explanation for this phenomenon as well. Corticotropin-releasing factor (CRF) is a neurotransmitter involved in CNS responses to stress; however, it also is involved in midbrain continence functions. Additionally, norepinephrine is also involved in both stress/anxiety and bladder/rectal function. Therefore, these are two neurochemicals that may help explain how stress can influence urinary continence by way of a neurotransmitter.

While some children have an unconscious and/or biochemical cause of psychologically related enuresis, other children might wet the bed volitionally (including a percentage of children with RAD). While revenge enuresis might be a rare cause of nocturnal enuresis, it nonetheless does occur with some frequency.

Diagnostic Approach

Reaching the proper diagnosis begins with a thorough history-taking (see Table 18.2). By the completion of the history and physical, one should be able to order further lab testing when indicated, treat, and/or make an appropriate referral.

A thorough history of the enuretic child addresses many questions, but perhaps the most important is: "Why now?" Why is the child being brought in for evaluation and treatment now? This question can give insight into (among other things) parental expectations.

The history should also focus on the following: child's age, onset of symptoms (primary/secondary), the timing (nocturnal/diurnal/both, during school, while playing or laughing, only during weekdays), and the frequency of symptoms (number of times per night, number of nights per week). A total urinary frequency of or exceeding eight times per day is considered too much whereas three or less is considered not enough. Urgency, hematuria, and child discomfort (abdominal pain, abnormal/painful voiding (dysuria), and anxiety) should also be ascertained during the initial evaluation.

It is important to inquire about straining, poor urine stream, the presence of dribbling, and unusual posturing. The pattern of fluid intake, family history of enuresis (including when it resolved), method of toilet training (rewards/punishments), sleeping habits, sleeping arrangement in the home, snoring, insomnia, and

Table 18.2 Useful Information in the evaluation of enuresis and encopresis.

Age

Onset of symptoms (primary vs secondary)

Pattern of symptoms (nocturnal/diurnal/both)

Frequency of accidents (no. of times per night/week)

Timing (during school, play, etc.)

Location (especially when evaluating encopresis)

Frequency of urination (≥ 8 or ≤ 3 per day are abnormal)

Urinary or fecal urgency

Child discomfort (anxiety, abdominal pain, dysuria, pain with defecation)

Quality of urination (unusual posturing, straining, poor urine stream, presence of dribbling)

Stool size and consistency

Presence of concurrent encopresis or enuresis

Pattern of fluid intake

Sleeping habits and arrangement

Sleep quality (snoring, insomnia, sleepwalking)

Family history of enuresis (including when it resolved)

Method of toilet-training (punishments/rewards)

Developmental history (including motor and language delays)

Secondary sexual characteristics

Psychological stressors (recent death, parental divorce, bullying, abuse, changes in the home, birth of sibling, recent injury, hospitalization, etc.)

Concurrent mental health disorder (depression, anxiety, attention-deficit hyperactivity disorder, etc.)

Current medications

Substance use (caffeine, alcohol, opioids, others)

Medical history (illness, past surgeries)

Prior treatment for enuresis (what has been tried, successes/failures, duration of past treatment)

---

sleepwalking may be revealing. The presence of constipation and encopresis, the developmental history (including a history of language/motor delays), and secondary sex characteristics may also aid in the diagnosis. Recent stressors (death of someone close to them, parental divorce, abuse/bullying, new school/home/sibling/caregiver, recent hospitalization/injury) should be determined. Questions regarding symptoms of a mental health disorder (ADHD, anxiety, depression, etc.), use of medications/caffeine/alcohol/illicit substances, current and previous medical ailments/surgeries, previous successes/failures of treatments for enuresis, and duration of treatments will also prove useful during the evaluation process.

A parent might say, "We've tried everything." However, this is rarely the case. Having them list the treatments and duration of each treatment is important in assessing whether the trial was of adequate duration.

When possible, a parent should complete an enuresis frequency/volume calendar for the 2 weeks preceding the intake appointment. Urine volume can be measured by weighing the diapers (and clothes/sheets if necessary). Not infrequently, keeping this 2-week calendar results in an improvement or resolution of symptoms. If enuresis is only occurring during school days/nights, this can help clarify the etiology.

As part of the history, one should assess the child's mental status. What is the child's level of distress concerning enuresis? What views and misconceptions do the parents and child have? At the beginning of the interview (so as not to skew their answer toward enuresis) ask the child, "If I gave you three wishes, what would you wish for? Bearing in mind that you can wish for things to have, but you can also wish for things to change." This may give some insight into how impairing the child finds her or his enuresis to be.

The primary care physician's comprehensive physical exam will focus on a neurological exam – including gait abnormalities, general strength testing, deep tendon reflexes (DTRs) (with special focus on the ankle reflexes), and coordination/motor/sensory functions at the ankles and feet because their neural loops enter the sacral cord in close proximity to the neural loops for the bladder and rectum.

A throat/neck exam evaluates tonsils and thyroid. The skin exam includes looking for tufts of hair and cutaneous lesions over the sacrum, a sacral dimple, and/or asymmetric gluteal cleft (the latter being suggestive of spinal dysraphism). During the abdominal exam, one should palpate for masses/large amounts of stool/discomfort). The rectal exam assesses for fecal impaction. A genital exam completes the physical examination.

It is suggested that all children with newly diagnosed enuresis should have a blood draw including a basic metabolic panel (BMP) to evaluate sodium (Na), glucose, blood urea nitrogen (BUN), and creatinine (Cr). The BMP can help determine if diabetes is an underlying etiology. If there is an acute onset of polyuria, the cause of enuresis may be diabetes mellitus (and in some cases a hemoglobin A1C (HbA1c) is indicated). The urinalysis (UA, mid-stream) helps to evaluate glucose and specific gravity, and to rule out a UTI and hematuria. It is recommended to do the UA first thing in the morning to accurately assess specific gravity at this time. This can help to predict a response to desmopressin (especially if specific gravity is below 1.015). A thyroid stimulating hormone (TSH) level is sometimes warranted.

While some have recommended a genitourinary (GU) system ultrasound scan for all children meeting diagnostic criteria for enuresis, this is not the current standard of care. Nonetheless, there are still clear instances where a consult to a pediatric urologist and an ultrasound of the GU system are indicated. This is particularly the case if there are recurrent UTIs or there is also a diurnal component (daytime wetting). The ultrasound may discover a thick bladder wall. This may indicate detrusor hypertrophy and overactivity. A thin bladder wall may indicate areflexia and urinary retention. Other studies may include a voiding cystourethrogram and a renal ultrasound.

Further evaluation might include a pediatric neurology consultation (including an electroencephalogram (EEG) if an underlying seizure disorder is suspected).

A sleep study may also be indicated if there is suspicion of a sleep disorder such as OSA. If OSA is then confirmed, a surgical consultation may be pursued. While there are mixed conclusions about whether a tonsillectomy and adenoidectomy (T&A) can be curative of nocturnal enuresis, there certainly are individual cases where a resolution of enuretic symptoms has occurred following a T&A. Conversely, surgery for urinary outflow tract problems is rarely recommended, but females with an ectopic ureter may benefit from surgical intervention.

Physical exam findings and laboratory results can help guide treatments and referrals. Given that psychological conditions (such as anxiety, depression, and ADHD) are frequently comorbid with enuresis, pediatricians often make referrals to mental health professionals.

Treatment Approach

Regrettably, 68% of children with clinical enuresis never see a physician for this disorder. For those who do present for evaluation, treatment can generally be thought of as comprising five categories: (i) education; (ii) watchful waiting; (iii) nonpharmacological management (including behavioral modification such as the bell and pad); (iv) medication management; and (v) other interventions (including psychodynamic psychotherapy, CBT, and acupuncture) (see Table 18.3).

With a 15% annual spontaneous remission rate, there are instances where a family may choose watchful waiting. This may be an appropriate modality in some cases. For those families that choose this option, it is the role of the clinician to educate the patient and parents about the natural history, available treatments, and prognosis for enuresis. When appropriate, emphasizing that it's not the patient's fault can be extraordinarily beneficial. Sometimes it is not until the evaluation that a child learns that Mom and Dad also struggled with

Table 18.3 Interventions for enuresis.

Advice/education
Reviewing and correcting parental expectations
Waiting until the child is ready for potty training
Ensuring there is no teasing/shame given for failures
Limiting caffeine and dairy products in evening hours
Limiting nighttime, but not daytime fluid intake
Nonpharmacological interventions (behavioral modifications)
Bell and pad
Ultrasonic bladder-volume alarm
Calendar chart noting frequency of enuresis
Pharmacological interventions
Nocturnal enuresis
Desmopressin [FDA indicated]
Imipramine [FDA indicated]
Other TCAs (desipramine, amitriptyline, nortriptyline)
SSRIs
Methylphenidate, dextroamphetamine
Indomethacin
Mesterolone
Diurnal enuresis
Oxybutynin [FDA indicated]
Tolterodine
Hyoscyamine
Terodiline
Propantheline
Methylphenidate
Other nonpharmacological interventions
Cognitive behavioral therapy (CBT)
Psychodynamic psychotherapy
Biofeedback
Acupuncture

continence. This normalization of their difficulties can alleviate some anxiety.

For those families that wish to pursue treatment, an analysis of the underlying etiology/etiologies will help determine which modalities will be the most successful. If there is an obvious underlying medical condition (diabetes, sleep apnea, hyperthyroidism, etc.), the first step is to treat that disorder appropriately. Surgery may be indicated to correct the following: ectopic ureter, neurogenic bladder, bladder calculus, and possibly T&A (for OSA). Surgery might be required in the removal of a foreign body that is causing obstruction and/or a UTI.

If there is no underlying general medical condition, then the clinician must assess whether a pharmacological approach is more appropriate than a non-pharmacological approach. In general, nonpharmacological approaches (such as the bell and pad) require a lot of time and familial effort. However, where there is motivation, the bell and pad has the best success rate (with the lowest relapse rate of all modalities). Yet, the bell and pad takes time. Parents who lack the motivation required for the bell and pad will often opt for pharmacological management. Also, when there is a need for a rapid cure (sleepover or camp), then this is usually a clear indication for medication.

Advice/Education

The first step in the treatment of enuresis is education. While discussing etiology, course, treatments, and prognosis, a clinician should review basic principles.

Advice can be curative. A clinician can reduce a family's guilt, anxiety, and frustration by:

(1) Reminding children that it is not their fault.
(2) Teaching parents that it takes time and that most children eventually achieve continence.
(3) Educating parents not to punish the child for enuresis.
(4) Reminding parents to be optimistic, but realistic (since there is no quick cure).
(5) Warning parents about the potential for relapse.

In order to give sound advice, it is beneficial to review what parents may have already heard or read. *What to Expect: The Toddler Years* recommends starting toilet training when the child signals her or his readiness. Summer is often an easier time of year to begin (since there are fewer clothes to remove), but if a child is signaling readiness in the winter, then winter it is. Parents should also teach children to learn to monitor their body signals (hunger, urination, defecation). Good behavior is best encouraged with small rewards such as stickers. Using potty training targets that children can aim at is often beneficial [26].

The book also contains a list of dos and don'ts of toddler toilet training. These include the following:

- Don't expect too much too soon (some children will achieve continence later than others and it does not occur overnight).
- Don't deny daytime fluids.
- Don't force the issue.
- Don't be a broken record.
- Don't turn toileting into a moral issue (e.g., "good boys don't wet the bed").
- Don't scold, punish, or shame.
- Don't discuss progress/regressions in front of the child.
- Don't take slow progress personally.
- Don't give up hope.

If the child is not ready for potty training, then it might be wise to put a hold on training until they demonstrate an interest. Ninety-nine percent of children will eventually figure it out.

Practical daily advice for the enuretic child begins with an understanding of fluid intake. A parent should not limit fluids during the day. A parent needs to know how much the child is drinking at school. If a child is too timid to ask to go to the bathroom, then they might decide to drink less during the day. This might lead them to drink more at night (causing nocturnal enuresis). Having the teacher discreetly remind the child to use the restroom might be a simple cure. Babysitters and daycare providers may not be giving enough fluids.

While limiting daytime fluid intake is not advised, limiting nighttime fluid intake does have a role. All fluids should be withheld 1 hour before bed. Dairy products (due to the potential for osmotic diuresis) should be stopped 4 hours before bed. Due to its long half-life, caffeine use should be limited to morning use. Some recommend limiting carbonated beverages and drinks high in citrus. All children should be encouraged to urinate before bed. A hallway nightlight can encourage the child to find the bathroom in the middle of the night. If the bathroom is far from the child's room, it might be beneficial to place a potty chair in his or her room. Parents should not allow siblings to tease the patient. The child should help in the cleaning/changing of soiled linens. Overall, the parents should remind the child that bedwetting is not his or her fault.

There are other cases of incontinence where simple but practical advice can be curative. Girls sometimes need to be reminded of ways in which to prevent recurrent UTIs (including wiping front to back). When there is daytime postvoid incontinence, it typically occurs in an overweight female who has vaginal reflux caused by an improper voiding posture. Simply telling her to keep her knees apart while urinating (instead of holding her legs together) is typically curative.

Nonpharmacological Interventions

The most common and most successful nonpharmacological intervention is the bell and pad. This behavioral modification technique relies on both classical conditioning and operant conditioning. The child typically sleeps on a pad (or has it affixed to their clothing). When the child begins to urinate, a sensor within the pad triggers an alarm (typically an audible alarm, but it may also be a vibratory alarm).

From a classical conditioning perspective, after repeated use of the bell and pad, the distention of the bladder and the sense to urinate become associated with the auditory signal. This leads to waking (the conditioned response). From an operant conditioning perspective, the child views the alarm as a punishment (which may awaken others in the house as well). The child therefore seeks to avoid triggering the alarm [2].

It typically takes several months for the bell and pad method to work. One month of dry nights is considered success. Studies indicate a success rate of 80–90% with the bell and pad if families stick with it. However, 48% of families prematurely terminate. When success is achieved, relapse rate approaches 40%. In those with a relapse, a reintroduction of the bell and pad can be recommended [27–29].

If the bell and pad has the best efficacy and lowest remission rate of all treatment modalities, then why is it not used more often? The answer is that some families find that it is expensive, time consuming, requires a lot of motivation on the part of the parents and the child, is cumbersome, and that some children may find it embarrassing (especially if parents require them to take it to sleepovers or siblings tease) [30].

When the child and the family can remain compliant with the bell and pad, success is frequently achieved. Failure often results where there is a lack of motivation on the part of parents and/or child. Other negative prognostic factors include: (i) elevated familial stress levels related to enuresis; and (ii) significant behavioral disturbance in the child.

The bell and pad method has been around for more than 100 years. In 1904, Pfaundler developed an alarm system that indicated when a child needed changing. Mowrer and Mowrer's publication in 1938 marked a significant contribution to the treatment of nocturnal enuresis in the United States [31]. The basic design of today's bell-and-pad systems closely resembles the design from Mowrer and Mowrer. Today, the bell and pad is commercially available at many pharmacies and from websites such as bedwettingstore.com and pottymd.com.

Although these systems typically cost between $60 and $100, many families find this to be a significant barrier (since these systems are not covered by private insurance or Medicaid). Understandably, there are some accessories to the units that require replacement. While some believe that the bell and pad can be cost-prohibitive, one study calculated the yearly cost of untreated bedwetting to be approximately 1000 USD. Parents may invest in waterproof mattress pads and covers, nighttime pull-up diapers, absorbable underwear (for sleepovers), and stain removers. It should be noted here that insurance companies sometimes pay for nighttime pull-ups if the child has mental retardation (MR)/autism with enuresis. Parents find this beneficial since some MR children may never be able to achieve continence. Overall, bedwetting can have many economic consequences including increased laundry and decreased parental sleep, thus affecting parents' work.

Another behavioral modification technique is the ultrasonic bladder-volume alarm. This is worn by the child. It senses when the bladder is nearing capacity. This has the added advantage of alerting the child before they wet.

As mentioned above, a simple calendar used for charting the frequency of enuretic symptoms can reduce symptoms. A star chart system is sometimes beneficial. Under this model, a child earns a star for each dry night. Some advocates recommend rewarding the child when certain levels have been achieved. While this provides a cure for only a small percentage of children, it is noninvasive and it also helps significantly in the tracking and reporting of symptoms.

Nightlifting (taking the child to the toilet in a semi-sleep state) has not been found to have good efficacy. Timed night awakening (such as every 2 hours) can be beneficial, but it requires significant parental investment. Conversely, as a treatment for diurnal enuresis, timed trips to the restroom are effective (with the simple investment in a digital watch with a countdown timer). Bladder training exercises are generally not very effective. Overlearning (by drinking a large amount of fluid and holding it as long as possible) can be effective, but this is often regarded as unpleasant and is therefore not recommended.

Pharmacological Interventions

The benefit of medications for enuresis is that they can work quickly. This can be beneficial for sleepovers and camp. If so desired, they can be used for these discrete periods of time or longer. Of the medications, only desmopressin and imipramine have US Food and Drug Administration (FDA) indications for the treatment of nocturnal enuresis in children. They are relatively ineffective in the treatment of diurnal enuresis. Conversely, oxybutynin (which has an FDA indication for overactive bladder in children) can be effective in the treatment of diurnal enuresis, but it has little to no effect in most cases of nocturnal enuresis. However, there may be cases when a combination of desmopressin and oxybutynin is indicated.

In addition to desmopressin and imipramine, a number of other medications have been successfully utilized in the treatment of nocturnal enuresis. These include: other tricyclic antidepressants (TCAs), SSRIs, psychostimulants, indometacin (a nonsteroidal anti-inflammatory drug, or NSAID), and mesterolone (an androgenic steroid).

Diurnal enuresis (as indicated above) can be treated with oxybutynin (an anticholinergic agent). Additionally, other anticholinergics and doxazosin (an alpha-adrenergic blocker) are also useful.

Methylphenidate is the only medication that has been found to have efficacy for giggle incontinence. For all medications, a tapering-off during discontinuation is recommended.

Nocturnal Enuresis

Desmopressin (DDAVP) is typically regarded as the first-line agent in the treatment of primary nocturnal enuresis. This is (at least in part) due to its more favorable safety profile compared with TCAs. Success rates with desmopressin range from 10% to 65% (with a relapse rate as high as 80%) [29–32].

Desmopressin is a long-acting synthetic form of argi-nine vasopressin (AVP) (also known as antidiuretic hormone, or ADH). AVP is produced in the hypothala-mus and stored in the posterior pituitary. While some AVP is released directly into the brain, most is released into the bloodstream. From there, it travels to the kidney where it acts on V2 receptors in the collecting ducts and distal tubules, causing them to take up free water (there-by reducing urine output).

Desmopressin (synthetic AVP) acts in the same way to reduce urine output. After administration, it takes ap-proximately 1 hour to reach efficacy, so it should be administered 2 hours before bed. The child should stop drinking 1 hour before administration of desmo-pressin (3 hours before bed) (and the child should not drink for at least 8 hours following its administration). Its duration of action is 10–12 hours. There is often a compensatory polyuria the next day when its effect has worn off.

Long-term use of desmopressin has not been associ-ated with a depression of endogenous AVP secretion. The general recommendation is to take desmopressin for 6 months and then stop for 2 months to see if a cure has been affected.

Desmopressin comes in an oral formulation. This medication can be crushed for easy administration in those children with pill-swallowing difficulties. In chil-dren older than 6 years of age, the typical starting dose is 0.2 mg by mouth at night. The maximum recommended FDA dose is 0.6 mg by mouth at night.

The intranasal formulation lost FDA approval for nocturnal enuresis in 2007 due to concerns regarding safety. There were reports of hyponatremia leading to seizures in some individuals using intranasal desmopres-sin. In two cases, the patients died (although a direct connection between the deaths and desmopressin was reported to be unclear) [33, 34].

While the oral formulation has retained its FDA indication, the recommendation is for monitoring of the patient's sodium level due to concerns of hypona-tremia. Further recommendations include withholding the medication during acute illnesses that may lead to fluid and/or electrolyte imbalances. If the patient has hyponatremia (or a history of hyponatremia), the use of desmopressin is contraindicated/cautioned. Younger children who are early in treatment with desmopressin are at the greatest risk for hyponatremia. While this is a concern, the risk is reportedly low, and desmopressin remains an effective treatment.

In addition to desmopressin, the only other medica-tion with an FDA indication for nocturnal enuresis in children is imipramine (a TCA). Imipramine (brand-name Tofranil) was a mainstay of treatment before desmopressin gained FDA approval. Cure rates range from 40% to 60%. As many as 80–90% may show some improvement in symptoms. Relapse is as high as 50% [21, 35, 36].

While it is accepted that desmopressin treats noctur-nal enuresis by a single mechanism (acting as a synthetic form of AVP), imipramine's effects are many. This might be one reason for its better overall success rate than desmopressin. As a TCA, it helps to treat comorbid anxiety and depression. Since it is also quite anticholin-ergic, it may therefore mediate relaxation of the bladder detrusor muscle. It also increases sphincter tone. Beyond this, imipramine also increases AVP release (thereby causing free water retention). A final proposed mecha-nism is that imipramine increases brain arousal during sleep and acts to suppress rapid eye movement (REM) sleep (making it easier for the child to awaken). These many actions work together to make imipramine effec-tive in the treatment of many of the causes of nocturnal enuresis. With so many mechanisms (including anticho-linergic effects), TCAs may show some efficacy in the treatment of diurnal enuresis as well.

Because of its multiple mechanisms of actions, a trial of imipramine may be warranted if a child fails to respond with desmopressin. An added benefit is that imipramine also has efficacy in the treatment of ADHD. As we have mentioned earlier, there is a high comorbid-ity between nocturnal enuresis and ADHD.

Interestingly, the amount of imipramine needed to treat nocturnal enuresis is often less than that needed to treat depression. Regarding treatment with imipramine, nocturnal enuresis also improves faster than depression.

The typical starting dose for a 6–12-year-old (for the treatment of nocturnal enuresis) is 10 mg by mouth at bedtime. The maximum dose is listed as 50 mg per night. For children older than 12 years of age, the starting dose is the same (10 mg), but the maximum FDA-recommended dose is listed as 75 mg by mouth per night.

The real problem with all TCAs is their side-effect profile and potential lethality in overdose. First, there is imipramine's black-box warning for increased suicidality risk in children, adolescents, and young adults with major depressive disorder or other psychiatric disorders. One must weigh the risk versus benefits since the medication can be deadly in overdose. While the concern is that a patient might intentionally overdose, there is also significant concern for accidental overdoses. Children, after all, often have magical thinking. "If two pills make me better tonight, then the whole bottle will cure me." There may also be younger children in the home who believe the medication is candy. There are reported cases of both instances leading to accidental death.

In overdose, the "Tri-Cs" of tricyclics are not uncommon. These are cardiac dysrhythmias, convulsions, and coma. Death may be the ultimate consequence. Even when taken appropriately, side effects are many. Roughly 10% of patients will have side effects. TCAs are anticholinergic [37]. Drowsiness, dry mouth, dizziness, constipation, difficulty starting urine stream, blurred vision, and palpitations are only a few of the common reactions that may occur. The mnemonic for anticholinergic syndrome is "red as a beet, dry as a bone, blind as a bat, mad as a hatter, and hot as a hare." The mnemonic refers to flushing, dry skin/mucous membranes, mydriasis with a loss of accommodation, altered mental status, and fever.

Before starting a TCA, a baseline electrocardiogram (ECG) is recommended. Due to the blackbox warning, close follow-up is also indicated. When imipramine is effective, most recommend that the medication be continued for 4–6 months before a taper is initiated. If symptoms return during the taper, simply increase the dose again and restart the taper at a later time.

While they might not have FDA indications for nocturnal enuresis in children, other TCAs (specifically desipramine, amitriptyline, and nortriptyline) are often effective as well.

SSRIs also lack an FDA indication for enuresis, but they can be effective. There are case reports where SSRIs have made nocturnal enuresis better and others where it caused nocturnal enuresis (or made symptoms worse).

Methylphenidate (Ritalin) and dextroamphetamine (Adderall) are best used in combination with behavioral therapy (bell and pad) for the treatment of nocturnal enuresis. The proposed mechanism is that they may reduce the depth of sleep thereby allowing the child to more easily awaken to the sense of a full bladder.

Further down the treatment algorithm are: indometacin (an NSAID) and mesterolone (an androgenic steroid). Both have showed some success. Indomethacin's proposed mechanism of action is that it enhances the effects of AVP.

Diurnal Enuresis

Anticholinergics are rarely effective for nocturnal enuresis, but they often do have efficacy for diurnal enuresis. Among them, only one currently has an FDA indication for children. This medication (oxybutynin) has an indication for overactive bladder.

Oxybutynin (brandnames: Ditropan, Ditropan XL, and Urotrol) is an anticholinergic agent. It relaxes bladder smooth muscle and inhibits involuntary detrusor muscle contractions. It comes in both tablet and liquid formulations. The starting dose for the immediate-release formulation (in children with overactive bladder who are older than 5 years) is 5 mg by mouth twice per day. For children ages 1 to 5, the starting dose is 0.2 mg/kg by mouth twice daily. The maximum dose for all children is a total of 15 mg per day. The extended-release form can be initiated (in children older than 6 years of age) at a dose of 5 mg by mouth once per day. The maximum dose is 20 mg per day. Even though anticholinergics are rarely effective for nocturnal enuresis, some children who fail desmopressin may respond to oxybutynin.

Tolterodine (brandnames Detrol and Detrol LA), hyoscyamine, terodiline, and propantheline are other anticholinergics that have some demonstrated efficacy due to their antispasmodic effects on smooth muscle. Doxazosin (brandname Cardura) (an alpha-adrenergic blocker) has also been useful in some cases of diurnal enuresis. Methylphenidate is the only reported treatment with efficacy for giggle incontinence.

Overall, combination therapy is sometimes indicated. This can take the form of behavioral modification plus medication (quicker to dry) or two medications (especially if a child has enuresis with multiple etiologies). Again, one example of this is desmopressin plus oxybutynin.

Other Treatments

Cognitive behavioral therapy and psychodynamic psychotherapy can significantly help secondary enuresis (especially when the cause is a psychological stressor). There is benefit in mentally practicing the routine of bladder continence (while addressing cognitive distortions).

Biofeedback (which is essentially pelvic floor physical therapy) can be advantageous. Kegel exercises may strengthen the pelvic floor musculature.

Acupuncture (especially over the sacral area where innervation for the bladder is) can be helpful, although the jury is still out [38]. [39], Dry bed training also has its supporters and detractors. There is also currently no empirical evidence to suggest the efficacy of hypnotherapy, dietary manipulation, or desensitization to allergens in the treatment of enuresis.

Course and Prognosis

Untreated, the yearly spontaneous remission rate for nocturnal enuresis is 15%. Behavioral and medication interventions can be curative. Treatment allows children to more easily participate in camps, sleepovers, and begin dating. Given the potential long-term ramifications of nocturnal enuresis, parents should seriously consider intervention by age 5. Some prefer to wait until age 6 or 7.

In the United States, 25% of children are punished for bedwetting. Parents with less education are more likely to discipline. Punishments often make symptoms of enuresis worse and the duration of symptoms longer. As indicated earlier, it is usually not bedwetting itself, but the reactions of parents, siblings, peers, and the child that determine whether a child's bedwetting has enduring implications. Bullies, teasing, and ostracizing by peers can make childhood a lonely and anxiety-filled experience.

Erikson noted that this is a time of Autonomy versus Shame and Doubt. By the end of toddlerhood, the successful child has achieved a mastery of elimination. A sense of autonomy arises out of this control of bodily sensations. When there is a failure to achieve continence, there may be mental health implications. Failure can lead the child to wonder if he or she is capable of meeting future challenges. Anxiety may arise from this. Some have postulated that obsessive-compulsive personality disorder (OCPD) has its origins here.

MacDonald and others have noted that a domino effect may lead from bedwetting to sociopathic behavior. However, in spite of peer taunting and parental abuse, many children who have suffered from some level of bedwetting do not meet criteria for anxiety, depression, or a personality disorder in adulthood. However, although they might not meet criteria for a disorder, many are still haunted by childhood bedwetting on some level. This underscores the importance of appropriate treatment.

CASE EXAMPLE 1

Brian, a 5-year old boy, is brought to his pediatrician for his well-child check and immunizations. A questionnaire of current symptoms reveals that he still regularly wets the bed at night. His parents express frustration and embarrassment that their 5-year-old is still not fully toilet trained. The pediatrician notes that the parents so far have tried a reward system by giving Brian stickers to place in a calendar chart each morning that he is dry. She also finds that they mark failures with a big sad-face on days that he is not. Though the parents push for medication treatment, an initial approach is taken where the pediatrician explains the need for positive reinforcement. It is then revealed that the child has been restricting water intake during the day in response to the shame he feels with his failures. This led him to drink more in the evening, compounding the problem. The parents eliminate their criticism based on the advice of the pediatrician and instead focus on his successes. After several weeks, they noted a marked improvement in his nocturnal symptoms.

CASE EXAMPLE 2

Nancy is a 7-year-old girl who is brought to her pediatrician by an exasperated mother. She had never had problems with enuresis as a young child, but 2 months ago she started to consistently wet the bed at night. In addition, she recently began to have accidents during the daytime, and has recently had two at school that led to significant teasing by her peers. Nancy, through tears, expresses that she does not want to return to school for fear of another accident. In gathering further history it is revealed that her mother recently returned to work due to financial stress in the home, and that her symptoms seemed to coincide with this change. Given Nancy's level of anxiety related to her mother's return to work (including concerns about family finances) and concerns about bullying and being ostracized at school, a combination therapy was recommended. Desmopressin was initiated and a referral to a psychologist was placed. The combination successfully treated both her daytime and nighttime incontinence. After several months the medication was discontinued, although Nancy continued to work with her therapist for continuing anxiety symptoms.

Encopresis

Of the elimination disorders, enuresis is the more common; however, encopresis may be more impairing and may have more enduring consequences. While watchful waiting may be a viable treatment alternative for enuresis, it is not for encopresis.

As mentioned above, the typical progression in toilet training is for bowel continence to be achieved before urinary continence. When bowel continence is not achieved by the age of 4, a diagnosis of encopresis may be made based upon DSM-IV-TR classification.

Encopresis is defined as the repeated passage of feces in inappropriate places (usually undergarments). This soiling is typically regarded as involuntary, although it may also be volitional. The etiology may be physiological and/or psychological.

Fecal incontinence due to medications and/or a general medical condition cannot be defined as encopresis according to the DSM-IV-TR unless constipation is involved. Some cases of encopresis persist into adulthood. Even though this chapter focuses on childhood elimination disorders, a brief mention of bowel incontinence in later life is valuable. While fecal incontinence becomes more common in the elderly population (for a variety of reasons), it is never considered a normal part of aging.

Definitions

Encopresis comes from the Greek word "kopros" meaning dung or feces. As with enuresis, the delineation between primary and secondary encopresis has value. *Primary encopresis* is soiling in a child who has never gained bowel continence for 6 months or more. *Secondary encopresis* is soiling in a child who had previously acquired bowel control. When secondary encopresis is due to psychological stress, it is sometimes termed *regressive encopresis*.

Encopresis according to the DSM-IV-TR is also broken into two categories: retentive and nonretentive. *Retentive encopresis* is also referred to as

encopresis "with Constipation and Overflow Incontinence." *Nonretentive encopresis* is therefore also known as encopresis "without Constipation and Overflow Incontinence."

Unlike enuresis, encopresis rarely occurs during sleep. When it does, it is usually a poor prognostic indicator.

Prevalence

By the age of 4 years, 95% of children have achieved bowel continence. As is true with bladder continence, boys tend to lag behind girls. More boys therefore meet diagnostic criteria for encopresis. Between the ages of 7 and 8, prevalence is reported to be 1.5%, with a 3:1 male to female ratio [2, 38].

Retentive encopresis (constipation with overflow incontinence) represents 80–95% of cases overall. Nonretentive encopresis comprises the remaining cases. Secondary encopresis (50–60%) is slightly more common than primary encopresis.

One study reported some degree of fecal incontinence in 9.8% of first graders and 5.6% of fourth graders. Although most did not meet full criteria for encopresis, isolated incidents can still have significant consequences (embarrassment and anxiety) and may lead to teasing/bullying [40].

Diagnostic Criteria

Criteria for encopresis according to the DSM-IV-TR include: [12]

- Repeated passage of feces into inappropriate places (e.g., clothing or floor) whether involuntary or intentional.
- At least one such event a month for at least 3 months.
- Chronological age of at least 4 years (or equivalent developmental level).
- Behavior that is not due exclusively to the direct physiological effects of a substance (e.g., laxatives) or a general medical condition except through a mechanism involving constipation.

Two subtypes are specified, with separate codes: With Constipation and Overflow Incontinence (787.6), with evidence of constipation on physical examination or a history of a stool frequency of less than three per week; and Without Constipation and Overflow Incontinence (307.7),with no evidence of constipation on physical examination or by history. Currently, no revisions for encopresis are being considered for inclusion in the DSM-V.

Etiology and Differential Diagnosis

As indicated above, bowel incontinence may be related to: a delay in the maturation of the elimination system; an underlying medical condition, a psychological or behavioral issue, and/or constipation.

Among the causes of bowel incontinence are: anismus (spastic pelvic floor syndrome), irritable bowel syndrome (IBS), rectal hypersensitivity, spinal cord trauma/injury, diarrheal diseases, Hirschsprung disease, chronic laxative use, pain medication use (such as Vicodin, which can slow gastrointestinal (GI) motility), lead poisoning, hypothyroidism, hypokalemia, hypercalcemia, diabetes, intestinal smooth muscle disorders (such as scleroderma), toilet phobia, and developmental delays.

When there is an underlying medical condition – e.g., spinal cord injury, *Clostridium difficile* (c-diff colitis, etc.) – causing bowel incontinence, a diagnosis of encopresis cannot be made according to DSM-IV-TR criteria (except through a mechanism involving constipation).

Since retentive encopresis (constipation with overflow incontinence) represents 80–95% of cases of encopresis, we will focus primarily on this mechanism here. Constipation may occur by a variety of methods. Children with constipation generally have infrequent bowel movements, large stools, and difficult and/or painful defecation. Often constipation is self-limited. However, a domino effect may occur leading eventually to encopresis.

The domino effect begins with the cause of constipation. The longer that stool is retained in the intestines, the more water is reabsorbed. With enough time, the stool becomes hard. This can make the passage of stool painful. In an effort to avoid this painful experience, the child withholds (delays bowel movements). Each painful stooling may cause the child to delay the next bowel movement for as long as possible in an effort to avoid the next painful experience. Unfortunately, this effort causes the next stool to become hardened. A cycle emerges as each painful stooling causes the next. The stool may eventually become too large to pass through the anus. The bowel may also distend as stool accumulates. With time, this may result in the child losing the ability to sense a full bowel. As stool continues to accumulate, liquid stool may leak around this blockage and cause soiling (encopresis with constipation and overflow incontinence). Breaking the cycle is key in the treatment of retentive encopresis.

Overall, the causes of constipation are many. Both poor fluid intake and poor nutrition (including insufficient fiber in the diet) are common causes of constipation. A child may also be anxious to use a public restroom. Other causes of constipation (including medications) have been listed above.

While enuresis and encopresis are often comorbid, one is advised against using TCAs in retentive encopresis (when encopresis is due to constipation with overflow incontinence). This is due to the fact that TCAs (and other medications with anticholinergic properties) can make constipation worse by slowing the GI tract. While TCAs may make retentive encopresis worse, TCAs are sometimes beneficial in the treatment of nonretentive encopresis (where there is no constipation).

The slow maturation of the elimination system is sometimes a significant cause of encopresis. This may make the child unable to retain feces at an age when most of their peers have attained control of their bowels (age 4). This delayed physical maturation is a common cause of primary retentive encopresis. Primary retentive encopresis is also sometimes the result of problematic and overly-harsh toilet training. This can take many forms including: starting training too early, forcing the child to sit on the toilet for very extended periods of time, and physical punishments/ridicule for failures.

Even when parents recognize that the child may not yet be ready for toilet training, they may nonetheless force the issue since keeping a child in diapers can be expensive. Additionally, the child may need to have some level of continence before a babysitter will consent to watch her or him. When parents need a child to be continent so that they can work, the economic pressure is clear. Conversely, some neglectful parents may never begin the process of potty training. These problematic toilet training experiences can cause the child significant anxiety leading to toilet phobia in some cases.

A parent's responses to elimination do not go unnoticed by the child. The young child may have difficulty flushing away the bowel movement because he is proud of his accomplishment. He had worked hard to use the toilet correctly, but now it must be discarded. He might also sense this flushing away of his feces as a loss of an important part of himself. Parents can aid their children in this process by praising them and waving goodbye as the toilet is flushed. A parent should not react in disgust to a child's bowel movement.

When parents attempt to control all facets of a child's life, the child may soon discover that he can withhold or deposit feces inappropriately. This may be conscious or unconscious, but the effect is the same: the child engages the parent in a battle over control of his or her own internal body processes. Therefore parental reactions can determine whether or not the child becomes successful with continence. Ultimately, the child who can master elimination further develops a sense of autonomy (that he or she can accomplish tasks and solve problems).

Secondary encopresis may arise in the face of new stressors (birth of a sibling, parental divorce, starting school, and/or sexual abuse). Bowel incontinence in response to the birth of a sibling or other stressors is considered regressive in nature.

Encopresis can be volitional in some cases. Children with oppositional defiant disorder (ODD) and conduct disorder (CD) may use soiling in inappropriate places as a form of retaliation and anger against parents and authority.

Many infants and very small children may find their feces interesting enough to smear it when given the opportunity. However, it has been our experience that most older children find this activity too repugnant to engage in. Among those older children who do engage in fecal smearing, many often have a diagnosis of MR/autism, psychosis, or RAD. While individuals with some Axis II pathology may engage in this behavior, it is certainly more rare. Some cases of fecal smearing may also result when an embarrassed child attempts to hide or clean up feces that were involuntarily passed. In many cases, the presence of fecal smearing can help to clarify the diagnosis.

Anal itching in children can have many causes including pinworms, yeast, hemorrhoids, diarrhea, irritants from foods (dairy products, spicy foods, nuts, caffeine), and genital warts (often from sexual trauma). Rectal digging is frequently associated with Prader–Willi syndrome.

Diagnostic Approach

Typically, the patient with encopresis presents to a primary care physician. The normal work-up consists of a history and physical, labs (when necessary), and appropriate referrals. Treatment is often indicated.

During the history-taking, the clinician seeks to learn: "Why now?" Why is the child being brought in now for evaluation and treatment? The clinician should also inquire about parental expectations.

The approach to history-taking is similar to that for enuresis (see Table 18.2). The history should focus on the following: child's age, onset of symptoms (primary/secondary), timing (occurring solely during the day/night/both or during school or play), and frequency of symptoms (number of soiling episodes per month). The location of soiling (clothes/on floor/etc.), overall frequency of bowel movements, stool size and consistency, melena/hematochezia, and presence of hemorrhoids are important factors.

A child's discomfort (anxiety, nausea/emesis, abdominal pain/distention, pain with defecation), fluid and dietary habits, height/weight (failure to thrive), presence of enuresis (due to a high comorbidity) [41], developmental history (including a history of language/motor delays), and secondary sex characteristics may help to direct treatment. Recent stressors (death of someone close to them, parental divorce, abuse, new school/home/sibling/caregiver) and symptoms of a mental health disorder (anxiety, depression, MR, autism, RAD, ODD, CD, etc.) may point toward a mental health referral. Current and previous medical ailments/surgeries, recent hospitalization/injury, current medications, use of alcohol and illicit substances, family history of constipation/encopresis (including when encopresis resolved), method of toilet training (rewards/punishments), previous successes/failures of treatments for encopresis, and duration of treatments will aid in the treatment of the encopretic child.

When possible, a parent should complete an encopresis frequency calendar to help clarify frequency and associated symptoms. As part of the history, one should assess mental status. What is the child's level of distress concerning encopresis? At the beginning of the interview (so as not to bias a child's answer toward encopresis) ask the child, "If I gave you three wishes, what would you wish for?" What views and misconceptions do the parents and child have?

The primary care physician's comprehensive physical exam will focus on a neurological exam – including gait abnormalities, general strength testing, DTRs, and (more specifically) ankle reflexes and coordination/motor/sensory functions at the ankles and feet because these neural loops enter the sacral cord in close proximity to the neural loops for the bladder and rectum. A skin exam includes looking for tufts of hair and cutaneous lesions over the sacrum, a sacral dimple, flat buttocks (may indicate sacral agenesis), and an asymmetric gluteal cleft (possibly suggestive of spinal dysraphism). The abdominal exam palpates for masses/large amounts of stool/discomfort. The rectal exam assesses rectal tone and the presence of fecal impaction.

A BMP to check glucose, potassium, and calcium levels is sometimes recommended. An abdominal X-ray may be beneficial during both the initial evaluation (to look for fecal impaction) and during treatment (to assess progress). Collecting stool for fecal fat, ova, parasites, and white blood cells is sometimes helpful in ruling out malabsorption and infection. Hemoccult testing may also be indicated. Rectal biopsy, anal manometry, and a barium enema are helpful if Hirschsprung disease is suspected. A TSH assay is warranted if one suspects hypothyrodism (since this can cause constipation).

Lead levels may also be indicated in some cases. If cystic fibrosis is suspected, then a sweat chloride is indicated. Tissue transglutaminase IgA may be elevated in celiac disease. Pelvic floor electromyography can assess pelvic floor functioning. A colonoscopy is also sometimes recommended.

At the end of the initial evaluation, the primary care physician may treat and/or decide to refer the child to a pediatric gastroenterologist. The physician may also make a referral to a mental health professional given that psychological conditions (such as anxiety and depression) are sometimes comorbid with encopresis.

Treatment Approach

An empty bowel cannot soil. This is the foundation upon which most treatment protocols rest. The goal of treatment is for the child to have one to three stools per day (without soiling). Interventions for encopresis often include: education, nonpharmacological, and pharmacological modalities (Table 18.4). More specifically the list includes: dietary changes, behavioral strategies, biofeedback, psychotherapy, and medications. However, before discussing the treatment of encopresis, it is again important to underscore the value of the history and physical, lab testing, and imaging studies. When an identifiable organic cause can be determined, this should be treated appropriately (antibiotics, surgery, biofeedback, etc.).

Table 18.4 Interventions for encopresis.

Advice/education
Dietary changes (foods high in fiber)
Increased fluid intake
Make toilet training nonthreatening
Make the toilet easily accessible for the child
Regular bathroom times
Nonpharmacological
Behavior rewards (star chart, etc.)
Cognitive behavioral therapy (CBT)
Psychodynamic psychotherapy
Biofeedback
Acupuncture
Pharmacological interventions
Fiber supplements
Stool softeners (docusate and mineral oil)
Osmotic laxatives (polyethylene glycol-electrolyte solution (PEG), lactulose, glycerine)
Stimulant laxatives (senna and bisacodyl)
TCAs (for nonretentive encopresis)

Advice, Education, and Nonpharmacological Interventions

For encopresis, parental education, psychological interventions, and behavioral therapy are the gold standards of initial treatment. Increasing both fluid intake and dietary fiber is often an effective recommendation. Reducing intake of dairy, peanuts, and bananas may be beneficial. Older children should be encouraged to exercise more frequently to help promote bowel motility.

Foods that are high in fiber include: fruits, vegetables, nuts, bread, and cereals. Fiber supplements are also commercially available (including chewable fiber Gummi bears). Dairy products should be limited (but not eliminated).

For the toddler, parents should be taught how to make toilet-training nonthreatening. They should attempt to demystify the process for the child. The bathroom should be a place that is easily accessible to them and safe for them. Simple interventions such as placing a step-stool in the bathroom can greatly improve the process. This can improve access to the toilet, and it also provides the child with a support while straining. Star charts and small rewards (stickers) are sometimes recommended, whereas punishment/shaming are inappropriate and frequently harmful. One study found that the daily timed sitting (in conjunction with rewards for successes) showed a 78% success rate. Children should assist in the cleaning of soiled clothing. Experts warn that care must be taken so that this does not become "too harsh."

For the child with anxieties, a warm bath may help calm them and make bowel movements easier. The value of routine should not be discounted. Regular bathroom times are recommended. The best times are after meals. A child may sit on the toilet for up to 15 minutes after each meal. After breakfast is typically regarded as the time when the colon is programmed for defecation.

If there is a comorbid mental health disorder (anxiety, depression, etc.), then that disorder should also be addressed (whether it is the cause of encopresis or the product of encopresis). This is underscored by the fact that encopretic children with comorbid mental health disorders/behavioral problems often have poorer outcomes with toilet-training protocols. CBT and psychodynamic psychotherapy can help decrease symptoms of anxiety and depression associated with encopresis [42, 43].

Biofeedback can be beneficial in the treatment of pelvic floor dysfunction. It can also teach the child sphincter control. The combination of biofeedback with another modality can have added benefits.

Pharmacological Interventions

For children with retentive encopresis (constipation with overflow bowel incontinence), increased fluid intake is important. Dietary changes (high-fiber foods and fiber supplements), laxatives, suppositories, and enemas help to break the cycle. Osmotic laxatives – polyethylene glycol (PEG), lactulose, and glycerine – stimulant laxatives (senna and bisacodyl), and stool softeners (docusate and mineral oil) have proven efficacy.

Mineral oil may be given after meals. While it is important for all children to take a multivitamin, it is of particular importance here since mineral oil can limit the absorption of fat-soluble vitamins (vitamins A, D, E, and K) from the diet [44]. Mineral oil may take weeks to restore normal bowel function. Once bowel movements are regular, it may be discontinued in a tapered fashion. For those children with an aspiration risk, mineral oil is contraindicated.

In cases with impaction, either oral or rectal medications may be used in the process of disimpaction. Oral medications are the first-line agents. While rectal medications may act faster, they are also more invasive than oral medications. The rectal route (enemas) may therefore worsen the child's anxiety. Also, repeated phosphate enemas may negatively affect both water and electrolyte balances.

After fecal disimpaction, the use of maintenance laxatives may be required for months to years in order to prevent relapse. However, one should consider the risks associated with chronic laxative use.

There are some cases where TCAs (such as imipramine) have been modestly effective in the treatment of encopresis (usually in nonretentive encopresis). While cases of improvement with imipramine do exist, one must also remember that the anticholinergic effects of TCAs may cause constipation or make it worse.

Loperamide (an opioid receptor agonist) may also be beneficial in cases of nonretentive encopresis. However, it should be used only when other interventions have failed. It can increase anal sphincter pressure (thereby reducing bowel incontinence).

Other emerging medications include: prucalopride (a serotonin receptor agonist with enterokinetic properties) and lubiprostone (a selective chloride channel-2 activator that increases fluid secretion in the intestine).

Other Treatments

Some literature does exist regarding acupuncture and hypnotherapy in the treatment of encopresis. However, these treatment modalities have unproven efficacy.

Course and Prognosis

Compared with enuresis, the long-term prognosis of encopresis is not as well studied, although the prevalence of the disorder declines with age. Encopresis rarely extends into adulthood.

Symptoms may spontaneously resolve in some cases. Despite a significant rate of spontaneous resolution, watchful waiting is not recommended. When a child meets criteria for the disorder, treatment of some form should be sought. At the very least, education and behavioral modifications are recommended. As is the case with enuresis, the reactions of parents, siblings, peers, and the child strongly influence the level of anxiety/shame/self-doubt that the child experiences. These factors often greatly influence the symptom duration and severity.

Despite the efficacy of treatments, not all children are afforded the opportunity to be evaluated. One study from The Netherlands looked at 11–12-year-old children. Only 27% of children with encopretic symptoms had ever been taken to a physician for an evaluation of those symptoms. When encopresis is left untreated, children may experience shame and self-doubt. They may avoid certain activities (school, sports, and camp) for fear of having an episode of bowel incontinence. The long-term ramifications of untreated symptoms can lead to significant psychopathology (anxiety, depression) in adulthood.

Acknowledgement

The authors and editors respectfully acknowledge the contribution of Daniel J. Feeney to this chapter: Feeney DJ. Elimination disorders: enuresis and encopresis. In: Klykylo WM, Kay J (eds) *Clinical Child Psychiatry*, 2nd edn. John Wiley & Sons, Ltd, 2005; pp. 327–341.

References

1. Gemelli R. *Normal Child and Adolescent Development*. Washington, DC: American Psychiatric Press, 1996; pp. 125, 217–218.
2. Lucas CP, Shaffer D. Childhood disorders: elimination disorders and childhood anxiety disorders. In: Tasman A, Kay J, Lieberman JA, First MB, Maj M (eds) *Psychiatry*, 3rd edn. John Wiley & Sons, Ltd, 2008; pp. 868–879.
3. Fritz G, Rockney R, Bernet W, *et al*. Practice parameter for the assessment and treatment of children and adolescents with enuresis. *J Am Acad Child Adolesc Psychiatry* 2004;**43**:1540–1550.
4. Foxman B, Valdez RB, Brook RH. Childhood enuresis: Prevalence, perceived impact, and prescribed treatments. *Pediatrics* 1986;**77**:482–487.

5. Bienenfeld D. *Psychodynamic Theory for Clinicians.* Philadelphia, PA: Lippincott Williams & Wilkins, 2006; pp. 13–14 and 59–62.

6. Brenner C. *An Elementary Textbook of Psychoanalysis.* New York: International Universities Press, 1965; p. 26.

7. Forsythe WI, Redmond A. Enuresis and spontaneous cure rate. Study of 1129 enuretics. *Arch Dis Child* 1974;**49**: 259.

8. Macdonald JM. The threat to kill. *Am J Psychiatry* 1963;**120**:125–130.

9. Somers S. *Keeping Secrets.* Warner Books, Inc., 1991.

10. Glicklich LB. An historical account of enuresis. *Pediatrics* 1951;**8**:859.

11. Gill D., Enuresis through the ages. *Pediatr Nephrol* 1994; **9**:120–122.

12. American Psychiatric Association. *Diagnostic and Statistical Manual of Mental Disorders, Fourth Edition (Text Revision)* (DSM-IV-TR). Washington, DC: American Psychiatric Association, 2000; pp. 116–121.

13. Mathew JL. Evidence-based management of nocturnal enuresis: An overview of systematic reviews. *Indian Pediatr* 2010;**47**:777–780.

14. Nunes VD, O'Flynn N, Evans J, Sawyer L. Management of bedwetting in children and young people: Summary of NICE guidance. *Brit Med J* 2010;**341**:c5399.

15. American Psychiatric Association. DSM-5 development. L 00 Enuresis (Not Due to a General Medical Condition). Available at: www.dsm5.org/ProposedRevisions/Pages/proposedrevision.aspx?rid=117 [accessed 31 March 2011].

16. Arnell H, Hjalmas K, Jagerall M. The genetics of primary nocturnal enuresis: Inheritance and suggestion of a second major gene on chromosome 12q. *J Med Genet* 1997;**34**: 360–365.

17. Eiberg H, Berendt I, Mohr J. Assignment of dominant inherited nocturnal enuresis (ENUR 1) to chromosome 13q. *Nat Genet* 1995;**10**:354–356.

18. von Gontard A, Eiberg H, Hollmann E, Rittig S, Lehmkuhl G. Molecular genetics of nocturnal enuresis: Linkage to a locus on chromosome 22. *Scand J Urol Nephrol* 1999;**202**:76–80.

19. von Gontard A, Schaumburg H, Hollmann E, Eiberg H, Rittig S. The genetics of enuresis: A review. *J Urol* 2001;**166**:2438–2443.

20. Karabiber H, Garipardic M, Uzel M, *et al.* Hand grip and pinch strength in patients with nocturnal enuresis: Is there a role of muscle strength in pathogenesis of enuresis? *Neurourol Urodyn* 2011; doi: 10.1002/nau.21027.

21. Kita H, Ohi M, Chin K, *et al.* The nocturnal secretion of cardiac natriuretic peptides during obstructive sleep apnoea and its response to therapy with nasal continuous positive airway pressure. *J Sleep Res* 1998;**7**:199–207.

22. Firoozi F, Batniji R, Aslan AR, Longhurst PA, Kogan BA. Resolution of diurnal incontinence and nocturnal enuresis after adenotonsillectomy in children. *J Urol* 2006;**175**:1885–1888.

23. Mikkelsen EJ, Rappaport JL, Nee L, Gruenau C, Mendelson W, Gillin JC. Childhood enuresis: Sleep patterns and psychopathology. *Arch Gen Psychiatry* 1980;**37**: 1139.

24. Cohen-Zrubavel V, Kushnir B, Kushnir J, Sadeh A. Sleep and sleepiness in children with nocturnal enuresis. *Sleep* 2011;**34**:191–194.

25. Ramadan MI, Khan AY, Weston WE. Response to SSRI-induced enuresis: A case report. *J Clin Psychopharmacol* 2006;**26**:99–100.

26. Murkoff H. *What to Expect: The Toddler Years.* New York: Workman Publishing, 1996; pp. 438–439, 539–556.

27. Jensen IN, Krisensen G. Alarm treatment: Analysis of response and relapse. *Scand J Urol Nephrol* 1999;**33**:73–75.

28. Houts AC, Berman JS, Abramson H. Effectiveness of psychological and pharmacological treatments for nocturnal enuresis. *J Consult Clin Psychol* 1994;**62**:737–745.

29. Forsythe WI, Butler RJ. Fifty years of enuretic alarms. *Arch Dis Child* 1989;**64**:879–885.

30. Elsayed ER, Abdalla MM, Eladl M, Gabr A, Siam AG, Abdelrahman HM. Predictors of severity and treatment response in children with monosymptomatic nocturnal enuresis receiving behavioral therapy. *J Pediatr Urol* 2011; 3 Feb [e-pub ahead of print].

31. Mowrer OH, Mowrer WM. Enuresis: A method for its study and treatment. *Am J Orthopsychiatry* 1938;**8**:346–359.

32. Reiner WG. Pharmacotherapy in the management of voiding and storage disorders, including enuresis and encopresis. *J Am Acad Child Adolesc Psychiatry* 2008;**47**:5.

33. Lee T, Suh HJ, Lee HJ, Lee JE. Comparison of effects of treatment of primary nocturnal enuresis with oxybutynin plus desmopressin, desmopressin alone or imipramine alone: A randomized controlled clinical trial. *J Urol* 2005;**174**:1084–1087.

34. Van de Walle J, Van Herzeele C, Raes A. Is there still a role for desmopressin in children with primary monosymptomatic nocturnal enuresis?: A focus on safety issues. *Drug Saf* 2010;**33**:261–271.

35. Evans J, Malmsten B, Maddocks A, Popli HS, Lottmann H. Randomized comparison of long-term desmopressin and alarm treatment for bedwetting. *J Pediatr Urol* 2011;**7**:21–29.

36. Brown ML, Pope AW, Brown EJ. Treatment of primary nocturnal enuresis in children: A review. *Child Care Health Dev* 2011;**37**:153–160.

37. Gepertz S, Neveus T. Imipramine for therapy resistant enuresis: A retrospective evaluation. *J Urol* 2004;**171**: 2607–2610.

38. Mikkelsen EJ. Enuresis and encopresis: Ten years of progress. *J Am Acad Child Adolesc Psychiatry* 2001;**40**: 1146–1158.

39. Bower WF, Diao M. Acupuncture as a treatment for nocturnal enuresis. *Auton Neurosci* 2010;**157**:63–67.

40. van der Wal MF, Benninga MA, Hirasing RA. The prevalence of encopresis in a multicultural population. *J Pediatr Gastroenterol Nutr* 2005;**40**(Suppl 3):345–348.

41. Loening-Baucke V. Urinary incontinence and urinary tract infection and their resolution with treatment of chronic constipation of childhood. *Pediatrics* 1997;**100**:2.

42. Gavanski M. Treatment of non-retentive secondary encopresis with imipramine and psychotherapy. *CMAJ* 1971;**104**:46–48.

43. von Gontard A, Baeyens D, Van Hoecke E, Warzak WJ, Bachmann C. Psychological and psychiatric issues in urinary and fecal incontinence. *J Urol* 2011;**185**: 1432–1437.

44. Polin RA, Ditmar MF. *Pediatric Secrets*, 4th edn. Philadelphia, PA: Elsevier Mosby, 2005; pp. 207–212, 421–424.

19

Sexual Development and the Treatment of Sexual Disorders in Children and Adolescents

James Lock, Jennifer Couturier

In this chapter, we review sexual development and discuss sexual disorders whose origins are in childhood. Although the central role of sexuality in theoretical models of psychological health and development originated with the psychoanalytic work of Sigmund Freud, sexuality has always played key roles in the biological and social activities of humans. These roles have varied significantly over time and across cultures. What seems natural and correct to the Balinese would likely astonish the Saudis, and what would be commonplace in ancient Greece would be stigmatized in modern Greece. Biology seems to have established a mandate for sexual behavior within humans, both for procreation and for pleasure, but the structure of this behavior is extremely varied and has an ongoing and lively interaction with historical and cultural beliefs and values.

It is important for the clinician to keep these historical [1] and cultural [2] factors in mind when working on issues of sexual behavior. Today, especially in regions where many cultures interface, variations between and among cultures can increase children's confusion about sexuality and sexual behavior. Parental attitudes, which are based in various cultural belief systems, can be at odds with the prevailing peer group attitudes of their children, thus adding to the confusion. Clinicians working with child and adolescent sexual problems need to be aware of these cultural belief systems to better facilitate solutions to conflicts that arise among family members in these areas. Although this chapter's perspective and approach largely draw from Western contemporary culture, it is hoped that most readers work primarily in this context themselves so will benefit from this perspective.

Sex and Gender Development

An understanding of the relationship between sexual development and gender development – which encap-

sulates the relationship between the biological and cultural aspects of sexuality – is central to the evaluation of sexual behavior. A review of the behavioral, cognitive, and biological dimensions of this topic provides a basis for understanding both normal and unusual sexual behavior within a developmental scheme.

Infancy and Early Childhood

During early infancy, both sexes enjoy the sensations associated with nursing, diapering, and the cleansing of the genitals. It is not unusual for infants to begin to play with their genitals in the first year of life. Boys are likely to discover the genitals earlier than girls. Masturbation develops from genital play gradually to the second year of life. Self-stimulation in girls is less frequent and less focused than in boys. Self-stimulation and pleasure contributes to feelings of autonomy, control, and mastery.

By age 2 years, self-stimulation is more focused, intense, and frequent. There is increased genital pride, which may be accompanied by exhibitionism. The child may begin to develop a primitive form of fantasy life associated with self-stimulation. In girls, masturbation usually involves indirect methods and may begin by using legs, thighs, or toys, for example. In the United States, sexual socialization of the 2-year-old mixes issues of autonomy, sexuality, and toileting and may create confusion in the child's mind by superimposing issues of control and autonomy over sexual pleasure and activity.

Erotic interests become more diverse as children develop. Games such as "mommy and daddy" or "playing doctor" are common, and by the age of 4 years, one-half of US preschoolers are involved in sex games or masturbation. Parental concerns with gender, and investment in gender behavior, are an important part of a child's perception of how to behave along these lines.

Clinical Child Psychiatry, Third Edition. Edited by William M. Klykylo and Jerald Kay.
© 2012 John Wiley & Sons, Ltd. Published 2012 by John Wiley & Sons, Ltd.

Both direct and subtle messages about self-worth are contained in these parental and familial messages. Achievement, competition, and the control of emotional expression are the norm for parents when raising boys, as is an intolerance of behaviors that deviate from the traditional male stereotype. Parents predict atypical outcomes (such as homosexuality) in boys with feminine behaviors more often than in girls with masculine behaviors.

Kohlberg postulated a series of sequential stages of gender development [3]. The first stage starts when children become aware that there are two sexes. Somewhat later, they become aware of differences between the sexes and can self-identify, but the difference has no meaningful content. In the next stage, children learn specific content regarding differences between the sexes. Children who master this stage can be said to have achieved gender identification. The next task for the child is to understand that gender is a stable and consistent aspect of their identity. Finally – usually in the early school-age years – they achieve the stage of gender constancy.

School-Age Years

When children enter school, significant behavioral changes occur to their family's interactions. Children tend to bathe alone as they grow older. It is uncommon for mothers to bathe with sons who are over 8 years old, or for fathers to bathe with daughters more than 9 years old. Although for children at about age 5 years there is some reduction in sexual activity and apparent erotic interest, children continue to be concerned with sexuality. In Kinsey's 1953 study, 57% of males and 48% of females who were interviewed as adults remembered sexual play occurring between the ages of 8 and 13 years [4]. Among males interviewed when they were prepubescent, 70% claimed that they engaged in some sex play. After age 7 years, relationships tend to be with same-sex peers. On the playground, sexual topics are common, especially among boys. By this time, children are well aware of adult prohibitions around sex and try not to be caught. Nonetheless, games of "truth or dare" or strip poker remain common.

During the school-age years, group behavior is divided clearly along gender lines. Those who do not engage in such behavior risk being ostracized and ridiculed. Boys are particularly intolerant of deviation from gender norms. Some studies, however, indicate that boys' peer groups (ages 9 to 11 years) use their group activities to achieve varying levels of sexual arousal and use all-male groups to practice using sexually oriented language, viewing erotic materials, and disparaging other

males with sexually laden terms, usually with negative homosexual content [4].

Adolescence

Although Offer [5] and others have argued persuasively against the *storm and stress* or *turmoil-ridden* notions of adolescence and have claimed that approximately 80% of teenagers report a generally smooth and uneventful passage through adolescence, many nonetheless experience difficulty and anxiety around sexual behavior and development. It is therefore important for the clinician working with sexual issues to conduct a brief review of pertinent biological and sexual behavioral norms in adolescents. Physical changes associated with puberty are the external marker of profound emotional changes that lead to the development of social and behavioral changes. When compared with other biological changes that occur over a lifetime, the changes associated with puberty are rapid and dramatic and second only to those in the first year of life. The most observable changes emerge over a 4-year period and begin and end approximately 2 years earlier for girls than for boys. Hormonal systems are established prenatally but are reactivated at puberty. It has been observed in both sexes that children reach a critical fat-to-lean ratio roughly represented by weight, that appears to be correlated with the onset of puberty.

Boys

The average age at which the first penis and testes growth begins is between 10 and 11 years. This is followed by the development of pubic hair about the age of 12 to 13 years. Rapid growth of the penis and testes occurs in the 13th and 14th years, followed by the development of axillary hair, down on the lip, and voice changes in the 14th to 15th years. By ages 15 to 16 years, boys have mature spermatozoa, and by age 16 to 17 years, facial hair and body hair are present. Improved health and nutrition are causing puberty to begin earlier. Studies of the psychological effects of the timing of puberty in boys indicate that those who mature early have an advantage, at least in the teen years, over those who mature late. In adolescence, the former are more athletic, socially valued, and are perceived to be leaders. Their maturity is generally perceived positively by adults, and they tend to experience less guilt, anxiety, or other emotional problems. In adulthood, they continue to hold leadership positions, but they also seem to take conventional approaches to problems, which sometimes limits their leadership and social relations. Boys who mature late, in contrast, are less confident, hold more negative self-concepts, and are viewed less positively by peers and adults. In adulthood, however, these men display greater intellectual curiosity, more social initiative, and are more creative problem-solvers. A recent study supports some of these views, finding that in early adulthood, young men who matured late had increased rates of disruptive behavior and substance use disorders during the transition to adulthood, but that early maturation was not linked to any lifetime or current disorders among young men [6].

Masturbation is the most common source of orgasm in boys. By age 14 years, 80% have masturbated, and by age 18 years, 90–98% have masturbated. At the same time, more than 50% of boys experience guilt in relation to this activity. Studies of first coitus in males show that by age 19 years, 79% have had intercourse. First intercourse at age 13 years is experienced by 5% of males. Approximately one-half of these experiences occur in the context of a romantic partnership, but one-third occur with friends or new acquaintances. About two-thirds of boys find this first experience to some degree satisfying; the remaining one-third are disappointed.

Girls

Puberty typically begins in girls between the ages of 9 and 14 years. It is initiated by the release of gonadotropin-releasing hormone, which is produced by the hypothalamus. Between the ages of 8 and 13 years, breast buds appear, and pubic hair begins to develop on the labia as breast buds enlarge. Later, when the breast areolae and nipples begin to form, menstruation first occurs. Menarche starts at an average age of 12.5 years. These first menstrual cycles are usually painless, because they are not accompanied by ovulation. During this time, asymmetry of breast development is common and vaginal secretions increase, both of which cause concern in some girls. Growth rate slows after the onset of menstruation, and most girls gain about 25 lb (11.3 kg) during puberty. The timing of maturation in girls also has an effect on social and sexual behaviors. In contrast to the trend in boys, girls who mature early are more likely than those who mature late to be viewed negatively by peers and adults, to initiate sexual interactions earlier, and to become pregnant in the teen years. In young adulthood, women who mature early report elevated lifetime rates of major depressive disorder, anxiety, and disruptive behavior disorder compared with those who mature on time [6]. They also report poorer quality of relationships as young adults. Girls who mature late do not appear to be at a disadvantage, and do not have elevated rates of disorder. In fact, women who are late maturers have been found to be more likely to complete college [6].

According to the few reports available, masturbation occurs less frequently in girls than in boys. Sexual intercourse is generally unplanned and unprotected. Adolescent sexual activity has steadily increased over the past five decades. Studies indicate that about 60% of girls have intercourse by age 18 years, and 47–53% of US teenage females engage in sexual intercourse; 58% of these girls have had two or more partners. Approximately 89% of US adult women have had sexual intercourse. However, the adolescent sexual climate appears to be changing with the advent of the internet. Adolescents have more privacy with this medium than ever before, which may aid the phenomenon of "hooking up" (sexual experimentation without dating), along with a shift to oral sex rather than intercourse [7].

A significant issue during adolescence is pregnancy. Every year in the United States, about 1 million adolescent girls become pregnant. Of these, one-half give birth, accounting for 18% of firstborns in the United States. The remainder obtain abortions (40%) or miscarry (10%). Birth rates among teens are rising. Medical complications of teenage pregnancy include inadequate or excessive weight gain, hypertension, anemia, sexually transmitted diseases, and cephalopelvic disproportion. Most of these complications are a result of poor nutrition and poor prenatal care. In comparison to other adolescent girls, those who become teenage mothers are more likely to receive less education, have lower adult incomes, and have higher rates of depression. They are also less likely to be with the father after 2 years. Developmental issues of adolescence may be so foreshortened that identity issues remain unresolved; this may result from a continued dependency on families of origin or from the loss of opportunities for peer relations.

Sexuality and the Developmental Tasks of Adolescence

Adolescence can be viewed as comprising three phases, each of which has a specific relationship to sexual development and behaviors. The first of these is the *early phase* (ages 12–14 years), which primarily involves the dramatic physical changes associated with puberty. The *middle phase* of adolescence (ages 14–16 years) is dominated by adolescents' increasing use of peers and abstracting abilities to distinguish themselves from parents. The *late phase* of adolescence (ages 16–19 years) is associated with setting patterns and plans for work and establishing patterns of more intimate interpersonal relationships.

In the early phase, the most significant issues involve the changes associated with puberty itself. These are specifically related to attractiveness, size, and maturation rate and the relationship of these issues to self-esteem and body image. As noted earlier, these issues are processed somewhat differently for boys than for girls, at least in our culture. Girls generally are more concerned with maturing too early, being overweight or too tall, and not being perceived as attractive. Boys, conversely, are more concerned with maturing late, being too small or too short, and not being strong enough.

In the middle phase, sexual issues intensify and more strongly affect peer relationships. General themes of these sexual issues include dating competence, sexual orientation, and exploratory sexual experiences. Other issues that can complicate sexual development in this period involve separation from one's family and can include guilt, fears of abandonment, and angry and rebellious feelings. Repression, avoidance, and the isolation of sexual impulses may be one approach to this difficulty, whereas acting out, promiscuity, and other reckless sexual behavior may be another. This phase is further complicated by increasing comparisons of oneself to the peer group. When these comparisons cause lowered self-esteem and self-worth, this can lead to problems with sexual development.

In the late phase of adolescence, sexual issues principally involve practicing for true sexual intimacy. This phase is characterized by increasing wishes and ability for emotional and sexual intimacy and fewer needs for a familial base. Sexual problems that might arise during this phase are derived from residual problems in these areas, such as continued excessive emotional or physical dependency on parents or family, continued anxiety about sexual abilities or body image, and anxiety about the meaning of personal intimacy in terms of procreation.

Medical Illness and Sexual Development

Physical illnesses affect sexual development and behavior in a variety of ways that include physical, social, and emotional components. For physically ill children, the type of problems with sexual issues experienced during the early phase of adolescence is governed largely by the impact their illness or its treatment has on their pubertal development. These effects might include influences on the timing of puberty and associated secondary sex characteristics, body size, or the development of dysmorphic physical features. There are several examples of medical illnesses that affect the timing of puberty, such as endocrinopathies and intersex genetic anomalies. In addition, medical treatments of a variety of illnesses can include agents such as steroids and can thus affect the timing of puberty. A secondary effect of changing the timing of puberty is the impact this may have on height and weight, which can also be affected by specific illnesses and medical treatments. For boys, especially at this

phase, body size is a significant source of sexual and gender role anxiety. Illnesses that make them shorter or thinner have a powerfully negative impact on their developing image of themselves as sexual and male. For girls, illnesses or treatments that cause weight gain or facial changes are particularly troubling during this phase.

During the middle phase, sexual problems arise as a result of impediments to the development of peer groups. Medically ill adolescents can experience difficulties in sexual development for many reasons that include dependency on family members and institutions for care, increased periods of isolation from peers due to physical illness, decreased capacities for sexual action due to acute or chronic health limitations (e.g., infections, injury, energy, and medication side effects), and increased shame surrounding illness and its impact on psychosocial functioning. If a genetic cause is suspected, increased familial guilt and patient anger can become particularly evident. These emotions can lead to a kind of angry enmeshed familial dynamic that effectively stifles the sexual emancipation and exploration that are key to working through this phase of adolescence.

Seizure disorders, chronic illnesses, and oncological disorders are examples of illnesses that can have a particularly negative effect on sexual development during the middle phase. Adolescents with seizure disorders are often ashamed of an illness that can cause them to lose bowel and bladder control at unpredictable times. In addition, the medications required can interfere with social activities, and their side effects can inhibit both physical and sexual functioning. These adolescents are sometimes not allowed to drive, which can interfere with social activities, especially dating, leading to avoidance or counterphobic sexual behavior. Teenagers with oncological illness demonstrate another aspect of difficulties during this developmental stage: these teens often have increased dependency on family members, become socially isolated from their peers because of hospitalization and shame, and experience side effects of treatment that alter appearance and can lead to body image distortions. As a result, these teens can exhibit avoidance, family enmeshment and infantilization of sexual drives, shame about their body, lower sexual self-esteem, higher sexual anxiety, and a reluctance to explore sexual intimacy.

In the late phase of adolescence, sexual issues are associated with an increasing need and desire for intimate personal relationships and decreasing emotional ties with the family. Key sexual issues for the medically ill adolescent include concern about decreased lifespan, fertility, transferring dependency needs from families to intimate partners, and the potential for the genetic transmission of illness. Because of chronic dependency on their family and then disability and pain, these teenagers experience extreme difficulty in finding and developing young adult roles for sexual intimacy. Families are often overprotective and infantilize them, which adds to the burden. In addition, some patients worry about the genetic transmission of their illness to their offspring, which may inhibit desire. Case One illustrates how hemophilia is an illness affecting the issues of this phase. For a comprehensive review of psychosexual development in adolescents with chronic medical illnesses see Lock [8].

CASE STUDY

Case One

Tony was an 18-year-old male with hemophilia who had experienced repeated hospitalizations for pain and bleeding throughout his adolescence. He had missed most of high school because of this, although he had completed an equivalent educational process at home. His father had abandoned the family when Tony was a boy, and Tony and his mother had developed a close, if sometimes turbulent, relationship that veered from overprotection to threats of abandonment. At age 18 years, Tony had no sexual experiences and had few friends. He was aware of his own anger at his parents for "giving me this illness," and he felt a deep ambivalence about procreation. He felt that he was unattractive and unlikely ever to find a mate. He was increasingly despondent and refused to interact with anyone whom he had not known for many years. The therapist working with Tony avoided talking to him about his sexual needs and development because of feeling unprepared about how to help him. With supervision and education, however, the therapist ultimately helped Tony discuss sexual issues and developed some strategies to help him with his questions and need for love and sexual interactions.

Disorders of Sex Development

The term "disorders of sex development" (DSD) includes congenital conditions with atypical development of chromosomal, gonadal, or anatomical sex [9]. A consensus statement derived by international experts in this area in 2006 proposed that DSD replace terms such as "intersex," "hermaphroditism,"

"pseudohermaphroditism," and "sex reversal," as these terms can be viewed as pejorative and are confusing to clinicians and parents [9]. A variety of medical conditions directly or indirectly affect sexual development via biological processes that control sexual maturity, sexual organs, and sexual capacities. Many of these disorders are inherited, but few systematic studies have examined the sexual behaviors and concerns of these patients. In the area of sex chromosome disorders, we do know that girls with Turner syndrome (karyotype 45, X) have greater problems with socialization and peer relationships leading to increased difficulties with sexual immaturity. Among boys with endocrinopathies, those with Klinefelter syndrome have been reported as experiencing significant psychosexual implications, including transsexualism, body image problems, and low sexual self-esteem.

In regard to DSD in females born with masculinized genitalia caused by virilizing congenital adrenal hyperplasia, these individuals have greater bodily concerns, higher androgyny scores, difficulties with gender identity, and delays in dating and sexual relations as adolescents and adults. Boys who are genetically males but who are born with agenesis of the penis or only partial genesis of the penis experience special problems. Many are surgically castrated and raised as females and are therefore socialized into female gender roles. Unfortunately, many do not accept this categorization and end up seeking sex reassignment during adolescence or young adulthood. For example, Reiner and Gearhart [10] studied 16 genetic males born with cloacalexstrophy, a defect in pelvic embryogenesis that results in severe genital inadequacy along with urological and gastrointestinal malformations. Of these 16 genetically male children, 14 were reassigned to female sex (two subjects were reared as males because the parents refused to have them reassigned). At the time of the study, subjects were 5 to 16 years old, and 6 of the 14 subjects reassigned female at birth had declared themselves male and were living as males. The sexual behavior and attitudes of all 16 subjects reflected strong male-typical characteristics. This research calls for a reconsideration of reassignment of genetically male infants to female sex, and suggests reassignment may only complicate already complex neonatal conditions [10].

Sex reassignment surgery creates great upheaval in families who may feel guilt about their original decision as well as anxiety about the life their child will lead after reassignment. For those boys who are brought up as males, other problems develop, mostly related to self-esteem, sexual anxiety, and inhibition. Surgical enhancement of the penis is possible, but this is only a cosmetic change and may lead to other frustrations.

These young men are ashamed of their genitalia and avoid any occasions on which others, even those they are attracted to, would see them. Naturally, this inhibits any sexual experimentation and seriously curtails even the social aspects of dating relationships. Therapeutic involvement is helpful and should focus on differentiating the concept of masculinity from the concrete presence or absence of a penis. With older adolescents, it may help to associate this condition with other males who because of injury, illness, or paralysis are no longer sexually functional. Peer support groups to parents and children can be extremely beneficial if started prior to adolescence, as once in the teen years, adolescents may resist attempts at peer support due to shame and embarrassment [9].

Fortunately, DSD are rare. However, there remains much controversy over the urgency of sex assignment in these conditions, and attitudes in the medical profession are changing after many individuals have condemned infant genital surgery [11]. In the 1960s, newborn penile size charts were used, and if the stretched penis was less than 2.5 cm, gender was likely to be assigned as female, and surgery performed within the first few months of life. It was thought that infants were gender neutral at birth and that gender development occurred by interaction with the environment, relying on appearance of the genitalia. Thus, early surgery was preferred in order to reduce parental anxiety and align genital appearance to sex of rearing [11]. However, no studies have confirmed that psychological functioning of parents or children is improved by early surgery. Surgical management should focus on functional outcome rather than cosmetic appearance [9].

A set of guidelines published by a multidisciplinary team working with children born with atypical genitalia concluded that none of the appearance-altering surgeries need to be done urgently, and that surgery to normalize appearance done without the consent of the patient lacks ethical justification [12]. This is in contrast to a document produced by the American Academy of Pediatrics suggesting that the birth of a child with ambiguous genitalia constitutes a social emergency and that a diagnosis and treatment plan be established as quickly as possible to minimize medical, psychological, and social complications [13]. However, waiting for surgery brings forth another ethical dilemma of whether the child should be raised as male, female, or an intersex person. There are many differing views on this subject as well. In any case, Frader et al [12]. suggest that the available data do not provide reasons for using surgery in most cases before the child has the capacity to participate in decision-making. They also suggest that the field undertakes a comprehensive assessment of practice, that rigorous follow-up studies are essential, that health professionals need considerably more education in this area, that children have

the right to know about their bodies in an age-appropriate fashion, and that families with children with a DSD require a comprehensive package of services immediately following diagnosis, including access to mental health professionals and support groups [12]. A recent consensus statement proposes that gender assignment in newborns must be avoided before experts have completed a comprehensive evaluation; however, all individuals should receive a gender assignment following this assessment. These guidelines also propose that evaluation and long-term management be undertaken at a center with multidisciplinary experience in this area, that open communication with patients and families and participation in decision-making is encouraged, and that confidentiality be maintained [9].

CASE STUDY

Case Two

Matt was a 17-year-old football star and straight A student referred to a psychiatrist by his urologist because of depression. Matt was tall, good-looking, and muscular. He had trouble making eye contact with the psychiatrist but described his problem as a "masculinity problem." Matt disclosed that his erect penis was only about one-and-a-half inches long and that he was ashamed of it. He described how even though he was an athlete, he had managed to avoid being seen by male peers all through high school. In addition, he had recently broken up with a girl that he loved because one evening she had attempted to touch him between the legs. He said he left her then and never spoke to her again. Matt was very depressed and felt hopeless about his situation. He understood his achievements were in many way attempts to compensate for his feeling of inadequacy, but he could see no way to feel better about himself.

Homosexuality

One of the most common issues of adolescence is a concern with sexual orientation. Data do not support the formulation of the world into homosexuals and heterosexuals. Kinsey's scale that rated sexual orientation from 1 to 6 – exclusive heterosexual to exclusive homosexual – found that a significant percentage fall in the 3 to 4 range [4]. In addition, the few existing studies suggest that many people, especially males, participate in homosexual behavior at some point. Solitary or group masturbation and same-sex sexual experiences are well-known components of male adolescent sexual histories. These activities seem to serve as a means of expressing manhood and masculinity, by demonstrating a capacity for, frequency of, and rapidity of ejaculation. Girls do not appear to use these strategies as boys do. Nonetheless, homosexual behavior and varying levels of heterosexual and homosexual desire may complicate a person's sense of their sexual orientation and gender role performance. Some adolescents, rather than experience this same-sex behavior as expressive of their masculinity or femininity, may experience increased anxiety about these issues and as a result develop homophobic avoidance and defensiveness. In other words, although homosexual activity is apparently naturally occurring and common, it may be difficult for some people to integrate it into their need to conform to gender and gender role expectations.

Adolescents who are gay or lesbian can develop significant problems secondary to *internalized homophobia* (the self-hatred that develops as a result of being a socially stigmatized person) or *externalized homophobia* (the irrational hatred of a person because he or she is believed to be homosexual). Estimates of the overall homosexual population range from 2–4% to more than 10%. Few studies have examined the impact of homophobia on gay and lesbian youth. One study of gay and lesbian youths aged 15 to 21 years found that, as a result of their sexual orientation, 80% had experienced verbal insults, 44% had been threatened with violence, 33% had had objects thrown at them, 31% had been chased or followed, and 17% had been physically assaulted [14]. Numerous studies have identified an increased rate of suicide attempts among gay and lesbian youth. Risk factors for suicide attempts before age 20 years in gay and lesbian youth include:

(1) Discovering same-sex preference early in adolescence.
(2) Experiencing violence due to gay or lesbian identity.
(3) Using alcohol or drugs to cope.
(4) Being rejected by family members as a result of being homosexual [15].

Other studies have reported increased high-school drop-out rates, substance abuse, and family discord among gay and lesbian youths and adolescents. In studies attempting to predict patterns of sexual acts among homosexual and bisexual youths, researchers have found that improved patterns of sexual risk-taking behaviors are associated with decreased levels of internalized homophobia, as demonstrated by high self-esteem and low levels of anxiety, depression, and

substance abuse [16]. Another study found self-acceptance, a corollary of decreased internalized homophobia, to be the single largest predictor of mental health – more important, for example, than either family support or victimization alone [17].

Adolescents and young adults often need assistance with problems that develop as a result of internalized homophobia. Therapeutic work with sexual minority youth has employed both individual and group approaches. Key elements of psychodynamic treatments include neutralizing internalized homophobia through education, interpreting anxieties about passivity, dependency, masculinity, and femininity, and using techniques that are supportive and affirm homosexual identity [18]. Group approaches for teens and young adults aim to diminish isolation, create supportive communities, and serve as psychoeducational forums [19]. Although intervention with families seems advisable, because of the lack of support provided by society as a whole, only limited clinical research has addressed the family factors that play a role in the difficulties faced by gay and lesbian youth. Overall, there is a lack of research specific to the needs of gay and lesbian youth. Reports do indicate, however, that they have been coming out at younger ages: 10 years ago the average age was 21 years in women and 19 in men, whereas the average ages are now 19 years in women and 16 years in men. Other studies have focused on the societal origins of homophobia and have attempted to provide prevention and intervention for gay and lesbian youth in high schools or community centers [20–22]. These approaches to the prevention of internalized and externalized homophobia have been difficult to develop and maintain, in large measure because of parental and societal fears about homosexuality.

Sex And Gender Disorders

Taking a Sexual History

One of the most neglected aspects of training, perhaps especially in child psychiatry, is the process of taking a sexual history. It is presumed that clinicians have learned to take an appropriate and detailed history, but more often than not clinicians are uncomfortable with taking a sexual history or have not determined how best to conduct such a history. An understanding of a patient's sexual history is especially important for those clinicians who work with children and adolescents who have sexual problems. Interviewing may be done face to face with patients and families and through the use of questionnaires. The clinician must be able to sensitively interview children and adolescents to determine if the child has been sexually abused or is at risk for such abuse. Unfortunately, the legal mandate to report such findings may contribute to some clinicians' hesitancy to take thorough sexual histories. In addition, since sexual behavior poses increased risk to general health, because of sexually transmitted diseases and human immunodeficiency virus (HIV), clinicians need to be aware of their adolescent patients' sexual behaviors to educate and help them manage these behaviors more safely.

To successfully interview children and adolescents, the clinician should approach the patient with an awareness of his or her developmental capacities. Questions should be straightforward, direct, and posed without embarrassment. The correct terminology for all body parts should be used. For younger children, anatomically correct dolls may be employed as an aid. Adolescents sometimes prefer a self-administered format that allows them to respond with less embarrassment. However, there are no self-report questionnaires on adolescent sexual behavior that are commonly used for clinical purposes. The Youth Risk Behavior Survey has been used in epidemiological studies [23]. Confidentiality of adolescent responses should be assured. Patience and support are also necessary, since children and adolescents may require extra time and encouragement to answer these types of inquiries.

Gender Identity Disorder (GID)

Definition

For a diagnosis of Gender Identity Disorder, the *Diagnostic and Statistical Manual of Mental Disorders, Fourth Edition, Text Revision* (DSM-IV-TR [24]. criteria require the presence of a strong and persistent cross-gender identification that is manifested by four of the following:

(1) Repeatedly stated desire to be of the other sex.
(2) In boys, a preference for cross-dressing or simulating female attire; in girls, insistence on wearing only stereotypical masculine clothing.
(3) Strong preference for cross-sex play and fantasies.
(4) Strong preference for playmates of the other sex.
(5) Intense desire to participate in games of the other sex.

This must be accompanied by persistent discomfort with one's own sex or gender role.

Epidemiology, Etiology, and Pathology

Sexual identity is the biological sex, *gender identity* is the identification of oneself as belonging to a gender, and *gender roles* are the behaviors associated with a particular sex within a culture or group. GID is concerned with each of these to a degree, but the principal problems psychologically are the dysphoria a child experiences with his or her biological sex and the behavioral manifestations of this dissatisfaction, most typically as gender role nonconformity.

Diagnostic criteria for GID have evolved, but there is still much debate surrounding them [25]. In early formulations, there was considerable variation between the criteria for boys and girls, which generally allowed girls more gender role variation than boys. The more recent criteria are gender neutral [24]. The referral rates for GID, however, continue to range from 6 to 30 boys for every girl. The sex ratio for referred adolescents appears less skewed, with a male-to-female ratio of 1.4:1 [26]. What may simply be increased concern by parents and social institutions about femininity in boys has led some to criticize this diagnostic category's scientific basis. Critics of the diagnostic criteria for GID contend that the behaviors such children exhibit are not in themselves psychopathological but are labeled as such from parental and social intolerance of them, and that distress results from such intolerance [27]. They suggest that cross-gender behavior may be a normal developmental pathway to later homosexuality and point out that there is very little research on the validity of this diagnosis [27]. A study of cross-gendered behaviors among children, in which mothers reported their perception of their son's wishes to be of the opposite sex, found that at age 4 to 5 years, about 15% of clinically referred boys wished to be of the opposite sex, compared to about 1% of nonreferred boys [28]. This study suggests that a substantial number of males without GID nonetheless experience opposite-gendered behavior during early childhood. The rates in this study were also higher for referred than for nonreferred girls but were stable at much lower rates of 4–8% [28].

There are no formal estimates of the prevalence of GID. If it is assumed that GID leads to adult transsexualism, it would constitute a rare disorder – 1 in 24 000 to 37 000 men and 1 in 103 000 to 150 000 women become transsexual [29]. Others assume that GID ultimately ends in homosexuality. Estimates of the homosexual population are also contested, however. In addition, although some homosexuals recall engaging in cross-gendered behavior, it is doubtful that most ever met the criteria for GID. One is left to conclude that cross-gendered behavior is common but that GID is relatively rare.

Etiological theories for GID fall into two major classes: biological and psychoanalytic. The biological theories cite genetic and hormonal studies or medical conditions that support a biological basis for GID. The support for a genetic etiology draws from studies that indicate a hereditary basis for homosexuality. The most compelling data on this issue are from Pillard and Bailey's study of 56 monozygotic twins, 54 dizygotic twins, and 57 genetically unrelated adopted brothers. The researchers found that 11% of the adoptive brothers, 22% of the dizygotic twins, and 52% of the monozygotic twins were concordant for homosexuality [30]. Other studies have indicated that up to 70% of the variation may be accounted for genetically [31]. Similar, though somewhat less dramatic, findings have also been found in lesbians. Nonetheless, the presumption that GID is genetically determined is a leap from these data because, as noted earlier, GID is not a precondition of homosexuality and does not itself necessarily lead to homosexuality.

Another etiological hypothesis is derived from studies of psychoendocrine research. This research examined sexual orientation in the context of psychosexual development as it is influenced by hormones. No association between systemic sex hormone levels during adolescence and adulthood and GID or homosexuality was found, however. More recent research is based only on a theory that prenatal exposure to androgens promotes the development of attraction to females whereas nonresponsiveness to androgens is associated with erotic attraction to males. Some support for this theory comes from studies on girls and women with congenital adrenal hyperplasia, in which female fetuses are exposed to increased levels of androgens *in utero*. These girls display some gender role behaviors that are more similar to those of boys. In addition, compared to control women, adult women with this condition have less heterosexual involvement and more homosexual fantasy (see review by Bradley and Zucke [26]). In boys, it has been hypothesized that some pregnant mothers expose the male fetus to risk of incomplete androgenization of the brain, resulting in homosexual attraction. Possible mechanisms for this include antibodies to testosterone from previous pregnancy with a male fetus, and androgen insufficiency caused by stress. Support for this hypothesis comes from studies that demonstrate later birth order for male homosexuals and an increased number of male older siblings [32], [33]. Problems arise with this hypothesis because of the genetic studies already cited and the lack of comparable data for female homosexuality. The tenuous link between homosexuality and GID also continues to be a limitation.

Brain anatomy studies attempting to find similarities between homosexual men and heterosexual women to support the prenatal exposure theory have been inconclusive and unreplicated. In addition, cognitive performance in untreated patients with GID has been investigated in order to support this theory. Results have been inconsistent. Haraldsen *et al* [34]. found that performance appears to be consistent with biological sex and not gender identity, while Cohen-Kettenis *et al* [35]. found that male patients with GID had an advantage in verbalization more similar to female controls. More recent studies are investigating the possibility that the brain begins to develop differently in males and females even before sex hormones come into play, and that perhaps in the future genes may be identified that predict the likely gender identity of an individual [36].

Psychoanalytic theories examine familial, especially parental, factors as the root cause of GID. Family studies have shown that fathers are absent in 34–85% of the families of boys with GID; and in those families with a father present, he spent notably less time than is typical interacting with the son in early childhood [37]. Mothers in these families were found to be hostile toward males and viewed their husbands as potentially violent and out of control. These mothers discouraged "rough and tumble" play and were often harsh and authoritarian disciplinarians [37]. Many of these mothers had themselves experienced traumatic experiences during the early years of their child's life (e.g., rape, or death of another child or parent). Another study found that mothers of boys with GID have higher levels of emotional overinvolvement and lower criticism than mothers of externalizing boys, mothers of community control boys, and mothers of community control girls [38]. Theoretically, then, mothers' anxiety about masculine violence, their poor management of stress, and their ambivalent and hostile relationship with the fathers could lead the parents to promote cross-gender behaviors in their sons. Conversely, the sons are anxious about maternal withdrawal and abandonment – over 60% meet criteria for separation anxiety disorder (SAD) – and identify with the mother to assuage the anxieties associated with separation and loss [37]. In accordance with a more behavioral theory, one of the strongest findings in children with GID is the lack of parental discouragement of cross-sex behavior [26].

Differential Diagnosis

The most important distinction to make in an assessment of GID is between predictable cross-gender exploration and play and cross-gendered behaviors that are rooted in persistent and intense distress about one's biological sex. An example of predictable cross-gendered play might involve a boy putting on a wig or a dress temporarily, whereas an elaboration of this play, along with enthusiasm and persistence, might be of more concern. The quality of persistence is best assessed by several factors, including the age of the child, the length of time the behavior or belief has existed, and the determination with which the behavior is maintained. In general, increased age of the child, duration of the cross-gendered behaviors, and resistance to changing the behaviors all indicate a more likely diagnosis of true GID. Factors such as familial stress, the death of a parent, the birth of a sibling, and other traumas may be associated with brief periods of cross-gendered behaviors. These adjustment factors should be considered in any assessment.

Course and Natural History

Studies of the outcome of boys with gender nonconformity in childhood are conflicting. In a study of existing longitudinal data, Kohlberg *et al.* found little or no correlation between childhood masculinity or femininity and heterosexuality in adulthood [39]. Studies have shown that a large proportion of boys referred for gender nonconformity grow up to become homosexuals; these studies, however, may represent a particular subset of homosexuals. Studies examining the childhood memories of adult homosexuals indicate that some degree of gender nonconformity may predict later homosexuality. A meta-analysis of retrospective literature found a very strong relationship between the extent of childhood cross-gender behavior and later homosexual orientation for both men and women [40].

The child with GID is likely to develop significant problems with peer relations. School-age children are anxious about gender role behavior and are often intolerant of variations from stereotypes. Thus children, especially boys, with GID are likely to be teased and harassed by their peers. This can result in school avoidance, truancy, and other behavior problems. They are also likely to develop lower self-esteem, which is to some degree dependent on social approval. Separation anxiety is a common confounding condition for those individuals with GID and can add to the burden of both familial and peer interactions. Zucker and Bradley [41]. found that children with GID had less social competence on the Child Behavior Checklist (CBCL), and that boys had a predominance of internalizing, as opposed to the typical externalizing behavioral difficulties seen in clinical samples of boys. Girls with GID had both internalizing and externalizing elevations on the CBCL. An international study found that boys with GID had even more problems with peer relations than girls with GID, and that poor peer relations were the strongest predictor of behavior problems [42]. A study found that 52% of children with GID meet criteria for one or more other psychiatric diagnoses, most commonly an anxiety

disorder (31%) [43]. When present, any comorbid conditions, such as depression and separation anxiety, should be treated in conjunction with the GID.

By the time gender identity-disordered children reach puberty and high school, approximately two-thirds of them are likely to have developed a homosexual orientation. A new set of social problems emerges as sexual and aggressive impulses of peers are now near adult levels. Exposure to this now physically threatening level of harassment leads to significant risk of depression, truancy, and substance abuse. In those families that are intolerant of homosexuality, runaway behavior and homelessness are common. For those adolescents who do not become homosexual as adults, harassment for continued cross-gendered behavior is likely to result, even though they are heterosexual, and may be similar to problems that homosexuals experience. Others with GID may become transsexuals and decide to live their lives as members of the opposite biological sex. Some of these individuals seek hormonal and surgical treatments to physically augment their psychological and behavioral cross-gender condition. A prospective follow-up study of 20 adolescents with GID who underwent hormone treatment and sex reassignment surgery over a 4–5-year period found that at one year post-surgery they were no longer gender dysphoric and were functioning well [44]. No one expressed regret about the surgery. The authors suggest that with careful diagnosis and strict criteria, earlier treatment may have some benefits over later treatment, including improved social and psychological functioning.

Treatment

Treatment for GID is a conflict-ridden area of child and adolescent psychiatric practice. As discussed earlier, some practitioners argue that children with gender nonconformity are treated inappropriately because the problem is not their behavior so much as others' responses to it. These practitioners argue that educating the parents and communities about the acceptability of these behaviors is preferable to teaching children to hide or change what comes naturally to them. More conventional approaches try to help the child find safe opportunities to play however he or she chooses, help parents understand their need to protect, support, and love their child, and help the child understand the reactions of peers and others. Other practitioners use a variety of psychoanalytic approaches, such as working with concepts of enmeshment and overidentification with the mother figure and trying to change core gender identity. No systematic data are available on the effectiveness of any of these treatments, whatever their explicit aims.

Goals and Phases of Treatment The principal goal of psychotherapeutic treatment for GID is to reduce the patient's anxiety and dysphoria. Often these problems are not associated with the cross-gendered behaviors themselves but with parental and social reactions to them. Thus, the first task is to address the family's reactions to the behavior of the gender-disordered child. This often involves a thorough assessment of the familial variables, including parental hostility, paternal avoidance, maternal dependence on the patient, and the identification of traumatic injuries in parents that remain unresolved and contribute to the child's difficulties. In addition, education about the prognosis and likely outcome of their child is an important part of the treatment. When the patient is male, involving the father in more interactions with him may be another important intervention. The goal is not to change the child's behaviors but rather to change the dynamics of familial issues. The reinforcement of cross-gendered behaviors should be limited, but punishment, ridicule, and other methods of criticizing the child should cease. Often it is helpful to provide the child with a safe alternative place to play and thereby to ultimately encourage the exploration of other less cross-gendered activities. This technique increases the likelihood that the child will find ways to better relate to peers and may thus assist the child in maintaining a positive self-image.

Some practitioners have used behavioral approaches to discourage cross-gendered behaviors. Although these approaches have not been studied systematically, some improvements have been noted on specific behaviors. A technical problem with this approach is that specific behavioral treatments do not generalize to other cross-gender behaviors (e.g., the cessation of cross-dressing does not lead to decreased play with dolls). Ethical problems with this treatment emerge if one considers that biological bases for these disorders exist in many cases. Efforts to partially modify these behaviors – without being able to ultimately change the overall disorder–can therefore add to the child's burden by reinforcing negative and judgmental appraisals of his or her interests and behaviors. This approach is generally not recommended. Many suggest that the focus of clinical work should be the dysphoria accompanying the gender identity rather than treating gender role behavior itself [27].

Common Problems in Management There are a variety of common problems that clinicians face when treating patients with GID. Resistance to change on the part of the family and the child are predictable. Embarrassment and shame, especially among fathers, is another common difficulty. Work with group childcare settings and schools, when appropriate, should also be undertaken to protect and support the child. Occasionally countertransference problems can contribute to an inability to empathize and assist children and families with this disorder. Religious and moral beliefs about sex roles and homosexuality, whether in families or therapists, may confound the treatment of these patients.

CASE STUDY

Case Three

Tommy's mother brought him in for an evaluation at her husband's insistence. Tommy was 4 years old and according to his mother was a wonderful child with an active interest in dolls, dressing up in her clothing, and playing with girls and an active disinterest in playing with other boys, whom he considered too rough and mean. During the interview, Tommy appeared developmentally appropriate on all measures. His appearance was noteworthy for wearing pink plastic sandals and carrying a tin lunch box with Cinderella on the cover. Tommy was polite and deferential to the male evaluator. As the evaluation proceeded, it became clear that Tommy's mother and father were having marital problems. He was an only child and languished in their discord. The father was an overworked physician who had little time or interest in his son and was clearly displeased with his feminine appearance and behaviors. Work with Tommy was supportive and consisted of play therapy intended to explore the meaning of his play interests. He was clearly anxious about both his parents. He wanted his father's attention, but his mother was the only parent consistently available to him. He both enjoyed her attention and felt anxious about her approval. The mother reported that she enjoyed her son's cross-gender play and in some ways encouraged it. The therapist began to work with her on being more neutral in her reaction to Tommy's behavior and also encouraged the family to develop opportunities for the father and son to interact more frequently. Although Tommy remained interested in many feminine things, over time he also clearly enjoyed a broader range of play. When he started kindergarten the following year, he was not teased or routinely harassed.

Paraphilias

Definition

The DSM-IV-TR lists the following paraphilias: exhibitionism, fetishism, transvestic fetishism, frotteurism, pedophilia, masochism, sadism, and voyeurism.

Epidemiology, Etiology, and Pathology

These disorders all share the diagnostic criteria that patients experience recurrent, intense, and sexually arousing fantasies, sexual urges, or behaviors for at least 6 months that lead to clinically significant distress or impairment in social, occupational, or other important areas of functioning. Although there are specific characteristics for each major subtype of paraphilia, general characteristics of paraphilias include the use of nonhuman objects, suffering, the humiliation of self or a sexual partner, or children, or nonconsensual sexual interactions.

Our scientific understanding of paraphilia is extremely limited. Paraphilias are rarely diagnosed clinically, but the large commercial market in paraphilia-related materials suggests that it is more prevalent than clinical samples indicate. Paraphilias, with the exception of sexual masochism, are only rarely diagnosed in females. The most common presenting paraphilias in clinical populations are pedophilia, voyeurism, and exhibitionism – but this may be simply a result of these patients coming to the attention of clinicians because of legal involvements resulting from these sexual behaviors. About 50% of the patients with paraphilia are married. Most paraphilias are chronic, lifelong disorders. They usually begin in childhood and adolescence and diminish in intensity with advancing age. Multiple paraphilias are the rule, not the exception. Most paraphilias are exacerbated with other psychiatric illness, stress, or additional free time. Personality disorders and depression are common among patients with a paraphilia.

The etiology of paraphilias is unclear. Paraphilias have been a part of the psychiatric literature since the time of Freud, but reports of paraphilic behaviors stretch back centuries. Psychoanalytic, behavioral, traumatic, and biological theories have all been suggested to explain the origin of paraphilias. The most developed theories are psychoanalytic. Freud thought that paraphilia was based on a childhood belief that women had penises, and that individuals with paraphilias were preoccupied with the fantasy that they would be castrated [45]. Stoller thought that hatred and hostility, which resulted from past humiliation, were eroticized in paraphilicbehaviors [46]. He preferred the term "perversion" rather than paraphilia, explaining that this term better represents the desire to harm, hurt, be cruel to, or humiliate someone. Cooper's related theory suggested that paraphiliacs attempt to manage a deeply traumatizing relationship with primary maternal figures through efforts to absolutely control sexual interactions [47]. Others have viewed paraphilia as the result of gender instability and a form of intimacy dysfunction [48]. Behavioral theorists contend that paraphilias are learned behaviors that are strongly reinforced by intermittent sexual rewards. Because there is considerable evidence that men with paraphilia have a high incidence of sexual abuse histories, often intrafamilial, some theories suggest that a specific trauma may lead to paraphiliac behavior.

The biological bases for paraphilia have been examined during the 1980s and 1990s. The original hypothesis was based on a theory of excessive testosterone in pedophiles, since castration, either chemical or physical, was found to be effective in curtailing pedophilic behaviors. Other studies have focused on the comorbid psychiatric conditions found among paraphiliacs, including depression, obsessive-compulsive disorders, anxiety disorders, and substance abuse, as the basis for biological origin. Evidence that paraphiliacs respond to selective serotonin reuptake inhibitors (SSRIs) suggests a neurotransmitter dysregulation of the serotonin system as the root cause of paraphilia [49], [50].

Diagnosis, Course, and Natural History of Specific Paraphilias

Exhibitionism

Exhibitionism is characterized by intense sexually arousing activities or fantasies that involve exposure of one's genitalia to strangers. Usually no other sexual activity is sought with these strangers. These urges to expose seem to occur in waves, perhaps associated with an increase in either free time or stress. Exhibitionism is rare in females. The typical exhibitionist has hundreds of exposures before seeking treatment. About 20% of adult females have been targets for exhibitionists or voyeurs.

Fetish and Transvestic Fetish

The fetishist uses a nonhuman object for sexual gratification but does not cross-dress whereas the transvestic fetishist finds the cross-dressing process itself sexually arousing. Most fetishes begin in adolescence and involve males. The fetishist may develop erectile difficulties without the fetish present. Most problems develop for the fetishist because they exclude their sexual partners in their erotic activities. Transvestic fetishists are usually heterosexual, but a few of them have had occasional homosexual experiences. Transvestic fetishes usually begin in childhood and progress in adolescence. Cross-dressing appears to not only be sexually arousing but also mitigates symptoms of anxiety and depression. Both of these disorders result in feelings of shame and guilt, which complicate their presentations and treatment.

Frotteurism

Frotteurism is rubbing or touching an unsuspecting person for sexual arousal. Most frotteurs operate in crowded situations, attempting to touch the body of a female through clothing with an erect penis. Most frotteurs are passive, nonassertive men. The behavior starts in adolescence and is most frequent when the patient is between the ages of 15 and 24 years. As with any of the paraphilias, frotteurism may not be considered pathological in some cultures, and the cultural context must be taken into account [24].

Pedophilia

Pedophilia elicits the most social disapproval of the paraphilias because the victims are children. Pedophilia generally involves older males engaging females in sexual acts – usually genital fondling or oral sex. Ninety-five percent of pedophiles are heterosexual, although they may engage in pedophiliac sexual interactions with either sex. Female victims are usually between the ages of 8 and 10 years, and male victims are usually slightly older. The primary motive behind these actions appears to be achieving sexual arousal and activity without the threat of an adult partner. Most pedophiles have low self-esteem and begin the behavior in adolescence. Recidivism is extremely high among pedophiles and can be predicted by a preference for male victims and an exclusive attraction to children. Ten to twenty percent of all children have been sexually molested by the age of 18 years.

Masochism

Sexual masochism is the only perversion for which females are also commonly diagnosed. Still, the male-to-female ratio is 20:1. Masochists are sexually stimulated by fantasies and activities that can include humiliation, the infliction of pain, and suffering. Examples of such activities include bondage, blindfolding, paddling, whipping, cutting, being urinated or defecated on, and being verbally abused. Two additional variations are *infantism*, in which the masochist is diapered and bottle fed, and *hypoxyphilia*, which involves near strangulation or oxygen deprivation. Approximately one-third of masochists have played the sadist role as well. Most sexual masochism begins in early adulthood.

Sadism

Most sexually sadistic behavior starts before the age of 18 years. Fantasies of sadistic activities, however, begin in childhood well before such behaviors. Sadists are sexually aroused by fantasies and behaviors that cause real suffering. Most sadists work with one or only a few partners, who may be consenting or nonconsenting. Sadists do not necessarily need to increase the level of suffering over time to achieve arousal and sexual satisfaction. About 8% of rapists have a sadistic sexual interest.

Voyeurism

Voyeurs find it sexually exciting to observe an unsuspecting person undressing or having sex. This is the earliest type of paraphilia to develop and usually begins before the age of 15 years. Usually the voyeur masturbates while others are undressing or engaged in sexual activity. Because there are few consequences of this behavior and victims are not likely to know they are being watched, it can go undetected for an extended period. This can reinforce the behavior and make it more difficult to treat. As with other paraphilias, voyeurism can also increase in waves associated with mood, stress, and available time.

Treatment

Most information about treating patients with paraphilias is derived from work with adults, because most patients are not identified until adulthood. There are three major approaches to working with patients with paraphilia. The oldest and most common approach uses psychotherapy, usually with a psychoanalytic base; the next is a behavioral approach; and the most recent is the use of medications. Combinations of treatments are also common, because the effectiveness of any of these approaches is limited.

Psychotherapy

The first assumption of the psychotherapies used to treat paraphilia is that the paraphilia serves a function in the patient's life. The goal is to find other ways to meet the need that the paraphilic behavior is masking. Paraphilia is, in this sense, a way to avoid insight. Paraphilias are perceived as a means of preventing the recall of past trauma, poor parenting relationships, or past victimization. Paraphilia may also temporarily help sexually insecure males with a fragile sense of masculinity. Other evidence suggests that paraphilias help these individuals manage emotional slates other than cognitive and developmental distortions – particularly anger, depression, anxiety, sadness, guilt, and loneliness. Thus, paraphilias can be seen as a means of avoiding the realities of life and the demands of intimacy and human relations. Therapeutic approaches to these issues include identifying underlying motivations behind the behaviors; clarifying the relationship of these behaviors to the patient's emotional states; interpreting any resistance to changing behaviors; and helping the patient progress into the often frightening areas of more intimate human relationships without depending on or relapsing into paraphilic behaviors and fantasies.

Specific approaches to working with adolescents with paraphilia require an awareness of the overall challenges of adolescent psychotherapeutic work. Adolescents have varying developmental capacities and motivations for psychotherapy. In addition, they are often more invested in erotic interest than older adults. Conversely, patterns of personal relationships and defensive management of emotional needs are not as fixed as in adults and may therefore be more malleable to treatment. The family may also play a part in the treatment of this age group. Because many of these patients only come to the attention of a psychiatrist if a victim has come forward – sometimes with the force of law – family members feel shame, anger, and guilt, and their wishes to punish and avoid the child often need to be addressed. In addition, since issues of relationships with parental figures are almost always a part of the history of these patients, the therapist will likely encounter significant efforts to deny or distort family dynamics. The younger the patient, the more important it is to keep the family involved.

One of the most important problems that therapists face when working with these adolescents is countertransference. It is often difficult for therapists to manage their own feelings of disgust, anger, and fear of the fantasies and behaviors of patients with paraphilias. Identification with the victims and their families is common and can limit the development of an empathic relationship with the patient. The younger the victim and the more physically aggressive the sexual assault, the more likely the therapist will experience these difficulties. Therapists may need to work to overcome these reactions. Those that do can find meaningful and rewarding work in developing a therapeutic relationship that not only assists the particular patient but also prevents further victimization.

Behavioral Treatment

Behavior therapy is used to interrupt a learned paraphilic behavioral pattern. Approaches include cogniti-

vebehavior therapy (CBT), social skills learning, and relapse-prevention strategies. A CBT approach aims to identify and elucidate the sequence of events that lead to paraphilic behavior. Usually, both an initial event and a sequence of subsequent events are required to support the ultimate expression of the paraphiliac behavior. By learning to identify these events and developing an increased awareness of the pattern, patients can identify opportunities to disrupt the ultimate behavioral outcome. Cognitive awareness is sometimes coupled with noxious stimuli, such as electric shocks and bad odors, to recondition the behavior and prevent its reinforcement. It is often helpful if these treatments can be self-administered, because it allows the patient to assess and interrupt the chain of events leading to paraphilic behavior when therapists are unavailable. Group cognitive work can support the individual cognitivebehavioral approach by adding a supportive element as well as providing the patient with perspectives from others with similar difficulties. Most of the research on these behavioral treatments is directed toward the treatment of pedophilia. No substantive empirical studies have been published on the behavioral treatment of adolescents with paraphilia.

Medication

Biological approaches to treating paraphilia have been developed for many years. The basic goal of the initial approaches was to decrease testosterone levels and thereby reduce the sexual drive and arousal that motivated paraphilic behaviors. Although castration is an effective method of limiting these behaviors, surgical castration is intrusive and irreversible. Chemical castration may be a reasonable alternative for treatment-resistant patients with severe paraphilia that results in the chronic victimization of others. In the early 1980s, medroxyprogesterone acetate (MPA; Depo-Provera) and cyproterone acetate (CPA) began to be used to treat paraphilia of a severe and persistent nature (e.g., constant masturbation, committing sex offenses, and high-risk sexual behaviors). MPA inhibits gonadotropin secretions whereas CPA antagonizes the effects of testosterone through competitive inhibition at androgen receptors. Weekly injection of MPA was highly successful in reducing these behaviors, but a significant number of patients experienced side effects of weight gain, hypertension, muscle cramps, and gynecomastia. In the late 1980s, oral MPA, in doses of 30 to 80 mg/day, was also found effective, and with fewer side effects. Currently, the intramuscular (IM) route of administration is only recommended for the most severe of cases often accompanied by treatment non-compliance [51].

More recently, studies using long-lasting luteinizing hormone-releasing hormone (LHRH) agonists have shown similar results, with decreases in paraphiliac behaviors paralleling the decrease of plasma testosterone levels. These agents (leuprolide, nafarelin, goserelin, triptorelin) work by exerting a continuous, rather than the physiological pulsatile effect, on the pituitary-gonadal axis thereby downregulating the gonadotroph cells. Although effective, these medications are not without serious side effects, including bone demineralization with osteoporosis, gynecomastia, erectile dysfunction, nausea, and depression [51]. Due to the side effects of MPA, CPA, and LHRH agonists, they are generally considered in adults for a moderate to severe disorder, or after other treatments have been tried (for review and treatment algorithm see Briken *et al* [51]). In adolescents, these drugs are rarely used due to these side effects [52]. In fact, psychotherapeutic interventions are commonly first-line treatments in adolescent patients.

The most recent breakthrough in psychopharmacological management is the use of SSRIs to treat paraphilia. In case reports in the 1980s and early 1990s as well as clinical trials currently being conducted, these agents are showing promising effects. Clomipramine, fluoxetine, fluvoxamine, paroxetine, and sertraline are all medications under investigation [49], [50]. In their algorithm of medication treatment for paraphilias in adults, Briken *et al* [51]. suggest that SSRIs be first-line treatments for adults with mild symptoms, or for those with comorbid depressive, anxious, or obsessive-compulsive symptoms, and that for moderate to severe symptoms with or without comorbid mood or anxiety symptoms, a combination of SSRIs and CPA, MPA, or LHRH could be used. They suggest that all pharmacological interventions should be accompanied by supportive or intensive psychotherapy. Another recent set of guidelines including a treatment algorithm for adults with paraphilias supports the use of psychotherapy, SSRIs at high doses (similar to obsessive-compulsive disorder), antiandrogens (CPA), and long-acting LHRH in various combinations depending on the intensity and type of paraphilic symptoms, risk of violence, and patient compliance [53]. The relationship between paraphilia, obsessive-compulsive disorder, and depression is also being explored, since the latter two are also responsive to SSRIs. Although these medications are promising, and perhaps safer in adolescents due to a better side-effect profile, rigorous studies of their effectiveness are not yet available.

CASE STUDY

Case Four

An 18-year-old male high-school senior was brought in by his professional father for an evaluation for a transvestic fetish. The boy described himself as hypermasculine, with interests in every sport and a wish to join the air force to become a pilot. Over the past 2 years, however, he had begun to cross-dress and masturbate. He felt ashamed of this behavior and wanted to end it so he could join the military. The onset of this behavior was after the divorce of his parents and his subsequent decision to live with his father, which he had made about 3 years prior to the evaluation. His father was a heterosexual man who was powerful, good-looking, charming, and seductive. From early childhood the boy had wished to be close to this man who was at once powerful and unavailable. Although the young man was heterosexual, his wish to have a closer relationship with his father, now that his mother was out of the picture, apparently increased and led to the transvestic fetish. Although there was clearly a sexual component, the real purpose of the transvestism was to allure and involve the father, who was both fascinated and overinvolved with his son during his treatment. This relationship during therapy allowed the son to control the father and reverse the dynamic that had been humiliating to the son. When the therapist gave the son permission to openly participate in his transvestic fetish, it apparently lost some of its appeal; he gave it up and joined the military. It is likely, however, that this paraphilia will return or another will take its place.

The Effect of Sexual Abuse on Sexual Development and Behavior

The subject of sexual abuse and its treatment are covered elsewhere in this book. However, some specific discussion of the impact of sexual abuse on sexual development and behavior is warranted here. As with any abuse, sexual abuse is likely to have the most severe effects on persons who are otherwise vulnerable or young, when the abuser is a close relative, or when the abuse is violent and ongoing.

Victim Psychological Responses

Although sexual abuse can assume many possible manifestations in later sexual development, two of the most hazardous are becoming an offender oneself and repeating the experience of being a sexual victim. Although there is no definitive rule, abused boys often take the former course and abused girls take the latter. Boys may be socially and otherwise conditioned to find the role of victim particularly ego dystonic. In other words, no matter how abused they may have been, it may seem that the best way to manage these painful experiences is to identify with the sexual aggressor. They thus become seemingly free from the past trauma. Girls may find the role of being a sexual aggressor less socially acceptable and may instead find a familiarity with the role of victim, which frees them from past traumas because these repetitions override past memories.

Either of these ways of managing sexual abuse can lead to abnormal sexual behaviors. Sexually abused children may initiate sexual activities earlier than others, seek out much older or much younger partners, and find sexual experiences to be dissociated from feelings of intimacy. As a result, they may struggle to achieve real emotional connection with their sexual partners. Some may find it impossible to have sexual relationships with people they love. Some sexually abused children grow up to be sexually avoidant and unusually anxious about sexual development; they, too, may be unable to achieve real emotional intimacy with those they love. Children who are sexually abused by someone of the same sex may feel that this predetermines their sexual orientation. Although this is not the case, this feeling can be reinforced by peers and by misinformation in the culture that supports this view.

Treatment of Sexually Abused Children

Assisting a child or adolescent with issues surrounding sexual abuse requires unusual sensitivity and patience on the part of therapists. Although medications might alleviate some aspects of post-traumatic experiences, medication has little to offer in the specific area of sexual development. A variety of approaches have been attempted, and include individual therapy aimed at revisiting the past trauma and group therapy aimed at reducing the child's or adolescent's feeling of isolation and shame. Clearly, the first goal is to ensure that the abuse has stopped and that the child is safe. It is also necessary to ensure that the possibility of contact with the abuser has ended. This sets a framework in which the therapist can establish safe parameters to conduct exploratory work. It is essential for the therapist to recog-

nize that sexual abuse is clearly about aggression and minimally about sex; sex is the vehicle for aggression. In the child's eye, sex and aggression are merged. This leads to both emotional and cognitive confusion that underlies many of the behavioral and emotional difficulties that may develop. The goals of therapy are to assist the child or adolescent with sexual difficulties that have resulted from abuse, to help them understand why this confusion exists, and to help them to change these feelings as much as possible.

Shame is another result of sexual abuse that can complicate later sexual functioning. Shame may result in feelings of being unlovable, damaged, and worthless, and different from peers because of this sexual experience. Helping a child or adolescent resolve this sexual shame requires addressing fundamental ideas of the self and how it has been damaged from abuse. Psychotherapeutic exploration of these issues is currently best formulated with techniques of empathy, mirroring, and other reflecting tools. Issues of provocative sexual behavior, dress, and language by sexually abused children should be anticipated as part of sexually abused children's therapy. Therapists need to be available and empathic, while also maintaining an extraordinary awareness of their boundaries to keep the patient safe from any hint of violation. Even the most experienced clinicians find it beneficial to get supervision with such cases.

Group treatments have been used in therapy for sexual abuse but have received mixed reviews. Some abused children find them helpful; others find that they are intrusive and increase their feelings of shame. When timed appropriately, these group treatments can be a helpful adjunct to individual work, because they allow for a level of peer support around sexual activity and exploration that is normative for peers. Although such groups are even used for younger children, this seems inadvisable because of the developmental limitation of younger peer groups to provide reliable support and guidance.

Sex Offenders

Sex offenders have sometimes been victims themselves. They have become perpetrators, perhaps in an effort to manage some of the anxieties that their own abuse continues to provoke. Becker summarized the data on male adolescent sexual assault: each year, between 200 000 and 450 000 sexual assaults using force occur [54]. About 20% of these are rapes, and 30–50% involve child abuse. About three-quarters of adolescent sex offenders have assaulted someone before their 12th birthday. Overall, about 2% of adolescent males engage in aggressive sexual assaults, and as many as 15% are estimated to engage in some type of forced sexual contact. Approximately one-third of females and one-tenth of males report sexual abuse before the age of 18 years.

Sex offenders have been described as loners, under-achievers, impulsive, having low frustration tolerance, and tending to rely on external regulators of behaviors. In comparison to other nonsexual violent offenders, sex offenders live more often with their birth parents, have lower self-reported delinquency, and use fewer drugs and alcohol; they do, however, have more familial violence and abuse, especially sexual abuse, and are more socially and sexually isolated. A history of childhood sexual abuse seems to be particularly high among those sex offenders whose victims are boys. Some studies have shown that there is also an increased rate of depressive symptomatology in this group [54]. Among incarcerated male teens who had been perpetrators of sexual assault, there were four predictors of sexual assault:living with violence at home, being a victim of sexual assault, parents encouraging violence, and knowing a role model for sexual assault [55]. There is evidence that the management of sexual aggression, considered a learned restraint, is mediated by family interaction patterns.

Treatment of Sex Offenders

Treatment of child and adolescent sex offenders includes individual, family, and group work and is aimed at preventing recurrence of the behavior. A review of treatment approaches for this group found a paucity of empirically based research [56]. To date there have only been two controlled outcome studies in this area, one on multisystemictherapy, and the other of a court-based sexual offender outpatient treatment program. Although the results from multisystemictherapy were encouraging, the sample size was small, and the study has not yet been replicated (see review by Becker and Hick [56]). There have been many other uncontrolled studies using various therapies including cognitive-behavioral interventions, relapse prevention models, group therapy, and family therapy. However, there is no clear evidence for the efficacy of any treatment approaches for adolescent sex offenders. Another critique of existing treatment studies concludes that the treatment outcome literature is still developing, although preliminary reports indicate that juvenile sex offenders appear responsive to treatment [57].

References

1. Yates A. Childhood sexuality. In: Lewis M (ed.) *Child and Adolescent Psychiatry: A Comprehensive Textbook.* Baltimore: Williams & Wilkins, 1991; pp. 195–214.
2. Currier RL. Juvenile sexuality in global perspective. In: Constantine LL, Marinson FM (eds) *Children and Sex:*

New Findings, New Perspectives. Boston: Little Brown & Co., 1981; pp. 9–19.
3. Kohlberg L. A cognitive developmental analysis of children's sex roles and attitudes. In: Maccoby EE (ed.) *The Development of Sex Differences.* Stanford: Stanford University Press, 1966; pp. 82–173.
4. Kinsey AC, Wardell BP, Martin CE. *Sexual Behavior in the Human Male.* Philiadelphia: WB Saunders, 1948.
5. Offer D. In defense of adolescents. *JAMA* 1987;**257**: 3407–3408.
6. Graber JA, Seeley JR, Brooks-Gunn J, Lewinsohn PM. Is pubertal timing associated with psychopathology in young adulthood. *J Am Acad Child Adolesc Psychiatry* 2004;**43**:718–726.
7. Denizet-Lewis B. Friends, friends with benefits and the benefits of the local mall. *NY Times Magazine,* May 30, 2004.
8. Lock J. Psychosexual development in adolescents with chronic medical illnesses. *Psychosomatics* 1998;**39**: 340–349.
9. Lee PA, Houk CP, Ahmed SF, Hughes IA. Consensus statement on management of intersex disorders. International Consensus Conference on Intersex. *Pediatrics* 2006;**118**:e488–500.
10. Reiner WG, Gearhart JP. Discordant sexual identity in some genetic males with cloacalexstrophy assigned to female sex at birth. *N Engl J Med* 2004;**350**:333–341.
11. Creighton SM, Liao LM. Changing attitudes to sex assignment in intersex. *Brit. J Urol Int* 2004;**93**: 659–664.
12. Frader J, Alderson P, Asch A, *et al.* Health care professionals and intersex conditions. *Arch Pediatr Adolesc Med* 2004;**158**:426–428.
13. American Academy of Pediatrics. Evaluation of the newborn with developmental anomalies of the external genitalia. *Pediatrics* 2000;**106**:138–142.
14. Pilkington NW, D'Augelli AR. Victimization of lesbian, gay, and bisexual youth in community settings. *Community Psychol* 1995;**23**:34–56.
15. Hammelman TL. Gay and lesbian youth: Contributing factors to serious attempts or considerations of suicide. *J Gay Lesbian Psychother* 1993;**2**:77–89.
16. Rotheram-Borus MJ, Rosario M, Reid H, Koopman C. Predicting patterns of sexual acts among homosexual and bisexual youths. *Am J Psychiatry* 1995;**152**: 588–595.
17. Hershberger SL, D'Augelli AR. The impact of victimization on the mental health and suicidality of lesbian, gay, and bisexual youth. *Dev Psychol* 1995;**31**:65–74.
18. Troiden RR. *Gay and Lesbian Identity.* Dix Hills, NY: General Hall, 1988.
19. Hetrick ES, Martin AD. Developmental issues and their resolution for gay and lesbian adolescents. *J Homosex* 1987;**14**:25–43.
20. Lasser J, Tharinger D. Visibility management in school and beyond: a qualitative study of gay, lesbian, bisexual youth. *J Adolesc* 2003;**26**:233–244.
21. Stanley JL. An applied collaborative training program for graduate students in community psychology: a case study of a community project working with lesbian, gay, bisexual, transgender, and questioning youth. *Am J Community Psychol* 2003;**31**:253–265.
22. Uribe V. Project 10: A school-based outreach to gay and lesbian youth. *High School Journal* 1993;**77**(Special issue): 108–112.

23. Brenner ND, Collins L, Kann L. Reliability of the youth risk behavior survey questionnaire. *Am J Epidemiology* 1995;**141**:575–580.

24. American Psychiatric Association. *Diagnostic and Statistical Manual of Mental Disorders*, 4th edn, Text Revision. Washington, DC: American Psychiatric Association, 2000.

25. Cohen-Kettenis PT, Pfafflin, F. The DSM diagnostic criteria for gender identity disorder in adolescents and adults. *Arch Sex Behav* 2009;**39**:499–513.

26. Bradley SJ, Zucker KJ. Gender identity disorder: a review of the past 10 years. *J Am Acad Child Adolesc Psychiatry* 1997;**36**:872–880.

27. Wilson I, Griffin C, Wren B. The validity of the diagnosis of gender identity disorder (child and adolescent criteria). *Clin Child Psychol Psychiat* 2002;**7**:335–351.

28. Zucker KJ. Cross-gender-identified children. In: Steiner BW (ed.) *Gender Dysphoria: Development, Research, and Management*. New York: Plenum Publishing, 1985; pp. 75–174.

29. Zucker KJ, Green R. Psychosexual disorders in children and adolescents. *J Child Psychol Psychiat* 1992;**33**:107–151.

30. Pillard RC. Kinsey scale: is it familial? In: McWhirter DP, Sanders SA, Reinisch JM (eds) *Homosexuality/Heterosexuality: Concepts of Sexual Orientation*. New York: Oxford University Press, 1990; pp. 88–100.

31. Meyer-Bahlburg HFL. Sex hormone changes during puberty and sexual behavior. In: Samson J (ed.) *Childhood and Sexuality*. Montreal: Éditions Études Vivantes, 1980; pp. 113–122.

32. Blanchard R. Fraternal birth order and the maternal immune hypothesis of male homosexuality. *Horm Behav* 2001;**40**:105–114.

33. Blanchard R, Zucker KJ, Bradley SJ, Hume C. Birth order and sibling sex ratio in homosexual male adolescents and probably prehomosexual feminine boys. *Dev Psychol* 1995;**31**:22–30.

34. Haraldsen IR, Opjordsmoen S, Egeland T, Finset A. Sex-sensitive cognitive performance in untreated patients with early onset gender identity disorder. *Psychoneuroendocrinology* 2003;**28**:906–915.

35. Cohen-Kettenis PT, van Goozen SHM, Doorn CD, Gooren LJG. Cognitive ability and cerebral lateralisation in transsexuals. *Psychoneuroendocrinology* 1998;**23**:631–641.

36. Dennis C. The most important sexual organ. *Nature* 2004;**427**:390–392.

37. Coates S, Person ES. Extreme boyhood femininity: isolated behavior or pervasive disorder? *J Am Acad Child Psychiatry* 1985;**24**:702–709.

38. Owen-Anderson AF, Bradley SJ, Zucker KJ. Expressed emotion in mothers of boys with gender identity disorder. *J Sex Marital Ther* 2010;**36**:327–345.

39. Kohlberg L, Ricks D, Snarey J. Childhood development as a predictor of adaptation in adulthood. *Genet Psychol Monogr* 1984;**110**:91–172.

40. Bailey JM, Zucker KJ. Childhood sex-typed behavior and sexual orientation: A conceptual analysis and quantitative review. *Dev Psychol* 1995;**31**:43–55.

41. Zucker KJ, Bradley SJ. *Gender Identity Disorder and Psychosexual Problems in Children and Adolescents*. New York: Guilford Press, 1995.

42. Cohen-Kettenis PT, Owen A, Kaijser VG, Bradley SJ, Zucker KJ., Demographic characteristics, social competence, and behavior problems in children with gender identity disorder: a cross-national, cross-clinic comparative analysis. *J Abnorm Child Psychol* 2003;**31**:41–53.

43. Wallien MS, Swaab H, Cohen-Kettenis PT. Psychiatric comorbidity among children with gender identity disorder. *J Am Acad Child Adolesc Psychiatry* 2007;**46**: 1307–1314.

44. Smith YL, van Goozen SH, Cohen-Kettenis PT. Adolescents with gender identity disorder who were accepted or rejected for sex reassignment surgery: a prospective follow-up study. *J Am Acad Child Adolesc Psychiatry* 2001;**40**:472–481.

45. Freud S. *Three Essays on the Theory of Sexuality*. Standard Edition, 7th edn. London: Hogarth, 1905; pp. 125–231.

46. Stoller RJ. *Observing the Erotic Imagination*. New Haven, CT: Yale University Press, 1985.

47. Cooper AM, Sack MH. Sadism and masochism in character disorder and resistance. In: Fogel GI, Myers WA (eds) *Perversions and Near Perversions in Clinical Practice: New Psychoanalytic Perspectives*. New Haven, CT: Yale University Press, 1991; pp. 17–25.

48. Kaplan LJ. *Female Perversions: The Temptations of Emma Bovary*. New York: Doubleday & Co., 1991.

49. Abouesh A, Clayton A. Compulsive voyeurism and exhibitionism: a clinical response to paroxetine. *Arch Sex Behav* 1999;**28**:23–30.

50. Kafka MP. Sertraline pharmacotherapy for paraphilias and paraphilia-related disorders: an open trial. *Ann Clin Psychiatry* 1994;**6**:189–195.

51. Briken P, Hill A, Berner W. Pharmacotherapy of paraphilias with long-acting agonists of luteinizing hormone-releasing hormone: a systematic review. *J Clin Psychiatry* 2003;**64**:890–897.

52. Gerardin P, Thibaut F. Epidemiology and treatment of juvenile sexual offending. *Paediatr Drugs* 2004;**6**:79–91.

53. Thibaut F, De La Barra F, Gordon H, Cosyns P, Bradford J. The World Federation of Societies of Biological Psychiatry (WFSBP) guidelines for the biological treatment of paraphilias. *World J Biol Psychiatry* 2010;**11**: 604–655.

54. Becker JV. Offenders: characteristics and treatment. *Future Child* 1994;**4**:176–197.

55. Morris RE, Anderson MM, Knox GW. Incarcerated adolescents' experiences as perpetrators of sexual assault. *Arch Pediatr Adolesc Med* 2002;**156**:831–835.

56. Becker JV, Hicks SJ. Juvenile sexual offenders: characteristics, interventions, and policy issues. *Ann N Y Acad Sci* 2003;**989**:397–410; discussion 441–445.

57. Walker DF, McGovern SK, Poey EL, Otis KE. Treatment effectiveness for male adolescent sexual offenders: A Meta-analysis and review. *J Child Sexual Abuse* 2005;**13**: 281–293.

Section III
Developmental Disorders

20

Learning and Communications Disorders

Pamela A. Gulley

Introduction

The American Psychiatric Association's 1987 decision to move from a single diagnostic criterion to multiaxial diagnostic criteria for psychiatric disorders afforded clinicians an opportunity to use a more holistic approach to determine pathology [1]. This was a particularly important change with respect to our current understanding of the nature of childhood psychiatric disorders. Pathology in children does not consist of a discrete series of behaviors that fit easily into designated areas. Rather, the child's difficulties are manifested as behaviors that could be mislabeled and misdiagnosed depending on the system that is used to first identify the a typical concerns.

The child who is slow to develop language skills, for example, may be classified as mentally retarded, but with further investigation, it may be discovered that a trauma occurred that resulted in elective mutism. This chapter discusses the educational aspects of clinical diagnosis as well as the impact of communication disorders on a "child's ability to function effectively in his or her environment."

Educational disorders coded on Axis I relate to reading, writing, and mathematical abilities as measured on individually administered achievement tests. A child is identified as having a disorder in an academic area if his or her academic achievement is not commensurate with the standards for the child's chronological age, measured cognitive ability, and age-appropriate education. The term learning disability has been used in the educational field since the early 1970s. Learning disorders appeared as a part of the clinical criteria of the *Diagnostic and Statistical Manual of Mental Disorders* (DSM) system in 1987. Much controversy has surrounded the definition and the diagnosis of children's learning problems. In the educational arena, the concept of learning disability has gone through several phases of definition, which are delimited as follows [2,3]:

- Foundation phase – involved basic research in the area of brain function and dysfunction that led to a definition of learning disabilities based on a neurological handicap.
- Transition phase – focused on the information processing aspect of the disorder. Learning disabilities were considered to be related to perceptual disorders; this led to many theories of the relationships among the various sensory systems – auditory, visual, tactile, and kinetic. If the sensory systems did not communicate effectively with each other, then a learning disability was identified.
- Integration phase – recognized that children with learning disorders would require specialized educational services to achieve better success in school. It also became evident that children with learning disorders were not fitting into categories for special educational services because they were not mentally retarded or behaviorally handicapped. Legislation enacted to rectify this problem (the 1969 Children with Specific Learning Disabilities Act) began the establishment of appropriate educational programs for children with learning disabilities [4].

With program options in place, other controversies ensued related to the definition, identification, and proper diagnosis of a learning disability. The term "learning disability" became a catch-all "diagnosis" for any child who had academic difficulties. Controversy also centered around methods for determining whether a child's learning problems are related to a disorder, a dysfunction, or behavioral, emotional, or environmental influences. Related issues included the reliability and validity of assessment measures as well as the professional training required to determine whether a person has a disability. The Education for All Handicapped Act of 1975 was enacted to provide federal guidelines clarifying the inconsistency and controversy created by the original law [5]. This law defined the various disabilities, established

Clinical Child Psychiatry, Third Edition. Edited by William M. Klykylo and Jerald Kay.
© 2012 John Wiley & Sons, Ltd. Published 2012 by John Wiley & Sons, Ltd.

the general provisions from which programs were developed, and determined the funding of such programs. In 1990, the Individuals with Disabilities Education Act (IDEA) amended the 1972 laws [6]. The entire language of the original law was amended to reflect "person-first" language and to establish the use of the term "disability." The term "handicapped" was dropped from the law. This was an important step for people with disabilities: they were recognized as individuals with many needs rather than as people who were placed into established categories in the name of available educational programming.

In 2004, the Improving Education Results for Children with Disabilities Act, which reformed the 1997 IDEA, raised the bar on accountability not only for those identified as having a disability, by including them in state assessment accountability systems, but also for those teaching in special needs settings, using highly qualified teacher standards [7]. In the United States, the federal definition of learning disabilities (Table 20.1) parallels the clinical diagnostic categories of the DSM-IV. Each state using the federal definition must develop specific definitions that are consistent and appropriate for determining educational services and interventions in the public school system. The funding of such programs is linked to an accurate interpretation and implementation of the IDEA. When determining an accurate diagnosis for a child, therefore, it is important that clinicians be aware of the specific laws of the state in which they work. It can create confusion if a parent or guardian is told that the child has a disability only to be informed by educational personnel that the child does not meet the appropriate criteria to receive services within the school setting. (See Table 20.1 for the IDEA's definition of specific learning disabilities.)

Diagnostic Categories

From a clinical viewpoint, the definition of specific learning disabilities translates into the following DSM-IV diagnostic categories [8].

- Mathematics Disorder   315.1
- Reading Disorder   315.00
- Disorder of Written Expression   315.2
- Learning Disorder Not Otherwise Specified   315.9

When coding any of these disorders, it is important to note on Axis III any sensory deficits or related medical conditions, such as a neurological disorder.

To determine the existence of an academically based disorder, the results of an individually administered achievement test are compared with the individual's expected academic aptitude. Achievement tests measure reading accuracy and comprehension, mathematics and calculation ability, and writing skills. A child's performance on such measures determines if he or she is performing "substantially below" what is expected given the individual's intelligence, which is measured on an individual standardized test, chronological age, and age-appropriate education. Such a discrepancy between a child's expected academic level and actual academic performance might result in impaired academic achievement or daily living skills [9].

The qualifier "substantially below" is typically defined as two standard deviations below the expected level of performance. Typically, 15 points represents one standard deviation in a quotient score. With an intelligence quotient (IQ) of 115, for example, a child would be eligible for special education services if he or she obtained a standard score of 85 or below on a measure of academic achievement. In most states this qualifier is

---

Table 20.1 Specific learning disability.

A disorder in one or more of the basic psychological processes involved in understanding or in using language, spoken or written, that may manifest itself in an imperfect ability to listen, think, speak, read, write, spell, or to do mathematical calculations. This includes such conditions as perceptual disabilities, brain injury, minimal brain dysfunction, dyslexia, and developmental aphasia. This does not apply to children who have learning problems that are primarily the result of visual, hearing, or motor disabilities, mental retardation, emotional disturbance, or environmental, cultural, or economic disadvantages.

Documentation must provide evidence of the following:
(1) A severe discrepancy between ability and achievement that is not correctable without special education and/or related services
(2) The determination that the discrepancy is not primarily the result of a visual, hearing, or motor impairment; mental retardation; emotional disturbance; or environmental, cultural, or economic disadvantage
(3) The relationship of observed behavior to the child's academic functioning

From Individuals with Disabilities Education Act of 1990. Public Law 91-230, Title 20, US Code Section 1401(a)15; 1997.

determined by the local education agency; it is important for clinicians to understand a particular state's criteria prior to diagnosing a learning disorder. A child with a learning disability may present behaviors such as sadness, irritability, anger, and nonmotivation, especially regarding activities related to school tasks. This disorder does not mean that the child cannot perform academically, however; it means that the child is not performing up to an expected academic level. This lack of achievement is first evident in an educational setting; therefore, unless associated developmental problems exist, a learning disability may not be identified until the child reaches school age and enters the educational arena.

This disorder is typically first manifest in a child as a reluctance to complete school work or homework, a disinterest in going to school, and possibly even school refusal. Acting out or oppositional behavior may also be evident. The child with a specific learning disability is aware that school is difficult and can feel much stigma because he or she cannot compete in the classroom. Children with learning disabilities are easily singled out as the subjects of a teacher's efforts to assist them with individual instruction, retention, or specialized programs. Although these interventions may be truly academically appropriate for the child, they can also lead to emotional and behavioral difficulties related to the frustration of the disorder and the social consequence of not being as competent as one's peers.

Learning disorders may also coexist with other disorders, such as attention-deficit hyperactivity disorder (ADHD), oppositional defiant disorder (ODD), conduct disorder, and depression. This complicates not only the diagnostic process but also treatment planning. Children with ADHD frequently have an associated learning disorder, even though learning disorders and attention-deficit disorders can exist by themselves. Except on the most difficult tasks, the academic performance of children with both a learning disability and ADHD may not differ from that of children with only a learning disability [10]. Children who have a diagnosis related to disruptive behaviors such as a conduct disorder or an ODD may also be found to have associated learning problems. In many of these instances, it is difficult to discern the primary diagnosis, since it is often unclear whether the behavior or the poor school performance was first present. However the behavior initially presented itself, it must be identified and appropriate treatment strategies implemented for the child to begin to change behavior and integrate more effectively into his or her environment [11].

Depression in childhood often presents in children with learning disabilities. It is frequently manifested as a lack of motivation, a pervasive sense of unhappiness, and a general apathy toward school.

Specific Learning Disabilities

Reading

To determine what a reading disorder is, the clinician must have a general understanding of the process of reading. Reading is a complex set of behaviors composed of many specific skills and an audiovisual task that involves obtaining meaning from symbols (letters and words) [9]. It involves two basic processes. The first process is understanding the relationship between a phoneme (a basic unit of sound) and a grapheme (a writing symbol) and then translating the printed symbols – words – into oral language. This basic process enables the individual to decode and then pronounce words correctly. The second process, comprehension, involves understanding the meaning of words both in the context of other words and in isolation. Reading is the integration of the two processes into a fluid application of these skills. Reading skills are critical to success in an educational environment. Difficulties in reading are the principal cause of school failure and strongly influence a child's self-concept and feelings of competency.

The best way to screen a child for the presence of reading difficulties is to ask him or her to read. First, observe the child's reaction to the task. If the child eagerly approaches a stack of children's books and begins to choose a favorite, chances are that reading is not a chore. If the child becomes oppositional or reluctant, this should be noted for further consideration. Second, listen to how the child reads. If the child struggles to pronounce every word or hesitates and needs assistance, an assessment of specific skills may be warranted. Mispronunciation, substitution of words, and insertion of words not on the printed page are also indicators of reading problems.

Older children often easily disclose academic difficulties in the process of the clinical interview. To determine if reading should be further assessed, it may help to ask children if they like to read, what they like to read, or to remember a favorite book. The education system is typically ahead of clinicians in detecting reading problems; therefore, the parents should request school records to provide to the clinician. Parents typically keep report cards and school group achievement results that can also be shared. If the child is presenting with a history of school difficulties, the results of a previous psychoeducational assessment by the school psychologist are often available.

Mathematics

This is a process that is based on logical structure. It involves skill development that occurs in a hierarchical manner from the ability to sort objects by size, to match objects, to compute, and to understand fractions, decimals, and percentages. A disability in mathematics usually involves an inability first to construct simple relationships and then to move on to more complex tasks. Particularly in mathematics, lower-level skills are essential for learning higher-order math skills [9]. The most effective way of recognizing a mathematics disability in a clinical setting is to review educational records or to conduct an interview or an assessment in mathematics.

Written Language

Written expression requires the use of a variety of cognitive activities. One must first conceive ideas, integrate the ideas into logical thought, and finally express the thoughts in written form. One's ability to use these cognitive activities to engage readers in a written format requires much more than the mechanical aspects of spelling, punctuation, capitalization, grammar, word use, penmanship, outlining, and organizational skills. Written expression also requires basic psychological processes such that if a disorder is present, the individual can be identified as having a learning disability in this specific area. To determine if a disability exists in written expression, the assessment should focus on the mechanics taught in an educational setting, such as spelling and sentence structure. Standardized instruments can be used; however, a careful review of a person's actual writing is the most effective screening measure. Writing a journal is frequently used as an effective technique in therapy. A review of both writing mechanics and content of the writing can indicate whether further assessment for a disorder in this area is warranted.

Learning Disorder Not Otherwise Specified

The DSM-IV provides a category to identify learning disorders that do not meet the criteria of any specific categories. This diagnosis is appropriate if a disability exists in all three areas and significantly interferes with the academic functioning of the individual. This diagnosis can be used even if performance on standardized tests is not substantially below the level expected for a given chronological age, intellectual level, and age-appropriate education. Making a diagnosis of learning disabilities not otherwise specified can also help the clinician indicate that the client as a learner has specific needs that must be considered in the treatment planning process.

Communication Disorders

The assessment and diagnosis of communication disorders are unfamiliar to many clinicians. These disorders are typically identified by family physicians, pediatricians, or school personnel if a child exhibits slow development in either the expression or reception of language. How a child develops oral language is crucial to his or her overall emotional health and can affect both the existence and treatment of a psychiatric disturbance. Communication disorders are frequently linked with additional educational disorders. When a child with a communication disorder exhibits a psychiatric disorder, the psychiatric disorder can be overlooked by mental health clinicians because of the child's inability to tell someone how he or she is thinking and feeling. Any behavior that exists because of a communication problem may be considered "treatable" in the realm of speech and language services without consideration of possible psychiatric needs; this follows the logic that if a child can understand and communicate language more effectively, the problematic behavior will diminish.

Communication disorders are categorized into difficulties with expressive language and difficulties with receptive language. Expressive language difficulties are manifest as a limited vocabulary, grammar errors (e.g., incorrect tense usage), and syntax errors (e.g., word recall and language structure). Receptive language disorders are manifest as an inability to understand the meaning of individual words, whole statements, or the relationships of specific words in a phrase (e.g., the relationship of the two words "Mommy's keys" means that these keys belong to Mommy) [10].

The diagnosis of a communication disorder typically follows a battery of standardized tests that measure whether a child is functioning substantially below the performance expected for a given chronological age and level of cognitive functioning. The federal definition of speech or language impairment is:

A communication disorder such as stuttering, impaired articulation, a language impairment, or a voice impairment that adversely affects a child's educational performance.

> Individuals with Disabilities Act; 1990.
> Public Law 91-230, Title 20,
> US Code Section 1401(a)15; 1997.

DSM-IV categories include expressive language disorder, mixed receptive-expressive disorder, phonological disorder, stuttering, and communication disorder not otherwise specified.

A phonological disorder exists when a child does not produce the developmentally appropriate speech sounds for his or her age and dialect. It is evident in a clinical setting when the child is difficult to understand and is reluctant to repeat a word or phrase when asked. A disorder in this area is typically evaluated and diagnosed early in a child's development, owing to a general awareness that the child is not speaking normally. Programs that typically screen for delays in articulation include Head Start programs and preschool and kindergarten programs. Speech intervention programs are also readily available to identified children through the IDEA [5].

Stuttering is a developmentally inappropriate interruption of the normal fluency and pacing of an individual's speech. It is categorized as the frequent occurrence of one or more of the following: sound and syllable repetition; sound prolongation; interjections; pauses within words; filled or unfilled pauses in speech (known as silent blocking); words produced with an excess of physical tension; and monosyllabic whole-word repetitions (e.g., 'my-my-my book').

Communication disorder not otherwise specified includes a voice disorder or other disorder that does not meet the criteria of the other communication disorder categories (Table 20.2).

When considered in relation to a psychiatric disorder, the critical aspect of a language disorder is that oral language is a behavior that enables individuals to generate ideas and to transmit those ideas to other people in their community. When a disruption occurs in this process and a person is not understood, an emotional component takes hold. If a person experiences a significant life stressor or trauma and because of a language disorder cannot tell others accurately or process the experience symbolically, there will be some effect on his or her psychic structure. Language disorders make it difficult to interview individuals not only because of

their inability to communicate but also because of their own awareness of not being understood. It may help to use alternative methods of collecting information regarding mental health needs. This could take the form of interviewing significant caretakers or using inventories and checklists such as the Children's Depression Inventory [12], the Incomplete Sentences test [13], and the Child Behavior Checklist [14].

Diagnostic Comorbidity

Comorbidity, defined as the coexistence of two or more distinct psychiatric diagnoses in the same individual, is of significant concern to clinicians when it is evident in individuals with learning or language disorders [15]. An understanding of the comorbidity between distinct diagnostic categories will assist clinicians in choosing an appropriate treatment approach, since individuals with comorbid disorders respond differently to specific therapeutic approaches.

Cantwell and Bake [16], demonstrated that approximately one-half of children identified with learning or language disorders also exhibited other behavioral characteristics that could lead to a psychiatric diagnosis, and in 1988 Camarata and colleagues reported a direct correlation between difficulties in oral language and behavior disorders [17]. ADHD, for example, has consistently been reported in the literature as having a high level of comorbidity with learning and language disorders. The degree of overlap has been measured as high as 92% and as low as 10%, with variation dependent on selection criteria, sampling, and measurement instruments as well as inconsistencies in the criteria used to define both ADHD and learning disorders [18,19].

Table 20.2 Features common to all communication disorders.

(1) Inadequate development of some aspect of communication
(2) Absence (in developmental types) of any demonstrable etiology of physical disorder, neurological disorder, global mental retardation, or severe environmental deprivation
(3) Onset in childhood
(4) Long duration
(5) Clinical features resembling the functional levels of younger normal children
(6) Impairments in adaptive functioning, especially in school
(7) Tendency to run in families
(8) Predisposition toward males
(9) Multiple presumed etiological factors
(10) Increased prevalence in younger ages
(11) Diagnosis requiring a range of standardized techniques
(12) Tendency toward certain specific associated problems, such as attention-deficit hyperactivity disorder
(13) Wide range of subtype and severity

Adapted from Baker L. Specific communication disorders. In: Garfinkel BD, Carlson GA, Weller EB (eds) *Psychiatric Disorders in Children and Adolescents*. Philadelphia: WB Saunders Co., 1990; p. 258.

Studies have shown that children with ADHD who also perform poorly in academic areas are more likely to require placement in special education programs and additional assistance to complete homework and meet the requirements of the grade-appropriate curriculum. Not all children with learning and language difficulties have ADHD, however.

There is also a correlation in children between learning or language disorders and disruptive behavior disorders. If a child is ineffective in the school environment, he or she may learn quickly to draw attention away from the learning difficulty and to his or her behavior. Comorbidities that exist between ODD, conduct disorder, and learning disorders complicate the clinician's efforts to discern the most effective course of treatment. Even if the child's behavioral symptoms are minimized through psychiatric intervention, educational issues may persist, and the child's behavior at school may not be affected by only one type of treatment. To address the multiple needs of the child, it may be necessary to involve many aspects of the child's environment, such as school, family, and community.

Comorbidity with mood disorders is more complicated. Depression is reported as a high-risk factor for children with psychiatric diagnoses of ADHD, ODD, and conduct disorder as well as learning or language disorders, thus making a diagnostic conundrum inevitable.

The following are basic principles that will help clinicians gather the information needed to make accurate diagnoses that will guide the treatment of children with learning and language disorders.

(1) Past historical information and traditional developmental data are especially important in the diagnostic assessment of children. The history needs to focus on behavioral observation and the child's history of approach to printed material, interest in books, interest in listening to stories, and making up stories. Information surrounding the child's first exposure to the educational environment should include whether the child was ever excited about going to school or played school either in pretend play or with peers or family members. The caregiver should also provide information about the child's initial reaction to the school experience. In general, children present a history of looking forward to school and being interested and enthusiastic about learning. When this is not apparent, a learning difficulty may be underlying the presenting symptoms.

(2) Current history regarding the child's reaction to the educational environment is helpful to determine if a child's behavioral symptoms are related to learning issues. If school performance has been typical and there is a sudden change in the child's reaction to

Table 20.3 Cognitive characteristics of school-age children.

Preschool-kindergarten (ages 5–6 years)
• Children begin to develop a theory of mind
• Children are becoming quite skillful with language
• Children may overgeneralize rules in using language
• Competence is encouraged by interaction, interest, opportunities, and signs of affection

Primary school (1st through 3rd grade)
• Children understand that there are different ways to know things and that some ways are better than others
• Children begin to understand that learning and recall are caused by cognitive processes that they can control
• Children of this age do not learn as efficiently as older children
• Talking aloud to oneself reaches a peak between the ages of six and seven

Elementary school (4th through 6th grade)
• Children can think logically, although such thinking is constrained and inconsistent
• On simple memory tasks, children this age can perform as well as adolescents or adults
• With more complex memory tasks, the performance of children this age is limited

Middle School (7th through 9th grade)
• Middle-school students need a classroom environment that is open, supportive, and intellectually stimulating
• Self-efficacy becomes an important influence on intellectual and social behavior

High school (10th through 12th grade)
• High-school students become increasingly capable of engaging in formal thought, but may not use this ability
• Between the ages of 12 and 16, political thinking becomes more abstract, liberal, and knowledgeable

Adapted from Snowman et al.[21]

school, learning disorders are less likely to be an underlying factor.

(3) Collateral information from educational personnel as well as school records will augment a caregiver's description of the child's behavioral symptoms. It is helpful for the clinician to have access to any papers that the child has completed and to ask the child to complete age-appropriate tasks. Materials such as workbook [20] that provide tasks appropriate for various age groups are available in most bookstores. Observing the child's reaction to being given an educationally based task can be not only an informational strategy but also an effective means of establishing rapport.

(4) Observation is one of the clinician's most effective diagnostic tools for evaluating a child. An understanding of the behaviors and reactions to learning of typical children can provide the benchmark for determining if learning is an issue. Beihler and Snowman have provided an excellent resource for characteristics that are related to age and grade-level expectation [21] (Table 20.3).

Objective assessments are the most common means of determining if a learning problem exists. Table 20.4 provides currently used assessment measures that can assist in diagnosing learning problems. School personnel can also help the clinician by obtaining specific assessment data through curriculum-based measurement techniques and learning style inventories.

To formulate an accurate diagnosis for children with learning disorders, the clinician must be conscious of many factors. The following basic rules for formulating a diagnosis can help clinicians decide what to treat first, plan further diagnostic efforts, and determine the likely prognosis [22]:

Table 20.4 Commonly used achievement tests (arranged by type).

Group Administered
California Achievement Test (CAT)
Comprehensive Test of Basic Skills (CTBS)
Iowa Test of Basic Skills (ITBS)
Tests of Academic Proficiency (TAP)
Metropolitan Achievement Test (MAT)
Stanford Achievement Test (SAT)

Individual Achievement Tests
Peabody Individual Achievement Test (PIAT)
Woodcock–Johnson Test of Achievement
Brigance Comprehensive Inventory of Basic Skills
KeyMath3™ Diagnostic Assessment
Diagnostic Assessment for Reading (DAR)

- disorders due to general medical conditions or cognitive disorders pre-empt all other diagnoses that could produce the same symptoms;
- use the fewest possible diagnoses to explain the presenting symptoms;
- consider first those disorders that have been present the longest;
- family history is a primary guide;
- start with the diagnosis that is the most treatable and has the best prognosis.

Taking all of these factors into consideration provides the foundation upon which the clinical decision-making process can be built. As children grow and their disorder become more complicated this basic strategy will continue to guide the clinical process.

References

1. American Psychiatric Association. *Diagnostic and Statistical Manual of Mental Disorders,* 4th edn, revised. Washington, DC: American Psychiatric Association, 2000.
2. Singh NN, Beale IL (eds). *Learning Disabilities: Nature, Theory, and Treatment.* New York: Springer-Verlag, 1992.
3. Swanson HL, Harris KR, Graham S (eds). *Handbook of Learning Disabilities.* New York: Guilford Press, 2003.
4. Children with Specific Learning Disabilities Act of 1969. Public Law 91-230. 91st US Congress, 1969.
5. Education for All Handicapped Children Act of 1975. Public Law 94-142. 94th US Congress, 1975.
6. Individuals with Disabilities Education Act of 1990. Public Law 91-230, Title 20, U.S. Code Section 1401(a)15; 1997.
7. Individuals with Disabilities Education Act of 2004. Public Law, Title, U.S.
8. American Psychiatric Association. *Diagnostic and Statistical Manual of Mental Disorders,* 4th edn. Washington, DC: American Psychiatric Association, 1997.
9. Lerner JW, Johns B. *Learning Disabilities and Related Mild Disabilities: Characteristics, Teaching Strategies and new Directions.* Boston: Houghton Mifflin, 2009.
10. Brown, Thomas E. *ADHD Comorbidities: Handbook for ADHD Complications in Children and Adults.* Washington, DC: American Psychiatric Publishing, 2009.
11. Mercer CD, Mercer AR. *Teaching Students with Learning Problems.* Columbus, OH: Charles E. Merrill, 2005.
12. Kovacs M. *Children's Depression Inventory (CDI).* New York: Multi-health Systems, Inc., 1992.
13. Lanyon BP, Lanyon R. *Incomplete Sentences Task: Manual.* Chicago: Stoelling, 1980.
14. Achenbach TM. *Child Behavior Checklist for Ages 4–16.* San Antonio, TX: The Psychological Corporation, 2001.
15. Bird HR, Gould MS, Staghezza BM. Patterns of diagnostic comorbidity in a community sample of children aged 9 through 16 years. *J Am Acad Child Adolesc Psychiatry* 1993;**32**:2.
16. Cantwell DP, Baker L. *Psychiatric and Developmental Disorders in Children with Communication Disorders.* Washington, DC: American Psychiatric Association, 1991.

17. Camarata SM, Hughes CA, Ruhl KL. Mild/moderate behaviorally disordered students: A population at risk for language disorders. *Lang Speech Hear Serv Schools* 1988;**19**:191–200.

18. Biederman J, Newcom J, Spich S. Comorbidity of attention-deficit disorder with conduct, depressive, anxiety and other disorders. *Am J Psychiatry* 1991;**148**:564–577.

19. Maser JD, Cloninger CR. Comorbidity of anxiety and mood disorders: Introduction and overview. In: Maser JD, Cloninger CR (eds) *Comorbidity of Mood and Anxiety Disorders.* Washington, DC: American Psychiatric Press, 1990.

20. The Original Workbook Series. Grand Rapids, MI: School Zone Publishing Co., 2011; available at: http://www.schoolzone.com/about-us.

21. Snowman J, Beihler RF, McCowan, R. *Psychology Applied to Teaching,* 12th edn. Boston: Houghton Mifflin, 2009.

22. Morrison J. *DSM-IV Made Easy: The Clinician's Guide to Diagnosis.* New York: Guilford Press, 2007.

21

The Autistic Spectrum Disorders

Russell Tobe, Young Shin Kim, Thomas B. Owley, Bennett L. Leventhal

Autism has long been the paradigmatic syndrome for a group of conditions most recently classified in the *Diagnostic and Statistical Manual of Mental Disorders, Fourth Edition* (DSM-IV) under the category of Pervasive Developmental Disorders. However, more recent considerations of this group of conditions suggest that a spectrum of symptoms more accurately reflects the nature of these disorders, leading to the current concept of Autism Spectrum Disorders (ASDs).

Autism and the ASDs come from a long history of confusion and stigma. Even before the syndrome was originally named by Leo Kanner in his 1943 paper, as a condition of "autistic disturbance of affective contact," the condition has been the focus of considerable confusion. Some of this confusion comes from the association of the term "autism" with the so-called "4 A's" that Eugen Bleuler used to characterize schizophrenia. This was compounded by descriptions of Victor, the Wild Boy of Aveyron who, after allegedly having been reared by wolves, was brought to Paris and trained by the French psychologist Itard. And, with the advent of the psychoanalytic era of psychiatric theories, Bettelheim's Empty Fortress and Margaret Mahler's "normal autistic phase" of development suggested that failures in parenting caused this pervasive and persistent disorder. This early work gave rise to notions about "refrigerator" mothers as the cause of such serious psychopathology and created an enormous burden and stigma for parents seeking to understand and care for their children. Sadly, some of these biases and misconceptions persist to this day, interfering with early diagnosis and treatment as well as scientific approaches to research on autism.

Today we understand ASDs to be a group of clinical syndromes that have varying degrees of two fundamental elements: developmental delays and developmental deviations. Two-thirds of cases have evidence of atypical development before 12 months, and one-third of cases have a regression in speech and language before 18 months. Onset occurs before 30 months for all but childhood disintegrative disorder. The core syndrome includes deficits in social interactions and communication, along with presence of stereotyped behaviors, activities, and interests. The prototypic ASD is autistic disorder. The other ASDs, including Rett's disorder, childhood disintegrative disorder, Asperger's disorder, and pervasive developmental disorder not otherwise specified (PDD NOS), share many of the core features of autistic disorder.

Epidemiology

By the standards of childhood onset disorders, ASDs have long been thought to be relatively common; however, there have been recent concerns about recurring reports of rising ASD prevalence and the possibility of an ASD epidemic. Studies of ASD, conducted since 1985, have reported progressively higher prevalence estimates, ranging from 0.07% to 1.8% [1–7], and an even higher rate of 2.64% from the most comprehensive, total population-based survey to date [8]. Review of studies across cultures reveals similar rates of autistic disorder and consistent phenomenology, and ASDs are seen throughout all socioeconomic levels [5, 9, 10]. Autistic disorder has been reported to be four times more prevalent in males than females [9, 11], but this has been questioned by more recent work [8]. The other ASDs seem to be similar to autistic disorder with a greater ratio of affected males, except in the case of Rett's disorder, which is diagnosed almost exclusively in females.

Historically, about one-half of children with autistic disorder are said to have an intellectual disability (ID; or mental retardation), with intelligence levels ranging from profoundly retarded to above average in autistic disorder and the other ASDs [9, 12]. A notable exception

Clinical Child Psychiatry, Third Edition. Edited by William M. Klykylo and Jerald Kay.
© 2012 John Wiley & Sons, Ltd. Published 2012 by John Wiley & Sons, Ltd.

may be childhood disintegrative disorder, in which all affected children are mentally retarded [13].

Follow-up studies of autistic disorder have suggested that, when present, ID persists from the time of diagnosis onward [14]. Intelligence quotients (IQs) tend to be stable over time and are felt to be one of the most important predictors of outcome in autism [15]. Individuals with ASD have been said to have relative strengths in visuospatial skills and rote memory skills [16]. A small number of individuals with ASD are reported to have phenomenal abilities in particular areas, such as in memory, calendar calculation, or artistic endeavors. These so-called "savant" talents are also seen in individuals with other developmental disorders [17].

As one looks closer at the issue of ASD prevalence, more recent data suggest that most of the ASD prevalence increases are attributable to a combination of factors, most likely including: greater public awareness; better case ascertainment; broadening of the ASD diagnostic construct; lower age at diagnosis; diagnostic substitution; and target study population [7]. This is best exemplified in a comprehensive, total population study that examined both the clinical samples that were the targets of previous studies as well as a general population. This landmark study by Kim et al. found an overall ASD prevalence of 2.64%. This number is striking, but even more striking was their finding that while 0.75% of the children were enrolled in special education schools, a disability registry and/or receiving psychiatric services, 2/3's or 1.79% although clearly clinically impaired, were attending regular education schools and had no prior psychiatric/developmental evaluations or services. There were two equally important findings: the male:female ratio in the group receiving services was 5 : 1, whereas it was 2.5 : 1 in the regular education group. IQs varied as well, with a mean IQ of 75 in the special education group and of 98 in the regular education group [8]. Taken together, these data indicate that sample selection and careful measurement play a big role in determining the prevalence and clinical phenotype in groups of individuals with ASD.

What remains uncertain is if increased ASD prevalence is even partially attributable to a true increase in incidence. While more than 40 surveys have been conducted to examine ASD prevalence in North America, Europe, and Asia, only a handful of studies have examined ASD incidence, reporting incidence rates ranging from 0.4 to 33.7/10,0000 [5, 18–27]. Furthermore, methodological limitations (such as retrospective case identification from available records and inconsistent use of various diagnostic criteria) do not allow for the examination of changes in ASD incidence over time. Accurate incidence estimates, measured in a prospective study of consecutive birth cohorts using systematic and standardized assessments, are essential for determining if the increasing ASD prevalence is even partly caused by increasing ASD incidence; such an increased incidence may suggest that some environmental factor(s) and their interactions with genetic vulnerability are possible risk mechanisms for ASD.

In conclusion, ASD prevalence is definitely increasing over time but there is no evidence of a so-called epidemic. However, it is still possible that small to modest increases in incidence may be accounting for a meaningful proportion of the reported prevalence rises. More study is urgently need to address this problem.

Etiology and Pathophysiology

At this time, the precise etiologies and pathogeneses of ASDs are unknown. Early biological hypotheses focused on neurotransmitter abnormalities as a cause of autistic disorder, starting with Freedman's early observation of hyperserotonemia in many individuals with autism [28]. This has been replicated numerous times [29], proving it to be one of the most enduring biological findings in psychiatry. Hyperserotonemia is most likely due to genetic variations leading to abnormalities in the functioning of proteins involved in serotonergic regulation, such as the serotonin transporter and serotonin 5-HT_{2A} receptor, which are expressed in both the developing brain and platelet [30, 31]. A range of 30% to 75% of autistic individuals have nonspecific neurological abnormalities including: poor coordination, hypo- or hypertonicity, choreiform movements, abnormal posture and gait, tremor, and myoclonic jerking [32]. About 25% of autistic individuals develop seizures by the end of adolescence or electroencephalographic (EEG) abnormalities [33]. This phenomenon has been highly correlated with mental retardation and may be more correlated with mental impairment than the presence of PDD or autism [33, 34]. Seizures with onset in adolescence often generalize, but are typically infrequent [35]. Though these early observations are historically relevant and give a unique insight into the neurobiology of ASDs, advances in the sensitivity of genomic and neuroimaging technologies, particularly in the past decade, have further contributed to overwhelming evidence for a strong, yet complex, neurodevelopmental disease process.

Autism spectrum disorders are arguably the most heritable psychiatric illnesses according to twin and family studies. Concordance in monozygotic twin pairs has ranged from 60% to over 90%, while dizygotic twin pairs in these studies have generally found a concordance rate similar to that found in siblings of unaffected children [36, 37]. When considered as a spectrum disorder, twin studies suggest that at least 92% of monozygotic twin pairs are concordant for at least milder but similar deficits in the social and communication realms, compared to a 10% rate in these studies for dizygotic twin pairs [36]. Since the ASDs are often associated with mental retardation, the search for etiology has included common factors. For example, individuals with fragile X syndrome are considered to have a higher prevalence rate of autism [38]. While fragile X syndrome may account for only a small number of cases of ASDs, most children with fragile X syndrome have an ASD [39]. Other genetic disorders have been associated with ASDs, including duplications of the proximal portion of the long arm of chromosome 15 [40, 41], phenylketonuria [42], and tuberous sclerosis [43]. A significant advance occurred with the ascertainment of a genetic basis for Rett's disorder; mutations in the gene, MECP2, encoding X-linked methyl-CpG-binding protein 2 (MeCP2) have been identified as the cause of more than 80% of classic cases of Rett's syndrome [44].

Though the above rare variant gene changes incur large effect sizes and therefore strong linkage with ASD, their allelic frequency is low and they ultimately account for only a small proportion of ASD cases. Replication of many of these findings has also proved challenging [45]. With the advent of microarray analysis and the capacity for detection of copy-number variation (CNV) paving the way for genome-wide association studies [46], investigation of common variant genes (those with greater allelic frequency but smaller effect sizes) has yielded some positive results: chromosome 5p14.1 [47], the MACROD2 locus [48], and semaphorin 5A [49]. However, despite the significant advance of microarray analyses, replication of common variant analyses has proved difficult given insufficient powering of studies [48]. As a result, rare variant analyses remain a primary source of genetic data in ASD. Among the most readily replicated include the X-linked NLGN4 and NLGN3 genes along with interaction genes Shank 3 and Neurexin 1 [45], which are involved in encoding proteins regulating maturation and signaling in the excitatory synapse [50]. Though studies into the genetic basis of ASDs have yielded replicable results, these collected data account for a minority of ASDs, with the majority stemming from unclear etiology to date. It is hoped that further investigation of rare variant genes will yield insights into the specific neurobiology and pathogenesis of these illnesses, while advancing genomic techniques and more adequately powered studies will highlight common variant risk genes that compound phenotypic risk [47].

Using direct neuroradiological or neuropathological evidence or well-documented lesions from other cases with specific neuroanatomical or neurophysiological abnormalities, there has been a search for a lesion that underlies autism. Arguments for very specific, highly localized deficits (e.g., in facial recognition or processing of gaze) have been made as well as those that propose broader deficits in information processing and cognition that have less clear implications for neurobiology. Whatever the primary deficit or deficits in autism, these deficits must affect the way in which a child acquires information and skills from very early in development. In addition, the hypothesized deficits must allow for relative sparing of some domains (e.g., early gross motor development, sequence of development of syntax and lexical semantics, object permanence).

There is evidence for neuropathological changes in ASDs. Post-mortem studies have shown abnormalities in the cerebellum [51, 52], hippocampus, and amygdala [52]. Small studies have found a reduction in the size of cortical minicolumns, as well as an increased number of these minicolumns in both subjects with autism [53] and Asperger's disorder [54].

In terms of structural studies of the brain in subjects with autism, a consistent finding is that young subjects with autism have larger brains than matched controls; more precisely, there appears to be an acceleration in brain growth that subsequently slows by late childhood [55]. Increased volume of the caudate nucleus in ASDs has been demonstrated and shown to correlate with the degree of restricted and repetitive behaviors [56]. Reductions in corpus callosum volume have also been demonstrated [57], as well as preliminary evidence for impaired neural connectivity of the corpus callosum and other white matter tracts via diffusion tensor imaging analyses [58]. Some magnetic resonance imaging (MRI) studies have demonstrated cerebellar vermal hypoplasia, but not all studies [59, 60]. This may be related partly to IQ effects on cerebellar morphology [61]. Other studies have found decreased cross-sectional area of the area dentata [62], increased amygdala volumes [55, 63, 64], as well as differences in cortical asymmetries [65]. MRI studies have revealed increased brain and lateral ventricular volume in autistic disorder [66].

Functional imaging studies, particularly fMRI, have had a profound impact on the understanding of autism neurobiology [67]. Though discussion of each series of findings is beyond the scope of this chapter, hypoactivation of the fusiform gyrus during face processing has been amongst the most reported findings [68]. Hypoactivation and impaired modulation of other complementary social brain regions, such as amygdala and the posterior superior temporal sulcus, have also been implicated [69]. Furthermore, those individuals with high-functioning autism have been demonstrated to have normal fusiform activation with familiar faces but impaired activation with unfamiliar faces, again hinting at the large phenotypic and neurobiological heterogeneity of autism spectrum disorders [70].

Positron emission tomography (PET) revealed generalized hypermetabolism in one [71] but not another study [72]. Investigations using PET scans on patients with infantile spasms found that 10 of 14 children who had bitemporal hypometabolism met criteria for an ASD at follow-up [73]. The same group [74] found asymmetries in serotonin synthesis in the brains of children with autism, as well as a global increase in cerebral serotonin synthesis capacity in children with ASDs (vs controls that show a steady decrease with age toward adult levels) [75]. Subjects with ASD show decreased activation in the amygdala while undergoing a facial processing task [76].Magnetic resonance spectroscopy (MRS) revealed decreased levels of phosphocreatine and αATP in the dorsolateral frontal cortex [77].

Diagnosis

Phenomenology

There is much controversy associated with the diagnosis of autism. This is somewhat surprising at times as this seems to be largely related to the concerns about the growing ASD prevalence. Some have argued that increasing prevalence is due to changing diagnostic criteria. It is a bit ironic since the DSM-IV criteria have been in place for 20 years. Further, autism is one of the few psychiatric disorders for which there is agreement between the DSM and International Classification of Diseases (ICD) diagnostic classification systems. In fact, despite the concerns, the reliability and stability of the diagnosis of ASD is well established through the use of the widely accepted Autism Diagnostic Inventory-Revised (ADI-R) and the Autism Diagnostic Observation Schedule (ADOS). These are internationally acknowledged as gold standard instruments for research and clinical practice.

The central feature of the autism spectrum disorders is a disturbance of social development, including difficulty in developing meaningful attachments and social reciprocity [78, 79]. There is clearly some variation in the clinical presentation. Typically, a child with ASD has atypical patterns of eye contact and facial expression. Children with ASD are less apt to engage in these behaviors and are seemingly less able to coordinate expressive and receptive social cues. They also seem to lack empathy or the ability to perceive others' moods or anticipate others' responses. This may lead the child to act in a socially inappropriate manner or lack the social responsiveness necessary for success in social settings. These difficulties may result in subsequent difficulty in developing close, meaningful relationships. However, some youths with ASD eventually develop warm, friendly relationships with family even though their relationships with peers lag behind considerably.

Another area of difficulty for many children with ASD is in the acquisition and proper use of language for communication. It was previously estimated that only about one-half of children with ASD develop functional speech, However, the percentages may be larger as more high-functioning individuals with ASD are identified. If a child with ASD does begin to speak, their babble is decreased in quantity and lacks vocal experimentation. Yet, some children with ASD are loquacious; however, their speech tends to be repetitious and focused on preoccupations rather than aimed at maintaining reciprocity or engagement in a dialogue. People with ASD may use stereotyped speech including immediate and delayed echolalia, pronoun reversal, and neologisms. This is especially the case when the level of speech is limited. Even in individuals with higher functioning, speech may be idiosyncratic, consist of concrete constructions, include grammatical anomalies, lack or include atypical social meaning, and lack inference and imagination. For these individuals, the delivery of speech frequently includes atypical tone, pitch, and prosody (accent and cadence).

Individuals with ASD frequently engage in unusual patterns of behavior. They may resist or have significant difficulty with new experiences or transitions, to an extent much greater than their typical peers. At younger mental ages, they may engage in stereotyped motor behaviors. Classically, this has included hand flapping, peculiar finger movements (often in the periphery of the visual field), or rocking. Some children with autism engage in self-injurious behaviors, including biting or striking themselves, or banging their heads. Self-injury is most likely to occur in children with autism with moderate, severe, or profound mental retardation, but is also found in children with autism without mental retardation [80].

The play of children with ASD does not usually involve traditional toys or uses toys in atypical fashion. Play is often repetitive and may involve unusual preoccupations.

Individuals with ASD may have unusual sensitivity to some sensory experiences. This may include sensitivity in any of the five senses but particularly sound and touch. It is not clear whether these sensitivities have a neural substrate, are unusual habits, or if they reflect a resistance to unique or unexpected experiences in the environment.

Other problems in autistic disorder and other ASDs include deficits in shifting of attention and "joint attention." [81, 82] "Joint attention," or the ability to share one's attention with another, typically develops by 12 months of age. At that developmental level, it is characterized by children shifting their gaze to follow verbal and nonverbal cues of the parent so they can share a visual experience. Children with ASD are often very delayed in developing joint attention, if they ever develop it all. Examples of joint attention include social exchanges that include pointing, referential gaze, and gestures showing interest. For those who do develop joint attention, the skill is usually not nearly as effective as it is in typical children.

Many children with ASD also have symptoms of hyperactivity and difficulty sustaining attention, but these must be distinguished from the joint attention deficits. It is not clear whether children with ASD can also have attention-deficit hyperactivity disorder (ADHD), although many children with ASD may meet diagnostic criteria for the latter condition.

For many years, it was thought that *Asperger's disorder* was a condition distinct from autistic disorder as they share many common features. When originally describing the condition, Hans Asperger remarked that the children he studied began to speak at about the same time as typical children and eventually gained a full complement of language and syntax. However, he also observed that his patients had an exhaustive focus on particular topics. Asperger also described that the children he studied had difficulty in social reciprocity, and focused on certain interests excessively [83]. A DSM-IV diagnosis of Asperger's disorder is made if criteria for social deficits and repetitive stereotyped interests and behaviors of autistic disorder are met, but language is normal at 3 years of age by history, and full criteria for autistic disorder are not met. Even with Asperger's observations in mind, it is difficult to make the distinction between Asperger's disorder and so-called "high-functioning autism." And, given that there are no known biological (including genetic or functional and neuroanatomical imaging) differences between the conditions, the value of such a nosology is being questioned.

Rett's disorder is a developmental disorder that occurs almost exclusively in females and typically differs substantially from autistic disorder after the toddler stage. Typically, the child with Rett's disorder has an uneventful prenatal and perinatal course that continues through at least the first 6 months. With onset of the disease, there is typically deceleration of head growth, usually between 5 months and 4 years of age. In toddlerhood, the manifestations of Rett's disorder can be similar to those of autistic disorder in that there is frequently impairment

in language and social development along with the presence of stereotyped motor movements. In particular, there is loss of acquired language, restricted interest in social contact or interactions, and the start of hand wringing, clapping, or tapping in the midline of the body. Purposeful hand movement is typically lost. Another common symptom is hyperventilation. The child with Rett's disorder actually may improve in social capabilities as time passes while progressively deteriorating in cognitive and motor function. The disorder is relatively easily differentiated from other ASDs after the child has reached the age of 4 or 5 years [84]. Mutations in the gene (*MECP2*) encoding X-linked methyl-CpG-binding protein 2 (MeCP2) have been identified as the cause of more than 80% of classic cases of Rett's syndrome [44, 85]. Different mutations are likely responsible for much of the phenotypic variation seen in the disorder [86], including cases with preserved speech and normal head circumference [87].

Childhood disintegrative disorder and autistic disorder have some similarities in that they both involve deficits in social interaction and communication, as well as repetitive behaviors. However, the symptoms of childhood disintegrative disorder appear abruptly or over a few months after 2 years or more of normal development. There is generally no prior serious illness or insult although a few cases have been linked to certain organic brain ailments such as measles, encephalitis, leukodystrophies, or other diseases. With the onset of childhood disintegrative disorder, the child loses previously mastered cognitive, language, and motor skills and regresses to such a degree that there is loss of bowel and bladder control [13, 88]. Children with childhood disintegrative disorder tend to lose abilities that would normally allow them to take care of themselves, and their motor activity contains fewer complex, repetitive behaviors than in autism. Some children with this disorder experience regression that occurs over a period of time and then becomes stable. Another group of children afflicted with childhood disintegrative disorder have a poorer outcome with onset of focal neurological findings and seizures, in the face of a worsening course and greater motor impairment [89]. The vast majority of children with this disorder deteriorate to a severe level of mental retardation with a few retaining selected abilities in specific areas. Differential diagnosis of childhood disintegrative disorder requires obtaining a particularly thorough developmental history, history of course of illness, and neurological evaluation to rule out disorders including acquired epileptic aphasia (see "Differential Diagnosis" below).

Pervasive developmental disorder not otherwise specified (PDD NOS), or atypical autism, should be reserved for cases in which there are qualitative impairments in reciprocal social development, communication, and imaginative and flexible interests, but criteria for a specific pervasive developmental disorder as described above are not met. It is important in the education of parents, teachers, and colleagues to be clear that PDD NOS is closely related to autistic disorder, since many families that have been given diagnoses of autistic disorder and PDD NOS have the mistaken impression that this represents strong diagnostic disagreement between clinicians.

At the present time, it would appear that among autistic disorder, Asperger's disorder, childhood disintegrative disorder, and pervasive developmental disorder, there is a distinction without a difference. That is, it is not clear that these are distinct entities. As a result, the current nomenclature appears to encompass all these conditions under the rubric of "autism spectrum disorder" (ASD) (Table 21.1).

Given that this is a "spectrum" disorder, it suggests the possibility that the symptoms of ASD fall along a spectrum from extreme to mild impairment. However, this model can be further elucidated by examining several spectra (Figure 21.1).

Differential Diagnosis

The diagnosis of ASD requires distinguishing amongst several disorders that consist of deviations in socialization, language, and play. One systematic approach would be to examine the course of the patient from birth and determine if there was ever a period of normal development. Disorders to be considered in the differential diagnosis include developmental language disorder, intellectual disability, acquired epileptic aphasia (Landau–Kleffner syndrome), schizophrenia, selective mutism, psychosocial deprivation, and other conditions, as listed in Table 21.2.

Children with developmental language delay and sensory deficits can appear to have symptoms related to ASD at early ages. Due to their language deficits, these children may seem to have communication problems, and may be socially immature. However, children with language delay use relatively normal patterns of language, engage in imaginative play, and demonstrate appropriate attachment behaviors and social interactions with family and friends [90]. These children do not tend to have obsessive interests, or restricted and repetitive behaviors like those seen in children with ASD. They also do not respond unusually to sensory experiences as children with autism frequently do [91].

Approximately one-half of severely and profoundly mentally retarded children have symptoms consistent with ASD; it is unclear whether this is due to a high rate of ASD in this group or a consequence of severe and profound mental retardation having some phenomenological overlap with ASD, at least in terms of the

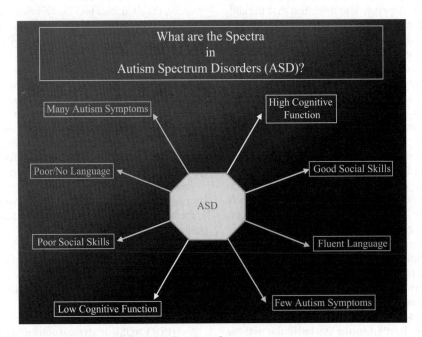

Figure 21.1   What are the Elements of the ASD Spectrum?

Table 21.1 DSM-IV diagnosis of autistic disorder and other pervasive developmental disorders.

	Autistic Disorder	Rett's Disorder	Childhood Disintegrative Disorder	Asperger's Disorder	Pervasive Developmental Disorder Not Otherwise Specified (PDD NOS)
Age of onset	Delays or abnormal functioning in social interaction, language, or play by age 3 years 6 of 12 of criteria below must be met at time of diagnosis	Apparently normal prenatal development; apparently normal motor development for first 5 months; normal head circumference at birth; deceleration of head growth between 5 months and 48 months	Apparently normal development for at least the first 2 years of birth; clinically significant loss of previously acquired skills before age 10	No clinically significant delay in language, cognitive development or development of age-appropriate self-help skills, adaptive behavior, and environment in childhood	This diagnosis is to be used in cases of pervasive impairment in social interaction and communication, with presence of stereotyped behaviors or interests when criteria for a specific PDD are not met
Social Interaction	Qualitative impairment in social interaction, as manifested by at least two of the following: a) marked impairment in the use of multiple nonverbal behaviors, i.e., eye-to-eye gaze, facial expression b) failure to develop peer relationships appropriate to developmental level c) lack of spontaneous seeking to share enjoyment, interests, or achievements with other people d) lack of social or emotional reciprocity	Loss of social engagement early in the course (although often social interaction develops later)	Qualitative impairment along with loss of social skills or adaptive behavior	Same as Autistic Disorder	

(*Continued*)

Table 21.1. (*Continued*)

	Autistic Disorder	Rett's Disorder	Childhood Disintegrative Disorder	Asperger's Disorder	Pervasive Developmental Disorder Not Otherwise Specified (PDD NOS)
Communication	Qualitative impairments of communication as manifested by at least one of the following: a) delay in, or total lack of, the development of spoken language (without attempt to compensate with gesture) b) marked impairment in initiating or sustaining a conversation with others in individuals with adequate speech c) stereotyped and repetitive use of language or idiosyncratic language d) lack of varied, spontaneous make-believe or imitative play appropriate to developmental level	Severely impaired expressive and receptive language development with severe psychomotor retardation	Qualitative impairment in communication along with loss of expressive or receptive language	No clinically significant delay in language (single words by age 2 and communicative phrases by 3 years)	

Restricted and repetitive interests	Restricted, repetitive, and stereotyped patterns of behavior, as manifested by one of the following: a) preoccupation with one or more stereotyped or restricted patterns of interest that is abnormal in either intensity or focus b) apparently inflexible adherence to nonfunctional routines or rituals c) stereotyped and repetitive motor mannerisms d) persistent preoccupation with parts of objects	Loss of previously acquired purposeful hand movements with the subsequent development of stereotyped hand movements; appearance of poorly coordinated gait or trunk movements	Restricted, repetitive and stereotyped patterns of behavior with loss of bowel or bladder control, play motor skills previously acquired	Same as Autistic Disorder
Exclusions	Disturbance not better accounted for by Rett's Disorder or Childhood Disintegrative Disorder	Disturbance not better accounted for by another PDD or Schizophrenia	Criteria are not met for another PDD or Schizophrenia

Table 21.2 Differential diagnosis of autistic disorder and other pervasive developmental disorders (PDDs).

Developmental language disorder
Mental retardation
Acquired epileptic aphasia (Landau–Kleffner syndrome)
Fragile X syndrome
Chromosome 15q11-13 duplication
Schizophrenia
Selective mutism
Psychosocial deprivation
Hearing impairment
Visual impairment
Traumatic brain injury
Dementia
Metabolic disorders (inborn errors of metabolism, e.g., phenylketonuria)

presence of developmental delays. Individuals with profound intellectual disability, without an ASD, usually have social skills consistent with their mental age, in sharp contrast to the individual with ASD, whose social skills are always delayed.

Acquired epileptic aphasia (Landau–Kleffner syndrome) is very rare compared to autistic disorder and other ASDs. A high index of suspicion for this disorder is raised by the loss of phrase speech after the age of 24 months, with EEG confirmation. Since the typical regression associated with ASD occurs before 18 months of age, children with language regression between 18 months and 30 months should also be evaluated by EEG, preferably with unmedicated sleep, to rule out an atypical acquired epileptic aphasia syndrome. The diagnosis of acquired epileptic aphasia is important because language may return after anticonvulsant or corticosteroid treatment [92].

Schizophrenia is differentiated from autism on the basis of symptom presentation. While some children with autism may have disorganized speech or behavior, they will not exhibit the hallucinations or delusions that characterize childhood schizophrenia. In terms of thought processes, higher functioning people with ASD tend to be ruminative, and may be so preoccupied as to appear illogical or thought disordered. Again, however, delusions and hallucinations will not be present, except in rare cases in which older adolescents or young adults with autism develop schizophrenia.

In selective mutism, the child is unable to speak in certain situations. As in ASD, the child may seem socially isolative and nonresponsive to environments outside the home. The child with selective mutism

usually can converse with family members and engage in imaginative play. Some selectively mute children do have articulation problems and/or language delay, but do not have deviations of speech such as those found in children with ASD [93].

Children with severe psychosocial deprivation can present with broad language deficiencies, stunted social development, and odd motor movements and habits [94]. However, this triad is qualitatively distinct from that seen in autistic disorder. Fortunately, many children subjected to extreme neglect, even over periods of years, can resume the developmental process at a rapid rate when exposed to nurturing and stimulating surroundings [95]. A child with a significant abuse and/or neglect history, as well as other children, should not be presumed to have ASD unless a diligent assessment, as described below, has been completed.

Course and Natural History

The general course of ASD is one of improvement over time. While the developmental trajectory may have a slope considerably less than that of a typically developing child, children with ASD do improve.

Assessing the course of ASD is complicated by co-morbidity, especially the presence of intellectual disability and language problems. As a result, development expectations or a prognosis must control for these issues. And, with the growing awareness of higher functioning individuals, it seems clear that the ultimate capacity for semi-independent or even independent living in the community is a real possibility.

Just because a child has ASD does not mean that they have stopped developing. Indeed, in general, as children with ASD grow older, some of the more "classical" symptoms of the disorder also change. Even those children with lower functional levels, who appear completely socially removed, with virtually no speech or only echolalic speech, motor stereotypies, and little ability to adapt to change, most often improve. As children with ASD enter the school years, the echolalic speech patterns lessen and more spontaneous communication begins to appear – this may even include spontaneous speech. In addition, there will likely be a growing tolerance of being around and even beginning to play with other children. Furthermore, social relationships, even if impaired or idiosyncratic, begin to appear.

As the child gets older, many of the bothersome behaviors appear to subside. These include a decrease in stereotyped movements such as rocking or spinning. However, as the child with ASD learns to adjust to the demands or expectations of daily living, frustration with being required to disrupt routines or a limited ability to communicate wants and needs, may lead to behavioral disruptions. This is exacerbated by the fact that idiosyncratic interests and ritualistic behaviors can and often do persist into adolescence and adulthood. In terms of language, receptive and expressive abilities can gradually improve over the adolescent years [35, 80, 96–99].

With the advent of adolescence comes a new set of challenges. Not only do the changes associated with puberty add new challenges to the child and family facing ASD, but increased body size and a more adult appearance make previous "childish" behaviors seem far more awkward or even dangerous. In some adolescents, however, there is an increase in aggression with the onset of puberty; if this occurs, a reassessment of the child is essential, including an EEG, as there is an increased possibility of seizures appearing in this age group, and significant regression may accompany this epileptic activity.

Aspects of puberty such as sexual drive and menstruation are complex but can be managed with appropriate educational and behavioral interventions. Many individuals with ASD do not understand the social implications of sexuality, such as masturbation, nudity, and touching, as well as other sexual behaviors. They are also more vulnerable to the sexual advances of predatory adolescents or adults. Therefore, anticipatory guidance and planning are important.

With maturity, and especially with the advent of adolescence, higher functioning individuals with ASD may become aware of the fact that they differ significantly from their peers. They often develop some interest in others and a desire to make friendships, but they often lack the "know-how" to accomplish this. This may lead to demoralization and even depression.

Previous follow-up studies of children with ASD (largely in children with "classical" or "Kanner" autism) into adulthood show that approximately two-thirds remain seriously impaired and are incapable of catering for their own needs. This earlier experience suggested that many of these individuals live in protected home-based or longer-term residential settings during their adult years, including community-based group homes. Between 5% and 17% of autistic adults are able to work with minimal support. In spite of social improvement in about one-half of children with autism over periods of years, most autistic individuals have abnormal social relationships. Outcome in autism is largely determined by IQ and language abilities, with IQ being the most powerful predictor. Good or fair outcomes are almost always associated with full-scale IQs of greater than 60. Acquisition of useful speech by 5 years of age is another important predictor of positive outcome. Even when an individual has an IQ and language abilities within a relatively normal range, there is nearly always residual social impairment that is persistent into adulthood.

There is a pressing need for follow-up studies on the newly identified, higher functioning individuals with ASD. Given recent reports that perhaps as many as two-thirds of ASD youth may live in the community and participate in regular education without services, the likelihood of a more successful, long-term adaptation is probable. However, even for higher functioning individuals with ASD, it is unusual for an autistic adult to marry or sustain a long-term sexual relationship. But, the possibility of having friends, a social life, and living independently is quite realistic.

Evaluation

As with all careful evaluations, the diagnostic process for an individual with a suspected ASD begins with careful history-taking, as well as the collection of data about behavior, cognitive abilities, and developmental functioning. Appropriate sources for this information include parents, teachers, and anyone who has had meaningful contact with the child. Other means of obtaining needed information include direct observation of the child and standardized assessment. A crucial step in evaluating developmental disorders lies in procuring a solid account of the developmental history. Special heed should be taken with regard to developmental phases of language, social interactions, and play [78]. Also, investigation of any chronic illnesses or illnesses with a neurological bearing in the child, as well as the medical history of the family, should be performed. Clinicians should inquire about family history of neurological disease, psychiatric disorder, history of developmental delay, and social, language, and learning problems.

Structured interviews are available for use in evaluating children specifically for autism, which help clinicians collect and organize historical information in a reliable manner. One such instrument is the Autism Diagnostic Interview-Revised (ADI-R), which is a standardized, semi-structured interview that can be administered to parents to help determine if the child has an ASD [79].

An essential piece of the overall evaluation is gained through direct observation of the child. Ideally, this should be done in a variety of settings to obtain an overall view of the child's behaviors and functioning under differing environmental conditions. The Autism Diagnostic Observation Schedule (ADOS) is recommended to structure observation of children, adolescents, and adults with suspected autism [100]. There are also a variety of other instruments available for evaluative purposes, including the Childhood Autism Rating Scale [101] and the Autism Behavior Checklist [102]. Another useful instrument is the Aberrant Behavior Checklist-Community Version (ABC-CV), which is useful for following responses of irritability and hyperactivity to interventions [103].

A complete physical examination, including a thorough neurological exam, is an essential component of any evaluation. It is important to identify and treat any medical and dental problems that contribute to or exacerbate a child's psychiatric symptoms. Overall physical health should be assessed and particular attention should be paid to those findings that could be related to ASD. For instance, cardiac and other congenital physical anomalies should be noted, and a skin (visual and Wood's lamp exam) and dysmorphology exam should be done to search for lesions consistent with genetic, metabolic, or structural disorders. All children with speech delay or articulation problems should have audiological testing, as even subtle hearing loss can adversely affect social and language development. Vision testing should be performed if there is any suggestion of visual deficit. There are no specific diagnostic laboratory tests for autism. A high index of suspicion should be maintained for seizure disorder. Specialized laboratory tests are warranted only with specific indications, but these might include chromosomal analysis, amino acid studies, and/or EEG. Although one-quarter of children have nonspecific findings on structural neuroimaging scans, MRI should only be performed if there are findings from the history and physical examination that suggest a potentially treatable structural lesion.

Chromosomal studies are indicated for children with a history and physical examination suggestive of fragile X syndrome or other specific chromosomal abnormalities. Although genetic counseling, including chromosomal analysis to exclude fragile X syndrome, interstitial 15q11q13 duplications, and other chromosomal anomalies, is most obviously indicated for families considering a subsequent pregnancy, 25% of the boys born to maternal aunts of children with fragile X syndrome will have fragile X syndrome. Currently, there is no specific treatment for fragile X syndrome or duplications of the Prader–Willi/Angelman syndrome region of chromosome 15, but chromosomal testing will have implications beyond genetic counseling if treatments are developed for these disorders in the future.

Complex neuroimaging studies, EEG, and other laboratory procedures have been recommended during the course of evaluation of an individual with ASD. In general, these are not indicated, unless there are specific clinical indicators for such evaluations (Table 21.3).

Psychological Testing

Psychological testing is a useful adjunctive procedure in the diagnosis of ASD. It provides details of the clinical picture that facilitate development of intervention programs while also providing benchmarks for monitoring developmental and treatment progress.

Psychological testing never stands alone as conclusive evidence of an individual's skills. The most useful measures are those that yield data about adaptive functioning, language skills, and intelligence. Testing can include the full spectrum of cognitive assessments, but since language deficits are so common in ASD, careful examinations should include both verbal and nonverbal cognitive measures – for example, Merrill-Palmer Scale [104], Leiter International Performance Scale [105], Bayley Scales of Infant Development [106], and Differential Abilities Scales [107]. The measures used depend on the individual being assessed, as well as the skill and experience of the examiner.

Other psychological testing may include assessments in other areas, including neuropsychological testing. For many children, examination for learning disabilities and comorbid psychopathology may be crucial. Since psychological testing instruments are not normed for use in individuals with ASD, the validity of the results of such testing must be considered before utilizing the data for diagnosis, treatment planning, or other purposes.

Objective measures of the capacity of an individual to utilize their skills to meet the demands of everyday life appear to be crucial in the assessment of individuals with ASD. Because cognitive and language measures may underestimate skills, reports of the skills necessary for self-care and daily living are very useful. While there are many instruments used in the assessment of so-called "adaptive skills" or "activities of daily living," the Vineland Adaptive Behavior Scales [108, 109] are the well-validated standard that provides valuable information about adaptive functioning so necessary for treatment planning and monitoring.

Goals of Treatment

The treatment of ASD has become progressively more complex. Historically, attempts were made to treat autism with psychoanalytic interventions. There remains little evidence that these psychoanalytic or other traditional insight-oriented psychotherapies are beneficial in the treatment of ASD. In more recent years, the treatment strategies have focused on the symptoms of ASD, and the goal of therapy has shifted from "cure" to optimizing adaptive functioning. As a result, behavioral treatments have had increasing prominence in the treat-

Table 21.3 Suggested components of an evaluation of suspected autism.

History

Sources: parents, teachers, other caregivers, anyone with regular meaningful contact

Developmental history – semi-structured interview with primary caregiver(s) strongly suggested: Autism Diagnostic Interview-Revised (ADI-R)

Past medical history

Family history

Examination

Direct observation of child's social, communication, and imaginative skills

Autism Diagnostic Observation Schedule (ADOS) suggested

Psychological testing (nonverbal and verbal intellectual testing)

Speech and language evaluation

Tests of adaptive functioning: e.g., Vineland Adaptive Behavior Scales

Vocational Assessment

Physical examination including particular attention to the neurological examination, dysmorphology examination, and examination of the skin (preferably with a Wood's lamp to rule out hypopigmented macules of tuberous sclerosis)

Audiological testing

Laboratory testing

Lead level

Quantitative urinary amino acids

Other tests depending on clinical situation

EEG if suspicion of history of possible seizures or speech regression after 24 months

Chromosomal analysis and fragile X DNA testing if dysmorphology, family history of chromosomal disorders, or as part of genetic counseling

MRI if findings in history or examination to suggest potential therapeutic yield

Other laboratory testing based on findings from history and physical examination (e.g., organic acids, thyroid function tests, etc.)

EEG, electroencephalogram; MRI, magnetic resonance imaging.

ment of ASD [110]. Unfortunately, behaviors learned by children with autism in one particular setting are not necessarily carried over to other contexts or retained well [111]. As a result, it appears that a group of interventions linked together appear to have the most promise for most individuals with an ASD.

Autism spectrum disorders are chronic disorders with a changing course requiring long-term intervention with implementation of various treatments at different points in time. Given that there is no current cure for ASD, treatment must be individualized and have both short-term and long-term goals for the individual and his/her family. Rutter has defined treatment in terms of four quintessential aims. These include the following:

(1) The advancement of development, particularly regarding cognition, language, and socialization.
(2) The promotion of learning and problem-solving.
(3) The reduction of behaviors that impede the learning process.
(4) The assistance of families coping with autism.

Since these aims are broad, it is useful to further differentiate them in terms of immediate and long-term needs. Each goal likely will require a distinct plan of its own and even a unique set of clinical skills to address the manifold complexities associated with ASD (Table 21.4). Most effective plans use community-based rather than residential treatment resources, as institutional settings tend to limit the experiences necessary to optimize functioning for living in a more typical social setting. This can usually be accomplished, except in

Table 21.4 Goals for treatment.

Advancement of normal development, particularly regarding cognition, language, and socialization

Promotion of learning and problem-solving

Reduction of behaviors that impede learning

Assistance of families coping with autistic disorder

Treatment of comorbid psychiatric disorders

times of extreme stress or need, when a child could benefit from respite care or brief hospitalization. Effective treatment often entails setting appropriate expectations for the child and adjusting the child's environment to foster success [78].

Approach to Treatment

Individuals with ASD require diverse treatments and services simultaneously, at various levels, and across the lifespan [112]. This complexity demands that a single individual becomes the primary clinician who serves as a coordinator of services. All too often this role is relegated to parents; however, even the most well-informed parent needs assistance in "directing the traffic." The primary clinician should have regular contact and visits with the child and his or her caretakers in order to assess the individual needs of the child while establishing a therapeutic alliance not only with the child but also the "team" invested in the child's (or adult's) care. An effective approach often calls for the services of a number of professionals working in a multidisciplinary, collaborative team. This group may include psychiatrists, pediatricians, psychologists, pediatric neurologists, special educators, speech and language therapists, behavior therapists, occupational therapists, physical therapists, social workers, and a myriad of other specialized therapists.

Psychosocial Interventions

Some of the most beneficial interventions for children with autism have been achieved through the educational process. With the passage in the United States of the Education for All Handicapped Children Act of 1975 (Public Law 94-142) and the subsequent IDEA (Individuals with Disabilities Education Act), all handicapped children, including those with ASD, are guaranteed the right to a free, appropriate public education in the least restrictive environment (LRE). This right is guaranteed notwithstanding the severity or nature of the child's disability. Improvement in the educational experience afforded children with ASD in recent years has resulted in fewer children requiring long stays in institutional settings [113]. With regard to lower functioning or severely intellectually disabled children with autism, no single educational approach has been identified as superlative in improving a specific area of weakness.

A debate has been ongoing during the last several years regarding the issue of mainstreaming of handi-

capped children within the schools. Although there has been a move toward implementation of mainstreaming, many children with ASD remain in specialized classrooms with children of similar need for intensive language and behavioral management services. Many children with ASD will be able to function academically or behaviorally at their best if placed totally within a regular classroom setting with no other supports. However, there can be distinct advantages in the placement of mild-to-moderately functioning children with ASD in a regular classroom for at least part of the day. These benefits include social exposure to typical children and greater intellectual stimulation.

Curricula that encourage and teach appropriate communications benefit the majority of children with ASD. This can be done individually with even very young children, and also can involve teaching parents and others how to foster effective communication in a child with ASD. Behavioral techniques derived from operant conditioning theory are used routinely by teachers and clinicians working with children with autism. Reinforcing positive behaviors, not reinforcing unwanted behaviors, and using simple techniques to replace an undesirable behavior with a more adaptive one are standard behavioral procedures. Organizing a milieu that is predictable and promotes understanding and learning for the child with ASD often alleviates the need for intensive behavior programs.

Success has been achieved in placing adults with ASD in jobs and workshops in the community. How successful one is in securing a job for an adult with ASD often depends on the resources in the community, and the ability of the adult's parents or others to advocate for them. Work placement and training as well as encouragement and consistent support on the job have contributed to success in the workplace for the individual with ASD.

Depending on the specific needs of the individual autistic child, a child can benefit from many different therapies or interventions. Among these are speech and language therapy, occupational therapy, and physical therapy. Some programs offer art and/or music therapy as a means of encouraging communication and self-expression. Brief individual psychotherapies – especially structured treatments like cognitive behavioral therapy (CBT) – may be helpful to those who are verbal and have a focused problem or are experiencing symptoms of anxiety or depression. Social skills groups or training may be especially beneficial for higher functioning children, adolescents, and adults. These interventions can serve to give the individual social experience in a positive, supportive setting.

Doctor-Patient Relationship

As with any clinical relationship, respect for the patient is the cornerstone of assessment and treatment. And while many patients with ASD have difficulty establishing and maintaining social relationships, they can and do benefit from relationships with their clinicians. It is incumbent upon the physician and other clinicians to come to understand the unique likes and dislikes of their patients and to be able to respond accordingly. Individuals with ASD can even have a sense of humor, albeit quirky, at times. Appreciating this and other unique qualities of each patient with ASD improves the overall relationship with the patient and the quality of care.

Many of the difficulties faced by persons with ASD are not a consequence of their own lack of empathy but the lack of sensitivity to the unique problems of ASD shown by those around them. In many ways, this stems from the adverse feelings that are all-too-often directed at individuals with culturally defined "defects." [114] Not only must the clinician be sensitive to these issues but also it is equally important that family members, teachers, and others help their community to have a proper perspective on individuals with ASD and not to respond out of fear or prejudice. Irrespective of the presence or absence of any diagnosis, we are all sensitive to how we are treated by others; this is true for most individuals with ASD. One must be cognizant that drives for mastery, development of autonomy, and acceptance are not reduced by the presence of an ASD.

Family Support

Having a child with ASD poses many complex challenges to all members of the family. As a result, even the strongest families will benefit from a broad spectrum of supports. Certainly, this support begins with the primary clinician and all the members of the clinical team; however, it should also include other members of the community. It is important to help families build bridges to community services in areas such as recreation and participation in religious activities. In many instances, families (both nuclear and extended) need to be taught about ASD and how to help a child (or adult) with ASD. In some cases, the stresses or demands on a family may be sufficiently destabilizing that some form of structured family therapy may be necessary. Helping families deal with frustration, disappointment, fear, and ambivalence with regard to their handicapped family member is essential. Other crucial steps include aiding families in arranging for special services or respite care in addition to providing behavior management techniques and emotional support. Many individuals with autistic

disorder and their families access support and services through local and national organizations. Such agencies include the Association for Retarded Citizens, Autism Society of America, Autism Speaks, and other community support groups. Books are also available to assist families [115] and peers [116] in learning about pervasive developmental disorders and to assist families in adapting to having a child with autistic disorder [117].

Pharmacotherapy

Even though ASD is considered to be a largely biological disorder, biological interventions in the form of medications have mostly proven to be of limited utility. Indeed, there is no pharmacotherapy that is specifically directed at treating the ASD syndrome. However, there are treatments that may be useful for the treatment of some of the symptoms of ASD and to help sustain behaviors to support other behavioral and environmental interventions. In short, pharmacotherapy is an adjunctive treatment for ASD.

For a long time the number of adequately controlled and powered psychopharmacological treatment trials in ASD has been limited. There are only two pharmacological agents with FDA-approved labeling specific for the treatment of ASD, and both target the "irritability" associated with ASD and not the specific syndrome itself. This is problematic, because many of the symptoms commonly seen in ASD (rituals, aggressive behavior, and hyperactivity) are also common in other individuals with developmental disorders such as intellectual disability without a pervasive developmental disorder. While these symptoms are clearly disruptive and problematic, they do not appear to be unique to ASD. As a result, some of the treatment strategies currently employed are derived from studies of other neuropsychiatric conditions with similar symptoms, including ADHD and OCD.

It is important to remember that the current state of the art is empirical treatment of target symptoms. Some parents and teachers of children with autistic disorder may have the misconception that medication can eliminate core social and cognitive dysfunction. There is no pharmacological substitute for appropriate educational, behavioral, communication, vocational, and recreational programming. It is essential to remember and remind parents, teachers, and others that medication should always be seen as an adjunct to the core interventions that address the primary developmental challenges associated with these disorders.

The use of medications to treat ASD appears to have significant potential as an adjunct to educational, environmental, and social interventions. Regrettably, there is no diagnosis-specific treatment at present. Nonetheless, individuals with ASD still have significant impairments as well as the all-too-often forgotten potential to gain skills and levels of functioning compatible with living in the community. It is a reasonable goal for clinicians to adopt the judicious use of psychopharmacological agents to assist in this adaptation. As one prepares for psychopharmacological treatment, we have found six principles to be useful:

(1) Environmental manipulations, including behavioral treatment, may be as effective, if not more effective, than medication for symptom treatment. Medications should be used as a part of an integrated environmental and medical treatment program.
(2) It is essential that the living arrangement for the individual being treated is capable of safely and consistently administering and monitoring the medication to be used.
(3) Individuals with ASD, when compared to the general population, are at as much, if not greater, risk for additional DSM-IV Axis I disorders/diagnoses. If a comorbid Axis I disorder is present, standard treatment for that disorder should be considered.
(4) There must be an established way of specifically monitoring the response to treatment over time. Side effects are common and mechanisms for identifying and reporting them must be established especially for those individuals with ASD least able to communicate them.
(5) A careful assessment of the risk-benefit ratio must be made before initiating treatment and, to the extent possible, the patient's caretakers *and* the patient must understand the risks and benefits of the treatment.
(6) The risk-benefit ratios change over time and thus must be regularly reassessed over the course of treatment.

Potent Selective Serotonin Reuptake Inhibitors (SSRIs)

This class of agents includes selective and potent serotonin reuptake inhibitors (fluoxetine, sertraline, paroxetine, fluvoxamine, citalopram, and escitalopram), as well as the less selective but potent clomipramine, a tricyclic antidepressant. This group of medications is most effective when insistence on routines or rituals is present to the point of manifest anxiety or aggression in response to interruption of the routines or rituals [118–122], or after the onset of another disorder such as major depressive disorder or obsessive-compulsive disorder [123]. The common side effects associated with SSRIs are motor restlessness, insomnia, elation, irrita-

bility, and decreased appetite, each of which may occur alone or, more often, together. These side effects are usually dose-related; however, for unclear reasons (perhaps having to do with the well-replicated findings of serotonergic dysmodulation in ASD), there is very wide variation in the dose that this population can tolerate before these side effects emerge [124]. Because many of the side effects may be present as symptoms in the often cyclical natural course of ASD when medication is not present, the emergence of new symptoms, a different quality of the symptom, and occurrence of these symptoms in a new cluster are clues that the symptoms are side effects of medication rather than part of the natural course of the disorder [118]. Until genetic variation or some other marker is discovered that allows us to predict the final dose, it is best to begin at a very low dose in this population, and raise the dose in a forced titration fashion. When the dose-related side effects are encountered, the dose should be decreased to the highest previously tolerated dose [124].

Stimulants

It was long considered that stimulants were not appropriate in the treatment of ASD in spite of the fact that attentional problems are quite common. Small but significant reductions in hyperactivity ratings may be seen in children with ASD in response to stimulants such as methylphenidate [125], dextroamphetamine, and pemoline. In a placebo-controlled crossover study, 8 of 13 subjects showed a reduction of at least 50% in ADHD symptoms when treated with methylphenidate [126]. More recent studies have suggested that methylphenidate is clearly effective in reducing hyperactivity and inattention in individuals with ASD – perhaps as effective as it is in treating ADHD, alone [127]. Of course, stimulants are not without side effects. It has been reported that stereotypies may worsen, and irritability and dysphoria may appear in association with the treatment with stimulants. Similarly, as with other patients treated with stimulants, sleep and appetite disturbances may appear or worsen – this is particularly problematic in ASD when these symptoms may already be problematic.

A key distinction in assessing attentional problems of children with autistic disorder is the distinction between poor sustained attention (characteristic of children with ADHD) and poor joint attention (characteristic of children with autistic disorder). Problems in joint attention require educational and behavioral interventions or treatment of compulsions or rituals with SSRIs. Problems in maintenance of attention of the type seen in ADHD are more likely to respond to stimulants.

It is not clear if there is any superiority of one stimulant over another in treating ASD. One report suggested that mixed amphetamine salts tend to be more effective than the methylphenidate products in ASD; [124] however, there are no direct comparison trials. In general, longer-acting agents are likely to be easier, and because swallowing capsules may be a challenge, medication that can be sprinkled may be more useful in ASD.

Sympatholytics

Sympatholytics have been considered for treatment of children with ASD because they are reportedly effective in treating attention and hyperactivity symptoms and because they cause some degree of sedation. The α_2-adrenoceptor agonist clonidine reduced irritability as well as hyperactivity and impulsivity in two double-blind, placebo-controlled trials [128, 129]. However, tolerance developed several months after initiation of the treatment in each child who was treated long term [129]. Tolerance was not prevented by transdermal skin patch administration of the drug. If tolerance does develop, the dose should not be increased because tolerance to sedation does not occur, and sedation may lead to increased aggression due to decreased cognitive control of impulses. Newer, long-acting forms of clonidine and guanfacine may prove to be more useful but they have not been studied in this patient population

Adrenergic receptor antagonists, such as propranolol and naldolol, have not been tested in double-blind trials in ASD. However, open trials have reported the use of these medications in the treatment of aggression and impulsivity in developmental disorders [130], including autistic disorder [131].

Neuroleptics

Typical Neuroleptics Because they were among the first classes of psychopharmacological drugs to be developed, typical neuroleptics have been among the most extensively studied drugs in ASD. Trifluoperazine, haloperidol, and pimozide have been studied in double-blind, controlled trials lasting from 2 to 6 months. Reduction of fidgetiness, interpersonal withdrawal, speech deviance, and stereotypies has been documented in response to these treatments [132–139]. However, patients with autistic disorder are as vulnerable to potentially irreversible tardive dyskinesia as any other group of young patients [140, 141]. Owing to the often earlier age at initiation of pharmacotherapy, patients with ASD treated with typical neuroleptics may be at higher risk because of the potential increased lifetime exposure.

Atypical Neuroleptics Because of the positive response of many children with autistic disorder to typical neuroleptics, similar medications with reduced risk of extrapyramidal symptoms must be considered. In addition, atypical neuroleptics are often effective in treating the negative symptoms of schizophrenia, which seem similar to several of the social deficits in autistic disorder. However, although atypical neuroleptics have seen increased use, they also have side effects that are highly undesirable.

Initially, both risperidone and olanzapine showed promise in open-label trials in reducing hyperactivity, impulsivity, aggressiveness, and obsessive preoccupations [142–145]. A large double-blind, placebo-controlled study found risperidone to be more effective than placebo in the treatment of repetitive behavior, aggression, and irritability [120, 146], and these gains appear to hold up over time [147]. Weight gain has been a significant problem in longer-term studies [148]. Open-label outcomes with olanzapine for similar target symptoms have been mixed, with positive results being found by some [142, 145], but not others; [149] weight gain was also a severe problem in these studies. The perceived effectiveness of these medications coupled with the problems with weight gain have led some to look at ziprasidone (which is not thought to cause weight gain) in this population. In one study [150], a retrospective chart review was undertaken of adult subjects who had been on an atypical agent and were then switched to the atypical ziprasidone. Seven of ten subjects did better or as well on ziprasidone, and there was a net weight loss. Another study with youths also found positive outcomes in 6 of 12 subjects with autism and also reported no weight gain. However, ongoing concern about QTc prolongation exists for ziprasidone without more safety data for children and adolescents in general and ASD more specifically. More recently, controlled trials of aripiperazole have shown promise in treating ASD. In a recent study, Owen et al reported on a 8-week double-blind controlled trial in 98 patients and controls. Aripiperazole showed a significant improvement in reducing irritability starting in week 1 and persisting through the 8 weeks. However, twice as many patients on active drug had adverse events and discontinuation (10.6% vs 5.9%), with extrapyramidal symptoms occurring in 14.9% of patients (cf. 8% on placebo). Further, there was a 2 kg weight gain in 8 weeks for the treatment group versus 0.8 kg in the placebo group [151].

The promises and challenges of using the atypical neuroleptics in the treatment of ASD are manifold. While they are quite effective in treating irritability and aggression and may work when nothing else seems to help, the side effects are legion and problematic in the long term. Therefore, these should be seen as agents used for short-term, focused interventions while behavioral and other strategies are put into place. If they must be used longer term, then careful monitoring for weight gain and metabolic syndrome are an essential part of the treatment.

Anticonvulsants

Seizures are reported in 25% to 33% of patients with ASD. As a result, a significant number of ASD patients may be on anticonvulsants at some point in time. However, in addition to their antiepileptic properties, the anticonvulsants are potent psychotropics that have been shown to stabilize mood in patients with mood disorders. Since problems with emotional/mood regulation may be present in ASD, the psychopharmacological management of patients with ASD may include anticonvulsants [33]. Unfortunately, very few studies have been undertaken in this area. In an open trial of divalproex, 10 of 14 patients responded favorably, including improvements in affective stability, impulsivity, and aggression [152].

Barbiturates (e.g., phenobarbital) should be avoided, when possible, because barbiturates have been associated with hyperactivity, depression, and cognitive impairment; they should be changed to an alternative drug, depending on the seizure type [153, 154]. In addition, phenytoin (Dilantin) is sedating and causes hypertrophy of the gums and hirsutism, which may contribute to the social challenges for people with ASD.

Carbamazepine and valproate may have positive psychotropic effects, particularly when cyclical irritability, insomnia, and hyperactivity are present. Several children with ASD were treated with valproic acid after electroencephalographic abnormalities were found. These children had an improvement in behavioral symptoms associated with autistic disorder after valproate treatment [155]. Oxcarbazepine may have some of the positive psychotropic effects of carbamazepine, with less risk of agranulocytosis, but concern about uncommon hyponatremia remains. Similarly, reports of side effects including polycystic ovary syndrome have been associated with valproate. As a result of these side effects, other, newer anticonvulsants have been proposed for ASD individuals. However, lack of adequate clinical trials and many side effects leave the assessment of risk-benefit of such treatment to the individual practitioner and patient.

Naltrexone

The opiate antagonist naltrexone was suggested as a specific treatment for ASD. However, double-blind trials have suggested that naltrexone has little efficacy in treating the core social and cognitive symptoms of autistic disorder [156]. Naltrexone has also been suggested for the treatment of self-injurious behavior in ASD, although the controlled data are equivocal [156, 157]. Controlled trials have shown a modest reduction in symptoms of hyperactivity and restlessness sometimes associated with ASD [156, 158, 159]. Potential side effects include nausea and vomiting. Naltrexone may have an adverse effect on the outcome of Rett's disorder, on the basis of a relatively large, randomized, double-blind, placebo-controlled trial [160].

Lithium

Adolescents and adults with ASD often exhibit symptoms in a cyclic manner and so there is much interest in how these patients might respond to agents typically used in bipolar disorder. A single open trial of lithium revealed no significant improvement in symptoms in patients with ASD without bipolar disorder [161].

Anxiolytics

Benzodiazepines have not been studied systematically in children and adolescents with ASD. However, their use to reduce anxiety in short-term treatment, such as before dental procedures, is similar to their use in the management of anxiety in people without ASD. One open-label study found a decrease in anxiety and irritability in patients receiving the anxiolytic buspirone [162].

Glutamatergic Antagonists

Interest in these agents has been sparked by the hypothesis that ASD may be a disorder of hypoglutaminergic activity [163]. In a double-blind, placebo-controlled study of the glutamatergic antagonist amantadine hydrochloride, there were substantial improvements in clinician-rated hyperactivity and irritability, although parental reports did not reach statistical significance (which may have been partially due to a strong placebo response) [164]. Further study of this medication and consideration of this hypothesis is warranted.

Pyridoxine and Dietary Supplements

Pyridoxine, the water-soluble essential vitamin B_6, has been used extensively as a pharmacological treatment in ASD. In the doses used for ASD, it is not being used as a cofactor for normally regulated enzyme function or as a vitamin; rather, it is used as a pharmacological agent to modulate the function of neurotransmitter enzymes, such as tryptophan hydroxylase and tyrosine hydroxylase. While Martineau (1988) [165] showed modest improvements in about 30% of children, subsequent reviews concluded that there were few data to support the claim that vitamin B_6 improves developmental course [166, 167].

Fenfluramine

Although fenfluramine originally showed promise in the treatment of ASD and associated cognitive dysfunction [168], double-blind controlled trials did not confirm an improvement in cognitive function or a reduction in core autistic symptoms [169, 170]. However, much like naltrexone, fenfluramine may reduce hyperactivity and impulsivity commonly present in autistic disorder and other developmental disorders [171]. The potential changes in neurochemical regulation after long-term administration [170], which *may* represent neurotoxic effects [172], and potential for acquired cardiac valvular disease when coadministered with phenteramine, suggests that fenfluramine should no longer be used in ASD.

Secretin

A case series of three ASD patients who showed improvement in core symptoms after receiving the gastrointestinal hormone secretin [173], led to a series of studies of this substance as a possible treatment for ASD. The results have been disappointing, with all studies done so far showing the substance to be no more useful than placebo [174–182]. These studies, along with the negative studies that followed initial excitement following open-label studies of naltrexone and fenfluramine, point to the necessity of performing double-blind, placebo-controlled studies of any putative treatments to ensure safety and establish effectiveness (Table 21.5).

Summary and Future Considerations

Autism spectrum disorder has had a long and complex history that has paralleled the evolution of psychiatry. From the mysterious notion of children being reared by wolves [183], to profound maternal deprivation, to the contemporary notion of a genetic disorder with environmental influences, ASD has become a well-recognized and highly studied clinical condition starting in early childhood. Despite the long history of these disorders, their specific etiology and treatments for the underlying pathophysiology have yet to be discovered. However, some things remain constant:

(1) As one more carefully explores the "autism spectrum" it is apparent that ASD is a relatively common condition, with a prevalence of 2–3%.

Table 21.5 Summary of treatment principles.

Psychosocial interventions
  Educational
  Curricula that target communication:
  – behavioral techniques
  – structured milieu
  – vocational training and placement
  – other specialized interventions such as speech and language therapy, physical, and occupational therapy
  Social skills training
  Individual psychotherapy for high-functioning individuals
Medical interventions
  Cohesive doctor-patient relationship
  Supportive measures for families coping with autistic disorder
  Behavioral treatment
  Pharmacotherapy to address problematic signs and symptoms

(2) The clinical picture of ASD remains complex with early onset and a range of severity from mild to severe with impairments in the domains of social, communicative, and flexible/adaptive behavior.
(3) The diagnosis can be made reliably and validly.
(4) Treatment is possible and leads to successful outcomes if it includes a coordinated, multidisciplinary approach that focuses on development of adaptive, social, and communicative functioning.
(5) Promising research is leading to a clearer picture of the ASD phenotype, and current studies are providing new insights into the neurobiology of this group of pervasive developmental disorders.

References

1. Gillberg C. Autistic children growing up: problems during puberty and adolescence. *Dev Med Child Neurol* 1984;**26**:125–129.
2. Baird G, Simonoff E, Pickles A, *et al.* Prevalence of disorders of the autism spectrum in a population cohort of children in South Thames: the Special Needs and Autism Project (SNAP). *Lancet* 2006;**368**:210–215.
3. CDC. Prevalence of autism spectrum disorders – Autism and Developmental Disabilities Monitoring Network, United States, 2006. *MMWR Surveill Summ* 2009;**58**:1–20.
4. Yeargin-Allsopp M, Rice C, Karapurkar T, Doernberg N, Boyle C, Murphy C. Prevalence of autism in a US metropolitan area. *JAMA* 2003;**289**:49–55.
5. Kawamura Y, Takahashi O, Ishii T. Reevaluating the incidence of pervasive developmental disorders: impact of

elevated rates of detection through implementation of an integrated system of screening in Toyota, Japan. *Psychiat Clin Neurosci* 2008;**62**:152–159.

6. Chakrabarti S, Fombonne E. Pervasive developmental disorders in preschool children. *JAMA* 2001;**285**:3093–3099.

7. Fombonne E. Epidemiology of pervasive developmental disorders. *Pediatr Res* 2009;**65**:591–598.

8. Kim YS. Leventhal BL. Koh YJ. Fombonne E. Laska E. Lim EC. Cheon KA. Kim SJ. Kim YK. Lee H. Song DH. Grinker RR. Prevalence of autism spectrum disorders in a total population sample. American Journal of Psychiatry. 168(9):904-12, 2011 Sep.

9. Fombonne E. The epidemiology of autism: a review. *Psychol Med* 1999;**29**:769–786*/*

10. Zahner G, Pauls D. Epidemiological surveys of infantile autism. In: Cohen D, Donnellan A (eds) *Handbook of Autism and Pervasive Developmental Disorders*. New York: John Wiley & Sons, Ltd, 1987; pp. 199–210.

11. Ritvo ER, Jorde LB, Mason-Brothers A, *et al.* The UCLA-University of Utah epidemiologic survey of autism: recurrent risk estimates and genetic counseling. *Am J Psych* 1989;**146**:1032–1036.

12. Volkmar F, Klin A, Siegel B, Szatmari P, *et al.* Field trial for autistic disorder in DSM-IV. *Am J Psychiatry* 1994;**151**:1361–1367.

13. Kurita H, Kita M, Miyake Y. A comparative study of development and symptoms among disintegrative psychosis and infantile autism with and without speech loss. *J Autism Dev Disord* 1992;**22**:175–188.

14. Freeman BJ, Ritvo ER, Needleman R, Yokota A. The stability of cognitive and linguistic parameters in autism: a five-year prospective study. *J Am Acad Child Psychiatry* 1985;**24**:459–464.

15. Venter A, Lord C, Schopler E. A follow-up study of high-functioning autistic children. *J Child Psychol Psychiat* 1992;**33**:489–507.

16. Rutter M. Cognitive deficits in the pathogenesis of autism. *J Child Psychol Psychiat* 1983;**24**:513–532.

17. Frith U. *Autism: Explaining the Enigma*. New York: Blackwell, 1989.

18. Powell JE, Edwards A, Edwards M, Pandit BS, Sungum-Paliwal SR, Whitehouse W. Changes in the incidence of childhood autism and other autistic spectrum disorders in preschool children from two areas of the West Midlands, UK. *Dev Med Child Neurol* 2000;**42**:624–628.

19. Davidovitch M, Holtzman G, Tirosh E. Autism in the Haifa area – an epidemiological perspective. *Isr Med Assoc J* 2001;**3**:188–189.

20. Lauritsen MB, Pedersen CB, Mortensen PB. The incidence and prevalence of pervasive developmental disorders: a Danish population-based study. *Psychol Med* 2004;**34**:1339–1346.

21. Icasiano F, Hewson P, Machet P, Cooper C, Marshall A. Childhood autism spectrum disorder in the Barwon region: a community based study. *J Paediatr Child Health* 2004;**40**:696–701.

22. Honda H, Shimizu Y, Imai M, Nitto Y. Cumulative incidence of childhood autism: a total population study of better accuracy and precision. *Dev Med Child Neurol* 2005;**47**:10–18.

23. Williams K, Glasson EJ, Wray J, *et al.* Incidence of autism spectrum disorders in children in two Australian states. *Med J Aust* 2005;**182**:108–111.

24. Barbaresi WJ, Katusic SK, Colligan RC, Weaver AL, Jacobsen SJ. The incidence of autism in Olmsted County, Minnesota, 1976–1997: results from a population-based study. *Arch Pediatr Adolesc Med* 2005;**159**:37–44.

25. Jick H, Beach KJ, Kaye JA. Incidence of autism over time. *Epidemiology* 2006;**17**:120–121.

26. Senecky Y, Chodick G, Diamond G, Lobel D, Drachman R, Inbar D. Time trends in reported autistic spectrum disorders in Israel, 1972–2004. *Isr Med Assoc J* 2009;**11**:30–33.

27. Wong VC, Hui SL. Epidemiological study of autism spectrum disorder in China. *J Child Neurol* 2008;**23**:67–72.

28. Schain RJ, Freedman DX: Studies on 5-hydroxyindole metabolism in autistic and other mentally retarded children. *J Pediatrics* 1961;**58**:315–320.

29. Anderson GM, Freedman DX, Cohen DJ, *et al.* Whole blood serotonin in autistic and normal subjects. *J Child Psychol Psychiat* 1987;**28**:885–900.

30. Cook E, Arora R, Anderson G, *et al.* Platelet serotonin studies in hyperserotonemic relatives of children with autistic disorder. *Life Sci* 1993;**52**:2005–2015.

31. Cook EH, Fletcher KE, Wainwright M, Marks N, Yan S-Y, Leventhal BL. Primary structure of the human platelet serotonin 5-HT$_{2A}$ receptor: Identity with frontal cortex serotonin 5-HT$_{2A}$ receptor. *J Neurochem* 1994;**63**:465–469.

32. Damasio AR, Maurer RG. A neurological model of childhood autism. *Arch Neurol* 1978;**35**:777–786.

33. Volkmar FR, Nelson DS. Seizure disorders in autism. *J Am Acad Child Adolesc Psychiatry* 1990;**29**:127–129.

34. Deykin EY, Macmahon B. The incidence of seizures among children with autistic symptoms. *Am J Psychiatry* 1979;**136**:1310–1312.

35. Rutter M, Greenfield D, Lockyer L. A five to fifteen year follow-up study of infantile psychosis. II. Social and behavioural outcome. *Brit J Psychiat* 1967;**113**:1183–1199.

36. Bailey A, Le Couteur A, Gottesman I, *et al.* Autism as a strong genetic disorder: evidence from a British twin study. *Psychol Med* 1995;**25**:63–77.

37. Bailey A, Bolton P, Butler L, Le Couteur A, Murphy M, Scott S,Webb T, Rutter M: Prevalence of the fragile X anomaly amongst autistic twins and singletons. *J Child Psychol Psychiatry* 1993; **34**(5):673–688.

38. Steffenburg S, Gillberg C, Hellgren L, *et al.* A twin study of autism in Denmark, Finland, Iceland, Norway and Sweden. *J Child Psychol Psychiat* 1989;**30**:405–416.

39. Reiss AL, Freund L. Fragile X syndrome, DSM-III-R, and autism. *J Am Acad Child Adolesc Psychiatry* 1990;**29**:885–891.

40. Gillberg C, Steffenburg S, Wahlström J, *et al.* Autism associated with marker chromosome. *J Am Acad Child Adolesc Psychiatry* 1991;**30**:489–494.

41. Cook E, Lindgren V, Leventhal B, *et al.* Autism or atypical autism in maternally but not paternally derived proximal 15q duplication. *Am J Hum Genet* 1997;**60**:928–934.

42. Knoblock H, Pasamanick B. Some etiologic and prognostic factors in early infantile autism and psychosis. *Pediatrics* 1975;**55**:182–191.

43. Smalley SL, Tanguay PE, Smith M, Gutierrez G. Autism and tuberous sclerosis. *J Autism Dev Disord* 1992;**22**:339–355.

44. Buyse IM, Fang P, Hoon KT, Amir RE, Zoghbi HY, Roa BB. Diagnostic testing for Rett syndrome by DHPLC and direct sequencing analysis of the MECP2 gene: identification of several novel mutations and polymorphisms. *Am J Hum Genet* 2000;**67**:1428–1436.

45. State MW. The genetics of child psychiatric disorders: Focus on autism and Tourette syndrome. *Neuron* 2010;**68**:254–269.

46. Cook EH, Scherer SW. Copy-number variations associated with neuropsychiatric conditions. *Nature* 2008;**455**:919–923.

47. Wang K, Zhang H, Ma D, Bucan M, *et al.* Common genetic variants on 5p14.1 associate with autism spectrum disorders. *Nature* 2009;**459**:528–533.

48. Anney R, Lambertus K, Pinto D, *et al.* A genome-wide scan for common alleles affecting risk for autism. *Hum Mol Genet* 2010;**19**:4072–4082.

49. Weiss LA, Arking DE, Gene Discovery Project of Johns Hopkins and the Autism Consortium, Daly MJ, Chakravarti A. A genome-wide linkage and association scan reveals novel loci for autism. *Nature* 2009;**461**:802–808.

50. Levinson JN, El-Husseini A. A crystal-clear interaction: relating neuroligin/neurexin complex structure to function at the synapse. *Neuron* 2007;**56**:937–939.

51. Ritvo ER, Freeman BJ, Scheibel AB, *et al.* Lower Purkinje cell counts in the cerebella of four autistic subjects: Initial findings of the UCLA-NSAC autopsy research report. *Am J Psychiatry* 1986;**143**:862–866.

52. Bauman M, Kemper T. Neuroanatomic observations of the brain in autism. In: Bauman M, Kemper T (eds) *The Neurobiology of Autism*. Baltimore: Johns Hopkins University Press, 1994; pp. 119–145.

53. Casanova MF, Buxhoeveden DP, Switala AE, Roy E. Neuronal density and architecture (Grey Level Index) in the brains of autistic patients. *J Child Neurol* 2002;**17**:515–521.

54. Casanova MF, Buxhoeveden DP, Switala AE, Roy E. Asperger's syndrome and cortical neuropathology. *J Child Neurol* 2002;**17**:142–145.

55. Sparks BF, Friedman SD, Shaw DW, *et al.* Brain structural abnormalities in young children with autism spectrum disorder. *Neurology* 2002;**59**:184–192.

56. Hollander E, Anagnostou E, Chaplin W, *et al.* Striatal volume on magnetic resonance imaging and repetitive behaviors in autism. *Biol Psychiatry* 2005;**58**:226–232.

57. Piven J, Bailey J, Ranson BJ, Arndt S. An MRI study of the corpus callosum in autism. *Am J Psychiatry* 1997;**154**:1051–1105.

58. Jou RJ, Jackowski AP, Papademetris X, Rajeevan N, Staib LH, Volkmar FR. Diffusion tensor imaging in autism spectrum disorders: preliminary evidence of abnormal neural connectivity. *Aust NZ J Psychiatry* 2011;**45**:153–162.

59. Courchesne E, Yeung CR, Press GA, Hesselink JR, Jernigan TL. Hypoplasia of cerebellar vermal lobules VI and VII in autism. *N Engl J Med* 1988;**318**:1349–1354.

60. Holttum J, Minshew N, Sanders R, Philips N. Magnetic resonance imaging of the posterior fossa in autism. *Biol Psychiatry* 1992;**32**:1091–1101.

61. Stanfield AC, McIntosh AM, Spencer MD, Philip R, Gaur S, Lawrie SM. Towards a neuroanatomy of autism: A systematic review and meta-analysis of structural magnetic resonance imaging studies. *Eur Psychiatry* 2008;**23**:289–299.

62. Saitoh O, Karns CM, Courchesne E. Development of the hippocampal formation from 2 to 42 years: MRI evidence of smaller area dentata in autism. *Brain* 2001;**124**:1317–1324.

63. Rojas DC, Smith JA, Benkers TL, Camou SL, Reite ML, Rogers SL: Hippocampus and amygdale volumes in parents of children with autistic disorder. *Am J Psychiatry* 2004;**161**:2038–2044.

64. Schumann CM, Hamstra J, Goodlin-Jones BL, *et al.* The amygdale is enlarged in children but not adolescents with autism; the hippocampus is enlarged at all ages. *J Neurosci* 2004;**24**:6392–6401.

65. Herbert MR, Harris GJ, Adrien KT, *et al.* Abnormal asymmetry in language association cortex in autism. *Ann Neurol* 2002;**52**:588–596.

66. Piven J, Arndt S, Bailey J, Havercamp S, Andreasen NC, Palmer P. An MRI study of brain size in autism. *Am J Psychiatry* 1995;**152**:1145–1149.

67. Minshew NJ, Keller TA. The nature of brain dysfunction in autism: functional brain imaging studies. *Curr Opin Neurol* 2010;**23**:124–130.

68. Schultz RT, Gauthier I, Klin A, *et al.* Abnormal ventral temporal cortical activity during face discrimination among individuals with autism and Asperger syndrome. *Arch Gen Psychiatry* 2000;**57**:331–340.

69. Pelphrey KA, Morris JP, McCarthy G, LaBar KS. Perception of dynamic changes in facial affect and identity in autism. *Soc Cogn Affect Neurosci* 2007;**2**:140–149.

70. Pierce K, Redcay E. Fusiform function in children with an autism spectrum disorder is a matter of 'who'. *Biol Psychiatry* 2008;**64**:552–560.

71. Rumsey JM, Duara R, Grady C, *et al.* Brain metabolism in autism: Resting cerebral glucose utilization rates as measured with positron emission tomography. *Arch Gen Psychiatry* 1985;**42**:448–455.

72. Herold S, Frackowiak RSJ, Le Couteur A, Rutter M, Howlin P. Cerebral blood flow and metabolism of oxygen and glucose in young autistic adults. *Psychol Med* 1988;**18**:823–831.

73. Chugani HT, Da Silva E, Chugani DC. Infantile spasms: III. Prognostic implications of bitemporal hypometabolism on positron emission tomography. *Ann Neurol* 1996;**39**:943–649.

74. Chugani DC, Muzik O, Rothermel R, *et al.* Altered serotonin synthesis in the dentatothalamocortical pathway in autism boys. *Ann Neurol* 1997;**42**:666–669.

75. Chugani DC, Muzik O, Behen M, *et al.* Developmental changes in brain serotonin synthesis capacity in autistic and nonautistic children. *Ann Neurol* 1999;**45**:287–295.

76. Pierce K, Muller RA, Ambrose J, Allen G, Courchesne E. Face processing occurs outside the fusiform "face area" in autism: evidence from functional MRI. *Brain* 2001;**124**:2059–2073.

77. Minshew N. In vivo brain chemistry in autism: ^{31}P magnetic resonance spectroscopy studies. In: Bauman M, Kemper T (eds) *The Neurobiology of Autism*. Baltimore: Johns Hopkins University Press, 1994; pp. 86–101.

78. Rutter M. Infantile autism. In: Shaffer D, Ehrhardt AA, Greenhill LL (eds) *The Clinical Guide to Child Psychiatry*. New York: The Free Press, 1985; pp. 48–78.

79. Lord C, Rutter M, Le Couteur A. Autism Diagnostic Interview – Revised: a revised version of a diagnostic interview for caregivers of individuals with possible per-

vasive developmental disorders. *J Autism Dev Disord* 1994;**24**:659–685.

80. Rumsey JM, Rapoport JL, Sceery WR. Autistic children as adults: psychiatric, social, and behavioral outcomes. *J Am Acad Child Psychiatry* 1985;**24**:465–473.

81. Mundy P, Sigman M. The theoretical implications of joint-attention deficits in autism. *Dev Psychopathol* 1989;**1**:173–183.

82. Kasari C, Sigman M, Mundy P, Yirmiya N: Affective sharing in the context of joint attention interactions of normal, autistic, and mentally retarded children. *J Autism Dev Disord* 1990;**20**:87–94.

83. Asperger H. Die 'Autistischen Psychopathen' kindesalter. *Arch Psychiatr Nervenkr* 1944;**117**:76–136.

84. Olsson B, Rett A. A review of the Rett syndrome with a theory of autism. *Brain Dev* 1990;**12**:11–15.

85. Amir RE, Van den Veyver IB, Wan M, Tran CQ, Francke U, Zoghbi HY. Rett syndrome is caused by mutations in X-linked MECP2, encoding methyl-CpG-binding protein 2. Nat Genet. 1999 Oct;23(2):185-8.

86. Naidu S, Bibat G, Kratz L, *et al.* Clinical variability in Rett's syndrome. *J Child Neurol* 2003;**18**:662–668.

87. Kim SJ, Cook EH Jr. Novel de novo nonsense mutation of MECP2 in a patient with Rett Syndrome. *Hum Mutat* 2000;**15**:382–383.

88. Volkmar F, Cohen D. Disintegrative disorder or "late onset" autism. *J Child Psychol Psychiat* 1989;**30**:717–724.

89. Corbett J, Harris R. Progressive disintegrative psychosis of childhood. *J Child Psychol Psychiat* 1977;**18**:211–219.

90. Bartak L, Rutter M, Cox A. A comparative study of infantile autism and specific developmental receptive language disorder. I: The children. *Brit J Psychiatry* 1975;**126**:127–145.

91. Ornitz E, Ritvo E. The syndrome of autism: a critical review. *Am J Psychiatry* 1976;**133**:609–621.

92. Lerman P, Lerman-Sagie T, Kivity S. Effect of early corticosteroid therapy for Landau–Kleffner syndrome. *Dev Med Child Neurol* 1991;**33**:257–260.

93. Kolvin I, Fundudis T. Elective mute children: psychological development and background factors. *J Child Psychol Psychiat* 1981;**22**:219–232.

94. Hoffman-Plotkin D, Twentyman C. A multimodal assessment of behavioral and cognitive deficits in abused and neglected preschoolers. *Child Dev* 1984;**55**:794–802.

95. Rutter M, Andersen-Wood L, Beckett C, *et al.* Quasi-autistic patterns following severe early global privation. English and Romanian Adoptees (ERA) Study Team. *J Child Psychol Psychiatry* 1999;**40**:537–549.

96. Brown J. Adolescent development of children with infantile psychosis. *Semin Psychiatry* 1969;**1**:79–89.

97. Kanner L, Rodriguez A, Ashenden B. How far can autistic children go in matters of social adaptation. *J Aut Child Schizo* 1972;**2**:9–33.

98. Lotter V. Social adjustment and placement of autistic children in Middlesex: a follow-up study. *J Aut Child Schizo* 1974;**4**:11–32.

99. Gillberg C. Infantile autism and other childhood psychoses in a Swedish urban region. Epidemiological aspects. *J Child Psychol Psychiat* 1984;**25**:35–43.

100. Lord C, Risi S, Lambrecht L, *et al.* The Autism Diagnostic Observation Schedule-Generic: a standard measure of social and communication deficits associated with the spectrum of autism. *J Autism Dev Disord* 2000;**30**:205–223.

101. Schopler E, Reichler RJ, Renner BR. *The Childhood Autism Rating Scale (CARS)*. Los Angeles, CA:Western Psychological Services, 1988.

102. Krug D, Arick J, Almond P: Behavior checklist for identifying severely handicapped individuals with high levels of autistic behavior. *J Child Psychol Psychiat* 1980;**21**:221–229.

103. Aman M. *Aberrant Behavior Checklist – Community Version*. East Aurora, NY: Slosson Educational Publications, 1994.

104. Stutsman R. *Merrill-Palmer Scale of Mental Tests*. New York: Harcourt, Brace, and World, 1948.

105. Shah A, Holmes N. The use of the Leiter International Performance Scale with autistic children. *J Autism Dev Disord* 1985;**15**:195–204.

106. Bayley N. *Manual for the Bayley Scales of Infant Development*. New York: Psychological Corporation, 1969.

107. Elliott C. *Differential Abilities Scales*. Pensacola, FL: Psychological Corporation, 1990.

108. Sparrow S, Balla D, Cicchetti D. *Vineland Scales of Adaptive Behavior, Survey Form Manual*. Circle Pines, MN: American Guidance Service, 1984.

109. Sparrow S, Cicchetti D, Balla D. *Vineland II: A Revision of the Vineland Adaptive Behavior Scales: II. Expanded Form*. Circle Pines, MN: Pearson Assessments, 2009.

110. Carr E. The motivation of self-injurious behavior: a review of some hypotheses. *Psychol Bull* 1977;**84**:800–816.

111. Lord C. The development of peer relations in children with autism. In: Morrison F, Lord C, Keating D (eds) *Applied Developmental Psychology*. New York: Academic Press, 1984; pp. 165–229.

112. Campbell M, Schopler E, Cueva J, Hallin A. Treatment of autistic disorder. *J Am Acad Child Adolesc Psychiatry* 1996;**35**:134–143.

113. Schopler E, Olley G. Comprehensive educational services for autistic children: the TEACCH model. In: Reynolds C, Gutkin T (eds) *The Handbook of School Psychology*. New York: John Wiley & Sons, Ltd, 1982; pp. 629–643.

114. Solnit A, Stark M. Mourning and the birth of a defective child. *Psychoanalytic Study of the Child* 1961;**16**:523–537.

115. Powers M. *Children with Autism: A Parent's Guide*. 1989 Woodbine House; 2 Sub edition (July 15, 2000).

116. Amenta C. *Russell is Extra Special: A Book about Autism for Children*. New York, Brunner/Mazel, 1992.

117. Siegel B, Silverstein S. *What About Me? Growing Up with a Developmentally Disabled Sibling*. New York: Plenum, 1994.

118. Cook E, Rowlett R, Jaselskis C, Leventhal B. Fluoxetine treatment of patients with autism and mental retardation. *J Am Acad Child Adolesc Psychiatry* 1992;**31**:739–745.

119. Gordon C, State R, Nelson J, Hamburger S, Rapoport J. A double-blind comparison of clomipramine, desipramine, and placebo in the treatment of autistic disorder. *Arch Gen Psychiatry* 1993;**50**:441–447.

120. McDougle CJ, Holmes JP, Carlson DC, Pelton GH, Cohen DJ, Price LH. A double-blind, placebo-controlled study of risperidone in adults with autistic disorder and other pervasive developmental disorders. *Arch Gen Psychiatry* 1998;**55**:633–641.

121. Posey DJ, Litwiller M, Koburn A, McDougle CJ. Paroxetine in autism. *J Am Acad Child Adolesc Psychiatry* 1999;**38**:111–112.

122. Namerow LB, Thomas P, Bostic JQ, Prince J, Monuteaux MC. Use of citalopram in pervasive developmental disorders. *J Dev Behav Pediatr* 2003;**24**:104–108.

123. Ghaziuddin M, Tsai L, Ghaziuddin N. Fluoxetine in autism with depression. *J Am Acad Child Adolesc Psychiatry* 1991;**30**:508–509.

124. Owley T. The pharmacological treatment of autistic spectrum disorders. *CNS Spectr* 2002;**7**:663–669.

125. Quintana H, Birmaher B, Stedge D, *et al.* Use of methylphenidate in the treatment of children with autistic disorder. *J Autism Dev Disord* 1995;**25**:283–294.

126. Handen BL, Johnson CR, Lubetsky M. Efficacy of methylphenidate among children with autism and symptoms of attention-deficit hyperactivity disorder. *J Autism Dev Disord* 2000;**30**:245–55.

127. RUPP. Randomized, controlled, crossover trial of methylphenidate in pervasive developmental disorders with hyperactivity. *Arch Gen Psychiatry* 2005;**62**:1266–1274.

128. Fankhauser MP, Karumanchi VC, German ML, Yates A, Karumanchi SD. A double-blind, placebo-controlled study of the efficacy of transdermal clonidine in autism. *J Clin Psychiatry* 1992;**53**:77–82.

129. Jaselskis CA, Cook EH, Fletcher KE, Leventhal BL. Clonidine treatment of hyperactive and impulsive children with autistic disorder. *J Clin Psychopharm* 1992;**12**:322–327.

130. Williams DT, Mehl R, Yudofsky S, Adams D, Roseman B: The effect of propranolol on uncontrolled rage outbursts in children and adolescents with organic brain dysfunction. *J Am Acad Child Psychiatry* 1982;**21**(2):129–135.

131. Ratey JJ, Mikkelsen E, Sorgi, P, Zuckerman HS, Polakoff S, Bemporad J, Bick P, Kadish W: Autism: the treatment of aggressive behaviors. *J Clin Psychopharmacol* 1987;**7**(1):35–41.

132. Anderson LT, Campbell M, Grega DM, Perry R, Small AM, Green WH. Haloperidol in the treatment of infantile autism: Effects on learning and behavioral symptoms. *Am J Psychiatry* 1984;**141**:1195–1202.

133. Anderson LT, Campbell M, Adams P, Small AM, Perry R, Shell J. The effects of haloperidol on discrimination learning and behavioral symptoms in autistic children. *J Autism Dev Disord* 1989;**9**:227–239.

134. Campbell M, Anderson LT, Meier M, et al. A comparison of haloperidol and behavior therapy and their interaction in autistic children. *J Am Acad Child and Adolesc Psychiatry* 1976;**17**:640–655.

135. Cohen IL, Campbell M, Posner D, Small AM, Triebel D, Anderson LT. Behavioral effects of haloperidol in young autistic children. An objective analysis using a within subject reversal design. *J Am Acad Child Psychiatry* 1980;**19**:665–677.

136. Ernst M, Magee HJ, Gonzalez NM, Locascio JJ, Rosenberg CR, Campbell M: Pimozide in autistic children. *Psychopharmacol Bull* 1992;**28**:187–191.

137. Fish B, Shapiro T, Campbell M. Long-term prognosis and the response of schizophrenic children to drug therapy: A controlled study of trifluoperazine. *Am J Psychiatry* 1966;**123**:32–39.

138. Naruse H, Nagahata M, Nakane Y, Shirahashi K, Takesada M, Yamazaki K. A multi-center double-blind trial of pimozide (Orap), haloperidol and placebo in children with behavioral disorders, using crossover design. *Acta Paedopsychiat* 1982;**48**:173–184.

139. Perry R, Campbell M, Adams P, Lynch N, Spencer EK, Curren EL, Overall JE: Long-term efficacy of haloperidol in autistic children: continuous versus discontinuous drug administration. *J Am Acad Child Adolesc Psychiatry* 1989;**28**(1):87–92.

140. Campbell M, Adams P, Perry R, Spencer EK, Overall JE. Tardive and withdrawal dyskinesia in autistic children: A prospective study. *Psychopharmacol Bull* 1988;**24**:251–255.

141. Campbell M, Armenteros JL, Malone RP, Adams PB, Eisenberg ZW, Overall JE: Neuroleptic-related dyskinesias in autistic children: a prospective, longitudinal study. *J Am Acad Child Adolesc Psychiatry* 1997;**36**(6): 835–843.

142. Malone RP, Cater J, Sheikh RM, Choudhury MS, Delaney MA. Olanzapine versus haloperidol in children with autistic disorder: an open pilot study. *J Am Acad Child Adolesc Psychiatry* 2001;**40**:887–894.

143. Masi G, Cosenza A, Mucci M, Brovedani P. Open trial of risperidone in 24 young children with pervasive developmental disorders. *J Am Acad Child Adolesc Psychiatry* 2001;**40**:1206–1214.

144. McDougle CJ, Holmes JP, Bronson MR, *et al.* Risperidone treatment of children and adolescents with pervasive developmental disorders: a prospective open-label study. *J Am Acad Child Adolesc Psychiatry* 1997;**36**:685–693.

145. Potenza MN, Holmes JP, Kanes SJ, McDougle CJ: Olanzapine treatment of children, adolescents, and adults with pervasive developmental disorders: an open-label pilot study. *J Clin Psychopharmacol* 1999;**19**:37–44.

146. McCracken JT, McGough J, Shah B, *et al.* Risperidone in children with autism and serious behavioral problems. *N Engl J Med* 2002;**347**:314–321.

147. G Masi, A Cosenza, M Mucci, and P Brovedani. A 3-year naturalistic study of 53 preschool children with pervasive developmental disorders treated with risperidone. *J Clin Psychiatry* 2003;**64**:1039-1047

148. Gagliano A, Germano E, Pustorino G, Impallomeni C, D'Arrigo C, Calamoneri F, Spina E: Risperidone treatment of children with autistic disorder: effectiveness, tolerability, and pharmacokinetic implications. *J Child Adolesc Psychopharmacol* 2004; **14**(1):39–47.

149. Kemner C, Willemsen-Swinkels SH, de Jonge M, Tuynman-Qua H, van Engeland H. Open-label study of olanzapine in children with pervasive developmental disorder. *J Clin Psychopharmacol* 2002;**22**:455–460.

150. Cohen SA, Fitzgerald BJ, Khan SR, Khan A. The effect of a switch to ziprasidone in an adult population with autistic disorder: chart review of naturalistic, open-label treatment. *J Clin Psychiatry* 2004;**65**:110–113.

151. Owen, R, Sikich, L, Marcus, RN, *et al.* Aripiperazole in the treatment of irritability in children and adolescents with autistic disorder. *Pediatrics* 2009;**124**:1533–1540.

152. Hollander E, Dolgoff-Kaspar R, Cartwright C, Rawitt R, Novotny S. An open trial of divalproex sodium in autism spectrum disorders. *J Clin Psychiatry* 2001;**62**:530–534.

153. Brent DA, Crumrine PK, Varma RR, Allan M, Allman C. Phenobarbital treatment and major depressive disorder in children with epilepsy. *Pediatrics* 1987;**80**:909–917.

154. Vining EPG, Mellits D, Dorsen MM, *et al.* Psychologic and behavioral effects of antiepileptic drugs in children: A double-blind comparison between phenobarbital and valproic acid. *Pediatrics* 1987;**80**:165–174.

155. Plioplys AV. Autism: electroencephalogram abnormalities and clinical improvement with valproic acid. *Arch Pediatr Adolesc Med.* 1994 Feb;**148**(2):220-2.

156. Campbell M, Anderson L, Small A, Adams P, Gonzalez N, Ernst M. Naltrexone in autistic children: Behavioral symptoms and attentional learning. *J Am Acad Child Adolesc Psychiatry* 1993;**32**:1283–1291.

157. Willemsen-Swinkels SHN, Buitelaar JK, Weijnen FG, Van Engeland H. Placebo-controlled acute dosage naltrexone study in young autistic children. *Psychiatry Res* 1995;**58**:203–215.

158. Willemsen-Swinkels SH, Buitelaar JK, van Berckelaer-Onnes IA, van Engeland H. Brief report: six months continuation treatment in naltrexone- responsive children with autism: an open-label case-control design. *J Autism Dev Disord* 1999;**29**:167–169.

159. Willemsen-Swinkels SHN, Buitelaar JK, Van Engeland H. The effects of chronic naltrexone treatment in young autistic children: A double-blind placebo-controlled crossover study. *Biol Psychiatry* 1996;**39**:1023–1031.

160. Percy AK, Glaze DG, Schultz RJ, *et al.* Rett syndrome: controlled study of an oral opiate antagonist, naltrexone. *Ann Neurol* 1994;**35**:464–470.

161. Campbell M, Fish B, Korein J, Shapiro T, Collins P, Koh C. Lithium and chlorpromazine: A controlled crossover study of hyperactive severely disturbed young children. *J Autism Child Schizophr* 1972;**2**:234–263.

162. Buitelaar JK, van der Gaag RJ, van der Hoeven J. Buspirone in the management of anxiety and irritability in children with pervasive developmental disorders: results of an open label study. *J Clin Psychiatry* 1998;**56**:56–59.

163. Carlsson ML. Hypothesis: is infantile autism a hypoglutamatergic disorder? Relevance of glutamate–serotonin interactions for pharmacotherapy. *J Neural Transm* 1998;**105**:525–535.

164. King B, Wright D, Handen B, *et al.* A double-blind, placebo-controlled study of amantidine hydrochloride in the treatment of children with autistic disorder. *J Am Acad Child Adolesc Psychiatry* 2001;**40**:658–665.

165. Martineau J, Barthelemy C, Cheliakine C, Lelord G, Brief report: an open middle-term study of combined vitamin B6-magnesium in a subgroup of autistic children selected on their sensitivity to this treatment. *Journal of Autism & Developmental Disorders.* **18**(3):435-47, 1988 Sep.

166. Kleijnen J, Knipschild P. Niacin and vitamin B6 in mental functioning: a review of controlled trials in humans. *Biol Psychiatry* 1991;**29**:931–941.

167. Pfeiffer SI, Norton J, Nelson L, Shott S. Efficacy of vitamin B6 and magnesium in the treatment of autism: a methodology review and summary of outcomes. *J Autism Dev Disord* 1995;**25**:481–493.

168. Geller E, Ritvo ER, Freeman BJ, Yuwiler A: Preliminary observations on the effect of fenfluramine on blood serotonin and symptoms in three autistic boys. *N Engl J Med* 1982;**307**(3):165–169.

169. Aman MG, Kern RA. Review of fenfluramine in the treatment of the developmental disabilities. *J Am Acad Child Adolesc Psychiatry* 1989;**28**:549–565.

170. Leventhal B, Cook E, Morford M, Ravitz A, Heller W, Freedman D. Fenfluramine: clinical and neurochemical effects in children with autism. *J Neuropsychiatry Clin Neurosci* 1993;**5**:307–315.

171. Aman MG, Kern RA, Arnold LE, McGhee DE. Fenfluramine and mental retardation. *J Am Acad Child Adolesc Psychiatry* 1991;**30**:507–508.

172. Schuster CR, Lewis M, Seiden LS. Fenfluramine: neurotoxicity. *Psychopharm Bull* 1986;**22**:148–151.

173. Horvath K, Stefanatos G, Sokolski KN, Wachtel R, Nabors L, Tildon JT. Improved social and language skills after secretin administration in patients with autistic spectrum disorders. *J Assoc Acad Minor Phys* 1998;**9**:9–15.

174. Chez MG, Buchanan CP, Bagan BT, et al. Secretin and autism: a two-part clinical investigation. *J Autism Dev Disord* 2000;**30**:87–94.

175. Coniglio SJ, Lewis JD, Lang C, *et al.* A randomized, double-blind, placebo-controlled trial of single-dose intravenous secretin as treatment for children with autism. *J Pediatr* 2001;**138**:649–655.

176. Dunn-Geier J, Ho HH, Auersperg E, *et al.* Effect of secretin on children with autism: a randomized controlled trial. *Dev Med Child Neurol* 2000;**42**:796–802.

177. Owley T, McMahon W, Cook EH, *et al.* Multi-site, double-blind, placebo-controlled trial of porcine secretin in autism. *J Am Acad Child Adolesc Psychiatry* 2001;**40**:1293–1299.

178. Roberts W, Weaver L, Brian J, *et al.* Repeated doses of porcine secretin in the treatment of autism: a randomized, placebo-controlled trial. *Pediatrics* 2001;107:E71.

179. Sandler AD, Sutton KA, DeWeese J, Girardi MA, Sheppard V, Bodfish JW. Lack of benefit of a single dose of synthetic human secretin in the treatment of autism and pervasive developmental disorder. *N Engl J Med* 1999;**341**:1801–1806.

180. Unis AS, Munson JA, Rogers SJ, Goldson E, Osterling J, Gabriels R, Abbott RD, Dawson G: A randomized, double-blind, placebo-controlled trial of porcine versus synthetic secretin for reducing symptoms of autism. *J Am Acad Child Adolesc Psychiatry* 2002;**41**(11):1315–1321.

181. Levy SE, Souders MC, Wray J, Jawad AF, Gallagher PR, Coplan J, Belchic JK, Gerdes M, Mitchell R, Mulberg AE: Children with autistic spectrum disorders. I: comparison of placebo and single dose of human synthetic secretin. *Arch Dis Child* 2003;**88**(8):731–736.

182. Molloy CA, Manning-Courtney P, Swayne S, Bean J, Brown JM, Murray DS, Kinsman AM, Brasington M, Ulrich CD 2nd: Lack of benefit of intravenous synthetic human secretin in the treatment of autism. *J Autism Dev Disord* 2002;**32**(6):545–551.

183. Lane H. *The Wild Boy of Aveyron.* Cambridge, MA: Harvard University Press, 1976.

22

Intellectual Disability (Mental Retardation)

L. Lee Carlisle, Bryan H. King, Arthur Maerlender

Introduction

Intellectual disability, or intellectual developmental disorder, describes a heterogeneous condition affecting a diverse population. There are no unique personality traits that define persons with intellectual disability, and insofar as generalizations are possible, it is worthwhile to remember that a person's IQ reveals about as much about that person's thought, behavior, and aspirations as does his or her age. Just as a group of 70-year-olds might include both the supervisors and the supervised, so, also, a group of persons with intelligence quotients of 70 will include persons representing an enormous range of talents and temperaments.

And just as we have always recognized individuals in the population whose intellectual development is impaired relative to most people, drawing boundaries around the disorder, and naming it, has always been a challenge as well. At the time of this writing the American Psychiatric Association's *Diagnostic and Statistical Manual of Mental Disorders*, 5th edition (DSM-5), is still a work in progress but it is highly likely that Mental Retardation, as a diagnostic term, is out and a new term, for example, Intellectual Disability or Intellectual Developmental Disorder, will be in [1]. Likewise, the DSM-5 will probably revisit how severity levels are assigned, using some combination or synthesis of IQ along with adaptive function rather than relying on IQ alone.

As the landscape regarding intellectual disability comes into clearer view, and we refine how we recognize and describe it, the terrain separating us from that elusive horizon of understanding also comes into greater focus.Thus, while new gene targets are identified, the complex interplay between genes, the timing of their onset and offset,and their regional variation in the brain, and their interplay with other genes and with the environment present a daunting to do list for science. Even so, as advances in our understanding mount, we are closer to the development of new therapeutics, and also have a growing appreciation for the important role that psychiatry can play in the understanding and care of persons with intellectual disability.

Definition of Intellectual Disability

The diagnostic requirements for mental retardation according to the DSM-IV-TR [2] require:

(1) A significant deficit in intellectual functioning, generally indicated by an IQ below 70.
(2) Concurrent deficits in adaptive functioning.
(3) Onset prior to age 18.

The diagnosis is further divided into mild, moderate, and severe categories based on IQ. Standardized tests, or scales, are used to evaluate items 1 and 2 above.

Intellectual Assessment

Most standard IQ tests are primarily geared toward testing IQs within a relatively narrow range on either side of normal. For individuals with IQs in the moderately severe and profound ranges they become unreliable and therefore of limited value when it comes to evaluating for intellectual disability. Additionally, persons with significant intellectual disability often have difficulty understanding and/or following the instructions on "normal" IQ tests. Additionally, there are few tasks available for them to demonstrate what they are able to do [3].

Some of the more common tests used for assessing intellectual ability are listed in Table 22.1.

Functional Assessment

In order to make a diagnosis of intellectual disability, the diminished mental abilities must cause a functional impairment, or a deficit in adaptive behavior. Several

Clinical Child Psychiatry, Third Edition. Edited by William M. Klykylo and Jerald Kay.
© 2012 John Wiley & Sons, Ltd. Published 2012 by John Wiley & Sons, Ltd.

Table 22.1 Common measures of intellectual ability in children and adolescents.

Name	Administration	Time	Measures	Age	Scores generated	Comments
Stanford–Binet Intelligence Scales-fifth edition (SB-V)	One-on-one administration by psychologist	45–75 min for full-scale IQ 15–20 min for abbreviated battery	Fluid reasoning Knowledge Quantitative reasoning Visual-spatial processing Working memory	2–89	Full-scale IQ and five composite scores	Latest version of gold-standard assessment instrument Extensive normative, reliability, and validity evidence
Wechsler Intelligence Scale for Children-fourth edition (WISC-IV)	One-on-one administration by psychologist		Verbal comprehension Perceptual reasoning Working memory Processing speed	6–16 years	Full-scale IQ and four composite scores	Less emphasis on acquired knowledge Instructions to children have been simplified
Wechsler Preschool and Primary Scale of Intelligence (WPPSI)	One-on-one administration by psychologist	Core subtests: Ages 2:6–3:11, 30–45 min Ages 4:0–7:3, 45–60 min	Verbal reasoning Concept formation Sequential processing Auditory comprehension Cognitive flexibility Social judgment Perceptual organization Processing speed	2.6–7.3	Scaled scores by age, IQs	
Differential Abilities Scales, 2nd Ed. (DAS-II)	One-on-one administration by psychologist	Core subtests: Ages 2:6– 6:11, 30-45 min; Ages 7:0 – 17:11, 45-60 min.	Early years measures nonverbal reasoning, basic oral language skills; School age measures nonverbal reasoning, visual-spatial skills, verbal reasoning	2:6–17:11	Global IQ and three (two) Composite Standard Scores, T-scores for subtests by age	Rasch scaling to reduce testing time; Overlap of age ranges allows more flexibility to drop down or move up in test forms

Table 22.2 Common measures of functional ability in children and adolescents.

Name	Administration	Age	Comments
Vineland Adaptive Behavior Scales, second edition (VABS-II)	Semistructured interview of caregivers	0–18	'Gold' standard for measuring adaptive behavior for children and adolescents with neurodevelopmental and other disorders
Adaptive Behavior Assessment System, second edition (ABAS-II)	Uses parents' and caregivers' reports of child functioning	0–89	Based upon recommendations of the American Association on Intellectual and Developmental Disabilities

factors can influence the assessment of adaptive behavior including the scale used, the age and sex of the child, the informant and the examiner, and the setting. Some of the more common tests used for assessing adaptive behavior are listed in Table 22.2.

Epidemiology

Prevalence rates for intellectual disability are highly fluid, ranging anywhere from fewer than 5 to more than 100 cases per 10,000 population, depending upon a plethora of variables that push and pull on it from every conceivable direction. In a meta-analysis of 52 studies from around the world published between 1980 and 2009 [4], Maulik, *et al.* found the prevalence of intellectual disability, across all studies, to be 10.37/10 000. The primary factors that affect rates include: the income group of the country of origin (lower country income level is correlated with higher prevalence rates); the age group (lower age group is correlated with higher prevalence rates); and study design.

Etiological Considerations

It is important to note that intellectual disability is not a disease in itself, but the developmental outcome of genetic influences, environmental causes, or combinations of the two. In the past, it has generally been accepted that the more severe a patient's intellectual disability, the higher the diagnostic yield would be from genetic testing. With continual improvements in our ability to both acquire and interpret data from a number of sources, including subtelometric screening, fluorescence *in situ* hybridization (FISH), and comparative genomic hybridization,this isno longer necessarily the case [5].

New causes of intellectual disability, or the genetic etiologies of formerly unspecified syndromes, continue to be identified at an extraordinary pace.In the previous version of this chapter, it was noted that a keyword search of "mental retardation" in the Online Mendelian

Inheritance in Man database [6] yielded 1231 entries. At the time of this writing the number has grown to 1740.

Behavioral Phenotypes

The explosion in medical genetics research over the last two decades has supported an ongoing interest in "behavioral phenotypes." While there is no universally agreed upon definition, a reasonable way to think of behavioral phenotype is as a specific and characteristic behavioral repertoire exhibited by individuals with a specific cause (most often genetic or chromosomal) for their disorder [7]. Stereotyped hand movements, for example, have been described in many contexts, but a particular form of stereotyped hand wringing is almost invariably seen in Rett's syndrome.Obesity is certainly nonspecific, but the probability of an individual with Prader–Willisyndrome becoming obese is nearly 100% without aggressive dietary management. Penrose [8] anticipated modern neuropsychological characterization when he observed that persons with Down's syndrome were typified by "…cheerful and friendly personalities.Their capacities for imitation and their memories for people, for music and for complex situations may be found to range far beyond their other abilities.They are incapable of abstract reasoning. They cannot do arithmetic although they may sometimes be able to read and write" (p. 206).

The ongoing process of identifying and clarifying behavioral phenotypes brings with it considerable benefit.Clinically, recognition of certain behavioral patterns may suggest a diagnosis, and thus provide valuable information regarding the course, prognosis, treatment, and expected areas of relative strength and difficulty associated with a syndrome. In addition, understanding a condition's behavioral phenotype can be helpful in sorting out or even anticipating symptoms.Is a certain behavior more likely part and parcel of the genetic abnormality or could it be due to some other, more remediable, disorder? From a research perspective, the elaboration of behavioral phenotypes is equally important. As basic and clinical sciences continue rapidly to advance, individuals with known genetic lesions and well-defined behavioral manifestations may provide scientists with critical insights into the complex interaction of nature and nurture. For example, behavioral phenotypes can teach us about gene-to-behavior pathways with potential far-reaching significance. For example, understanding the mechanisms of hyperphagia in Prader–Willi syndrome may be relevant to appetite control in the general population [9].

As noted above, there are several hundred genetic conditions that are linked to intellectual disability. Table 22.3 provides a mere overview of the conditions for which behavioral phenotypes have been fairly well established.

Intellectual Disability and Comorbid Psychopathology

The presence of intellectual disability does not preclude the presence of one or more psychiatric disorders. To the contrary, the prevalence of emotional and behavioral problems in children and adolescents with intellectual disabilities is three to four times higher than in typically developing youths [10]. In the case of Down's syndrome, the risk for externalizing problems – attention-deficit hyperactivity disorder (ADHD), oppositional defiant disorder (ODD), conduct disorder (CD), and aggressive behaviors – is higher than for internalizing problems. Children with Down's syndrome are at a lower risk for developing psychiatric disorders than are other children with intellectual disability (ID), but their risk is still higher than the general population [11].

While it is clear that intellectual disability is a significant risk factor for mental disorders, the problem of what to consider a mental disorder and how to diagnose it is one that has long challenged psychiatrists in this field. How does one diagnose psychosis in a patient who cannot endorse hallucinations or delusions? How does depression or anxiety manifest itself when these feelings cannot be communicated verbally? When is a behavior problem evidence of a mental disorder and not a downstream consequence or a manifestation of the underlying condition causing the intellectual disability?

The approach to these challenges is similar to the approach child psychiatrists utilize in evaluating young patients who similarly may be unable to understand or articulate feelings, and whose behavior may even be attributed to their young age by parents or careproviders. When it comes to children with intellectual disability, clinicians must determine how a particular symptom or pattern of behavior relates to what could be expected from a person of a given developmental age, and to appreciate how certain subjective feeling states might be communicated in the context of a limited repertoire for such expression.

Adaptation of diagnostic criteria

Since the last revision of this text the *Diagnostic Manual – Intellectual Disability (DM-ID): A Textbook of Diagnosis of Mental Disorders in Persons with Intellectual Disability*, along with its companion text, a condensed version called *Diagnostic Manual – Intellectual Disability*: A Clinical Guide for Diagnosis of Mental Disorders in Persons with Intellectual Disability, have been published and are now available. The DM-ID was developed by the National Association for the Dually Diagnosed (NADD) in association with the American Psychiatric Association (APA) and was specifically designed to facilitate an accurate DSM-IV-TR diagnosis in persons who have intellectual disabilities [12]. Still relatively new, having been published in 2007, the DM-ID should become a valuable resource for clinics that specialize to any significant degree in the care of persons with ID. What follows is not meant to be a recapitulation of the DM-ID but a supplemental overview of the most common disorders that come into play as "dually diagnosed" or co-occurring conditions with intellectual disability.

Disruptive Behavior Disorders (DBD)

Attention-Deficit Hyperactivity Disorder (ADHD)

For persons with ID the diagnosis of ADHD currently requires that symptoms are excessive compared with a child of comparable intellectual and chronological age rather than with a younger, typically developing, child of comparable developmental age. Individuals given the diagnosis of ADHD in this context should, in comparison to their peers with similar levels of disability, exhibit unusually short attention span (even for activities of interest), excessive psychomotor activity level, remarkable impulsivity, and so on. Another important adaptation concerns the age requirement for onset of symptoms. If an early developmental history is unavailable, the requirement that symptoms causing impairment be present before age 7 is dropped [12].

The clinician may encounter situations in which an individual does not evidence remarkable psychomotor activity or attention difficulties and yet is unusually impulsive. In these situations, most commonly exemplified by an individual who might inexplicably strike out at a peer in the absence of any identifiable environmental

Table 22.3 Intellectual disability and representative behavioral phenotypes.

Pathogenic features	Clinical features	Behavioral phenotype
Angelman syndrome (AS)		
Deletion in 15q11-15q13 (same region as for Prader–Willi syndrome, PWS) but of maternal origin (70%). Some cases of paternal uniparental-disomy (3%), and intragenic mutations. Approximately 20% of cases have an unknown genetic etiology. As with PWS, many candidate genes could contribute to aspects of the phenotype. Involvement of a gamma-aminobutyric acid receptor subunit gene may be important in the pathogenesis of epilepsy in AS. Estimated incidence is 1 in 20 000 live births. Prevalence in populations of individuals with severe mental retardation is 1.4%	Fair hair and blue eyes (66%), dysmorphic-facies including wide mouth, thin upper lip, pointed chin, epilepsy (90%) with characteristic EEG, ataxia, small head circumference, 25% microcephalic	Happy disposition, paroxysmal laughter, hand flapping, clapping, sleep disturbance with nighttime waking Developmental delay, which becomes apparent by 6–12 months of age, severely impaired expressive language, ataxic gait, tremulous-ness of limbs, and a typical behavioral profile, including a happy demeanor, hypermotoric behavior, and short attention span. Receptive language somewhat better than expressive, in part due to oral-motor dyspraxia
Cornelia de Lange syndrome		
Deletion in *NIPBL* gene (human homolog of *Drosophila* "Nipped-B" gene) at 5p13.1. Similar phenotype has been associated with other chromosomal deletions including one at 3q26.3. Prevalence is estimated to be as high as 1:10 000	Continuous eyebrows, thin downturning upper lip, microcephaly, short stature, small hands and feet, small upturned nose, anteverted nostrils, malformed upper lips, failure to thrive.	Language delays, avoidance of being held, stereotypic movements, twirling behaviors Degree of mental retardation from borderline (10%), through mild (8%), moderate (18%), and severe (20%) to profound (43%). A wide variety of symptoms occur frequently, notably hyperactivity (40%), self-injury (44%), daily aggression (49%), and sleep disturbance (55%). These behaviors correlate closely with the presence of an autistic-like syndrome and with the degree of mental retardation. The frequency and severity of disturbance, continuing beyond childhood, is important when planning the amount and duration of support required by parents
Cri du chat syndrome		
Autosomal dominant deletion in chromosome 5p15.2, probably involving the adherens junction protein, delta-catenin (*CTNND2*). This protein is expressed early in neuronal development and plays a role in cell motility. Estimated prevalence is between 1:15 000 and 1:45 000 live births	Round face; moderate to severe intellectual disability (ID); significantly better receptive language than expressive (but still delayed). Abnormal ears, hand webbing, microcephaly.	High-pitched cat-like cry; excessive drooling.

(Continued)

Table 22.3. (*Continued*)

Pathogenic features	Clinical features	Behavioral phenotype
Down's syndrome Trisomy 21, most often associated with nondisjunction (95%); the remainder are generally translocations involving chromosome 21. Frequency of occurrence is 1:1000 live births, but increases dramatically with maternal age to 1:2500 in women <30 years old, 1:80 <40 years old	Some level of impaired cognitive development. Children with mosaicism tend to have higher IQ scores than those with trisomy 21. Visual short-term memory better than auditory	Cognitive development declines with age. Children with mosaicism tend to score higher on IQ tests than those with trisomy 21. Some indication of average visual-perceptual skills in mosaicism children as well. Evidence that cognitive development and learning can continue beyond adolescence and into adulthood, particularly with appropriate learning experiences
Fetal alcohol syndrome Maternal alcohol consumption (third trimester > second > first trimester), 1 in 3000 live births in Western countries (most common preventable cause of mental retardation). As many as 1:300 children may have Fetal Alcohol Effects (FAE)	Microcephaly, short stature, midface hypoplasia, short palpebral fissure, thin upper lip, retrognathia in infancy, micrognathia in adolescence, hypoplastic long and smooth philtrum	Mental retardation is possible; often learning disabilities, attention deficits, hyperactivity, memory loss and conduct problems due to poor awareness of consequences of behavior. Irritability, decreased abstracting ability, impulsivity, speech and language delays; fetal alcohol effects = incomplete syndrome
Fragile X syndrome Inactivation of *FMR-1* gene at Xq27.3 is generally due to >200 CCG base repeats and associated methylation. Inheritance is recessive. Frequency of occurrence is 1:1000 male births and 1:3000 female. FraX accounts for 10–12% of MR in males and remains the most common heritable cause of MR	Strengths in verbal memory; executive dysfunction including attention deficits, short attention span, hyperactivity	Perseverative behaviors; females with normal IQ often have learning disabilities, attention and organizational problems, and math difficulties; characteristic hand-clapping
Galactosemia Autosomal recessive defect in galactose-1-phosphate uridylyltransferase gene located at 9p13. The disorder is quite rare, occurring in as few as 1:62 000 births (slightly more common in Caucasians)	Mental retardation is a diagnostic feature. In children with galactosemia, cognitive outcome appears to relate to genotype rather than metabolic control. Poor feeding and jaundice; There is evidence that variability in neurocognitive outcome is at least in part dependent on allelic heterogeneity	ADHD: tend to be socially withdrawn; autistic behavior; frequently irritable

Hunter's syndrome		
Rare deficiency in iduronatesulfatase, located at Xq28. Estimated prevalence is 1:111 000 births	Normal infancy; symptom onset at 2–4 years; typical coarse facies with flat nasal bridge, flaring nostrils, hearing loss, ataxia, hernia common, enlarged liver and spleen, joint stiffness, recurrent infections, growth retardation, cardiovascular abnormalities; death in first or second decade	Hyperactivity; MR evident by age 2 years; speech delay, loss of speech at age 8–10 years; restless, aggressive, inattentive, abnormal sleep; apathetic, sedentary with disease progression
Hurler's syndrome		
Rare autosomal recessive deficiency in alpha-L-iduronidase, located at 4p16.3. Estimated prevalence is 1:144 000 births	Decline in cognition after first year; sensory impairments with language delays secondary to hearing loss. Loss of skills by age 3 years. CNS deterioration accompanied by hydrocephalus	Early onset, short stature, hepatosplenomegaly, hirsutism, corneal clouding, death before 10 years of age; dwarfism, coarse facial features, recurrent repiratory infections. Moderate to severe MR, anxious, fearful, rarely aggressive
Lesch–Nyhan syndrome (LNS)		
Single gene defect in hypoxanthine guanine phosphoribosyltransferase (Xq26-27.2) with possible secondary dopamine supersensitivity in the striatum. LNS is recessive, and rare, with incidence estimated to be 1:38 000	Variability in cognitive compromise with the majority below 70 IQ: difficulty with multi-step reasoning and working memory demands; also cognitive flexibility, sequential skills, and environmental monitoring. Focused attention seems strong. Motor skills are impaired, with visual-motor integration less so. Some indication that visual-spatial skills are a strength. Severe (compulsive) self-biting behavior is common; aggression and anxiety are also frequent	Ataxia, spasticity, chorea, kidney failure, gout; progressive decline likely

(Continued)

Table 22.3. (*Continued*)

Pathogenic features	Clinical features	Behavioral phenotype
Monosomy 1p36 1p36 is a contiguous gene syndrome with estimated incidence 1:5000 to 1:10 000, and it may account for 0.5–0.7% of idiopathic mental retardation	Clinical features include hypotonia, severe developmental delay, seizures, growth retardation, obesity, microcephaly, cardiac malformations, cardiomyopathy, hypothyroidism, sensorineural hearing loss, and ophthalmological anomalies Craniofacial dysmorphic features include large anterior fontanelle, prominent forehead, deep-set eyes, flat nasal bridge, midface hypoplasia, ear asymmetry, pointed chin, and orofacialclefting. Also, hydrocephalus with a posterior interhemispheric ventricular cyst, focal polymicrogyria of the cerebral hemispheres, and marked cerebellar hypoplasia	High percentage have severe-to-profound mental retardation; moderate to mild in remaining samples. Expressive language absent in most. Behavior disorders present in almost 50%, including self-biting of hands and wrists, temper tantrums, reduced social interaction. Less frequently seen arestereotypies such as holding hands in front of face, hand washing or flapping, head shaking or banging and rocking, tendency to smell, or beating or rolling objects in a repetitive and purposeless way, and hyperphagia
Neurofibromatosis Type 1 (NF1) One of the most common autosomal dominant disorders in humans, located at 17q11.2, and affecting 1 in 3000 individuals. *NF1* is a large gene that encodes neurofibromin. Loss of *NF1* gene expression results in enhanced cell proliferation and tumor formation. NF2 is much rarer, estimated to occur in 1:33 000, and the majority of these cases are asymptomatic. The gene for NF2 appears to be at chromosome 22q12.2	Full-scale IQs range from 70 to 130 among children with NF1 and from 99 to 139 among unaffected sibs. Scores of parents with NF1 range from 85 to 114 compared to 80 to 134 in unaffected parents Compared to sibs, children with NF1 may show significant deficits in language and reading abilities, but not in mathematics. They also can have impaired visuospatial and neuromotor skills	A statistically significant correlation has been found between lowering of IQ and visuospatial deficits and the number of foci seen on MRI scan Speech difficulties, verbal IQ > performance IQ, distractible, impulsive, hyperactive, anxious; possible association with increased incidence of mood and anxiety disorders Variable physical manifestations may include *café au lait* spots, cutaneous neurofibromas, Lisch nodules, short stature, and macrocephaly
PTEN hamartoma tumor syndromes Include: Bannayan–Zonana syndrome; Riley–Smith syndrome; Ruvalcaba–Myhre–Smith syndrome Gene map locus: 10q23.31	Clinical features include macrocephaly, lipomatosis, and angiomatosis, pseudopapilledema	Delayed motor development with incoordination, delayed speech development, and mild mental retardation. Drooling is often a problem in children. The disorder is apparently autosomal dominant, but some suggest that about 80% of affected persons are male

The *PTEN*(phosphatase and tensin homolog) gene encodes a ubiquitously expressed tumor suppressor dual-specificity phosphatase that antagonizes the phosphatidylinositol 3-kinase (PI3K) signaling pathway through its lipid phosphatase activity and negatively regulates the mitogen-activated protein kinase (MAPK) pathway through its protein phosphatase activity

Phenylketonuria (PKU)

Autosomal recessive defect in phenylalanine hydroxylase (PAH) located at 12q.24.1, or cofactor (biopterinsynthetase, 11q22.3–q23.3), with toxic accumulation of phenylalanine. The prevalence is approximately 1:12 000.

While early-treated PKU children exhibit IQ levels with in the normal range, itappears that they do not reach level spredicted by parent and sibling levels. Declines possible, particularly with poor dietary control

Symptoms absent neonatally, later development of seizures (25% grand mal), fair skin, blue-eyes, blond hair, rash
Untreated: mild to profound MR, languagedelay, destructiveness, self-injury, rage attacks, hyperactivity
Treated: possible increase in hyperactivity and anxiety

Rett's syndrome

Caused by mutations in the methyl-CpG-binding protein-2 gene; X-linked dominant
Magnetic resonance spectroscopy (MRS) findings: decreased *N*-acetylaspartate (NAA)/creatinine (Cr) ratio and increased myoinositol/Cr ratio with age, suggestive of progressive axonal damage and astrocytosis. The NAA/Cr ratios decreased with increasing clinical severity score.The findings indicated that Rett's syndrome is associated with mild white matter pathology.
Prevalence: 1:10 000–1:15 000 female births

Occurs almost exclusively in females, characterized by arrested development between 6 and 18 months of age, regression of acquired skills, loss of speech, stereotypical movements (classically of the hands), microcephaly, seizures, and mental retardation
EEG abnormalities include slow waking background, intermittent rhythmical slowing (3–5 Hz), epileptiform discharges and seizures
Also gait ataxia and apraxia, truncal ataxia, dystonia, cortical atrophy (frontal area)

Behavioral manifestations include autistic behaviors, hand stereotypies (e.g., hand wringing), sleep disturbance, bruxism, breath holding

(Continued)

Table 22.3. (*Continued*)

Pathogenic features	Clinical features	Behavioral phenotype
Prader–Willi syndrome (PWS) Deletion in 15q11-15q13 region of paternal origin (75%). Some cases of maternal uniparental disomy (22%) and imprinting errors and translocations (3%). A number of genes within the critical region may contribute to specific features of the phenotype. Incidence of PWS ranges from 1:10 000 to 1:25 000 live births	Hypotonia, often failure to thrive in infancy, later obesity, small hands and feet, microorchidism, cryptorchidism, short stature, almond-shaped eyes, fair hair, light skin, flat face, scoliosis, orthopedic problems, prominent forehead, and bitemporal narrowing	Obsessive-compulsive disorder (OCD) iscommon Relative strengths in spatial-perceptual organization and visual processing (puzzles); relative weaknesses in short-term processing. Considerable variability in profiles Findings support the reports of cognitive differences between deletion and disomy genetic subgroups, with higher verbal abilities in those with chromosome 15 disomy, while those with deletions are similar to the general learning disability (LD) group A new finding is that the disomy groups have particular difficulty with graphomotor control
Rubinstein–Taybi syndrome (RTS) Autosomal dominant deletion involving the cyclic adenosine monophosphate (cAMP) response element binding (CREB) protein gene (CBP) located at 16p13.3. Estimated prevalence is 1:10 000 live births and RTS may account for approximately 0.2% of individuals with mental retardation in institutional settings	Short stature and microcephaly, broad thumb and big toes; prominent nose, broad nasal bridge, hypertelorism, ptosis, frequent fractures, feeding difficulties in infancy, congenital heart disease, EEG abnormalities in 75%, seizures in 25%	Poor concentration, distractible, expressive language difficulties, Performance IQ > Verbal IQ; anecdotally happy, loving sociable, responsive to music, self-stimulating behavior; older individuals with mood lability and temper tantrums
Sanfilipo syndrome type A, B, C, and D Autosomal recessive (1:24 000 live births); heparin-N-sulfatase deficiency (type A); chromosome 12q is implicated in type D	Normal early development, recurrent ear, nose, throat, and bowel problems; CNS deterioration by age 6 years, hearing loss, mild skeletal abnormalities, death in second or third decade	Poor concentration, distractible, expressive language difficulties, PIQ > VIQ; anecdotally happy, loving sociable, responsive to music, self-stimulating behavior; older individuals with mood lability and temper tantrums

Smith–Lemli–Opitz syndrome
Caused by mutations in the gene encoding sterol delta-7-reductase, which maps to chromosome 11q12-q13

Autosomal recessive multiple congenital malformation and mental retardation syndrome. The syndrome constitutes a clinical and biochemical continuum from mild to severe
Clinical signs include microcephaly, mental retardation, hypotonia, incomplete development of the male genitalia, short nose with anteverted nostrils

Characteristic behavioral profile of cognitive delay, sensory hyper-reactivity, irritability, language impairment, sleep-cycle disturbance, self-injurious behavior, syndrome-specific motor movements, and autism spectrum behaviors (autism spectrum disorder is frequently diagnosed)

Smith–Magenis syndrome (SMS)
Most cases of SMS have a large deletion within chromosome 17p11.2. Several candidate genes have been suggested. Disturbed melatonin secretion may be implicated in the sleep disturbance associated with this syndrome. Estimated prevalence is approximately 1:25 000 live births

Broad face, flat midface, short, broad hands, small toes, and hoarse, deep voice

Severe self-injury including hand biting, head banging, and pulling out finger and toe nails; autistic features; initial and middle insomnia

The measured IQ ranges between 20 and 78, most patients falling in the moderate range of mental retardation (40–54), although scores in the mild or borderline range are not uncommon. Simultaneous processing is generally stronger than sequential processing. A strength in visual-gestalt closure and reading/decoding has been identified. Expressive vocabulary is stronger than receptive vocabulary. Relative weaknesses in arithmetic and in under standing riddles have also been identified. Longer-term memory processes appear to be relatively stronger than short-term processes, which also impact attentional functioning. Hyperactivity in 75%

Tuberous sclerosis complex (TSC) 1, 2
Autosomal dominant disorder caused by a mutation in either the *TSC1* gene (hamartin) on chromosome 9q34 or the *TSC2* gene (tuberin) on chromosome 16p13. These proteins form a TSC1-TSC2 tumor suppressor complex, providing an explanation for the similar phenotype in individuals with mutations in either of these genes. Prevalence is approximately 1:6000 individuals, TSC1 (50%) and TSC2 (50%), but TSC1 may be associated with a milder phenotype

Epilepsy; autism is common (as many as 40% of individuals), hyperactivity, impulsivity, aggression

The spectrum of MR ranges from none (30%) to profound. Self-injurious behaviors, sleep disturbances including nightmare waking and early morning waking have all been described

Velocardiofacial syndrome (VCFS), DiGeorge syndrome, CATCH 22

(Continued)

Table 22.3. (*Continued*)

Pathogenic features	Clinical features	Behavioral phenotype
Several candidate genes have been identified at the 22q11.2 locus for VCFS including the T-box gene, *TBX1*. T-box genes are transcription factors involved in the regulation of developmental processes. The catechol-*O*-methyltransferase gene, *COMT*, is also located at the 22q11.2 region, and its importance in the catabolism of catecholamines, including the neurotransmitters dopamine, epinephrine, and norepinephrine, may be important in the high incidence of psychosis associated with VCFS. Prevalence is 1:4000. VCFS is the second most common cause of congenital cardiac anomalies after Down's syndrome	VCFS is the most common MR syndrome to have palatal anomalies as a major feature. Cleft palate, cardiac anomalies, typical facies. Less frequent features include microcephaly, mental retardation, short stature, slender hands and digits, minor auricular anomalies, and inguinal hernia. Prominent tubular nose, narrow palpebral fissures, and slightly retruded mandible. Ophthalmological abnormalities including tortuous retinal vessels, small optic discs, or bilateral cataracts (70%). Neonatal hypocalcemia requiring treatment may occur (13%)	Higher verbal than nonverbal IQ scores, assets in verbal memory, and deficits in the areas of attention, story memory, visuospatial memory, arithmetic performance relative to other areas of achievement, and psychosocial functioning. Learning disabilities characterized by difficulty with abstraction, reading comprehension, and mathematics. Children with VCFS may have characteristic personality features of blunt or inappropriate affect, with a greater than expected number of children developing severe psychiatric illnesses as they approach adolescence
	Cardiac pathology, most commonly tetralogy of Fallot, ventricular septal defect, interrupted aortic arch, pulmonary atresia/ventricular septal defect, and truncusarteriosus	
Williams' syndrome		
Hemizygous (autosomal dominant) deletion in chromosome 7q11.23, often including the gene for elastin (*ELN*).Prevalence may be as high as 1:7500, or 6% of individuals with identifiable genetic causes for mental retardation	Short stature, unusual facial features including broad forehead, depressed nasal bridge, stellate pattern of the iris, widely space dteeth, full lips; renal and cardiovascular abnormalities, hypercalcemia	ADHD, poor peer relationships, loquaciousness, excessive anxiety, sleep disturbance, increased mimicry, socially outgoing and disinhibited
		Verbal abilities typically better than non verbal. Visuospatial construction very weak, with improvement over time, but more protracted development rarely reaching average levels. Auditory rote memory better than might be expected given overall cognitive ability. Oral language skills are relative strengths. Overall IQ scores variable, but typically below average

stressor, the diagnosis of Intermittent Explosive Disorderor Impulse Control Disorder should be entertained. The value in rendering such a diagnosis is that it indicates that other disorders (for which criteria are arguably better established) like depression, anxiety, and so on, have been considered and ruledout.The diagnosis of a specific disorder of impulse control also identifies a target for intervention beyond ID.

Oppositional Defiant Disorder/Conduct Disorder

The DSM-IV-TR diagnosis of oppositional defiant disorder or conduct disorder also requires comparisons to be made with others of similar mental age.In addition, both diagnoses assume some degree of willfulness on the part of the individual in question (e.g., disobedience motivated by spite or resentment), which can be very difficult to discern in nonverbal subjects with profound cognitive deficits.This point also has been made by Reid [13]. As with many psychiatric illnesses in this context, the certainty with which the disorder is diagnosed will tend to evaporate with greater severity of intellectual disability.

The adaptations in DM-ID for ODD remind one to rule out other reasons for oppositional behavior such as underlying mood disorders or medical conditions. There is also a reminder to evaluate language and cognition to rule out "comprehension and specific cognitive difficulties that might otherwise explain the noncompliance." Similar to the case with ADHD, caution is advised when the diagnosis of ODD is being considered in cases of severe ID due to the child's potential lack of understanding. Again, it is required to use individuals of comparable age and severity of ID when assessing frequency and severity of symptoms [14].

In conduct disorder, one is cautioned when looking at criteria of physical cruelty to people and animals to ascertain that the individual displaying the behavior has understood the significance and impact of his or her actions. When looking at criteria regarding theft one is cautioned to establish that the individual has mastered the concept of a sense of ownership. When looking at serious violation of rules one is instructed to carefully examine the home environment and the reasons why the individual is running away and staying out at night. The child psychiatrist should consider neglect and abuse, which arecertainly risk factors for these behaviors in children with ID.

Impulse Control Disorder

In contrast to normally developing children, impulse control disorder is a helpful diagnosis for children who have ID because they are more likely to present with aggressive behavior for which neither an antecedent event nor identifiable psychiatric disorder can be identified. Criteria have been adapted in the DM-ID: for example, "Frequent episodes lasting at least two months" replaces "several discrete episodes" of failure to resist aggressive acts or destruction of property. The aggressiveness expressed during the episodes should be grossly out of proportion to any precipitating psychosocial stressors and to the level of ID. Clinicians should also be sure the aggressive episode is not better accounted for by another diagnosis. For example, a person with a mild specific phobia and severe aggression not confined to the phobic situation should receive the additional diagnosis of Impulse Control Disorder [15].

Anxiety Disorders

Anxiety disorders are probably more often overlooked than many other mental illnesses in this population, but there is clear evidence that the full range of anxiety disorders can occur in the context of intellectual disability [16–19]. Specific anxiety disorders like separation anxiety, overanxious disorder, obsessive-compulsive disorder, panic disorder, generalized anxiety disorder, and so on, rely heavily on an individual's ability to describe subjective symptoms of anxiety. According to DSM-IV-TR, concurrent pervasive developmental disorder specifically trumps the diagnosis of most of these disorders as well. Nevertheless, many children with autism spectrum disorders in particular, and intellectual disability in general, are referred with constellations of signs and symptoms that best are captured in the anxiety disorder spectrum.

Children and adolescents who are clearly avoidant, who exhibit autonomic arousal in the face of stimuli that most of their peers would not find aversive, who present with other features of anxiety might be given a diagnosis of anxiety disorder not otherwise specified (NOS) when they cannot articulate their subjective states. In some cases individuals engage in behavior that appears compulsive or driven, and even ego-alien. The diagnosis of obsessive-compulsive disorder NOS might be considered under such circumstances.

Several instruments have been developed to assist in the assessment of mood and anxiety symptoms in persons with ID. The Anxiety, Depression, and Mood Scale(ADAMS) [20] is an empirically derived, behaviorally based instrument with established reliability. The Glasgow Anxiety Scale for people with ID demonstrates good discriminant reliability and validity as well [21]. The anxiety disorders section of the Diagnostic Interview Schedule for Children [22, 23] and The Early Child Inventory and Child Symptoms Inventory [24, 25] have also been useful. The Fear Survey for Children-Revised was used by Dykens [26] in a study comparing youths with Williams' syndrome to a control group of mixed ID etiology. These investigators found that the Williams' syndrome youth reported more fears than their parents appreciated, and significantly more fears than the control group. Thus, Williams' syndrome in particular is associated with high rates of anxiety even relative to ID.

In a recent study of adults with ID a strong correlation between anxiety and tantrums was found [27].

Post-Traumatic Stress Disorder (PTSD)

In the DM-ID, PTSD is highlighted as separate from other anxiety disorders due to its complexity and importance [28]. Studies of PTSD and ID are rare and the empirical strength of the few studies is low [29]. The adapted PTSD symptoms in the DM-ID are thus based primarily upon clinical consensus. Events that in a typically developing youth may not usually be considered traumatic can be so in the setting of ID. Thus, missed developmental milestones, residential placement, and consensual sexual experiences may be experiences that lead to post-traumatic reactions in some individuals with ID. The range of potentially traumatizing events may be even greater for individuals with lower developmental age, though no hard data are available [30].

There is a proposed revision for the DSM-5 of a new childhood disorder, Posttraumatic Stress Disorder in Preschool Children, which may be helpful in the diagnosis of youths that are developmentally at a preschool level. As is the case for other diagnoses, the peer group by which they should be compared should comprise individuals of similar age and severity of ID. The proposed criteria stipulate that "spontaneous and intrusive memories may not necessarily appear distressing and may be expressed as play reenactment." This may also present beyond the preschool years in children with ID who are functioning at a preschool level. The proposed criteria generally lower the number of symptoms necessary to diagnose PTSD for preschool children. In addition there are several new items under consideration for the new DSM-5 category including "reckless or self-destructive behavior" and "substantial increased frequency of negative mood states." The adaptive criteria in DM-ID are similar to the adaptive criteria in DSM-IV-TR for children. These included fear presenting as disorganized and agitated behavior. Re-experiencing in the most severely affected individuals with ID may involve behavioral acting out of the traumatic experience and may be associated with self-injurious behavior (SIB). Dreams may be present and frightening without recog-

nizable content. In the avoidance criteria, caregivers might report avoidance as noncompliance, especially if an individual is unable to verbally express post-traumatic desires to avoid activities. The criterion on inability to recall aspects of trauma could be very difficult to discern depending upon developmental age and would take careful assessment. Diminished interest might also be confused with noncompliance. The sense of a foreshortened future is also very challenging to ascertain in the setting of ID where individuals may not have normative expectations of the future due to defects in abstract thought [31].

Obsessive-Compulsive Disorder (OCD)

The diagnosis of OCD in mild-moderate levels of ID is relatively straightforward with DSM-IV-TR diagnostic criteria. With severe and profound levels of ID, however, there is a definite need for adaptation as language deficits can be a major stumbling block when attempting to ascertain an individual's obsessive thoughts or attempts to suppress such thoughts. Repetitive behaviors may be observable in these patients, and yet the language deficits and cognitive impairments make it extremely difficult to connect them to obsessive thoughts or to understand their function. The patient may not recognize the excessiveness or unreasonableness of their thoughts. Instead of marked distress, which may not occur, happiness or intense preoccupation may be present. Aggression and SIB may be associated with perseveration and compulsions. There is a need to distinguish compulsive behavior from stereotypes and insistence on sameness. Drug-induced movement disorders must also be considered and ruled out to make this diagnosis [32].

Repetitive behaviors are not uncommon in persons with mental retardation. These behaviors should not be equated with compulsions necessarily. For example, a child may quite enjoy flipping light switches on and off or swinging in a swing. These behaviors may be innately reinforcing for sensory or other reasons, and would not satisfy an anxiolytic or "ego-alien" criterion thought to be at the core of OCD. Such behaviors are perhaps better viewed on a continuum with stereotyped movements, but in some cases may be more goal directed. The discrimination between repetitive behaviors in terms of their etiology and their treatment (if appropriate) should be a focus of additional research in this population.

Another form of repetitive behavior includes self-injury. For some of these individuals, there may also be evidence of self-restraint. They may, for example, secure their extremities in their clothing or hold on to objects such that their hands are functionally unavailable. Alternatively, they might cling to their parents or care-providers – seemingly to prevent self-injurious behaviors [32]. In these cases, the self-injury appears to be compulsive, or "driven," and a diagnosis of OCD might be considered.

Mood Disorders

Depression in mild to moderate ID is also fairly straightforward using DSM-IV-TR criteria. The most useful criteria are sadness, irritability, decreased social interaction, regression in skill levels, sleep disturbance, diurnal variation, and aggression. Modified criteria have been recommended for severe ID with the use of observational data [33]. In the DM-ID these adapted criteria focus on observations by caregivers of behaviors that are change from baseline, including sad facial expressions, flat affect or absence of emotional expression, rare smiles or laughs, and crying or tearfulness. Additional behaviors of interest include irritability, grouchiness or anger, or an increase in agitation (assaults, SIB, spitting, swearing, disruptive or destructive behaviors) accompanied by an angry affect. In autism spectrum disorders individuals with high rates of baseline stereotypies, ritualistic or repetitive behaviors may experience an increase in these behaviors with irritability. The Self-Report Depression Questionnaire (SRDQ) was reviewed by Esbensen and colleagues for adult patients from several studies, and reliability and validity were good in patients with adequate verbal skills [34]. Another self-reported mood instrument, the Intellectual Disability Mood Scale, demonstrated validity in an adolescent ID population and used a unique adaptation of a five-point Likert scale with pictures of buckets filled with increasing amounts of fluid to correspond to the scale [35]. Esbensen studied adults with mild ID using the SR DQ and the Children's Attribution Styles Questionnaire among other measures and found that depressed patients with ID demonstrated responses consistent with Beck's cognitive triad such as more automatic thoughts, more negative attribution styles, and lower self-esteem. The results supported intervention with cognitive behavioral therapy (CBT) in mild ID with depression [36]. A study of 60 adults with ID using the Semi-structured ICD-10, Adaptive Testing, Reiss Screen for Maladaptive Behavior, and the American Association of Mental Deficiency (AAMD) Adaptive Behavior Scale Part II found that individuals in the affective group demonstrated the highest aggression scores on the Reiss screen and highest rebellious behaviors on the AAMD scale. Kishore and colleagues'

results are consistent with aggression as a behavioral equivalent of a symptom for mood disorder [37]. In a recent study of 181 adults from Norway with ID using the Aberrant Behavior Checklist (ABC), the investigators found that SIB had low correlation with most psychiatric symptom subscales but did correlate with depression and mania in mild-to-moderate ID. In severe-to-profound ID, there was a correlation between aggression and also with screaming and depression and mania. The study showed a strong relationship between behavior problems and psychiatric problems in individuals with ID. More symptoms of psychiatric disorders were found in mild-to-moderate ID than in severe-to-profound ID [38].

Psychosis

Approximately 10–20% of youths diagnosed with schizophrenia have premorbid histories of intellectual disability [39–42]. However, the diagnosis of schizophrenia essentially requires that a patient relate the experience of delusions or hallucinations. As has been suggested by others [43–45], persons with profound mental retardation and limited communicative ability pose particular problems when it comes to diagnosing classic schizophrenia. Nonetheless, the display of presumptive evidence of response to hallucinations (e.g., striking or shouting at empty space, throwing imaginary peers from furniture) or the adoption of catatonic postures can appear to be psychotic in origin. In these cases the diagnosis of psychosis NOS should be considered if these signs exist in the absence of sufficient evidence to warrant the diagnosis of a supervening mood disorder.

In DM-ID, the challenges of recognizing positive symptoms of schizophrenia in verbal patients are considered similar to the difficulties of diagnosing any mental illness in ID. The negative symptoms, however, are more problematic even in mild ID. The insidious onset of changes in affect, volition, and speech can be difficult to elicit and interpret [46].

Sleep disorders

Sleep disturbances are a common reason for referral for treatment or evaluation, and have received relatively little study in this population. Ultimately, they require the subjective input of the patient regarding the adequacy of rest, occurrence of nightmares, and so on, and given the frequent history of abuse reported for people with intellectual disability as a group, one should not overlook the possibility of PTSD when sleep disturbance is a presenting problem.

Provisional Diagnoses

Comorbidity is common. Additionally, some individuals may have psychiatric symptoms that significantly interfere with function, but that do not allow for a clear distinction between diagnoses. An impulse control disorder NOS, perhaps characterized by an individual who engages in impulsive aggressive acts, versus an anxiety disorder NOS, perhaps suggested by an individual who strikes out in the context of a stressor that would go unnoticed by most people, may be very difficult to discriminate from one another. The clinician should always make a best effort at a working diagnosis, and be prepared to make modifications as indicated by data gathered through collateral sources and from increasing familiarity with a particular patient. It should be acknowledged that the diagnostic process is a "work in progress," and the certainty with which a clinician comes to a diagnosis will in most cases be inversely proportional to the patient's degree of disability [47].

Eating Disorders

The diagnoses of anorexia nervosa and bulimia are effectively precluded for individuals with severe or profound ID because of the near total reliance of diagnostic criteria upon the subjective experience of the patient with the eating disorder. For example, it would be a challenge at best to identify classic distortions in body image, or guilt feelings associated with bingeing in nonverbal subjects. Food refusal or self-induced vomiting would have to be viewed as atypical eating disorders if such symptoms were to occur in the absence of other diagnosable disorders (e.g., depression, rumination). Pica is likely to be among the most common of the eating disorders diagnosed among persons with ID; however, psychogenic overeating, vomiting, rumination, and simple food refusal may be relatively common [48].

As suggested in the DM-ID [49], in mild ID the criteria for anorexia nervosa and bulimia nervosa are more easily adapted. Though individuals with ID may not be able to verbalize fear of gaining weight, they may still manifest their fear through an avoidance of food.

Disorders Associated with a General Medical Condition

Strictly speaking, one might submit that everyone with ID has some "organic" cerebral dysfunction, by definition, and thus any psychiatric illness should be regarded as organic or associated with a general medical condition. Importantly, in his study of psychiatric illness in a sample of institutionalized patients with Down's syndrome, Menolascino [50] argued that psychiatric nosology did not have to be reinvented to accommodate individuals with a "tissue diagnosis." Moreover, patients with so called "dual diagnoses" of mental illness and Down's syndrome need to be distinguished from others with Down's syndrome alone. Thus, the application of the diagnoses of organic mental syndromes and disorders is probably best approached as if patients do not have mental retardation. The same principle should apply to Axis II personality disorders. The diagnosis of "organic" personality disorder is best reserved for individuals whose pre-existing personality was altered in a pathological way by some additional cerebral insult. In essence, this category (due to a medical condition) is best reserved for patients whose mental retardation is acquired and results in a change in personality, usually secondary to CNS trauma experienced in childhood or early adolescence.

Approach to Maladaptive Behavior

As with child psychiatry in general, there is little specificity that can be attached to a given symptom. Persons with ID will typically be referred for evaluation because of self-injurious, aggressive, impulsive, or hyperactive behavior. Because of the lack of diagnostic specificity for each of these symptoms, a diagnostic decision tree with any utility cannot be constructed. Instead, it is perhaps more useful to ask a series of questions about the expression of a particular behavior. If the behavior is of recent onset, one is more likely to consider an acute medical or psychiatric etiology. If the behavior is highly situational, occurring primarily in the context of the stress of task demands, the likelihood of a psychosis or mood disorder is probably reduced. If attempts are made to avoid the behavior by self-restraint, the inference of some compulsive features may be tenable. Assessing the sum of these and collateral data will lead the clinician to a presumptive diagnosis that will form the basis for a treatment plan.

For self-injurious and other maladaptive behavior, if the behavior becomes the focus of a treatment intervention, a diagnosable psychiatric disorder is present by definition. On the other hand, a given behavior, in and of itself, does not constitute grounds for a diagnosis. Just as "shopping" may be normal in most contexts, unrestrained buying may come to be recognized as harmful to an individual. In the absence of any other clear psychopathology, excessive shopping will likely be diagnosed as a disorder of impulse control. The same principle applies for many behaviors in the context of ID.

Treatment

Our ability to diagnose the underlying condition causing a child's intellectual disability is rapidly improving. The child psychiatrist, however, is rarely – if ever –called upon for this purpose. Rather, it is generally the purview of pediatricians and genetic specialists. We, as child psychiatrists, are left with an arguably more daunting task: the diagnosis and treatment of psychiatric disorders and especially disruptive behaviors within this patient population. And, for the most part, we are asked to see these patients when behaviors have, more or less, escalated to the point where they are out of control. Therefore, the child psychiatrist often is in a position where the ability to help the patient may well determine if the patient stays at home, in an independent or semi-independent environment, or requires the support of an institutional environment.

The formal study of comorbid psychopathology in persons with intellectual disability is still a relatively recent phenomenon, and the literature in this area, especially in regard to controlled data, is scarce. Likewise, there are currently no practice parameters or specific guidelines for evidence-based treatment in this area. As such, the child psychiatrist's approach to psychiatric and especially behavioral problems in patients with intellectual disability is primarily based on empirical data, experience, and clinical consensus.

On the other hand, progress is being made on all fronts. The following sections reviewpsychosocial therapeutic approaches, medication approaches, and holistic or ecological approaches. What follows is not a laundry list of every treatment modality available, but an attempt to focus on integrating treatments that seem to be the most pertinent and well grounded.

Ecological Approach

Like the foundation of a home, ecological aspects are perhaps the least glamorous of the issues to be discussed and yet what they provide are vital, the basis for a successful treatment program. It seems intuitively obvious that the environmental milieu of the patient's everyday life must certainly influence any psychopathology. Yet, until recently, quality of life issues received little to no attention. While these *ecological* characteristics, or factors, are important for patients of all abilities their significance is even more acute for patients with intellectual disabilities. First, individuals with intellectual disability are more susceptible to environmental shortcomings, and are more subject to abuse in all forms. Furthermore, persons with intellectual disability may have little control over their environments or lack of resources, internally and externally, to change their circumstances. Finally, even reporting their living conditions can be problematic.

Gathering ecological data is both difficult and time-consuming and requires a multidisciplinary approach. It is, however, vital if one's goal is to provide the best possible care. For example, how effective is instructing a patient in clinic to turn negative thoughts into positive thoughts when he goes home to what is in reality an overwhelmingly negative environment with little or no support? How can one expect to have an impact on aggressive behaviors in light of ongoing physical abuse? How can one expect a patient's depression to respond if her environment is woefully bereft of light and stimulation? Even if she is instructed in certain activities or exercise to aid her treatment, will she be able to implement the plan onher own?

Family/Caregiver

There are several different ways to involve the parent(s)/caregiver(s) in the patient's therapy. These typicallyfall into two general divisions: in one the parents/caregivers and patients are actually in therapy together, whereas the other consists of several types of parental training. Often these are combined in certain programs.

In a meta-analysis consisting of over 1400 patients, Dretzke *et al* [51]. looked into the cost-effectiveness and care effectiveness of parent training/education programs for the treatment of conduct disorder including oppositional defiant disorder in children. They concluded that these programs appeared to not only be effective in treating the patient, but potentially cost-effective for children with conduct disorder. In a randomized clinical trial of a new behavioral family intervention called Stepping Stones Triple P, for preschoolers with developmental and behavior problems, Roberts and colleagues [52] found the intervention to be associated with fewer child behavior problems, improved maternal parenting style, and decreased maternal stress. Additionally, these positive effects were maintained at a 6-month follow-up.

A very promising therapeutic approach for behavior problems in children with ID is parent-child interaction therapy (PCIT). PCIT is a highly individualized form of therapy aimed at helping parents learn better behavioral skills. It is performed in two sections, a child-directed portion and a parent-directed portion. All sessions are conducted with a "bug in the ear" so the therapist, who is on the other side of a one-way mirror, can direct the parent's interaction with the child. In a randomized, controlled trial, PCIT was shown to be effective in treating disruptive behavioral problems in children with ID [53]. It was additionally noted that no change had to be made in the protocol of the PCIT program from that which is used with typically developing children.

Another recent study evaluated parent training and medication versus medication alone in treating children with pervasive developmental disorder and serious behavior difficulties. Parent training plus medication outperformed medication alone in this study [54].

Functional Behavioral Analysis (FBA)

Functional behavioral analyses are used to determine the function of aggressive and disruptive behaviors. These behaviors are often socially mediated with predictable antecedent and reinforcing events; that is, there is a goal and a reward for the behavior. FBAs use both direct and indirect observation methods to determine what the antecedent event(s) and reinforcement(s) of the targeted behavior are, and should inform most treatment programs [55]. Importantly, an FBA may help lead to the identification of important medical considerations for the treatment of behavior disturbance, for example, a child with episodic SIB who only engaged in SIB during times when he had otitis media [56].

Cognitive Behavioral Therapy (CBT)

Cognitive behavioral therapy is a well-established, highly validated treatment for many childhood psychiatric disorders. It is well known to be effective in childhood post-traumatic stress disorder and obsessive-compulsive disorder; and more recently in the Child/Adolescent Anxiety Multimodal Study (CAMS) for separation anxiety disorder, generalized anxiety disorder, and social phobia the combination of CBT and sertraline was significantly better than sertraline alone – 81% responders compared to 55%, respectively. CBT alone had 60% responders and placebo was at 24% [57]. In this context, while there are few controlled studies in children with ID, there is evolving research in this area. There are, of course, limitations for these patients, especially ones with more severe ID. Several studies have looked at ways to screen patients to predict if they would be able to respond to CBT [58]. At present, it seems best to ensure that the patient can, at a minimum, verbally express his or her feelings.

In addition to assessing the patient's ability to participate in CBT, therapy should be adapted based on assessment of the patient's needs [58]. It is important when administering CBT for children with ID to use therapeutic techniques tailored to their abilities and circumstances. A related challenge, for example, is that a 15-year-old functioning at a 6-year-old intellectual level likely has experiences – sexual development, for instance – that most 6-year-olds and their families will not have accumulated and these must be appreciated as well.

Disruptive Behaviors

The treatment of aggressive behavior, including SIB, warrants further discussion. It is a frequent problem in the care of patients with ID and a common cause for referral to a child psychiatrist. As with any medical investigation, it is important to determine, if possible, the underlying cause of the disruptive or aggressive behaviors. For example, patients with fragile X syndrome (FXS) have a high incidence of ADHD. If untreated, some of the symptoms may present as aggression. In these cases, treating the ADHD often improves the disruptive/aggressive behavior as well. Another example would be autism spectrum disorders where social anxiety may be responsible for the unwanted behaviors, and treatment of the anxiety, specifically, will be critical for reducing the maladaptive behavior.

Several disorders within the spectrum of intellectual disability, such as Lesch–Nyhan syndrome and Smith–Magenis syndrome, are particularly prone to disruptive/aggressive/self-injurious behaviors. Additionally, certain comorbid psychiatric diagnoses are associated with aggressive/disruptive behavior including mood disorders, anxiety disorders (especially PTSD and OCD), and disruptive behavioral disorders (ADHD, ODD, and CD).

Behavioral Treatments for Disruptive Behaviors in Patients with ID

In addition to CBT, several forms of behavioral therapy have been studied in patients with ID and shown to be useful. At the present time it seems prudent to recommend a complete evaluation of the patient including his or her environment, as discussed above. Treatment should then be tailored to a behavior program that matches the patient's strengths and weaknesses to the best advantage. Pharmacological treatment is generally not a solo treatment in regard to treating behavioral disorders in children with ID but is used in conjunction with other approaches [59].

Treatment of Disruptive Behaviors in Patients with ID with Psychotropic Medication

At present the mainstay of pharmacological treatment for disruptive behavior disorders in children with ID is risperidone. A number of studies have demonstrated risperidone to be effective in reducing aggression, irritability, hyperactivity, and other disruptive behaviors [60, 61]. A study by Aman *et al.* showed that risperidone plus parent training was better than risperidone alone in treating these individuals [62]. On the other hand, a recent review of the literature expresses concerns about the lack of long-term efficacy and safety with the use of psychotropic medications in treating pediatric patients with behavior problems [59]. Indeed, even for the studies that show efficacy for psychotropic medicines in this group of patients the effect can be quite modest [63].

Self-Injurious Behavior (SIB) in People with Intellectual Disability

The overall incidence of SIB in ID is approximately 10%. Lesch–Nyhan syndrome is perhaps the prototype disorder for SIB. These individuals virtually always engage in SIB, most commonly in the form of finger biting and lip biting, though a myriad of other injurious behaviors including head banging have been reported. In a review of behavioral treatment for SIB in Lesch–Nyhan syndrome [64], the most common form of treatment was the use of restraints – a negative form of behavior modification – and yet it was far from being the most effective. Some studies have demonstrated that these symptoms are more effectively controlled with positive behavioral approaches.

Perhaps the most promising treatment for SIB is preventative in nature. A major part of this strategy, of course, is developing reliable ways to predict SIB, or risk factors for SIB, and to target these for intervention.

Attention-Deficit Hyperactivity Disorder (ADHD)

Attention-deficit hyperactivity disorder is a relatively well-studied common comorbidity for patients with ID. Stimulants are the mainstay of treatment, as in typically developing youths. However, the response rate has been reported at 45–66%, which is lower than that for the general population with ADHD [65]. Although less well studied, atomoxetine and alpha-antagonists are typically considered for second-line treatment. There are also data to support an effect of atypical antipsychotics (e.g., risperidone and aripiprazole) for hyperactivity in some developmental disorders, but the side-effect profile of this class would clearly make it a less desirable option for ADHD symptoms.

Side effects from stimulants may be more common in patients with ID, particularly adverse behavioral symptoms like irritability, impulsivity, and hyperactivity. Adverse effects from stimulants may also include symptoms such as weight loss, loss of appetite, insomnia, possible growth suppression and, particularly in this group of patients, the development of tics can be problematic [66].

Mood Disorders

Mood disorders are common in patients with ID. Because internalized "feelings" of depression may be hard to access in this group, diagnosis depends on collateral information from others and observation of patient behaviors as well as a search for any triggering causes [67]. As always with assessing patients with ID their developmental level needs to be taken into consideration. Changing caregivers, a recent move or change in environment, or medication effects such as a akathisia or irritability can exacerbate mood disorders in these patients. Mood disorders can sometimes manifest as aggressive behavior. Thus, a marked increase in aggressive behaviors or new aggressive behaviors should be evaluated in this context [68]. Treatment for depression in patients with ID is similar to that in typically developing youths with the caveat that side effects from the medication can be more prominent in patients with ID [69].

Anxiety Disorders

Cognitive behavioral therapy and other forms of behavior intervention have been useful for anxiety disorders in patients with ID. SSRIs are most often used to treat anxiety in this patient population as with typically developing youths. Caution is advised with the use of some anxiolytic medications, particularly benzodiazepines, as they may cause agitation and paradoxical excitement [70].

Post-traumatic stress disorder is common in children with ID and one must keep in mind that a traumatic event for a child with ID may be different than that for the typically developing child.

Schizophrenia and Other Psychotic Disorders

Treatment for psychosis is similar to that in typically developing children though relatively lower doses of antipsychotic medication may be sufficient. Risperidone is the most widely studied antipsychotic medication for use in children with ID. Weight gain can be significant and metabolic effects should be monitored. Somnolence is a common sideeffect and may be more problematic in the setting of ID.

Use of Antipsychotic Medications in Children with ID

At present, four second-generation antipsychotics – risperidone, olanzapine, aripiprazole, and quetiapine –

have been approved for use in schizophrenia for children aged 13 to 17. Risperidone and aripiprazole have also been approved for treatment of irritability associated with autistic disorder in children and adolescents aged 5–16 years, including symptoms of aggression toward others, deliberate self-injuriousness, temper tantrums, and quickly changing moods. Historically, however, antipsychotic medications have been used for a multitude of purposes in children with ID. Progress is occurring in the areas of targeting which patients may or may not benefit from the use of antipsychotic medications.

The Child Psychiatrist as Consultant

As a result of advances in such diverse fields as molecular biology, pharmacology, and psychology, clinicians are increasingly able to make a difference in the lives of patients with intellectual disability and of their families. Along with these advances has come a steadily expanding role for the child psychiatrist. The therapeutic nihilism long associated with psychiatric diagnosis and treatment of patients with intellectual disability has given way to a clear understanding of the important role such consultation must play in the careful identification and management of intellectual disability syndromes and their associated behavioral phenotypes, in the recognition and treatment of comorbid psychiatric disorders, and the astute use of medications to augment behavioral, psychotherapeutic, and ecological treatments. The multidisciplinary approach for patients with intellectual disability is the state of the art, and the child psychiatrist is an essential member of that team.

References

1. American Psychiatric Association. DSM-5 Development. A 00 Intellectual Developmental Disorder. 2010. Available from: http://www.dsm5.org/ProposedRevisions/Pages/proposedrevision.aspx?rid=384.

2. American Psychiatric Association.*Diagnostic and Statistical Manual of Mental Disorders*, 4th edn, Text Revision. Washington, DC: American Psychiatric Association, 2000.

3. Toth K, King BH. Intellectual disability (mental retardation). In: Dulcan MK (Ed.) *Dulcan's Textbook of Child and Adolescent Psychiatry*. Chicago: American Psychiatric Publishing, 2010; pp. 153–154.

4. Maulik PK, Mascarenhas MN, Mathers CD, Dua T, Sexena S. Prevalence of intellectual disability: a metavanalysis of population-based studies. *Res Dev Disabil* 2011;**32**:419–436.

5. Battaglia A, Bianchini E, Carey JC. Diagnostic yield of the comprehensive assessment of developmental delay/mental retardation in an institute of child neuropsychiatry. *Am J Med Genet*1999;**82**:60–66.

6. McKusick VA.*Mendelian Inheritance in Man: a Catalog of Human Genes and Genetic Disorders*, 12th edn. Baltimore,

MD:Johns Hopkins University Press, 1998; available at: http://www.ncbi.nlm.nih.gov/omim/.

7. Flint J. Behavioral phenotypes: conceptual and methodological issues. *Am J Med Genet*1998;**81**:235–240.

8. Penrose LS. *The Biology of Mental Defect*. London: Sidgwick & Jackson, Ltd. 1963.

9. Einfeld SL. Behavior phenotypes of genetic disorders. *Curr Opin Psychiatry* 2004;17:343–348.

10. Gray KM, Mohr C. Mental health problems in children and adolescents with intellectual disability. *Curr Opin Psychiatry* 2004;17:365–370.

11. Dykens EM. Annotation: Psychopathology in children with intellectual disability. *J Child Psychol Psychiat* 2000;**41**:407–417.

12. Fletcher R, Loschen E, Stavrakaki C, First M(eds). *Diagnostic Manual – Intellectual Disability (DM–ID): A Textbook of Diagnosis of Mental Disorders in Persons with Intellectual Disability*. Kingston, NY: NADD Press, 2007.

13. Reid AH. Psychiatric disorders in mentally handicapped children: A clinical and follow-up study. *J Ment Def Res* 1980;**24**:287–298.

14. Fletcher R, Loschen E, Stavrakaki C, First M (eds). *Diagnostic Manual – Intellectual Disability: A Clinical Guide for Diagnosis of Mental Disorders in Persons with Intellectual Disability*. Kington, NY: NADD Press, 2007; p 93.

15. Fletcher R, Loschen E, Stavrakaki C, First M (eds).*Diagnostic Manual – Intellectual Disability: A Clinical Guide for Diagnosis of Mental Disorders in Persons with Intellectual Disability*. Kington, NY: NADD Press, 2007; p. 293.

16. Stavrakaki C, Lunsky Y, Bouras N, *et al*. Depression, anxiety and adjustment disorders in people with intellectual disabilities. In:Bouras N, Holt G (eds) *Psychiatric and Behavioral Disorders in Intellectual and Developmental Disabilities*, 2nd edn. New York: Cambridge University Press, 2007; pp. 113–131.

17. Saulnier C, Volkmar F, Bouras N, *et al*. Mental health problems in people with autism and related disorders. In: Bouras N, Holt G (eds) *Psychiatric and Behavioral Disorders in Intellectual and Developmental Disabilities*, 2nd edn. New York: Cambridge University Press, 2007; pp. 215–225.

18. Schlauch RC, Gordon KH, Schmidt NB, *et al*.The assessment, diagnosis, and treatment of psychiatric disorders in individuals with a dual diagnosis: The co-occurrence of developmental disorders and psychiatric disorders. In: Buckner JD, Castro Y, Holm-Denoma JM, Joiner TE (eds)*Mental Health Care for People of Diverse Backgrounds*. Abingdon,UK: Radcliffe Publishing, 2007; pp. 101–121.

19. Masi G, Favilla L, Mucci M. Generalized anxiety disorder in adolescents and young adults with mildmental retardation. *Psychiatry* 2007;**63**:54–64.

20. Esbensen AJ, Rojahn J, Aman MG, Ruedrich S. Reliability and validity of an assessment instrument for anxiety, depression, and mood among individuals with mental retardation. *J Autism Dev Disord* 2003;**33**:617–629.

21. Mindham J, Espie CA. Glasgow anxiety scale for people with an intellectual disability (GAS-ID):development and psychometric properties of a new measure for use with people with mild intellectual disability. *J Intell Disabil Res* 2003;**47**:22–30.

22. Muris P, Steerneman P, Merckelbach H, *et al*. Comorbid anxiety symptoms in children with pervasive developmental disorders. *J Anxiety Disord* 1998;**12**:387–393.

23. Dekker MC, Koot HM. DSM-IV disorders in children with borderline to moderate intellectual disability. I: prevalence and impact. *J Am Acad Child Adolesc Psychiatry* 2003;**42**:915–922.

24. Weisbrot DM, Gadow KD, DeVincent CJ, *et al.* The presentation of anxiety in children with pervasive developmental disorders. *J Child Adolesc Psychopharmacol* 2005; **15**:477–496.

25. Gadow KD, DeVincent CJ, Pomeroy J, *et al.* Psychiatric symptoms in preschool children with PDD and clinic and comparison samples. *J Autism Dev Disord* 2004;**34**: 379–393.

26. Dykens EM. Anxiety fears and phobias in persons with Williams syndrome. *DevNeuropsychol* 2003;**23**:291–316.

27. Myrbakk E, Tetzchner S. Psychiatric disorders and behavior problems in people with intellectual disability. *Res Dev Disabil* 2007;**29**:316–332.

28. Fletcher R, Loschen E, Stavrakaki C, First M (eds). *Diagnostic Manual – Intellectual Disability: A Clinical Guide for Diagnosis of Mental Disorders in Persons with Intellectual Disability.* Kington, NY:NADD Press, 2007; p. 215.

29. Mevissen L, Jongh A. PTSD and its treatment in people with intellectual disabilities: A review of the literature. *ClinPsychol Rev* 2010;**30**:308–316.

30. Fletcher R, Loschen E, Stavrakaki C, First M (eds). *Diagnostic Manual – Intellectual Disability: A Clinical Guide for Diagnosis of Mental Disorders in Persons with Intellectual Disability.* Kington, NY: NADD Press, 2007; p. 220.

31. Fletcher R, Loschen E, Stavrakaki C, First M (eds). *Diagnostic Manual – Intellectual Disability: A Clinical Guide for Diagnosis of Mental Disorders in Persons with Intellectual Disability.* Kington, NY: NADD Press, 2007; pp. 220–224.

32. Fletcher R, Loschen E, Stavrakaki C, First M (eds). *Diagnostic Manual – Intellectual Disability: A Clinical Guide for Diagnosis of Mental Disorders in Persons with Intellectual Disability.* Kington, NY: NADD Press, 2007; pp. 209–214.

33. Janowsky DS, Davis JM. Diagnosis and treatment of depression in patients with mental retardation. *Curr Psychiatry Rep* 2005;**7**:421–428.

34. Reynolds WM, Baker JA. Assessment of depression in persons with mental retardation. *Am J Ment Retard* 1988; **21**:331–347.

35. Argus GR, Terry PC, Bramston P, Dinsdale SL. Measurement of mood in adolescents with intellectual disability. *Res Dev Disabil* 2004;**25**:493–507.

36. Esbensen AJ, Benson BA. Cognitive variables and depressed mood in adults with intellectual disability. *J Intellect Disabil Res* 2005;**49**:481–489.

37. Kishore MT, Nizamine SH, Nizamine A. The behavioural profile of psychiatric disorders in persons with intellectual disability. *J Intell Disabil Res* 2005;**49**:73–85.

38. Myrbakk E, Tetzchner S. (2007) Psychiatric disorders and behavior problems in people with intellectual disability. Res Devl Disabil 29,316–332.

39. Green WH, Padron–Gayol M, Hardesty AS, *et al.* Schizophrenia with childhood onset: a phenomenological study of 38 cases. *J Am Acad Child Adolesc Psychiatry* 1992; 31:968–976.

40. McClellan J, McCurry C. Neurodevelopmental pathways in schizophrenia. *Semin Clin Neuropsychiat* 1998;**3**:320–332.

41. McClellan J, Werry JS, Ham M. A follow-up study of early onset psychosis: comparison between outcome diagnoses of schizophrenia, mood disorders, and personality disorders. *JAutism DevDisord* 1993;**23**:243–262.

42. Werry JS, McClellan JM, Chard L. Childhood and adolescent schizophrenia, bipolar, and schizoaffective disorders: a clinical and outcome study. *J Am Acad Child Adolesc Psychiatry* 1991;**30**:457–465.

43. Reid AH. Psychoses in adult mental defectives:II. Schizophrenic and paranoid psychoses. *Br J Psychiatry* 1972; **120**:213–218.

44. Wright EC. The presentation of mental illness in mentally retarded adults.*Br J Psychiatry* 1982;**141**:496–502.

45. Sovner R. Limiting factors in the use of DSM-III criteria with mentally ill/mentally retarded persons. *Psychopharmacol Bull* 1986;**22**:1055–1059.

46. Fletcher R, Loschen E, Stavrakaki C, First M (eds). *Diagnostic Manual – Intellectual Disability: A Clinical Guide for Diagnosis of Mental Disorders in Persons with Intellectual Disability.* Kington, NY: NADD Press, 2007; p. 144.

47. Rush AJ, Frances A (eds). Expert Consensus Guideline Series: treatment of psychiatric and behavioral problems in mental retardation. *Am J Ment Retard* 2000; **105**:159–226.

48. Gravestock S. Diagnosis and classification of eating disorders in adults with intellectual disability:the diagnostic criteria for psychiatric disorders for use with adults with learning disabilities/mental retardation (DC-LD) approach. *J Intell Disabil Res* 2003;**47**(Suppl 1):72–83.

49. Fletcher R, Loschen E, Stavrakaki C, First M (eds). *Diagnostic Manual – Intellectual Disability: A Clinical Guide for Diagnosis of Mental Disorders in Persons with Intellectual Disability.* Kington, NY: NADD Press, 2007; pp. 277–279.

50. Menolascino FJ. Down's syndrome: Clinical and psychiatric findings in an institutionalized sample. In: Menolascino FJ (ed.) *Psychiatric Approaches to Mental Retardation.* New York: Basic Books,1970.

51. Dretzke J, Frew E, Davenport C, *et al.* The effectiveness and cost-effectiveness of patient training/education programs for the treatment of conduct disorder, including oppositional defiant disorder in children. *Health Technology Assessment* 2005;**9**:77.

52. Roberts C, MazzucchelliT, Studman L, Sanders MR. Behavioral family intervention for children with developmental disabilities and behavioral problems. *J Clin Child Adolesc Psychol* 2006;**35**:180–193.

53. Bagner DM, Eyberg SM. Parent-child interaction therapy for disruptive behavior in children with mental retardation: a randomized controlled trial. *JClin Child Adolesc Psychol* 2007;**36**:418–429.

54. Aman MG, McDougle C, Schhill L, *et al.* Medication and parent training in children with pervasive developmental disorders and serious behavior problems: results from a randomized clinical trial. *J Am Acad Child Adolesc Psychiatry* 2009;**48**:1143–1154.

55. Brosnan J, Healy O. A review of behavioral interventions for the treatment of aggression in individuals with developmental disabilities. *Res Devel Disabil* 2011; **32**:437–446.

56. O'Reilly MF. Functional analysis of episodic self-injury correlated with recurrent otitis media. *J Appl Behav Anal* 1997; **30**:165–167.

57. Compton SN, Walkup JT, Albano AM, *et al*. Child/adolescent anxiety multimodal study. *Child Adolesc Psychiatry Ment Health* 2010;**4**:1–15.

58. Johoda A, Dagnan D, Stenfert-Kroese B, Pert C, Trower P. Cognitive behavioural therapy: from face to face interactions to a broader contextual understanding of change. *J Intell Disabil Res* 2009; **53**:759–771.

59. Nevels RM, Dehon EE, Alexander K, Gontkovsky ST. Psychopharmacology of aggression in children and adolescents with primary neuropsychiatric disorders: a review of current and potentially promising treatment options. *Exp Clin Psychopharmacol* 2010;**18**:184–201.

60. Aman MG, Smedt GD, Derivan A, Lyons B, Findling RL. Double-blind, placebo-controlled study of risperidone for the treatment of disruptive behaviors in children with subaverage intelligence. *Am J Psychiatry* 2002;**159**: 1337–1346.

61. Read SG, Rendall M. An open-label study of risperidone in the improvement of quality of life and treatment of symptoms of violent and self-injurious behavior in adults with intellectual disability. *J Appl Res Intellect Disabil* 2007;**20**:256–264.

62. Aman MG, McDougle C, Schhill L, *et al*. Medication and parent training in children with pervasive developmental disorders and serious behavior problems: results from a randomized clinical trial. *J Am Acad Child Adolesc Psychiatry* 2009; **48**:1143–1154.

63. Matson JL, Neal, D. Psychotropic medication use for challenging behaviors in persons with intellectual disabilities: an overview. *Res Dev Disabil* 2009;30:572–586.

64. Olson L, Houlihan D. A review of behavioral treatments used for Lesch-Nyhan syndrome. *Behav Modif* 2000; **20**:202–222.

65. Aman MG, Collier-Crespin A, Lindsay RL. Pharmacotherapy of disorders in mental retardation. *Eur Child Adolesc Psychiat* 2000;**9**(Suppl 1):198.

66. Handen BL, Benjamin L, Gilchrist R. Practitioner review: Psychopharmacology in children and adolescents with mental retardation. *J Child Psychol Psychiat* 2006; **47**:871–882.

67. Fletcher R, Loschen E, Stavrakaki C, First M (eds). *Diagnostic Manual – Intellectual Disability: A Clinical Guide for Diagnosis of Mental Disorders in Persons with Intellectual Disability*. Kington, NY: NADD Press, 2007; pp. 158–159.

68. Hurley D. Mood disorders in intellectual disability. *Curr Opin Psychiatry* 2006;19:465–469.

69. Shea SS. Mental retardation in children ages 6 to 16. *Semin Pediatric Neurol* 2006;**13**:262–270.

70. Davis E, Saeed SA, Antonacci DJ. Anxiety disorders in persons with developmental disabilities: empirically informed diagnosis and treatment. *Psychiatry* 2000;**79**: 249–263.

23

Movement Disorders: Tics and Tourette's Disorder

Kevin Lam, Barbara J. Coffey

Introduction

Tics are stereotyped, rapid, recurring motor movements or vocalizations that are nonrhythmic, involuntary, and sudden in onset [1]. According to the *Diagnostic and Statistical Manual for Mental Disorders, Fourth Edition, Text Revision* (DSM-IV-TR) [1], tic disorders include transient tic disorder, chronic motor tic disorder, chronic vocal tic disorder, and Tourette's disorder [1]. Transient tic disorder, which can include both motor and vocal symptoms that last more than 4 weeks but less than a year, is the most common of the tic disorders; the prevalence is estimated to be up to 20% of school-age children [2]. Chronic tic disorders are clinically important conditions that have gained increasing recognition in recent years; Tourette's disorder (TD), also known as Tourette's syndrome (TS), is the most complex of the chronic tic disorders. Tourette's disorder is characterized by multiple, waxing and waning, motor and at least one vocal tic lasting greater than 1 year, with onset in childhood.

A community-based study reported that about 3% of school-age children meet criteria for TD. Although TD is thought to be lifelong, information on its longitudinal course is limited and somewhat contradictory. Studies suggest that while tics may often persist into adulthood, tic severity often declines significantly in adolescence [3, 4]. The past two decades have been marked by significant progress in the understanding of the clinical phenomenology, epidemiology, and psychiatric comorbidity of TD.

Comorbidity with psychiatric disorders such as attention-deficit hyperactivity disorder (ADHD) and obsessive-compulsive disorder (OCD) is common in clinically referred individuals [5–10]. In addition, mood disorders, and non-OCD anxiety disorders such as separation anxiety disorder and generalized anxiety disorders are not uncommon [5]. Explosive outbursts have been reported in a substantial minority of clinically referred patients, particularly in the context of comorbid ADHD and OCD.

The past two decades have been marked by significant progress in the understanding of the etiology, genetics, and epidemiology of tic disorders. Treatment studies proliferated, focusing initially on the use of neuroleptic agents, and alternatives such as the α_2-adrenergic agonists clonidine and guanfacine [11–14]. Treatment studies expanded to include the atypical neuroleptics and targeted combined pharmacotherapy [15]. Nevertheless, TD and tic disorders continue to pose many challenges, especially in the areas of pathophysiology, genetics, developmental neuroscience, psychopathology, and treatment.

Classification and Clinical Phenomenology

Tics typically involve one muscle or a group of muscles and may be characterized by their anatomical location, number, frequency, duration, and complexity [16]. They can be classified as simple (involving one muscle or sound), or complex (slower, more purposeful movements involving multiple muscle groups, or multiple sounds). Examples of simple motor tics are eye blinking, shoulder shrugging, and head turning; complex motor tics include touching objects, jumping, or rotating (Table 23.1). Examples of simple vocal tics are throat clearing, coughing, and sniffing; complex vocal tics include repeating syllables, words, phrases, or echolalia (repeating others' words). According to the DSM-IV-TR [1], tic disorders can be classified as transient (i.e., duration of at least 4 weeks but less than 1 year) or chronic (i.e., duration greater than 1 year).

Stress, excitement, and anxiety can exacerbate tics. Tics are experienced as irresistible, but can be suppressed

Clinical Child Psychiatry, Third Edition. Edited by William M. Klykylo and Jerald Kay.
© 2012 John Wiley & Sons, Ltd. Published 2012 by John Wiley & Sons, Ltd.

Table 23.1   Some examples of tics.

Motor		Vocal	
Simple	Complex	Simple	Complex
Eye blinking	Touching objects or self	Throat clearing	Syllables or words
Nose twitching	Squatting or jumping	Coughing	Phrases
Shoulder shrugging	Hand gestures	Sniffing	Swearing, grunting

for varying periods of time [17–21]. A common perception is that following a period of voluntary suppression, tics will have a "rebound" effect; however, studies of tic suppression do not support this [22–24]. Many patients with TD characterize their tics as a voluntary response to an uncomfortable feeling or urge that precedes them. These feelings, or premonitory sensations, have been described by the majority of Tourette's patients; these sensations can be localized or general, and physical or mental in nature [17, 18, 25–28].

Clinical Course

The typical course of TD is characterized by the onset of facial, head, or neck tics at about age 5 or 6 years, followed by a rostral-caudal progression of motor tics over several years (Table 23.2). Vocal tics typically start 1–2 years after; more complex tics often begin later, as do obsessive-compulsive symptoms at about age 11 or 12 [3, 4, 21, 29–31]. As many as half of clinically referred TD patients may show signs of ADHD, such as hyperactivity, impulsivity, and distractibility, prior to the onset of tics [20, 29, 32, 33]. Tics tend to stabilize over time, and some patients have lengthy periods during

which most or all manifestations diminish or remit. Recent studies indicate that tic severity usually peaks early during the second decade of life, with many patients showing a marked reduction in severity by the end of adolescence [3, 4, 34, 35]. Chronic motor and vocal tic disorders usually have a similar natural history and are considered closely related conditions or variants of TD [19, 20], but there are considerably fewer data regarding their course and outcome (Table 23.2).

Epidemiology

Prevalence estimates for Tourette's disorder vary. As in all population-based studies, results may be influenced by a variety of factors, including diagnostic criteria, methods of sampling and inquiry, the gender and age distributions in the study population, or the size of the sample. Lifetime rate estimates vary from 1 to 10 per 1000, and a common prevalence figure for individuals meeting criteria for TD is 1 per 200 for the full spectrum of chronic tic disorders.

Based on data from the 2007 National Survey of Children's Health (NSCH), the estimated prevalence of a lifetime diagnosis of TD by parent report was 3.0 per

Table 23.2   Diagnostic features of Tourette's disorder.

Diagnostic features	Classification of tic disorders[*]		
	Tourette's disorder	Chronic motor or vocal tic disorder	Transient tic disorder
Tic type	Multiple motor and one or more vocal tics (not necessarily concurrently)	Single or multiple motor or vocal tics, but not both	Single or multiple motor and/or vocal tics
Onset	Before 18 years of age	Before 18 years of age	Before 18 years of age
Duration	Many times a day nearly every day or intermittently for a period of more than 1 year, no tic-free period >3 consecutive months	Many times a day nearly every day or intermittently for a period of more than 1 year, no tic-free period >3 consecutive months	Many times a day, nearly every day for at least 4 weeks but < 1 year

[*]Based on the DSM-IV-TR classification [1].

1000 [36]. A population-based epidemiological study of lifetime prevalence of Tourette's disorder in Israel yielded a point prevalence of 4.3 ± 1.2 (mean ± SE) per 10 000 in 16- and 17-year-olds [19, 37, 38]. Subsequently, prevalence rates were estimated to be as high as 4% in a community-based study when all tic disorders are included [39], and 3% in a survey of middle-school youths in the United Kingdom [40]. Kurlan and colleagues reported rates of TD as high as 7% in special education classes in a school-based community survey, and about 4% in regular classrooms [2]. Studies in both children and adults suggest that males are at least three to four times more likely than females to manifest TD [36, 41].

Psychiatric Comorbid Disorders

The scientific relationship between Tourette's disorder and frequently observed psychiatric comorbid disorders has not yet been disentangled. Obsessive-compulsive symptoms, developmentally inappropriate motoric hyperactivity and inattention, anxiety, and aggressive dyscontrol frequently have been described in association with TD [4, 6, 8, 10, 42–46]. Motor, vocal, behavioral, cognitive, and emotional dysfunction may all represent manifestations of the underlying central disinhibition problem [47, 48].

Developmentally inappropriate hyperactivity, inattention, and impulsivity are also problematic for many TD patients. Some investigators have reported that 50–75% of TD patients also meet criteria for ADHD [6, 41, 49–51]. The nature of the scientific relationship between ADHD and TD is not firmly established, although their comorbidity may reflect common underlying neurobiological circuits and substrates [52, 53].

There appears to be a bidirectional relationship between TD and OCD in most patient cohorts [54–57]. Twenty to forty percent of TD patients have been reported to meet full criteria for OCD, and up to 90% have been reported to have subthreshold symptoms, such as repetitive counting, touching, or symmetry needs. Family studies indicate that OCD is found at a higher rate in close relatives than in controls, which further supports this finding [58–61].

In addition to OCD, mood and non-OCD anxiety disorders have been described in clinically referred TD patients, including major depression, bipolar disorder, separation anxiety disorder, panic disorder, and simple and social phobias [5, 10, 57, 62–64]. Furthermore, a substantial minority of youths with TD evaluated in clinical settings may meet criteria for intermittent explosive disorder manifest by explosive outbursts, or rage attacks [42]. Whether these dysregulated emotions are primary (i.e., related to the underlying pathophysiology

of TD) or secondary to the demoralization and/or impairment related to having a chronic illness remains to be clarified. Gorman and colleagues reported that nearly one-third of older adolescents with TD had a lifetime diagnosis of major depressive disorder, independent of ADHD and/or OCD, and suggested that depression could be inherently linked to TD, independent of the burden of chronic illness [63]. A review also suggests that approximately 6% of autistic patients meet criteria for TD and the prevalence is higher if chronic tics are included [65].

Recent studies have indicated that the quality of life can be negatively impacted in individuals with TD, particularly with regard to comorbid conditions, which are reported to be significant in determining which aspects of quality of life are most affected, including burden on social, school, and family functioning [35, 63, 66–72]. Poorer psychosocial outcomes in youth leading into adulthood were associated with greater ADHD, OCD, and tic severity [63, 66, 67, 73–76]. OCD symptoms in children with TD were found to become more severe at a later age and were more likely to persist than tic symptoms [76].

Genetic Findings

Genetic data have derived historically from family pedigree and twin studies. TD, chronic tic disorders, and OCD cluster in families. Twin studies have shown a high concordance rate for tic disorders among monozygotic (MZ) pairs (ranging from about 50% to 90%) in contrast to a relatively low rate among dizygotic twins (often around 20%) [77]. Other studies have reported that first-degree relatives of TD patients have a higher percentage of TD, chronic tics, and OCD than normal controls [58, 59, 77]. Historically, genetic analyses were thought to be consistent with an autosomal dominant mode (with incomplete penetrance) of inheritance; [58, 59, 61] some investigators argued that a semi-dominant, semi-recessive pattern could also exist [78–80]. However, older studies were confounded by relatively high rates of bilineality and complexity of the phenotype [81, 82]. Family genetic studies have also reinforced the view that TD and some forms of OCD and ADHD are etiologically related. In a heritability analysis of a large sibling-pair sample, OCD and ADHD were highly heritable, and there were significant genetic correlations between TD and OCD and between OCD and ADHD, but not between TD and ADHD; [83] this finding was also corroborated in linkage studies [84].

Linkage strategies have proposed a major gene locus in combination with other genes and/or environmental factors. To date, no unique locus has been specifically identified for TD. A systematic genome scan with 76 affected sibling-pair families with 110 sib-pairs demonstrated that 4q and 8p were chromosomal regions of interest, with lod scores of 2.38 and 2.09, respectively. In addition, four other regions on chromosomes 1, 10, 13, and 19 had lod scores greater than 1. Nonparametric studies through the Tourette Syndrome Association International Consortium for Genetics have been inconclusive to date; a genome-wide association study is currently underway.

Recent studies have begun to focus on rare sequence variants, such as the gene for SLITRK1, a single-pass transmembrane protein, which may play a role in axonal repulsion and dendritic patterning [85–87]. Other genes that are being investigated include the glutamate transporter genes [88, 89], gamma-aminobutyric acid- (GABA), and acetylcholine-related genes [89], and the HDC gene encoding L-histidine decarboxylase [90].

Etiology and Pathophysiology

The etiology and pathophysiology of TD and other tic disorders remain unknown. Considerable data accumulated during the past two decades from neuroanatomical and neurochemical studies of TD point to a diffuse process in the brain involving cortico-striato-thalamo-cortical pathways in the basal ganglia, striatum, and frontal lobes [47, 91–103]. Several neurotransmitters and neuromodulators have been implicated, including dopamine, serotonin, and endogenous opioids [91, 92, 98, 104–122], and more recent genetic findings have suggested a role for histaminergic transmission [90]. Striatal GABAergic interneurons have also been investigated and may play a role in the inhibitory motor control circuits that are believed to be abnormal in TD [65, 123, 124]. Although a specific animal model has not been identified, some parallels may exist with horses that display spontaneous motor tics accompanied by vocalizations as in crib biting [125], dogs with acral lick syndrome [126], and rodents with paroxysmal idiopathic dystonia [122].

Neuroimaging studies employing cerebral blood flow and glucose metabolism parameters – e.g., positron emission tomography (PET) and single photon emission tomography (SPECT) – suggest altered activity (increased or decreased, and at times unilaterally) in various areas of brain (e.g., frontal and orbital cortex, striatum, putamen) in TD patients compared to controls or across brain regions within TD patients [93–95, 113, 127–129]. In one study, metabolic patterns of TD patients were reported to be correlated with OCD, as characterized by reduced activity of the anterior cingu-late and dorsolateral prefrontal cortical regions associated with relative increases in primary motor cortex and precuneus [129].

Magnetic resonance imaging (MRI) studies have indicated volume or asymmetry abnormalities in caudate, thalamic, or lenticular nuclei in subjects with TD compared to controls [130, 131]. Volumetric magnetic resonance spectroscopy studies have shown a loss of the normal asymmetry of the basal ganglia [94, 132, 133]. Cerebellar morphology may also be affected in TD patients [134]. Functional connectivity studies are becoming more important in helping to define the circuits involved in TD and comorbid disorders. The author (B.J.C.) and her colleague F.X. Castellanos are currently using functional MRI and diffusion tensor imaging (DTI) to investigate the changes in neural networks associated with TD.

A study in monozygotic twins concordant for TD but discordant for severity demonstrated abnormalities in D2 dopamine receptors in the caudate area in the more severely afflicted twin [96]. In 10 pairs of monozygotic twins, the right caudate was smaller in the more severely afflicted individuals, supporting evidence for the role of environmental components [135]. Amat and colleagues reported that a childhood diagnosis of TD, OCD, or ADHD significantly increased the likelihood of detecting cerebral hyperintensities, particularly in the subcortex [136]. This may support the notion that subcortical injury, perhaps due to autoimmune processes, may play a role in the pathophysiology of these conditions.

Pediatric Autoimmune Neuropsychiatric Disorders Associated with *Streptococcus* (PANDAS)

Swedo and colleagues have described a putative subgroup of children with a lifetime history of tic disorder and/or OCD and antecedent group A beta-hemolytic *Streptococcus* (GABHS) infection who have symptom onset and/or exacerbation precipitated by *Streptococcus* infection – pediatric autoimmune disorders associated with *Streptococcus*, or PANDAS [137]. They describe specific diagnostic criteria for PANDAS, including prepubertal onset, sudden, explosive onset and/or exacerbations and remissions, and a temporal relationship between symptoms and GABHS [138, 139].

Recent studies have demonstrated mixed results in supporting the association of GABHS and tic/OCD symptom exacerbation. In a prospective longitudinal study, Leckman and colleagues found no evidence for a temporal association between GABHS infections and tic/obsessive-compulsive (OC) symptom exacerbations in children who had met the published PANDAS diagnostic criteria [140]. They reported that out of the 51 cases of newly diagnosed GABHS infection, only six (12%) of cases were followed by an exacerbation of tic and/or OC symptoms within 2 months. Lin and colleagues also found no exacerbation of tic and OC symptoms after every new GABHS infection [141]. Kurlan and the Tourette Syndrome Study Group, in a prospective cohort study, reported that PANDAS patients represent a subgroup of those with chronic tic disorders and OCD who may be vulnerable to GABHS as a precipitant of symptom exacerbation; however, GABHS was not the only, or even the most common, antecedent event associated with exacerbations for these patients [142].

A double-blind, placebo-crossover study of administering prophylactic oral penicillin in an attempt to reduce recurrences of tic/OCD exacerbations failed to show any difference between drug and placebo [143]. There is still a lack of conclusive evidence regarding the benefit of antibiotic and immunomodulatory treatments in children with PANDAS [144]. The role of immune-mediated responses, particularly in the area of the basal ganglia, continues to be investigated in patients with TD [145–152]. Taken together, the relationship between GABHS and tic disorders/OCD remains controversial, as do diagnosis and treatment [149, 153]. There appears to be no evidence for the utility of prophylactic antibiotic treatment to date.

Differential Diagnosis

Differential diagnosis of TD and other tic disorders can be challenging. Diagnosis is made on clinical grounds, primarily based on characteristic features of the history (Table 23.3). No specific laboratory tests are confirmatory. Many patients will suppress their symptoms during the initial office visit; the diagnosis can still be made provisionally.

Diagnostic hallmarks of tic disorders include onset in childhood or adolescence, and the characteristic natural history of waxing and waning of symptoms. Other movement disorders to be considered in the differential diagnosis include:

(1) Sydenham's chorea, a neurological complication of streptococcal infection in which choreiform, writhing, and truncal movements are observed.
(2) Huntington's disease, an autosomal dominant disorder presenting with chorea and dementia and with an onset typically in the fourth or fifth decade.
(3) Parkinson's disease, typically a late life disorder, characterized by flat facies, gait disturbance, rigidity, cogwheeling, and "pill rolling" resting tremor.
(4) PANDAS (see above).

In psychiatric settings, patients who have been exposed to neuroleptics are at risk for neuroleptic-related dyskinesias, including tardive and withdrawal dyskinesias. Dyskinesias can also occur in TD patients secondary to neuroleptic treatment, but may be easily overlooked [154, 155]. Repetitive and compulsive behaviors observed in pervasive developmental disorder (PDD) and OCD also need to be differentiated from tic symptoms [156–159].

Clinical Evaluation

A comprehensive, detailed history with observations derived from multiple sources is the cornerstone of the clinical evaluation of patients with tic disorders. Since TD is a diagnosis made primarily on the basis of its unique history, reliable sources of information are essential. This is particularly important, because in many patients tics may be suppressed during the initial examinations.

Historical inquiry should include detailed medical and developmental information, medication history

Table 23.3 Differential diagnosis of movement disorders.

Descriptive terms	Observable movement pattern(s)
Akathisia	Motor restlessness (an unpleasant need to move), usually in the lower extremities
Athetosis	Slow, writhing movements, usually in the hands and fingers
Ballismus	Large-amplitude jerking, shaking, flinging
Chorea	Irregular, spasmodic, usually limbs or face
Dyskinesia	Choreiform or dystonic, stereotyped and not suppressible
Dystonia	Sustained, tonic contraction that progresses to abnormal postures
Myoclonus	Sudden, brief, clonic, shock-like jerks or spasms, usually involving the limbs
Periodic movements of sleep	Periodic dorsiflexion of the foot and flexion of the knee, occurring during sleep
Stereotypy	Repetitive, usually meaningless, gestures, habits, or automatisms

(including substances of abuse or recreation), educational and occupational data, social and interpersonal history, and a thorough family pedigree covering at least three generations. A careful, descriptive, longitudinal assessment of the movement disorder is important. The physical examination should include height, weight, presence or absence of dysmorphic features, posture, gait, reflexes, and a systematic rating of current abnormal movements. The Abnormal Involuntary Movement Scale (AIMS) is a systematic assessment procedure (and rating form) that can be adapted for use with children. Videotaped standardized interviews and evaluation procedures are used in some research studies; these could also be used in the clinical setting. However, absence of observed tics on initial examination does not preclude the diagnosis of a tic disorder.

Psychiatric evaluation should include a formal assessment of the behavioral and emotional symptoms known to clinically cluster with TD, including OCD, ADHD, other anxiety disorders, mood disorders, and manifestations of impaired or dysregulated affect (e.g., impulsivity, explosive outbursts). The use of structured or semi-structured diagnostic interviews, such as the Diagnostic Interview Schedule for Children (DISC) or the Children's Schedule for Affective Disorders and Schizophrenia (K-SADS), can improve classification and the assessment of comorbidity [160–162]. Since rating instruments can provide quantifiable baseline data, such as frequency and intensity of tics, these data can also be used to measure treatment response. Standardized rating scales developed specifically for assessment of tic domains used in research studies can also be helpful in clinical care. The Yale-Global Tic Severity Scale (Y-GTSS) [163, 164], the "gold standard" of quantitative tic assessment, is a clinician-administered semi-structured interview rating tic domains including number, frequency, intensity, complexity, and interference on a scale of 0 to 50, and tic-related impairment (school, social, family functioning, and self-esteem) on a 0 to 50 scale. Specific rating scales for OCD (the Children's Yale Brown Obsessive Compulsive Scale, or C-YBOCS [165, 166]) and ADHD (Iowa Parent and Teacher Conners or Swanson, Nolan and Pelham (SNAP)) [167–169] can also be utilized.

Auxiliary data from outside sources are essential. Pediatric and medical records may document developmental and medical history, adequacy of medication trials and responses, hospitalization(s), or laboratory findings. A review of school records is advised for children, as many TD patients manifest difficulties in school settings. Report cards can document academic performance; direct phone contact with teachers may provide data about attentional functioning and social and emotional competencies. Neuropsychological or speech and language testing may be indicated for patients with impairments in school or occupational functioning. Areas of social reasoning, executive functioning, and nonliteral language can be affected in patients with TD and may have an impact on social functioning [170–175]. Recent studies suggest that the neuropsychological deficits in response inhibition and visual-motor integration in children with TD are secondary to comorbid ADHD and not due to TD alone [176, 177]. Identified areas of strength and weakness are subsequently conveyed to appropriate educational personnel for inclusion into educational or vocational planning.

Treatment

General Guidelines

Overall treatment goals for patients with tic disorders are to reduce symptoms, support adaptive functioning and strengths, and enhance overall developmental progress. The decision to treat tic and/or comorbid symptoms should be based on a comprehensive evaluation. Patients with symptoms that significantly interfere with adaptation to family, school, or work life, peer relationships, or developmental progress should be treated. Patients who suffer significant emotional distress or inadvertently cause significant distress to key persons in their lives may also be candidates for treatment, even when symptoms are relatively mild. Most patients with very mild symptoms need only monitoring, education, guidance, and support. Moderate to severe symptoms usually should be treated aggressively.

Self-esteem at all times should be supported, as most patients with tic disorders will have at least some sense of personal and emotional vulnerability. Early on, education as to the phenomenology and natural history of TD is essential. Accurate diagnosis and identification of comorbid conditions is an essential step toward appropriate treatment for patients with TD [178, 179]. In patients with comorbid ADHD, OCD, depression, or bipolar disorder, treatment of the comorbid condition first may diminish tic severity.

Clarification that the patient's symptoms are not voluntary in most situations eases psychological burdens for both patients and families. This is especially important since families observe that tics, at times, can be suppressed. Struggles over whether the symptoms are tics or "negative behavior" are pointless and should be curtailed; a more practical goal involves personal management of, and responsibility for, symptoms and behavior, regardless of their origin.

Active management and containment is a cornerstone of treatment. Even with use of effective treatments, it is rare for tics to remit completely. Use of a "tic room" or a "time-out" area provides an opportunity to contain problematic tics or compulsions and to "destimulate." Since emotional conflicts and stress frequently increase symptom intensity and frequency, time-limited withdrawal from stressful situations can be beneficial.

Support for parents and families and advocacy can be facilitated, in the United States, by referral to the national Tourette Syndrome Association (TSA) (www.tsa-usa.org; 718-224-2999). Most states have local chapters of the TSA that may provide educational information, support groups, and referrals for services with experienced providers.

Behavioral Therapy

Behavioral paradigms may be beneficial in many tic disorder patients. Simple behavioral approaches can be used with the majority of TD patients to "destimulate" and contain the symptoms. In a recent 10-week randomized controlled trial in 126 children, aged 9–17 years, with TD or chronic tic disorder, comprehensive behavioral intervention for tics (CBIT), or habit reversal therapy, led to a greater reduction of tics compared with supportive therapy and education [180]. The treatment effect size of 0.68 was comparable to that of the most effective medications. Benefit of treatment was maintained for at least 6 months follow-up [180].

Habit reversal training (HRT) – isometric muscle tensing to oppose motor tics – appears to have utility in the treatment of tic disorders. HRT draws upon the patient's development of awareness of pre-tic urges or sensations, known as premonitory sensations. These urges or sensations can be quantified using the Premonitory Urge for Tics Scale (PUTS) [28]. The patient is taught to contract opposing muscles following the urge to tic. This competing response theoretically prevents the emergence of the tic through reduction of or accommodation to the premonitory urge [181]. Similarly, Wilhelm and colleagues conducted a randomized controlled trial comparing efficacy of HRT with supportive psychotherapy (SP) in adult patients with TD. They reported that HRT, but not SP, significantly reduced tic severity. Follow-up data indicated that patients remained significantly improved at the 10-month follow-up [181]. A larger, multicenter study is currently underway.

Currently, given the positive results and a lack of significant adverse effects, HRT may be considered a first-line treatment for youths aged 9–17 years with mild–moderate tics. Scientific evidence regarding the combination of behavior therapy and medication is not yet available.

Other behavioral interventions, such as massed negative practice (i.e., self-imposed forceful repetition of the tic) for a period of time (with intervals for rest), may be beneficial for some patients. The ensuing tiredness theoretically produces a decrease in tic frequency. About half of the published studies on massed negative practice have found this technique to be beneficial [182]. Anger control training has also been shown to improve disruptive behaviors in a randomized controlled study of adolescents with TD and disruptive behavior [183].

Specific paradigms, such as exposure and response prevention, are indicated for obsessions, and compulsions. Relaxation techniques, such as deep breathing, guided imagery, and use of relaxation tapes, can be useful for the anxious or stressed TD patient.

Pharmacotherapy

Before initiation of medication, a clinical work-up is essential. A complete physical examination and neurological screening, psychiatric evaluation, vital signs, height, weight, body mass index (BMI), waist circumference, and a baseline assessment for abnormal movements, such as the Abnormal Involuntary Movement Scale (AIMS), should be undertaken for all patients. Basic laboratory screening (including a complete blood count with differential, urinalysis, and a blood chemistry screen including liver and thyroid tests, fasting blood glucose, and metabolic screen including cholesterol and triglycerides), and an electrocardiogram (ECG) are recommended before initiation of most medications.

Generally, medication should be initiated at the lowest possible dose and titrated upward gradually (Table 23.4). In TD patients most maximum doses will be low (compared to dosages needed for other indications for these same medications). When possible, a single medication (monotherapy) should be used initially. At times more than one agent will need to be prescribed simultaneously (targeted combined pharmacotherapy) when monotherapy has not been efficacious, or has resulted in limiting side effects, or tics and a comorbid disorder are being treated.

Determining an adequate duration for a medication trial for patients with tics can be quite challenging, since the natural history of TD is waxing and waning of symptoms over time. A baseline observation period before initiation of treatment is recommended, if feasible. In general, it is best to incorporate a waiting period after changing a dose before making any conclusions about therapeutic response. External stressors must be taken into account at all times as potential determinants of increased symptomatology during medication trials.

Table 23.4 Pharmacotherapies for Tourette's and tic disorders.

Class/medication	Typical range (mg)	Starting dose (mg)	Maximum[1] dose (mg)	Common side effects
Neuroleptics				
Haloperidol	0.25–5.0	0.25–0.5	5.0	Sedation, weight gain, dysphoria, extrapyramidal effects
Pimozide	1.0–10	0.5–1.0	15–20	Sedation, weight gain, ECG changes
Risperidone	1.0–3.0	0.25–0.5	4–6	Weight gain, sedation
Aripiprazole	2.5–15	1.25–2.5	20	Akathisia, sedation, agitation
Partial α_2-adrenergic agonists				
Clonidine	0.05–0.45	0.025–0.05	0.45	Sedation, headaches, insomnia, stomach aches, hypotension
Guanfacine	1.0–3.0	0.25–0.5	3–4	Sedation, headaches, hypotension
Tricyclic antidepressants				
Desipramine	25–300	10–25	250–300	Sedation, dry mouth, weight gain, tachycardia, prolongation of QTc
Clomipramine	50–200	10–25	250–300	Sedation, dry mouth, weight gain, tachycardia, prolongation of QTc
Selective serotonin reuptake inhibitors (SSRIs)[2]				
Fluoxetine	5.0–40	2.5–10	60–80	Insomnia, anxiety, weight loss, headaches, gastrointestinal distress, sexual dysfunction; suicidality
Sertraline	25–200	12.5–25	200–300	Insomnia, activation, gastrointestinal distress, sexual dysfunction; suicidality
Paroxetine	10–40	5–10	50–60	Same as above
Fluvoxamine	50–300	12.5–25	300	Same as above
Citalopram	5–40	2.5–5	60	Same as above
Escitalopram	2.5–20	2.5	20	Same as above

1 These are usual maximum doses for adults.
2 These medications have been found to be effective in patients with obsessive-compulsive disorder.

Alpha-Adrenergic Agonists

The alpha-adrenergic agents are recommended as first-line pharmacotherapy for most patients with mild–moderate tics. Clonidine, an α_2-adrenergic (presynaptic) agonist, has been used for more than two decades for treatment of TD [12, 14, 184, 185]. Given in low doses, it is postulated that presynaptic noradrenergic effects mediate the observed clinical improvement in motor and vocal tics. In addition, clonidine also reduces disinhibition, impulsivity, inattention, and hyperactivity, which are often present in young TD patients.

Clonidine should generally be started at 0.025 mg daily to b.i.d. for children, and can be increased by 0.025 mg every 4–7 days. Prepubertal patients will generally need t.i.d. to q.i.d. dosing. Adolescents or adults can be started on 0.05 mg daily and increased by 0.05 mg increments to b.i.d. dosing. A recommended target total daily dose is usually 0.1 mg to 0.45 mg (i.e., up to 8.0 µg/kg). The most commonly observed adverse effects include sedation, headaches, or stomach aches. Sedation,

the most common and sometimes limiting adverse effect, usually attenuates or abates over several weeks; when it does not, dosage reduction may be helpful. Hypotensive effects are minimal in this dosage range, but blood pressure, pulse, and ECG should be monitored at baseline and follow-up visits. A newer, extended-release version has recently become available, indicated for ADHD in children and adolescents, but has not been studied in tic disorders to date.

Guanfacine, an α_2-adrenergic agonist, has also been reported to be efficacious for hyperactivity, impulsivity, and tics [13, 186]. Some data suggest that guanfacine may also have anxiolytic effects, which may be helpful in patients with tic disorders. It is thought to be somewhat more tolerable than clonidine, given its longer half-life and less frequent dosing, and also perhaps less sedation. Prepubertal patients are typically started on 0.25 mg daily and increased by 0.25 mg increments given twice daily; older patients and adults are typically started on 0.5 mg daily and increased by 0.5 mg increments to a recommended target total daily dose of 3–4 mg daily. The most commonly observed adverse effects include sedation, headaches, or stomach aches. Sedation, the most common and sometimes limiting adverse effect, usually abates over several weeks; when it does not, dosage reduction may be helpful. Hypotensive effects are minimal in this dosage range, but blood pressure, pulse and ECG should be monitored at baseline and follow-up visits, as with clonidine. A newer, extended-release guanfacine has become available recently, although data regarding efficacy and tolerability for tic disorders are not yet available.

Neuroleptics (Antipsychotics)

Since the late 1960s when haloperidol was first introduced as a treatment for TD patients, haloperidol and pimozide have been the only US Food and Drug Administration (FDA) labeled, formally approved agents for treatment of TD [155, 187–201]. These medications block D2 (dopamine) receptors and are generally effective in tic reduction; however, considerable variation exists in clinicians' use and patients' thresholds for acceptance. The decision to use a neuroleptic may be guided by both symptom severity and quality of life concerns. In general, neuroleptic agents are not recommended for mild tics.

Neuroleptics should generally be initiated at the lowest possible dose and then increased very gradually. For haloperidol, children are typically started at 0.125–0.25 mg daily to b.i.d. and increased by 0.125–0.25 mg increments weekly or biweekly. Adults are usually started on 0.5 mg, with weekly or biweekly increases of 0.5 mg. Pimozide is an alternative D2-blocking agent, which may cause fewer side effects than haloperidol. However, because pimozide also has calcium channel blocking properties, normal cardiac function (ascertained from cardiac assessment and an ECG) is a prerequisite to its use. Approximately half as potent as haloperidol, pimozide should be started at 0.5–1.0 mg for children, and at about 1.0 mg for adolescents or adults. Most patients will require less than 10 mg daily.

The newer, atypical agents have gained more recent acceptance as first-line pharmacotherapy when a neuroleptic is indicated for moderate to severe tics. These agents, which block both dopamine and serotonin receptors, have the potential advantage of fewer extrapyramidal side effects. Randomized controlled trials have demonstrated that risperidone is efficacious for tics compared to a placebo. Risperidone is typically started at 0.125–0.25 mg daily to b.i.d. and titrated upward to about 1–2 mg daily in prepubertal children; adolescents

are typically started on 0.25 mg daily to b.i.d. Doses are typically in the 1–3 mg range [189, 193]. Additional studies of the atypicals in TD have included ziprasidone and olanzapine [202, 203].

Aripiprazole, a novel atypical neuroleptic with partial agonist-antagonist effects on the dopamine and serotonin system, may be useful in some patients who have not responded to more established treatments. Several small, open-label studies have suggested that aripiprazole may be both beneficial and tolerable, and may also address comorbid explosive outbursts [204–210]. Lyon and colleagues conducted a systematic, open-label trial of aripiprazole in youths with TD and reported that aripiprazole was effective in reducing tics at low–moderate doses (mean daily dose was 4.5 mg). Aripiprazole was also reasonably well tolerated, with the most common side effects including appetite increase, weight gain, sedation, and mild extrapyramidal side effects, such as akathisia [201].

Common adverse effects of neuroleptics include weight gain, sedation, muscle cramps, and stiffness. Dosage reduction or switching to an alternative medication is the recommended approach to address these adverse effects. Fortunately, extrapyramidal side effects (EPS) do not appear to be common sequelae from neuroleptic use at the usual dosages in tic disorder patients; nevertheless, clinicians should be alert to the possibility of their occurrence, and consider appropriate interventions (e.g., antiparkinsonian agents, dosage reduction) on a case-by-case basis. EPS are generally less common with the atypical agents than with the typicals. Tardive dyskinesia, while probably not common, has been described in patients with TD and may be difficult to differentiate from tics [154].

Weight gain is likely with both typical and atypical neuroleptics, but the risk appears to be greater with use of the atypical agents such as olanzapine and risperidone. The possibility of weight gain should be addressed proactively in all youths who are candidates for neuroleptics [211]. At treatment initiation, education regarding the need for a healthy diet and regular exercise is recommended; at times nutritional consultation may be indicated.

Serotonin Reuptake Inhibitors (SRIs)

Serotonergic agents such as fluoxetine, fluvoxamine, and sertraline may be beneficial for obsessive-compulsive symptoms in children and adolescents with TD [212, 213]. Complex motor tics such as repetitive squatting and touching may be very similar phenomenologically to compulsive rituals. Fluoxetine has been most studied in TD, but efficacy of SRIs is likely to be comparable.

Choice typically rests with consideration of the adverse effects and pharmacokinetic profiles of the agents.

When obsessions or compulsions are of moderate to severe intensity or impair adaptive functioning, SRIs are indicated. The recommended starting dose of fluoxetine is 2.5–5.0 mg daily for children and 5.0–10 mg for adolescents. Fluoxetine in combination with a neuroleptic can be useful for both tics and obsessive-compulsive symptoms; neuroleptic dosages may require reduction or adjustment because of the oxidative enzyme inhibiting properties of fluoxetine. Common adverse effects include activation, insomnia, headaches, anorexia, and weight loss.

Clomipramine may be started at 10–25 mg for children and 25–50 mg for adolescents or adults. Total dosage ranges are typically 100–300 mg daily; clomipramine blood levels may be obtained for monitoring, but at present no therapeutic range has been established. Common adverse effects are those reported in other tricyclic antidepressants, including sedation, dry mouth, constipation, blurring of vision, weight gain, and ECG changes.

Sertraline, fluvoxamine, citalopram, and escitalopram may also be beneficial, but experience with them is still limited. There are more data available on the use of clomipramine in OCD, but the adverse effects may be more problematic [214].

Tricyclic Antidepressants

Some studies of desipramine have suggested potential efficacy for the treatment of tics in patients with comorbid ADHD [215–217]. Dosages are not established, but may parallel doses used in ADHD without tics. Careful cardiovascular monitoring must take place, including blood pressure, pulse, and baseline and follow-up ECGs.

Benzodiazepines

Another class of medications that may be beneficial is the benzodiazepines (e.g., clonazepam). Some studies suggest a reduction in tics independent of anxiolytic effects [218]. This effect may also reflect a reduction in anxiety that, in turn, could reduce tic frequency. In addition, benzodiazepines can be used to treat the comorbid anxiety symptomatology or panic attacks that can also occur in TD patients. Dosages are not established, but are often quite low (0.125 mg daily to b.i.d.). Adverse effects of particular concern in younger patients are sedation, cognitive impairment, and disinhibition.

Stimulants

There has been a controversy in the past decade about the role of stimulants in TD; however, recent studies have demonstrated that some TD patients with significant ADHD may be candidates for methylphenidate when no other treatments have been effective [219, 220]. In one study, behavior improved and tics did not worsen at moderate dosages of 0.1–0.5 mg/kg. A randomized controlled study of clonidine and methylphenidate in ADHD and chronic tics reported that the combination, and each drug alone, was more effective than placebo in reduction of both tics and ADHD symptoms. Increase in tics did not occur in the methylphenidate group to any extent more significantly than in the placebo group [15]. Adverse effects include insomnia, appetite suppression, and weight loss. In a double-blind controlled trial, Gadow and colleagues found that immediate-release methylphenidate effectively suppressed ADHD, oppositional defiant disorder, and peer aggression behaviors without altering the severity of tic disorder or OCD behaviors [221]. Lyon and colleagues reported that relative to the no-medication condition, tics were reduced when children with ADHD and TD were given a single dose of dexmethylphenidate. Behavioral reinforcement of tic suppression resulted in lower rates of tics compared to baseline, but dexmethylphenidate did not enhance this suppression [222]. Further investigation is underway with a pilot study comparing the effects of methylphenidate alone to methylphenidate plus habit reversal therapy in children and adolescents with ADHD and chronic tic disorders.

Nonstimulant ADHD Treatment

Atomoxetine   Atomoxetine, a selective norepinephrine inhibitor, is approved for treatment of ADHD in children, adolescents, and adults, and it has also been studied in youths with ADHD and chronic tics. In children with ADHD and TD, atomoxetine was effective in improving symptom measures of ADHD and reducing tic severity [223, 224]. It is dosed based on bodyweight, and titrated gradually from a starting dose of 0.5 mg/kg/day to 1–1.5 mg/kg/day. The therapeutic response, unlike stimulants, takes a few weeks. Adverse effects include headache, nausea, fatigue, and stomach aches.

Other Alternatives   Many other medications have been used in TD patients. Opioid antagonists (e.g., naltrexone) may be an alternative for those patients with self-injurious behaviors [109–111, 118, 225]. The dosage range for naltrexone may be approximately 25–75 mg/day. Nicotine, both in gum and in a transdermal form, has also been studied in TD [226–228]. Pergolide, a dopamine agonist, was reported to be more effective than placebo in a randomized controlled trial in 24 youths with TD [229]. Botulinum toxin has been used in several studies [230, 231]. In retrospective case studies of 24 patients with TD, mecamylamine, a nicotine antagonist, in doses of 2.5 mg daily, reduced tic severity and improved irritability and mood [232, 233]. However, in a double-blind, controlled trial in 61 subjects with TD at doses up to 7.5 mg daily, mecamylamine was found to be no more effective than placebo [234]. Metoclopramide, an antiemetic with D2 dopamine receptor antagonist properties, was reported to reduce total tic severity scores by 39% after 8 weeks in a randomized, double-blind, placebo-controlled trial in patients with TD [235]. Tetrabenazine, a presynaptic dopamine-depleting agent, more commonly used for the treatment of hyperkinetic movement disorders, has also been suggested as a possible novel treatment of TD [236, 237].

Baclofen, a GABAergic muscle relaxant, has been studied in one large open-label and one controlled trial [238, 239]. In the open-label trial, at mean dose of 30 mg/day (range 10–80 mg/day), tics improved significantly [238]. In the controlled trial, there was no difference between drug and placebo in total tic score, but baclofen was superior to placebo with regard to tic-related impairment on the Yale Global Tic Severity Scale (YGTSS) [239]. Levetiracetam, an anticonvulsant with an atypical GABAergic mechanism of action, has also been studied in open-label trials, with improvement in tic severity at doses of 800–2000 mg/day; [240, 241] however, a randomized controlled trial did not find it more beneficial than placebo in suppressing tics in patients with TD [242]. Topiramate, another anticonvulsant that enhances the inhibitory activity of GABA, has been studied in a single randomized, double-blind, placebo-controlled trial. The study showed that patients with TD (mean age 16.5 years) treated with topiramate (mean dose 118 mg) demonstrated a significant improvement in total tic score on the YGTSS; overall, it was well tolerated [243].

Gabbay and colleagues recently conducted a controlled trial of omega-3 fatty acids (O3FA), derived from fish oil, in youths with TD. The mean YGTSS-Global endpoint score was significantly lower in the O3FA-treated group than in the placebo group. Significantly more subjects were considered responders in the O3FA treatment group than the placebo group on the YGTSS-Global Severity measure (and on the YGTSS-Impairment measure but not on the YGTSS-Tic measure). Findings suggested that O3FA may be beneficial for some children and adolescents with TD through the reduction of tic-related impairment (V. Gabbay, personal communication).

Targeted combined pharmacotherapy, or the specific combination of two or more medications at one time to address two or more different symptom clusters or disorders [244], is often used in clinical practice. Since there are very few data for this approach, ideally this should be utilized only after adequate trials of monotherapy have failed. However, many patients with TD also have comorbid ADHD or OCD – often both – and frequently monotherapy addresses one problem but not the other(s). An example is the combination of methylphenidate and clonidine to target tics and ADHD symptoms in patients with ADHD and chronic tic disorders [15]. Judicious use of SRIs plus neuroleptics for TD and comorbid OCD is another example of this approach; in some patients with OCD and tics, this approach may be more effective than monotherapy [245].

Nonmedication Treatment

Stereotaxic neurosurgical techniques have been used in a few cases of severely impaired adults [246, 247]. To date, deep brain stimulation has been used in 50–55 adult patients with intractable symptoms [248]. However, given the significant medical risks for these procedures, there is no indication for use of these techniques in youths at this time. In a case report of an adolescent boy with TD and self-injurious behavior (SIB), cingulotomy and subsequent limbic leucotomy reduced the severity and frequency of his SIB [249].

Transcranial magnetic stimulation is an experimental study tool and therapy that may effect long-term changes in cortical excitability, which is thought to be affected in TD [250].

Psychotherapy

Individual, group, and family therapies are supportive adjuncts to evidence-based treatment. Individual supportive therapy may be indicated for patients having adjustment difficulties, or difficulties with school or occupational functioning. Evidence-based therapy, such as cognitive behavioral treatment of OCD or depression, may also be helpful.

Family work or therapy may be useful to address the many complex interpersonal and family issues that arise for children with TD. At a minimum, each parent should be seen at least once as part of the initial evaluation, to assess parenting styles, family stressors, and coping abilities. Ideally, family members can be sources of support and nurture. Family therapy is indicated when family development (i.e., growth and maturation) has slowed or halted because of the focus on the patient with the tic disorder, in the context of maladaptive reactions from or to siblings, or with specific symptoms that are affecting the entire family.

Group therapy, specifically social skills therapy, is another important adjunct [251, 252].

School and Occupational Interventions

Learning problems and classroom difficulties occur commonly in patients with tic disorder. Specific developmental disorders and ADHD- or OCD-related symptoms may interfere with academic performance [253].

Consultation, guidance, and education for teachers or employers of patients with tic disorders is often indicated, and perceived as helpful. Useful special educational interventions include creating moderate, task-oriented structure in the classroom, preferential seating, one-to-one support, or individualized educational or work plans. Flexibility is a key element in educational and occupational intervention. To promote tic control, there may be a need for optional "time-outs" from class or work settings. Time limits may have to be extended or eliminated for exams. Some patients also may benefit from writing aides, such as silent typewriters and computers. Silent typewriters allow patients with handwriting difficulties to take notes in class without disturbing others. Adaptive, as contrasted to regular, physical education can be particularly helpful for children with TD. This form of physical education can be arranged through special education departments in local schools. Programs can be tailored to each child's needs, strengths, and weaknesses.

Specific workplace interventions include structured tasks, organization of tasks into smaller units, flexible time limits, and ample physical space.

Summary

Tourette's disorder is a complex neuropsychiatric disorder with a heterogeneous phenotype characterized by core disinhibition mediated by the cortico-striato-thalamo-cortical tracts. TD is genetically determined in most cases. There is a growing appreciation and understanding of the role of psychiatric comorbidity in the diverse clinical presentation and impact on quality of life in those affected. Treatment interventions should be multimodal in nature, and include psychoeducation, referral (in the United States) to the Tourette Syndrome Association for support and advocacy, comprehensive behavioral intervention for tics, pharmacotherapy, educational monitoring/consultation, and, where indicated, family intervention. Prospective longitudinal studies and randomized clinical trials have advanced our understanding of several models of pathogenesis and our evidence base regarding novel treatment options. However, further investigation is needed to better understand the phenomenology, developmental psychopathology, and treatment. Until then, as Dr Georges Gilles de la Tourette originally described in 1885, Tourette's disorder remains as its "character equivocal, cause unknown, and treatment problematical." [254]

References

1. American Psychiatric Association. *Diagnostic and Statistical Manual of Mental Disorders*, 4th edition, Text Revision (DSM-IV-TR). Washington DC: APA Press, 2000.
2. Kurlan R, McDermott MP, Deeley C, *et al.* Prevalence of tics in schoolchildren and association with placement in special education. *Neurology* 2001;**57**:1383–1388.
3. Leckman JF, Zhang H, Vitale A, *et al.* Course of tic severity in Tourette syndrome: the first two decades. *Pediatrics* 1998;**102**:14–19.
4. Coffey BJ, Biederman J, Geller D, *et al.* Reexamining tic persistence and tic-associated impairment in Tourette's Disorder: findings from a naturalistic follow-up study. *J Nerv Ment Dis* 2004;**192**:776–780.
5. Coffey BJ, Biederman J, Spencer T, Geller DA, Faraone SV, Bellordre CA. Informativeness of structured diagnostic interviews in the identification of Tourette's disorder in referred youth. *J Nerv Ment Dis* 2000;**188**:583–588.
6. Comings DE, Comings BG. A controlled study of Tourette syndrome. I. Attention-deficit disorder, learning disorders, and school problems. *Am J Hum Genet* 1987;**41**:701–741.
7. Comings DE, Comings BG. A controlled study of Tourette syndrome. II. Conduct. *Am J Hum Genet* 1987;**41**:742–760.
8. Comings DE, Comings BG. A controlled study of Tourette syndrome. IV. Obsessions, compulsions, and schizoid behaviors. *Am J Hum Genet* 1987;**41**:782–803.
9. Comings DE, Comings BG. Tourette's syndrome and attention deficit disorder with hyperactivity. *Arch Gen Psychiatry* 1987;**44**:1023–1026.
10. Robertson MM, Channon S, Baker J, Flynn D. The psychopathology of Gilles de la Tourette's syndrome. A controlled study. *Br J Psychiatry* 1993;**162**:114–117.
11. Leckman JF, Cohen DJ, Detlor J, Young JG, Harcherik D, Shaywitz BA. Clonidine in the treatment of Tourette syndrome: a review of data. *Adv Neurol* 1982;**35**:391–401.
12. Leckman JF, Hardin MT, Riddle MA, Stevenson J, Ort SI, Cohen DJ. Clonidine treatment of Gilles de la Tourette's syndrome. *Arch Gen Psychiatry* 1991;**48**:324–328.
13. Scahill L, Chappell PB, Kim YS, *et al.* A placebo-controlled study of guanfacine in the treatment of children with tic disorders and attention deficit hyperactivity disorder. *Am J Psychiatry* 2001;**158**:1067–1074.
14. Du YS, Li HF, Vance A, *et al.* Randomized double-blind multicentre placebo-controlled clinical trial of the clonidine adhesive patch for the treatment of tic disorders. *Aust N Z J Psychiatry* 2008;**42**:807–813.
15. Tourette's Syndrome Study Group. Treatment of ADHD in children with tics: a randomized controlled trial. *Neurology* 2002;**58**:527–536.
16. Shapiro A. Proposed nosology, criteria, and differential diagnosis. In: Shapiro A, Shapiro E, Young JG, Feinberg T (eds) *Gilles de la Tourette Syndrome*. New York: Raven Press, 1988; pp. 343–380.
17. Lang A. Patient perception of tics and other movement disorders. *Neurology* 1991;**41**:223–228.

18. Leckman JF, Walker DE, Cohen DJ. Premonitory urges in Tourette's syndrome. *Am J Psychiatry* 1993;**150**: 98–102.

19. Shapiro A. Epidemiology. In: Shapiro A, Shapiro E, Young JG, Feinberg T (eds) *Gilles de la Tourette Syndrome*. New York: Raven Press, 1988; pp. 45–60.

20. Shapiro A. Signs, symptoms, and clinical course. In: Shapiro A, Shapiro E, Young JG, Feinberg T (eds) *Gilles de la Tourette Syndrome*. New York: Raven Press, 1988; pp. 169–193.

21. Leckman JF, Bloch MH, King RA, Scahill L. Phenomenology of tics and natural history of tic disorders. *Adv Neurol* 2006;**99**:1–16.

22. Verdellen CW, Hoogduin CA, Keijsers GP. Tic suppression in the treatment of Tourette's syndrome with exposure therapy: the rebound phenomenon reconsidered. *Mov Disord* 2007;**22**:1601–1606.

23. Himle MB, Woods DW. An experimental evaluation of tic suppression and the tic rebound effect. *Behav Res Ther* 2005;**43**:1443–1451.

24. Meidinger AL, Miltenberger RG, Himle M, Omvig M, Trainor C, Crosby R. An investigation of tic suppression and the rebound effect in Tourette's disorder. *Behav Modif* 2005;**29**:716–745.

25. Cohen AJ, Leckman JF. Sensory phenomena associated with Gilles de la Tourette's syndrome. *J Clin Psychiatry* 1992;**53**:319–323.

26. Miguel EC, Coffey BJ, Baer L, Savage CR, Rauch SL, Jenike MA. Phenomenology of intentional repetitive behaviors in obsessive-compulsive disorder and Tourette's disorder. *J Clin Psychiatry* 1995;**56**:246–255.

27. Steinberg T, Shmuel Baruch S, Harush A, *et al.* Tic disorders and the premonitory urge. *J Neural Transm* 2010;**117**:277–284.

28. Woods DW, Piacentini J, Himle MB, Chang S. Premonitory Urge for Tics Scale (PUTS): initial psychometric results and examination of the premonitory urge phenomenon in youths with tic disorders. *J Dev Behav Pediatr* 2005;**26**:397–403.

29. Bruun RD, Budman CL. The natural history of Tourette syndrome. *Adv Neurol* 1992;**58**:1–6.

30. Jankovic J. Tourette's syndrome. *N Engl J Med* 2001; **345**:1184–1192.

31. Luo F, Leckman JF, Katsovich L, *et al.* Prospective longitudinal study of children with tic disorders and/or obsessive-compulsive disorder: relationship of symptom exacerbations to newly acquired streptococcal infections. *Pediatrics* 2004;**113**:e578–585.

32. Bruun RD, Shapiro AK, Shapiro E, Sweet R, Wayne H, Solomon GE. A follow-up of 78 patients with Gilles de la Tourette's syndrome. *Am J Psychiatry* 1976;**133**: 944–947.

33. de Groot CM, Bornstein RA, Spetie L, Burriss B. The course of tics in Tourette syndrome: a 5-year follow-up study. *Ann Clin Psychiatry* 1994;**6**:227–233.

34. Kerbeshian J, Burd L, Klug MG. Comorbid Tourette's disorder and bipolar disorder: an etiologic perspective. *Am J Psychiatry* 1995;**152**:1646–1651.

35. Bloch MH, Leckman JF. Clinical course of Tourette syndrome. *J Psychosom Res* 2009;**67**:497–501.

36. Centers for Disease Control and Prevention (CDC). Prevalence of diagnosed Tourette syndrome in persons aged 6–17 years – United States, 2007. *MMWR Morb Mortal Wkly Rep* 2009;**58**:581–585.

37. Apter A, Pauls DL, Bleich A, *et al.* An epidemiologic study of Gilles de la Tourette's syndrome in Israel. *Arch Gen Psychiatry* 1993;**50**:734–738.

38. Apter A, Pauls DL, Bleich A, *et al.* A population-based epidemiological study of Tourette syndrome among adolescents in Israel. *Adv Neurol* 1992;**58**:61–65.

39. Costello EJ, Angold A, Burns BJ, *et al.* The Great Smoky Mountains Study of Youth. Goals, design, methods, and the prevalence of DSM-III-R disorders. *Arch Gen Psychiatry* 1996;**53**:1129–1136.

40. Mason A, Banerjee S, Eapen V, Zeitlin H, Robertson MM. The prevalence of Tourette syndrome in a mainstream school population. *Dev Med Child Neurol* 1998;**40**:292–296.

41. Shapiro A, Shapiro E, Young JG, Feinberg T. Patient characteristics. In: Shapiro A, Shapiro E, Young JG, Feinberg T (eds) *Gilles de la Tourette Syndrome*. New York: Raven Press, 1988; pp. 61–126.

42. Budman CL, Bruun RD, Park KS, Lesser M, Olson M. Explosive outbursts in children with Tourette's disorder. *J Am Acad Child Adolesc Psychiatry* 2000;**39**:1270–1276.

43. Comings BG, Comings DE. A controlled study of Tourette syndrome. V. Depression and mania. *Am J Hum Genet* 1987;**41**:804–821.

44. Comings DE, Comings BG. A controlled study of Tourette syndrome. III. Phobias and panic attacks. *Am J Hum Genet* 1987;**41**:761–781.

45. Erenberg G, Cruse RP, Rothner AD. The natural history of Tourette syndrome: a follow-up study. *Ann Neurol* 1987;**22**:383–385.

46. Coffey BJ, Rapoport J. Obsessive-compulsive disorder and Tourette's disorder: where are we now? *J Child Adolesc Psychopharmacol* 2010;**20**:235–236.

47. Leckman JF, Pauls DL, Peterson BS, Riddle MA, Anderson GM, Cohen DJ. Pathogenesis of Tourette syndrome. Clues from the clinical phenotype and natural history. *Adv Neurol* 1992;**58**:15–24.

48. Cohen DJ, Leckman JF. Developmental psychopathology and neurobiology of Tourette's syndrome. *J Am Acad Child Adolesc Psychiatry* 1994;**33**:2–15.

49. Comings D. ADHD in Tourette syndrome. In: Comings D (ed.) *Tourette Syndrome and Human Behavior*. Duarte, CA: Hope Press, 1990; pp. 99–104.

50. Shapiro A, Shapiro E, Young JG, Feinberg T. Psychology, psychopathology, and neuropsychology. In: Shapiro A, Shapiro E, Young JG, Feinberg T (eds) *Gilles de la Tourette Syndrome*. New York: Raven Press, 1988; pp. 195–252.

51. Spencer T, Biederman J, Harding M, Wilens T, Faraone S. The relationship between tic disorders and Tourette's syndrome revisited. *J Am Acad Child Adolesc Psychiatry* 1995;**34**:1133–1139.

52. Plessen KJ, Royal JM, Peterson BS. Neuroimaging of tic disorders with co-existing attention-deficit/hyperactivity disorder. *Eur Child Adolesc Psychiatry* 2007;**16** (Suppl 1):60–70.

53. Stewart SE, Illmann C, Geller DA, Leckman JF, King R, Pauls DL. A controlled family study of attention-deficit/hyperactivity disorder and Tourette's disorder. *J Am Acad Child Adolesc Psychiatry* 2006;**45**:1354–1362.

54. Grad LR, Pelcovitz D, Olson M, Matthews M, Grad GJ. Obsessive-compulsive symptomatology in children with Tourette's syndrome. *J Am Acad Child Adolesc Psychiatry* 1987;**26**:69–73.

55. Leonard HL, Swedo SE, Rapoport JL, *et al.* Tourette syndrome and obsessive-compulsive disorder. *Adv Neurol* 1992;**58**:83–93.

56. Pauls DL, Hurst CR, Kruger SD, Leckman JF, Kidd KK, Cohen DJ. Gilles de la Tourette's syndrome and attention deficit disorder with hyperactivity. Evidence against a genetic relationship. *Arch Gen Psychiatry* 1986; **43**:1177–1179.

57. Pitman RK, Green RC, Jenike MA, Mesulam MM. Clinical comparison of Tourette's disorder and obsessive-compulsive disorder. *Am J Psychiatry* 1987; **144**:1166–1171.

58. Pauls DL. The genetics of obsessive compulsive disorder and Gilles de la Tourette's syndrome. *Psychiatr Clin N Am* 1992;**15**:759–766.

59. Pauls DL. Issues in genetic linkage studies of Tourette syndrome. Phenotypic spectrum and genetic model parameters. *Adv Neurol* 1992;**58**:151–157.

60. Pauls DL, Pakstis AJ, Kurlan R, *et al.* Segregation and linkage analyses of Tourette's syndrome and related disorders. *J Am Acad Child Adolesc Psychiatry* 1990;**29**: 195–203.

61. Pauls DL, Raymond CL, Stevenson JM, Leckman JF. A family study of Gilles de la Tourette syndrome. *Am J Hum Genet* 1991;**48**:154–163.

62. Coffey B, Frazier J, Chen S. Comorbidity, Tourette syndrome, and anxiety disorders. *Adv Neurol* 1992;**58**: 95–104.

63. Gorman DA, Thompson N, Plessen KJ, Robertson MM, Leckman JF, Peterson BS. Psychosocial outcome and psychiatric comorbidity in older adolescents with Tourette syndrome: controlled study. *Br J Psychiatry* 2010;**197**:36–44.

64. Schneider J, Gadow KD, Crowell JA, Sprafkin J. Anxiety in boys with attention-deficit/hyperactivity disorder with and without chronic multiple tic disorder. *J Child Adolesc Psychopharmacol* 2009;**19**:737–748.

65. Swain JE, Scahill L, Lombroso PJ, King RA, Leckman JF. Tourette syndrome and tic disorders: a decade of progress. *J Am Acad Child Adolesc Psychiatry* 2007;**46**: 947–968.

66. Eddy CM, Rizzo R, Gulisano M, *et al.* Quality of life in young people with Tourette syndrome: a controlled study. *J Neurol* 2011;**258**:291–301.

67. Eddy CM, Cavanna AE, Gulisano M, *et al.* Clinical correlates of quality of life in Tourette syndrome. *Mov Disord* 2011;**26**:735–738.

68. Conelea CA, Woods DW, Zinner SH, *et al.* Exploring the impact of chronic tic disorders on youth: results from the Tourette Syndrome Impact Survey. *Child Psychiatry Hum Dev* 2011;**42**:219–242.

69. Zinner SH, Coffey BJ. Developmental and behavioral disorders grown up: Tourette's disorder. *J Dev Behav Pediatr* 2009;**30**:560–573.

70. Bernard BA, Stebbins GT, Siegel S, *et al.* Determinants of quality of life in children with Gilles de la Tourette syndrome. *Mov Disord* 2009;**24**:1070–1073.

71. Storch EA, Merlo LJ, Lack C, *et al.* Quality of life in youth with Tourette's syndrome and chronic tic disorder. *J Clin Child Adolesc Psychol* 2007;**36**:217–227.

72. Lin H, Katsovich L, Ghebremichael M, *et al.* Psychosocial stress predicts future symptom severities in children and adolescents with Tourette syndrome and/or obsessive-compulsive disorder. *J Child Psychol Psychiatry* 2007;**48**:157–166.

73. Pringsheim T, Lang A, Kurlan R, Pearce M, Sandor P. Understanding disability in Tourette syndrome. *Dev Med Child Neurol* 2009;**51**:468–472.

74. Scahill L, Sukhodolsky DG, Williams SK, Leckman JF. Public health significance of tic disorders in children and adolescents. *Adv Neurol* 2005;**96**:240–248.

75. Denckla MB. Attention deficit hyperactivity disorder: the childhood co-morbidity that most influences the disability burden in Tourette syndrome. *Adv Neurol* 2006;**99**: 17–21.

76. Bloch MH, Peterson BS, Scahill L, *et al.* Adulthood outcome of tic and obsessive-compulsive symptom severity in children with Tourette syndrome. *Arch Pediatr Adolesc Med* 2006;**160**:65–69.

77. Pauls DL, Leckman JF. The inheritance of Gilles de la Tourette's syndrome and associated behaviors. Evidence for autosomal dominant transmission. *N Engl J Med* 1986;**315**:993–997.

78. Comings DE, Comings BG. Alternative hypotheses on the inheritance of Tourette syndrome. *Adv Neurol* 1992;**58**:189–199.

79. Comings DE, Muhleman D, Dietz G, Dino M, LeGro R, Gade R. Association between Tourette's syndrome and homozygosity at the dopamine D3 receptor gene. *Lancet* 1993;**341**:906.

80. Comings DE, Comings BG. A controlled family history study of Tourette's syndrome, I: Attention-deficit hyperactivity disorder and learning disorders. *J Clin Psychiatry* 1990;**51**:275–280.

81. Lichter DG, Dmochowski J, Jackson LA, Trinidad KS. Influence of family history on clinical expression of Tourette's syndrome. *Neurology* 1999;**52**:308–316.

82. Kurlan R, Eapen V, Stern J, McDermott MP, Robertson MM. Bilineal transmission in Tourette's syndrome families. *Neurology* 1994;**44**:2336–2342.

83. Mathews CA, Grados MA. Familiality of Tourette syndrome, obsessive-compulsive disorder, and attention-deficit/hyperactivity disorder: heritability analysis in a large sib-pair sample. *J Am Acad Child Adolesc Psychiatry* 2011;**50**:46–54.

84. O'Rourke JA, Scharf JM, Yu D, Pauls DL. The genetics of Tourette syndrome: a review. *J Psychosom Res* 2009;**67**:533–545.

85. Stillman AA, Krsnik Z, Sun J, *et al.* Developmentally regulated and evolutionarily conserved expression of SLITRK1 in brain circuits implicated in Tourette syndrome. *J Comp Neurol* 2009;**513**:21–37.

86. O'Roak BJ, Morgan TM, Fishman DO, *et al.* Additional support for the association of SLITRK1 var321 and Tourette syndrome. *Mol Psychiatry* 2010;**15**:447–450.

87. Abelson JF, Kwan KY, O'Roak BJ, *et al.* Sequence variants in SLITRK1 are associated with Tourette's syndrome. *Science* 2005;**310**:317–320.

88. Adamczyk A, Gause CD, Sattler R, *et al.* Genetic and functional studies of a missense variant in a glutamate transporter, SLC1A3, in Tourette syndrome. *Psychiatr Genet* 2011;**21**:90–97.

89. Tian Y, Gunther JR, Liao IH, *et al.* GABA- and acetylcholine-related gene expression in blood correlate with tic severity and microarray evidence for alternative splicing in Tourette syndrome: A pilot study. *Brain Res* 2011;**1381**:228–236.

90. Ercan-Sencicek AG, Stillman AA, Ghosh AK, *et al.* L-histidine decarboxylase and Tourette's syndrome. *N Engl J Med* 2010;**362**:1901–1908.

91. Singer HS. Neurochemical analysis of postmortem cortical and striatal brain tissue in patients with Tourette syndrome. *Adv Neurol* 1992;**58**:135–144.

92. Singer HS, Hahn IH, Moran TH. Abnormal dopamine uptake sites in postmortem striatum from patients with Tourette's syndrome. *Ann Neurol* 1991;**30**:558–562.

93. Singer HS, Wong DF, Brown JE, *et al*. Positron emission tomography evaluation of dopamine D-2 receptors in adults with Tourette syndrome. *Adv Neurol* 1992;**58**:233–239.

94. Singer HS, Reiss AL, Brown JE, *et al*. Volumetric MRI changes in basal ganglia of children with Tourette's syndrome. *Neurology* 1993;**43**:950–956.

95. Stoetter B, Braun AR, Randolph C, *et al*. Functional neuroanatomy of Tourette syndrome. Limbic-motor interactions studied with FDG PET. *Adv Neurol* 1992;**58**:213–226.

96. Wolf SS, Jones DW, Knable MB, *et al*. Tourette syndrome: prediction of phenotypic variation in monozygotic twins by caudate nucleus D2 receptor binding. *Science*;**273**:1225–1227.

97. Cohen DJ, Friedhoff AJ, Leckman JF, Chase TN. Tourette syndrome. Extending basic research to clinical care. *Adv Neurol* 1992;**58**:341–362.

98. Gilbert DL, Christian BT, Gelfand MJ, Shi B, Mantil J, Sallee FR. Altered mesolimbocortical and thalamic dopamine in Tourette syndrome. *Neurology* 2006;**67**:1695–1697.

99. Franzkowiak S, Pollok B, Biermann-Ruben K, *et al*. Altered pattern of motor cortical activation-inhibition during voluntary movements in Tourette syndrome. *Mov Disord* 2010;**25**:1960–1966.

100. Mazzone L, Yu S, Blair C, *et al*. An FMRI study of frontostriatal circuits during the inhibition of eye blinking in persons with Tourette syndrome. *Am J Psychiatry* 2010;**167**:341–349.

101. Heise KF, Steven B, Liuzzi G, *et al*. Altered modulation of intracortical excitability during movement preparation in Gilles de la Tourette syndrome. *Brain* 2010;**133**:580–590.

102. Makki MI, Govindan RM, Wilson BJ, Behen ME, Chugani HT. Altered fronto-striato-thalamic connectivity in children with Tourette syndrome assessed with diffusion tensor MRI and probabilistic fiber tracking. *J Child Neurol* 2009;**24**:669–678.

103. Marsh R, Maia TV, Peterson BS. Functional disturbances within frontostriatal circuits across multiple childhood psychopathologies. *Am J Psychiatry* 2009;**166**:664–674.

104. Anderson GM, Pollak ES, Chatterjee D, Leckman JF, Riddle MA, Cohen DJ. Brain monoamines and amino acids in Gilles de la Tourette's syndrome: a preliminary study of subcortical regions. *Arch Gen Psychiatry* 1992;**49**:584–586.

105. Bornstein RA, Baker GB. Urinary amines in Tourette's syndrome patients with and without phenylethylamine abnormality. *Psychiatry Res* 1990;**31**:279–286.

106. Bornstein RA, Baker GB. Urinary indoleamines in Tourette syndrome patients with obsessive-compulsive characteristics. *Psychiatry Res* 1992;**41**:267–274.

107. Bornstein RA, Baker GB, Carroll A, King G, Ashton S. Phenylethylamine metabolism in Tourette's syndrome. *J Neuropsychiat Clin Neurosci* 1990;**2**:408–412.

108. Braun AR, Stoetter B, Randolph C, *et al*. The functional neuroanatomy of Tourette's syndrome: an FDG-PET study. I. Regional changes in cerebral glucose metabolism differentiating patients and controls. *Neuropsychopharmacology* 1993;**9**:277–291.

109. Chappell PB, Leckman JF, Riddle MA, *et al*. Neuroendocrine and behavioral effects of naloxone in Tourette syndrome. *Adv Neurol* 1992;**58**:253–262.

110. Chappell PB. Sequential use of opioid antagonists and agonists in Tourette's syndrome. *Lancet* 1994;**343**:556.

111. Chappell PB, Leckman JF, Scahill LD, Hardin MT, Anderson G, Cohen DJ. Neuroendocrine and behavioral effects of the selective kappa agonist spiradoline in Tourette's syndrome: a pilot study. *Psychiatry Res* 1993;**47**:267–280.

112. Cohen DJ, Shaywitz BA, Young JG, *et al*. Central biogenic amine metabolism in children with the syndrome of chronic multiple tics of Gilles de la Tourette: norepinephrine, serotonin, and dopamine. *J Am Acad Child Psychiatry* 1979;**18**:320–341.

113. Demeter S. Structural imaging in Tourette syndrome. *Adv Neurol* 1992;**58**:201–206.

114. Gillman MA, Sandyk R. The endogenous opioid system in Gilles de la Tourette syndrome. *Med Hypotheses* 1986;**19**:371–378.

115. Leckman JF, Riddle MA, Berrettini WH, *et al*. Elevated CSF dynorphin A [1-8] in Tourette's syndrome. *Life Sci* 1988;**43**:2015–2023.

116. Riddle MA, Leckman JF, Anderson GM, *et al*. Plasma MHPG: within- and across-day stability in children and adults with Tourette's syndrome. *Biol Psychiatry* 1988;**24**:391–398.

117. Sandyk R. The opioid-noradrenergic link in Gilles de la Tourette's syndrome. *Clin Pharm* 1985;**4**:494.

118. Sandyk R, Bamford CR. Opioid-serotoninergic dysregulation in the pathophysiology of Tourette's syndrome. *Funct Neurol* 1988;**3**:225–235.

119. Singer HS, Butler IJ, Tune LE, Seifert WE Jr, Coyle JT. Dopaminergic dsyfunction in Tourette syndrome. *Ann Neurol* 1982;**12**:361–366.

120. Jijun L, Zaiwang L, Anyuan L, *et al*. Abnormal expression of dopamine and serotonin transporters associated with the pathophysiologic mechanism of Tourette syndrome. *Neurol India* 2010;**58**:523–529.

121. Steeves TD, Ko JH, Kideckel DM, *et al*. Extrastriatal dopaminergic dysfunction in Tourette syndrome. *Ann Neurol* 2010;**67**:170–181.

122. Leckman JF, Bloch MH, Smith ME, Larabi D, Hampson M. Neurobiological substrates of Tourette's disorder. *J Child Adolesc Psychopharmacol* 2010;**20**:237–247.

123. Kalanithi PS, Zheng W, Kataoka Y, *et al*. Altered parvalbumin-positive neuron distribution in basal ganglia of individuals with Tourette syndrome. *Proc Natl Acad Sci U S A* 2005;**102**:13307–13312.

124. Llinas R, Urbano FJ, Leznik E, Ramirez RR, van Marle HJ. Rhythmic and dysrhythmic thalamocortical dynamics: GABA systems and the edge effect. *Trends Neurosci* 2005;**28**:325–333.

125. Dodman NH, Shuster L, Court MH, Dixon R. Investigation into the use of narcotic antagonists in the treatment of a stereotypic behavior pattern (crib-biting) in the horse. *Am J Vet Res* 1987;**48**:311–319.

126. Dodman NH, Shuster L, White SD, Court MH, Parker D, Dixon R. Use of narcotic antagonists to modify stereotypic self-licking, self-chewing, and scratching behavior in dogs. *J Am Vet Med Assoc* 1988;**193**:815–819.

127. Riddle MA, Rasmusson AM, Woods SW, Hoffer PB. SPECT imaging of cerebral blood flow in Tourette syndrome. *Adv Neurol* 1992;**58**:207–211.

128. Sieg KG, Buckingham D, Gaffney GR, Preston DF, Sieg KG. Tc-99m HMPAO SPECT brain imaging of Gilles de la Tourette's syndrome. *Clin Nucl Med* 1993;**18**:255.

129. Pourfar M, Feigin A, Tang CC, et al. Abnormal metabolic brain networks in Tourette syndrome. *Neurology* 2011;**76**:944–952.

130. Miller AM, Bansal R, Hao X, et al. Enlargement of thalamic nuclei in Tourette syndrome. *Arch Gen Psychiatry* 2010;**67**:955–964.

131. Bloch MH, Leckman JF, Zhu H, Peterson BS. Caudate volumes in childhood predict symptom severity in adults with Tourette syndrome. *Neurology* 2005;**65**:1253–1258.

132. Peterson B, Riddle MA, Cohen DJ, et al. Reduced basal ganglia volumes in Tourette's syndrome using three-dimensional reconstruction techniques from magnetic resonance images. *Neurology* 1993;**43**:941–949.

133. Peterson BS, Leckman JF, Tucker D, et al. Preliminary findings of antistreptococcal antibody titers and basal ganglia volumes in tic, obsessive-compulsive, and attention deficit/hyperactivity disorders. *Arch Gen Psychiatry* 2000;**57**:364–372.

134. Tobe RH, Bansal R, Xu D, et al. Cerebellar morphology in Tourette syndrome and obsessive-compulsive disorder. *Ann Neurol* 2010;**67**:479–487.

135. Hyde TM, Stacey ME, Coppola R, Handel SF, Rickler KC, Weinberger DR. Cerebral morphometric abnormalities in Tourette's syndrome: a quantitative MRI study of monozygotic twins. *Neurology* 1995;**45**:1176–1182.

136. Amat JA, Bronen RA, Saluja S, et al. Increased number of subcortical hyperintensities on MRI in children and adolescents with Tourette's syndrome, obsessive-compulsive disorder, and attention deficit hyperactivity disorder. *Am J Psychiatry* 2006;**163**:1106–1108.

137. Swedo SE, Leonard HL, Garvey M, Mittleman B, Allen AJ, Perlmutter S, et al. Pediatric autoimmune neuropsychiatric disorders associated with streptococcal infections: clinical description of the first 50 cases. *Am J Psychiatry* 1998;**155**:264–271.

138. Kiessling LS, Marcotte AC, Culpepper L. Antineuronal antibodies in movement disorders. *Pediatrics* 1993;**92**:39–43.

139. Allen AJ, Leonard HL, Swedo SE. Case study: a new infection-triggered, autoimmune subtype of pediatric OCD and Tourette's syndrome. *J Am Acad Child Adolesc Psychiatry* 1995;**34**:307–311.

140. Leckman JF, King RA, Gilbert DL, et al. Streptococcal upper respiratory tract infections and exacerbations of tic and obsessive-compulsive symptoms: a prospective longitudinal study. *J Am Acad Child Adolesc Psychiatry* 2011;**50**:108–118.e3.

141. Lin H, Williams KA, Katsovich L, et al. Streptococcal upper respiratory tract infections and psychosocial stress predict future tic and obsessive-compulsive symptom severity in children and adolescents with Tourette syndrome and obsessive-compulsive disorder. *Biol Psychiatry* 2010;**67**:684–691.

142. Kurlan R, Johnson D, Kaplan EL, and the Tourette Syndrome Study Group. Streptococcal infection and exacerbations of childhood tics and obsessive-compulsive

143. Garvey MA, Perlmutter SJ, Allen AJ, et al. A pilot study of penicillin prophylaxis for neuropsychiatric exacerbations triggered by streptococcal infections. *Biol Psychiatry* 1999;**45**:1564–1571.

144. Martino D, Defazio G, Giovannoni G. The PANDAS subgroup of tic disorders and childhood-onset obsessive-compulsive disorder. *J Psychosom Res* 2009;**67**:547–557.

145. Krause D, Matz J, Weidinger E, et al. Association between intracellular infectious agents and Tourette's syndrome. *Eur Arch Psychiatry Clin Neurosci* 2010;**260**:359–363.

146. Morer A, Chae W, Henegariu O, Bothwell AL, Leckman JF, Kawikova I. Elevated expression of MCP-1, IL-2 and PTPR-N in basal ganglia of Tourette syndrome cases. *Brain Behav Immun* 2010;**24**:1069–1073.

147. Kawikova I, Grady BP, Tobiasova Z, et al. Children with Tourette's syndrome may suffer immunoglobulin A dysgammaglobulinemia: preliminary report. *Biol Psychiatry* 2010;**67**:679–683.

148. Zykov VP, Shcherbina AY, Novikova EB, Shvabrina TV. Neuroimmune aspects of the pathogenesis of Tourette's syndrome and experience in the use of immunoglobulins in children. *Neurosci Behav Physiol* 2009;**39**:635–638.

149. Gabbay V, Coffey BJ, Babb JS, et al. Pediatric autoimmune neuropsychiatric disorders associated with streptococcus: comparison of diagnosis and treatment in the community and at a specialty clinic. *Pediatrics* 2008;**122**:273–278.

150. Gabbay V, Coffey BJ, Guttman LE, et al. A cytokine study in children and adolescents with Tourette's disorder. *Prog Neuropsychopharmacol Biol Psychiatry* 2009;**33**:967–971.

151. Rizzo R, Curatolo P, Gulisano M, Virzi M, Arpino C, Robertson MM. Disentangling the effects of Tourette syndrome and attention deficit hyperactivity disorder on cognitive and behavioral phenotypes. *Brain Dev* 2007;**29**:413–420.

152. Chang YT, Li YF, Muo CH, et al. Correlation of Tourette syndrome and allergic disease: nationwide population-based case-control study. *J Dev Behav Pediatr* 2011;**32**:98–102.

153. Schrag A, Gilbert R, Giovannoni G, Robertson MM, Metcalfe C, Ben-Shlomo Y. Streptococcal infection, Tourette syndrome, and OCD: is there a connection? *Neurology* 2009;**73**:1256–1263.

154. Silva RR, Magee HJ, Friedhoff AJ. Persistent tardive dyskinesia and other neuroleptic-related dyskinesias in Tourette's disorder. *J Child Adolesc Psychopharmacol* 1993;**3**:137–144.

155. Bruun RD. Subtle and underrecognized side effects of neuroleptic treatment in children with Tourette's disorder. *Am J Psychiatry* 1988;**145**:621–624.

156. Worbe Y, Mallet L, Golmard JL, et al. Repetitive behaviours in patients with Gilles de la Tourette syndrome: tics, compulsions, or both? *PLoS One* 2010;**5**:e12959.

157. Roberts E, Rostain AL, Samar S, Coffey BJ. Obsessional and atypical tic symptoms in an adolescent with complex Tourette's disorder and atypical pervasive developmental disorder not otherwise specified. *J Child Adolesc Psychopharmacol* 2010;**20**:219–223.

158. Nass R, Coffey BJ. Compulsive spitting in a child with pervasive developmental disorder and Tourette's

symptoms: a prospective blinded cohort study. *Pediatrics* 2008;**121**:1188–1197.

disorder: tic or compulsion? *J Child Adolesc Psychophar-macol* 2010;**20**:71–73.

159. Kotcher L, Wieland N, Coffey B. Trichotillomania and co-morbid psychiatric disorders in a 10-year-old boy. *J Child Adolesc Psychopharmacol* 2007;**17**:137–141.

160. Robins LN, Helzer JE, Croughan J, Ratcliff KS. National Institute of Mental Health Diagnostic Interview Schedule. Its history, characteristics, and validity. *Arch Gen Psychiatry* 1981;**38**:381–389.

161. Orvaschel HPJ. *Schedule for Affective Disorders and Schizophrenia for School-age Children: Epidemiologic 4th Version*. Fort Lauderdale, FL: Nova University, Center for Psychological Study, 1987.

162. Debes NM, Hjalgrim H, Skov L. The presence of comorbidity in Tourette syndrome increases the need for pharmacological treatment. *J Child Neurol* 2009;**24**: 1504–1512.

163. Leckman JF, Riddle MA, Hardin MT, *et al*. The Yale Global Tic Severity Scale: initial testing of a clinician-rated scale of tic severity. *J Am Acad Child Adolesc Psychiatry* 1989;**28**:566–573.

164. Cohen D, Leckman J, Shaywitz B. The Tourette syndrome and other tics. In: Scaffer D, Ehrhardt AA, Greenhill LL (eds) *The Clinical Guide to Child Psychiatry*. New York: Free Press, 1985; pp. 3–28.

165. Goodman WK, Price LH, Rasmussen SA, *et al*. The Yale-Brown Obsessive Compulsive Scale. I. Development, use, and reliability. *Arch Gen Psychiatry* 1989;**46**:1006–1011.

166. Goodman WK, Price LH, Rasmussen SA, *et al*. The Yale-Brown Obsessive Compulsive Scale. II. Validity. *Arch Gen Psychiatry* 1989;**46**:1012–1016.

167. Loney J, Milich R. Hyperactivity, inattention, and aggression in clinical practice. In: Routh DK (ed.) *Advances in Behavioral Pediatrics*. Greenwich, CT: JAI Press, 1982; pp. 113–147.

168. Pelham WE, Milich R, Murphy DA, Murphy HA. Normative data on the IOWA Conners teacher rating scale. *J Clin Child Psychol* 1989;**18**:259–262.

169. Swanson JM. *School Based Assessments and Interventions for ADD Students*. Irvine, CA: K.C. Publishing, 1992.

170. Eddy CM, Mitchell IJ, Beck SR, Cavanna AE, Rickards H. Social reasoning in Tourette syndrome. *Cogn Neuropsychiatry* 2011 Jan 18:1–22 [epub ahead of print].

171. Eddy CM, Mitchell IJ, Beck SR, Cavanna AE, Rickards HE. Impaired comprehension of nonliteral language in Tourette syndrome. *Cogn Behav Neurol* 2010;**23**:178–184.

172. Eddy CM, Mitchell IJ, Beck SR, Cavanna AE, Rickards HE. Altered attribution of intention in Tourette's syndrome. *J Neuropsychiatry Clin Neurosci* 2010;**22**: 348–351.

173. Khalifa N, Dalan M, Rydell AM. Tourette syndrome in the general child population: cognitive functioning and self-perception. *Nord J Psychiatry* 2010;**64**:11–18.

174. Marcks BA, Berlin KS, Woods DW, Davies WH. Impact of Tourette Syndrome: a preliminary investigation of the effects of disclosure on peer perceptions and social functioning. *Psychiatry* 2007;**70**:59–67.

175. Lavoie ME, Thibault G, Stip E, O'Connor KP. Memory and executive functions in adults with Gilles de la Tourette syndrome and chronic tic disorder. *Cogn Neuropsychiatry* 2007;**12**:165–181.

176. Sukhodolsky DG, Landeros-Weisenberger A, Scahill L, Leckman JF, Schultz RT. Neuropsychological functioning in children with Tourette syndrome with and without attention-deficit/hyperactivity disorder. *J Am Acad Child Adolesc Psychiatry* 2010;**49**:1155–1164.

177. Schwartz SJ, Sharma KC, Coffey BJ. Executive function deficits, attention-deficit/hyperactivity disorder, tics, and obsessive-compulsive disorder in an adolescent. *J Child Adolesc Psychopharmacol* 2009;**19**:585–588.

178. Scahill L, Erenberg G, Berlin CM Jr, *et al*. Contemporary assessment and pharmacotherapy of Tourette syndrome. *NeuroRx* 2006;**3**:192–206.

179. Gilbert D. Treatment of children and adolescents with tics and Tourette syndrome. *J Child Neurol* 2006;**21**:690–700.

180. Piacentini J, Woods DW, Scahill L, *et al*. Behavior therapy for children with Tourette disorder: a randomized controlled trial. *JAMA* 2010;**303**:1929–1937.

181. Wilhelm S, Deckersbach T, Coffey BJ, Bohne A, Peterson AL, Baer L. Habit reversal versus supportive psychotherapy for Tourette's disorder: a randomized controlled trial. *Am J Psychiatry* 2003;**160**:1175–1177.

182. Azrin N, Peterson A. Behavioral therapy for Tourette's syndrome and tic disorders. In: Cohen D, Bruun R, Leckman J (eds) *Tourette's Syndrome and Tic Disorders: Clinical Understanding and Treatment*. New York: John Wiley & Sons, Ltd, 1988; pp. 237–576.

183. Sukhodolsky DG, Vitulano LA, Carroll DH, McGuire J, Leckman JF, Scahill L. Randomized trial of anger control training for adolescents with Tourette's syndrome and disruptive behavior. *J Am Acad Child Adolesc Psychiatry* 2009;**48**:413–421.

184. Cohen DJ, Young JG, Nathanson JA, Shaywitz BA. Clonidine in Tourette's syndrome. *Lancet* 1979;**ii**: 551–553.

185. Shapiro AK, Shapiro E, Eisenkraft GJ. Treatment of Gilles de la Tourette's syndrome with clonidine and neuroleptics. *Arch Gen Psychiatry* 1983;**40**:1235–1240.

186. Chappell PB, Riddle MA, Scahill L, *et al*. Guanfacine treatment of comorbid attention-deficit hyperactivity disorder and Tourette's syndrome: preliminary clinical experience. *J Am Acad Child Adolesc Psychiatry* 1995;**34**:1140–1146.

187. Boris M. Gilles de la Tourette's syndrome: remission with haloperidol. *JAMA* 1968;**205**:648–649.

188. Bruun RD. Gilles de la Tourette's syndrome. An overview of clinical experience. *J Am Acad Child Psychiatry* 1984;**23**:126–133.

189. Bruun RD, Budman CL. Risperidone as a treatment for Tourette's syndrome. *J Clin Psychiatry* 1996;**57**:29–31.

190. Cohen DJ, Riddle MA, Leckman JF. Pharmacotherapy of Tourette's syndrome and associated disorders. *Psychiatr Clin North Am* 1992;**15**:109–129.

191. Colvin CL, Tankanow RM. Pimozide: use in Tourette's syndrome. *Drug Intell Clin Pharm* 1985;**19**:421–424.

192. Goetz CG, Tanner CM, Klawans HL. Fluphenazine and multifocal tic disorders. *Arch Neurol* 1984;**41**:271–272.

193. Lombroso PJ, Scahill L, King RA, *et al*. Risperidone treatment of children and adolescents with chronic tic disorders: a preliminary report. *J Am Acad Child Adolesc Psychiatry* 1995;**34**:1147–1152.

194. Moldofsky H, Brown GM. Tics and serum prolactin response to pimozide in Tourette syndrome. *Adv Neurol* 1982;**35**:387–390.

195. Sallee FR, Sethuraman G, Rock CM. Effects of pimozide on cognition in children with Tourette syndrome: interaction with comorbid attention deficit hyperactivity disorder. *Acta Psychiatr Scand* 1994;**90**:4–9.

196. Sandor P, Musisi S, Moldofsky H, Lang A. Tourette syndrome: a follow-up study. *J Clin Psychopharmacol* 1990;**10**:197–199.

197. Shapiro AK, Shapiro E. Treatment of Gilles de la Tourette's syndrome with haloperidol. *Br J Psychiatry* 1968;**114**:345–350.

198. Shapiro AK, Shapiro E, Fulop G. Pimozide treatment of tic and Tourette disorders. *Pediatrics* 1987;**79**:1032–1039.

199. Shapiro E, Shapiro AK, Fulop G, *et al.* Controlled study of haloperidol, pimozide and placebo for the treatment of Gilles de la Tourette's syndrome. *Arch Gen Psychiatry* 1989;**46**:722–730.

200. Shapiro AK, Shapiro E, Eisenkraft GJ. Treatment of Gilles de la Tourette syndrome with pimozide. *Am J Psychiatry* 1983;**140**:1183–1186.

201. Lyon GJ, Samar S, Jummani R, *et al.* Aripiprazole in children and adolescents with Tourette's disorder: an open-label safety and tolerability study. *J Child Adolesc Psychopharmacol* 2009;**19**:623–633.

202. Budman CL, Gayer A, Lesser M, Shi Q, Bruun RD. An open-label study of the treatment efficacy of olanzapine for Tourette's disorder. *J Clin Psychiatry* 2001; **62**:290–294.

203. McCracken JT, Suddath R, Chang S, Thakur S, Piacentini J. Effectiveness and tolerability of open label olanzapine in children and adolescents with Tourette syndrome. *J Child Adolesc Psychopharmacol* 2008;**18**: 501–508.

204. Murphy TK, Mutch PJ, Reid JM, *et al.* Open label aripiprazole in the treatment of youth with tic disorders. *J Child Adolesc Psychopharmacol* 2009;**19**:441–447.

205. Budman C, Coffey BJ, Shechter R, *et al.* Aripiprazole in children and adolescents with Tourette disorder with and without explosive outbursts. *J Child Adolesc Psychopharmacol* 2008;**18**:509–515.

206. Winter C, Heinz A, Kupsch A, Strohle A. Aripiprazole in a case presenting with Tourette syndrome and obsessive-compulsive disorder. *J Clin Psychopharmacol* 2008;**28**: 452–454.

207. Seo WS, Sung HM, Sea HS, Bai DS. Aripiprazole treatment of children and adolescents with Tourette disorder or chronic tic disorder. *J Child Adolesc Psychopharmacol* 2008;**18**:197–205.

208. Ben Djebara M, Worbe Y, Schupbach M, Hartmann A. Aripiprazole: a treatment for severe coprolalia in "refractory" Gilles de la Tourette syndrome. *Mov Disord* 2008;**23**:438–440.

209. Constant EL, Borras L, Seghers A. Aripiprazole is effective in the treatment of Tourette's disorder. *Int J Neuropsychopharmacol* 2006;**9**:773–774.

210. Kastrup A, Schlotter W, Plewnia C, Bartels M. Treatment of tics in Tourette syndrome with aripiprazole. *J Clin Psychopharmacol* 2005;**25**:94–96.

211. Pringsheim T, Pearce M. Complications of antipsychotic therapy in children with Tourette syndrome. *Pediatr Neurol* 2010;**43**:17–20.

212. Kurlan R, Como PG, Deeley C, McDermott M, McDermott MP. A pilot controlled study of fluoxetine for obsessive-compulsive symptoms in children with Tourette's syndrome. *Clin Neuropharmacol* 1993;**16**: 167–172.

213. Riddle MA, Hardin MT, King R, Scahill L, Woolston JL. Fluoxetine treatment of children and adolescents with Tourette's and obsessive compulsive disorders: prelimi-

214. Leonard H, Swedo S, Rapoport JL, Coffey M, Cheslow D. Treatment of childhood obsessive compulsive disorder with clomipramine and desmethylimipramine: a double-blind crossover comparison. *Psychopharmacol Bull* 1988;**24**:93–95.

215. Riddle MA, Hardin MT, Cho SC, Woolston JL, Leckman JF. Desipramine treatment of boys with attention-deficit hyperactivity disorder and tics: preliminary clinical experience. *J Am Acad Child Adolesc Psychiatry* 1988;**27**: 811–814.

216. Singer HS, Brown J, Quaskey S, Rosenberg LA, Mellits ED, Denckla MB. The treatment of attention-deficit hyperactivity disorder in Tourette's syndrome: a double-blind placebo-controlled study with clonidine and desipramine. *Pediatrics* 1995;**95**:74–81.

217. Spencer T, Biederman J, Kerman K, Steingard R, Wilens T. Desipramine treatment of children with attention-deficit hyperactivity disorder and tic disorder or Tourette's syndrome. *J Am Acad Child Adolesc Psychiatry* 1993;**32**:354–360.

218. Gonce M, Barbeau A. Seven cases of Gilles de la Tourette's syndrome: partial relief with clonazepam: a pilot study. *Can J Neurol Sci* 1977;**4**:279–283.

219. Gadow KD, Nolan EE, Sverd J. Methylphenidate in hyperactive boys with comorbid tic disorder: II. Short-term behavioral effects in school settings. *J Am Acad Child Adolesc Psychiatry* 1992;**31**:462–471.

220. Gadow KD, Sverd J. Stimulants for ADHD in child patients with Tourette's syndrome: the issue of relative risk. *J Dev Behav Pediatr* 1990;**11**:269–271; discussion 272.

221. Gadow KD, Sverd J, Nolan EE, Sprafkin J, Schneider J. Immediate-release methylphenidate for ADHD in children with comorbid chronic multiple tic disorder. *J Am Acad Child Adolesc Psychiatry* 2007;**46**:840–848.

222. Lyon GJ, Samar SM, Conelea C, *et al.* Testing tic suppression: comparing the effects of dexmethylphenidate to no medication in children and adolescents with attention-deficit/hyperactivity disorder and Tourette's disorder. *J Child Adolesc Psychopharmacol* 2010;**20**:283–289.

223. Spencer TJ, Sallee FR, Gilbert DL, *et al.* Atomoxetine treatment of ADHD in children with comorbid Tourette syndrome. *J Atten Disord* 2008;**11**:470–481.

224. Allen AJ, Kurlan RM, Gilbert DL, *et al.* Atomoxetine treatment in children and adolescents with ADHD and comorbid tic disorders. *Neurology* 2005;**65**:1941–1949.

225. Sandyk R. Naloxone abolishes obsessive-compulsive behavior in Tourette's syndrome. *Int J Neurosci* 1987;**35**:93–94.

226. McConville BJ, Fogelson MH, Norman AB, *et al.* Nicotine potentiation of haloperidol in reducing tic frequency in Tourette's disorder. *Am J Psychiatry* 1991;**148**:793–794.

227. McConville BJ, Sanberg PR, Fogelson MH, *et al.* The effects of nicotine plus haloperidol compared to nicotine only and placebo nicotine only in reducing tic severity and frequency in Tourette's disorder. *Biol Psychiatry* 1992;**31**:832–840.

228. Silver AA, Sanberg PR. Transdermal nicotine patch and potentiation of haloperidol in Tourette's syndrome. *Lancet* 1993;**342**:182.

229. Gilbert DL, Dure L, Sethuraman G, Raab D, Lane J, Sallee FR. Tic reduction with pergolide in a randomized controlled trial in children. *Neurology* 2003;**60**:606–611.

230. Jankovic J. Botulinum toxin in the treatment of dystonic tics. *Mov Disord* 1994;**9**:347–349.

231. Scott BL, Jankovic J, Donovan DT. Botulinum toxin injection into vocal cord in the treatment of malignant coprolalia associated with Tourette's syndrome. *Mov Disord* 1996;**11**:431–433.

232. Sanberg PR, Shytle RD, Silver AA. Treatment of Tourette's syndrome with mecamylamine. *Lancet* 1998;**352**:705–706.

233. Silver AA, Shytle RD, Sanberg PR. Mecamylamine in Tourette's syndrome: a two-year retrospective case study. *J Child Adolesc Psychopharmacol* 2000;**10**:59–68.

234. Silver AA, Shytle RD, Sheehan KH, Sheehan DV, Ramos A, Sanberg PR. Multicenter, double-blind, placebo-controlled study of mecamylamine monotherapy for Tourette's disorder. *J Am Acad Child Adolesc Psychiatry* 2001;**40**:1103–1110.

235. Nicolson R, Craven-Thuss B, Smith J, McKinlay BD, Castellanos FX. A randomized, double-blind, placebo-controlled trial of metoclopramide for the treatment of Tourette's disorder. *J Am Acad Child Adolesc Psychiatry* 2005;**44**:640–646.

236. Porta M, Sassi M, Cavallazzi M, Fornari M, Brambilla A, Servello D. Tourette's syndrome and role of tetrabenazine: review and personal experience. *Clin Drug Investig* 2008;**28**:443–459.

237. Lopez Del Val LJ, Lopez-Garcia E, Martinez-Martinez L, Santos-Lasaosa S. Therapeutic use of tetrabenazine. *Rev Neurol* 2009;**48**:523–533.

238. Awaad Y. Tics in Tourette syndrome: new treatment options. *J Child Neurol* 1999;**14**:316–319.

239. Singer HS, Wendlandt J, Krieger M, Giuliano J. Baclofen treatment in Tourette syndrome: a double-blind, placebo-controlled, crossover trial. *Neurology* 2001;**56**:599–604.

240. Fernandez-Jaen A, Fernandez-Mayoralas DM, Munoz-Jareno N, Calleja-Perez B. An open-label, prospective study of levetiracetam in children and adolescents with Tourette syndrome. *Eur J Paediatr Neurol* 2009;**13**:541–545.

241. Awaad Y, Michon AM, Minarik S. Use of levetiracetam to treat tics in children and adolescents with Tourette syndrome. *Mov Disord* 2005;**20**:714–718.

242. Smith-Hicks CL, Bridges DD, Paynter NP, Singer HS. A double blind randomized placebo control trial of levetiracetam in Tourette syndrome. *Mov Disord* 2007;**22**:1764–1770.

243. Jankovic J, Jimenez-Shahed J, Brown LW. A randomised, double–blind, placebo-controlled study of topiramate in the treatment of Tourette syndrome. *J Neurol Neurosurg Psychiatry* 2010;**81**:70–73.

244. Wilens TE, Spencer T, Biederman J, Wozniak J, Connor D. Combined pharmacotherapy: an emerging trend in pediatric psychopharmacology. *J Am Acad Child Adolesc Psychiatry* 1995;**34**:110–112.

245. McDougle CJ, Goodman WK, Leckman JF, Lee NC, Heninger GR, Price LH. Haloperidol addition in fluvoxamine-refractory obsessive-compulsive disorder. A double-blind, placebo-controlled study in patients with and without tics. *Arch Gen Psychiatry* 1994;**51**:302–308.

246. Babel TB, Warnke PC, Ostertag CB. Immediate and long term outcome after infrathalamic and thalamic lesioning for intractable Tourette's syndrome. *J Neurol Neurosurg Psychiatry* 2001;**70**:666–671.

247. Maciunas RJ, Maddux BN, Riley DE, *et al.* Prospective randomized double-blind trial of bilateral thalamic deep brain stimulation in adults with Tourette syndrome. *J Neurosurg* 2007;**107**:1004–1014.

248. Hariz MI, Robertson MM. Gilles de la Tourette syndrome and deep brain stimulation. *Eur J Neurosci* 2010;**32**:1128–1134.

249. Anandan S, Wigg CL, Thomas CR, Coffey B. Psychosurgery for self-injurious behavior in Tourette's disorder. *J Child Adolesc Psychopharmacol* 2004;**14**:531–538.

250. Orth M. Transcranial magnetic stimulation in Gilles de la Tourette syndrome. *J Psychosom Res* 2009;**67**:591–598.

251. Murphy T, Heyman I. Group work in young people with Tourette Syndrome. *Child Adolesc Ment Health* 2007;**12**:46–48.

252. Lambert S, Christie D. A Social skills group for boys with Tourette's syndrome. *Clin Child Psychol Psychiatry* 1998;**3**:267–277.

253. Debes N, Hjalgrim H, Skov L. The presence of attention-deficit hyperactivity disorder (ADHD) and obsessive-compulsive disorder worsens psychosocial and educational problems in Tourette syndrome. *J Child Neurol* 2010;**25**:171–181.

254. Gilles de la Tourette G. Étude sur une affection nerveuse caractérisée par de l'incoordination motrice, acompagnée d'écholalie et de coprolalie (jumping, latah, myriachit). *Arch Neurol (Paris)* 1885;**9**:158–200.

24

Psychotic Disorders

Michael T. Sorter, Daniel A. Vogel

Introduction

The difficulties of the child or adolescent identified as suffering from childhood psychosis are frequently the most challenging the child and adolescent psychiatrist must manage, the most devastating for families and patients, and the most costly for society and communities [1]. These children demonstrate serious difficulties in all developmental lines. Although varied in their presentations, they struggle with simple adaptive functioning and suffer with cognitive, emotional, perceptual, and interpersonal difficulties.

Psychosis has various definitions, all of which have a common thread of severe impairment of mental functioning with disturbance in reality testing. Reality testing is the ability to evaluate the nature of the external environment, to tell the difference between one's internal and external worlds, and to accurately evaluate the relationship between oneself and the environment. Reality testing requires functioning of accurate perception, organization of thought processes, and adaptive flexibility of thought and behavior, including interpersonal interaction. Hallucinations and delusions, along with impairments in reality testing are the classical characteristics of psychosis [2].

The *Diagnostic and Statistical Manual of Mental Disorders, Fourth Edition, Text Revision* (DSM-IV-TR) from the American Psychiatric Association identifies psychotic disorders to include schizophrenia, schizophreniform disorder, schizoaffective disorder, delusional disorder, brief psychotic disorder, shared psychotic disorder, psychotic disorder due to general medical condition, substance-induced psychotic disorder, and psychotic disorder not otherwise specified (NOS) [3]. Psychotic symptoms are a prominent manifestation of these illnesses. Associated psychotic features may also be demonstrated in disorders such as mood disorders, trauma-related disorders, pervasive developmental disorders, and personality disorders. In these disorders, psychosis is not the primary or predominant characteristic of these illnesses. Early-onset schizophrenia will be the primary topic considered in this text.

Historical Perspective

In 1906, the term *dementia praecoccissima* was proposed by DeSanctis to identify a group of children with bizarre behavior, language abnormalities, social isolation, inappropriate affect, intellectual deficits, and developmental delays [4]. These children were likened to adults described by Kraeplin as having *dementia praecox*. Kraeplin later noted that some cases of dementia praecox began in childhood [5]. Following these early descriptions of children with multiple pervasive impairments, childhood psychosis was often equated with childhood-onset schizophrenia.

The diagnosis and classification of childhood and adolescent psychoses have been controversial. Both narrow and broad definitions have been applied to the diagnosis of schizophrenia in children, and the exact relationship between adult schizophrenia and childhood psychoses has been the center of debate. In the past, inclusive definitions were used such that children with autism and other forms of pervasive developmental disorders fell under the diagnosis of childhood schizophrenia. Psychiatrists such as Bender [6] and Fish [7] considered the presentations of children with pervasive developmental delays, such as difficulties in emotional and social functioning, intellectual deficits, disturbances in affect, social isolation, and bizarre behavior, to be similar to the difficulties seen in adult patients suffering with schizophrenia.

Kanner [8], Kolvin [9], and others challenged this inclusive definition and instead identified specific characteristics that appear to differentiate the child with autism from the child with schizophrenia. Kanner identified a group of children he regarded as distinct from those with childhood schizophrenia: these children were

Clinical Child Psychiatry, Third Edition. Edited by William M. Klykylo and Jerald Kay.
© 2012 John Wiley & Sons, Ltd. Published 2012 by John Wiley & Sons, Ltd.

severely disturbed and demonstrated a powerful desire to be alone and to maintain "sameness." [8] Later work by Kolvin [9] and Rutter [10] suggested that childhood psychoses could be differentiated into separate groups, based on clinical characteristics, family history, and central nervous system (CNS) functioning. They described a group with very early onset that was characterized by a higher prevalence of mental retardation, seizures, electroencephalogram (EEG) abnormalities but that rarely developed hallucinations, delusions, or thought disorder. A group with later onset demonstrated more prominent hallucinations, delusions, thought disorder, and a family history of schizophrenia. This latter group was thought to resemble those patients diagnosed with schizophrenia in adulthood.

Data from these studies led to the classification of childhood psychoses in the *Diagnostic and Statistical Manual of Mental Disorders, Third Edition* (DSM-III) [11]. The separate diagnostic category of *childhood*

schizophrenia was eliminated. Schizophrenia in childhood was defined using adult criteria, and separate criteria were used for infantile autism and childhood-onset pervasive developmental disorder. Subsequent research has reinforced the continuity and validity of diagnostic criteria between children and adults [12, 13].

This trend to differentiate schizophrenia in childhood from the pervasive developmental disorders has continued. In the DSM-IV-TR, the current edition, the same criteria used for the diagnosis of adult schizophrenia are applied to children, and the pervasive developmental disorders have been differentiated into several separate entities (see Box 24.1) [3]. These include autistic disorder, Asperger's disorder, childhood disintegrative disorder, and Rett's disorder, all of which are marked by a symptom complex of difficulties in social relatedness, communication skills, and the presence of stereotyped behavior, interests, and activities [3].

BOX 24.1   DSM-IV-TR DIAGNOSTIC CRITERIA FOR SCHIZOPHRENIA

Characteristic symptoms: Two (or more) of the following, each present for a significant portion of time during a 1-month period (or less if successfully treated):

delusions
hallucinations
disorganized speech (e.g., frequent derailment or incoherence)
grossly disorganized or catatonic behavior
negative symptoms, i.e., affective flattening, alogia, or avolition

Note: Only one Criterion A symptom is required if delusions are bizarre or hallucinations consist of a voice keeping up a running commentary on the person's behavior or thoughts, or two or more voices conversing with each other.

Social/occupational dysfunction: For a significant portion of the time since the onset of the disturbance, one or more major areas of functioning such as work, interpersonal relations, or self-care are markedly below the level achieved prior to the onset (or when the onset is in childhood or adolescence, failure to achieve expected level of interpersonal, academic, or occupational achievement).

Duration: Continuous signs of the disturbance persist for at least 6 months. This 6-month period must include at least 1 month of symptoms (or less if successfully treated) that meet Criterion A (i.e., active-phase symptoms) and may include periods of prodromal or residual symptoms. During these prodromal or residual periods, the signs of the disturbance may be manifested by only negative symptoms or two or more symptoms listed in Criterion A present in an attenuated form (e.g., odd beliefs, unusual perceptual experiences).

Schizoaffective and Mood Disorder exclusion: Schizoaffective Disorder and Mood Disorder With Psychotic Features have been ruled out because either (1) no Major Depressive, Manic, or Mixed Episodes have occurred concurrently with the active-phase symptoms; or (2) if mood episodes have occurred during active-phase symptoms, their total duration has been brief relative to the duration of the active and residual periods.

Substance/general medical condition exclusion: The disturbance is not due to the direct physiological effects of a substance (e.g., a drug of abuse, a medication) or a general medical condition.

Relationship to a Pervasive Developmental Disorder: If there is a history of Autistic Disorder or another Pervasive Developmental Disorder, the additional diagnosis of Schizophrenia is made only if prominent delusions or hallucinations are also present for at least a month (or less if successfully treated).

Prevalence and Epidemiology

Owing to the changes in classification and our understanding of schizophrenia and childhood psychosis, studies using strict diagnostic criteria are limited. Research indicates that prepubertal onset of schizophrenia is exceedingly rare but is somewhat more prevalent in individuals after they reach puberty [13].

Most studies examining the prepubertal rates of schizophrenia compare the prevalence of childhood schizophrenia with that of autism. Autism appears to be more prevalent than childhood schizophrenia [9]. Using DSM-III criteria, Burd and Kerbeshian found the prevalence of prepubertal schizophrenia to be approximately 2 cases per 100 000 [14]. Most studies indicate the male-to-female ratio of schizophrenic children to be from 1.5 : 1 to 2.5 : 1 [15, 16].

The diagnosis of schizophrenia is much more frequently made in adolescents than in children, with the incidence rate in adolescents approaching that of adults [13]. Adolescent schizophrenia differs from childhood-onset schizophrenia in affecting males and females more equally [17]. In adult populations, the incidence of schizophrenia is the same between the sexes, with men having an earlier age of onset [18]. Emergence of the psychotic symptoms of schizophrenia most often occurs in late adolescence or early adulthood with peak ages of onset from 15 to 30 years [19].

Schizophrenia shows a lifetime prevalence of about 1%, and in adults an annual incidence of 0.2 to 0.4 per 1000 [20]. While early studies supported a role for puberty in age of onset of symptoms, more recent studies have not [21]. Meta-analyses have shown that the male to female lifetime risk ratio is 1.4 : 1, making male gender a risk factor for the development of schizophrenia [22, 23].

Clinical Description: Premorbid Functioning

Numerous studies have attempted to examine the children who later develop schizophrenia. Investigators have focused on high-risk populations such as the offspring of schizophrenic parents and have also conducted follow-up studies, which examine the past history and condition of patients diagnosed as schizophrenic and review past clinical records, school reports, and similar data to understand premorbid conditioning. Both types of studies have indicated that a variety of difficulties appear to be more prevalent in children who later develop schizophrenia, but no clear indicative pattern of symptoms or functioning has been found [16, 24, 25]. These prospective high-risk and follow-back studies have suggested numerous premorbid vulnerabilities, including higher rates of abnormal physical and perceptual motor development [7], impaired attention and information processing, lower intelligence quotient (IQ), academic problems, delayed or disturbed language, excessive anxiety, social withdrawal, and isolation [24, 26–31]. Childhood-onset cases appear to have higher rates of premorbid abnormalities [32].

McClellan [33], in a study comparing youths with early-onset psychotic disorders found that youths with schizophrenia had significantly higher rates of premorbid social withdrawal and global impairment and tended to have fewer friends than those with bipolar disorder or psychosis not otherwise specified.

Research groups have attempted to define criteria that would identify individuals at high risk for the development of psychosis. Intervention strategies for these ultra-high-risk individuals are currently being studied to see what treatment strategies may prevent or delay conversion to full expression of psychotic symptoms or mitigate the severity of future illness [34, 35]. Ultra-high-risk studies will be described later in this chapter.

Symptoms of Schizophrenia

The onset of the disorder is usually insidious and is followed by a slow deterioration in functioning [9, 36]. Acute onset with no premorbid signs of disturbance and an acute exacerbation of symptoms in patients with insidious illness have also been described [9, 15]. Symptoms of schizophrenia include positive, negative, cognitive, and mood symptoms. Positive symptoms include formal thought disorder, delusions, and hallucinations. Negative symptoms refer to paucity of thought and speech, flattened affect, alogia, abulia, and apathy [2, 19, 37].

Cognitive deficits in early-onset schizophrenia (EOS, onset prior to 18 years old) include lower intelligence scores in EOS compared to normal controls, with several studies showing a decline in intelligence measures occurring roughly 2 years prior to the onset of psychotic symptoms and persisting for 2 years after the onset [38]. Intelligence then remains stable thereafter [39]. Earlier estimates indicate 10–20% of patients with early-onset schizophrenia have borderline IQ or mental retardation [37, 40]. The frequency of mental retardation may be significantly higher due to the exclusion of these patients from studies. Meta-analysis of studies of adult-onset schizophrenia have revealed the existence of memory deficits [41]. General and verbal memory are especially impaired in EOS compared to normal controls [38]. Although there are fewer studies supporting deficits in EOS, attentional deficits are fairly well established in adult-onset schizophrenia [42]. Executive functioning has also been demonstrated to be impaired in EOS [43].

Because of the previous lack of rigid diagnostic criteria for schizophrenia in childhood and adolescence, there is a paucity of studies that examine the exact nature of this thought disturbance. Some studies do indicate that auditory hallucinations, which are usually present in over 75% of patients, are the most common symptom presentation [16, 44]. Auditory hallucinations may be persecutory in nature or may be command hallucinations, and they usually are simple rather than complex, often consisting of brief phrases or sentences [45]. In children, these auditory hallucinations may be a voice that is strange to them or one that is well known from family or frightening characters. The voices often tell the patient to do bad things or speak to them in a mean manner or curse. The voices may converse or make ongoing commentary about the child. Visual and somatic hallucinations are not rare but are less frequent than auditory hallucinations [44]. Visual hallucinations may be manifest as ghosts, threatening animals, or vague frightening entities [45].

Delusions appear to be common in children with schizophrenia, with prevalence rates ranging from 50% to 85% [9, 44, 46]. Delusions include a variety of presentations, such as persecutory thoughts, feelings of being tormented, somatic concerns, or grandiose perceptions or religious ideation. Delusional beliefs in young people are less likely to be the organized systemic delusions that are commonly found in adults [47]. The emotional and cognitive developmental level may influence the expressed content of thought disturbance: younger children more frequently have disturbances regarding animals, ghosts, or monsters, whereas disturbances in adolescents more often have abstract themes, such as paranoia or mind control, that more closely resemble those found in adults [48].

Formal thought disorder may be difficult to assess in children, owing to a variety of other disorders first evident in childhood that may present with disorganized speech or behavior. Formal thought disorder may present as magical irrational thinking, tangentiality, illogicality, and a loosening of associations; occasionally, there may be sustained periods of incoherence [45]. Negative symptoms such as a low energy, apathy, social withdrawal, inattention, and flat affect may also be present [17, 37].

Overall, the clinical picture of children with schizophrenia supports the observation that childhood-onset schizophrenia has the same manifestations as adolescent- and adult-onset schizophrenia [37, 45].

Etiology

Schizophrenia is considered a neurodevelopmental disorder, with high rates of premorbid abnormalities that include neurological, cognitive, and social findings [37, 40, 49]. The etiology of schizophrenia remains unknown; many investigators regard schizophrenia as a final common disease state perhaps with multiple possible etiologies [50]. Investigations have extended into several aspects of illness, including neurobiological, genetic, and psychological processes, and environmental, family, and interpersonal dynamics.

Genetic Factors

Schizophrenia is strongly heritable, with genetic factors conferring roughly 80% of the liability to develop the disease [51, 52]. Adoptive and twin studies indicate that the risk is genetic [49, 53]. There is a 10-fold increase in morbid risk for schizophrenia in the relatives of an affected first-degree family member [53, 54]. Morbid risk increases to near 50% in offspring when both parents are affected [55]. Reviews of twin studies indicate a significant genetic component, with higher concordance rate in monozygotic twins (50%) than in dizygotic twins (17%) [53, 56]. Similarly, adoption studies have shown that the offspring of schizophrenic parents raised by nonschizophrenic adoptive parents demonstrate a much higher rate of schizophrenia than do the early-adopted offspring of nonschizophrenic biological parents [57]. The prevalence of schizophrenia in the biological offspring of schizophrenics who were later adopted did not differ significantly from that of offspring reared by a schizophrenic biological parent [58]. Children born to nonschizophrenic biological parents but adopted into a family in which a parent became psychotic tended not to develop schizophrenia [59].

Since the penetrance of schizophrenia found in twin studies of childhood-onset schizophrenia is much higher than that of adult-onset schizophrenia, it has been theorized that childhood-onset schizophrenia represents a more virulent form of illness, with more complete penetrance [60–62]. In a comparison of child-onset schizophrenia and adult-onset schizophrenia [63], parents of the patients with childhood-onset schizophrenia were found to have a morbid risk of schizophrenia spectrum disorders of nearly 25%. Parents of adult-onset patients had a morbid risk of 11%, while parents of comparison groups had a morbid risk of 1.5%. This may indicate a stronger familial association in childhood-onset schizophrenia. Schizophrenia studies indicate that the liability for schizophrenia is genetically mediated but not genetically determined, and results from an interaction of genes and environment. Genome scan strategies have provided multiple chromosomal regions of interest that may contain one or more susceptibility genes for schizophrenia [53].

Identifying a genetic "cause" for schizophrenia has proven difficult with considerable genetic heterogeneity and small effect sizes of multiple genes or chromosomal regions linked to schizophrenia [50]. Copy number variations (CNV) are structural variants that have been associated with COS as compared to adult-onset schizophrenia [64]. Structural chromosomal abnormalities of interest include deletions in 22q11 that cause velocardiofacial syndrome and a high degree of schizophrenia and other psychiatric disorders and may represent a significant endophenotype of COS [65, 66]. Susceptibility genes associated with adult-onset schizophrenia include *COMT* (catechol-*O*-methyltransferase), *DISC1* (disrupted in schizophrenia 1), *DRD1* to *DRD4* (dopamine receptors 1–4), *DTNBP1* (dysbindin), and *NRG1* (neuregulin 1). *NRXN1* (neurexin 1) is a presynaptic signal mediator with a strong association with schizophrenia, mental retardation, and autism [67]. Sex chromosome abnormalities may also occur more in younger-onset cases of schizophrenia [66]. Cytogenetic abnormalities have been found to be more prevalent in COS than in adult-onset schizophrenia [68]. Finally, large trinucleotide repeats of CAG/CTG were identified in males with COS [69].

Neurobiological Deficits

There is no clear premorbid personality profile for children and adolescents who develop schizophrenia. Children who develop schizophrenia are more apt to have a premorbid history of social anxiety, withdrawal, academic difficulties, poor peer relationships, clingy withdrawn behavior, and suspiciousness [28]. There also may be a higher preponderance of deficits in language and communication functioning, causing early language to be delayed or disturbed [25, 28, 70, 71]. It is unclear whether personality characteristics predispose patients to vulnerabilities associated with schizophrenia. Findings about neurobiological abnormalities in youths with schizophrenia are similar to those in the adult literature, and include smooth-pursuit eye movement, autonomic responsivity, and abnormal smooth-pursuit eye movement, autonomic responsivity and cognitive deficits. [37].

Schizophrenia has been viewed as a neurodevelopmental disorder [49]. Psychosis emerges after many years of early structural brain changes [72]. The same patterns of structural abnormalities are found in first-degree family members [73], suggesting shared familial risk. Histological studies indicate abnormalities in neuronal migration, resulting in cellular disorganization,

anomalous cortical development, and irregularities in laminar distribution of neurons [49, 74]. The absence of glial reactions suggests that neuropathological changes are prenatal rather than postnatal [75]. Individuals with schizophrenia have a significantly higher frequency of morphological brain abnormalities [76–78].

The most consistent neuroimaging findings in adult-onset schizophrenia are the enlargement of the ventricular system [76] and overall reduction in cortical gray matter and brain volume [77]. Decreased volumes of multiple structures have also been indicated in adult schizophrenia. These include frontal lobes, amygdala, hippocampus, parahippocampus, thalamus, cingulate gyrus, superior temporal gyrus, and medial temporal lobe [49, 76, 78, 79]. Patients with childhood-onset schizophrenia have similar findings in regard to smaller brain and enlarged lateral ventricles [80, 81]. It is unclear to what degree brain volume changes are due to synaptic pruning or decreased myelination [82].

The National Institute of Mental Health COS study has contributed to our understanding of gray matter volume changes in COS. During adolescence, patients with childhood-onset schizophrenia demonstrate loss of cortical gray matter progressing from parietal to frontal regions, with greater loss in COS subjects compared to controls [83]. This cortical thinning involves frontal, parietal, and temporal regions with loss slowing as the subjects approach adult age [80, 84, 85].

Preliminary studies also indicated alteration in brain white matter integrity in adolescents with early-onset schizophrenia, similar to findings in adults with chronic schizophrenia [86]. Diffusion tensor imaging (DTI) has been used to study white matter tract integrity in schizophrenia, with abnormalities found in the corpus callosum, cingulum, arcuate fasciculus, and uncinate fasciculus [87]. Decreased fornix volume without DTI abnormalities has been observed in COS [88].

Family Factors

Numerous studies have investigated the families of patients with schizophrenia, but the majority were conducted prior to the use of strict diagnostic criteria. Most studies have examined aberrant communication patterns, which were once believed to lead to schizophrenia. Communication deviances usually refer to a confusing and unclear communication style that precipitates a disruption in the focus of attention [89]. These communication deviances have been found to be more prevalent in parents of children with schizophrenia and schizotypal disorder than in parents of children with depressive disorders, and are thought to be more genetic traits than causal factors [90]. Other investigators have focused on the levels of expressed emotion, the harshness of criticism, and parents' excessive negative response to the child's negative or disruptive behavior. These patterns of interaction do negatively influence relapse rates [19, 61]. Findings are inconclusive, and it remains unclear whether parent behavioral style promotes the child's pathology or is a response to it [91]. Communication deviances in parents have been associated with a higher risk for adolescents to develop schizophrenia in adulthood [92]. High expressed emotion as evidenced by critical comments, hostility, or emotional overinvolvement has been shown to be a robust predictor of relapse in adults with schizophrenia [93].

A positive family environment predicted improvement in symptoms in social functioning in adolescents at imminent risk for onset of psychosis, with positive remarks from caregivers associated with decreased negative symptoms [94]. In adults, higher scores on family interpersonal warmth were associated with decreased relapse rates [95]. The cultural context of expressed emotion may also have an impact on the relationship between family functioning and potential relapse rates. In African American families, high expressed emotion was not a predictor of relapse [96].

Environment

Low socioeconomic status has been associated with higher rates of schizophrenia [97]. It remains unclear, however, whether the lower socioeconomic level predisposes people to developing schizophrenia, is a result of the schizophrenic patient being unable to maintain the parent's socioeconomic level, or if the lower socioeconomic status is a result of underlying parental psychopathology [49]. Adverse life events such as the death of a parent or rejection of the child may be associated with the onset of a schizophrenic disorder. Little research has focused on environmental effects in childhood, and the effects are more thoroughly described in adult patients [98]. The relationship of socioeconomic status to child-onset schizophrenia remains unclear as most studies have had an inpatient bias and contradictory results [37]. In adult studies of schizophrenia, diverse prevalence and incidence rates have been reported among various cultural groups, but studies using strict criteria have indicated the incidence and clinical syndrome to be similar in a variety of cultural settings [20, 49, 99, 100].

Maternal infection and poor nutrition in the first and early second trimesters have been linked to an increased risk for developing schizophrenia [101, 102]. Maternal influenza is most often implicated, but rubella, toxoplasmosis, measles, polio, and herpes simplex have been associated with increased risk, leading to the hypothesis that infection-induced disruption of early prenatal brain development predisposes for long-lasting structural and functional brain abnormalities leading to psychopathology in later life [103]. Other factors linked to increased risk of schizophrenia include older paternal age, birth in late winter and early spring months, obstetric and perinatal complications, and social contexts of urbanicity and migration [104].

Assessment

To ensure adequate diagnostic evaluation and treatment planning, the proper assessment of a child or adolescent with psychosis requires an evaluation of all areas of functioning. The diagnostic process is often prolonged and usually requires multiple informants. Since the families are often under extreme stress from the child's illness and deterioration, early in the diagnostic evaluation the clinician must be aware of the need to enhance the alliance with the family. Family members provide the majority of the data required for assessment and are the most important agents in the eventual care of the patient.

The evaluation of psychosis in children and adolescents requires a detailed history, including the age of onset, the nature of symptoms and their course, premorbid functioning, school and psychosocial adaptive skills, precipitants of trauma preceding the illness, and a biological family history of psychiatric disorders. The family assessment must include current adaptive functioning and any specific family or cultural beliefs regarding psychiatric illness. Substance abuse history should investigate past patterns of use and its effects, and also assess whether any intoxication or withdrawal syndrome is present. The developmental history must elucidate any deficits or delays in speech or language or in cognitive, sensory, and motor function. The medical history and review of systems must include any evidence of CNS insult or general medical conditions that may precipitate mental status changes.

A clinician conducting a mental status examination may require several sessions with the child. In the first encounter, the clinician must have special awareness of any fluctuations in the level of consciousness or impairments in orientation, since these may indicate delirium and organic processes requiring more immediate attention. Clinicians should evaluate any hallucinations, delusions, thought disorders, and the presence or absence of negative symptoms to assist in clarifying phenomenology. If prominent and significant in duration, mood disturbance may indicate affective disorder with secondary psychotic symptoms. An assessment of suicidal or homicidal ideation must be performed on initial contact and, if required, appropriate safeguards enacted.

A medical evaluation that includes a complete physical and neurological examination is important to detect the presence of any physical disorders that might precipitate psychotic symptoms. Special attention must be paid to any abnormal neurological history or functioning, the results of which may assist in determining if any special procedures or evaluation are required. Owing to the common occurrence of substance abuse and its propensity to cause psychotic symptoms, drug screening should be conducted on all patients.

Psychological testing often helps to assess the nature and severity of impairment in patients with psychosis. Projective testing may help clinicians to evaluate the severity and nature of psychotic thinking. Investigations into cognitive ability, educational achievement, and adaptive living skills often identify the strengths and weaknesses of an individual patient and initial directions for intervention.

Many well-researched and validated psychiatric interview schedules help to assess psychotic symptoms and provide a systematic coverage of symptoms to ensure that all key symptom areas are probed [105]. Some of the schedules have an ease of use that allows them to be used in clinical work. Examples include the Schedule for Positive Symptoms (SAPS), which reviews hallucinations, delusions, bizarre behavior, and formal thought disorder, and the Schedule for Negative Symptoms, which examines flat affect anergy, avolition, asociality, and inattention [106]. The Kiddie PANNS is a modification of the Adult Positive and Negative Syndrome Scale [105, 107].

Speech and language evaluations are often helpful, especially with young children for whom psychosis is suspected. Patients with communication difficulties may present with extremely disorganized speech that is suggestive of underlying psychosis or schizophrenia. (for a summary of assessment procedures, see Table 24.1).

Differential Diagnosis

An organic etiology must be considered for all children and adolescents presenting with psychosis. Multiple substance-related disorders may present with psychotic symptomatology: substance intoxication from cocaine, amphetamines, hallucinogens, cannabis, phencyclidine, solvents, or alcohol; or withdrawal syndromes such as those from alcohol, barbiturates, benzodiazepines, and other sedatives. Both the frequency of a substance-related disorder that produces psychotic symptoms and the condition of comorbid substance abuse in a patient with schizophrenia underlie the importance of initial and perhaps serial toxic screening, The associated physical findings of many of the substance-use disorders and the persistence of

Table 24.1 Assessment and evaluation.

History and development
History of current difficulties
Age of onset
Course and nature of symptoms
Premorbid functioning
School and cognitive skills
Psychosocial adaptive skills
Precipitants
History of trauma
Family history of psychiatric disorders
Family adaptive functioning
Family and cultural beliefs concerning illness
Substance use history
Developmental history
Communication/speech and language functioning

Mental status examination
Level of consciousness and orientation
Hallucinations and delusions
Thought disorder and negative symptoms
Affective symptoms
Assessment of dangerous, impulsive activity
Suicidality and homicidality

Psychological evaluation
Projective testing for evaluation of thought disturbance, hallucinations, etc.
IQ and formal educational testing for assessment of achievement
Assessment of adaptive skills
Assessment of communication/speech and language

Medical and neurological history and evaluation
Physical examination for associated medical conditions
Toxicology screen for evaluation of substance abuse
Neurological consultation, including EEG

Adapted from Volkmar FR [44].

symptoms seen in a primary psychotic illness often assist in differentiating these two disorders [108].

Other entities that must be excluded through careful medical and neurological evaluation include metabolic disorders, heavy metal intoxication, CNS trauma, neoplasia, neurodegenerative disorders, seizure disorders, and delirium. Infectious diseases such as encephalitis and meningitis must be excluded, with special attention given to risk factors for human immunodeficiency virus (HIV) infection. HIV infection in adolescents is not uncommon [109], and the often chaotic, difficult backgrounds of these patients may be similar to those of patients most at risk for schizophrenia [110]. The high-risk behaviors of substance abuse and dangerous sexual activity are indicators for HIV testing.

Patients with schizophrenia and psychotic mood disorders often present with a wide variety of mood and psychotic symptoms [111]. Owing to similarities in presentation, patients later diagnosed with bipolar disorder are frequently previously misdiagnosed as having schizophrenia [112]. Bipolar disorder in adolescents is much like that in adults, although psychotic features appear to be more common in adolescents [113, 114]. Early episodes may show many schizophrenic features such as bizarre delusions, hallucinations, paranoid ideation, and ideas of reference [113]. Younger children are more likely to present with irritability, emotional lability, and aggression, often with poor demarcation of discrete episodes [115]. Symptom overlap creates difficulties in diagnosis. In a study of youths with schizophrenia, bipolar disorder, and psychotic disorder NOS, no differences were found in measures of positive symptoms, behavioral difficulties, or dysphoria. Measures of negative symptoms differentiated the patients with schizophrenia from the other two groups [111]. Patients with early-onset schizophrenia appear to have more difficulties in premorbid functioning, with more social withdrawal, impaired global functioning, and fewer friends than those with bipolar disorder [33]. The presence of features such as grandiosity, euphoria, pronounced irritability, pressured speech, and hyperactivity may be indicators of the affective nature of the disorder. Due to the frequent overlay of affective and psychotic symptoms, schizoaffective disorder, with its requirements for distinct mood and psychotic periods, has been difficult to diagnose in a reliable, predictable way in youths [112]. Longitudinal reassessment is frequently required to confirm the accuracy of the diagnosis.

Patients with the pervasive developmental disorders characteristically present with severe deficits in language and social relatedness. Typically, they do not present with the characteristic symptoms of delusions and hallucinations. When delusions and hallucinations are present, however, they are usually temporary and not the predominant manifestation of the illness; they are also distinguished by their early age of onset and the absence of normal development [9]. It is possible that both illnesses may coexist, in which case the onset of the schizophrenia is significantly later than that of autism [37]. Asperger's syndrome and childhood disintegrative disorder differ from autism in their absence of language deficits and in having a later onset, respectively. They also lack the pervasive hallucinations, delusions, and thought disorder characteristics of schizophrenia. Patients with significant communication disorders such as receptive and expressive language disorders are often difficult to assess, since the communication difficulties often resemble those of children with primary thought disorder. In younger children, normal fantasy and a distortion of communication through speech and language deficits exacerbate the task of proper diagnosis [116]. Prolonged, serial assessments are often required to determine the presence or absence of the hallucinations and delusions that are indicative of schizophrenia. The often illogical perseverative thoughts of the patient with obsessive-compulsive disorder (OCD) may resemble those of thought disorder seen in patients with psychotic illness. In severe cases of OCD, the perception that the obsessions are irrational may be intermittent or lacking, thus making it difficult to differentiate from true delusions. Patients with schizophrenia may have significant obsessive thoughts and compulsive behavior. The lack of hallucinations and delusions and more constricted nature of symptomatology of OCD frequently help to distinguish it from schizophrenia.

A history of abuse or neglect in a child is often associated with reports of psychotic symptoms [117]. Investigations into children with psychotic disorder NOS reveal significant symptom overlap with schizophrenia, but they have significantly higher rates of abuse histories and post-traumatic stress disorder (PTSD) [33]. Psychological trauma may produce dissociative phenomena similar to a psychotic state.

Patients with borderline and schizotypal personality disorders may exhibit symptoms of transient hallucinations and near delusional thinking [25]. They lack the delusions and formal thought disorder of patients with schizophrenia and also show differences in relationship skills: the relationships of children with borderline personality disorders are chaotic and intense, whereas children with schizophrenia are often socially isolated and awkward [108].

Transient hallucinations may occur in preschool-age nonpsychotic children [118]. These hallucinations are often visual and tactile, frequently with onset at night, and are thought to be relatively benign. In young children, there may be magical thinking, fantasy figures, and a poor notion of adult rules of logic or reality. Their presentation may resemble those of a thought disorder, but it is the persistence of such symptoms into school age that is indicative of pathology [44, 119]. Differential diagnosis is summarized in Table 24.2.

Treatment

The treatment of schizophrenia requires a comprehensive multimodal approach, with the goals of decreasing the characteristic psychotic symptomatology, returning the child to more appropriate lines of development, and

Table 24.2   Differential diagnosis of schizophrenia.

Disorder	Differentiating diagnostic features
Autistic spectrum disorders (Asperger's disorder, autistic disorder, childhood disintegrative disorder, pervasive developmental disorder NOS)	Differentiated by developmental history indicating deficits in social relatedness, activities, interest, and/or language Hallucinations/delusions not the predominant manifestation
Psychosis associated with mood disorder (bipolar disorder, major depressive disorder)	In major depression and bipolar disorder, history of psychosis is associated with significant mood changes – though not always reliable. Relative lack of negative symptoms may differentiate bipolar disorder from schizophrenia
Other psychotic disorders (psychotic disorder NOS, schizoaffective disorder)	Schizophrenia is associated with more prominent negative symptoms and less association with trauma than psychotic disorder NOS. Diagnosis of schizoaffective disorder is poorly understood with unreliable predictability in children
Obsessive-compulsive disorder (OCD)	In severe cases, obsessions and compulsions may be seen as irrational. OCD typically lacks the hallucinations and delusional characteristics of schizophrenia
Post-traumatic stress disorder; dissociative disorder	Global impairment, negative symptoms, and chronic course more characteristic of schizophrenia
Personality disorders (schizotypal, schizoid, borderline, paranoid)	May have periods of transient hallucinations and delusions, but not the chronic course and differing pattern of relationships.
Communication disorders	May present with disorganization in speech and communication that resemble formal thought disorder. Do not have typical hallucinations, delusions, or negative symptoms characteristic of schizophrenia
Substance-induced psychosis (amphetamines, cocaine, phencyclidine, marijuana, hallucinogens, alcohol hallucinosis, solvents, sedative withdrawal); toxic encephalopathy due to medications or toxins (corticosteroid, anticholinergics, heavy metals)	Clinical manifestations of acute, often transient psychosis, associated physical findings, toxic screening, and lack of negative symptomatology aid in differentiation from schizophrenia
Medical conditions (delirium, epilepsy, CNS trauma or neoplasm, infectious diseases, human immunodeficiency virus infection, herpes encephalitis, neurosyphilis, encephalitis meningitis, neurodegenerative disease, metabolic disorders)	Comprehensive, medical, and neurological evaluation and monitoring required. Demands close attention to rule out medical emergency. Consider neuroimaging, EEG, and laboratory assessment. Lack of blunted or flattened affect or presence of alterations in consciousness, disorientation, memory impairment, or other physical findings suggests psychosis secondary to medical condition or delirium

reintegrating the child into his or her home and community. Treatment requires a variety of medical, psychiatric, and community resources along with supportive and educational intervention by the family. Limited studies have been conducted on the efficacy of treatment for childhood- and adolescent-onset schizophrenia; treatment parameters result from these limited findings and extrapolation from adult studies [37, 108].

Although there are numerous studies documenting the efficacy of neuroleptics in adults with schizophrenia, there are few parallel studies in adolescents and children. These latter studies do indicate, however, that the antipsychotic medications are superior to placebo in reducing symptoms of hallucinations and delusions [45, 120]. However, many of these patients had limited response, continued to demonstrate symptoms, and had significant rates of adverse events. The Treatment of Early Onset Schizophrenia Spectrum Disorders Study (TEOSS) compared the efficacy and safety of olanzapine, risperidone, and molindone in the treatment of early-onset schizophrenia and schizoaffective disorder, and showed no superiority of the atypical agents over molindone. Side effects included more akathisia associated with molindone and significant weight gain associated with the second-generation agents, more so with olanzapine [121]. Carlisle and McClellan reviewed studies of randomized controlled trials of antipsychotics in children and adolescents, and found positive findings for both first-generation (loxapine, haloperidol, thiothixene, thioridazine, and molindone) and second-generation medications (clozapine, risperidone, olanzapine, aripiprazole) [122]. In a randomized double-blind comparison study of clozapine and haloperidol, improvement in multiple assessments was found to be significantly greater with clozapine than haloperidol [123, 124]. In open-label studies examining adolescents and younger children, clozapine has been found to improve the positive and negative symptoms of schizophrenia, with the most frequent adverse events including drowsiness, weight gain, nonspecific changes in EEG, and hypersalivation [125, 126]. An open trial of clozapine in adolescents found a mean weight gain of 15.4 lb (7 kg) in 6 weeks, a faster increase than that found in adults [125]. Open-label studies of risperidone have indicated improvement in both positive and negative symptoms in adolescents. Common side effects have included weight gain, sedation, and extrapyramidal symptoms (EPS) [124, 127, 128]. In initial open-label trials, olanzapine produced equivocal results regarding improvement in both positive and negative symptoms [128]. Subsequent investigation demonstrated improvement in positive and negative symptom scores. However, treatment was characterized by increased appetite and sedation as the most common adverse events [124, 129]. Quetiapine has also been found in open-label trials to be effective in the treatment of adolescents with psychotic disorders [130]. An open-label extension trial demonstrated that in adolescents with psychoses, quetiapine was well tolerated in the long term, with sustained symptom improvement [131]. Oral paliperidone has also been approved by the US Food and Drug Administration for treatment of EOS.

Because of the long-term side effects that result from using antipsychotics, careful practice parameters must be followed. As in all areas of treating this disorder, the clinician should extensively educate the family about the potential side effects and benefits of these agents. The informed consent of the guardian and, if appropriate, the patient should be obtained. A baseline physical and the use of structured evaluations such as the Abnormal Involuntary Movement Scale are necessary to document the presence or absence of any abnormal movements [132]. Careful monitoring and frequent re-evaluation are required to detect potential side effects of medication, such as extrapyramidal side effects, excessive sedation, cognitive blunting, tardive dyskinesia, and neuroleptic malignant syndrome. Atypical antipsychotics, because of their unique side-effect profiles – including sedation, weight gain, impaired glycemic control, hyperlipidemia, prolactin elevation, and hematological changes – require ongoing monitoring of height, weight, body mass index, and, as required, review of hematological and serum chemistry values, along with glucose, prolactin, lipids, thyroid hormones, and baseline ECG [133].

Psychosocial treatments must address the needs of the individual rather than the specific diagnosis of schizophrenia. All environmental and psychological factors that may complicate recovery must be explored. The treatment plan must be well integrated and the intervention adapted to the developmental level of the child. Prospective investigations of this population are limited, and most treatment recommendations stem from data gathered in studies of adults. Supportive psychotherapy may benefit some children with schizophrenia [134]. Intensive traditional insight-oriented psychotherapies have not been clearly demonstrated as helpful and are usually not recommended in the acute phases of the illness [37, 108].

In adult studies, the combinations of psychoeducational family treatment, medication therapy, and social skills training and cognitive behavioral therapy have decreased relapse rates [135–137]. These recommendations have been extended to children and adolescents [37, 108]. The initial focus of therapy is to support the patient and family during acute crises and to provide information. Using a psychoeducational approach, the causes for schizophrenia and its prognosis, symptoms, and effects on development are shared with the family and the patient. Supportive and cognitive behavioral strategies are used to improve adaptive functioning. The adult literature gives strong support for improving neurocognition and processing speed with the use of cognitive enhancement therapy [138, 139]. Individual and group interventions focus on improving conflict resolution, social skills, problem solving, and the activities of daily living. The clinician must work to establish a stable therapeutic relationship with the patient and his or her family. The family usually remains the strongest advocate for these children, and the clinician acts as their guide in negotiating the obstacles of obtaining the extensive care their child requires. Intervention with families is primarily psychoeducational, but supportive therapy can be required to help families manage the grief and loss that are experienced with their child's illness. Advocacy and educational groups are also beneficial, since they may reduce the sense of stigma and isolation experienced by families.

Children and adolescents with schizophrenia typically struggle in a standard classroom setting: ongoing work with the school is required. Typically, special education is required to maintain the child in an educational facility and to address developmental and learning problems. Frequently, the psychiatrist must conduct ongoing consultation with contact people at the school, since they are often unfamiliar with the difficulties of such students and are ill-equipped to manage all their needs.

During the acute phase of the illness, psychiatric hospitalizations may be required. Once initial stabilization in the hospital is complete, transfer to a day or partial hospital program may ease the transition to the home or community environment. Community services can help in maintaining the patient outside the hospital. Case management, in-home therapeutic care, therapeutic recreation, and vocational rehabilitation may be offered by community mental health programs and are frequently required to meet the long-term needs of these patients.

Outcome

There are few data on the course of childhood schizophrenia, and most studies do not use the current restrictive criteria. Eggers reviewed the outcomes of 57 children with an onset of schizophrenia prior to age 14 years [48, 140]. Low IQ and poor premorbid functioning were associated with poor outcome. The least reliable predictor of outcome was the onset of the illness early in life (i.e., before age 10 years). Of the 57 patients studied, approximately 25% were described as in remission, 25% improved, and 50% showing severe deficits. In a follow-up study, Werry and colleagues reported a more severe course, with higher rates of early death from suicide or accidents and low levels of gainful employment or education [112]. Many patients (90%) continued to receive neuroleptics, and the majority exhibited severe levels of impairment [112]. Asarnow reported similar outcome figures to those seen in Eggers' study [48], but with higher rates of remission and better outcome [61, 141]. In this study, however, there were high rates of multiple rehospitalizations and placement in residential treatment centers, often due to disruptive, out-of-control behaviors [61, 141].

Predictors of poor outcome appear to be poor premorbid adjustment, nonacute insidious onset, and early age of onset; better outcomes are associated with the presence of affective symptoms, acute and older age of onset, and better premorbid adjustment [62, 142]. In a study by Hafner and Nowotny [143] comparing child onset cases of schizophrenia to adult onset, earlier onset was associated with more dramatic social con-

sequences than adult onset, and they postulated that it was due to more disturbance in cognitive and social development at earlier developmental stages. Other studies have indicated that the best predictor of social and functional outcome was premorbid functioning. In the Maudsley Early Onset Schizophrenia Study, early-onset subjects were followed over 4 years. Unlike earlier studies, age of onset was not associated with outcomes but childhood premorbid functioning was the best predictor, with poor childhood premorbid functioning and the severity of negative symptoms at baseline associated with worse global functioning and social adaptation [144].

The length of time of untreated psychosis has also been implicated in determining outcomes [145]. The duration of untreated psychosis (DUP) is defined as the time interval between onset of psychosis and initiation of treatment. In a meta-analysis of first episode schizophrenia, a shorter duration of untreated psychosis was associated with a better response to antipsychotic treatment as measured by the severity of global psychopathology positive and negative symptoms and functional outcomes. The duration of untreated psychosis at treatment initiation was associated with the severity of negative symptoms, but not neurocognitive function, severity of positive symptoms, or general psychopathology [146]. The study highlighted that the duration of untreated psychosis may be a prognostic factor available to improved interventions.

Ultra-High-Risk Syndrome

Over the last decade and a half, there have been intensive research efforts to identify individuals in the prodromal phase of schizophrenia. Research centers in the United States, Australia, Germany, and elsewhere have developed criteria to identify those individuals at highest risk of developing psychosis. Differing terminology has been utilized for these groups, including: ultra-high-risk [35], clinical high risk (CHR) [147], or at-risk mental state (ARMS) [148]. Patients included in these high-risk groups fall into three categories:

(1) Attenuated psychotic symptom group, where patients have experienced subthreshold, attenuated positive psychotic symptoms during the past year.
(2) Brief limited intermittent psychotic symptoms, where patients have experienced episodes of frank psychotic symptoms, but not lasting longer than a week, and have remitted spontaneously.
(3) The risk factor group, composed of patients with first-degree relatives with psychotic disorders, or individuals identified with a schizotypal personality

disorder who have experienced a significant decrease in functioning during the previous year.

This classification has led to identification of a high-risk group of patients who have an enhanced risk for development of psychosis, more than several hundredfold higher than the general population [35].

A complementary approach has been utilized to identify these high-risk individuals based on a German concept of basic symptoms [149]. These symptoms are subjectively self-perceived cognitive and perceptual deficits, or basic symptoms, that are thought to be close to the underlying disturbances found in schizophrenia. Some of these symptoms have been found to be predictive of schizophrenia in clinical samples [150]. Examples of these symptoms include: the inability to divide attention; thought interference; thought pressure; thought blockages; disturbances of receptive and expressive speech; difficulties in abstract thinking; and unstable ideas of reference [151]. These concepts of basic symptoms have been integrated with the ultra-high-risk criteria to identify high-risk groups for development of psychosis [34]. Identification of these individuals is allowing current investigation into potential biomarkers, characterization of outcomes other than schizophrenia, and intervention. Intervention studies in these ultra-high-risk and psychosis-risk syndrome individuals have the goals of: preventing or delaying transition to psychosis; treating current comorbid illness, such as depression or anxiety; engaging in treatment; and attempting to minimize the duration of untreated psychosis. Studies have included the use of cognitive behavioral therapy, antipsychotics, and antidepressants and other pharmacological intervention. Some studies demonstrate diminished conversion rates or delay in conversion to a psychotic state compared to controls. In randomized controlled trials, cognitive behavioral therapy, low-dose olanzapine, cognitive behavioral therapy with risperidone, omega-3 fatty acids, and amisulpride demonstrated decreased conversion rates to psychosis as compared to controls [152–156]. However, in available studies with extended observation, the effect of these interventions appeared to diminish, with active treatment groups showing no significant difference in level of symptomatology or functioning [34, 35].

CASE STUDY

Tom, aged 8 years, was initially brought to the Emergency Department by his mother after he was found in the street kicking moving cars. The mother reported that Tom had had in-

creasing difficulties getting along with children at school and intermittently would complain about a "ghost's hand" hitting him. She reported that he would frequently turn his head and yell, "stop the devil!" Tom reported that he felt "devils" were hitting him in the head. They would push him in the back and yell bad things at him. He reported that he saw the devil in cars passing his house and that he went out to kick the cars to make the devil leave his house.

On examination, Tom would stare blankly, interrupted by yelling at the spirits to go away and leave him alone. On later evaluations, he was found in a panic, screaming and rubbing his stomach. He later described that a ghost's hand had entered his mouth and he could see it coming out of his stomach with his bowels in the hand of the ghost. He reported wanting to die because he was "bad."

Tom's school reported that he was at the bottom of his class but was not a behavior problem. Over the past year, they had noted a deterioration in his performance, marked by his frequently not completing work and staring blankly at the floor or at other members of the class. They had not previously observed him demonstrating overtly delusional behavior or hallucinations.

The family history revealed that his maternal grandfather had been diagnosed with schizophrenia and that Tom's mother had mild mental retardation. The mother rarely left the house and frequently deteriorated to a state in which she needed assistance from her children to care for the home.

Tom was placed in the hospital, where medical evaluation failed to reveal a cause for his mental status changes. The use of antipsychotic medication risperidone decreased the intensity of the auditory, visual, and tactile hallucinations.

After hospitalization, Tom was placed in a more tightly structured special education setting. A case manager was assigned to assist in administering medication and ensuring compliance with appointments. Psychological testing revealed a full-scale IQ of 79 and marked impairments in adaptive functioning. At the 5-year follow-up, Tom had remained out of the hospital but continued to believe that the devil hit him and lived outside his home. He rarely left his home, except for school and a therapeutic day camp. Due to poor response, multiple attempts were made to augment his risperidone, including substitution with alternative atypical antipsychotics. A clozapine trial failed due to his inability to comply with blood draws. The addition of the typical antipsychotic haloperidol helped decrease some of his positive symptoms; however, his impairment remained severe.

References

1. McGuire T. Measuring the economic costs of schizophrenia. *Schizophr Bull* 1990;**17**:375–388.
2. Sadock BJ, Kaplan HI, Sadock VA. *Synopsis of Psychiatry: Behavioral Sciences/Clinical Psychiatry,* 10th edn. Lippincott Williams & Wilkins, 2007; pp. 272–284.
3. American Psychiatric Association. *Diagnostic and Statistical Manual of Mental Disorders,* 4th edn, Text Revision (DSM-IV-TR). Washington, DC: American Psychiatric Association, 2000.
4. DeSanctis S. Sopra alcune varieta della demenzi precoce. *Rev Sper D Fen Med Leg* 1906;**32**:141–165.
5. Kraeplin E, Barclay RM (trans.). *Dementia Pecos and Paraphernalia.* Edinburgh: Livingstone, 1919.
6. Bender L. Childhood schizophrenia. *Am J Orthopsychiatry* 1947;**17**:40–56.
7. Fish B. Neurobiologic antecedents of schizophrenia in children: Evidence for an inherited, congenital neurointegrative defect. *Arch Gen Psychiatry* 1977;**34**:1297–1313.
8. Kanner L. Autistic disturbances of affective contact. *Nerv Child* 1943;**2**:217–250.
9. Kolvin I. Studies in childhood psychoses: I. Diagnostic criteria and classification. *Br J Psychiatry* 1971;**118**:381–384.
10. Rutter M, Lockyer L. A five- to fifteen-year follow-up study of infantile psychosis: I. Description of sample. *Br J Psychiatry* 1967;**113**:1169–1182.
11. American Psychiatric Association. *Diagnostic and Statistical Manual of Mental Disorders,* 3rd edn. Washington, DC: American Psychiatric Association, 1980.
12. Beitchman JH. Childhood schizophrenia: A review and comparison with adult-onset schizophrenia. *Psych Clin N Am* 1985;**8**:793–814.
13. Werry JS. Child and adolescent (early-onset) schizophrenia: A review in light of DSM-IIIR. *J Autism Dev Disord* 1992;**22**:601–624.
14. Burd L, Kerbeshian J. A North Dakota prevalence study of schizophrenia presenting in childhood. *J Am Acad Child Adolesc Psychiatry* 1987;**26**:347–350.
15. Green WH, Campbell M, Hardesty AS, *et al.* A comparison of schizophrenic and autistic children. *J Am Acad Child Adolesc Psychiatry* 1984;**23**:399–409.
16. Russel AT, Bott L, Sarnmons C. The phenomenology of schizophrenia occurring in childhood. *J Am Acad Child Adolesc Psychiatry* 1989;**28**:399–407.
17. Remschmidt HE, Schulz E, Martin M, *et al.* Childhood-onset schizophrenia: History of the concept and recent studies. *Schizophr Bull* 1994;**20**:727–745.
18. Murray RM, Van Os J. Predictors of outcome in schizophrenia. *J Clin Psychopharmacol* 1998;**18**(Suppl 1):2S–4S.
19. American Psychiatric Association. Practice guideline for the treatment of patients with schizophrenia. *Am J Psychiatry* 1997;**154**(4, Suppl):1–63.
20. Jablensky A. The 100 year epidemiology of schizophrenia. *Schizophr Res* 1997;**28**:111–125.
21. Frazier JA, Alaghband-Rad J, Jacobsen L, *et al.* Pubertal development and onset of psychosis in childhood onset schizophrenia. *Psychiatry Res* 1997;**70**:1–7.
22. Aleman A, Kahn RS, Selten JP. Sex differences in the risk of schizophrenia: evidence from meta-analysis. *Arch Gen Psychiatry* 2003;**60**:565–571.
23. McGrath J, Saha S, Welham J, *et al.* A systematic review of the incidence of schizophrenia. *BMC Med* 2004;**2**:13.
24. Cantor S. *Childhood Schizophrenia.* New York: Guilford, 1988.
25. King RA, Noshpitz JD. *Pathways of Growth: Essentials of Child Psychiatry, Vol. II: Psychopathology.* New York: John Wiley & Sons, Ltd, 1991.
26. Cornblatt BA, Erlenrneyer-Kirnling L. Global attentional deviance as a marker of risk for schizophrenia: Specificity and predictive validity. *J Abnorm Psychol* 1985;**94**:470–486.
27. Green WH, Deutsch SI: Biological studies of schizophrenia with childhood onset. In: Deutsch SI (ed.) *Application of Basic Neuroscience to Child Psychiatry.* New York: Plenum Medical, 1990; pp. 217–229.
28. Watkins JM, Asarnow RF, Tanguay PE. Symptom development in childhood onset schizophrenia. *J Child Psychol Psychiatry* 1988;**29**:865–878.
29. Schaeffer JL, Ross RG. Childhood-onset schizophrenia: premorbid and prodromal diagnostic and treatment histories. *J Am Acad Child Adolesc Psychiatry* 2002;**41**:538–545.
30. Lewis R. Should cognitive deficit be a diagnostic criterion for schizophrenia? *Rev Psychiatr Neurosci* 2004;**29**:102–113.
31. Isohanni M, Jones PB, Moilanen K, *et al.* Early developmental milestones in adult schizophrenia and other psychoses. A 31-year follow-up of the Northern Finland 1966 birth cohort. *Schizophr Res* 2001;**52**:1–19.
32. Alaghband-Rad J, McKenna K, Gordon CT, *et al.* Childhood-onset schizophrenia: the severity of premorbid course. *J Am Acad Child Adolesc Psychiatry* 1995;**34**:1273–1283.
33. McClellan J, Breiger D, McCurry C, Hlastala S. Premorbid functioning in early onset psychotic disorders. *J Am Acad Child Adolesc Psychiatry* 2003;**42**:666–672.
34. Correll CU, Huaser M, Auther AM, Cornblatt BA. Research in people with psychosis risk syndrome: a review of the current evidence and future directions. *J Child Psychol Psychiat* 2010;**51**:390–431.
35. Yung AR, Nelson B. Young people at ultra high risk for psychosis: a research update. *Early Intervention in Psychiatry* 2011;**5**(Suppl 1):52–57.
36. Asarnow JR, Ben-Meir S. Children with schizophrenia spectrum and depressive disorders: A comparative study of onset patterns, premorbid adjustment, and severity of dysfunction. *J Child Psychol Psychiatry* 1988;**29**:477–488.
37. Practice Parameter for the Assessment and Treatment of Children and Adolescents with Schizophrenia. *J Am Acad Child Adolesc Psychiatry* 2001;40(7 Suppl):4S–23S.

38. Kravariti E, Morris RG, Rabe-Hesketh S, Murray RM, Frangou S. The Maudsley Early Onset Schizophrenia Study: cognitive function in adolescents with recent onset schizophrenia. *Schizophr Res* 2003;**61**:137–48

39. Gochman PA, Greenstein D, Sporn A, *et al*. IQ stabilization in childhood-onset schizophrenia. *Schizophr Res* 2005;**77**:271–7.

40. McClellan J, McCurry C. Neurocognitive pathways in the development of schizophrenia. *Semin Clin Neuropsychiatry* 1998;**3**:320–332.

41. Heinrichs RW, Zakzanis KK. Neurocognitive deficit in schizophrenia: a quantitative review of the evidence. *Neuropsychology* 1998;**12**:426–445.

42. Bilder RM, Goldman RS, Robinson D, *et al*. Neuropsychology of first episode schizophrenia: initial characterization and clinical correlates. *Am J Psychiatry* 2000;**157**: 549–559.

43. Kravariti E, Morris RG, Rabe-Hesketh S, Murray RM, Frangou S. The Maudsley Early Onset Schizophrenia Study: cognitive function in adolescent-onset schizophrenia. *Schizophr Res* 2003;**65**:95–103.

44. Volkmar FR. Childhood and adolescent psychosis: A review of the past 10 years. *J Am Acad Child Adolesc Psychiatry* 1996;**35**:843–851.

45. Spencer EK, Campbell M. Children with schizophrenia: Diagnosis, phenomenology, and pharmacotherapy. *Schizophr Bull* 1994;**20**:713–725.

46. Volkmar FR, Cohen DJ, Hoshino Y, *et al*. Phenomenology and classification of the childhood psychoses. *Psychol Med* 1988;**18**:191–201.

47. Russell AT. The clinical presentation of childhood-onset schizophrenia. *Schizophr Bull* 1994;**20**:631–646.

48. Eggers C. Course and prognosis in childhood schizophrenia. *J Autism Childhood Schizophr* 1978;**8**:21–36.

49. Mueser KT, McGurk SR. Schizophrenia. *Lancet* 2004; **363**:2063–2072.

50. Tandon R, Keshavan MS, Nasrallah HA. Schizophrenia, "Just the Facts": What we know in 2008, Part I: Overview. *Schizophr Res* 2008;**100**:4–19.

51. Cardno A, Marshall E, Coid B, *et al*. Heritability estimates for psychotic disorders: the Maudsley twin psychosis series. *Arch Gen Psychiatry* 1999;**56**:162–168.

52. Farmer AE, McGuffin P, Gottesman II. Twin concordance for DSM-III schizophrenia. Scrutinizing the validity of the definition. *Arch Gen Psychiatr* 1987;**44**:634–640.

53. Riley B. Linkage studies of schizophrenia. *Neurotoxicity Res* 2004;**6**:17–34.

54. Kendler KS, Diehl SR. The genetics of schizophrenia, a current, genetic-epidemiologic perspective. *Schizophr Bull* 1993;**19**:261–285.

55. McGuffin P, Own MJ, Farmer AE. Genetic basis of schizophrenia. *Lancet* 1995;**346**:678–682.

56. Cardno AG, Gottesman II. Twin studies of schizophrenia, from bow-and-arrow concordances to Star Wars Mx and functional genomics. *Am J Med Genet* 2000;**97**: 12–17.

57. Lowing PA, Mirsky AF, Pereira R. The inheritance of schizophrenic spectrum disorders: A reanalysis of the Danish adoptee study data. *Am J Psychiatry* 1983;**140**: 1167–1171.

58. Higgins J. Effects of child rearing by schizophrenic mothers: A follow-up. *J Psychiatr Res* 1976;**13**:1–9.

59. Wender PH, Rosenthal D, Kety SS, *et al*. Crossfostering: A research strategy for clarifying the role of genetic and experimental factors in the etiology of schizophrenia. *Arch Gen Psychiatry* 1974;**30**:121–128.

60. Rosenthal D. *Genetic Theory and Abnormal Behavior*. New York: McGraw-Hill, 1970.

61. Asarnow JF. Childhood-onset schizophrenia. *J Child Psychol Psychiatry* 1994;**35**:1345–1371.

62. Zeitlin H. The natural history of psychiatric disorder in children. *Inst Psychiatry Maudsley Monogr* 1986;**29**.

63. Nicolson R, Brookner BF, Lenane M, *et al*. Parental schizophrenia spectrum disorders in childhood-onset and adult-onset schizophrenia. *Am J Psychiatry* 2003;**160**: 490–495.

64. Walsh T, McClellan JM, McCarthy SE, *et al*. Rare structural variants disrupt multiple genes in neurodevelopmental pathways in schizophrenia. *Science* 2008;**320**: 539–543

65. Sporn A, Addington A, Reiss AL, *et al*. 22q11 deletion syndrome in childhood onset schizophrenia, an update. *Mol Psychiatry* 2004;**9**:225–226.

66. Rapoport JL, Addington AM, Frangou S. The neurodevelopmental model of schizophrenia: update 2005. *Mol Psychiatry* 2005;**10**:434–449.

67. Rujescu D, Ingason A, Cichon S, *et al*. Disruption of the neurexin 1 gene is associated with schizophrenia. *Hum Mol Genet* 2008;**17**:458–465.

68. Nicolson R, Giedd JN, Lenane M, *et al*. Clinical and neurobiological correlates of cytogenetic abnormalities in childhood-onset schizophrenia. *Am J Psychiatry* 1999; **156**:1575–1579.

69. Burgess CE, Lindblad K, Sidransky E, *et al*. Large CAG/CTG repeats are associated with childhood onset schizophrenia. *Mol Psychiatry* 1998;**3**:321–327.

70. Baltaxe CAM, Simmons JQ III. Speech and language disorders in children and adolescents with schizophrenia. *Schizophr Bull* 1995;**21**:677–692.

71. Caplan R. Communication deficits in children with schizophrenia spectrum disorders. *Schizophr Bull* 1994;**20**:671–674.

72. Allin M, Murray R. Schizophrenia: A neurodevelopmental or neurodegenerative disorder? *Curr Opin Psychiatry* 2002;**15**:9–15.

73. McDonald C, Grech, A, Touloupoulou T, *et al*. Brain volumes in familial and non-familial schizophrenic probands and their unaffected relatives. *Am J Med Genet Neuropsych Genet* 2002;**114**:616–625.

74. Akbarian S, Vinuela A, Kim JJ, Potkin SG, Bunney WEJ, Jones EG. Distorted distribution of nicotinamide-adenine dinucleotide phosphate-diaphorase neurons in temporal lobe of schizophrenics implies anomalous cortical development. *Arch Gen Psychiatry* 1993;**50**:178.

75. Weinberger DR, Marenco S. Schizophrenia as a neurodevelopmental disorder. In: Hirsch SR, Weinberger DR (eds) *Schizophrenia*, 2nd edn. Oxford: Blackwell Publishing, 2003; pp. 326–348.

76. Wright IC, Rabe-Hesketh S, Woodruff PWR, *et al*. Meta-analysis of regional brain volumes in schizophrenia. *Am J Psychiatry* 2000;**157**:16–25.

77. Andreasen NC, Flashman L, Flaum M, *et al*. Regional brain abnormalities in schizophrenia measured with magnetic resonance imaging. *JAMA* 1994;**272**:1763–1769.

78. Byne W, Buchsbaum MS, Mattiace LA, *et al*. Postmortem assessment of thalamic nuclear volumes in subjects with schizophrenia. *Am J Psychiatry* 2002; **159**:59–65.

79. Lawrie SM, Abukmeil SS. Brain abnormality in schizophrenia: a systematic and quantitative review of volumetric magnetic resonance imaging studies. *Br J Psychiatry* 1998;**172**:110–120.

80. Gogtay N, Giedd J, Rapoport JL. Brain development in healthy, hyperactive, and psychotic children. *Arch Neurol* 2002;**59**:1244–1248.

81. Sowell ER, Levitt J, Thompson PM, *et al.* Brain abnormalities in early-onset schizophrenia spectrum disorder observed with statistical parametric mapping of structural magnetic resonance images. *Am J Psychiatry* 2000;**157**:1475–1484.

82. Toga AW, Thompson PM, Sowell ER. Mapping brain maturation. *Trends Neurosci* 2006;**29**:148–159.

83. Thompson PM, Vidal C, Giedd JN, *et al.* Mapping adolescent brain change reveals dynamic wave of accelerated gray matter loss in very early onset schizophrenia. *Proc Natl Acad Sci USA* 2001;**98**:11650–11655.

84. Sporn AL, Greenstein DK, Gogtay N, *et al.* Progressive brain volume loss during adolescence in childhood-onset schizophrenia. *Am J Psychiatry* 2003;**160**:2181–2189.

85. Greenstein D, Lerch J, Shaw P, *et al.* Childhood-onset schizophrenia: cortical brain abnormalities as young adults. *J Child Psychol Psychiatry* 2006;**47**:1003–1012.

86. Kumra S, Ashtari M, McMeniman M, *et al.* Reduced frontal white matter integrity in early-onset schizophrenia: a preliminary study. *Biol Psychiatry* 2004;**55**: 1138–1145.

87. Kubicki M, McCarly R, Westin CF, *et al.* A review of diffusion tensor imaging studies in schizophrenia. *J Psychiatric Res* 2007;**41**:15–30.

88. Kendi M, Kendi AT, Lehericy S, *et al.* Structural and diffusion tensor imaging of the fornix in childhood and adolescent onset schizophrenia. *J Am Acad Child Adolesc Psychiatry* 2008;47:826–832.

89. Singer MT, Wynne LC. Thought disorder and family relations of schizophrenics. IV. Results and implications. *Arch Gen Psychiatry* 1965;**12**:201–209.

90. Asarnow JR, Goldstein MJ, Ben-Meir S. Parental communication deviance in childhood onset schizophrenia spectrum and depressive disorders. *J Child Psychol Psychiatry* 1988;**29**:825–838.

91. Hooley JM, Campbell C. Control and controllability: beliefs and behaviour in high and low expressed emotion relatives. *Psychol Med* 2002;**32**:1091–1099.

92. Goldstein MJ. The UCLA high risk project. *Schizophr Bull* 1987;**13**:505–514.

93. Butzlaff, RL, Hooley JM. Expressed emotion and psychiatric relapse: a meta-analysis. *Arch Gen Psychiatry* 1998;**55**:547–552.

94. O'Brien MP, Gordon JL, Bearden CE, *et al.* Positive family environment predicts improvement in symptoms and social functioning among adolescents at imminent risk for onset of psychosis. *Schizophr Res* 2006;**81**: 269–275.

95. Briedborde NJ, Lopez SR, Wickens TD, *et al.* Toward specifying the nature of the relationship between expressed emotion and schizophrenic relapse: the utility of curvi-linear models. *Int J Methods Psychiatr Res* 2007;**16**:1–10.

96. Rosenfarb IS, Bellack AS, Aziz N. Family interactions and the course of schizophrenia in African American and White patients. *J Abnorm Psychol* 2006;**115**: 112–120.

97. Bruce MLK, Takeuchi DT, Leaf PJ. Poverty and psychiatric status: longitudinal evidence from the New Haven epidemiologic catchment area study. *Arch Gen Psychiatry* 1991;**48**:470–474.

98. Rabkin JG. Stressful life events in schizophrenia: A review of the research literature. *Psychol Bull* 1980;**87**: 408–425.

99. US Institute of Medicine. *Neurological, Psychiatric, and Developmental Disorders: Meeting the Challenges in the Developing World.* Washington, DC: National Academy of Sciences, 2001.

100. Jablensky A. Sartorius N, Emberg G, Anker M, Korten A, Cooper JE. Schizophrenia: manifestations, incidence, and course in different cultures – a World Health Organization ten-country study. *Psychol Med Monograph Suppl* 1992;**20**:1–97.

101. Penner JD, Brown AS. Prenatal infectious and nutritional factors and risk of schizophrenia. *Expert Rev Neurotherapeutics* 2007;**7**:797–805.

102. Meyer U, Yee BK, Feldon J. The neurodevelopmental impact of prenatal infections at different times in pregnancy: the earlier the worse. *Neuroscientist* 2007;**13**: 241–266.

103. Meyer U, Feldon J. Neural basis of psychosis-related behaviour in the infection model of schizophrenia. *Behav Brain Res* 2009;**204**:322–334.

104. Tandon R, Keshavan MS, Nasrallah HA. Schizophrenia, "Just the Facts," What we know in 2008. 2. Epidemiology and etiology. *Schizophr Res* 2008;**102**:1–18.

105. Reimherr JP, McClellan JM. Diagnostic challenges in children and adolescents with psychotic disorders. *J Clin Psychiatry* 2004;**65**(Suppl 6):5–11.

106. Andreasen NC, Olsen S. Negative v positive schizophrenia: definition and validation. *Arch Gen Psychiatry* 1982;**39**:789–794.

107. Fields JH, Grochowski S, Lindenmayer JP, *et al.* The assessment of affective disorders in children and adolescents by semistructured interview: test-retest reliability of the schedule for affective disorders and schizophrenia for school-age children, present episode version. *Arch Gen Psychiatry* 1985;**42**:696–702.

108. McClellan JM, Werry JS. Practice parameters for the assessment and treatment of children and adolescents with schizophrenia. *J Am Acad Child Adolesc Psychiatry* 1994;**33**:616–635.

109. American Academy of Pediatrics Task Force on Pediatric AIDS. Adolescents and human immunodeficiency virus infection: The role of the pediatrician in prevention and intervention. *Pediatrics* 1993;**92**:626–630.

110. *Report of the Presidential Commission on the Human Immunodeficiency Virus Epidemic.* Washington, DC: Government Printing Office, 1988.

111. McClellan J, McCurry C, Speltz ML, *et al.* Symptom factors in early-onset psychotic disorders. *J Am Acad Child Adolesc Psychiatry* 2002;**41**:791–798.

112. Werry JS, McClellan JM, Chard L. Childhood and adolescent schizophrenia, bipolar and schizoaffective disorders: A clinical and outcome study. *J Am Acad Child Adolesc Psychiatry* 1991;**30**:457–465.

113. Ballenger JC, ReusVI, Post RM. The "atypical" clinical picture of adolescent mania. *Am J Psychiatry* 1982;**139**:602–606.

114. Rosen LN, Rosenthal NE, Van Dusen PH, *et al.* Age at onset and number of psychotic symptoms in bipolar I and

schizoaffective disorder. *Am J Psychiatry* 1983;**140**: 1523–1524.

115. Carlson GA. Bipolar affective disorders in childhood and adolescence. In: Cantwell DP, Carlson GA (eds) *Affective Disorders in Childhood and Adolescence: An Update.* New York: Spectrum Publications, 1983; pp. 61–84.

116. Baker L, Cantwell DP. Disorders of language, speech, and communication. In: Lewis M (ed.) *Child and Adolescent Psychiatry: A Comprehensive Textbook.* Baltimore: Williams & Wilkins, 1991; pp. 516–521.

117. Famularo R, Kinscherff R, Fenton T. Psychiatric diagnoses of maltreated children: preliminary findings. *J Am Acad Child Adolesc Psychiatry* 1992;**31**:863–867.

118. Rothstein A. Hallucinatory phenomena in childhood: A critique of the literature. *J Am Acad Child Adolesc Psychiatry* 1981;**20**:623–635.

119. Caplan R. Thought disorder in childhood. *J Am Acad Child Adolesc Psychiatry* 1994;**33**:605–615.

120. Kydd RR, Werry IS. Schizophrenia in children under 16 years. *J Autism Dev Disord* 1982;**12**:343–357.

121. Sikich L, Frazier JA, McClellan J, *et al.* Double blind comparison of first- and second-generation antipsychotics in early-onset schizophrenia and schizo-affective disorder: findings from the Treatment of Early Onset Schizophrenia Spectrum Disorders (TEOSS) Study. *Am J Psychiatry* 2008;**165**:1420–1431.

122. Carlisle LL, McClellan J. Psychopharmacology of schizophrenia in children and adolescents. *Pediatr Clin N Am* 2011;**58**:205–218.

123. Kumra S, Frazier JA, Jacobsen LK, *et al.* Childhood-onset schizophrenia: a double-blind clozapine-haloperidol comparison. *Arch Gen Psychiatry* 1996;**53**:1090–1097.

124. Findling RL, McNamara NK. Atypical antipsychotics in the treatment of children and adolescents: clinical applications. *J Clin Psychiatry* 2004;**65**(Suppl 6):30–44.

125. Frazier JA, Gordon CT, McKenna K, *et al.* An open trial of clozapine in 11 adolescents with childhood-onset schizophrenia. *J Am Acad Child Adolesc Psychiatry* 1994;**33**:658–663.

126. Turetz M, Mozes T, Toren P, *et al.* An open trial of clozapine in neuroleptic-resistant childhood-onset schizophrenia. *Br J Psychiatry* 1997;**170**:507–510.

127. Armenteros JL, Whitaker AH, Welikson M, *et al.* Risperidone in adolescents with schizophrenia: an open pilot study. *J Am Acad Child Adolesc Psychiatry* 1997;**36**: 694–700.

128. Kumra S, Jacobsen LK, Lenane M, *et al.* Childhood-onset schizophrenia: an open label study of olanzapine in adolescents. *J Am Acad Child Adolesc Psychiatry* 1998;**37**: 377–385.

129. Findling RL, McNamara NK, Youngstrom EA, *et al.* A prospective, open-label trial of olanzapine in adolescents with schizophrenia. *J Am Acad Child Adolesc Psychiatry* 2003;**42**:170–175.

130. Shaw JA, Lewis JE, Pascal S, *et al.* A study of quetiapine: efficacy and tolerability in psychotic adolescents. *J Child Adolesc Psychopharmacol* 2001;**11**:415–424.

131. McConville B, Carrero L, Sweitzer D, *et al.* Long-term safety, tolerability, and clinical efficacy of quetiapine in adolescents: an open-label extension trial. *J Child Adolesc Psychopharmacol* 2003;**12**:73–80.

132. National Institute of Mental Health. Abnormal Involuntary Movement Scale. *Psychopharmacol Bull* 1985;**18**: 515–541.

133. McConville BJ, Sorter MT. Treatment challenges and safety considerations for antipsychotic use in children and adolescents with psychoses. *J Clin Psychiatry* 2004;**65** (suppl 6):20–29.

134. Cantor S, Kestenbaum C. Psychotherapy with schizophrenic children. *J Am Acad Child Adolesc Psychiatry* 1986;**25**:623–630.

135. Asarnow, JR, Tompson MC, McGrath EP. Annotation: childhood-onset schizophrenia: clinical and treatment issues. *J Child Psychol Psychiatry* 2004;**45**:180–194.

136. Patterson TL, Leeuwenkamp OR. Adjunctive psychosocial therapies for the treatment of schizophrenia. *Schizophr Res* 2008;**100**:108–119.

137. McGurk SR, Twamley EW, Sitzer DI, *et al.* A meta-analysis of cognitive remediation in schizophrenia. *Am J Psychiatry* 2007;**164**:1791–1802.

138. Hogarty GE, Flesher S, Ulrich R, *et al.* Cognitive enhancement therapy for schizophrenia: effects of a 2-year randomized trial on cognition and behavior. *Arch Gen Psychiatry* 2004;**61**:866–876.

139. Eack SM, Greenwald DP, Hogarty SS, *et al.* Cognitive enhancement therapy for early-course schizophrenia: effects of a two-year randomized controlled trial. *Psychiatr Serv* 2009;**60**:1468–1476.

140. Eggers C. Schizoaffective disorders in childhood: A follow-up study. *J Autism Dev Disord* 1989;**19**:327–342.

141. Asarnow JR, Tompson MC. Childhood onset schizophrenia: A follow-up study. *Eur J Child Adolesc Psychiatry* 1999;**8**:9–12.

142. Werry JS, McClellan JM. Predicting outcome in child and adolescent (early onset) schizophrenia and bipolar disorder. *J Am Acad Child Adolesc Psychiatry* 1992;**31**: 147–150.

143. Hafner H, Nowotny B. Epidemiology of early-onset schizophrenia. *Eur Arch Psychiatry Clin Neurosci* 1995; **245**:80–92.

144. Vyas NS, Hadjulis M, Vourdas A, Byrne P, Frangou S. The Maudlsey Early Onset Schizophrenia Study. Predictors of psychosocial outcome at 4-year follow-up. *Eur Child Adolesc Psychiatry* 2007;**15**:465–470.

145. Bottlender R, Sato T, Jager M, *et al.* The impact of the duration of untreated psychosis prior to first psychiatric admission on the 15-year outcome in schizophrenia. *Schizophr Res* 2003;**62**:37–44.

146. Perkins DO, Gu H, Boteva K, Lieberman JA. Relationship between duration of untreated psychosis and outcome in first-episode schizophrenia: a critical review and meta-analysis. *Am J Psychiatry* 2005;**162**:1785–1804.

147. Cornblatt B, Lencz T, Obuchowski M. The schizophrenia prodrome: treatment and high-risk perspectives. *Schizophr Res* 2002;**54**:177–186.

148. Broome MR, Woolley JB, Johns LC, *et al.* Outreach and Support in South London (OASIS): implementation of a clinical service for prodromal psychosis and the at risk mental state. *Eur Psychiatry* 2005;**20**:372–378.

149. Huber G, Gross G. The concept of basic symptoms in schizophrenic and schizoaffective psychoses. *Recent Prog Med* 1989;**80**:646–652.

150. Klosterkotter J, Hellmich M. Steinmeyer EM, Schultze-Lutter F. Diagnosing schizophrenia in the initial prodromal phase. *Arch Gen Psychiatry* 2001;**58**:158–164.

151. Klosterkotter J, Gross G, Huber G, Wieneke A, Steinmeyer EM, Schultze-Lutter F. Evaluation of the 'Bonn Scale for the Assessment of Basic Symptoms – BSABS' as

an instrument for the assessment of schizophrenia proneness: a review of recent findings. *Neurol Psychiatry Brain Res* 1997;**5**:137–50.

152. Morrison AP, Frnech P, Walford L, *et al.* Cognitive therapy for the prevention of psychosis in people at ultra-high risk: randomised controlled trial. *Br J Psychiatry* 2004;**185**:291–297.

153. McGlashan TH, Zipursky RB, Perkins D, *et al.* Randomized double-blind trial of olanzapine versus placebo in patients prodromally symptomatic for psychosis. *Am J Psychiatry* 2006;**163**:790–799 [see comment].

154. McGorry PD, Yung AR, Phillips LJ, *et al.* Randomized controlled trial of interventions designed to reduce the risk of progression to first-episode psychosis in a clinical sample with sub-threshold symptoms. *Arch Gen Psychiatry* 2002;**59**:921–928.

155. Amminger GP, Schafer MR, Papageorgiou K, *et al.* Long-chain omega-3 fatty acids for indicated prevention of psychotic disorders: a randomized, placebo-controlled trial. *Arch Gen Psychiatry* 2010;**67**: 146–154.

156. Ruhrmann S, Bechdolf A, Kuhn KU, *et al.* Acute effects of treatment for prodromal symptoms for people putatively in a late initial prodromal state of psychosis. *Br J Psychiatry* 2007;**51**(Suppl):s88–s95.

25

Neuropsychological Assessment and the Neurologically Impaired Child

Scott D. Grewe, Keith Owen Yeates

Introduction

This is an exciting time in our understanding of brain-behavior relationships in children. Researchers have not only provided fascinating insights into the workings of the developing central nervous system [1, 2] but also increasingly have clarified the behavioral and cognitive sequelae associated with the various medical conditions that affect it [3, 4]. A number of factors are responsible for our increased ability to articulate the nature of and relationship between developing neuropsychological organization in children and deficits in functioning. These include both advances in neuroscience research [5–8] and increased survival rates for children suffering neurological trauma [9, 10]. For example, the death rate for children with brain tumors decreased from 1/100 000 to 0.7/100 000 between 1975 and 2001, while 5-year survival improved from rates of about 50% during the early 1970s to typically 75–80% in the late 1990s [11].

The purpose of this chapter is to introduce neuropsychology and neuropsychological assessment of children, with a focus on neurologically impaired children. Thus, we begin with a brief historical overview of the concept of neurological impairment and neuropsychological assessment in children, and delineate the role of a neuropsychologist in diagnosis and assessment. Next, we offer a set of conceptual principles for neuropsychological assessment, review its related methods and procedures, and describe the differences in purpose and scope of evaluations conducted by school psychologists, clinical child psychologists, and neuropsychologists. After that, we review the neuropsychological outcomes associated with several of the more common childhood neurological disorders. Finally, we examine a neuropsychological management approach and related intervention techniques used to help neurologically impaired children adapt to and compensate for their difficulties.

Historical Overview

The field of child neuropsychology has been influenced by several related disciplines. Indeed, child neuropsychological assessment has involved not only the downward extension of the methods of adult neuropsychological assessment [12], but also incorporated advances in child psychiatry, clinical child psychology, developmental psychology, developmental pediatrics, and pediatric neurology. The history of child neuropsychological assessment can be divided into three distinct eras.

The first era developed as an outgrowth of early research on brain-injured soldiers in Europe during World War I. These severely brain-damaged individuals were described as stimulus bound (e.g., lacking in cognitive spontaneity and flexibility), perseverative, concrete, and emotionally labile. The application of these findings led to inferences about cognitive and emotional characteristics of intact adults and, later, of children.

Brain damage became an explanation for behavioral and educational problems in children following the epidemic of von Economo's encephalitis in 1918. These post-encephalitic children were described as antisocial, irritable, impulsive, and hyperkinetic. Additionally, other professionals working with mentally retarded children observed in their subjects many of the behaviors common to the brain-injured soldiers from World War I, and inferred underlying brain damage. Thus, the cardinal features of brain injury were originally elucidated as hyperkinesis, impulsivity, distractibility, emotional lability, and perseveration. This clinical picture became widely construed as *prima facie* evidence of brain injury despite the lack of clear documentation of such.

However, the advances of this era were limited by the anecdotal nature of clinical reports. Additionally, considerable professional resistance existed regarding

Clinical Child Psychiatry, Third Edition. Edited by William M. Klykylo and Jerald Kay.
© 2012 John Wiley & Sons, Ltd. Published 2012 by John Wiley & Sons, Ltd.

attempts to correlate behavior with specific brain regions. Indeed, such luminaries as Henry Head [13] argued that these and similar approaches were little more than revised phrenology, an argument that was not totally unfounded.

The second era of child neuropsychological assessment began around the time of World War II with the collaborative efforts of Strauss, Lehtinen, and Werner. They introduced experimental techniques for studying the behavior of children with purported brain injuries, and coined the term "minimal brain injury" to describe the cluster of behaviors they believed were characteristic of brain-injured children [14, 15]. Their work was very influential, and resulted in the popularity of the notion of "minimal brain dysfunction" in the conceptualization of learning disorders [16]. Again, one of the major shortcomings of this second era was the often made but unwarranted assumption that the presence of cognitive or behavioral deficits in children without any known injury was indicative of brain dysfunction.

Interestingly, modern neuroimaging technology and advances in cognitive neurosciences have made feasible the third, and current, era of child neuropsychology. This era has involved a more sophisticated approach to the study of brain-behavior relationships in children with neurological disease, as well as in those with other systemic medical illnesses, developmental disorders, psychiatric disorders, and normal developmental status [17–19]. Moreover, it has seen the establishment of scientific journals specifically focused in child and/or pediatric neuropsychology.

The transition to the most recent era of child neuropsychology also has been driven by attempts to ground child neuropsychological assessment in broader conceptual models [20–25], which help facilitate our understanding of neurobehavioral development through research and clinical practice. The goal of neuropsychological assessment, therefore, is not simply to document the presence of cognitive or behavioral deficits and their possible association with known or suspected brain damage. Rather, the goal is ultimately to enhance children's present and future adaptation by describing their cognitive, behavioral, and social functioning, relating their functioning to biological, developmental, and contextual variables, anticipating their unique struggles to typical developmental "stress points," and providing recommendations and interventions to insure children meet these developmental demands.

What is a Neuropsychologist?

Much as child neuropsychological assessment went through a period of development, so has the general profession of neuropsychology. Indeed, although such individuals as Paul Broca, Carl Wernicke, John Hughlings Jackson, Henry Head, and Kurt Goldstein were laying the foundation for neuropsychology in the nineteenth century, it was not until the mid-twentieth century that the term "neuropsychology" began appearing in the professional literature [26, 27]. Currently, neuropsychologists are licensed psychologists who have earned a doctorate in psychology, which typically includes formal coursework and practice in neuropsychology, and a predoctoral internship with additional neuropsychology training. However, for many neuropsychologists, the bulk of their specialized training occurs during a 2-year postdoctoral fellowship. Indeed, professional guidelines [28] support postdoctoral training as an entry-level educational requirement for all new graduates. Following postdoctoral training, more advanced Diplomate status can be achieved through a board-certification process, although not all practicing neuropsychologists are board-certified.

The specialty of neuropsychology includes individuals functioning in various capacities within clinical, research, administrative, and academic settings. Additionally, within this broader field are those who share an interest in facilitating the adaptive outcomes of children with genetic, medical, environmental, behavioral, and social problems; namely, the child, or pediatric, neuropsychologist.

General Principles

Neuropsychological assessment of children is based on various models that have conceptual foundations and knowledge bases cogently articulated by Bernstein and Waber [20, 21], Taylor and Fletcher [22], Rourke and his colleagues [23], and Yeates and Taylor [29]. These various assessment models highlight and stress different aspects and units of analysis in their respective approaches. However, the application of these knowledge bases is consistently grounded in understanding brain-behavior relationships across the developmental spectrum, all for the primary purpose of enhancing children's adaptation.

Adaptation

The primary focus of assessment is to promote the current and future adaptation of the child, rather than simply to document the presence or location of brain damage or dysfunction. Adaptation results from the interactions of children and their environments or contexts. Failures in adaptation, such as academic or behavioral difficulties, are usually the presenting problems that bring children to the attention of neuropsychologists. In this respect, neuropsychological assessment is optimally useful when it helps to explain those difficulties, provides avenues for intervention, and facilitates successful future outcomes. Indeed, the goals of assessment extend beyond facilitating learning and behavior in the present to include promoting future adaptation to the demands of adult life.

Brain and Behavior

The second principle is that insight into children's adaptation can be gained through an analysis of brain-behavior relationships. Advances in the neurosciences over the past several decades have yielded clearer understandings of the relationships between brain and behavior. Old notions regarding the localization of functions have been replaced by more dynamic models involving the interaction of multiple brain regions [30–32]. Although most of these models concern adults, recent advances in functional neuroimaging and related techniques are providing opportunities to determine if similar models apply to children. Future research should, therefore, eventually yield major advances in our understanding of the brain-behavior relationships in children.

Context

The third principle is that environmental contexts are influential in constraining, amplifying, and determining behavior, and, subsequently, affecting brain development and functioning. Indeed, the brain does not function in isolation. Thus, a neuropsychological assessment must carefully examine the influences of environmental or contextual variables on a child's behavior. The reasons for examining these factors are to assess the nature of environmental and situational demands, or even stressors, being placed on the child and assist in the process of explaining a child's adaptive difficulties. In this regard, neuropsychological assessment is designed not only to measure a child's specific cognitive, behavioral, and social skills, but also to determine how a child applies those skills in particular environments. Examining children's cognitive and behavioral profiles and how their profiles match the contextual demands of their environments allows the neuropsychologist to highlight the developmental risks facing children and make informed recommendations for intervention [21].

Development

The final guiding principle is that assessment involves the measurement of change, or development, across multiple levels of analysis. Developmental neuroscience has highlighted the multiple processes that characterize brain development (e.g., cell differentiation and migration, synaptogenesis, dendritic arborization and pruning, myelinization), and the timing of those processes [33]. Although less research has been conducted concerning developmental changes in children's environments, there is, nevertheless, a continuity and predictability to the environments of most children in our society, particularly when considering the academic, behavioral, and social demands they will face [34].

Consequently, neuropsychological assessment of children requires close scrutiny of the developmental changes that occur in brain, behavior, and context, because the interplay of these variables determines ultimate adaptational outcomes. Indeed, failures in adaptation often reflect a clash between different timetables (e.g., biological and environmental) that result in a lack of fit between children and the contexts within which they function.!

Methods of Assessment

The four general principles outlined above serve as the foundation for specific methods used by many child neuropsychologists. Neuropsychological assessment is usually equated with the administration of a battery of tests. However, in practice, neuropsychologists draw on multiple sources of information, rather than relying solely on the results of psychological tests. The most common combination of methods involves the collection of relevant historical information, focused behavioral observations, and psychological testing. Together, they permit a comprehensive examination of neuropsychological functioning.

History

The collection of a thorough history is a critical component in any neuropsychological assessment and its importance cannot be overstated. Indeed, a thorough history helps in the process of clarifying the nature, onset, and source of a child's presenting problems.

Birth and Developmental History

The information collected regarding a child's early development usually begins with the mother's pregnancy and extends to the attainment of developmental milestones. This information is useful in identifying early risk factors and indicators of anomalous development. Indeed, the presence of early risk factors or developmental anomalies helps makes a case for a

Table 25.1 Perinatal risk factors.

Risk factor	Associated outcomes
Maternal age < 17 years	General cognitive and motor deficits
Maternal cigarette consumption	Developmental delays, learning disabilities
Maternal alcohol consumption	Fetal alcohol syndrome/effects (FAS/FAE)
Maternal cocaine and/or methamphetamine use	Developmental delays, attention and executive function deficits
Maternal stress during pregnancy	Developmental and behavioral difficulties
Viral infections	Mental retardation, learning disabilities
Hypoxic events	Cerebral palsy, cognitive deficits
Extremely low, very low and low birthweight (ELBW, VLBW, LBW)	Graded IQ and neuropsychological function; improvement with increasing birthweight
Peri- and intraventricular hemorrhage (PVH/IVH)	Motor, perceptual, cognitive deficits

primary biological rather than environmental basis for a child's failures in adaptation.

Perinatal risk factors (Table 25.1) are of particular importance, because maternal illness during pregnancy, exposure to teratogens during gestation, complications during delivery, and early environmental deficiencies can affect later neuropsychological functioning.

The early development of the child also deserves consideration, including language skills, gross- and fine-motor skills, attentional and behavioral functions, social interactions, eating and sleeping patterns, and development of hand preference, as delays in these domains are often precursors of later learning and behavior problems [35].

Medical History

A child's medical history often contains predictors of neuropsychological dysfunction, the most obvious being a documented brain abnormality or injury. Indeed, closed head injuries during childhood can compromise cognitive and behavioral functions, and seizure disorders are frequently associated with neuropsychological deficits.

Another critical piece of medical information is whether the child is taking any medications. All medications have the potential to affect a child's neuropsychological functioning, including their performance on tests of cognitive skills (Table 25.2). However, those that are especially likely to do so are certain anticonvulsant, stimulant, and psychotropic medications [36–38].

Family and Social History

Genetic variation, although intrinsically linked with environment in the eventual expression of any inherent biological risk, plays an important role in the etiology of learning problems. Consequently, information about a family's history of academic difficulties, psychiatric disorders, and neurological illness helps to indicate a potential biological foundation for later neuropsychological deficits [39].

A review of family history must also examine socioeconomic factors. Although there is not a direct

Table 25.2 Commonly used medications and their potential neuropsychological side effects.

Medication	Associated adverse effects
Stimulants (dextroamphetatime, methylphenidate, pemoline, amphetamine compounds)	Lowered seizure threshold, potential worsening of tics
Antipsychotics (clozapine, haloperidol, loxapine, thioridazine, thiothixene, olanzapine, risperidone)	Cognitive slowing from sedation, memory and attention difficulties
Anxiolytics (benzodiazepine class)	Learning-related memory difficulties
Anticonvulsants (phenobarbital, phenytoin primidone, valproate, zonisamide), especially polytherapy	Inattention, motor and cognitive slowing, and memory deficits

relationship, parental education and occupation help gauge the stimulation and learning opportunities that a child has received, which, in turn, help predict later childhood intellectual competence [40]. Indeed, socio-economic disadvantage is one of the primary risk factors for mental retardation [41].

Information regarding a child's social history is also informative. Questions regarding peer relationships and friendships are important in neuropsychological assessment because poor peer relationships are typical for children with various developmental and psychiatric disorders, and in some cases suggest nonverbal learning problems [42]. In other instances, problems with peer relationships may signal psychological stress and poor self-esteem related to academic difficulties.

Educational History

A complete school history includes information about a child's current grade placement, any grade repetitions or special education involvement, and school placement changes. Information about school history is typically elicited from parents or guardians, although school personnel are often contacted to validate parent reports and to obtain additional descriptions of a child's academic and behavioral difficulties at school. More specifically, teachers and other school personnel can provide information on a child's ability to meet educational and social demands and how the child compares to peers.

For children who have been evaluated for or received special educational services in the past, the timing of those services provides insights about the nature of the underlying learning problems [34]. In addition, the results of prior testing can be compared to the child's current test performance, providing evidence of change or stability in neuropsychological functioning.

Details of prior and current educational interventions, often delineated in Individualized Education Programs (IEPs) through formal special education or Section 504 Plans, are also valuable. They help to characterize not only the academic demands a child is expected to meet, but also the amount and type of intervention and/or support that has been provided. If prior services have been ineffective, information about other resources is needed to make practical recommendations.

Behavioral Observations

Behavioral observations of the child are a second source of information for the neuropsychologist, and an area that often does not receive the attention it deserves. Observations are important, not only in interpreting the results of neuropsychological testing, but also because they provide a more naturalistic measure of social, communicative, problem-solving, and sensorimotor skills. Behavioral domains to which neuropsychologists routinely attend include mood and affect; thought processes; motivation and cooperation; social interaction and pragmatics; attention and activity level; response style; speech, language, and communication; sensory and motor skills; and physical appearance.

The first two domains listed can enormously affect the entire assessment process. If children are upset, they are likely to be less motivated and cooperative. While lack of cooperation does not automatically invalidate the results of an assessment, it must be taken into account in interpreting findings. Even subtle disturbances in motivation or cooperation are noteworthy. Indeed, the child who is compliant and follows directions, but is generally unenthused and does not initiate many actions spontaneously, may be demonstrating "frontal" symptomatology (e.g., flattened affect, poor self-initiation of behavior, impaired planning/problem-solving) [43]. Conversely, a lack of enthusiasm or outright resistance to testing may suggest anxiety and avoidance characteristic of children with learning disabilities when they are presented with school-like tasks [44]. Notably, a developing body of research in child neuropsychology is beginning to clarify not only the effects of effort and motivation on the assessment process but also to provide insight into the larger issue of symptom validity [45–47].

Observations of social interactions are also useful. A child who is antagonistic with parents but more appropriate with the examiner may not be managed very effectively at home. Conversely, a child who is consistently oppositional may be experiencing a more generalized behavioral disturbance. Similarly, a child who is appropriate with his or her parents and other adults, but is socially awkward or even inappropriate with the examiner and peers, may have a more subtle learning problem or developmental disorder [48, 49].

The capacity to regulate attention and activity level deserves close observation. Indeed, observations of inattention and motor disinhibition during an evaluation provide important information regarding children's capacity to modulate their behavior under performance demands.

Similarly, a child's response style provides a wealth of information regarding potential neuropsychological deficits. Qualitatively different errors (e.g., naming difficulties, retrieval problems, perseveration), for instance, have been associated with different types of brain dysfunction [50]. In general, the rate and organization of responses provide insight about a child's cognitive deficits and use of compensatory strategies (Table 25.3).

Table 25.3 Response errors and potential attributions to brain regions.

Response error	Associated brain region
Perseveration, reduced verbal and nonverbal fluency, motor programming and problem-solving deficits	Dorsolateral prefrontal cortex
Confabulation, social disinhibition, impulsivity, emotional lability	Orbitofrontal cortex
Decreased spontaneity, stimulus-boundedness, apathy	Medial frontal cortex

Speech, language, and communication skills also deserve close observation. Language disturbances are presumed to cause many failures in acquisition of basic academic skills, such as reading and writing. Thus, neuropsychologists monitor numerous aspects of children's speech and language skills, including spontaneous conversation, language comprehension and expression, and the occurrence of more pathognomonic errors, such as anomia and paraphasia.

Nonverbal aspects of communication are also important to observe. These typically include pragmatics (e.g., eye contact, reciprocity, topic maintenance, and supposition), discourse skills, and appreciation of paralinguistic features such as intonation, prosody, gesture, and facial expression. Difficulties in these areas provide qualitative information about behavioral and communicative regulation, which often mirror reports from other sources about social interactions.

Disturbances in sensory and motor functioning are also noteworthy because they may interfere with the standardized administration of psychological tests, and because of the asserted but not consistently proven association between neurological "soft signs" and cognitive functioning [51]. Moreover, asymmetries in sensory and motor functions can often assist with the lateralization and localization of brain dysfunction and, thereby, provide support for the notion that a child's difficulties have a primary neurological basis.

The final category of observation is physical appearance. Some physical anomalies are indicative of genetic syndromes and acquired neurodevelopmental disorders, which may be associated with specific neuropsychological profiles [52–54]. However, dress and hygiene also deserve consideration, because deviation from the "norm" can suggest mild neuropsychological deficits, such as poor social awareness or adaptive behavior deficits.

Psychological Testing

Psychological testing is the third source of information about the child, and the one most often equated with neuropsychological assessment. Animated and contentious debate continues regarding the merits of standardized test batteries versus more flexible approaches to assessment. However, most child neuropsychologists administer a variety of tests that sample numerous cognitive domains. The administration of a comprehensive group of tests provides an accurate portrayal of a child's overall profile of functioning in the domains of general cognitive ability, verbal abilities, nonverbal abilities, learning and memory, attentional and executive functions, sensory and motor functions, academic skills, behavioral and emotional adjustment, and adaptive behavior.

As discussed earlier, these domains are assessed through review of a child's relevant history and through behavioral observations, as well as by formal testing. In the following sections, we give examples of measures, and briefly examine the rationale and limitations of measurement, in each domain.

General Cognitive Ability

General cognitive ability is typically assessed using intelligence tests. Intelligence tests are standardized measures that assess a variety of cognitive skills and provide an estimate of a child's overall cognitive functioning (Table 25.4). However, intelligence tests are not, as is often suggested, measures of innate learning potential. Indeed, intelligence tests fail to measure many important skills, and were designed primarily to predict academic achievement. Thus, intelligence tests are only one, albeit significant, piece of a neuropsychological assessment.

Verbal Abilities

The field of neuropsychology owes much to the early researchers of aphasia and other acquired language disorders. Indeed, when testing verbal abilities, neuropsychologists commonly draw from aphasia batteries. Tests of verbal abilities are relevant for neuropsychological assessment because language skills are significant contributors to academic success and social compe-

Table 25.4 Commonly used intelligence tests.

Test	Comments
Bayley Scales of Infant Development-Third Edition (BSID-III)	Commonly used preschool measure
Differential Ability Scales-Second Edition (DAS-II)	Preschool and school-aged versions
Kaufman Adolescent and Adult Intelligence Test (KAIT)	
Kaufman Assessment Battery for Children-Second Edition (KABC-II)	
Kaufman Brief Intelligence Test, Second Edition (KBIT-2)	Screening measure
Mullen Scales of Early Learning	Commonly used preschool measure
Stanford-Binet Intelligence Scales, Fifth Edition (SB-V)	Commonly used school-aged measure
Wechsler Preschool and Primary Scale of Intelligence-Third (WPPSI-III)	Commonly used preschool Edition measure
Wechsler Intelligence Scale for Children-Fourth Edition (WISC-IV)	Most widely used test for school-age children
Wechsler Adult Intelligence Scale-Fourth Edition (WAIS-IV)	Most widely used test for older adolescents and adults
Wechsler Abbreviated Scale of Intelligence (WASI)	Screening measure
Woodcock–Johnson Test of Cognitive Abilities, Third Edition (W-J III-Cognitive)	

tence. As with intelligence tests, however, performance on language measures often reflects skills in addition to those for which the procedures were designed. Indeed, many of the tests routinely employed by neuropsychologists are not "pure" measures of any one skill or ability; rather, they are typically multifactorial (Table 25.5). Consequently, the interpretation of language test performance must take into account performance in other domains.

Nonverbal Abilities

Tests of nonverbal abilities typically fall into two categories – those that draw on visuoperceptual abilities, and those that demand constructional skills and, hence, motor control and planning (Table 25.6). Assessment of nonverbal skills is important because nonverbal deficits are often associated with poor performance in certain academic skills, particularly arithmetic, as well as with a heightened risk for psychosocial maladjustment. In addition, nonverbal deficits are particularly common in children with acquired neurological insults, suggesting that nonverbal skills are especially vulnerable to brain damage in children. As with language tests, however, most tests of nonverbal abilities also draw on other skills. Consequently, test interpretation, again, requires an appreciation for a child's overall neuropsychological profile rather than

the tacit assumption that observed difficulties represent "nonverbal" deficits.

Learning and Memory

Learning and memory difficulties are a frequent cause of referral to child neuropsychologists. However, despite the importance of learning and memory for children's adaptation, and especially their school performance, it is only recently that there have been instruments available for assessing these skills (Table 25.7). Performance on tests of memory and learning, however, is multiply determined. Performance on tests of verbal memory, for example, is affected by children's language abilities and attentional functions. A further limitation of measurement in this domain is that current tests of children's learning and memory do not necessarily reflect recent advances in the neuroscience of memory [55–57].

Attentional and Executive Functions

From a neuropsychological perspective, attention is a multidimensional construct that overlaps with "executive" functions. Neuropsychological assessment of attention, therefore, usually involves evaluation of numerous aspects, such as sustained, selective, and divided attention; working memory, or the ability to

Table 25.5 Commonly used verbal tests.

Test	Comments
Boston Naming Test	Core aphasia screening measure
Clinical Evaluation of Language Fundamentals Preschool-Second Edition (CELF Preschool-2)	Comprehensive measure
Clinical Evaluation of Language Fundamentals-Fourth Edition (CELF-4)	Comprehensive school-age measure
Expressive One-Word Picture Vocabulary Test & Receptive One-Word Picture Vocabulary Test	
Halstead–Wepman Aphasia Screening Test	
NEPSY-Second Edition (NEPSY-II)	Assesses receptive and expressive domains
Peabody Picture Vocabulary Test, Fourth Edition (PPVT-IV)	Commonly used receptive language screen
Preschool Language Scales, Fifth Edition (PLS-5)	Comprehensive preschool measure
Rapid Automatized Naming Test	Helpful adjunct when assessing for dyslexia
Sentence Repetition Test	
Token Test for Children	
Word Fluency Test	Commonly used measures of retrieval

internalize verbal and nonverbal task sequencing; the ability to shift set; and cognitive efficiency.

Attention problems are among the more common reasons for referral to a child neuropsychologist, and are central to the diagnosis of attention-deficit hyperactivity disorder. Unfortunately, the relationship between formal tests of attention and the attentional behaviors about which parents and teachers complain is equivocal [58, 59]. Nevertheless, because attentional functioning moderates performance on many psychological tests, it will remain an important component of neuropsychological assessment (Table 25.8).

Executive functions are those involved in the planning, organization, regulation, and monitoring of goal-directed behavior [43, 60, 61], and play a critical role in determining a child's adaptive functioning. Indeed, executive function deficits are a hallmark of the child who demonstrates neuropsychological impairment, whether as a result of focal brain dysfunction or in association with developmental learning disorders.

Table 25.6 Commonly-used nonverbal tests.

Test	Comments
Benton Facial Recognition Test	
Clock Drawing	Measures planning and organization skills
Developmental Test of Visual-Motor Integration, Fifth Edition (VMI)	Commonly used constructional test
Hooper Visual Organization Test	
Judgment of Line Orientation Test	
Motor-Free Visual Perception Test-Third Edition (MVPT-III)	
NEPSY-II	Assesses visual perceptual and constructional skills
Rey–Osterrieth Complex Figure (ROCF)	Measures constructional, planning and organizational skills
Test of Nonverbal Intelligence, Fourth Edition (TONI-4)	
VMI-Tests of Visual Perception and Motor Coordination	
Wide Range Assessment of Visual Motor Abilities (WRAVMA)	Comprehensive measure of visual perceptual constructional skills

Table 25.7 Commonly-used learning and memory tests.

Test	Comments
Benton Visual Retention Test	
California Verbal Learning Test-Children's Version (CVLT-C)	Commonly used measure of verbal learning and memory
California Verbal Learning Test-Second Edition (CVLT-II)	Adult version of the CVLT
Children's Memory Scale (CMS)	Comprehensive measure of verbal/nonverbal memory
NEPSY	Screening of verbal and nonverbal memory
Rey–Osterrieth Complex Figure (ROCF)	Measure of nonverbal memory
Test of Memory and Learning, Second Edition (TOMAL-2)	Comprehensive measure of verbal and nonverbal memory
Verbal Selective Reminding Test (VSRT)	Commonly used measure of verbal learning and memory
Wechsler Memory Scale-Fourth Edition (WMS-IV)	Comprehensive older adolescent and adult measure of verbal/nonverbal memory
Wide Range Assessment of Learning and Memory, Second Edition (WRAML2)	Comprehensive measure of verbal/nonverbal memory

Although considerable research and theorizing has been devoted to clarifying the construct of executive function in children and to assessing its various dimensions, the exact nature of executive function remains uncertain [62–64]. This is due, in part, to the uncritical assumption that all skills subsumed under the executive function rubric are mediated by frontal brain systems, as well as to the paucity of studies demonstrating the dissociability of these various functions in the test setting and the subsequent ecological validity of purported measures of executive function [65, 66].

Table 25.8 Commonly used attention and executive function tests.

Test	Comments
Behavior Rating Inventory of Executive Function (BRIEF)	Parent, teacher, and self-report forms
Cancellation Tests	Measure of visual attention
Category Test	Commonly used measure of reasoning
Children's Paced Auditory Serial Attention Test (CHIPASAT)	
Consonant Trigrams	
Contingency Naming Test	
Delis–Kaplan Executive Function System (D-KEFS)	Comprehensive measure for children and adults
Fluency Tests	
Gordon Diagnostic System	Computerized measure of inhibition and attention
Matching Familiar Figures Test	
Rey–Osterrieth Complex Figure (ROCF)	Measure of planning and organization
Stroop-Color Word Test	
Test of Everyday Attention for Children (TEA-Ch)	Comprehensive measure of attentional functions
Test of Variables of Attention (TOVA)	Computerized measure of inhibition and attention
Tower of Hanoi	Measure of planning and problem-solving
Tower of London	Measure of planning and problem-solving
Trail Making Test	Measure of visuomotor scanning and psychomotor speed
Wisconsin Card Sorting Test (WCST)	Commonly used measure of problem-solving

Table 25.9 Commonly used sensorimotor tests.

Test	Comments
Sensory-Perceptual Examination	Commonly used series of measures for children and adults
Finger Sequencing	
Finger Tapping Test	Measure of simple motor speed
Fist-Edge-Palm Test	
Grip Strength Test	
Grooved Pegboard	Measure of motor speed and coordination
Hand Pronation-Supination Test	
Lateral Dominance Examination	
Purdue Pegboard	
Timed Motor Examination	Commonly used series of motor tests for 5–10-year-olds

Sensory and Motor Functions

Tests of sensory and motor functions usually involve standardized versions of various components of the traditional neurological examination (Table 25.9). Relevant sensory skills include sensory suppression, finger localization, graphesthesia, stereognosis, and left-right orientation, while those in the motor domain relate to speed and dexterity. In addition, tests of oculomotor control, motor overflow, alternating and repetitive movements, and other related skills are often used to assess "soft" neurological status.

Tests of sensory and motor functions are useful because they are sensitive to acute and chronic neurological disorders and can provide confirmatory evidence for localized brain dysfunction. Tests of sensory and motor functions also may help to predict learning problems in younger children and to differentiate older children with different types of learning disorders [67]. Unfortunately, especially for young children and those with significant behavioral/ emotional difficulties, the assessment of sensory and motor functions is often compromised by lapses in attention or motivation, and the results of sensory and motor testing do not always carry obvious implications for treatment.

Academic Skills

Academic underachievement is one of the most common reasons for a child to be referred for neuropsychological assessment. Hence, testing of academic skills is typically critical in understanding a child's academic functioning. Indeed, academic skill assessment offers information about the nature and severity of underachievement, provides evidence of specific learning disabilities, is often used to determine whether a child is eligible for special education services, and is helpful in developing specific academic remediation approaches (Table 25.10). However, achievement tests also suffer from the same multifactorial issues as many of the cognitive tests. Thus, knowledge of the specific task demands of any given achievement test is required to accurately interpret a child's performance beyond a standard score or grade equivalent.

Behavioral and Emotional Adjustment, and Adaptive Behavior

Children referred for neuropsychological assessment often demonstrate psychological distress, inappropriate behavior, or other deficits in adaptive functioning. The central goal of neuropsychological assessment is to promote overall adaptation, so assessment of behavioral and emotional adjustment, as well as of adaptive functioning, is crucial (Table 25.11). In this respect, formal ratings of behavior from parents and teachers are helpful in clarifying variations in behavioral comportment between and among settings [68]. Additionally, because awareness of deficits in adjustment and adaptive behavior can help to identify a mismatch between children's neuropsychological profiles and their environmental demands, self-reports of adjustment from children are also often helpful.

However, relationships between neuropsychological skills and adjustment problems or deficits in adaptive behavior are not always straightforward. Indeed, some premorbid behavioral characteristics (i.e., impulsivity, aggression, attention-seeking behavior) actually increase the risk of mild brain injury and associated neuropsychological deficits [69], and other behavioral difficulties or adaptive deficits may be a direct manifestation of a specific neuropsychological deficit [70].

Types of Assessment Compared

School psychologists, clinical psychologists, and child neuropsychologists employ similar measures when

Table 25.10 Commonly used academic achievement tests.

Test	Comments
Bracken Basic Concept Scale, Third Edition (BBCS-III)	Measure of academic readiness for preschoolers
Comprehensive Test of Phonological Processing (CTOPP)	Helpful adjunct when assessing for dyslexia
Kaufman Tests of Education Achievement, Second Edition (KTEA-II)	Comprehensive measure of academic skills
Key Math, Third Edition (KeyMath3)	Comprehensive measure of math skill
Nelson–Denny Reading Test (NDRT)	
Peabody Individual Achievement Test-Revised (PIAT-R)	Comprehensive measure of academic skills
Wechsler Individual Achievement Test-Third Edition (WIAT-III)	Comprehensive measure of academic skills
Wide Range Achievement Test-Revision 4 (WRAT-4)	Commonly used academic screener
Woodcock–Johnson Tests of Achievement-Third Edition (WJ-III)	Comprehensive measure of academic skills
Woodcock Reading Mastery Test-Revised (WRMT-R)	

evaluating behavior – that is, they use psychological and other tests to examine how a child is functioning in comparison to his or her age-mates. Thus, any of these providers could use an intelligence test, academic achievement test, or test of a child's behavioral and emotional adjustment. Despite this clear overlap in instrumentation, the services offered by each discipline are quite different.

Assessments conducted by school psychologists typically address eligibility for special education or other school-related services and focus on evaluating a child's functioning in relationship to academic expectations and success. Assessments conducted by clinical psychologists often focus on the psychological/emotional functioning of the child, though they can examine almost any aspect of the child's cognitive or behavioral status. However, school and clinical psychological assessments generally emphasize skills, functions, or psychological processes, without explicitly referencing brain structures or mechanisms.

Table 25.11 Commonly used behavioral/emotional adjustment and adaptive behavior tests.

Test	Comments
ADHD Rating Scale-IV	Symptom checklist
Behavior Assessment System for Children-Second Edition (BASC-2)	Comprehensive measure with parent, teacher, and self-report versions
Child Behavior Checklist (CBC)	Commonly used parent screener
Child Depression Inventory (CDI)	
Conners' Rating Scales-Revised (CRS-R)	
Personality Inventory for Children, Second Edition (PIC-2)	Comprehensive, parent-completed measure
Personality Inventory for Youth (PIY)	Comprehensive, self-report measure
Minnesota Multiphasic Personality Inventory-Adolescent (MMPI-A)	Comprehensive, self-report measure for adolescents
Revised Children's Manifest Anxiety Scales, Second Edition (RCMAS-2)	
Reynolds Adolescent Depression Scale, Second Edition (RADS-2)	
Scales of Independent Behavior-Revised (SIB-R)	Comprehensive measure of adaptive behavior
Teacher Report Form (TRF)	Commonly used teacher screener
Vineland Adaptive Behavior Scales, Second Edition (Vineland-II)	Comprehensive measure of adaptive behavior
Youth Self-Report (YSR)	Commonly used self-report screener

In contrast, since one focus of a *neuro*psychological assessment is to examine the integrity of various brain systems, these assessments comprehensively examine neurocognitive and neurobehavioral functioning, in addition to psychosocial adjustment and academic achievement. By definition, knowledge about brain-behavior relationships informs neuropsychological assessments. Thus, whether an assessment is neuropsychological in nature is *not* determined by the use of traditional "neuropsychological" tests. Rather, an assessment becomes neuropsychological when a properly trained child neuropsychologist invokes the developmental brain-behavior knowledge base, particularly as it relates to the child's context or environment, to evaluate, diagnose, and intervene with a particular child.

Childhood Neurological Disorders

The previous section delineated the various domains relevant to child neuropsychological assessment, the psychological tests used to assess them, and the differences among three types of child assessment. The relevant research provides a solid overview of the typical cognitive and behavioral sequelae associated with various neurological disorders in children; the following section highlights the neuropsychological outcomes associated with three of the more common, and commonly researched, neurological disorders.

Head Injury

Head injuries are a leading cause of death and disability in children and adolescents. Although estimates of the rate of such injuries vary from study to study, the average incidence across studies is approximately 180/100 000 [71]. However, most researchers agree that the precise estimate depends on the type and severity of the injury, in part because many children with milder head injuries and no obvious sequelae often do not receive much formal medical attention [72]. Moreover, children sustain traumatic brain injuries in various ways including bicycle accidents, sports-related injuries, motor vehicle accidents, falls, and child abuse, some of which may decrease the likelihood of the children receiving medical care.

Children sustain head injuries in a number of settings, with rates varying according to the chronological age of the child. Infants, toddlers, and young children sustain their head injuries primarily through falls, pedestrian versus motor vehicle accidents, bicycle versus motor vehicle accidents, and child abuse. By late childhood and adolescence, the leading causes of head injuries include motor vehicle and sports-related accidents.

Motor vehicle-related injuries are often the most severe and account for a high proportion of fatal injuries among pediatric cases.

Neuropsychological Outcomes in Head Injury

The neuropsychological outcomes of head injuries in children vary greatly. Among the most important variables in determining outcome, however, are the nature and severity of the injury, the age and premorbid functioning of the child who sustains the injury, and the environmental context to which the child returns after the injury [73–75].

In general, children who sustain head injuries demonstrate deficits in overall IQ [76, 77], and the magnitude of the decline is closely related to the severity of the injury. Although these children typically demonstrate significant recovery over time, their performance continues to be impaired relative to premorbid levels, particularly for children who sustain moderate to severe injuries. Long-term deficits are especially common on nonverbal subtests, presumably because they are novel and require speeded, motor performance. However, recent research indicates that performance on verbal subtests, which has traditionally been considered resistant to disruption because it involves retrieval of previously acquired knowledge and has minimal motor demands, is also likely to be impacted (Table 25.12).

Overt aphasic disorders are less common in children post-head injury, but more subtle difficulties do occur. Indeed, long-term deficits have been identified in such areas as object identification and description, sentence

Table 25.12 Neuropsychological outcome in closed head injury.

- Declines in measured intelligence, particularly in nonverbal domains and with increased injury severity
- Subtle but pervasive language deficits, including pragmatics and discourse
- Significant nonverbal deficits, especially on timed tasks and those with substantial organizational demands
- Attention problems, particularly regarding response modulation and reaction time
- Pervasive memory deficits, particularly regarding explicit memory and with increased injury severity
- Generalized executive dysfunction
- Academic difficulties, typically including grade retention and/or special education involvement
- Behavior and personality changes (e.g., increased irritability, impulsivity, aggression, and hyperactivity), and difficulties in personal/social adaptation

repetition, comprehension, and verbal fluency [78]. Additionally, deficits in language pragmatics and discourse are commonly observed. In contrast, long-term deficits in nonverbal skills are relatively frequent, and the deficits are especially pronounced on timed tasks involving fine motor skills but also extend to those tasks with substantial organizational demands [67].

Attention problems are common for children following head injury. Indeed, although there are very few studies that have comprehensively assessed attention based on current theoretical models, those that have been completed tend to show deficits on measures of continuous performance. Moreover, these deficits tend to reflect poor response modulation and slowed reaction time [73].

Memory deficits are also quite common in children following head injury, and the magnitude of the observed deficits is dependent upon the severity of the injury [79]. Many studies have identified deficits in verbal and nonverbal memory, using learning, selective reminding, recall, and recognition formats. Additionally, studies have also addressed the question of differences between explicit and implicit memory, indicating that implicit memory is much more resistant to disruption [73, 80, 81].

Deficits in executive functions are nearly ubiquitous following head injury in children. Unfortunately, research in this area has been less common, partly because measurement of complex reasoning and problem-solving skills is more difficult. However, research has demonstrated difficulties in planning, problem-solving, verbal fluency, concept formation, cognitive flexibility, and organization [82].

Given the numerous cognitive difficulties outlined above, it is not surprising that children who sustain head injuries often experience academic difficulties. Interestingly, although academic skills often initially return to premorbid levels, subsequent performance frequently suffers, with growing discrepancies between the children with head injuries and their peers. Indeed, the vast majority of children who sustain a severe brain injury either fail a grade or qualify for special education services by 2 years post-injury [83]. However, it is unclear whether the placement in special education services results from academic skills deficits or from behavioral disturbance and overall neuropsychological functioning.

Behavioral difficulties are a final area of difficulty for children who sustain head injuries. Post-head injury behavioral problems include changes in temperament, increased irritability, impulsivity, aggression, and hyperactivity, as well as difficulties in personal/social adaptation. Behavioral changes may occur even in cases of minor and mild head injury, but these tend to be transient and short-lived, although the insensitive nature of typical rating scales may account for some of the apparent lack of persistent symptomatology [84]. In general, severely head-injured children are at the greatest risk for long-term problems in social adjustment [79].

The behavioral difficulties demonstrated by children who sustain head injuries are not attributed exclusively to injury-related factors, though. Indeed, these children must also cope with significant psychological stress resulting from acute and potentially permanent changes in function, reactions of family members, and subsequent changes in family interaction patterns [61]. Additionally, the type of behavioral difficulties may differ according to the child's age at the time of injury and at subsequent times in the future. Just as age-related factors influence the expression of cognitive difficulties following head injuries in children, they also affect the expression of behavioral difficulties.

In general, outcome research following head injury suggests that children who sustain mild head injuries typically return to or approach premorbid levels of functioning. In contrast, children who sustain moderate to severe head injuries generally suffer significant, long-term cognitive and behavioral sequelae. Specifically, these children are at increased risk for overall intellectual difficulties, as well as nonverbal, memory, and executive function deficits. Behavioral changes are also common, and may be exacerbated depending on the nature of the injury, premorbid characteristics, and social-environmental supports.

Epilepsy

Epilepsy refers to the recurrent convulsive or nonconvulsive seizures caused by local or generalized epileptogenic discharges in the brain. The prevalence of epilepsy in the pediatric population has been estimated at between 4.3 and 9.3 per 1000 [36]. Seizures in infancy and childhood differ in many respects from those in adulthood. Most importantly, they occur far more frequently in individuals under the age of 15 than in adults, and are considered by some experts to be a "disorder of childhood" differing in type and etiology from the adult disorders. Indeed, at least 75% of all individuals with epilepsy develop their initial symptoms before the age of 20 [36].

Although trauma has been suggested as the primary identified cause of epilepsy, a full complement of pre-, peri-, and post-natal disorders have also been considered. Moreover, an underlying etiology for epilepsy is identified in only 30% of the cases [36], and includes structural brain anomalies, metabolic derangement,

Table 25.13 Neuropsychological outcome in epilepsy.

- Attention problems
- Language deficits, particularly when concomitant academic difficulties are present
- Inconsistent verbal and nonverbal memory deficits, generally related to lateralization of seizure activity
- Academic difficulties, commonly including grade retention and/or special education involvement
- Behavioral and adjustment difficulties (e.g., low self-esteem, depression and anxiety, and external locus of control), resulting from neurological and psychosocial sources

birth anoxia, cerebrovascular insults, and central nervous system infections and/or neoplasms.

Neuropsychological Outcomes in Epilepsy

Many factors influence the outcome of children with epilepsy, including the etiology of seizure activity, age of onset, degree of seizure control, and associated neurological abnormalities. Consequently, adaptive difficulties in cognitive and behavioral domains are often encountered in children with epilepsy (Table 25.13).

In general, the distribution of IQ scores in children with epilepsy is similar to that found in the general pediatric population. Although some epileptic syndromes are associated with poorer cognitive outcomes (i.e., Lennox–Gastaut syndrome, West's syndrome), most children with epilepsy perform within the average range of intelligence and do not differ from their siblings. Additionally, when IQ declines have been observed, medication toxicity has often been implicated [85, 86].

Although children with epilepsy typically have average levels of intellectual functioning, specific cognitive deficits may be present. Indeed, research findings consistently suggest a disruption of attentional functions in children with epilepsy [36]. Language skills have been identified as areas of difficulty, particularly when there are concomitant academic difficulties. Memory deficits have also been reported, but not as consistently as disruption of attentional functions [87, 88]. More specifically, verbal and nonverbal memory deficits have been documented depending on the lateralized nature of the seizure activity, although other researchers [89] have failed to demonstrate seizure focus-specific cognitive dysfunction.

Academic achievement difficulties are common in children with epilepsy. Indeed, children with epilepsy are twice as likely as are their peers to repeat a grade or qualify for special education services [90]. Moreover, Dodrill [91] reported that adults whose seizures contin-

ued from childhood experienced lowered educational and occupational outcomes.

Specific academic difficulties do not appear to be associated with seizure focus, however. Indeed, when academic skills are examined, difficulties have been observed in all general skill areas. The etiology of these difficulties has been difficult to determine, but appears to relate more to socioeconomic and cultural variables than to seizure-specific factors [36].

Behavioral difficulties are also present in many children with epilepsy. Indeed, children with epilepsy have higher rates of psychiatric difficulties than do children in the general population or those with chronic illness [92]. Both neurological and psychosocial factors appear to contribute to the increased risk for psychological difficulties. However, most authorities agree that behavioral difficulties result from brain dysfunction. Indeed, behavioral and emotional difficulties appear to be closely linked to cognitive deficits [89, 93].

Some studies have suggested that children with focal electroencephalogram (EEG) abnormalities and temporal lobe epilepsy demonstrate a higher rate of psychiatric disorder. However, the preponderance of research provides negligible empirical support for a specific behavioral syndrome, personality disorder, or increased aggression in individuals with temporal lobe epilepsy [36, 92].

In general, children with epilepsy are prone to lower self-esteem, increased episodes of depression and anxiety, and an external locus of control. These difficulties appear to stem from the confluence of several factors including underlying brain impairment, increased seizure frequency, and psychosocial sources. Additionally, family variables, sociocultural attitudes, and level of knowledge about epilepsy are critical determinants of overall psychological functioning [36, 94].

When considering the cognitive and behavioral difficulties experienced by children with epilepsy, consideration must be given to the impact of antiepileptic drug (AED) treatment. Although the effects of AEDs have been difficult to isolate, they seem to exert their effect on attention and concentration, memory functions, processing and motor speed, and behavioral and emotional regulation [36].

Carbamazepine has been associated with few cognitive side effects. Indeed, although carbamazepine in moderate dosage has been found to affect memory functions, it seems to have minimal effects on sustained attention [95]. Valproate also appears to have minimal cognitive side effects, although effects may be significantly associated with dose level. Additionally, the fewest behavioral side effects have been noted with carbamazepine and valproate.

Phenytoin appears to have the most detrimental cognitive side effects of the AEDs. Indeed, phenytoin may result in a progressive encephalopathy with deterioration of intellectual function, particularly in children with already poor intellectual functions or neurological abnormalities [96]. Interestingly, phenytoin does not appear to have significant behavioral side effects [96].

Studies of phenobarbital have been equivocal in terms of cognitive side effects. Short-term memory difficulties have been reported when comparing phenobarbital to valproate. In contrast, phenobarbital has consistently been associated with behavioral side effects such as hyperactivity, irritability, and sleep disturbances. Indeed, phenobarbital appears to exacerbate existing behavioral problems, particularly in children with lowered cognitive functions [36].

One consistent finding concerning AED effects is the negative impact of polytherapy compared to monotherapy on cognition and behavior, effects that appear to be independent of drug type. Specifically, monotherapy in children has been associated with improvements in both cognitive and behavioral functions [96]. However, consideration must also be given to the possibility that children who are on more than one AED have more intractable seizures and/or underlying brain pathology.

In general, AEDs may result in cognitive and behavioral side effects that are exacerbated by higher serum levels and by polypharmacy. However, a child's response to AEDs is highly individualistic and established therapeutic ranges may not insure maximum seizure control and minimum side effects.

Hydrocephalus and Myelomeningocele

Hydrocephalus involves an imbalance in the production and absorption of cerebrospinal fluid (CSF). When normal pathways are interrupted or impaired, a progressive accumulation of fluid results, which exerts pressure on surrounding brain structures. Hydrocephalus is often associated with myelodysplasias, which refer to any of several malformations of the spinal cord and meninges. Myelodysplasias can range from reasonably benign pilonidal cysts to severe cases of spina bifida cystica. Myelomeningocele is one type of spina bifida cystica, and occurs with a frequency ranging from 1 to 5 per 1000 live births [97].

Neuropsychological Outcomes in Hydrocephalus and Myelomeningocele

Many factors influence the outcome of children with hydrocephalus and myelomeningocele, including the etiology of the hydrocephalus, duration, severity, timing of initiation of treatment, shunt complications, and associated neurological abnormalities. Consequently, adaptive difficulties in cognitive and behavioral domains are often encountered by children with hydrocephalus.

In general, children with hydrocephalus, particularly those with concomitant motor difficulties, have lower overall IQ scores than their peers, although the bulk of this lowered score is accounted for by nonverbal difficulties. However, research conclusions reflect group results and, as suggested above, the simple presence of hydrocephalus does not predict an individual child's intellectual performance [96], and the performance of such children is actually more variable than that observed in their peers [98].

While frank language disorders are relatively uncommon in children with hydrocephalus (i.e., problems with syntax, lexicon, and phonology), the literature contains many references to clinical descriptions of "cocktail party" speech. However, this phenomenon of superficial and perseverative social speech patterns is more commonly seen in children with below-average intellectual abilities. More typically, children with hydrocephalus show deficits reflecting difficulties with higher-order inferential language, inference, and discourse [99], which appear to be relatively independent of the overall level of cognitive ability.

In addition to having problems with tasks found in nonverbal sections of intelligence tests, children with hydrocephalus may have particular difficulty with tasks involving visuoperceptual and constructional skills. Not surprisingly, there seems to be an association between intelligence and perceptual motor skills, with lower IQ scores associated with lower scores on visuomotor tasks. Recent research suggests that these difficulties are associated with not only the speed and motor demands but also the perceptual and organizational demands of such tasks [100].

Relatively few studies have specifically addressed memory functioning of children with hydrocephalus, despite the knowledge that an enlarging ventricular system may directly affect structures and pathways that subserve encoding and retrieval of information. Moreover, the handful of studies available has yielded equivocal findings regarding verbal and nonverbal memory deficits [81, 98]. This is due not only to the nature of memory demands (implicit vs explicit) embodied in the research tasks, but also to the multiple cognitive demands necessary to perform well on memory tasks. Indeed, children with hydrocephalus often have difficulty with verbal memory tasks because of the language demands, while perceptual, constructional, and organizational demands can interfere with performance on nonverbal memory tasks. In general, however, when difficulties are observed, they reflect problems with learning, organization of stimuli, and subsequent retrieval; [98, 101] although research suggests that the discrepancy between intact implicit memory and impaired explicit memory is critical to understanding memory functioning in children with congenital brain disorders [81].

Attentional and executive functions in children with hydrocephalus have been relatively unexamined. However, parents of children with shunted hydrocephalus commonly report problems pertaining to attention difficulties, distractibility, and concentration [101], as well as generalized executive dysfunction [102]. Moreover, more severe medical involvement is associated with more impairment of attentional functions [103]. These difficulties are similar to those found in children diagnosed with an attention-deficit hyperactivity disorder of the predominantly inattentive type.

Motor dysfunction is common in children with hydrocephalus, and this dysfunction typically affects fine and gross motor abilities. Fine motor problems may be expressed as difficulties with copying, handwriting, writing speed, or in fine-motor coordination, speed, and dexterity, while gross motor difficulties are often expressed in poor standing balance and gait abnormalities, independent of the level of spinal lesion in myelomeningocele. It is not surprising, therefore, that performance on cognitive measures that depend on visuomotor skills or on motor speed is frequently impaired in children with hydrocephalus [98].

Academic skills in children with hydrocephalus have been poorly researched. The few studies completed show a general pattern favoring basic language-based over mathematics skills. More specifically, word reading and decoding, as well as spelling skills, are typically intact, but reading comprehension, written expression, and mathematics skills are much more deficient [104].

The behavioral difficulties experienced by children with hydrocephalus have also been poorly chronicled. However, the completed studies suggest that the adjustment problems displayed by children with hydrocephalus are generally not as severe as those displayed by children referred for mental health services. Indeed, the majority of children with hydrocephalus are relatively well adjusted, at least according to parent ratings [105].

Although children with spina bifida do not display an extremely high rate of psychopathology or behavior problems, they are vulnerable to more subtle adjustment problems, such as declines in self-esteem. Indeed, research to date has shown that children with hydrocephalus are prone to symptoms of depression and anxiety [101, 106] and disruptive behavior problems, although treatment, family, and social-environmental factors are also contributory in the adjustment of these children, particularly during adolescence [107].

Hydrocephalus, with or without associated myelodysplasias, places a child at risk for a number of cognitive and behavioral difficulties. Cognitive deficits are most apparent in nonverbal, memory, and sensorimotor domains. However, higher-level language skills, as well as various aspects of attention and executive function, are also susceptible to disruption. Additionally, various behavioral and emotional difficulties are common in children with hydrocephalus. Indeed, limitations in functions and issues regarding body integrity and self-esteem are ever-present stresses for children with hydrocephalus.

Neuropsychological Management

As can be seen from the preceding section, there is no clear cognitive or behavioral phenotype for the neurologically impaired child. Indeed, neurologically impaired children demonstrate neuropsychological deficits consistent with the nature of their injury or disorder, which are further influenced by numerous factors, including the etiology, injury or disorder severity, age at onset, rapidity and efficacy of treatment, and associated medical complications. However, using the conceptual framework elucidated earlier, it is possible to develop a coherent management strategy that addresses the various cognitive, behavioral, academic, and social difficulties of these children. Indeed, from that conceptual framework, the historical assumption that neurologically impaired children suffer from "organic" difficulties that are not amenable to therapeutic intervention is unjustified [108].

The first step in the management process is to evaluate the relevant history, behavioral observations, and test results with reference to levels and patterns of performance. The second step involves determining relevant *diagnostic behavioral clusters* [21], which are groups of findings that, although not necessarily content- or domain-specific, are consistent with our knowledge of brain function in children and the nature of cognitive-behavioral relationships across development. For instance, delays in language acquisition, relative deficits in language and reading tests, configurational approaches on constructional tasks, and right-sided sensorimotor deficits, within the context of otherwise normal functioning, might be construed as implicating the left hemisphere, without assuming that there is any focal brain lesion or dysfunction. Thus, diagnostic behavioral clusters are defined in terms of presumed neural substrates, but are not assumed to reflect underlying brain damage (Table 25.14).

Table 25.14 Common diagnostic behavioral clusters.

Diagnostic behavioral cluster	Neuropsychological assessment results
Left-hemisphere cluster	Delays in language acquisition, deficits on language and reading tests, right-sided sensorimotor deficits, configurational approach on constructional tasks, otherwise normal functioning
Right-hemisphere cluster	Relative nonverbal deficits, part-oriented approach on constructional tasks, left-sided sensorimotor deficits, arithmetic deficits, social pragmatics and skills deficits
Frontal brain regions cluster	Behavioral dysregulation, expressive language and constructional deficits, problem-solving deficits, poor abstract reasoning, motor deficits

Treatment recommendations follow logically from this approach, with particular attention to risks for future difficulties, given an individual child's neuropsychological profile. However, the assessment of risks faced by a specific child takes into account not only the child's neuropsychological profile, but also the particular characteristics of the child's environment, including home, school, and community [109, 110]. In other words, recommendations for management arise from the integration of historical information, behavioral observations, and test results in light of the four general principles outlined earlier. Recommendations typically fall into three categories: remediation, accommodation, and compensation. The focus in remediation is to correct a child's weaknesses, while the focus in accommodation is to structure the environment and demands so that they are more consistent with a child's skill set. The focus in compensation is to develop self-awareness and management on the part of the child as they individually address their struggles, with an appreciation of their strengths and weaknesses. Consequently, interventions to address a child's specific neuropsychological profile are employed across a number of settings.

Educational interventions are paramount because of the impact of academic attainment on future outcomes. Although only limited empirical support exists for specific educational interventions, there is support for several general principles that can guide the development of an effective educational program. These principles typically address context- and content-specific issues, and relate to maximizing direct instructional time, providing structure and direction in the instructional process, individualizing instruction and teaching to mastery, promoting generalization and transfer of learning across settings, providing incentives contingent on performance, and teaching to all deficits [111].

In general, the more instruction children receive the better they achieve. Thus, children should be provided with as much instruction as possible, and classroom activities should be organized to maximize instructional time. Instructional time must not only be increased, though, but also be structured and directed for the child. Step-by-step and repeated presentations, modeling, and concrete aides are often helpful regardless of the content domain being taught; children typically learn more easily, if they can see it, touch it, or do it.

The application of such instructional techniques must be individualized to a particular child's needs. More specifically, instructional techniques should be applied with reference to a child's particular pattern of neuropsychological strengths and weaknesses. To accomplish this, instruction often needs to occur in one-to-one or small-group settings.

Interventions must also stress generalization and transfer of learning to new settings and subjects. Indeed, academic instruction is often incomplete, where students have to "fill in the blanks" themselves, largely based on conceptual understanding they have from related information. They may understand what is "taught" but have difficulty generalizing the new learning to different situations and content. Thus, helping such children with generalization and "brainstorming" of alternative solutions and approaches is often a critical component of their intervention plan. In turn, reinforcements and consequences that are tied directly and logically to academic subjects are useful in keeping such children motivated and in promoting progress.

The final general principle stresses the need to teach to all areas of deficit. More specifically, specialized educational programs must address as many of a child's difficulties as possible. Remedial programs emphasize development of basic academic skills, tutorial programs provide assistance in learning regular curriculum content, and compensatory approaches teach children how to manage or adapt to the curriculum independently.

This last principle raises two issues about treatment strategies for children with neurological impairments. The first issue, cognitive remediation or rehabilitation, typically arises in the context of acutely brain-injured individuals. In general, research findings have not supported the notion that cognitive rehabilitation across groups of brain-injured subjects can result in restoration, or remediation, of cognitive functions to their pre-injury status. However, there is support for interventions that address environmental accommodations and teach compensatory skills to individuals [111–114], an approach consistent with the conceptual framework espoused throughout this chapter.

The second issue, alternative therapies, such as auditory integration training and sensory integration therapy, arises most commonly in the context of children with various developmental or learning difficulties. However, given the cognitive and behavioral struggles experienced by children with neurological impairments, "fad" interventions are often quite alluring. Unfortunately, research findings continue to identify such therapies as not only unproven, but also ineffective, remedial treatment for learning disabilities and other disorders [114–118]. Neurofeedback has some preliminary evidence to support it as a potentially promising alternative therapy but the available research continues to suffer from significant methodological shortcomings [119].

Obviously, incorporating various academic interventions and modifications into a regular educational classroom may be difficult. Fortunately, special education services are available for children with neuropsychological impairments, assuming their difficulties are having an adverse academic affect and require specialized designed instruction. There are several different categories in the special education system; the names of the specific categories vary from state to state but effectively are the same. Additionally, there exists a continuum of services ranging from tutorial assistance in the regular education classroom to full-time special education placement in a separate school or facility. Debate persists regarding the optimal provision of special education services (i.e. "inclusion" programs in the regular education classroom vs "pull-out" programs in separate classrooms), as federal law mandates that children receive a free and appropriate public education in the least restrictive setting possible, often resulting in a trend toward more regular classroom and less special classroom education. However, the primary benefit of special education services for neurologically impaired children is the requirement of an Individualized Educational Program (IEP) that makes explicit the interventions to be utilized in instruction and how the efficacy of those interventions will be determined.

A Section 504 Plan, which is a regular education approach, is another education vehicle to provide academic accommodations for such children. This approach is often utilized when a specific child's difficulties are not felt to require the intensity or specificity of intervention generally associated with formal special education. However, the vast majority of Section 504 Plans are vague and loosely structured, often limiting their effectiveness for such children.

Social interventions are also imperative, considering the psychosocial risk factors for neurologically impaired children. These interventions are typically focused on specific child difficulties, as well as relevant family issues. Behavior management interventions are the most common approaches, and allow for consistency between different environments (i.e. home and school). Indeed, such children typically benefit from classrooms and home environments that incorporate clear, brief, and more visible and external modes of presentation of behavioral requirements than is required for their peers. Consequences must also be more swift, immediate, frequent, and consistent than is necessary for their peers. Similarly, more frequently changing or rotating reinforcers or rewards helps maintain their salience and reward-generating qualities. Finally, incentives or motivators must be present (i.e., "rewarding early and often") before punishment can be implemented, because such children typically respond less robustly to response cost measures or time-out if the availability of reinforcement is relatively low. Indeed, such children typically behave least appropriately in settings in which the opportunity for reinforcement is low or when the reinforcement-consequence ratio weighs heavily in the direction of consequences.

In many cases, neurologically impaired children present with psychosocial difficulties resulting from numerous factors. Moreover, family members of neurologically impaired children often suffer significant grief and loss as they confront the reality of adaptive changes in their child, and as they navigate the ongoing recovery and/or developmental process [120–123]. Consequently, individual, group, and family therapies are important because they help individuals and families become more active participants in their ongoing adjustment. These approaches also help family members become appropriate in their expectations, as well as become active advocates for their child.

Psychopharmacological medications are another worthy intervention. However, such interventions with neurologically impaired children have been woefully underinvestigated. The available research has often been methodologically poor in quality, making the studies difficult to interpret; single-case reports and non-blind trials do not yield sufficient information for informed psychopharmacological interventions. Moreover, these studies have suffered from numerous methodological flaws including reporting bias, poor reliability of testing, retrospective and anecdotal reports, and the concurrent use of other psychotropic medications.

With these concerns in mind, several research models for assessing the efficacy of psychopharmacological interventions have been proposed, and seem to share several common features. These include the use of placebo controls and double-blind methodology, randomization of dose order across subjects, inclusion of multiple assessment measures, collection of assessment data when medication effects are most prominent, and evaluation of side effects during medication and non-medication conditions [124]. Additionally, Phelps and her colleagues provided a model approach for collaborative medication management, which details assessment of behavioral and emotional problems, identification of treatment goals, selection of empirically supported interventions, assessment of readiness for change, development and interpretation of medication-monitoring protocols, and coordination of the intervention team [125]. Such an approach would allow the comprehensive evaluation of medication effects on relevant symptomatology, while minimizing side effects on cognitive and behavioral functioning.

A final area of intervention is the ongoing education of families of neurologically impaired children. Over the past few decades, numerous agencies and organizations have been established to advocate on behalf of children with cognitive, academic, and behavioral difficulties. Moreover, the resources provided by these organizations often help families identify and marshal the diverse resources highlighted above (see Appendix 25.1).

Summary

The present chapter has provided an overview of the neuropsychological assessment of children, focusing on children with various forms of neurological impairment. The historical context of neuropsychological assessment in children bears consideration, as advances in related disciplines have spurred ongoing progress in the articulation of conceptual principles for neuropsychological assessment.

The model for child neuropsychological assessment espoused in this chapter considers adaptation, brain-behavior, context, and development to be dynamic factors that differentially influence any given child. Additionally, the relative importance of these factors changes over time, necessitating a developmental perspective to child neuropsychological assessment. Not surprisingly, child neuropsychological assessment has its roots in developmental neuroscience and developmental psychology. Consequently, contributions from those disciplines will forge clearer pictures of brain-behavior relationships in children and set the stage for clearer determinations of the ecological validity of neuropsychological assessment across adaptive areas [126–128].

As stated previously, there is no phenotype for neurologically impaired children, largely because of the myriad factors that influence outcome, although an outcome algorithm offered by Maureen Dennis may help in characterizing the unique influence of these various factors [17]. Head injuries, seizure disorders, and hydrocephalus are only three of the neurological conditions common in children. However, they serve to highlight the various cognitive and behavioral deficits associated with neurological impairment, and also make the case for considering specific injury- and disorder-related variables in the neuropsychological management of neurologically impaired children.

When neuropsychological management is viewed from the aforementioned contextual model, intervention techniques are logical extensions of specific diagnostic behavioral clusters. Indeed, they are developed with respect to the specific neuropsychological profile of a child, as well as with attention to relevant environmental demands, all in the context of development. In the future, however, clinicians and researchers will need to consider more closely the factors that influence success and failure of specific interventions. Examination of these factors will allow a more precise determination of their efficacy, as well as facilitate the application of interventions across groups of neurologically impaired children.

Appendix 25.1   Advocacy Organizations for Children and Their Families

Brain Injury Association of America: (800) 444-6443, www.biausa.org

The Spina Bifida Association of America: (800) 621-3141, www.sbaa.org

The Epilepsy Foundation of America: (800) 332-1000, www.epilepsyfoundation.org

Children and Adults with Attention Deficit/Hyperactivity Disorder (CHADD): (301) 306-7070, www.chadd.org

The Learning Disabilities Association of America (LDA): (412) 341-1515, www.ldanatl.org

LD Online: www.ldonline.org

Council for Learning Disabilities: (913-491-1011), http://www.cldinternational.org

International Dyslexia Association: (410) 296-0232, www.interdys.org

National Dissemination Center for Children with Disabilities (NICHCY): (800) 695-0285, www.nichcy.org

References

1. Schwaab DF. Relation between maturation of neuro-transmitter systems in the human brain and psychosocial disorders. In: Rutter M, Casaer P(eds) *Biological Risk Factors for Psychosocial Disorders*. Cambridge, UK: Cambridge University Press, 1991; pp. 50–66.

2. Bjorklund A, Hokfelt T, Tohyama M. *Handbook of Chemical Neuroanatomy*. Elsevier Science Publishers, 1992.

3. Nemeroff CB. Fostering foster care outcomes: Quality of intervention matters in overcoming early adversity. *Arch Gen Psychiatry* 2008;**65**:623–624.

4. Anderson V, Bond L, Catroppa C, Grimwood K, Keird E, Nolan T. Childhood bacterial meningitis: Impact of age at illness and acute medical complications on long term outcome. *J Int Neuropsychol Soc* 1997;**3**:147–158.

5. Fletcher JM, Dennis M. *Spina bifida and hydrocephalus*. In: Yeates KO,Ris MD,Taylor HG, Pennington BF (eds) *Pediatric Neuropsychology: Research, Theory, and Practice*, 2nd edn. New York: Guilford Press, 2010; pp. 3–25.

6. Shaywitz SE, Shaywitz BA. Paying attention to reading: The neurobiology of reading and dyslexia. *Dev Psychopathol* 2008;**20**:1329–1349.

7. Lange N, Froimowitz MP, Bigler ED, Lainhart JE. Associations between IQ, total and regional brain volumes, and demography in a large normative sample of healthy children and adolescents. *Dev Neuropsychol* 2010;**35**:296–317.

8. Giedd JN, Blumenthal J, Jeffries NO, *et al.* Brain development during childhood and adolescence: A longitudinal MRI study. *Nat Neurosci* 1999;**2**:861–863.

9. Aylward GP. Neurodevelopmental outcomes of infants born prematurely. *J Dev Behav Pediatrics* 2005;**26**:427–440.

10. Stanford LD, Dorflinger JM. Pediatric brain injury: Mechanisms and amelioration.In:ReynoldsCR,Fletcher-Janzen E (eds) *Handbook of Clinical Child Neuropsychology*, 3rd edn. New York: Springer Science, 2009; pp. 169–186.

11. Howlader N, Noone AM, Krapcho M, *et al.* (eds). *SEER Cancer Statistics Review*. Available at: http://seer.cancer.gov/csr/1975_2008/.

12. Benton AL. Foreword. In: Yeates KO,RisMD, Taylor HG (eds) *Pediatric Neuropsychology: Research, Theory, and Practice*. New York: Guilford Press, 2000; p. XV.

13. Head H. *Aphasia and Kindred Disorders of Speech*. New York: Macmillan, 1926.

14. Strauss AA, Lehtinen L. *Psychopathology and Education of the Brain-Injured Child*. New York: Grune & Stratton, 1947.

15. Strauss AA, Werner H. The mental organization of the brain–injured mentally defective child. *Am J Psychiatry* 1941;**97**:1194–1203.

16. Taylor HG. MBD: Meaning and misconceptions. *J Clin Neuropsychol* 1983;**5**:271–287.

17. Dennis M. Childhood medical disorders and cognitive impairment: Biological risk, time, development, and reserve. In: Yeates KO,Ris MD, Taylor HG (eds) *Pediatric Neuropsychology: Research, Theory, and Practice* New York: Guilford Press, 2000; pp. 3–24.

18. Dennis M, Barnes M. Developmental aspects of neuropsychology: Childhood. In: Zaidel D (ed.) *Handbook of Perception and Cognition*. New York: Academic Press, 1994; pp. 219–246.

19. Waber DP, de Moor C, Forbes PW, *et al.* The NIH MRI study of normal brain development: Performance of a population based sample of healthy children aged 6 to 18 years on a neuropsychological battery. *J Int Neuropsychol Soc (Special issue: Reviews)* 2007;**13**:729–746.

20. Waber DP. *Rethinking Learning Disabilities: Understanding Children who Struggle in School*. New York: Guilford Press, 2010.

21. Bernstein JH, Waber DP. Developmental neuropsychological assessment: The systemic approach. In: Boulton AA,Baker GB, Hiscock M (eds) *Neuromethods: Vol. 17, Neuropsychology*. New York: Humana Press, 1990; pp. 311–371.

22. Taylor HG, Fletcher JM. Neuropsychological assessment of children. In: Goldstein G, Hersen M(eds) *Handbook of Psychological Assessment*, 2nd edn. New York: Pergamon Press, 1990.

23. Rourke BP, Bakker DJ, Fisk JL, Strang JD. *Child Neuropsychology: An Introduction to Theory, Research, and Clinical Practice*. New York: Guilford Press, 1983.

24. Anderson V, Northam E, Hendy J, Wrennall J. *Developmental Neuropsychology: A Clinical Approach*. Hove, UK: Psychology Press, 2001.

25. Baron IS. *Neuropsychological Evaluation of the Child*. New York: OxfordUniversity Press, 2004.

26. Hebb DO. *The Organization of Behavior: A Neuropsychological Theory*. New York: John Wiley& Sons, Ltd, 1949.

27. Kluver H. *Behavior Mechanisms in Monkey*. Chicago: University of Chicago Press, 1957.

28. Hannay HJ, Bieliauskas L, Crosson BA, Hammeke TA, Hamsher K deS, Koffler S (eds). Proceedings of the Houston Conference on Specialty Education and Training in Clinical Neuropsychology. *Arch Clin Neuropsychol* 1998;**13**:157–250.

29. Yeates KO, Taylor HG. Neuropsychological assessment of older children. In: Goldstein G,Nussbaum P, Beers SR (eds) *Handbook of Human Brain Function: Vol III, Neuropsychology*. New York: Plenum Press, 1998; pp. 35–61.

30. Cummings JL. Frontal-subcortical circuits and human behavior. *Arch Neurology* 1993;**50**:873–880.

31. Middleton FA, Strick PL. Revised neuroanatomy of frontal-subcortical circuits. In: Lichter DG, Cummings JL (eds) *Frontal-Subcortical Circuits in Psychiatric and Neurological Disorders*. New York: Guilford Press, 2001; pp. 44–58.

32. Derryberry D, Tucker DM. Neural mechanisms of emotion. *J Clin Consult Psychol* 1992;**60**:329–338.

33. Nowakowski RS. Basic concepts of CNS development. *Child Dev* 1987;**58**:568–595.

34. Holmes JM. Finding common ground to promote dialogue and collaboration: Using case material to jointly observe children's behavior. In:Fischer KW, Bernstein JH, Immordino-Yang MH (eds) *Mind, Brain, and Education in Reading Disorders*. New York: Cambridge University Press, 2007; pp. 181–195.

35. Satz P, Taylor HG, Friel J, Fletcher JM. Some developmental and predictive precursors of reading disabilities: A six year follow-up. In: Benson AL,PearlD(eds) *Dyslexia: An Appraisal of Current Knowledge*. New York: OxfordUniversity Press, 1978; pp. 313–347.

36. Westerveld M. Childhood epilepsy. In: Yeates KO, Ris MD, Taylor HG, Pennington BF (eds) *Pediatric Neuropsycholo-*

gy: *Research, Theory, and Practice*, 2nd edn. New York: Guilford Press, 2010; pp. 71–91.

37. Brown RT, Daly BP. Neuropsychological effects of stimulant medication on children's learning and behavior. In: Reynolds CR, Fletcher-Janzen E(eds) *Handbook of Clinical Child Neuropsychology*, 3rd edn.New York: Plenum Press, 2009; pp. 529–580.

38. Cepeda ML. Nonstimulant psychotropic medication: Desired effects and cognitive events. In: Reynolds CR, Fletcher-Janzen E (eds) *Handbook of Clinical Child Neuropsychology*, 3rd edn. New York: Plenum Press, 2009; pp. 581–598.

39. Rutter M, Silberg JL, O'Connor TG, Simonoff E. Genetics and child psychiatry: II. Empirical research findings. *J Child Psychol Psychiatry* 1999;**40**:19–55.

40. Yeates KO, MacPhee D, Campbell FA, Ramey CT. Maternal IQ and home environment as determinants of early childhood intellectual competence: A developmental analysis. *Dev Psychology* 1983;**19**:731–739.

41. Duyme M, Dumaret AC, Tomkiewicz S. How can we boost IQs of "dull children"? A late adoption study. *Proc Natl Acad Sci USA* 1999;**96**:8790–8794.

42. Rourke BP. Introduction: The NLD syndrome and the white matter model. In: Rourke BP (ed.) *The Syndrome of Nonverbal Learning Disabilities: Neurodevelopmental Manifestations.*New York:Guilford Press,1995;pp.1–26.

43. Goldberg E. *The Executive Brain.* New York: Oxford University Press, 2002.

44. Spreen O. The relationship between learning disability, emotional disorders, and neuropsychology: Some results and observations. *J Clin ExpNeuropsychol* 1989;**11**:117.

45. Blaskewitz N, Merten T, Kathmann N. Performance of children on symptom validity tests: TOMM, MSVT, and FIT. *Arch Clin Neuropsychol* 2008;**23**:379–391

46. Donders, J. Performance on the Test of Memory Malingering in a mixed pediatric sample. *Child Neuropsychol* 2005;**11**:221–227.

47. Heilbronner RL, Sweet JJ, Morgan JE, Larrabee GJ, Millis SR. American Academy of Clinical Neuropsychology Consensus Conference Statement on the neuropsychological assessment of effort, response bias, and malingering. *Clin Neuropsychol* 2009;**23**:1093–1129.

48. Rourke BP, Tsatsanis KD. Nonverbal learning disabilities and Asperger syndrome. In: Klin A,Volkmar FR, Sparrow SS (eds) *Asperger Syndrome.* New York: Guilford Press, 2000; 231–253.

49. Ozonoff S. Autism spectrum disorders. In: YeatesKO, Ris MD,Taylor HG, Pennington BF (eds) *Pediatric Neuropsychology: Research, Theory, and Practice,* 2nd edn. New York: Guilford Press, 2010; pp. 418–446.

50. Kaplan E. A process approach to neuropsychological assessment. In: Boll T, Bryant BK (eds) *Clinical Neuropsychology and Brain Function: Research, Measurement, and Practice.* Washington, DC: American Psychological Association, 1988; pp. 125–168.

51. Shaffer D, O'Connor PA, Shafer SQ, Prupis S. Neurological "soft signs": Their origins and significance. In: Rutter M (ed.) *Developmental Neuropsychiatry.* New York: Guilford Press, 1983; pp. 144–163.

52. White BJ. The Turner syndrome: Origin, cytogenetic variants, and factors influencing the phenotype. In: Broman SH, Grafman J (eds) *Atypical Cognitive Deficits in Developmental Disorders: Implications for Brain Function* Hillsdale, NJ: Erlbaum, 1994; pp. 183–195.

53. Fuerst KB, Dool CB, Rourke BP. Velocardiofacial syndrome. In: Rourke BP (ed.) *The Syndrome of Nonverbal Learning Disabilities: Neurodevelopmental Manifestations.* New York: Guilford Press, 1995; pp. 119–137.

54. Mattson SN, Vaurio L. Fetal alcohol spectrum disorders. In: Yeates KO,Ris MD,Taylor HG, Pennington BF (eds) *Pediatric Neuropsychology: Research, Theory, and Practice,* 2nd edn. New York: Guilford Press, 2010; pp. 265–296.

55. Nelson CA. The ontogeny of human memory: A cognitive neuroscience perspective. *Dev Psychology* 1995;**31**: 723–738.

56. Butters N, Delis DC. Clinical assessment of memory disorders in amnesia and dementia. *Ann Rev Psychology* 1995;**46**:493–523.

57. Cowan NC, Hulme C. *The Development of Memory in Childhood.* Hove, East Sussex: Psychology Press, 1997.

58. Barkley RA. The ecological validity of laboratory and analogue assessment methods of ADHD symptoms. *J Abnorm Child Psychol* 1991;**19**:149–178.

59. Teicher MH, Polcari A, McGreenery CE.Utility of objective measures of activity and attention in the assessment of therapeutic response to stimulants in children with attention-deficit/hyperactivity disorder. *J Child Adolesc Psychopharmacol* 2008;**18**:265–270.

60. Denckla MB. Measurement of executive function. In: Lyon GR (ed.) *Frames of Reference for the Assessment of Learning Disabilities.* Baltimore: Paul H. Brookes Publishing, 1994; pp. 117–142.

61. Stuss DT, Benson DF. *The Frontal Lobes.* New York: Raven Press, 1986.

62. Lezak M. *Neuropsychological Assessment,* 3rd edn. New York: Oxford University Press, 1995.

63. Nigg JT. On inhibition/disinhibition in developmental psychopathology: Views from cognitive and personality psychology and a working inhibition taxonomy. *Psychol Bull* 2000;**126**:220–246.

64. Bernstein JH,Waber DP. Executive capacities from a developmental perspective. In:MeltzerL (ed.) *Executive Function in Education: From Theory to Practice.* New York: Guilford Press, 2007; pp. 39–54.

65. Archibald S, Kerns KA. Identification and description of new tests of executive functioning in children. *Child Neuropsychol* 1999;**5**:115–129.

66. Gioia GA, Isquith PK. Ecological assessment of executive function in traumatic brain injury. *Dev Neuropsychol* 2004;**25**:135–158.

67. Casey JE, Rourke BP. Disorders of somatosensory perception in children. In: Rapin I, Segalowitz SJ (eds) *Handbook of Neuropsychology, Vol. 6: Child Neuropsychology.* Amsterdam: Elsevier Science Publishers, 1992; pp. 477–494.

68. Achenbach TM. Commentary: Definitely more than measurement errors: But how should we understand and deal with informant discrepancies? *J Clin Child Adolesc Psychol* 2011;**40**:80–86.

69. Rutter M, Chadwick O, Shaffer D. Head injury. In: Rutter M (ed.) *Developmental Neuropsychiatry.* New York: Guilford Press, 1983; pp. 83–111.

70. Rourke BP, Fuerst DR. *Learning Disabilities and Psychosocial Functioning.* New York: Guilford Press, 1991.

71. Kraus JF. Epidemiological features of brain injury in children: Occurrence, children at risk, causes and manner of injury, severity, and outcomes. In: Broman SH,

Michel ME (eds) *Traumatic Head Injury in Children*. New York: Oxford University Press, 1995; pp. 55–69.

72. Bowman SM, Bird TM, Aitken ME, Tilford JM. Trends inhospitalizations associated with pediatric traumatic brain injuries. *Pediatrics* 2008;**122**:988–993.

73. Yeates KO. Traumatic brain injury. In:Yeates KO, Ris MD, Taylor HG, Pennington BF (eds) *Pediatric Neuropsychology: Research, Theory, and Practice*, 2nd edn. New York: Guilford Press, 2010; pp.112–146.

74. Taylor HG, Yeates KO, Wade SL, Drotar D, Stancin T, Burant C. Bidirectional child-family influences on outcome of traumatic brain injury in children. *J Int Neuropsychol Soc* 2001;**7**:755–767.

75. Stancin T, Wade SL, Walz NC, Yeates KO, Taylor HG. Familyadaptation18monthsaftertraumaticbraininjuryin early childhood. *J Dev Behav Pediatrics* 2010;**31**:317–325.

76. Anderson VA, Catroppa C, Rosenfeld J, Haritou F, Morse SA. Recovery of memory function following traumatic brain injury in pre-school children. *Brain Injury* 2000;14:679–692.

77. Catroppa C, Anderson VA. Recovery in memory function in the first year following TBI in children. *Brain Injury* 2002;**16**:369–385.

78. Ewing-Cobbs L, Levin HS, Eisenberg HM, Fletcher JM. Language functions following closed-head injury in children and adolescents. *J Clin Exp Neuropsychol* 1987;**9**:575–592.

79. Donders J. Traumatic brain injury. In: Farmer JE, Donders J, Warschausky S (eds) *Treating Neurodevelopmental Disabilities: Clinical Research and Practice*. New York: Guilford Press, 2006; pp. 23–41.

80. Yeates KO, Blumenstein E, Patterson CM, Delis DC. Verbal learning and memory following pediatric closed-head injury. *J Int Neuropsychol Soc* 1995;**1**:78–87.

81. Yeates KO, Enrile BG. Implicit memory in children with congenital and acquired brain disorder. *Neuropsychology* 2005;**19**:618–628.

82. Mangeot S, Armstrong K, Colvin AN, Yeates KO, Taylor HG. Long-term executive function deficits in children with traumatic brain injuries: Assessment using the Behavior Rating Inventory of Executive Function (BRIEF). *Child Neuropsychol* 2002;**8**:271–284.

83. Miller LJ, Donders J. Prediction of educational outcome after pediatric traumatic brain injury. *Rehabil Psychol* 2003;**48**:237–241.

84. Yeates KO. Mild traumatic brain injury and postconcussive symptoms in children and adolescents. *J Int Neuropsychol Soc* 2010;**16**:953–960.

85. Corbett JA, Trimble MR,Nichol TC. Behavioral and cognitive impairments in children with epilepsy: The long-term effects of anticonvulsant therapy. *J Am Acad Child Psychiatry* 1985;**24**:17–23.

86. Agarwal NB, Agarwal NK, Mediratta PK, Sharma KK. Effect of lamotrigine, oxcarbazepine and topiramate on cognitive functions and oxidative stress in PTZ-kindled mice. *Seizure* 2011;20:257–262.

87. Dunn DW, Johnson CS, Perkins SM,*et al*. Academic problems in children with seizures: Relationships with neuropsychological functioning and family variables during the 3 years after onset. *Epilepsy Behav* 2010;**19**:455–461.

88. Conant LL, Wilfong A, Inglese C, Schwarte A. Dysfunction of executive and related processes in childhood absence epilepsy. *Epilepsy Behav* 2010;**18**:414–423.

89. Camfield PR, Gates R, Ronen G, *et al*. Comparison of cognitive ability, personality profile, and school success in epileptic children with pure right versus left temporal lobe EEG foci. *Ann Neurol* 1984;**15**:122–126.

90. Dodson WE. Epilepsy and IQ. In: Dodson WE, Pellock JM (eds) *Pediatric Epilepsy: Diagnosis and Therapy*. New York: Demos, 1993; pp. 373–385.

91. Dodrill CB. Neuropsychological aspects of epilepsy. *Psychiat Clin N Am* 1992;**15**:383–394.

92. Gonzalez-Heydrich J, Dodds A, Whitney J, *et al*. Psychiatric disorders and behavioral characteristics of pediatric patients with both epilepsy and attention-deficit hyperactivity disorder. *Epilepsy Behav* 2007;**10**:384–388.

93. Austin JK, Fastenau PS. Are seizure variables related to cognitive and behavior problems? *Dev Med Child Neurol* 2010;**52**:5–6.

94. Austin JK, Caplan R. Behavioral and psychiatric comorbidities in pediatric epilepsy: Toward an integrative model. *Epilepsia* 2007;**48**:1639–1651.

95. Forsythe I, Butler R, Berg I, McQuire R. Cognitive impairment in new cases of epilepsy randomly assigned to carbamazepine, phenytoin, and sodium valproate. *Dev Med Child Neurol* 1991;**33**:524–534.

96. Glauser TA. Behavioral and psychiatric adverse events associated with antiepileptic drugs commonly used in pediatric patients. *J Child Neurol* 2004;**19**:S25–S38

97. Fishman MA. *Pediatric Neurology*. Orlando, FL: Grune & Stratton, 1986.

98. Fletcher JM, Dennis M. Spina bifida and hydrocephalus. In: Yeates KO, Ris MD, Taylor HG, Pennington BF (eds) *Pediatric Neuropsychology: Research, Theory, and Practice*, 2nd edn. New York: Guilford Press, 2010; pp. 3–25.

99. Dennis M, Jacennik B, Barnes MA. The content of narrative discourse in children and adolescents after early onset hydrocephalus and in normally developing age peers. *Brain Lang* 1994;**46**:129–165.

100. Yeates KO, Loss N, Colvin AN, Enrile BG. Do children with myelomeningocele and hydrocephalus display nonverbal learning disabilities? An empirical approach to classification. *J Int Neuropsychol Soc* 2003;**9**:653–662.

101. Yeates KO, Fletcher JM, Dennis M.. Spina bifida and hydrocephalus. In: Morgan JE, Ricker JH (eds) *Comprehensive Textbook of Clinical Neuropsychology*. Lisse, The Netherlands: Swets & Zeitlinger, 2008; pp. 128–148.

102. Mahone EM, Zabel TA, Levey E, Verda M, Kinsman S. Parent and self-report ratings of executive function in adolescents with myelomeningocele and hydrocephalus. *Child Neuropsychol* 2002;**8**:258–270.

103. Loss N, Yeates KO, Enrile B. Attention in children with myelomeningocele. *Child Neuropsychol* 1998;**4**:7–20.

104. Barnes MA,Dennis M. Reading in children and adolescents after early hydrocephalus and in normally developing age peers: Phonological analysis, word recognition, word comprehension, and passage comprehension skill. *J Pediatr Psychol* 1992;**17**:445–465.

105. Donders J, Rourke BP, Canady AI. Emotional adjustment of children with hydrocephalus and their parents. *J Child Neurol* 1992;**7**:375–380.

106. Helder EJ, Austria E, Lacy M, Frim DM. Behavioral outcome in congenital shunted hydrocephalus without spina bifida. *J Pediatric Neurol* 2011;**9**:41–47.

107. Holler KA, Fennell EB, Crosson B, Boggs SR, Mickle JP. Neuropsychological and adaptive functioning in younger

versus older children shunted for early hydrocephalus. *Child Neuropsychol* 1995;**1**:63–73.

108. Belsky J, Pluess M. Beyond diathesis stress: Differential susceptibility to environmental influences. *Psychol Bull* 2009;**135**:885–908.

109. Kanne SM, Grissom MO, Farmer JE. Interventions for children with neuropsychological deficits. In: Yeates KO, Ris MD, Taylor HG, Pennington BF (eds) *Pediatric Neuropsychology: Research, Theory, and Practice,* 2nd edn. New York: Guilford Press, 2010; pp. 499–520.

110. Farmer JE, Drewel EH. Systems interventions for comprehensive care. In: Farmer JE, Donders J, Warschausky S (eds) *Treating Neurodevelopmental Disabilities: Clinical Research and Practice.* New York: Guilford Press, 2006; pp. 269–288.

111. Taylor HG. Learning disabilities. In: Mash EJ, Terdal LG (eds) *Behavioral Assessment of Childhood Disorders,* 2nd edn. New York: Guilford Press, 1988; pp. 402–450.

112. Semrud-Clikeman M. *Traumatic Brain Injury in Children and Adolescents: Assessment and Intervention.* New York: Guilford Press, 2001.

113. Ylvisaker M, Chorazy AJL, Feeney TJ, Russell ML. Traumatic brain injury in children and adolescents: Assessment and rehabilitation. In: Rosenthal M, Griffith ER, Kreutzer JS, PentlandB (eds) *Rehabilitation of the Adult and Child with Traumatic Brain Injury,* 3rd edn. Philadelphia: F.A. Davis Co., 1999;pp. 356–392.

114. Braga LW, de Paz AC. Neuropsychological pediatric rehabilitation. In: Christensen A, Uzzell BP (eds) *International Handbook of Neuropsychological Rehabilitation.* Dordrecht, The Netherlands: Kluwer Academic Publishers, 2000; pp. 283–295.

115. Hoehn TP, Baumeister AA. A critique of the application of sensory integration therapy to children with learning disabilities. *J Learning Disabil* 1994;**27**:338–350.

116. Dawson G, Watling R. Interventions to facilitate auditory, visual, and motor integration in autism: A review of the evidence. *J Autism DevDisord* 2000;**30**: 415–421.

117. Smith T, Mruzek DW, Mozingo D. Sensory integrative therapy. In: Jacobson JJ, Foxx RM, Mulick JA (eds) *Controversial Therapies for Developmental Disabilities: Fad, Fashion, and Science in Professional Practice.*

Mahweh, NJ: Lawrence Erlbaum Associates, 2005; pp. 341–350.

118. Mudford OC, Cullen C. Auditory integration training: A critical review. In: Jacobson JJ, Foxx RM, Mulick JA (eds) *Controversial Therapies for Developmental Disabilities: Fad, Fashion, and Science in Professional Practice.* Mahweh, NJ: Lawrence Erlbaum Associates, 2005; pp. 351–362.

119. Hartmut H, Gevensleben H, Strehl U. Annotation: Neurofeedback–train your brain to train behaviour. *J Child Psychol Psychiat* 2007;**48**:3–16.

120. Ylven R, Bjorck-Akesson E, Granlund M. Literature review of positive functioning in families with children with a disability. *J Policy Pract Intellect Disabil* 2006; **3**:253–270.

121. Thompson RJ, Gustafson KE. *Adaptation to Chronic Childhood Illness.* Washington, DC: American Psychological Association, 1996.

122. Scorgie K, Wilgosh L, McDonald L. Stress and coping in families of children with disabilities: An examination of recent literature. *Dev Disabil Bull* 1998;**26**:22–42.

123. Brown RT. Chronic illness and neurodevelopmental disability. In:Farmer JE, Donders J, Warschausky S (eds) *Treating Neurodevelopmental Disabilities: Clinical Research and Practice.* New York: Guilford Press, 2006; pp. 98–118.

124. DuPaul GJ, McGoey KE, Mautone JA. Pediatric pharmacology and psychopharmacology. In: Roberts MC (ed.) *Handbook of Pediatric Psychology,* 3rd edn. New York: Guilford Press, 2003; pp. 234–252.

125. Phelps L, Brown RT, Power TJ. *Pediatric Psychopharmacology: Combining Medical and Psychosocial Interventions.* Washington, DC: American Psychological Association, 2002.

126. Sbordone RJ, Long CJ (eds). *Ecological Validity of Neuropsychological Testing.* Delray Beach, FL: St Lucie Press, 1995.

127. Silver CH. Ecological validation of neuropsychological assessment in childhood traumatic brain injury. *J Head Trauma Rehabil* 2000;**15**:973–988.

128. Bush SS, Ruff RM, Troster AI, *et al.* Symptom validity assessment: Practice issues and medical necessity NAN policy & planning committee. *Arch Clin Neuropsychol* 2005;**20**:419–426.

26

The Somatoform Disorders

Patricia I. Ibeziako, David Ray DeMaso

Overview

Pediatric psychosomatic medicine deals with the relationship between physiological and psychological factors in the causation or maintenance of disease states [1]. It is well known that general medical conditions are not simply caused by biological conditions alone, but are also significantly influenced by a child's emotions, thoughts, and environment. Somatization is the tendency to experience and communicate somatic symptoms, which are not fully accounted for by pathological findings [2]. Somatization can coincide with another emotional illness and when it occurs in conjunction with a physical illness, the symptoms and impairment are in excess of what would be expected from the known illness or findings [2].

Unlike the child mental health settings where physical symptoms are generally not the primary complaints [3], it is common in pediatric health-care settings for youngsters to present with troubling somatic symptoms that are unexplained by a physical disease or pathophysiological processes [4]. While many of these physical complaints represent transient symptoms that are resolved with the pediatrician, there are some youngsters whose symptoms become disabling and functionally impairing resulting in increased health-care utilization [5]. In these situations, the diagnosis and management of psychosomatic symptoms present enormous challenges to primary care clinicians and pediatric subspecialists [6, 7].

The most prevalent unexplained somatic symptoms in childhood involve pain, fatigue, and neurological and gastrointestinal complaints [8]. In early childhood, recurrent abdominal pain is the most common pain presentation, with headaches becoming more common in older children and adolescents. Neurological symptoms (pseudoseizures, numbness, blindness) and fatigue also tend to emerge later in childhood [2]. Multiple somatic complaints can be present in a single patient, with

surveys showing that youngsters report a mean of two somatic symptoms in the 2 weeks before a pediatric examination [3]. There is a gender disparity in the prevalence of somatic symptoms during adolescence (11% in girls and 4% in boys), which persists into adulthood [2].

While youngsters who are experiencing disabling and medically unexplained somatic symptoms are generally described from a biomedical or pediatrics perspective as having functional somatic symptoms or syndromes, from the psychiatric perspective they are diagnosed as having a somatoform disorder [9]. These disorders comprise a group of DSM-IV-TR (*Diagnostic and Statistical Manual of Mental Disorders, Fourth Edition, Text Revision*) emotional illnesses characterized by the production of physical symptoms that cannot be fully explained by a known general medical condition and cause clinically significant distress or impairment in functioning [10]. The overall prevalence of somatoform disorders in the general population is estimated to be 12% [11].

It must be noted that DSM-IV is currently under revision. The current DSM-V Workgroup on Somatoform Disorders is proposing renaming the classification to Somatic Symptom Disorders.

Furthermore, since Somatization, Hypochondriasis, and Pain Disorders share common somatic symptom and cognitive distortions, they have also proposed grouping these disorders under a new diagnostic classification named Complex Somatic Symptom Disorders [12]. Conversion disorders would remain a separate diagnostic entity. Since DSM-V has not been finalized at this time, this chapter will use the DSM-IV criteria.

As these patients can present with bewildering combinations of physical and emotional symptoms, they often pose a complex and challenging dilemma to even the most astute mental health clinician. A wide differ-

Clinical Child Psychiatry, Third Edition. Edited by William M. Klykylo and Jerald Kay.
© 2012 John Wiley & Sons, Ltd. Published 2012 by John Wiley & Sons, Ltd.

Table 26.1 DSM-IV-TR somatoform disorders in order of frequency of psychiatric consultation in a pediatric teaching hospital.

Pain Disorder
Conversion Disorder
Undifferentiated Somatoform Disorder
Somatization Disorder
Body Dysmorphic Disorder

ential must be considered as well as the frequent comorbidity of general medical conditions and other psychiatric disorders. This chapter presents the DSM-IV-TR somatoform disorders in the order most often faced by child and adolescent psychiatrists when consulted by pediatricians (Table 26.1). The aim is to provide a practical understanding and approach to pediatric patients presenting with unexplained somatic complaints.

Pain Disorders

> ### CASE STUDY
>
> Jake is a 9-year-old boy who was admitted to the Medical Service to evaluate recurrent abdominal pain of 5-month duration. A thorough workup had failed to reveal a medical etiology for his chronic pain and nausea, so a psychiatric referral was made. On examination, Jake presented as a temperamentally anxious boy who was under a great deal of pressure to excel academically by his professional parents. He met full DSM-IV criteria for an anxiety disorder. A comprehensive treatment program, including cognitive-behavioral techniques to reduce his anxiety, guidance for his parents, and ongoing medical follow-up, resulted in a rapid reduction in Jake's symptoms of abdominal pain.

Definition

Pain is a complex phenomenon consisting of a sensory experience originating in traumatized tissues and an emotional (affective) experience. In addition to tissue damage and noxious body stimulation, subjective representations of pain can be evoked and modified by a variety of factors such as emotional states, thoughts, beliefs, suggestion, and memories of past injuries, as well as by the emotional state of close others [13].

The DSM-IV criteria for a pain disorder include pain of sufficient severity to warrant clinical attention in which psychological factors are deemed to play an important role in the onset, severity, exacerbation, or maintenance of the symptoms [10]. The pain is not intentionally produced or feigned, nor can the pain be better accounted for by another psychiatric disorder. In addition, the pain must cause clinically significant distress or impairment in social, school, or home functioning.

Pain Disorders are divided into two DSM-IV subtypes:

(1) Pain Disorders associated with psychological factors, in which emotional factors alone are judged to play a major role.
(2) Pain Disorders associated with psychological factors and a general medical condition, in which both together are deemed to have important roles in the onset, severity, exacerbation, or maintenance of the pain [10].

Each subtype is further classified as either acute (duration <6 months) or chronic (duration >6 months). Pain that is entirely related to a general medical condition is not considered a psychiatric disorder and is coded on DSM-IV's Axis III.

Epidemiology

Pain disorders are the most prevalent of all the somatoform disorders, with studies indicating pain complaints in up to 70% of patients with somatoform disorders [11]. Chronic pain without an identifiable organic basis occurs in 4–15% of the normative adolescent population and represents a substantial proportion of referrals to adolescent medicine and adolescent rheumatology clinics [14].

Recurrent Abdominal Pain (RAP) falls within the DSM-IV criteria and is commonly defined as three or more pain episodes severe enough to affect the child's activities over a period longer than 3 months [15]. There is generally complete recovery between episodes. RAP is the most common recurrent childhood pain complaint [15], affecting 8% to 25% of children aged 9-12 years. RAP accounts for 2–4% of pediatric office visits, with the prevalence being greater in girls. The largest risk for these children is that they may undergo unnecessary and potentially risky hospitalizations, tests, and procedures [15].

The prevalence of pediatric headache increases from 8.3% for children aged under 10 years to up to 20% for ages 10 and older [16]. Other types of pain (e.g., limb pain or chest pain) occur with increasing prevalence in adolescence [2].

Etiology

Biological Factors

Imaging studies demonstrate a close relationship between pain and emotions in that many of the neural structures activated by pain (e.g., anterior cingulate cortex and insula) are also involved in the processing of affective states (e.g., fear, anger, or sadness) [13]. The combination of glial cell activation from psychological stress and neural firing from nociceptive pain input may lead to pain sensitization and long-term structural changes in pain-processing regions of the brain [17]. Negative affects (e.g., worry, fear, or sadness) can significantly influence how the brain processes pain and can result in heightening the pain experienced by the child [13].

Children with RAP exhibit hyper-reactive sympathetic nervous system arousal in response to environmental stressors, and hypervigilance to internal and external pain cues [18]. Other biological factors associated with unexplained abdominal pain include changes in intestinal wall sensory receptors, modulation of sensory transmissions, cortical perceptions, family history of pain, and pain memories [1].

The neurobiological components of pain involve complex interactions between ascending and descending pain pathways within the central and peripheral nervous systems. Endorphins and biogenic amine neurotransmitters such as serotonin and norepinephrine play important modulating roles in descending analgesic tracts. Studies have shown that the concentrations of serotonin and endorphin metabolites are reduced in the spinal fluid of patients with chronic pain [19]. Drugs that potentiate the central effects of biogenic amines (e.g., antidepressants) have been useful in producing analgesia by increasing their concentrations in these descending pathways.

Psychological Theories

Psychodynamic theory holds that the defense mechanism of conversion underlies medically unexplained pain. The pain is viewed as symbolically representing unconscious conflicts and can serve the unconscious goal of removing the individual from a conflictual situation. Additionally, there is considerable evidence from attachment studies that points to an association between insecure attachment and chronic pain, with patients with somatoform pain disorders demonstrating higher insecure attachment patterns [20].

Learning Theory

Social learning theory suggests that the pain symptoms are a result of "modeling" or "observational learning"

within the family. Somatizing children often live with family members who complain of strikingly similar physical symptoms and, as such, appear as a "symptom model." [2]

Classical and operant conditioning can lead to the perpetuation of pain-related behaviors long after the initial noxious stimulus has been removed. Classical conditioning results from repeated pairing of a neutral or conditioned stimulus with an unconditioned stimulus that evokes a response such that the neutral stimulus eventually comes to evoke the response. For example, settings that have been associated with pain may alone trigger pain-related behavior (sometimes referred to as "memory pain").

Operant conditioning holds that behaviors that are rewarded will increase in strength or frequency, while behaviors that are inhibited or punished will decrease. In some households physical complaints in children are more easily noticed and more acceptable than the expression of feelings (e.g., anxiety, fear, jealousy, and anger). In these environments, a child may obtain more attention and sympathy for somatic symptoms than for their emotional distress [2]. The increase in attention and decrease in responsibilities as well as the euphoric effects of analgesic medications may reinforce pain-related behaviors. If these behaviors or responses are reinforced early in the course of a pain disorder, it is likely that the behaviors will continue even after removal of the original painful stimulus. Conversely, health-related behaviors will diminish as they are no longer subject to systematic reinforcement [21].

Family Systems

Somatic preoccupation, recurrent pain complaints, alcohol abuse, and psychiatric disorders (i.e., anxiety and depression) are all factors within families that have been found to be associated with pain disorders [22]. Parental behaviors have also been suggested to contribute to the development of pain disorders and other somatic symptoms [1]. Parental overprotection has been found to be significantly associated with worse health outcomes in youngsters with functional somatic symptoms. When a family's focus is on their child's illness such that it allows for avoidance of conflict within the family, the child's illness behavior can become reinforced [8]. Parental responses to a child's pain and the parents' ongoing daily stressors have been found to be important in exacerbating and maintaining pain symptoms in children [1].

Sociocultural Factors

Studies investigating the effects of ethnicity on pain tolerance and behavior have provided mixed results.

For example, some empirical studies report that Irish and Anglo-Saxons have greater pain tolerance than individuals of southern Mediterranean ethnicity, while others have found no significant differences among ethnic groups [19]. In China, stress and unhappiness are known to manifest as psychosomatic symptoms in children, with the most commonly documented symptoms being headache and abdominal pain [23].

Diagnosis

Clinical Interview

In all somatoform disorders, thorough psychiatric interviews of the patient and family should be performed. The assessment should provide the information necessary for the clinician to generate a developmentally informed biopsychosocial formulation capable of informing management. The components of the AACAP (American Academy of Child and Adolescent Psychiatry) Practice Parameters for the Psychiatric Assessment and Management of Physically Ill Children and Adolescents are applicable to youngsters with somatoform disorders [24].

Close attention should be paid to current and past psychosocial stressors, in particular noting whether pain seems to be situation-dependent or temporally related to a stressor. The history of prior episodes of pain in the patient as well as of pain syndromes in other family members should be obtained [1]. The mental health clinician should aim to assess if these problems are comorbid with a physical disorder or exist independently and are etiological to the pain syndrome.

Physical Examination

The symptoms are neuroanatomically inconsistent with known pathways or are in significant excess of what would be expected from the physical findings. If physical findings are present they are often secondary to pathological changes associated with immobilization. Chronic pain often causes decreased mobility and poor posture, which may result in pathological changes such as osteoporosis, contractures, and circulatory disturbances, which contribute to progressive deterioration in functioning [19].

Studies

Infrared thermography may be helpful in identifying changes in temperature and vascular flow associated with certain disorders that can cause chronic pain [19]. Despite the fact that there are no specific laboratory abnormalities associated with somatoform pain disor-

ders, invasive procedures are more frequently performed in patients with these disorders than in patients with nociceptive or neuropathic pain [11].

Differential Diagnosis

General Medical Conditions

Every child and adolescent has a psychological reaction to experienced pain. The diagnosis of pain disorder is made when the response is out of proportion to the general medical condition and when deficits or impairment in emotional and behavioral functioning occur.

Important physical causes of pain that can be confused with psychogenic pain disorders include abdominal migraines, headache syndromes, neuropathy, or tumors. Reflex sympathetic dystrophy (or complex regional pain syndrome) is characterized by pain that spreads beyond the area of injury along a dermatomal pattern resulting in a regional area of involvement. The pain is often accompanied by autonomic dysfunction, edema, movement difficulties, and dystrophy. While not thought to be causative, psychosocial stressors generally accompany and may exacerbate these disorders.

Depressive and Anxiety Disorders

Several studies have found a strong relation between RAP and anxiety disorders in children, with the prevalence of anxiety disorders in these children ranging from 42% to 85% [15]. RAP is also strongly associated with depressive symptoms, anxious temperaments, other pain syndromes (i.e., headache, limb pain, or chest pain) as well as other somatic symptoms (i.e., fatigue, dizziness, weakness, and numbness) [25]. While it is generally acknowledged that the most common etiology is unknown it is increasingly held that RAP and anxiety disorders may share a common risk factor or are different aspects of a single causal process [25]. Generalized anxiety disorder, specific phobia, social phobia, and separation anxiety disorder have all been associated with RAP. Anxiety disorders have also been associated with children with chronic daily headaches, and with musculoskeletal pains [15, 26].

Depression is a common comorbid condition with pain disorders. In a comparison between children with and without RAP disorders, depression was found in 43% of those with pain versus 8% of the controls [25]. It was also noted that only a small minority of these children had depression alone, while the majority of patients had either an anxiety disorder alone or a mixed anxiety depression presentation [25].

Pain disorders should only be diagnosed if the symptoms cannot be better accounted for by the anxiety or mood disorder, since physical symptoms are often part of the criteria for some anxiety disorders. For example, "repeated complaints of physical symptoms (such as headaches, stomachaches, nausea, or vomiting) when separation from major attachment figures occurs or is anticipated" is part of the DSM-IV definition of Separation Anxiety Disorder.

Other Somatoform Disorders

Pain symptoms commonly occur in somatization disorders. The latter are diagnosed usually in adulthood with a history of symptom development often beginning in adolescence. Conversion disorders are medically unexplained deficits in motor and sensory functioning often accompanied by pain symptoms. Conversion and pain symptoms commonly occur together in patients.

Factitious Disorder

These disorders are characterized by physical symptoms, which are intentionally produced or feigned in order to assume the sick role. These disorders of illness falsification are generally described in adults though some cases in older children and adolescents have been reported [27]. The most common conditions falsified or induced are fevers, ketoacidosis, purpura, and infections.

Factitious disorder by proxy (or Münchausen syndrome by proxy) is the production of symptoms in another person who is under the individual's care; [10] younger children are more commonly affected although it can sometimes occur with older children [28]. The motivation for the perpetrator's behavior has been hypothesized to be a psychological need to assume a sick role or relationship with a caring physician.

Malingering

Malingering involves the intentional production or feigning of symptoms. The motivation for the behavior is the conscious goal of gaining or avoiding something in the environment, such as avoiding criminal prosecution or securing financial gain. Generally, this diagnosis is rarely seen in pediatrics though occasionally an older adolescent with conduct or antisocial traits may present with somatic symptoms.

Course

Children and adolescents with pain disorders can progress to having significant functional impairment with high utilization of medical services and substantial school absences [3]. The course of illness has been related to associated psychopathology, duration of pain, and extent of environmental reinforcement. Follow-up studies with patients with RAP found that 25–50% continue to suffer abdominal discomfort in adulthood [29]. Roughly 30% of patients with somatoform pain disorders abuse analgesics [30]. There is also evidence regarding a specific association between childhood abdominal pain and anxiety in young adulthood [31].

Conversion Disorders

CASE STUDY

Julie was a previously physically healthy 14-year-old girl who, over a period of 1 month, developed the inability to walk. Repeated physical examinations were normal, as were X-rays of her legs. Consultation with specialists from orthopedics and neurology found normal examinations. The presenting symptoms were not explained by a general medical condition. A psychiatric consultation was requested.

A psychiatric interview with Julie and her parents revealed a premorbidly emotionally healthy girl with a tendency to have frequent somatic complaints. Significant losses in this same time period included the separation of her parents along with the death of her close maternal grandmother. Her grandmother had been unable to walk for the last 6 months of her life due to complications of diabetes mellitus.

The prior history of somatic complaints, temporally related family stresses, and symptom model combined with symptoms unexplained by a general medical condition supported the diagnosis of a conversion disorder.

Definition

In DSM-IV Conversion Disorders are characterized by one or more symptoms affecting voluntary motor or sensory function that suggest a neurological or other general medical condition [10]. Psychological factors are judged to be associated with the symptom because conflicts or stressors precede the initiation or exacerbation of the symptom. The symptom is not intentionally produced or feigned. After appropriate investigation, the symptom cannot be fully explained by a general medical condition, by the direct effects of a substance, or as a culturally sanctioned behavior or experience. The disorder causes clinically significant distress or impairment in psychological functioning. A conversion disorder is not diagnosed when symptoms are limited to pain alone.

Typical sensory losses include blindness, deafness, loss of touch, pain sensation, and diplopia. Motor symptoms include paralysis, ataxia, aphonia, dysphagia, and urinary retention along with alterations in consciousness to produce seizures and unconsciousness. Pseudoseizures, unexplained falls, and fainting are the most common abnormalities, followed by gait and sensory deficits [29].

Epidemiology

The incidence of childhood conversion disorder varies among studies because of different patient populations and diagnostic criteria. In most studies the incidence varies between 0.5% and 10% [32]. This disorder is three times more common in adolescents than in children and rarely occurs under age 5 years [32]. Females predominate among adolescents with conversion disorders, while equal numbers of boys and girls are generally found in childhood.

Conversion presentations include paresthesia, paralysis, syncope, visual disturbances, headache, tremors or other disorders of movement, disorders of gait, and seizures [33]. Studies indicate episodic losses of consciousness (e.g., syncope or pseudoseizures) and motor functioning (particularly abnormal gait or inability to walk) are the most frequently reported symptoms of conversion disorder in childhood [6].

Etiology

Biological Factors

It has been hypothesized that patients with pseudoseizures have increased activity of neurobiological stress systems, which can be measured using serum cortisol levels [34]. Although basal hypercortisolism may be present in some patients with pseudoseizures, the level of cortisol has also been shown to be elevated after generalized and partial seizures, making it a poor differentiating diagnostic tool [34].

Psychological Theories

The term conversion derives from the psychoanalytical concept that the somatic symptom is the result of an unconscious resolution of a psychological conflict in which the mind "converts" psychological distress into a physical symptom [32]. Primary gain is obtained by keeping the conflict from consciousness and minimizing anxiety. The symptom can provide secondary gain by providing an escape from unwanted consequences or responsibilities.

A typical concept is one of good, compliant children from families with high expectations who are in intolerable situations they cannot escape or communicate about, and sometimes their fears of parental rejection or displeasure are manifested through conversion symptoms. This minimizes the hostility in attachment relationships and allows for maximum physical and psychological closeness and safety [35]. In attachment theories, insecure-avoidant attachment behavior is associated with a predisposition for increased complaints of physical symptoms, whereas secure attachment correlates with health-maintaining behavioral patterns [11].

Learning Theory

In a study of conversion disorders, a significant proportion of patients had family members who were reported to have medical conditions with similar presentations (e.g., migraines, headaches, seizures) [33]. Physical symptoms have been called a form of body language for children who have difficulty expressing emotions verbally and whose emotions are transformed into a bodily communication of their distress (these children are sometimes referred to as "body talkers"). These youngsters appear to be very attuned to the nonverbal communications of health professionals, thus making them adept "body readers" and skilled at picking up on negative attitudes [3, 14].

Common communication problems include difficulties with disclosing sexual abuse or expressing anger toward parents, and high-achieving children who cannot admit they are under too much pressure. A child may quickly learn the benefits of assuming the sick role and may be reluctant to give up the symptoms. Increased parental attention and avoidance of unpleasant school pressures only further reinforce the symptom.

Family Systems

Family systems play important roles in the initiation and maintenance of symptoms in the same manner as described earlier for pain disorders. Recent family stress, unresolved grief reactions, and family psychopathology occur at a higher frequency in cases of conversion symptoms [1]. Adjustment difficulties to changes in family situation (e.g., birth of a sibling or parental divorce) are commonly associated with development of conversion disorders [33].

Sociocultural Factors

School stress (e.g., fear of going to school, fear of exams or extracurricular activities, bullying by schoolmates) has been found to be a common external environmental factor in the presentation of a conversion symptom [33]. Stress in the school setting has been shown to be significantly associated with psychosomatic symptoms in school-age children in Norway, Sweden, Finland, and China [23].

Adolescence has been characterized as a stressful period of development. Emerging literature indicates the risk of conversion disorder may be higher in adolescents who have anxiety related either to sexual behaviors, orientation, or gender identity. Youngsters who recognize same-sex attraction in early adolescence undergo a unique "internal and interpersonal" stress, with difficulty communicating their struggles due to fear of parental rejection, peer isolation, stigmatization, and victimization; somatization may be an attempt to resolve what is perceived as an unacceptable but unavoidable feeling [36].

The use of nonverbal body language as a way of communication or expression of self in response to interpersonal conflicts may represent a culturally determined and socially learned behavior and is more common in certain cultures [6]. Spells or visions are common aspects of culturally sanctioned religious and healing rituals, while falling down with loss or alteration in consciousness is a feature in a variety of culture-specific syndromes. The form of symptom reflects local cultural ideas about acceptable and credible ways to express distress.

Diagnosis

Clinical Interview

As with pain disorders, the assessment should provide the information necessary for the clinician to generate a developmentally appropriate biopsychosocial formulation capable of informing management. A temporal relationship between psychological stress or conflict and the development of the conversion symptom is sought in thorough psychiatric interviews of the patient and family (Table 26.2). Prior history of conversion disorders or recurrent somatic complaints and the presence of a symptom model (e.g., family member with similar deficits) are especially helpful in making the diagnosis [19].

Some patients with pseudoseizures or nonelectrical seizures have been found to have significant prior histories of trauma (especially sexual abuse), though histories of family or school stressors are more common [4]. La belle indifference and histrionic personality traits

Table 26.2 Interview criteria important for diagnosis of a conversion disorder.

Psychological stress temporally related to symptom
Prior history of conversion symptoms
Prior history of recurrent somatic complaints
Dissociative and/or somatization disorders
Family stress and/or psychopathology
Symptom model

commonly cited in adult studies have not proven to be reliable diagnostic criteria in children and adolescents.

The diagnosis is not one of exclusion. The presence of biopsychosocial risk factors described above should be elicited as positive symptoms. If the consultant is unable to elicit any of the diagnostic criteria except for the motor or sensory symptoms, then the possibility of an underlying general medical condition should be reconsidered.

Physical Examination

The symptoms do not conform to known anatomical pathways and physiological mechanisms. If physical findings are present they may relate to either disuse atrophy or to sequelae of medical procedures.

The use of sensory stimuli can aid in the diagnosis of pseudoseizures or nonelectrical seizures. Eliciting a pain response with sternal rub or nailbed pressure and use of a noxious olfactory stimulus, may possibly terminate an episode of nonepileptic seizures [34]. Maneuvers such as placing a cotton swab in the nose, passively opening the patient's eyes, testing the corneal reflex, and the drop test are often met with resistance in a patient with nonelectrical events but not in a patient with epileptic seizures. Some patients are highly suggestible and respond to verbal suggestions to both induce and terminate events [34].

Studies

There are no specific laboratory studies associated with conversion disorders. An elevated serum prolactin level has been shown to be predictive of generalized tonic-clonic and complex partial seizures but not in nonepileptic seizures. The elevation in serum prolactin levels is thought to be caused by a disruption in the hypothalamic regulation of pituitary hormone release after stimulation from temporal lobe epileptic foci [34].

Video-EEG monitoring is the gold standard in diagnosing nonepileptic seizures and helps parents to comprehend the emotional, nonelectrical nature of these events as the seizures occur in the absence of electrical activity [37]. Neuroimaging such as head magnetic resonance imaging (MRI) or computed tomography (CT) scans are helpful for the evaluation of symptoms of sensory and motor loss.

Drug-assisted interviews (e.g., amytal, thiopental, or methohexital) have been found to be useful in some youngsters as the symptom may disappear transiently or even permanently following a drug-assisted interview; [38] however, there is scant recent literature about the use of this in children.

Differential Diagnosis

General Medical Conditions

The major diagnostic concern is the exclusion of neurological or physical conditions. Migraine syndromes, temporal lobe epilepsy, and central nervous system tumors have presented difficult diagnostic dilemmas. Multiple sclerosis, myasthenia gravis, and other myopathies are important additional considerations. The mental health clinician must also be alert to the dual existence of a physical condition and a conversion disorder (e.g., epileptic and nonepileptic seizures) in the same patient.

Psychological Factors Affecting Medical Conditions

The essential DSM-IV feature is the presence of one or more specific psychological or behavioral factors that adversely affect a general medical condition [10]. A mental disorder, personality traits, coping style, maladaptive health behaviors, or stress-related physiological responses are different psychological factors that can impact on a diagnosable general medical condition. This contrasts with conversion disorders, where no general medical condition exists to completely account for the symptoms produced.

Depressive and Anxiety Disorders

As stated earlier, depressive disorders can present with somatic symptoms in children and adolescents. Acute stress and post-traumatic stress disorders can present with symptoms suggestive of a conversion disorder. However, a conversion disorder should not be diagnosed if the symptoms are better accounted for by these disorders.

Somatoform Disorders

Conversion symptoms can occur in the course of a somatization disorder. The multiple symptom pattern of a somatization disorder contrasts with the mono-symptomatic and often time-limited presentations of conversion disorders. Pain disorder is diagnosed if the symptoms are limited to pain. Hypochondriasis usually begins in adulthood and is characterized by a preoccupation with having a serious disease. Body dysmorphic disorder does not involve motor or sensory deficits, but rather a preoccupation with defect in appearance.

Dissociative Disorders

More common in adults, these disorders share symptoms that may suggest neurological dysfunction and may occur in the same individual. Both diagnoses are made if conversion and dissociative symptoms appear in the same individual.

Malingering and Factitious Disorder

As described previously, these disorders involving the intentional or feigned production of symptoms, and are important in the differential for any somatoform disorder.

Course

Conversion symptoms typically occur suddenly and tend to be of short duration. Pediatricians are most likely to see transient reactions while psychiatric consultation occurs in more difficult cases. Symptoms may become chronic or recurrent, especially when the precipitating stress is persistent or repetitive, when there is associated significant psychopathology, or when the symptom has significant secondary gain [19]. Patients with pseudoseizures are more likely to have recurrences than are patients with paralysis or aphonia [39, 40].

Early studies reported high percentages of youngsters with an initial diagnosis of conversion disorder who were subsequently found to have a medical illness while other samples have revealed a more modest risk (<10%) of faulty diagnosis in children and adolescents [25].

The outcomes of conversion disorders vary with the type of presentation; for example, some studies show that children with paralysis tend to have a better outcome than those with seizures [33].

Somatization and Undifferentiated Somatoform Disorders

CASE STUDY

Jill was a 16-year-old girl who had not felt well for over 3 years. She presented with symptoms of generalized weakness and fatigue. She had shown evidence for a "strep throat" at the beginning of her illness but subsequent evaluations were normal. Additional medical workups by nearly half a dozen specialists found no general medical condition that could account for her symptoms.

Prior to her symptoms, Jill was described as a remarkable girl with excellent grades as well as outstanding performances as a gymnast and violinist. She was noted to have good friendships though she was often viewed as intensely competitive. A conflicted relationship between her professional parents had improved at the same time that her symptoms had continued. Jill's mother had a long history of multiple somatic complaints involving multiple organ systems.

The long-standing unexplained somatic complaints and positive family history for recurrent somatic complaints, combined with the possible secondary gains of avoiding high expectations and lowering parental conflict supported the diagnosis of an undifferentiated somatoform disorder.

Definition

Somatization disorder is characterized by a chronic pattern of multiple physical complaints causing clinically significant impairment in functioning that cannot be explained by any known physical condition [10]. Onset must be before age 30 years, and symptoms usually occur over a period of several years. Symptoms must include four pain symptoms, two gastrointestinal symptoms other than pain, one sexual or reproductive symptom as well as one pseudoneurological symptom [10]. This disorder was originally called Briquet's syndrome.

Obviously, the number of symptoms required over a several-year time period and the inclusion of criteria that are appropriate only for postpubertal and/or sexually active patients, mitigate against the diagnosis in children. Children and adolescents are more likely to meet DSM-IV criteria for an Undifferentiated Somatoform Disorder with criteria requiring only one or more unexplained physical complaint/s, functional impairment, and a duration of 6 months. Symptoms of less than 6 months duration are coded in DSM-IV as a Somatoform Disorder Not Otherwise Specified (NOS).

Epidemiology

While somatic complaints in childhood and adolescence are common, the diagnosis of somatization disorder is rarely made before adulthood. Lifetime prevalence rates range from 0.2% to 2% among women, and less than 0.2% among men [10]. Women have a five-fold to ten-fold greater lifetime risk of the disorder compared to men [32]. In the majority of cases, the symptoms begin during adolescence. Low socioeconomic, occupational, and educational status have been shown in adult studies to be more common in this disorder [19].

Etiology

Psychological, Learning, and Family System Theories

The psychodynamic, learning, and family system theories discussed earlier in relation to pain and conversion disorders influence the severity and frequency of the somatic symptoms.

Biological Factors

Genetic factors may contribute to the development of this disorder; [32] somatization disorder is observed in 10–20% of female first-degree relatives of probands with the disorder. Having a male or female relative with antisocial personality increases the risk for development of somatization disorder [10].

A "hysterical" information-processing pattern characterized by distractibility, difficulty distinguishing target and nontarget stimuli, and impaired verbal communication has been found in individuals with somatization disorder [19]. This pattern or deficit has been postulated to underlie the frequent physical complaints along with the vague and circumstantial processing of social and personal problems. This pattern has not been shown in child or adolescent patients.

Diagnosis

Clinical Interview

Again, the importance of an assessment that generates a developmentally informed biopsychosocial formulation that informs management is critical in approaching these disorders. The key interview finding is a medical history involving recurrent unexplained physical complaints involving multiple systems, with pain, gastrointestinal, sexual, and pseudoneurological complaints. There often is a history of concurrent treatment from many physicians. Comorbid anxiety and depressive symptoms are common. On mental status examination, circumstantial, imprecise, and vague thinking may be prominent given the "hysterical" information-processing deficit described earlier.

In an undifferentiated somatoform disorder, a similar clinical picture is elicited though without the required DSM-IV symptom criteria. "Neurasthenia," which is characterized by fatigue and weakness and is quite similar to "chronic fatigue syndrome," is classified in DSM-IV-TR as an undifferentiated somatoform disorder.

Physical Examination

As with conversion disorders, the symptoms do not conform to known physiological mechanisms. If physical signs are present they relate most often to the sequelae of medical procedures.

Studies

The paucity of laboratory findings is characteristic. Psychological testing may be useful in understanding underlying psychological traits but not to confirm a diagnosis. The Children Somatization Inventory (CSI) is a standardized self-rated scale for adolescents detailing 35 common physical symptoms experienced over the previous 2-week period. The CSI has been used in numerous studies of pediatric patients in different countries, including patients with chronic abdominal pain, headaches, chronic fatigue syndrome, and factitious disorder [9]. The Illness Attitudes Scale has been adapted for use in youngsters, and the Soma Assessment Interview is a validated parental interview to assess functional somatic symptoms in children [3]. Functional disability scales are also useful to determine the degree of impairment the symptoms have had on the child.

Differential Diagnosis

General Medical Conditions

The mental health clinician faces the challenge of identifying somatization disorder early in its course. Illnesses with vague and multiple somatic symptoms (e.g., infectious mononucleosis, Lyme disease, or multiple sclerosis) need to be ruled out.

Depressive and Anxiety Disorders

As noted previously, depressive disorders can be accompanied by multiple somatic complaints. Recurrent panic attacks and generalized anxiety disorder may be difficult to distinguish from somatization disorders. Symptoms associated with depressive and anxiety disorders encompass a broader range of emotional complaints. In contrast, somatization disorders have a more focused concern with somatic complaints. Nevertheless, these disorders may be comorbid with somatization disorder.

Chronic Fatigue Syndrome

This syndrome is characterized by chronic, incapacitating physical and mental fatigue that is not relieved by rest. Fatigue is exacerbated by physical or mental exertion and is accompanied by impaired memory and concentration, unrefreshing sleep, muscle and joint pain, and other symptoms [41]. There are no diagnostic clinical signs or laboratory markers although certain viral infections may precipitate chronic fatigue syndrome in children [3]. The syndrome is most likely a result of multiple etiologies of which one is an undifferentiated somatoform disorder; depression and anxiety-related symptoms are common in this syndrome.

Hypochondriasis

Hypochondriasis is a DSM-IV-TR somatoform disorder characterized by a preoccupation with fears of having, or the idea that one has, a serious disease based on a misinterpretation of one or more bodily signs or symptoms [10]. It is often associated with medical care dissatisfaction, deteriorating interpersonal relationships, and the risk of iatrogenic complications from excessive diagnostic procedures [42]. As a childhood symptom, hypochondriasis can occur as described in this chapter's overview, but the disorder develops far more commonly in adults. There is very poor supporting literature for this diagnosis in childhood [43].

Psychotic Disorders and Schizophrenia

Multiple somatic delusions need to be differentiated in some cases. Family history is important to elicit as there is no familial aggregation of the two disorders [19].

Malingering and Factitious Disorders

The additional presence of intentionally produced symptoms is common in somatization disorder. However, the majority of symptoms are not consciously produced, unlike in either malingering or factitious disorders.

Personality Disorders

The presence of personality disorders is very common, with histrionic, borderline, and antisocial personality disorders all having been reported to occur in adults with somatization disorder [10].

Course

Somatization disorder is a chronic illness, with fluctuation in the frequency and diversity of symptoms but without complete remission [44]. Patients often have a history of concurrent treatment from several physicians, resulting in fragmented care, mixed messages, and inconsistent treatment plans [32].

In childhood the full criteria for this disorder are rarely seen. However, there are children and more commonly adolescents who do experience multiple, significant, and disabling somatic complaints. These may represent the early presentation of the full illness seen later as adults. The diagnosis of these children is generally consistent with DSM-IV's criteria for an undifferentiated somatoform disorder. Headache and abdominal pain are most common among prepubertal children, while limb pain, muscle aches, fatigue, and other symptoms increase in frequency with age, resulting in diagnosis of syndromes such as fibromyalgia, postural orthostatic tachycardia syndrome, or irritable bowel syndrome [32].

It is important to realize that significant impairment and disability can occur if symptoms are not adequately treated. These can range from development of contractures and disuse atrophy in patients with difficulty walking, to the placement of gastric tubes in children with difficulty with eating; less positive outcomes are seen with more chronic symptoms.

Body Dysmorphic Disorder

CASE STUDY

Alexa was a lovely 17-year-old girl who was seen in the hospital's Craniofacial Clinic due to concerns about wanting to remove a disfiguring facial scar. The plastic surgeon found the scar to be minimal or even nonexistent. The psychiatric consultant who worked in the clinic found Alexa to have a persistent and excessive concern that her scar was readily apparent to others.

Definition

Body dysmorphic disorder as characterized by DSM-IV refers to a preoccupation with an imagined bodily defect or flaw in a normally appearing person [10]. If a physical anomaly is present, the concern and degree of distress exhibited by the individual is grossly out of proportion to the degree of the defect. This preoccupation causes significant distress and/or interferes with social or occupational functioning, is not better accounted for by another psychiatric disorder, and is not of psychotic proportions. Currently this disorder is under consideration by the DSM-V work group for possible reclassification with anxiety and obsessive-compulsive disorders.

The intense preoccupation regarding a bodily defect may involve any part of the body; however, it most often involves imagined or slight flaws of the face or head such as acne, scars, paleness/redness of complexion, thinning hair, facial asymmetry, or excessive facial hair. The preoccupation is frequently very distressing and difficult to resist. Associated behaviors, for instance, frequent mirror checking, questioning and reassurance seeking, or avoidance of photographs, can be very time-consuming. Social avoidance, embarrassment, and ideas of reference are not uncommon.

Epidemiology

Childhood epidemiological data on body dysmorphic disorder are limited; however, studies indicate a prevalence of 1.9–12% in adult populations [45]. The onset seems to occur during adolescence, with close to equal proportions of males and females [32]. Most patients are secretive about their symptoms and are reluctant to seek psychiatric treatment, but many have had consultations with surgeons and dermatologists. Reports in the literature suggest that patients wait a mean of 6 years before seeking psychiatric intervention [46].

Etiology

Psychological Theories

Psychodynamic theories have described the "unconscious displacement of sexual or emotional conflict or feelings of inferiority, guilt, or poor self-image onto a body part." [46] In one study of 75 patients with body dysmorphic disorder, over 70% reported a history of childhood maltreatment, such as physical, sexual, and emotional abuse or physical neglect [47].

Biological Factors

Body dysmorphic disorder has many similarities with obsessive-compulsive disorder, and a link between the two disorders has been suggested [48].

Diagnosis

Clinical Interview

A high index of suspicion is needed as individuals with this disorder are generally embarrassed by their "defect" and may be reluctant to discuss their concerns. Within the context of the interview, it can be difficult to distinguish between the "overvalued idea" of body dysmorphic disorder and the fixed false belief of a delusional disorder. The patient has persistent and excessive concern that these "defects" are readily apparent to others.

Physical Examination

The physical examination does not conform to the bodily complaints.

Differential Diagnosis

Normal Appearance Concerns

Adolescence is a time of physical and emotional change, as well as a time when a great deal of attention is paid to appearance. As such, heightened concern about physical appearance is considered to be a normal part of adolescence. The disorder is differentiated by its greater distress and increased severity of symptoms.

Obsessive-Compulsive Disorder

Preoccupation with imagined bodily defects and their associated behaviors are similar to obsessions and compulsions. In obsessive-compulsive disorder the symptoms are not limited to concern about appearance.

Depressive Disorder

In depressive illnesses, mood congruent ruminations about physical appearance occur only during the episode of mood disturbance.

Anorexia Nervosa

There is intense preoccupation with fatness in anorexia nervosa. Individuals with body dysmorphic disorder do not demonstrate the dissatisfaction of generalized body image seen in eating disorders, although patients with eating disorders may also have preoccupations with certain body parts.

Gender Identity Disorder

In this disorder, the patient's preoccupation is related to feelings of discomfort with primary and secondary sexual characteristics.

Avoidant Personality Disorder/Social Phobia

This is a pervasive pattern of feelings of inadequacy and hypersensitivity to negative evaluation. Symptoms are usually present in a variety of contexts, and specific concerns about physical defects are not as prominent, distressing, or time-consuming as in body dysmorphic disorder.

Delusional Disorder – Somatic Type

This psychotic disorder may include delusions that the individual has some physical defect (DSM-IV-TR).

The intensity with which the belief is held differentiates this disorder from body dysmorphic disorder.

Course

The onset may be abrupt or gradual and the diagnosis may not be made for years. As a result, although onset is said to occur in adolescence, patients rarely present before adulthood. Patients tend to initially seek treatment from dermatologists and plastic surgeons [32], who usually refer patients for mental health intervention when there are associated comorbid symptoms like depression or anxiety or significant impairment in functioning.

Without treatment, body dysmorphic disorder is a chronic condition that persists for years and perhaps decades. The body part(s) of concern may remain the same or shift over time. Many patients have poor insight and frequently seek cosmetic treatments to address their appearance-related distress, although such treatments are rarely beneficial [49].

Treatment of Somatoform Disorders

An Integrated Medical and Psychiatric Approach

The evaluation of somatoform disorders should include an assessment of biological, psychological, social, and developmental realms both separately and in relation to each other [50]. Physical illnesses have accompanying emotional symptoms, while psychiatric illnesses commonly have associated somatic or physical symptoms. Given the common "diagnostic uncertainty" of psychosomatic disorders, with frequent dual medical/psychiatric diagnoses, it is critical for health-care providers to avoid the dichotomy in which diseases are considered as being either organic or psychologically based, and instead utilize an integrated medical and psychiatric approach [50] (Table 26.3).

Beginning with the pediatrician (or physician primarily responsible) the evaluation should include both medical and psychosocial histories. This integrated approach allows for the exploration of both physical and psychological factors, which may be contributing to the clinical presentation.

Patients and family with somatoform disorders often present with the belief that there is a medical cause for their problem and mental health referral is often resisted. Following exhaustive medical investigations, which yield normal results, labeling the unexplained symptoms as "psychiatric" can effectively shift the search for the cause onto family functioning, resulting in patients and parents feeling blamed for the symptoms [14]. In some cases, reassurance and suggestion

Table 26.3 Psychiatry consultation in pediatric somatoform disorders – guidelines to an integrated medical and psychiatric approach.

Complete a psychiatric assessment
- Review histories, examinations, and studies by pediatrician and pediatric specialists
- Perform patient and family interviews
- Elicit diagnostic criteria
- Develop a developmental biopsychosocial formulation of the patient and family
- Facilitate a better understanding of experience by the patient and family

Convey developmental biopsychosocial formulation to pediatrician
- Remember somatoform illness is not a diagnosis by exclusion
- Remember symptoms can be in significant excess of what would be expected from the physical findings that are present
- Remember that physical findings may have accounted for early symptoms, but may no longer be the etiology for the current symptoms

Convene informing conference between pediatrician and family
- Convey integrated medical and psychiatric findings to family
- As family has medical model as their frame of reference, help reframe this understanding of symptoms into a developmental biopsychosocial formulation

Implement interventions in *both* medical and psychiatric domains
- Consider the following medical interventions:
  - set up ongoing pediatric follow-up appointments
  - physical therapy or other face-saving remedies may be added depending on symptoms
  - psychopharmacology (assess for target symptoms for psychotropic medications)
- Consider the following psychiatric interventions:
  - individual psychotherapy (i.e., cognitive-behavioral intervention or other modalities)
  - parent psychoeducation (advice, guidance, behavioral recommendations, etc.) family therapy
  - system intervention (i.e., school recommendations)
  - consider extended evaluation (rather than treatment) in situation of diagnostic uncertainty

---

from the pediatrician that the symptom will improve is helpful; however, in many instances a message of implied feigning may be heard [51].

Presenting the mental health consultation as part of a comprehensive evaluation will minimize the stigma and distrust, while emphasizing coping and support. Therefore it is preferable not to wait until all investigations are determined to be negative before introducing mental health consultation, but rather have the psychiatry consultation concomitantly with the medical workup when feasible [6]. Often, families worry that a mental health referral or the diagnosis of a somatoform disorder will be followed by abandonment by their physician. The pediatrician should directly communicate to the family that he or she will continue to integrate the psychiatric results together with the physical findings to develop a more complete understanding of the child's symptomatology. The scheduling of regular follow-up visits with the pediatrician can be important for maintaining the family's alliance and investment in mental health treatment and prevent potential doctor shopping

The mental health clinician should take a full history and mental status examination, being alert to the areas highlighted in the previous clinical interview sections. This assessment should include both the patient and parents (or caretakers). In addition, close attention during the interviews to the patient's and the family's "narrative" or "story" is important. This process of narration alone will frequently allow the family to better understand and gain perspective on their current experience. It will allow the mental health clinician the opportunity later to help the family "make meaning" of their experience by understanding and using the "family's own words."

The formulation and understanding of the problem is crucial. The narrow medical view of the problem needs to be reframed to a developmental biopsychosocial formulation. Once the psychiatric assessment is complete, the mental health clinician should begin by communicating this formulation to the pediatrician. The mental health clinician should be alert to countertransference reactions, sometimes engendered in physicians who feel frustrated by the time consumed in caring for patients and the never-ending recurrent complaints in individuals who might be perceived as "not really being sick." [2] A common reaction is a tendency to avoid or spend less time with these patients, but studies indicate that allocating sufficient time for communicating the diagnosis to the patient and family and showing respect for the patient's own illness perception are of great importance [52].

With acceptance of the formulation by the pediatrician, the next step is an "informing conference" that includes both the physician and family. In a supportive and nonjudgmental manner, the pediatrician should present the patient and the family with both the medical and psychosocial findings. The family should be told that many important things have been discovered, for example: "We have good news; we have ruled out a number of serious illnesses…." Statements such as "We couldn't find anything… It's in your mind… The symptoms are not real…" should be avoided. Close attention to the "family's words" allows them to be integrated into the biopsychosocial formulation, thereby facilitating family acceptance. The mental health clinician may or may not attend this meeting depending on the comfort and expertise of the pediatrician. Some pediatricians prefer to have the mental health clinician present especially if they have first-hand knowledge of the family's narrative of the illness from the psychiatric assessment.

Following an acceptance of a new formulation of the problem, the pediatrician and mental health clinician together can facilitate the formation of an integrated medical and psychiatric team. This team supports both the pediatrician's ongoing monitoring and treatment for possible physical illness and the mental health clinician's interventions [2].

Management and Treatment

Psychoeducation is the first intervention to help families move from searching for an underlying medical cause to focusing on coping and rehabilitation [14]. Characteristics of treatments reported to have good outcome include close liaison between mental health and pediatric professionals, an attitude of belief in the child's symptoms, moving the family toward a psychological understanding, and instituting a multidisciplinary rehabilitative approach including physical therapy [14]. The pediatrician can provide ongoing follow-up and may initiate benign face-saving remedies – lotions, vitamins, slings, heating pads, etc. – during the acute phase [42] while avoiding unnecessary medical investigations and procedures.

Psychiatric treatment is directed toward understanding the child and family's dynamics and reasons for assuming the sick role; understanding and adhering to treatment regimens; and enhancing communication with treating professionals. Cognitive behavioral therapy (CBT) has been helpful in addressing and overcoming the internal conflicts and underlying stressors [53]. The intervention is aimed at reinforcing health-related behaviors and diminishing pain or physical complaints. Strategies incorporated into rehabilitation approaches include activity scheduling, establishment of a sleep routine, and modification of negative thought patterns [14].

Techniques such as hypnosis, biofeedback, and relaxation training can be used to teach the patient the control he or she can have over certain physiological processes such as autonomic system activity [42]. Active coping strategies (e.g., problem-solving, emotional expression and modulation), result in a decline in somatic symptoms [1]. Psychodynamic therapy may be helpful in children with high levels of "psychological insight" to identify unconscious conflicts, which may be maintaining symptoms. Expression of feelings can be facilitated, and more adaptive coping mechanisms encouraged.

Parental involvement (e.g., family therapy and/or parent guidance) is an important component of any treatment program. A CBT family intervention study found that children receiving CBT experienced a higher rate of pain elimination, lower levels of relapse at follow-up, and lower levels of interference with their activities than children receiving standard pediatric care [8]. Studies have shown that children reported significantly more complaints when their parents gave attention to their complaints, than when parents distracted them from their complaints. Furthermore, parental overprotection may prevent adolescents from developing active coping strategies [8]. Family interventions discourage interactions that reinforce pain symptoms while teaching ways of providing positive reinforcement for improvement of functioning. This involves helping the children abandon their sick role through the encouragement of developmentally appropriate activities. Family therapy can explore ways in which the child's symptoms may serve to stabilize the system (i.e., a focus on the symptoms allows for the avoidance of conflict).

It is not uncommon for families to remain resistant to psychiatric intervention. In these cases it is helpful for the mental health clinician to remain a consultant to the pediatrician, by advising alternative ways in which the physician can decrease reinforcement for the sick role as well as encouraging mobilization of the patient. The mental health clinician can also help advise regarding the need for social service intervention around possible parental neglect, namely, seeking multiple unnecessary medical procedures.

Children with profound and pervasive withdrawal, including refusal to eat, drink, talk, walk, and engage in any form of self-care, will likely need more intensive treatment [3]. Inpatient multidisciplinary rehabilitation settings have a great deal to offer these patients as they are designed to support both physical and psychological recovery. Families feel reassured that staff can continue to monitor symptoms, thus ensuring that misdiagnoses will be recognized quickly.

Multidisciplinary rehabilitation approaches acknowledge the reality of the symptoms, emphasize the necessary involvement of both mind and body in the recovery process, but allow youngsters to "save face" through promoting physical recovery as the primary goal [14]. Studies have suggested that the treatment of patients on medical-psychiatric units leads to a decrease in medical service utilization and an appropriate increase in psychiatric interventions [54].

Pharmacotherapy

Psychopharmacological interventions are usually not the first line of treatment for somatoform disorders. However, judicious use of psychopharmacological treatment may be considered when other psychiatric disorders are co-occurring (e.g., depressive or anxiety disorders) [2].

For chronic pain disorders, tricyclic and serotonergic antidepressants have been effective in adult populations [55–57]. While there is an extensive literature on the use of analgesics for the treatment of acute pediatric pain [58], there are significant limitations in the existing data for the use of these medications for childhood pain disorders. For instance, while 84% of 25 children with recurrent abdominal pain responded to a citalopram trial, the study was limited by its open trial methodology and small sample size [59]. Clinical experience would suggest that the mental health clinician and pediatrician must be alert not to undertreat pain in the context of a presentation that has both psychological and physical contributing factors. Medication targeting the pain associated with the specific general medical condition should be an important consideration in an integrated medical and psychiatric intervention program. It is important for physicians to be alert to the use of analgesics to treat pain due to a general medical condition. Undertreated physical pain will only exacerbate any associated psychological factors, maintain functional disability, and undermine the treatment alliance.

The pediatric literature regarding the psychopharmacological treatment of body dysmorphic disorder is sparse; however, in adult studies, the selective serotonin reuptake inhibitors, in combination with CBT, have been judged to be effective in treating body dysmorphic disorder, with reductions in preoccupation about appearance and improvement in functioning [48].

Conclusion

Unexplained somatic complaints in children and adolescents represent a significant challenge to consulting mental health clinicians and their pediatric colleagues. The economic costs of somatization are great, in terms of loss of patient and family productivity and the negative impact on health-care costs and the delivery of services [5, 42]. The continuity of these disorders from childhood through adulthood is in need of further study to help the early identification of those "at risk" for chronic disabling illness. Clinical outcome studies are needed to assess the impact of integrated medical and psychiatric treatment interventions in children and adolescents.

References

1. Bursch B, Lester P, Jiang L, et al. Psychosocial predictors of somatic symptoms in adolescents of parents with HIV: a six-year longitudinal study. *AIDS Care* 2008; **20**:667–676.
2. Silber TJ. Somatization disorders: diagnosis, treatment, and prognosis. *Pediatr Rev* 2011;**32**:56–64.
3. Garralda ME. Unexplained physical complaints. *Child Adolesc Psychiatr Clin N Am* 2010;**19**:199–209, vii.
4. Kelly C, Molcho M, Doyle P, et al. Psychosomatic symptoms among schoolchildren. *Int J Adolesc Med Health* 2010;**22**:229–235.
5. Sumathipala A, Siribaddana S, Hewege S, et al. Understanding the explanatory model of the patient on their medically unexplained symptoms and its implication on treatment development research: a Sri Lanka Study. *BMC Psychiatry* 2008;**8**:54.
6. Coskun M, Zoroglu S. Long-lasting conversion disorder and hospitalization in a young girl: importance of early recognition and intervention. *Turk J Pediatr* 2009;**51**:282–286.
7. Spratt EG, Thomas SG. Pediatric case study and review: is it a conversion disorder? *Int J Psychiatry Med* 2008; **38**:185–193.
8. Janssens KA, Oldehinkel AJ, Rosmalen JG. Parental overprotection predicts the development of functional somatic symptoms in young adolescents. *J Pediatr* 2009;**154**:918–923.
9. Walker LS, Beck JE, Garber J, et al. Children's Somatization Inventory: psychometric properties of the revised form (CSI–24). *J Pediatr Psychol* 2009;**34**:430–440.
10. American Psychiatric Association. *Diagnostic and Statistical Manual of Mental Disorders*, 4th edn, Text Revision (DSM-IV-TR). Washington, DC: American Psychiatric Association, 2000.
11. Nickel R, Ademmer K, Egle UT. Manualized Psychodynamic Interactional Group Therapy for the treatment of somatoform pain disorders. *Bull Menninger Clin* 2010;**74**:219–237.
12. Schulte IE, Petermann F. Somatoform disorders: 30 years of debate about criteria! What about children and adolescents? *J Psychosom Res* 2011;**70**:218–228.
13. Kozlowska K, Rose D, Khan R, MA, Kram S, Lane L, Collins J. A conceptual model and practice framework for managing chronic pain in children and adolescents. *Harv Rev Psychiatry* 2008;**16**:136–150.
14. Griffin A, Christie D. Taking the psycho out of psychosomatic: using systemic approaches in a paediatric setting for the treatment of adolescents with unexplained physical symptoms. *Clin Child Psychol Psychiatry* 2008; **13**:531–542.

15. Dufton LM, Dunn MJ, Compas BE. Anxiety and somatic complaints in children with recurrent abdominal pain and anxiety disorders. *J Pediatr Psychol* 2009;**34**:176–186.

16. Groholt EK, Stigum H, Nordhagen R, *et al.* Recurrent pain in children, socio-economic factors and accumulation in families. *Eur J Epidemiol* 2003;**18**:965–975.

17. Borkum JM. Chronic headaches and the neurobiology of somatization. *Curr Pain Headache Rep* 2010;**14**:55–61.

18. Di Lorenzo C, Youssef NN, Sigurdsson L, *et al.* Visceral hyperalgesia in children with functional abdominal pain. *J Pediatr* 2001;**139**:838–843.

19. Cloninger CR. Somatoform and dissociative disorders. In: Winokur G, Clayton PJ (eds) *The Medical Basis of Psychiatry*, 2nd edn. Philadelphia: WB Saunders Co, 1994; p 169.

20. Meredith PJ, Ownsworth T, Strong J. A review of the evidence linking adult attachment theory and chronic pain: Presenting a conceptual model. *Clin Psychol Rev* 2008;**28**:407–429.

21. Stiles TC, Wright D. Cognitive behavioral treatment of chronic pain conditions. *Nord J Psychiatry* 2008;**62**(Suppl 47): 30–36.

22. Bursh B. Pediatric pain. In: Shaw RJ, DeMaso DR (eds) *Textbook of Pediatric Psychosomatic Medicine: Mental Health Consultation with Physically Ill Children*. Washington, DC: American Psychiatric Press, Inc., 2010; pp. 141–154.

23. Hesketh T, Zhen Y, Lu L, *et al.* Stress and psychosomatic symptoms in Chinese school children: cross-sectional survey. *Arch Dis Child* 2010;**95**:136–140.

24. American Academy of Child and Adolescent Psychiatry. Practice parameter for the psychiatric assessment and management of physical ill children and adolescents. *J Am Acad Child Adolesc Psychiatry* 2009;**48**:213–233.

25. Campo JV, Bridge J, Ehmann M, *et al.* Recurrent abdominal pain, anxiety, and depression in primary care. *Pediatrics* 2004;**113**:817–824.

26. Seshia SS, Phillips DF, von Baeyer CL. Childhood Chronic Daily Headache: a biopsychosocial perspective. *Dev Med Child Neurol* 2008;**50**:541–545.

27. Libow J. Beyond collusion: active illness falsification. *Child Abuse Negl* 2002;**26**:525–536.

28. Squires JE, Squires RH Jr., Munchausen syndrome by proxy: ongoing clinical challenges. *J Pediatr Gastroenterol Nutr* 2010;**51**:248–253.

29. Campo JV, Fritsch SL. Somatization in children and adolescents. *J Am Acad Child Adolesc Psychiatry* 1994;**33**:1223–1235.

30. Nickel R, Hardt J, Käppis B, Schwab R, Egle UT. Somatoform disorders with pain as the predominant symptom: Results to distinguish a common group of disease. *Schmerz* 2009;**23**:392–398.

31. Campo JV, Di Lorenzo C, Chiappetta L, *et al.* Adult outcomes of pediatric recurrent abdominal pain: Do they just grow out of it? *Pediatrics* 2001;**108**:e1.

32. Shaw RJ, Spratt EJ, Bernard RS, DeMaso DR. Somatoform Disorders. In Shaw RJ, DeMaso DR (eds) *Textbook of Pediatric Psychosomatic Medicine: Mental Health Consultation with Physically Ill Children*. Washington, DC: American Psychiatric Press, Inc., 2010; pp. 121–139.

33. Teo WY, Choong CT. Neurological presentations of conversion disorders in a group of Singapore children. *Pediatr Int* 2008;**50**:533–536.

34. Siket MS, Merchant RC. Psychogenic seizures: A review and description of pitfalls in their acute diagnosis and management in the emergency department. *Emerg Med Clin North Am* 2011;**29**:73–81.

35. Kozlowska K. Good children presenting with conversion disorder. *Clin Child Psychol Psychiat* 2001;**6**:575–591.

36. Johnson KB, Harris C, Forstein M, Joffe A. Adolescent conversion disorder and the importance of competence discussing sexual orientation. *Clin Pediatr (Phila)* 2010;**49**:491–494.

37. Bujoreanu IS, Ibeziako PI, DeMaso DR. Psychiatric concerns in pediatric epilepsy. *Child Adolesc Psychiatric Clin N Am* 2010;**19**:371–386.

38. Weller EB, Weller RA, Fristad MA. Use of sodium amytal interviews in pre-pubertal children: indications, procedure, and clinical utility. *J Am Acad Child Psychiatry* 1985;**24**:747–749.

39. Hafeiz HB. Hysterical conversion: a prognostic study. *Br J Psychiatry* 1980;**136**:548–551.

40. Weintraub MI. *Hysterical Conversion Reactions: A Clinical Guide to Diagnosis and Treatment.* New York: Spectrum, 1983.

41. Lin JM, Resch SC, Brimmer DJ, *et al.* The economic impact of chronic fatigue syndrome in Georgia: direct and indirect costs. *Cost Eff Resour Alloc* 2011;**9**:1.

42. Fritz GK, Fritsch S, Hagino O. Somatoform disorders in children and adolescents: A review of the past 10 years. *J Am Acad Child Adolesc Psychiatry* 1997; **36**:1329–1338.

43. Ibeziako PI, Shaw J, DeMaso DR. Psychosomatic illness. In: Kliegman RM, Stanton BF, St. Geme J, *et al.* (eds) *Nelson Textbook of Pediatrics*. Philadelphia: Elsevier, 2011, 67–70.

44. Guze SB, Cloninger CR, Martin RL, *et al.* A follow-up and family study of Briquet's syndrome. *Br J Psychiatry* 1986;**149**:17–23.

45. Allen A, Hollander E. Body dysmorphic disorder. *Psychiatr Clin North Am* 2000;**23**:617–628.

46. Phillips KA. Body dysmorphic disorder: the distress of imagined ugliness. *Am J Psychiatry* 1991; **148**:1138–1149.

47. Didie ER, Tortolani CC, Pope CG, *et al.* Childhood abuse and neglect in body dysmorphic disorder. *Child Abuse Negl* 2006;**30**:1105–1115.

48. Bjornsson AS, Didie ER, Phillips KA. Body dysmorphic disorder dialogues. *Clin Neurosci* 2010;**12**:221–232.

49. Sarwer DB, Crerand CE, Magee L. Body dysmorphic disorder in patients who seek appearance-enhancing medical treatments. *Oral Maxillofac Surg Clin North Am* 2010;**22**:445–453.

50. Shaw RJ, DeMaso DR. Somatoform disorders. In: Shaw RJ, DeMaso DR (eds) *Clinical Manual of Pediatric Psychosomatic Medicine*. American Psychiatric Publishing Inc., 2006; pp. 143–168.

51. Kanaan RA, Armstrong D, Wessely SC. Neurologists' understanding and management of conversion disorder. *J Neurol Neurosurg Psychiatry* 2011;**82**:961–966.

52. Karterud HN, Knizek BL, Nakken KO. Changing the diagnosis from epilepsy to PNES: patients' experiences and understanding of their new diagnosis. *Seizure* 2010;**19**:40–46.

53. Masia Warner C, Reigada LC, Fisher PH, *et al.* CBT for anxiety and associated somatic complaints in pediatric medical settings: an open pilot study. *J Clin Psychol Med Settings* 2009;**16**:169–177.

54. Leue C, Driessen G, Strik JJ, *et al.* Managing complex patients on a medical psychiatric unit: an observational study of university hospital costs associated with medical service use, length of stay, and psychiatric intervention. *J Psychosom Res* 2010;**68**:295–302.

55. Ansari A. The efficacy of newer antidepressants in the treatment of chronic pain: A review of the current literature. *Harv Rev Psychiatry* 2000;**7**:257–277.

56. Carter GT, Sullivan MD. Antidepressants in pain management. *Curr Opn Investig Drugs* 2002;**3**:454–458.

57. Goldstein DJ, Lu Y, Detke MJ, Hudson J, Iyengar S, Demitrack MA. Effects of Duloxetine on painful physical symptoms associated with depression. *Psychosomatics* 2004;**45**:17–28.

58. Berde CB, Sethna NF. Analgesics for the treatment of pain in children. *N Engl J Med* 2002;**347**:1094–1103.

59. Campo JV, Perel J, Lucas A, *et al.* Citalopram treatment of pediatric recurrent abdominal pain and comorbid internalizing disorders: An exploratory study. *J Am Acad Child Adolesc Psychiatry* 2004;**43**:1234–1242.

27

Sleep Disorders

Martin B. Scharf, Christine V. Wellborn

Introduction

After the birth of our first child 24 years ago, I [M.B.S.] experienced a clinical awakening, when on the first night home from the hospital my daughter wouldn't sleep or stop crying. Few things can disrupt a healthy family like a sleepless child. The cacophonous screaming was upsetting us all and adding to our frustration. When Grandma awoke, came downstairs, and took the child, it was if the Marines had landed: Rosalyn instantly quieted and went to sleep.

Few things can disrupt a healthy family like a sleepless child. Sleep is preponderant during the first few months of life and is important for growth, development, and good health. Disordered sleep can be an indication of a multitude of problems, both physiological and psychological, and can cause, contribute to, or exacerbate medical and psychiatric conditions.

Unfortunately, most physicians, even those earning their degrees as recently as the early 1990s, have throughout their medical training been exposed to less than 2 hours of didactic material regarding sleep [1]. Although adult psychiatrists have a better appreciation for insomnia because of its ubiquity in their patients, little is generally taught regarding childhood sleep disorders. Our goal in this chapter is to familiarize the reader with the nuances of normal sleep and to provide insight into the array of childhood sleep disorders and their diagnosis, management, and treatment.

Normal Sleep

Normal sleep is characterized by recurring cycles of non-rapid-eye-movement (NREM) sleep followed by rapid-eye-movement (REM) sleep, each cycle lasting on average between 70 and 90 minutes in adults. NREM sleep is divided into three stages. Stage 1 is the lightest stage and is generally a transient state; it is the stage associated with falling asleep and usually also occurs in association with body movements and arousals. Individuals can be easily awakened from stage 1 sleep and their eyes move slowly under the eyelids. Heart rate and breathing tend to slow down, and thought patterns are still associated with daytime activity. Individuals awakened from this stage of sleep often state that they were not sleeping and indicate an awareness of things occurring around them, although they may even have been snoring. Stage 2 is a deeper stage of sleep characterized by electroencephalogram (EEG) patterns known as sleep spindles and K-complexes. Eye movements are absent, and the heart rate continues to slow, as does respiration. Individuals awakened from this stage of sleep generally have little or no recall. Stage 3 is the deepest stage of sleep, in which high-voltage slow waves are a prominent component of EEG patterns. This stage includes the slowest rates of breathing and heart activity and the highest frequency of night sweats. Recall is difficult to obtain from this sleep stage, in part because individuals are very slow to awaken.

In REM sleep, eyes move rapidly under the eyelids. Heart rate and breathing become irregular and more rapid. There is a loss of muscle tone resulting in a generalized paralysis, except for twitches of small peripheral muscles. Watching a dog or cat sleeping – seeing it twitch its paws, move its whiskers, and make yelping noises – one can appreciate that even pets dream; we wonder what they think they are chasing. The paralysis observed in REM sleep seems to allow a safe expression of dream material by preventing people from acting out their dreams [2].

Newborns do not experience adult-like sleep stages until sometime during their first year. Newborn sleep is described as quiet, active, or indeterminate. Quiet sleep consists of NREM sleep, but with marked differences from that of adults. NREM sleep is undifferentiated, and newborns show no loss of muscle tone, and as a result, their REM sleep is more obvious and is referred to as active sleep, because of the eye movements, grimacing

Clinical Child Psychiatry, Third Edition. Edited by William M. Klykylo and Jerald Kay.
© 2012 John Wiley & Sons, Ltd. Published 2012 by John Wiley & Sons, Ltd.

and sucking activity, twitching and writhing body movements, and an increased level of physiological activity.

Newborn infants sleep approximately 16 hours per day in polyphasic, short bursts of 2–4 hours. REM, or active, sleep occupies the majority of total sleep time (Figure 27.1) [3–5]. Infants usually experience REM periods with the onset of sleep, unlike adults, whose *REM latency* (time from sleep onset to the first REM period) is 70–90 minutes [6]. Newborns' sleep time decreases over the course of the first year, and they continue to nap regularly until the age of about 2 or 3 years. Between the ages of 2 and 5 years, sleep is consolidated and reduced to a 10-hour period, with most children giving up daytime naps between 3 and 5 years of age [7–10].

By the end of their third month, infants typically exhibit the three distinct stages of NREM sleep as well as regular patterns of REM and NREM sleep, with little or no indeterminate sleep. The overall sleep cycle lasts approximately 40–60 minutes at this age and will gradually lengthen to 60–70 minutes in children, and to 90 minutes in adolescence and adulthood; total sleep time gradually decreases. The longest sleep period now tends to occur at night, and most children sleep through the night by 6 months of age [7–10].

Sleep patterns at all ages alternate through cycles that are generally 90 minutes in length; 5–10% of the night is spent in stage 1, 50% in stage 2, 20% in stage 3 sleep, and 20% in REM sleep. Young children spend more time in *slow wave* (stage 3) sleep than do adults. Children between 2 and 5 years of age usually obtain as much as 2 hours of slow-wave sleep over the course of a night. This is particularly significant because the preponderance of the 24-hour total growth hormone is released during these slow-wave sleep phases. Indeed, when sleep is moved to a different time of the 24-hour day, the timing of growth hormone secretion changes accordingly [3, 4]. As sleep cycles repeat throughout the night, REM sleep occupies a greater portion of each cycle, becoming as long as 40–60 minutes within the latter REM periods.

Dreams

Dreams occur in both REM and NREM sleep, but their characteristics are quite different. In NREM sleep, dream phenomena are concrete and more logical; recall is less elaborate and tends to be related to activities that normally occur during the day. Dreams occurring in REM sleep are less logical, are more elaborate, are associated with emotional experiences, and generally are more memorable [11–14].

Several theories exist regarding the function and purpose of dreams. Some researchers have hypothesized that dreams play a role in information processing and learning; they may function to consolidate newly acquired information, thereby reconciling new information with existing memories [15, 16]. The increased protein synthesis that occurs during REM sleep seems to support this view [17]. Protein buildup in some synapses has been shown to strengthen those synapses, increasing their influence on postsynaptic neurons and cumulatively serving to reorganize the neural pathways [18]. Crick and Mitchison have proposed that dreams may be important in unlearning faulty information and processing, making the subjective experience of dreaming merely a byproduct of this "waste removal" process [19].

Dreams in childhood tend to be shorter than those in adult life. The age of the child influences the subject matter: By about 12 to 18 months of age, the subject matter of children's dreams likely mirrors that of their waking fears [20]. Children's reports of their dreams are less elaborate, have less of a storyline, and involve more intense imagery and emotion. It is possible that since sleep is so much deeper in children than in adults, the delay in coming to full alertness allows the dream content to escape recall.

According to Golbin [21], there are recognizable stages in the development of dreams. Children between 3 and 5 years of age have easily identifiable negative images, which are generally singular. By 5 years of age, their dreams become more complex and can symbolically reflect real situations such as family conflict. Children become active participants in their dreams, trying

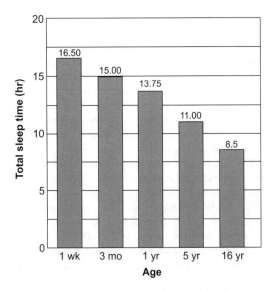

Figure 27.1 Age progression of total sleep time from newborn to 16 years.

Table 27.1 The progression of dream content in children.

Age	Dream content
0–12 months	Shorter periods than adults; content unknown
12–18 months	Association with waking fears
2 years	Recall begins; content usually related to emotionally significant events of the previous day
3–5 years	Easily identifiable negative images
5 years	Increased complexity that may reflect reality
10–12 years	Experiences such as pleasure, smell, and touch
Adolescence	Content increasingly repetitive or continuous

to run away, escape, or defend themselves. By 7 or 8 years of age, concrete images become rich, with some elaborate and bizarre recounts (Table 27.1).

Children don't only experience frightening nightmares but can become heroes and experience pleasant sensations in their dreams. By 10 to 12 years of age, children often experience movements and other sensations in their dreams that can be indistinguishable from hallucinations; they can experience senses of smell, feel, and touch. By adolescence, dreams can become repetitive or continuous. One only remembers the dreams from which one awakens. Thus, when patients report frequent dreaming, they may be describing the last dream of the night from which they awoke, or may also be providing an indication that frequent awakenings are occurring [22].

Sleep Hygiene

Sleep hygiene is a term used to describe the set of behaviors that influence a person's ability to initiate and maintain sleep. Good sleep hygiene can facilitate the development of normal sleep and stable sleep patterns, and prevent some behaviorally caused sleep disorders, whereas poor hygiene can serve to initiate or antagonize some sleep disorders. The exact behaviors of sleep hygiene may vary with a person's age, time constraints, and individual preferences, and they generally center on the themes of forming and adhering to a consistent pre-bedtime routine, maximizing comfort, and avoiding counterproductive habits.

Sleep Hygiene in Infants

Given the changes in sleep continuity that occur during infancy, optimal sleep hygiene behaviors vary even within this age group. Parents should generally not attempt to change the neonate's sleep patterns, because the highly fragmented nature of neonate sleep is a part of their natural development. Babies alternate between NREM and REM sleep, and sleep periods may last from a few hours to only a few minutes. Although it may be frustrating to parents at times, they can be reassured by the fact that severe sleep fragmentation typically does not last beyond the first 3 to 6 months. If an infant's sleep patterns must be modified to accommodate transient time constraints, such as while traveling, it is typically more effective to facilitate the change by waking the child from sleep than attempting to force sleep at normally non-sleeping times. As the infant's sleep begins to consolidate, sleep hygiene can facilitate the natural transition. In fact, this is a good time to start providing external cues that will help orient the child's sleep/wake patterns to an adaptive cycle [22–24].

Although the nutritional need for nighttime feedings is gone by 6 months of age, such feedings may persist. Problems arise when the child associates feeding with sleep; the child must then feed to return to sleep, which results in an excessive intake of fluid. The resulting bladder distention causes frequent awakenings, producing a circular pattern of arousals followed by feeding. The child's diapers are typically soaked by morning. If this pattern of feeing persists, it may prevent the child from developing a mature sleep/wake cycle by reinforcing an altered circadian rhythm. Since the child no longer has a biological need for nighttime feedings, treatment of this disorder consists of gradually decreasing and then ceasing feedings over 1–2 weeks [22, 25–27].

Routines

Routines serve to facilitate consistency in sleep patterns. Bedtimes and wake times should remain as constant as possible. When sleep begins to consolidate, an infant typically begins to respond to external cues that indicate when to sleep. It may be necessary at this time to supplement natural cues with parental cues. If, for example, an infant over 6 months of age tends to sleep more during the day than at night, it may be necessary to gradually shorten the daytime sleep period by waking the child early from his or her daytime sleep; this process should result in a lengthening of nocturnal sleep. Feeding and changing at night should be quiet, and it may help to reduce the amount of light during these times. It may also help to use loosely fitting clothing on the child at night, so changing diapers involves less activity and stimulation [22–24].

Prior to evening bedtime, it is important to begin a bedtime ritual. Although the particular activities may vary among individuals, they should follow some guidelines. The bedtime ritual should involve activities that minimize physical activity and elicit a calming response that prepares the infant for sleep. Often, pre-sleep rituals for infants involve parents giving them a warm bath; changing them into pajamas; reading, humming, or singing to them; changing their diapers; and feeding and burping them (not necessarily in that order). At this point in development, the content of the reading or singing is not as important as the sound of the parent's voice and contact with the parent. The routine should remain constant from night to night: Repeating the same activities in succession at the same time each night provides additional cues that bedtime is approaching. After a good bedtime ritual, an infant should be more relaxed and mentally prepared to sleep [22–24].

Infants, like adults, learn to associate certain environmental surroundings with sleep. Specific environmental cues (such as our bedrooms, our beds) alert us to the proper time and place to sleep. Even though we occasionally awaken during the night, these cues are available to reassure us that everything is as it should be and allow us to return to sleep, often without the awareness of having wakened. Anders and Keener [28] reported that even at 2 months of age, 50% of infants' nocturnal awakenings require no parental attention. Disorders arise, however, when sleep is associated with environmental characteristics that are no longer available in subsequent nocturnal awakenings. If a child is consistently rocked to sleep, for example, the child begins to associate sleep with rocking and may have difficulty falling asleep without it. This becomes more of a problem for parents during nocturnal awakenings, because the child cannot return to sleep without active parental participation. Problematic activities include consistently moving the child after the onset of sleep or holding the child until he or she is asleep, because the child cannot re-establish these conditions without some assistance. The distinguishing feature of this particular problem is that once the "required" conditions are re-established, the onset of sleep occurs rapidly. Note that the problem lies not in abnormal awakenings but rather in an inability to return to sleep, which abnormally prolongs the awakenings.

New associations with the onset of sleep can be established without parental participation. A child must learn to go to sleep in his or her own bed alone. To facilitate this learning process, parents must remove themselves from the environment to the furthest extent possible. The child should be placed in the crib, and the parent should leave the room while the child is still awake. In the case of crying, parents should return to

the room only after a predetermined period (usually no less than 15 minutes), and they should make only visual contact. This return allows the parent to show the child that he or she has not been abandoned but reaffirms that the task of falling asleep is the child's own responsibility. The length of time between the initiating of crying and the parental response should be gradually increased. If the problem is properly diagnosed, this treatment will typically result in dramatic improvements within the first few days. Since the treatment depends on parental commitment, parents should be involved in deciding the appropriate schedule [21, 24, 29–32].

Maximizing Comfort

Several steps can be taken to maximize comfort during sleep, which may help to eliminate some of the disruptions that can occur during nighttime awakenings. Although increasing infant comfort is helpful at any time, it is particularly appropriate if several nocturnal awakenings are accompanied by fussing rather than a quiet return to sleep. Infants should be placed in bed awake but drowsy in a position that seems to be the most comfortable for them. It is not imperative that they be placed in a bed awake every night, however; allowing infants to fall asleep on their own while drowsy conveys to them a sense of self-ownership of the task of falling asleep. An infant may therefore be less likely to demand the attention of an adult during each nighttime arousal and may instead learn to fall back to sleep independently [21]. Making the crib more comfortable by warming the sheets with a heating pad (be sure to check the temperature by hand before placing the infant in bed). An article of the parent's clothing may also be placed securely in the crib to make the crib smell more familiar [22].

Nocturnal congestion may affect an infant's breathing and sleep, given their physical propensity for obligate nose breathing. Sleep position may have an effect on the infant's ease of breathing, and it is commonly recommended to place babies on their backs. Using a humidifier may also be beneficial, as might the use of an external nasal dilator (e.g., Breathe Right). In a pilot study conducted in our laboratory, we demonstrated a marked reduction in obstructive breathing events in infants suffering nasal congestion, after applying Breathe Right strips, cut to size [33].

Younger children may experience an allergy to the cow's milk found in formula, resulting in frequent nocturnal awakenings and a shorter total sleep time than that of normal age cohorts [34]. Pain from otitis media is another reported source of younger childhood sleep disturbances [24].

Colic

A first major concern for 20% of parents is colic, which develops during the second or third week after birth [35]. Colic consists of extended spells of extreme fussiness, including inconsolable crying [36] and a hypertonic state characterized by clenched fists, twisting, writhing, batting, flapping, facial grimaces, and a sensitivity to light [36]. The exact cause of colic is unknown, but it may include immaturity of the central nervous system, a need to exercise the lungs [37], an allergy to cow's milk, pain from excess gas, and decreased progesterone levels [38]. Evidence suggests that colic may serve some adaptive purpose, but the negative impact on the parents' sleeping pattern and ability to cope with the child may have future deleterious effects.

Studies suggest that although colic itself usually subsides by 4 months of age, post-colic infants have a greater tendency toward disturbed sleep and are also more likely to develop a "difficult" temperament (Table 27.2). Weissbluth and colleagues reported that 76% of post-colic infants experience problems with frequent nocturnal awakenings and generally show a shorter sleep duration [38]. Some post-colic infants are also very sensitive to changes in the sleep/wake schedule such as might occur during vacations or illnesses. Parental mismanagement of sleep patterns in post-colic infants has been implicated as a major source of later sleep problems. To avoid future sleep problems, parents should set and adhere to strict sleep/wake schedules immediately after colic has subsided. Unfortunately, the nurturing behavior and over-responsiveness learned by parents during the colic phase may create a tendency toward overstimulating children during the post-colic phase. The resulting child behaviors may include irregular sleep (settling problems and prolonged awakenings), crankiness, easy frustration, and impatience. In contrast, adherence to a sleep/wake schedule combined with good sleep hygiene can lead to a more positive infant mood, more flexible behavior, and a calmer expression of emotion [35–37, 39–41].

Sleep Hygiene in Older Children

As children learn to comprehend and use language, the process of sleep hygiene should evolve to incorporate these changes. Once children can understand language, it becomes easier for parents to understand their needs and for children to understand the parents' expectations.

Routines

As a child gets older, poor sleep may result from a failure to set appropriate parental limits. Children presenting with this problem typically report no consistent bedtime routine. Parents may give in to a child's demands to read one more story or stay awake to watch a television program. The onset of sleep frequently occurs in atypical places such as in front of the television, resulting in poor sleep onset associations. Parental inconsistency reinforces the child's attempts to make demands, eventually resulting in a nightly power struggle. Difficulties in setting limits may concurrently manifest in other areas of the parent-child relationship.

Disordered routine modification focuses first on the parents. They should be educated about the use of bedtime rituals and the importance of being consistent and persistent in setting limits for their children. The creation of and adherence to a bedtime ritual that uses constant reminders to set expectations for the child can help turn bedtime into a positive experience for both

Table 27.2 Pediatric medical associations of sleeplessness.

Condition	Features
Colic	Inconsolable fussiness in late afternoon or evening, with manifestations such as clenched fists, twisting, writhing, batting, and facial grimaces Usually presents in the third or fourth week of life Usually subsides by 3 to 4 months of age
Sleep onset-association disorder	Child depends on specific caretaker behaviors (such as rocking) to initiate or reinitiate sleep
Feeding-related disorder	Child must feed on awakening to return to sleep
Limit-setting disorder	Failure by parents to exercise appropriate limits to child's behavior
Medical factors	Otitis media, gastroesophageal reflux, respiratory difficulties that may or may not meet the criteria for obstructive sleep apnea syndrome
Medication effects	All medications must be considered a possible cause, either by their intended effects, side effects, or withdrawal effects

parents and children. When the agreed bedtime arrives, the child must go to bed without exception. It may be necessary at first to place barriers to keep the child in his or her bedroom, but this tactic must always be used in conjunction with proximal parent supervision.

It is important when establishing limits that parents distinguish legitimate nighttime fears from a child's attempt to stay awake by professing fears; treating legitimate nighttime fears by setting strict limits may result in serious emotional problems [22, 24].

Routines can become more stable once a child's sleep has consolidated. Bedtimes and wake times can be more regular and should continue to be enforced. Bedtime rituals continue to prepare a child's body and mind for sleep, but the activities change as the child becomes older. The bedtime ritual should be discussed with the child, and the length of time should be agreed on before the ritual is used. Examples of appropriate ritual activities at the age of 5 years include quiet play, preparing for bed (brushing teeth, changing into pajamas, etc.), reading stories in bed, and spending time quietly discussing the day's events. The child should know the progression of events and the time at which each activity should occur. This child should also be occasionally reminded of the planned progression throughout the ritual (e.g., "Remember, it will be time to change into your pajamas in 5 minutes"). Such reminders will help avert struggles over when to go to bed and will make bedtime a pleasurable experience for the child, rather than one of uncertainty [22]. Activities should include relaxing behaviors and should provide a sense of closure for the day. A quiet time to talk about the day's events, for example, may provide the child with a chance to voice concerns and worries, which may prevent extensive brooding and a lack of sleep after the ritual is completed [22, 24].

Counterproductive Habits

Children should not be allowed to stay up as they wish. Bedtime and wake time should be consistent and determined by the parent. Bedtime rituals are employed in part to make the parentally imposed bedtime more acceptable to the child. Children should not be allowed to routinely fall asleep in rooms other than their own bedrooms or in front of a television. If a child begins to get drowsy, he or she may go to bed early. Activities in a child's bedroom should be restricted to sleeping and bedtime rituals only, so that the child associates going to his or her bedroom with going to sleep.

Changing the child's environment after he or she has fallen asleep should be avoided. Examples of changes include moving the child to a different room or a parent leaving the room after the child has fallen asleep. Such changes may confuse the child when he or she next awakens and may make returning to sleep more difficult. These changes can be avoided by planning a bedtime ritual that places the child in his or her bedroom alone before initiating sleep.

Counterproductive habits include anything that may interfere with the routines and comforts explained in the previous two sections. Some specifics include the following:

(1) Avoid permitting the child to dictate his or her sleep schedule after 3–6 months of age. Instead, actively provide cues that allow the child to adapt to the new sleep schedule.
(2) Avoid regularly sleeping with the child. Everyone's sleep is more disturbed from the extra movement of an additional person, and sleeping alone may reduce later separation anxiety [22, 24].
(3) Avoid engaging in physically stimulating activity immediately prior to bedtime. This is most easily accomplished by planning a bedtime ritual and adhering to it.

Avoid behaviors that make the child dependent on parents to fall asleep. Examples are consistently rocking the child to sleep or lying with the child until he or she is asleep. These behaviors become associated with falling asleep and can be counterproductive: Because children associate parents and parental behavior as a necessary part of falling asleep, if they awake during the night, they may need the sleep onset associations to be back to sleep [22, 24].

Problems of Childhood Sleep

Both transient and persistent insomnias exist in children of all ages. Although the onset of adult-like insomnia in childhood is rare (and even more rarely diagnosed), social, environmental, psychological, medical, and chronophysiological factors and parasomnias can interfere with a child's normal pattern of sleep [25]. One primary difference between the presentation of childhood and adult sleep disorders, however, is that it is typically the parents, not the patient, who have the complaints. Although when children are professionally treated, parents' subjective responses are generally more positive than childrens' [42]. Disordered sleep habits that keep the parents awake at night or influence the child's performance at school are more likely to be recognized than those that simply bring discomfort to the child (as might be more the case in adult insomnia) [22, 24].

When sleep problems occur in children, they tend to evoke pain and discomfort in the family, often raising more concern by the parents than by the child. Children and adolescents with insomnia most often report difficulty falling asleep, rather than difficulty maintaining sleep. Pre-sleep arousal, also referred to as *sleep onset anxiety*, is common in children after a day of stressful events or trauma or simply results from difficulty in establishing healthy bedtime routines.

Circadian rhythm disturbances (which can also cause difficulty in falling asleep) can result in severe daytime sleepiness, which affects school performance and self-image. Parasomnias, such as chronic bedwetting, sleepwalking, night terrors, and nightmares, can affect children's opportunities to socialize and can ultimately affect their self-image and self-esteem. In addition, sleep apnea, a condition most usually associated with middle-aged and older adults who are overweight, can occur in children, especially those with enlarged tonsils or nasal airway deformities. Recognizing how poor sleep can affect mood, daytime function, and overall development is an important responsibility of parents, physicians, and especially psychiatrists. Sleep laboratory evaluations are rarely necessary in children with a history of insomnia, sleepwalking, night terrors, or enuresis; however, when sleep apnea is suspected, home or laboratory recording is important. Often an overnight oximetry screen precedes the polysomnogram. Our preference is to record children in their home environment whenever possible to minimize the anxiety of being away from home and to make the recording less "hospital-like."

Disordered sleep can be an indication of other problems, both physiological and psychological, and can also contribute to and exacerbate medical and psychiatric conditions. Children typically "settle" into mature sleeping patterns between the ages of 6 and 12 months [43]. Disturbed sleep may recur throughout early childhood, however. Reports on the prevalence of disordered sleep continue to range between approximately 25% and 33% until children reach school age [22, 24]. One study of 60 children aged 15 to 48 months found that 42% had experienced some sleep problems [29]. Many of the earlier behavioral causes of troubled sleep contribute to the difficulty in navigating this transition into mature and normative sleep habits.

Childhood disruptions in sleep are often a source of serious frustration to parents, and they may trigger child abuse [40]. Therapy tends to focus on correcting the presenting complaint rather than determining the original cause. In most of these disorders, the child–parent interaction is a crucial part of the therapy, regardless of the underlying cause. But since children often respond differently to family authority figures, consulting a physician or a sleep specialist may be helpful. Interestingly, parents and children may assess sleep problems quite differently, making self-reports necessary when feasible. Parents may under-report their child's sleep difficulty and may not associate or fully comprehend the daytime challenges their child faces as a result of sleeplessness [42].

Medications

Medications may interfere with a child's ability to sleep. Paradoxically, sedating antihistamines may actually cause insomnia. Major sedatives, antihistamines, and short-acting benzodiazepines all have the potential for residual grogginess the next day, which may negate the effects of any improvements in sleep. Other medications, such as antibiotic preparations or nonprescription combination cold remedies, have also been noted to disturb sleep in children. If a medication is causing sleeplessness, it should be discontinued if possible. If discontinuation is not an option, the treatment should focus on examining the dosing regimen; changing the dose or the time the medication is taken may ameliorate the symptoms, as may changing to another drug of the same class [39].

Psychological Factors Related to Sleep Disorders

A range of psychological factors may also influence a child's quality of sleep. It is important to properly diagnose and address these issues to prevent their evolution into even more serious emotional disturbances. Childhood affective disorders tend to negatively affect sleep continuity. Children in a depressed mood frequently experience early morning awakenings, sleep onset problems, and more frequent nighttime arousals [44–47]. Maternal depression is also associated with sleep problems in children [39]. Emotional stressors such as family tension or grieving the death of a family member are associated with disrupted sleep. Five specific stressors have been found to be more prevalent in children with sleep disorders than in other children. These include:

(1) an accident or illness in the family;
(2) the unaccustomed absence of the mother during the day;
(3) a depressed mood of the mother;
(4) co-sleeping (i.e., sleeping with a parent); and
(5) maternal attitude of ambivalence toward the child [22, 24, 25, 45].

Nighttime fears and anxieties are a substantial psychological contributor to sleep disruption. The experience of fears and anxieties is normal in children but can become problematic if quality sleep is prevented. Typical topics include issues the child is currently facing, such as sibling rivalry, a fear of death or separation from a parent, and anxieties about negotiating the socialization process. The greatest treatment for these fears, even if they become excessive, is often parental understanding. Setting strict limits is not advised for this particular problem, but a change in bedtime or in the bedtime ritual may help alleviate some of the fears. For example, if children experience a phase delay (i.e., their actual sleep schedule falls behind their expected sleep schedule; see next section) but are put to bed early, the resulting hours awake in bed before the onset of sleep may produce some imaginative fears. The revised bedtime ritual for a child with excessive nighttime fears should include parental involvement and a gradual rather than abrupt withdrawal of the parent from the environment at bedtime [22, 24, 25].

Chronophysiological Factors

The influence of circadian rhythm on the human sleep/wake cycle is first evident between 6 weeks and 3 months of age [7, 48]. Infants' entrainment cues are initially related more to their feeding schedule than to light/dark cues. As entrainment shifts to light/dark cues, individual differences in the chronological distribution of circadian rhythms, or sleep phases, become apparent: Some people are more active in the early morning, whereas others seem to prefer being active at night. These individual differences are normal and become the source of sleep disturbance only when they conflict with a person's social, work, or school schedule. In childhood, problems may also arise if children's circadian rhythms conflict with their parents' schedule. Four basic problems associated with circadian rhythm may emerge: phase delay, phase advance, regular but inappropriate schedule, and irregular schedule (Table 27.3).

Phase delay occurs when a child's sleep schedule falls behind his or her expected sleep schedule [49–52]. A child with phase delay is physiologically ready for sleep later and naturally arises later than is expected or desired by the parents. Phase delay may result from the practice of going to bed later or from an inherited predisposition to sleep later. It occurs more in adoles-

cents than in younger children and often begins after a summer of late bedtimes and "sleeping in." Since the human circadian rhythm follows a 25-hour cycle without external cues, phase delay may occur quite easily [22, 25, 28]. The presenting complaint for phase delay is frequently insomnia associated with the onset of sleep or morning sluggishness [49–51, 53]. These children struggle to achieve sleep at bedtime because they are not physiologically ready; as a result, they may lie in bed for hours or struggle with parents at bedtime. Mornings are difficult for them, and they typically sleep late whenever possible to "catch up." If forced to awaken before they are ready (e.g., for school), they may experience sleep deprivation.

Proper diagnosis of phase delay is best accomplished by keeping a sleep diary for 23 weeks, including both weekdays and weekends (vacations too, if possible).

A clue to the diagnosis lies in weekend sleep behavior: Often the children stay up and sleep in late and feel much better than during the week when they are getting up at a time inconsistent with their optimal arising time. Diaries typically show that sleep onset occurs at approximately the same time regardless of bedtime (insomnia disappears on weekends or when the child is allowed to stay up later).

The treatment of *phase delay* should focus on accomplishing a phase advance that will synchronize the child's clock with his or her environment (Table 27.4). First, the child should be allowed to go to bed at the physiologically appropriate time (this effectively eliminates insomnia complaints). Next, the child should be awakened progressively earlier and prevented from taking excess naps. The resulting sleep deprivation will eventually function to advance the child's phase. In severe cases of phase delay, it may be more effective to allow the child's circadian clock to "free run," thereby delaying around the clock until it reaches the appropriate phase. Intense exposure to light at the appropriate times may facilitate the phase adjustment by providing additional external cues. When diagnosing symptoms as phase delay, it is important to be aware of a problem with similar symptoms called *motivational phase delay*. A child with motivational phase delay has trouble waking in the mornings

Table 27.3 Chronophysiological factors associated with sleep disorders.

Transition from feeding cues to light/dark cues (infants only)
Constitutional factors – Owl versus lark (i.e., naturally more alert in the morning vs evening)
Phase delay – Individual does not become sleepy until late; is difficult to awaken for school; exhibits no intrasleep problem
Phase advance – Individual becomes sleepy too early and awakens too early
Irregular schedule – Free-running lifestyle with no regular sleep/wake schedule

Table 27.4 Treatment of sleep phase disorders.

Phase delay	Awaken the child progressively earlier
	Prevent excessive napping
	Consider augmentation with bright light
Phase advance	Keep the child awake progressively later
	Prevent compensatory napping
	Delay dinner

The initial treatment of both types of sleep phase disorders involves adjusting the child's bedtime to his or her current sleep phase.

and going to sleep at night owing to school avoidance rather than a maladjusted biological clock. Children with this disorder may feel ambivalent toward treatment programs that address the phase problems because they really want to be told that they cannot go to school. In these instances, the reason for avoidance should be the initial focus of treatment [51].

Phase advance results when children go to bed early and wake early. It is less common than phase delay [22, 24, 52]. Children with phase advance may feel sleepy before their regular bedtime, and they frequently experience early morning awakenings. Again, the symptoms are related to the child's physiological readiness for sleep at a certain time. Often their entire schedule is advanced, including meals and naptimes as well as sleep onset and awakening. The symptoms may go unnoticed by parents if the child's schedule fits well with their own. Treatment involves adjusting the sleep/wake schedule to a later time by gradually (e.g., 30–60 minutes/day) adjusting the child's bedtime forward and allowing no extra napping during the day (see Table 27.4). Often it helps to delay dinner, making sure that the child is not eating an excessive number of snacks. Rest assured; despite the complaints, the child will not miss a meal but will likely stay awake longer to enjoy it. Since the human circadian rhythm naturally runs 25 hours, treating phase advance is typically easier than treating phase delay [51, 52].

Children with irregular sleep/wake patterns have time cues that are either inconsistent or completely lacking [24]. Their lives are often characterized by a lack of routine and possibly social instability. They may eat meals at irregular times and receive no appropriate cues to help orient their sleep/wake patterns. Children experiencing this problem often live in homes with little structure, in which some type of family dysfunction may coexist. Treatment should focus on teaching the parents to provide the appropriate structure that allows their children to form a consistent sleep/wake schedule.

Some children may simply sleep less and apparently need less sleep than other children. These *short sleepers* have less total sleep time but are otherwise normal, so long as there are no associated complaints. They may present with no bedtime struggles or early awakenings.

Attention-Deficit Hyperactivity Disorder (ADHD), Periodic Limb Movement Disorder (PLMD), and Restless Leg Syndrome (RLS)

Several medical conditions may result in childhood sleep difficulties. Children with ADHD often report restlessness and frequent awakenings, although sleep latency and total sleep time are typically normal [44, 54]. It has been documented that sleepy children, unlike sleepy adults, can become hyperactive and show decreases in attention span and increases in activity level [44, 45]. Studies involving experimental sleep restriction in children show resultant ADHD-like behavior and reduced cognitive performance [47]. Another study showed that 5–10-year-old boys diagnosed with ADHD were sleepier than controls [55]. This was confirmed in a study comparing Multiple Sleep Latency Tests (MSLT) in ADHD children to controls, suggesting that the attention deficits and hyperactivity may, at least in part, be due to insufficient or disordered nighttime sleep.

Picchietti has suggested that children with ADHD have a higher prevalence of PLMS [56–58]. This is reasonable given the impact of PLMS on subsequent daytime function. PLMS presents differently in children than in adults. Children with PLMS may have nonspecific symptoms like growing pains, restless sleep, or complaints of insomnia, and often many of these issues go unrecognized by parents of family members. In many cases the movements are just amusing and topics of discussion among family and friends but never meet the ears of the clinician.

Another disorder associated with PLMS is restless legs syndrome (RLS). In adults with restless legs, patients describe a sensory discomfort in their legs during periods of quiescence [59]. The majority of patients with restless legs also experience PLMS during sleep [60]. In children with restless legs the symptoms may manifest with "growing pains." [61] These are limb discomforts that do not meet the criteria for alternative diagnoses, such as arthritis or other types of joint pathology. While the cause of "growing pains" is unknown a recent review of the literature suggests that many children with growing pains meet the criteria for restless legs syndrome [61].

The Internal Restless Leg Syndrome Study Group have recently provided revised criteria for this diagnosis: [62]

(1) An urge to move the legs usually accompanied or caused by uncomfortable and unpleasant sensations in the legs. (Sometimes the urge to move is present without the uncomfortable sensations and sometimes the arms or other body parts are involved in addition to the legs.)

(2) The urge to move or unpleasant sensations begin or worsen during periods of rest or inactivity such as lying or sitting.

(3) The urge to move or unpleasant sensations are partially or totally relieved by movement, such as walking or stretching, at least as long as the activity continues.

(4) The urge to move or unpleasant sensations are worse in the evening or night than during the day or only occur in the evening or night. (When symptoms are very severe, the worsening at night may not be noticeable but must have been previously present.)

Many chronic conditions are also the cause of disrupted sleep, including migraine headaches, asthma, diabetes, gastroesophageal reflux, seizures, and neurological deficits and disorders [25, 39, 40]. In most of these instances, therapy involves treatment of medical problems and concurrently applying good sleep hygiene principles.

Parasomnias

Several seemingly different disorders are categorized as parasomnias [63–75]. These disorders include dramatic, sometimes bizarre symptoms and may cause distress for the observing parent, and are more frequent in childhood than adolescence [76]. Treatments may work only temporarily, but the disorders are often benign and end with spontaneous remission at the onset of puberty. Although the pathological prevalence of parasomnias is unknown, most of the normal population occasionally experience some of these symptoms, and the infrequent parasomnia event is generally not perceived to be problematic. Parasomnias are less frequently the cause of referral to a sleep-related specialist than are other sleep disorders, and they may be perceived as more normal in preadolescent children. Parasomnias may be considered more problematic in older children when they begin to curtail the child's participation in social events such as camps or sleepover. For patients who are referred, it is important for the clinician to be able to recognize when therapeutic intervention is necessary; often the best therapy is to merely reassure the parents that their child's behavior is normal and will most likely cause him or her no harm. The key to determining whether a given child's symptoms are normal or abnormal and in need of treatment lies in the frequency

and persistence of events over time and, in some instances, the amount of danger or health risk that results from the events [22, 24, 28].

The most common parasomnias are *sleepwalking, night terrors, nightmares, jactatio capitis nocturna*, and *sleep-related enuresis* (Table 27.5). In 1968, Broughton proposed calling these four disorders *disorders of arousal*, since electrophysiological features were common to each, including an arousal that most often occurs during slow-wave sleep [77]. Other features of these disorders include frequent body movements during sleep, autonomic activation, automatic and sometimes repetitive motor activity, mental confusion and disorientation, and relative unresponsiveness to external stimuli. In most instances, there is generalized amnesia to the episode, with little recall of mental activity during the event. These features are seen most consistently in sleepwalking and night terror episodes.

Sleepwalking episodes are characterized by a flurry of motor behavior that typically originates during the deep slow-wave sleep of the first third of the night [78]. It occurs most commonly in pubescent children and can persist into adulthood. Its pathogenesis is unknown, but psychological and physiological stress can precipitate episodes. Although usually benign, serious injury and

Table 27.5 Common parasomnias in children and their treatment.

Sleepwalking and night terrors (pavor nocturnus)

Occur primarily in slow-wave sleep (stages 3 and 4)

Most frequent in young children

Usually outgrown by adolescence

Can be precipitated by sleep deprivation or excessive fatigue

Treatment: Increased total nocturnal sleep time or late afternoon naps; benzodiazepine may help by lightening deep sleep

Occur at any age, but most common during preadolescence

Can be precipitated by traumatic events (even a frightening movie) or separation anxiety

Treatment: Reassurance and/or counseling usually helpful; recurring dreams may be extinguished by the daytime rehearsal of an acceptable ending

Sleep-related enuresis

Primary enuresis in 90% of patients; secondary in 10%

Family history of enuresis common

Most children dry by the age of 4 years, but 10% of 6-year-olds still wet

Spontaneous dryness achieved at rate of 15% a year

Treatment: Behavioral approaches most helpful

---

even death can result from the behavior. Episodes typically begin most commonly within the first 60 minutes after the onset of sleep. The individual sits up in bed and may perform a number of repetitive movements such as picking at the bed covers. Rarely, the individual performs behaviors that require complex motor function and cognitive ability, such as driving, talking on the telephone, or playing a musical instrument. Usually verbalization is rare unless a night terror is occurring. Individuals can hurt themselves during these episodes, for example, by stumbling or banging into furniture or by exiting open windows or climbing onto fire escapes. Occasionally, violent behavior can be a part of sleepwalking, although it is unusual for aggressive behavior to be directed toward specific individuals. Attempts at restraining the sleepwalker can be met with resistance and even a primitive level of ferocity, however [64, 65]. The following case studies involve sleepwalking in which destructive behavior occurred.

CASE STUDY

Case One

A young man began experiencing violent and destructive sleepwalking events – kicking in doors and walls and attacking anything in sight. He continued this behavior throughout his teenage years. In the episode that resulted in his referral to our sleep disorders center, his father attempted to restrain him. The child attacked his father with such ferocity that the father had to be hospitalized.

CASE STUDY

Case Two

A 14-year-old presented with a lengthy history of sleepwalking and night terrors that had begun with the divorce of his parents at the age of 5 years. His behavior during a recent episode was destructive, including breaking windows, walls, doors, and anything in his path. On two occasions he had thrown his mother across the room when she attempted to stop his sleepwalking. The events were controlled with a low dose of diazepam (Valium), but his compliance with the regimen was poor. At age 24 years, after spending 18 hours

working, he attended a wine festival, where he stayed up until early morning and then fell asleep outside in a chair. The police later found him wandering through the woods screaming that someone was trying to kill him. When confronted, he had difficulty answering questions and pleaded to be allowed to sleep. The next day he was told that someone matching his description had attacked an elderly couple and beat them viciously. He claimed absolutely no recall of having participated in this event. The victims lived directly across from where he had been sleeping.

Fifteen to thirty percent of healthy children have at least one episode of sleepwalking; 2–3% have more frequent episodes. Peak prevalence occurs at 12 years of age, and most children outgrow the behavior by 15 years of age. Fewer than 1% of adults exhibit sleepwalking. Some researchers have suggested a genetic component to the disorder, with a recessive mode of inheritance and incomplete penetrance. There is no evidence for racial or cultural differences, however. Sleep deprivation, excessive fatigue, sedatives, hypnotics, and even episodes of obstructive sleep apnea can precipitate sleepwalking. Sleepwalking in children is considered benign and is not usually associated with psychopathology [79].

Sleepwalking can be distinguished from psychogenic fugue in that the latter tends to occur in people with severe psychopathology and typically lasts for hours or days. REM behavior disorder, although similar to sleepwalking, tends to occur more in the elderly, rarely occurs in children, and is associated with more elaborate recall.

Treatment of sleepwalking involves securing the patient's bedroom to prevent injury and placing either an alarm or wind chime on the patient's door. Psychotherapy, relaxation therapy, and hypnosis all are reported to be equally effective. Benzodiazepines can be helpful, and we have obtained positive results with antidepressant therapy such as the use of desipramine.

Night Terrors

Night terrors, which are termed *pavor nocturnus* in children and *pavor incubus* in adults, are characterized by a person's arousal within the first third of the night usually from deep (stage 3 or 4) sleep [65, 66]. The episode may begin with a loud, piercing scream usually accompanied by an intense autonomic response, and is followed by a sense of anxiety and panic. Sleep terrors can precipitate or be associated with sleepwalking events. The person typically sits up in bed, seems frightened, and may be sweating and experiencing rapid breathing and tachycardia. Heart rate changes can occur precipitously to rates as high as 160 beats per minute. Patients may be inconsolable until the intense agitation dissipates (usually within 15 minutes). There is little if any recall of dream imagery, although there may be a sense of doom or impending death. In adults, there have been reports of cursing with night terrors. Polysomnographs indicate events similar to those occurring with sleepwalking. The severity of the episodes is proportional to the duration of the preceding stage of slow-wave sleep, and individuals with repetitive sleep terrors tend to show many brief awakenings from these stages of sleep [53].

Recurrent episodes of night terror are experienced by 1–6% of pubescent children. The peak prevalence occurs between 5 and 7 years of age, and the prevalence in adults is less than 1%. There is no evidence for racial or cultural differences in the prevalence of sleep terrors, but there is an increased familial incidence, with up to 96% of individuals having at least one family member with the condition [64].

Night terrors can be precipitated by stress, fatigue, and febrile illness. Accurate labeling of night terrors is important. Christopher Carranza categorizes night terrors as two distinct conditions. The temporary condition that is relatively common in childhood and ultimately resolves itself is "Type A Night Terror," while the rarer, extreme-trauma-related condition (which may begin either in childhood or adulthood) that has routinely resisted treatment for the entire lifetime of the individual is called "Type B Night Terrors." The disorder in adults more typically indicates some pathology and has been reported to occur as a symptom of post-traumatic stress disorder. Because of the necessity to address Type B, it is critical to distinguish between the two. Benzodiazepines can be helpful in treating night terrors, and very low doses of diazepam (2–5 mg) can reduce or ameliorate the condition; these doses can ultimately be given only on alternate nights. Imipramine has also been reported to be helpful. The disorder should be distinguished from dream anxiety attacks (nightmares), which tend to occur during REM sleep rather than deep sleep and are less likely to be associated with intense autonomic activity. Individuals experiencing dreaming anxiety attacks are usually awake and not amnesiac for the events.

Nightmares

Nightmares are vivid dreams of disturbing and often frightening content. They are a common sleep-related experience in both children and adults and are distinctly different from night terrors. Nightmares generally take place during REM sleep when general paralysis is present, preventing harm, and are not indicative of underlying psychosis or emotional trauma. Nightmares often awaken the patient and can be recounted, whereas night terrors generally cannot. In childhood, nightmares occur equally in both genders, are especially common in children between the ages of 3 and 6 years, and commonly occur in the second half of an extended period of sleep [24, 25].

Jactatio Capitis Nocturna

Rhythmic movement disorders before and during sleep, termed jactatio capitis nocturna, may include head banging, body rocking, and head rolling. Although they may persist into adulthood, they are most prevalent in infants and children, and generally occur during the transition to sleep but can also appear later in the sleep cycle. They are not necessarily benign: Injuries to the head or limbs can occur, especially with head banging. Head banging involves a rhythmic, forceful ramming of the head into a pillow or, less frequently, into a rigid surface such as a wall or a headboard. It typically occurs while the person is in a prone or supine position [67–70].

Body rocking is typically characterized by an individual positioned on hands and knees rocking his or her entire body in an anterior-posterior motion. When a child is in a crib, the body rocking may cause the crib to move all over the room and bang into the wall. These episodes tend to occur on a nightly basis and may last up to an hour. Head banging generally occurs in association with stressful situations, whereas body rocking typically occurs in conjunction with more pleasurable activities such as listening to music or getting ready for bed. Children rarely cry when exhibiting these behaviors, even when the movements are violent.

Polysomnographic studies show that jactatio capitis nocturna events occur primarily during wakefulness and in sleep stages 1 and 2. Head banging occurs in approximately 4% of children, typically with onset during the infant's first year at about 6–8 months of age; it rarely develops after 18 months of age. Head-rolling activity has been reported to occur in 6% of healthy children. The prevalence of this disorder declines rapidly with age: although more than 50% of infants exhibit some form of this activity, fewer than 25% of 2-year-olds and fewer than 10% of 4-year-olds exhibit this disorder. Head banging tends to occur more frequently in boys than in girls, but no gender differences have been noted for other rhythmic movement disorders. The behavior is more prevalent in individuals with mental retardation.

One explanation for the cause of bedtime rhythmic activity is that the child is attempting to comfort his or herself by reproducing the parents' cradling or rocking motions. Other hypotheses involve the rhythm of the mother's heartbeat or respiratory rhythm as a model for imitation. More recently, a model of self-stimulation has been suggested, in which rhythmic activity gives a rise to pleasurable sensations and reinforcement. Rhythmic body movements should be distinguished from seizure disorder or *spasms nutans*, which consists of fine head oscillations that are more commonly seen during wakefulness. In most cases, rhythmic movement disorders require no treatment other than providing reassurance to the family that injury is unlikely. When particularly violent activity occurs, however, such as in a child with mental retardation, more caution should be exercised; the use of extra padding, and in some instances protective helmets, may be needed to prevent injury. Some studies have shown that replacing the rhythmic activity with a frequency-matched metronome placed next to the bed at night can be helpful. Others have suggested allowing the opportunity for vigorous rocking in a rocking chair or a rocking horse before bedtime may reduce the behavior.

Nocturnal Enuresis (NE)

From earliest recorded history in primitive and civilized societies, NE (bedwetting) has been a source of unhappiness and embarrassment. Shame and ridicule have often been used to deter bedwetting. Even today in our society, it is not unusual for patients to shame the enuretic child by hanging soiled bedsheets outside the child's window or by threatening to rub the child's face into wet clothing and sheets. Fortunately, these attitudes appear to be giving way to more enlightened approaches [72].

Enuresis is technically defined as an involuntary discharge of urine, but it is usually used to denote bedwetting in children old enough to have acquired control of the urinary bladder. The age at which complete bladder control is attained (usually 4–5 years) depends on developmental, social, and cultural factors, the personality of the child, the general emotional climate in the home, and parental attitudes toward toilet training. There are two distinct subgroups of enuresis: primary and secondary. In *primary enuresis*, the child has never been consistently dry for more than 1 or 2 weeks at a time. Primary enuresis generally involves developmental and maturational factors and a strong genetic component. Psychological and medical factors usually play a minimal role in primary enuresis. In *secondary enuresis*, the child begins to wet again after an extended period of dryness. Psychological and medical factors are usually a major cause of secondary enuresis. Studies have variously estimated that primary enuresis constitutes 67–90% of all cases and secondary enuresis only 10–33%.

It is generally agreed that between five and seven million people in the United States have enuresis. The disorder affects all cultures, and boys are twice as likely than girls to be affected. Some studies have suggested that approximately 15% of all 6-year-olds wet their beds, and the spontaneous cure rate thereafter is about 15% per year. The current view is that enuresis does not ordinarily reflect any abnormality of sleep. Early studies suggested that enuresis was one of the disorders of arousal that occurred during deep stages of sleep. We have concluded, however, that there is no unique correlation between slow sleep and enuretic episodes: The frequency of enuretic episodes in each stage of sleep is proportional to the amount of time spent in each stage. The predominance of episodes during slow-wave sleep, therefore, appears to be related to the time of night at which this type of sleep occurs. In studies controlling for sleep stages, auditory arousal thresholds of children presenting with NE are often higher than those without NE, particularly in male subjects [80, 81]. As auditory arousal thresholds reduce with age, this evidence has been interpreted as a manifestation of neurodevelopmental delay [80, 82].

Researchers have investigated the possibility that enuresis is directly correlated to dreaming, since bedwetters frequently describe dreams of wetting or being wet. Studies have shown that children who are awakened and given dry clothing immediately after micturition do not report any dreams of wetness. Those children who were not awakened after micturition, then, may have incorporated a sense of wetness into a subsequent dream and on awakening may have believed that wetting actually occurred during a dream [72].

In sleep laboratory tests, people with enuresis recorded more frequent and intense contractions of the primary detrusor muscle – both spontaneous and evoked – as well as greater bladder pressure than control subjects [83]. In addition, non-REM sleep arousals were found to provoke primary bladder contractions in people with enuresis. Genetic factors may play a role in primary enuresis: A family history has been reported in 70% of enuretic children, which suggests that a maturation component may underlie the disorder [84].

The maturation of bladder function and control may be premature or delayed in people with enuresis. Studies have shown that these individuals experience more bladder irritation than do control subjects. This partially accounts for the smaller bladder capacity in children with enuresis: If their bladder is of normal size but their functional bladder capacity is smaller, they will have a decreased ability to tolerate a full bladder.

In patients with primary enuresis, emotional problems are usually a consequence of the disorder rather than any biological factor. Although enuresis has generally been described in the psychiatric literature as an expression of the need to regress and receive excessive attention and care – particularly following stresses such as the birth of a sibling or a family illness – such scenarios relate more significantly to secondary enuresis.

A causal factor often overlooked in both primary and secondary enuresis is sleep apnea. Studies have reported that in some instances the removal of tonsils to alleviate obstructed nocturnal breathing resulted in significant improvement or the resolution of enuresis [75, 85]. According to Weissbach et al., enuresis is resolved in 55–77% of children following adenotonsillectomy.

The most important component of evaluating a child with enuresis is obtaining a clear history (Table 27.6). The evaluation should include a thorough general history with specific attention to the bedwetting, a physical examination, and urinalysis. A more complete urological workup is indicated only when the history of physical examination suggests a urological disorder. Cystoscopy and intravenous pyelogram should be avoided unless there is a strong suspicion of urinary tract infection or blockage [83].

Most pediatricians tend to suggest a treatment approach of benign neglect: Do nothing and allow nature to eventually solve the problem. This approach can lead to considerable frustration for parents and children, however.

The sleep of children with enuresis and their parents may be fragmented due to the events, leading to complaints about daytime function and sleepiness. In such cases behavior modification therapies are warranted.

The use of behavior modification to treat enuresis is well established. Use of the bedwetting alarm has a demonstrated success rate of 60–75%. Unfortunately,

relapse just after conditioning is high, ranging from 35% to 80%. However, the disorder can be treated quickly and permanently with subsequent reconditioning and reapplication of the alarm. In recent years, we have instituted a comprehensive treatment program for childhood enuresis, combining some of the treatment paradigms described here. The program employs five methods:

(1) bladder-stretching exercises;
(2) stream interruption;
(3) counseling for motivation and responsibility;
(4) visual sequencing; and
(5) conditioning therapy.

Each of these techniques has been used alone or in some combination by other practitioners to treat enuresis. In our program, however, the methods have been modified slightly and organized into a paradigm that also incorporates a current understanding of sleep physiology. Our method relies heavily on personal contact between the clinic and the patient, motivation by the clinicians, and the active involvement of the child and his or her parents.

The effectiveness of this treatment program was evaluated in 100 children with primary enuresis. Children averaged 11.5 wet nights during the first 2-week period and decreased to 4.3 wet nights at the end of 16 weeks. Ninety-one percent of the children entering the program showed significant improvement by the end of 30 weeks. Most of the individual approaches used in our treatment program have been reported in the literature to be effective on their own. Stream interruption and bladder-stretching exercises have been reported to ameliorate enuresis in up to 30% of patients, and 29% of people with enuresis have been reported to respond to motivation and responsibility counseling. As many as 65–75% of children respond favorably to the use of conditioning alarms. These results suggest that enuresis should be considered a treatable condition whose resolution can be extremely gratifying for the patient, the family, and the clinician [71].

Obstructive Sleep Apnea Syndrome (OSAS)

Obstructive sleep apnea syndrome is the most common form of apnea in childhood. In older children and adults, the main feature of the syndrome is loud snoring associated with gasping, snorting, and respiratory pauses (Table 27.7). Sleep is often restless, and there may be concurrent nightmares and night terrors [86–88]. During the day, adults complain of excessive daytime fatigue and sleepiness. In children, the symptoms are more insidious, often being associated with increased irrita-

Table 27.6 Key points in taking of history of enuresis.

Primary vs. secondary enuresis (has the patient every been dry?)
Age
Current medications
Known ailments
Any signs or symptoms of obstructive sleep apnea syndrome (snoring, snorting, gasping)
Fluid intake pattern (quantity and time)

Table 27.7 Sleep apnea symptoms in children.

While sleeping at night
  Snore loudly and regularly
  Have pauses, gasps, and snorts and may stop
  breathing, disrupting sleep
  Restless or sleep in abnormal positions with the head
  in unusual positions
  Sweat heavily

Daytime consequences
  Difficult to wake up
  Social and behavioral problems
  Diagnosis of ADHD
  Report headaches during the day, especially in the
  morning
  Irritable, agitated, aggressive, and cranky
  May fall asleep or daydream

bility and a shortened attention span. There may be behavioral difficulties, morning headaches, obesity, a failure to thrive, or symptoms of cor pulmonale [86–88]. In children, the main causes of obstructive sleep apnea are hypertrophy of the tonsils and adenoids, craniofacial abnormalities such as micrognathia or retrognathia, abnormalities of the long soft palate, cleft palate repair, and macroglossia. This syndrome is common in patients with Down's syndrome. In addition, obesity can contribute to obstructive sleep apnea, as can neuromuscular disorders such as the Arnold–Chiari malformation, syringobulbia, cerebral palsy, myotonic dystrophy, and bulbar poliomyelitis.

Whereas in adults the snoring is often interrupted by pauses, children with sleep apnea usually snore continuously. Nasal obstructions such as polyps, enlarged turbinates, and a deviated septum may cause sleep apnea and should be treated with antihistamines or topical preparations. Enlarged tonsils and adenoids should be removed. These treatments generally result in a resolution of all symptoms. Nasal continuous positive airway pressure is a treatment of choice for obstructive sleep apnea syndrome in adults and can be effective for children as well. Long-term compliance is questionable, however. Another effective treatment for snoring and apnea in adults is a recently developed dental prosthesis that is worn like a boxer's mouthguard and stabilizes the jaw and tongue. Similar appliances can be fitted for children and simply require patent nasal airway. We frequently recommend the use of an external nasal dilator (Breathe Right) in children who snore or have nasal obstruction. These can be quite effective, and the national exposure given to the use of these devices by athletes has aided their acceptance by children.

CASE STUDY

Case Three

A 2½-year-old boy presented with difficulty falling asleep and with an inability to maintain sleep for more than 50 minutes at a time without awakening and disturbing his parents. He was unwilling to sleep in his own bed and upon awakening in the morning was extremely cranky and exhibited what his parents referred to as "energy-sucking" behavior. The parents were exhausted and extremely frustrated. A neurological examination showed no significant abnormalities but some suspicious findings in the frontal EEG leads resulting in the child being placed on Tegretol. The Tegretol was somewhat helpful and decreased the number of nocturnal awakenings by half (previously 15 to 20). After an afternoon nap the child seemed completely normal and calm. Examination of his nose and throat showed hypertrophic tonsils. He was a mouth breather and unable to maintain nasal airway patency. He had frequent upper airway infections and one could hear his tonsils vibrating while awake. During sleep, sucking noises and snoring punctuated his breathing. The parents were informed that a 50-minute sleep cycle is not unusual for a child of this age but that he is likely to be experiencing obstructive sleep apnea. A polysomnogram confirmed this. A Breathe Right nasal strip was utilized to maintain nasal airway patency and he was provided with melatonin at bedtime. This improved his ability to fall and stay asleep and markedly reduced his "energy sucking behavior." However, his polysomnogram also revealed the presence of 15 apnea and hypopnea events per hour, with oxygen desaturation levels reaching 79% of maximum – clear obstructive sleep apnea. Otolaryngological evaluation resulted in the removal of his tonsils and adenoids and a dramatic improvement in his sleep and waking behavior.

In patients with obstructive sleep apnea, attempts at breathing are compromised by a collapsing airway. Patients with central sleep apnea, however, suffer from a lack of respiratory effort [86]. During sleep, respiration is controlled by a metabolic respiratory control system.

A defect at any point in this system can contribute to central sleep apnea. The causes include encephalitis, cervical cordotomy, brainstem infarction, tumor, and bulbar poliomyelitis. Certain neuromuscular disorders such as neuromyopathy, myotonic dystrophy, muscular dystrophy, myasthenia gravis, diaphragmatic paralysis, and postpolio syndrome can also contribute to central sleep apnea. Finally, thoracic restrictive disorders such as kyphoscoliosis have also been associated with the condition. Patients with central sleep apnea exhibit normal voluntary respiration function during wakefulness but abnormal automatic control of ventilation. There is no response to hypocarbia during wakefulness or sleep, indicating that chemoreceptor abnormalities may be critical factors in this disorder. Patients also exhibit a blunted response to hypoxia and hypoventilation during sleep. Treatment for central sleep apnea can involve diaphragmatic pacing, mechanical ventilatory support, and negative pressure ventilation [86].

Sleeplessness in Childhood and Adolescence: Cognitive and Emotional Consequences

The importance of identifying and treating sleep disorders in childhood and adolescence is underscored by a number of associated consequences of sleep deprivation. Marked deficits in academic performance and cognitive function are experienced by children who report sleeping problems [28, 85, 89, 90]. Elementary and middle school students who got an additional hour of sleep exhibited improved attentiveness and reduced impulsivity [91, 92], improved memory function, and behavioral inhibition [42].

In sleep-deprived children there is a much greater likelihood of developing problems with behavior and emotional control, and at every age, including childhood and adolescence, depression has been linked to disturbances in normal sleep patterns and may present as insomnia or hypersomnia. Liu *et al.* reported that although the relationship between sleep disturbances and depression may be bidirectional, sleep-disturbed children were more severely depressed than children without sleep disturbance, and more likely to have comorbid anxiety disorders; each of these two groups demonstrated different depressive symptom profiles [93]. Inadequate sleep has been repeatedly shown to play a role in the development of depression and anxiety. Shorter sleep duration and chronic sleep deficit has been correlated with increased risk of suicidal ideation in adolescents [42, 93].

Adolescence represents a gradual change from childhood to adulthood, and is fraught with physical, emotional, and social challenges, as well as involvement in employment and extracurricular activities. Parental involvement in dictating sleep times is generally more limited and some emerging sleep problems of adolescence may reflect this transition. At least two-thirds of adolescents complain of sleep onset or sleep maintenance issues [42], sleep onset issues being the more common. Adolescents are more likely to exhibit symptoms of adult-like insomnia or to adjust their sleep patterns to reflect a more adult-like total sleep time, even though they may still biologically need more sleep than adults. Academic workload in middle and high school increases; hence, adolescents frequently stay up later than children but must wake for earlier school start times. This adjustment frequently results in sleep deprivation or phase delay. Adolescents as a group seem to exhibit several symptoms of disturbed sleep, including difficulty awakening, excessive daytime sleepiness, and irritability [90]. Additional serious consequences of daytime sleepiness include increased incidence of motor vehicle accidents, the leading cause of death among young adults [90].

Regardless of age, the importance of maintaining normal sleep cannot be overemphasized and parental involvement in healthy sleep hygiene practice and setting bedtimes is warranted [42]. Even modest manipulation of sleep may lead to improved memory, reaction time, improved attention, and behavioral regulation.

References

1. Rosen RC, Rosekind M, Rosevear C, *et al.* Physician education in sleep and sleep disorders: A national survey of U.S. medical schools. *Sleep* 1993;**16**:249–254.
2. Hartmann E, Baekeland R, Zwilling G. Psychological differences between long and short sleepers. *Arch Gen Psychiatry* 1972;**26**:463–468.
3. Aserinsky E, Kleitman N. Regularly occurring periods of eye motility, and concomitant phenomena during sleep. *Science* 1953;**118**:273–274.
4. Carskadon MA, Dement WC. Normal human sleep: An overview. In: Kryger MH, Roth T, Dement WC (eds) *Principles and Practice of Sleep Medicine*. Philadelphia: WB Saunders, 1994; pp. 16–25.
5. Carskadon MA, Rechtschaffen A. Monitoring and staging human sleep. In: Kryger MH, Roth T, Dement WC (eds) *Principles and Practice of Sleep Medicine*. Philadelphia: WB Saunders, 1994; pp. 943–960.
6. Roffwarg HP, Muzio IN, Dement WC. Ontogenetic development of the human sleep-dream cycle. *Science* 1996;**152**:604–619.
7. Anders TF, Keener M. Developmental course of nighttime sleep-wake patterns in fullterm and premature infants during the first year of life. I. *Sleep* 1985;**8**:173–192.
8. Anders TF, Keener MA, Kraemer H. Sleep-wake organization, neonatal assessment and development in premature infants during the first year of life. II. *Sleep* 1985;**8**:193–206.
9. Anders TF. Night-waking in infants during the first year of life. *Pediatrics* 1979;**63**:860–864.

10. Anders TF, Carskadon MA, Dement WC. Sleep and sleepiness in children and adolescents. *Pediatr Clin North Am* 1980;**17**:29–43.

11. Synder F. The phenomenology of dreaming. In: Madow L, Snow L (eds) *The Psychodynamic Implications of the Physiological Studies on Dreams.* Springfield, IL: Charles C. Thomas, 1970; pp. 124–151.

12. Foulkes D. Dream reports from different stages of sleep. *J Abnorm Psychol* 1962;**65**:14–28.

13. Foulkes D, Vogel G. Mental activity at sleep onset. *J Abnorm Psychol* 1965;**70**:231–243.

14. Dement W, Kleitman N. The relation of the eye movements during sleep to dream activity: An objective method for the study of dreaming. *J Exp Psychol* 1957;**53**:339–346.

15. Dewan EM. The P (programming) hypothesis for REMS. *Psychophysiology* 1968;**5**:365–366.

16. Greenberg R, Dewan E. Aphasia and dreaming: A test of the P-hypothesis. *Psychophysiology* 1968;**5**:203–204.

17. Levental M, Susie V, Rusic M, Rakic L. Rapid eye-movement (REM) sleep deprivation: Effect on acid mucopolysaccharides in rat brain. *Arch Int Physiol Biochim* 1975;**83**:221–232.

18. Shashoua V. The role of extracellular proteins in learning and memory. *Am Sci* 1985;**73**:364–370.

19. Crick F, Mitchison G. The function of dream sleep. *Nature* 1983;**304**:111–114.

20. Foulkes D. Longitudinal studies of dreams in children. In: Masserman J (ed.) *Science and Psychoanalysis.* 9. New York: Grune & Stratton, 1971; pp. 60–62.

21. Golbin AZ. *The World of Children's Sleep.* Salt Lake City, UT: Michaelis Medical Publishing Corp.; 1994.

22. Ferber R. Sleeplessness in the child. In: Kryger MH, Roth T, Dement WC (eds) *Principles and Practices of Sleep Medicine.* Philadelphia: WB Saunders, 1989; pp. 633–639.

23. Lansky V. *Getting Your Child to Sleep and Back to Sleep: Tips for Parents of Infants, Toddlers and Preschoolers.* Derphaven, MN: Bood Peddlers, 1991.

24. Ferber R. *Solve Your Child's Sleep Problems.* New York: Simon and Schuster, 1985.

25. Guilleminault C (ed.). *Sleep and Its Disorders in Children.* New York: Raven Press, 1987; pp. 243–252.

26. Van Tassel EB. The relative influences of child and environmental characteristics on sleep disturbances in the first and second years of life. *J Dev Behav Pediatr* 1985;**6**:81–86.

27. Ferber R, Boyle MP. Nocturnal fluid intake: A cause of, not treatment for, sleep disruption in infants and toodlers. *Sleep Res* 1983;**12**:243.

28. Anders TF, Keener M. Developmental course of nighttime sleep-wake patterns in full-term and premature infants during the first year of life. I. *Sleep* 1985;**8**:173–192.

29. Kataria S, Swanson MS, Trevathan GE. Persistence of sleep disturbances in preschool children. *J Pediatr* 1987;**110**:642–646.

30. Younger JB. The management of night waking in older infants. *Pediatr Nurs* 1982;**8**:155–158.

31. Jones DPH, Verdyn CM. Behavioral management of sleep problems. *Arch Dis Child* 1983;**58**:442–444.

32. Cuthbertson J, Schevill S. *Helping Your Child Sleep Through the Night.* Garden City, NY: Doubleday, 1985.

33. Scharf MB, Berkowitz DV, McDannold MD, Stover R, Brannen DE, Reyna R. Effects of an external nasal dilator on sleep and breathing patterns in congested and non-congested newborns. *J Pediatrics* 1996;**129**:804–808.

34. Anders TF. Night-waking in infants during the first year of life. *Pediatrics* 1979;**63**:860–864.

35. Weisbluth M. Sleep in the colicky infant. In: Guilleminault C (ed.) *Sleep and Its Disorders in Children.* New York: Raven Press, 1987; pp. 129–138.

36. Wessel MA, Cobb JC, Jackson EB, *et al.* Paroxysmal fussing in infancy, sometimes called "colic." *Pediatrics* 1954;**14**:421–434.

37. Jorup S. Colonic hyperperistalisis in neurolabile infants: Studies in so-called dyspepsia in breast infants. *Acta Paediatr* 1952;**85**:1–92.

38. Weissbluth M, Green OC. Plasma progesterone concentrations in infants: Relation to infantile colic. *J Pediatr* 1983;**103**:935–936.

39. Sheldon SH, Spire JP, Levy HB. *Pediatrics Sleep Medicine.* Philadelphia: WB Saunders, 1992.

40. Bax MCO. Sleep disturbance in the young child. *Brit Med J* 1980;**280**:1177–1179.

41. Darwin C. *The Expression of Emotions in Man and Animals.* London: Murray, 1889.

42. Gangwisch J, Babiss L, Malaspina D, *et al.* Earlier parental set bedtimes as a protective factor against depression and suicidal ideation. *Sleep* 2010;**33**:97–106.

43. Weissbluth M, Davis AT, Poncher J. Night waking in 4- to 8-month-old infants. *J Pediatr* 1984;**104**:477–480.

44. Greenhill L, Puig-Antich J, Goetz R, *et al.* Sleep architecture and REM sleep measures in prepubertal children with attention-deficit disorder with hyperactivity. *Sleep* 1993;**6**:91–101.

45. Chervin RD, Dillon JE, Bassetti C, Ganoczy DA, Pituch KJ. Symptoms of sleep disorders, inattention, and hyperactivity in children. *Sleep* 1997;**20**:1185–1192.

46. Dahl RE, Holttum J, Trubnick L. A clinical picture of child and adolescent narcolepsy. *J Am Acad Child Adolesc Psychiatry* 1994;**33**:834–841.

47. Fallone G, Acebo C, Arndt JT, Seifer R, Carskadon MA. Effects of acute sleep restriction on behavior, sustained attention, and response inhibition in children. *Percept Mot Skills* 2001;**93**:213–229.

48. Coons S, Guilleminault C. Development of consolidated sleep and wakeful periods in relation to the day/night cycle in infancy. *Dev Med Child Neurol* 1984;**26**:169–176.

49. Horne JA, Ostberg O. Individual differences in human circadian rhythms. *Biol Psychol* 1979;**5**:179–190.

50. Weitzman ED, Czeisler CA, Coleman RM, *et al.* Delayed sleep phase syndrome: A chronobiologic disorder with sleep onset insomnia. *Arch Gen Psychiatry* 1981;**38**:737–746.

51. Ferber R, Boyle MP. Delayed sleep phase syndrome versus motivated sleep phase delay in adolescents. *Sleep Res* 1983;**12**:239.

52. Loxoff B, Wolf AW, Davis NS. Sleep problems seen in pediatric practice. *Pediatrics* 1985;**75**:477–483.

53. Anders TF. State and rhythmic processes. *J Am Child Psychiatry* 1978;**17**:401–420.

54. Busby K, Firestone P, Pivik RT. Sleep patterns in hyperkinetic and normal children. *Sleep* 1981;**4**:366–383.

55. Randazzo AC, Muehlbach MJ, Schweitzer PK, Walsh JK. Cognitive function following acute sleep restriction in children ages 10–14. *Sleep* 1998;**21**:861–868.

56. Picchetti D, Walters A, Underwood D, *et al.* Periodic limb movement disorder in attention-deficit hyperactivity disorder in children. *Sleep Res* 1997;**26**:469.

57. Picchietti DL, England SJ, Walters AS, Willis K, Verrico T. Periodic limb movement disorder and restless legs syndrome in children with attention-deficit hyperactivity disorder. *J Child Neurol* 1998;**13**:588–594.

58. Picchietti DL, Underwood DJ, Farris WA, *et al.* Further studies on periodic limb movement disorder and restless legs syndrome in children with attention-deficit hyperactivity disorder. *Mov Disord* 1999;**14**:1000–1007.

59. Walters AS, Picchietti DL, Ehrenberg BL, Wagner ML. Restless legs syndrome in childhood and adolescence. *Pediatr Neurol* 1994;**11**:241–245.

60. Picchietti DL, Walters AS. Moderate to severe periodic limb movement disorder in childhood and adolescence. *Sleep* 1999;**22**:297–300.

61. Walters AS. Is there a subpopulation of children with growing pains who really have restless legs syndrome? A review of the literature. *Sleep Med* 2002;**52**:297–302.

62. Walters AS. Toward a better definition of the restless legs syndrome. The International Restless Legs Syndrome Study Group. *Mov Disord* 1995;**10**:634–642.

63. Ferber R. Sleep, sleeplessness, and sleep disruptions in infants and young children. *Ann Clin Res* 1985;**17**:227–237.

64. Kales A, Soldatos CR, Bixler ED, *et al.* Hereditary factors in sleepwalk night terrors. *Br J Psychiatry* 1980;**137**:111.

65. Kales JD, Kales A, Soldatos CR, *et al.* Night terrors: Clinical characteristics and personality patterns. *Arch Gen Psychiatry* 1980;**37**:1414–1417.

66. Kales JD, Kales A, Soldatos CR, Chamberlin K, Martin ED. Sleepwalking and night terrors related to febrile illness. *Am J Psychiatry.* 1979 Sep;136(9):1214–1215.

67. deLissovoy V. Head banging in early childhood: A study of incidence. *J Pediatr* 1961;**58**:803.

68. Kravitz H, Rosenthal V, Teplitz Z. A study of head-banging in infants and children. *Dis Nerv Syst* 1960;**21**:203:

69. Sallustro MA, Atwell CW. Body rocking, head banging, and head rolling in normal children. *J Pediatr* 1978;**93**:704.

70. Thorpy AJ, Glovinsky P. Jactatio capitis nocturne. In: Kryger M, Roth T, Dement WC (eds) *Principles and Practice of Sleep Medicine.* Philadelphia: WB Saunders, 1989; pp. 648–654.

71. Scharf MB. *Waking Up Dry: How to End Bedwetting Forever.* Cincinnati, OH: Writers Digest, 1986.

72. Agarwal A. Enuresis. *Am Fam Physician* 1982; **25**:203–207.

73. McLain LG. Childhood enuresis. *Curr Probl Pediatr* 1979;**9**:1–36.

74. Gerard MW. Enuresis: A study in etiology. *Am J Orthopsychiatry* 1933;**9**:48–58.

75. Welder DJ, Hauri PI. Nocturnal enuresis in children with upper airway obstructions. *Int J Pediatr Otorhinolaryngol* 1985;**9**:173–182.

76. Mason T, Pack A. Pediatric parasomnias. *Sleep* 2007; **30**:141–151.

77. Broughton R. Sleep disorders: Disorders of arousal? *Science* 1968;**59**:1070–1078.

78. Kales A, Soldatos CR, Caldwell AB, *et al.* Somnambulism: Clinical characteristics and personality patterns. *Arch Gen Psychiatry* 1980;**37**:1413–1417.

79. Association of Sleep Disorders Centers' Sleep Disorders Classification Committee, Roffward HP, chair. Diagnostic classification of sleep and arousal disorders. *Sleep* 1979;**2**:1–137.

80. Cohen-Zrubavel V, Kushnir B, Kushnir J, Sadeh A. Sleep and sleepiness in children with nocturnal enuresis. *Sleep* 2011;**34**:191–194.

81. Wolfish NM, Pivik RT, Busby KA. Elevated sleep arousal thresholds in enuretic boys: clinical impressions. *Acta Paediatrica* 1997;**86**:381–384.

82. Guilleminault C, Winkle R, Korobkin R, Simmons B. Children and nocturnal snoring: Evaluation of the effects of sleep related respiratory resistive load and daytime functioning. *Eur J Pediatr* 1982;**139**:165–171.

83. Starfield B. Functional bladder capacity in enuretic and nonenuretic children. *J Pediatr* 1967;**70**:777–781.

84. Frary LG. Enuresis: A genetic study. *Am J Dis Child* 1935;**49**:557–578.

85. Mitru G, Millrood D, Mateika J. The impact of sleep on learning and behavior in adolescents. *Teachers College Record* 2002;**104**:704–726.

86. Ariago RL. Development of respiratory control. In: Korobkin R, Guilleminault C (eds) *Advances in Perinatal Neurology.* New York: Spectrum Publications, 1979; pp. 249–280.

87. Rigatto H. Apnea. *Pediatr Clin North Am* 1982; **29**:1105–1116.

88. Guilleminault C, Korobkin R, Winkle R. A review of 50 children with obstructive sleep apnea syndrome. *Lung* 1981;**159**:275–287.

89. Weissbach A, Leiberman A, Tarasiuk A, Goldbart A, Tal A. Adenotonsillectomy improves enuresis in children with obstructive sleep apnea syndrome. *Int J Pediatr Otorhinolaryngol* 2006;**70**:1351–1356.

90. Millman R. Excessive sleepiness in adolescents and young adults: causes, consequences, and treatment strategies. *Pediatrics* 2005;**115**:1774–1786.

91. Sadeh, A, Gruber R, Raviv A. The effects of sleep restriction on school-age children: What a difference an hour makes. *Child Dev* 2003;**74**:444–455.

92. Lufi D, Tzischinsky O, Hadar S. Delaying school starting time by one hour: Some effects on attention levels in adolescents. *J Clin Sleep Med* 2011;**7**:137–143.

93. Liu X, Buysse D, Gentzler AL, *et al.* Insomnia and hypersomnia associated with depressive phenomenology and comorbidity in childhood depression. *Sleep* 2007; **30**:83–90.

Section IV
Special Problems in Child and Adolescent Psychiatry

28

Loss: Divorce, Separation, and Bereavement

Jamie Snyder

Introduction

Almost every young person will experience loss of some type before they reach adulthood. It may be as common as a friend who moves away or the death of a pet. It may involve witnessing the violent death of a parent or sibling, the loss of innocence of a sexually or physically abused child, or the loss of an intact family in divorce. Children (defined for the purposes of this chapter as persons below the age of 18) of different developmental stages experience and cope with loss in different ways. Their response depends not only on the severity of the loss, but their age, support system, coping skills, and numerous other factors.

We will discuss in some detail the specific losses of separation/divorce and bereavement, epidemiology and recent research in these areas, clinical diagnoses that may arise, and recommended treatment approaches.

Separation/Divorce

In 2010, the US Census Bureau [1] reported 22.9 million children living in single-parent households (or with neither parent). As large numbers of children continue to grow up in disrupted families, it is important to take into account the impact of divorce, both sociologically and individually. "The higher incidence of divorce reflects, and, in turn, influences the changing relationships between men and women [and] has significantly raised levels of anxiety…." [2]. On an individual basis, divorce may exacerbate a pre-existing condition or be a causative agent in a new condition. For example, a child might present to a child psychiatry clinic with symptoms of behavioral disturbance beginning at the time he or she was told of a pending parental separation or divorce, or a child with a previously stable condition (such as attention-deficit hyperactivity disorder) might present with an intensification of symptoms.

Research

The impact of divorce on a child's development, once thought of as a short-lived crisis, has over the past three decades been recognized as a significant long-term stressor. Many longitudinal studies of the long-term effects of divorce have been published within the last thirty years (Table 28.1). Kalter and Rembar found a greater representation of divorced children presenting to child and adolescent psychiatric clinics as compared with intact families, and the *Diagnostic and Statistical Manual of Mental Disorders, Fourth Edition, Text Revision* (DSM-IV-TR) recognizes divorce (on Axis IV) as a problem that may affect the diagnosis, treatment, and prognosis of mental disorders [3].

Although many of the studies examine separation and divorce as part of the same process, one study elucidated the effect of geographical separation from a parent as a separate issue. While geographical separation alone is a only a small part of the potential impact of divorce, several studies examine the loss of one parent as part of the divorce process and attempt to delineate the effect of this variable alone. Geographical separation due to a military deployment may add some insight to this clinical presentation [4]. Children geographically separated from one parent (generally the father) experienced elevated self-reported symptom levels of depression, as did the parent who was left behind. Furthermore, these families reported higher levels of stress during the year prior to separation, compared with a control group who did not undergo separation. These differences held up even after applying statistical controls for such things as children's age and parent's military rank. Although the elevated levels of depression did not reach statistical significance, this was attributed to inadequate statistical power. Geographical separation infrequently provoked a pathological level of symptoms: only 6% of the studied children had symptoms severe enough to warrant treatment. A somewhat higher effect of separation

Table 28.1 Summary of representative research on the impact of divorce on children.

Investigators	Title	Sample and design	Variables assessed	Summary of findings
Guidubaldi and Perry [42]	Divorce and mental health sequelae for children: a 2-year follow-up of a nationwide sample	2-year follow-up of 110 (of 699) elementary school boys and girls in divorced and intact families. Average time since divorce was 6 years at follow-up	Academic functioning School behavior Peer acceptance Locus of control General mental health	Children from divorced families performed at levels below those of children of intact families; boys showed more negative effects than girls
Hetherington and colleagues [43]	Long-term effects of divorce and remarriage on the adjustment of children	6-year follow-up of 124 (of 144) middle-class families, including 60 divorced and 64 intact families; mean age of children at time of follow-up was 10.1 years	Behavioral observation of home adjustment Academic performance Teacher and peer evaluation	Divorce has more adverse effects for boys, whereas remarriage is more difficult for girls
Kalter and Rembar [44]	The significance of a child's age at the time of parental divorce	144 children of divorced families ranging between 7 and 17 years of age who presented for evaluation in a child psychiatry outpatient clinic	Level of family stress Social competence Locus of control Presenting complaints, overall degree of emotional adjustment based on clinical evaluation	When divorce occurs in a child's life it is unrelated to the overall level of adjustment, but associated with characteristic patterns of problems at different stages of development
Wallerstein and Kelly [45]	Surviving the break-up: how children and parents cope with divorce	60 middle-class families with 131 children 2 to 18 years of age who participated in divorce counseling at time of divorce and were evaluated again at 18 months postseparation and at 5 years postdivorce	Assessment of child's response to 'and experience' of divorce, parent–child relationships, and support systems outside the home (including school)	The initial decision to divorce is associated with acute distress, including anxiety, depression and anger at parents; preadolescent boys seem to have the most difficulty adjusting at home and school; 30% of children present as clinically depressed at their 5-year evaluation; good adjustment depends on the quality of life in the postdivorce family
Wallerstein [46]	Children of divorce: preliminary report of a 10-year follow-up of	40 young adults between 19 and 29 years of age who were between 9 and 19, years of age at time of divorce	Clinical evaluation of young adults (continuation of the earlier study)	Subjects continue to view divorce as a major influence on their lives; most are committed to a lasting

Author	Focus	Method / Sample	Variables	Findings
			older children and adolescents	marriage, but women tend to fear repeating parents' mistakes
Fergusson, Horwood, and Lynskey [47]	Parental separation adolescent psychopathology, and problem behavior	15-year longitudinal study of 935 children	Exposure to parents' separation during childhood Measurements of adolescent psychopathology and problem behaviors at 15 years old Confounding factors	When confounding variables are accounted for, there remains a small but detectable increase for adolescent conduct disorder, mood disorder, and substance use disorders
Black and Pedro-Carroll [48]	Role of parent-child relationships in mediating the effects of marital disruption	Self-administered questionnaire from 288 college students, 60 of whom were children of divorce	Current and past levels of interparental conflict Current affective quality of parent-child relationships Present adjustment	Effects of interparental conflict mediate to parent-child relationships For women, parental divorce affects adjustment indirectly (via disrupting father-daughter relationship)
Kurtz [49]	Psychosocial coping resources in elementary school-age children of divorce	61 children of divorce compared with a nondivorced control group matched for gender, age, and parents' education	Self-perception Family environment Beliefs about parents' divorce Coping behaviors Family demographics	Children of divorced parents have lower levels of self-efficacy, self-esteem and social support and a less effective coping style
Bolgar, Zweig-Frank and Paris [50]	Childhood antecedents of interpersonal problems in young adult children of divorce	605 students awaiting routine medical exam (125 from a separated or divorced family, 467 with parents still married) completing an inventory of interpersonal problems and a family demographic questionnaire	Family demographics Level of current interpersonal problems Level of preseparation hostility Level of interference between parents on child's relationship with other parent Frequency of contact with noncustodial parent	Young adult children of divorce experience more problems with submission and over-control More interpersonal problems develop when mother never remarries, remarries numerous times, or in cases of high levels of parental discord

on boys compared to girls and particularly among young boys was found. This may be because the great majority of the absent parents were fathers and as has been suggested in several studies, young boys may be more vulnerable to the loss of a male figure in the home [5]. There was also a correlation between the number and severity of symptoms in the studied child and symptoms in the parent left behind to care for the child/children. Findings did not suggest that the parent's distress caused the child's symptoms but that the functioning of the parent and child are closely intertwined.

Clinical Course

While most studies of divorce begin with the separation or legal divorce of the parents, one naturalistic study by Block et al [6, 7]. was able to examine antecedent processes of 41 families participating in a 10-year study of personality and cognitive development of children. They found that by the time the marriage breaks down, many children have spent years in a conflict-ridden home, often feeling relatively unsupported or ill-tended by their parents. Undercontrolled, impulsive behaviors described as characteristic of boys during and after the divorce seem continuous with their behavior over many years in the pre-divorce family. There is a strong possibility that behaviors identified by researchers and clinicians as acute and reactive to the stress of a separation may well have existed long before the actual breakup. Of course there may be an exacerbation of the behaviors at the time of the separation as well.

Block et al. also examined the nature of the pre- and post-separation parent-child relationships. They documented:

(1) long-term and very early disengagement of fathers;
(2) unreliable paternal behavior toward their sons;
(3) anger of both parents at their sons; and
(4) a more modulated response by both parents to their daughters.

These findings contrast with the common belief that disengagement and withdrawal by the father occurs at the time of the divorce as a response to the anger of the mother toward the father. This study did not explore the link between a troubled marital relationship and deteriorating parenting within the still-intact family, that is, whether disagreements regarding parenting were causative or resulted from the marital problems.

At least two recent studies [8, 9] have examined possible genetic factors impacting both the divorce and the post-divorce deterioration in the children's behavior. The theory under evaluation is that genetic factors that might affect children's behavior after the divorce could be manifest in the parents and be causative in the divorce itself. However, the study by Burt et al [9]. firmly supported the view that it is not the genetic factors that impact the child's behavior as much as the environmental factors.

Most studies report a childhood crisis at the time of the permanent separation and often at the time of the actual divorce decree, usually manifested as high emotional distress and severe behavioral problems. Table 28.2 summarizes characteristic responses based on the child's developmental stage.

Several long-term studies identified a deterioration in parent-child relationships after the divorce, with both the custodial and noncustodial parent, especially among boys. In Hetherington's studies [10], three groups were examined: a nonremarried mother-custody group, a remarried mother-stepfather group, and a nondivorced group. The target children were 30 sons and 30 daughters within these three groups. At the time of the legal divorce they were 4 years old. At the 6-year follow-up, the divorced, nonremarried mother-son dyad showed more negative features than any other parent-child dyad in the study, with the exception of the stepfather-daughter relationship in the newly remarried timeframe. By contrast, nonremarried mother-daughter relationships differed little from a nondivorced mother-daughter dyad. In remarried families, by 2 years after remarriage boys were doing significantly better than girls. In the first 2 years after remarriage, mother-daughter conflict was high. Their behavior improved over time but they were more antagonistic and disruptive overall than other relationships. When the remarriage occurred before adolescence boys were also very difficult initially, but by 2 years post-remarriage were no more aggressive or noncompliant than boys in nondivorced families. Although both early adolescent boys and girls exhibited many behavioral problems 2 years after remarriage, stepfathers saw greater improvement among stepsons and greater involvement and warmth with them than with stepdaughters.

There seems to be a second peak of problems in late adolescence/early adulthood when the young person begins to confront issues regarding love, commitment, and marriage. In the California Children of Divorce Study [2], young people 19 to 29 years old, 10 years after their parents' divorce, acknowledged their parents' divorce as the major formative experience of their lives. Many appeared to be troubled and underachieving. Many young women who had initially coped well became very frightened of failure. Almost all expressed significant anxiety regarding love, commitment, and marriage, fearing betrayal and abandonment. As a

Table 28.2 Summary of characteristic responses to divorce at different developmental stages.

Developmental stage	Cognitive understanding	Emotional and behavioral responses (0–2 years after divorce)	Long-term sequelae (2 years after divorce)
Preschool to kindergarten	**4–5-year olds**	**3–5-year-olds**	**Separation or divorce occurring when child 0–2.5 years of age**
Infancy (0–2 years)	Understand divorce in terms of physical separation	Fear	Increased separation-related difficulties during latency
Preschool (3–5 years)	Perceive divorce as temporary	Regression	Nonaggression with parents by both boys and girls
	Are confused by parents' positive and negative feelings about each other	Separation anxiety	Aggression with peers in elementary school-aged girls
		Macabre fantasy	
		Bewilderment	Nonaggression with peers and academic problems in adolescent boys [44]
	Understand divorce in linear terms and believe they can cause behavior of parents	Replaceability-fear of own	**Separation or divorce occurring when child 3–5 years of age**
	Are cognitively unable to separate parental motives from their own	Fantasy denial	Increased subjective symptoms in elementary school boys
		Disruption or inhibition of play	Increased aggressive behavior with parents in adolescent boys and girls
		Increased aggression	Increased academic problems in adolescent girls [44]
		Inhibited aggression	
		Guilt	Increased externalizing behavior in elementary school boys and girls who were aggressive as preschoolers [43]
		Emotional neediness [45]	
Elementary school age	**6–8-year-olds**	**6–8-year-olds**	**School-age children and early adolescents**
Early (6–8 years)	Understand the finality of divorce	Grief	Both girls and boys from divorced families emerge as performing more poorly on mental health measures than children from intact families [42]
Late (9–12 years)	Appreciate psychologic and, physical effects of parental conflict	Fear leading to disorganization	
		Feeling of deprivation	Boys' performance significantly worse than girls'; boys experience more behavior problems in school and at home [42,43]
	Are unable to tolerate ambivalent feelings; usually blame one parent	Yearning for departed parent	
		Inhibition of aggression	Girls living in single mother custody homes as well adjusted as girls living in intact homes 6 years after divorce [43]
	May interpret divorce egocentrically and believe their behavior affects parental decision	Anger at custodial mother	
		Fantasies of responsibility and reconciliation	Girls living in remarriage families experience more difficulty adjusting than boys, who show good adjustment 2 years after remarriage [43]
		Conflicts in loyalty	*(Continued)*

Table 28.2. (*Continued*)

Developmental stage	Cognitive understanding	Emotional and behavioral responses (0–2 years after divorce)	Long-term sequelae (2 years after divorce)
	9–12-year-olds Understand psychologic motives for divorce Appreciate each parent's perspective of divorce Less likely than younger children to blame themselves Believe cessation of conflict will be a benefit of divorce for themselves	**9–12-year-olds** Initially superficially well defended Attempt mastery by activity and play Anger Shaken sense of identity Somatic symptoms Alignment with one parent Identity issues; environment important	Father's absence seems to contribute more significantly to cognitive development in boys than in girls [51]
Adolescence Early adolescence (12–14 yr) Late adolescence (15–18 yr)	**12–14-year-olds** Appreciate complexity of communication and can recognize incongruence, between verbal and nonverbal cues Understand stability of personality characteristics Express concern about parental intention and believe that negative responses result from malevolent motives **15–18-year-olds** Explain divorce in terms of parental incompatibility and feel it was a mature decision Detach from parental conflict and focus on personal concerns [52,53]	**13–18-year-olds** Change in parent-child relationships Worry about sex and marriage Mourning Anger and aggression Changing perceptions Loyalty conflicts Strategic withdrawal Greater maturity and moral growth possible than in children of nondivorced parents Changed responsibilities within the family	**13–18-year-olds** Adolescent girls and young women appear to be vulnerable to problems with feminine self-esteem and heterosexual development [46,54,55]

consequence, many young people either threw themselves counterphobically into short-term sexual relationships or avoided relationships altogether. While most subjects reported being ideologically committed to the ideals of a lasting marriage, romantic love, and fidelity, they were terrified of repeating their parents' mistakes and inflicting their pain on their own future children. Early results from the 15-year follow-up found many of these subjects working hard to resolve issues around male-female relationships, with a significant number entering psychotherapy.

Bereavement

According to the US Census Bureau in March 2010, there were 7,87,000 children (under 18 years of age) living with a widowed parent. This particular statistic includes only those children still living with one parent and does not account for children who have lost both parents, or children whose parents were never married (3,041,000 children live with neither parent.

Bereavement, as defined in DSM-IV-TR, consists of the reaction one has to the death of a loved one. For purposes of clarity, the majority of the studies conducted on children and adolescents examine a young person's reaction to the death of a parent.

Grief is mostly the *affect* resulting from bereavement; mental suffering or distress over affliction of loss, sorrow or regret. *Mourning* is the psychological process begun by the loss of a loved one; grief is the parallel subjective state.

Research

It was once believed that bereavement was not possible in children because they lack a mature personality structure [11]. Likewise, it was not until 1975 that a meeting of researchers concluded that depression can exist in children and adolescents [12]. Both of these views had an impact on many of the early studies of children undergoing losses of various types.

Many of the earlier studies of bereavement suffered from the following methodological flaws:

(1) Retrospective studies [13–16] examined the frequency of childhood loss in child and adult patients and these were prone to underestimate or overestimate the frequency of bereavement in a "normal" population. Moreover, they did not account for environmental variables such as the stability of the home environment prior to the loss, or the response and adaptation of the remaining parent.

(2) Prospective studies [17–19] followed bereaved and normal adolescents into adulthood. These three studies examined the same group of adolescents but assessed them at different ages. The first two studies found a higher rate of legal involvement (the first in tenth graders and the second when the sample was in their early 20s) compared to matched controls. The third study (with the sample in their 30s) found no relationship between bereavement and criminal behavior, but this study found higher rates of serious medical illness and emotional distress. Limitations in these studies included the lack of information regarding the duration, frequency, and type of symptoms experienced by bereaved adolescents, as well as the age of the child at bereavement, cause of parent's death, and coping ability of the surviving parent.

(3) Studies of psychiatric patients [11, 20, 21] are problematic in that sample size is limited. They focus on extreme grief reactions and do not reflect normal grief processes. Subjectivity of the ratings employed in these studies limits their generalizability.

(4) Studies of bereavement in normal children [22–25] also examined a small number of children. Two studies used subjects from a kibbutz, which make comparisons difficult with children in "average" American families. Studies often rely more on teacher or parent reports than on information obtained directly from the child. Many researchers question the reliability of child informants, assume that parents know more about their children, are more reliable, and easier to interview. It is more difficult to interview children, especially prepubertal age groups: establishing rapport is more difficult, and questions must be framed in an age-appropriate manner. Although parents accurately report overt signs and symptoms of behavioral changes in their children, they are frequently unaware of subjective symptoms such as sleep disturbance, anxiety, guilt, and suicidal thoughts [26]. Often the child tries to conceal such symptoms from the parent, especially if the child perceives the parent as being stressed.

Later studies tried to address some of the above questions. Weller *et al* [27]. conducted a study on 38 nonreferred prepubertal children who had recently experienced the death of one but not both of their parents. The comparison group consisted of 38 hospitalized, depressed children individually matched to each bereaved subject for age, sex, and socioeconomic status. Each child and their surviving parent was independently evaluated using the parent and child versions of the Diagnostic Interview for Children and Adolescents (DICA-C/P). Family histories and other demographic data were also obtained. When using both parent- and child-reported symptoms, 37% of the bereaved children met DSM-III-R criteria for a major depressive episode. When parent-reported symptoms were used exclusively the number dropped to 8%. The factors associated with increased depressive symptoms were: (i) the mother as the surviving parent; (ii) pre-existing untreated psychiatric disorder in the child; (iii) family history of depression; and (iv) high socioeconomic status.

Using the same sample, another study [28] examined anxiety symptoms in bereaved children. This study also included a control group of 19 normal children and added the Grief Interview to the DICA-C/P. While no bereaved children met DSM-III-R criteria for an anxiety disorder, anxiety symptoms were reported in 55% of bereaved children immediately after parental death and in 63% approximately 8 weeks later. Anxiety typically focused around the fear of other family members dying. Despite this finding, bereaved children did not report significantly more anxiety symptoms in this 8-week period than normal comparison children, and had significantly fewer symptoms than depressed children. Bereaved children with the most anxiety symptoms were also likely to have a depressive disorder. Age and sex of child, sex of surviving parent, anticipation of death, and family history of anxiety or depressive disorders were not significantly associated with increased anxiety. The major limitation of these studies is relatively small sample size and therefore the possibility of a type II statistical error (i.e., not finding a statistically significant difference when one actually exists).

Cerel's [29] study of 360 parent-bereaved children, when compared to 110 depressed children and 128 controls, found bereaved children more impaired than controls in the 2 years following the death, but less impaired than the depressed children. Higher socioeconomic status and lower level of parental depression were protective.

Brent et al. [30] found higher rates of major depression and alcohol or substance abuse among bereaved offspring compared to a nonbereaved control group. They also found the incidence of post-traumatic stress disorder (PTSD) was elevated in the bereaved group for the first 9 months after the death but not at the 21-month follow-up.

The study by Kaplow et al. [31] is based on a subsample of children from a longitudinal epidemiological study, so data were available on the youths and their families prior to the death of their parent. The early loss of a parent was associated with poverty and previous substance abuse problems, and greater functional impairment even before the loss (compared to nonbereaved controls), suggesting that pre-existing risk factors may play a role in the parental death as well as in the bereavement symptoms in the children. The bereaved youths were more likely to show symptoms of separation anxiety and depression around the time of the bereavement (compared to non-

bereaved controls). At an average of 1.5 years after the death, bereaved youths were more likely to exhibit symptoms of conduct disorder and substance abuse and to show greater functional impairment.

Clinical Course

Classic models of the grief process emphasized different stages of grief, such as numbness, protest, despair, and detachment [32–34]. While this type of model is very descriptive, it can lead to oversimplification, and is often unhelpful in conceptualizing treatment. More recently the concept of "tasks" of grief has been used by several authors in their understanding of bereavement [21, 35, 36]. These tasks are time-specific. Early tasks involve gaining an understanding of what has happened, as well as guarding against the full emotional impact of the loss. Middle tasks include accepting and reworking the loss, and coping with the intense psychological pain. Late tasks include consolidation of the child's identity and resumption of age-appropriate developmental progress. A timing model can be useful in guiding clinical work as interventions can be planned according to which tasks the child is trying to master. It also promotes a more adaptive view of grief behaviors as related to certain goals, providing a useful alternative to pathology-based models that identify individuals as "stuck" in grieving [37].

Early Tasks

Children struggling with the early tasks of grieving focus on understanding the fact that someone has died and the meaning of this. They are preoccupied with protecting themselves and their families. In order to understand death and its implications, children need information about death in general as well as information about the particular death at hand. Children listen carefully and watch others intently, ask questions, and act out conflicts through play. Gaps in their information are often filled by fantasy. However, even with accurate information they can rarely grasp events entirely and only gradually understand and integrate what they have been told. For preschool children particularly there are cognitive limitations to how well they can understand death, which is why it is important to provide them with accurate information in age-appropriate language. This information is often the foundation for the child's struggle to understand the meaning of their loss [37].

Children must feel secure in their environment in order to accomplish the difficult tasks of grieving. They commonly fear that they too may die, or that their families will disintegrate. Children and their families engage in denial, distortion, and emotional or physical isolation in order to protect themselves and avoid affective overstimulation. They put much of their energy into protecting other family members. Adults will sometimes withhold information from their children about death in their own attempts at self-protectiveness [37].

Middle Tasks

Three main tasks characterize this stage: accepting and emotionally acknowledging the reality of the loss; re-evaluating the relationship with the lost loved one; and facing and learning to bear the psychological pain that comes with the realization of the loss. These middle-phase tasks were described by Freud as a process of detachment, but several studies of normal bereavement [35, 38, 39] have found that an internal attachment to the lost loved one continues long after the death, and may be a sign of health and recovery. During this period the child must deal with their ambivalence and guilt regarding their lost loved one and their anger at the deceased for abandoning them. Open acknowledgment of these difficult feelings may be very threatening to the children as they fear losing their positive connection with their deceased loved one. Often these relationship issues are played out with the therapist, friends, a transitional object, or through fantasies about the dead person. Children often maintain a fantasy that the dead person is alive or will return. This reflects denial on the child's part, but it may also serve an adaptive function, especially in the case of parental death. The child's fantasy allows a slow step-by-step separation from the lost parent. Children may have a lower tolerance for psychological pain and often they may need more time during this middle phase to approach the pain gradually, in order not to become overwhelmed. Preschool children who have not fully developed their ability to test reality, may not fully accept the reality of a loved one's death until they are several years older [37].

Late Tasks

This stage involves a reorganization of the child's sense of self and of significant relationships in his or her life. The child must develop a new identity that includes, but is not limited to, the experience of the loss and some identifications with the deceased person. This allows the child to re-engage in his or her environment. The child needs to develop new relationships without an excessive fear of loss and without constantly comparing the new relationship to that with the deceased. The child must maintain an enduring internal relationship to the lost loved one. Like adults, they must resume the age-appropriate developmental tasks and activities that were interrupted by the emotional loss and be able to tolerate the periodic return of their pain, typically at points of developmental transition, specific anniversaries, or holidays. Sometimes these "anniversary reactions" may occur years after the death and the child may not directly connect their current feelings with a loss that occurred some time ago. This may also be true of their surviving parent, who perceives the child to have "gotten over" his or her loss long ago. Conflicts may arise between different tasks in this later phase, such as the need for new relationships conflicting with the development of the strong internal attachment to the lost loved one. This can be especially problematic if a new member is added to the family, either the birth of a new sibling after a sibling loss, or a new step-parent after a parental loss. Significant limitations may arise in this phase of grief if other members of the family have become arrested in the grieving process. For instance, a parent in a state of chronic, unresolved grieving may heighten the child's sense of loyalty making it difficult for them to pursue new relationships outside the family [37].

Differential Diagnosis

Adjustment Disorder

The most likely symptoms that arise from a loss of any type are typically compatible with an adjustment disorder. The DSM-IV-TR defines Adjustment Disorder as:

(1) The development of emotional or behavioral symptoms in response to an identifiable stressor(s) occurring within 3 months of the onset of the stressor(s).
(2) These symptoms or behaviors are clinically significant as evidenced by either of the following:
  (a) marked distress that is in excess of what would be expected from exposure to the stressor;
  (b) significant impairment in social or occupational (academic) functioning.
(3) The stress-related disturbance does not meet the criteria for another specific Axis I disorder and is not merely an exacerbation of a pre-existing Axis I or Axis II disorder.
(4) The symptoms do not represent Bereavement.
(5) Once the stressor (or its consequences) has terminated, the symptoms do not persist for more than an additional 6 months.

Adjustment disorder subtypes are specified according to the predominant symptoms, namely:

(A) With Depressed Mood
(B) With Anxiety
(C) With Mixed Anxiety and Depressed Mood
(D) With Disturbance of Conduct
(E) With Mixed Disturbance of Emotions and Conduct
(F) Unspecified.

This diagnosis can encompass both acute and chronic disturbances ("Chronic" would be related to a chronic stressor or one with enduring consequences), as well as numerous symptom presentations. This can be a challenging distinction to make in the case of divorce, especially if divorce is considered a chronic stressor as most of the longitudinal studies seem to show. Another confounding variable is the possibility (discussed by Block *et al.* [6,7]) that by the time of the divorce, the children have often spent years in a conflict-ridden home and that some of the behaviors often identified as reactive to the divorce may have been chronic prior to the breakup. The clinical question then becomes "When is the termination of the stressor in the case of divorce?" The differential diagnoses of adjustment disorder would include bereavement, major depression, anxiety disorders, and disruptive behavior disorders. In rare cases, a child who has experienced a loss might present with symptoms of PTSD, acute stress disorder, or one of the somatoform disorders.

Bereavement

As mentioned above, bereavement is the deprivation due to loss or death. Feelings of sadness, insomnia, poor appetite, and weight loss, although characteristic of a major depressive disorder, are not diagnosed as such in the context of bereavement unless they persist, generally for more than 2 months. The expression of bereavement varies considerably in different cultural groups, and this should be taken into consideration when making this diagnosis. The DSM-IV-TR describes symptoms not considered "normal" during bereavement:

(1) Guilt about things other than actions taken or not taken by the survivor at the time of death.
(2) Thoughts of death other than the survivor feeling that he or she would be better off dead or should have died with the deceased person.
(3) Morbid preoccupation with worthlessness.
(4) Marked psychomotor retardation.
(5) Prolonged and marked functional impairment.
(6) Hallucinatory experiences other than thinking that he or she hears the voice of, or transiently sees the image of, the deceased person.

If any of these symptoms are seen, the diagnosis of bereavement may be complicated by a major depressive episode. In some cases bereavement may be complicated by an anxiety disorder, a disruptive behavior disorder, a PTSD, or a somatoform disorder.

Major Depressive Episode

Any child who has suffered a significant loss may show some symptoms of depression. If the loss is due to the death of a significant person, then the most appropriate initial diagnosis would be bereavement. If the symptoms are severe enough (or persist long enough) to meet criteria for a major depressive episode, then this diagnosis could be given as well. Symptoms of guilt/worthlessness and fatigue (both more common in depressed subjects) best discriminate bereaved from depressed subjects [27]. By relying on these two symptoms, 74% of bereaved children and 82% of depressed children could be correctly identified. Even so, 21% of bereaved children endorsed feelings of worthlessness/guilt. While 61% of bereaved children reportedly had suicidal ideation, none had actually attempted suicide. In contrast, 89% of depressed subjects reportedly had suicidal ideation and 42% had at least one suicide attempt. Weller hypothesized that suicidal ideation in bereaved children may represent a reunion fantasy rather than the devaluation of one's own life. This explanation was given by several subjects who reported suicidal ideation and may account for the lack of suicide attempts and the less frequent reports of worthlessness by the bereaved children.

Children experiencing a divorce may also suffer a major depressive episode. One must primarily decide if their symptoms exceed those more characteristic of adjustment disorder with depressed mood, or are severe and persistent enough to meet criteria for a major depressive episode. Consistent with the findings of the long-term effects of divorce, some consideration might need to be given to a diagnosis of dysthymia or chronic adjustment disorder if less severe symptoms persist over time.

Anxiety Disorders

Anxiety symptoms are commonplace when a child has experienced a loss. Typically there are concerns regarding further loss. For instance, a child of divorce may be upset that not only has a parent moved out, but they may fear that they will never see the parent again, or that the parent won't love them anymore. A child who has lost a loved one through death often fears losing other loved ones, especially the surviving parent. Sometimes this results in separation anxiety. If symptoms are time-limited, and of expected intensity given the stressor, adjustment disorder with anxiety would be the most appropriate diagnosis. If the symptoms persist for longer than 6 months, are more severe, or represent an exacerbation of a previously diagnosed anxiety disorder, then the appropriate specific anxiety disorder should be diagnosed.

Disruptive Behavior Disorders

Disruptive behaviors are a common response to loss in children. Young children are less able to express their feelings verbally, tending to act out or express emotional conflicts through disruptive behaviors. For children who have lost a parent to death or divorce, their environment is also likely to be more chaotic, at least temporarily, until the remaining parent is able to optimize his or her coping skills and access support systems. Although some children respond to a chaotic environment by becoming caretakers (i.e., the pseudomature child in an alcoholic household), many more respond with disruptive behaviors. Even within a single family unit, often both styles of coping and their variations are present. The pseudomature caretaker may actually need as much help as the child with disruptive behavior, although the focus of treatment for the parent is likely to center on the disruptive child. In the case of recent loss from death or divorce, the diagnosis of a disruptive behavior disorder should only be made if an adjustment disorder (with disturbance of conduct or with mixed disturbance of emotions and conduct) diagnosis would no longer be appropriate given the severity of symptoms or their chronicity.

Post-Traumatic Stress Disorder/Acute Stress Disorder

These diagnoses would primarily be applicable if the child witnessed the *traumatic* death of a loved one and is experiencing the specific constellation of symptoms characteristic of these disorders. If the extreme stressor is present but the symptoms do not meet diagnostic criteria for one of the above disorders, a diagnosis of adjustment disorder would still be appropriate.

Somatoform Disorders

Sometimes children who have experienced a loss will express their emotional pain with physical symptoms, especially if they come from a family that tends to be somatic. Their symptoms are often vague, center on abdominal complaints or headaches, or have numerous sites of origin. An example would be a child who develops physical symptoms that keeps him or her home from school after a parent's funeral. One study [40] of persistently somatizing adult patients found that those who experienced childhood loss of a parent had the poorest treatment outcome and a group with recent loss (within the past 2 years) had the best treatment outcome. The first point of contact for this child is usually the primary care physician. If the physician is aware of the recent loss or is astute enough to ask about recent stressors, the problem may be correctly identified and treated as a symptom of the child's emotional distress. Many good primary care physicians will give parents appropriate initial interventional strategies. If these are unsuccessful the physician often refers the child to a psychiatry clinic for evaluation/treatment.

Treatment

As is the case with any referral to a behavioral health practitioner, the treatment plan must be developed to meet the individual needs of a particular patient and their family. It must take into account the availability of various forms of treatment, the nature and severity of the presenting symptoms, the family's recognition of the symptoms as problematic, and the family's emotional and financial resources.

Often family therapy is the treatment of choice during the crisis immediately following a loss. Whether the loss is due to death or divorce, it is sure to have affected all of the family members. Many times there is an "identified patient," and the first task of the therapist is to reframe the problem in terms of optimizing *family* functioning, and engaging the family in treatment. The remaining/custodial parent may be so wrapped up in their own grieving process that little thought has been given to the needs of the child and the therapist may need to guide the parent in order to help the child/children. This is especially true in the case of younger children who lack the emotional resources to cope with the loss by themselves but depend upon the structure provided by others. In certain situations the parent may require a referral for their own individual therapy, particularly if he or she has features of a major depressive disorder.

Historically, psychodynamically oriented individual therapy was the treatment of choice for children and adolescents, especially if they continued to experience psychiatric symptoms or developmental inhibition some years after the loss. While this remains the treatment of choice in an ideal world, with all the changes in our medical system the emphasis has shifted to short-term and/or group treatments. The increased emphasis on short-term treatments has led to a resurgence in cognitive behavioral therapy. This treatment focuses on helping the child to develop a realistic appraisal of their situation and to modify their behavior to optimize their functioning within that situation through effective problem-solving and communication skills. Groups have become more available in recent years. Often schools conduct support groups for children of divorce, and in many communities, the hospice organization conducts groups for bereaved children and their families. A recent study by Velez *et al.* [41] of a randomized trial of parenting-focused preventive intervention in situations of divorce showed improvement in children's coping skills both in the short and long term.

When the experience of loss is complicated by a major depressive episode or an anxiety disorder, some consideration should be given to the use of appropriate medication. In the case of a disruptive behavior disorder, medication should only be considered if there has been no response to therapy or if behavior is dangerous to the patient or others.

Very little systematic research has been done to evaluate treatment modalities and their outcomes with regard to the issue of loss. In order for us to be successful advocates for children and adolescents, this field must address these challenges.

References

1. U.S. Bureau of the Census, Current Population Reports, "Living Arrangements of Children under 18, and Marital Status of Parents: March 2010," and earlier reports.
2. Wallerstein JS. The long-term effects of divorce on children: A review. *J Am Acad Child Adolesc Psychiat* 1991;**30**:349–360.
3. American Psychiatric Association. *Diagnostic and Statistical Manual of Mental Disorders*, 4th edn, Text Revision. Washington, DC: American Psychiatric Association, 2000.
4. Jensen PS, Martin D, Watanabe H. Children's response to parental separation during Operation Desert Storm. *J Am Acad Child Adolesc Psychiatry* 1996;**35**:433–441.
5. Blount BW, Curry A Jr, Lubin GI. Family separations in the military. *Mil Med* 1992;**157**:76–80.
6. Block JH, Block J, Gjerde PF. The personality of children prior to divorce. *Child Dev* 1986;**57**:827–840.
7. Block J, Block JH, Gjerde PF. Parental functioning and the home environment in families of divorce. *J Am Acad Child Adolesc Psychiatry* 1988;**27**:207–213.
8. D'Onofrio B, Turkheimer E, Emery RE, Maes HH, Silberg J, Eaves LJ. A Children of Twins Study of parental divorce and offspring psychopathology. *J Child Psychol Psychiatry* 2007;**48**:667–675.
9. Burt SA, Barnes AR, McGue M, IaconoWG. Parental divorce and adolescent delinquency: ruling out the impact of common genes. *Dev Psychol* 2008;**44**:1668–1677.
10. Hetherington EM. Coping with family transitions: Winners, losers, and survivors. *Child Dev* 1989;**60**:1–14.
11. Wolfenstein M. How is mourning possible? *Psychoanal Study Child* 1966;**21**:92–123.
12. Schulterbrandt JG, Raskin A. *Depression in Childhood: Diagnosis, Treatment, and Conceptual Models*. New York: Raven Press, 1977.
13. Barry H Jr, Lindeman E. Critical ages for maternal bereavement in psychoneuroses. *Psychosom Med* 1960;**22**:166–181.
14. Beck AT, Sethi BB, Tuthill RW. Childhood bereavement and adult depression. *Arch Gen Psychiatry* 1963;**9**:295–302.
15. Caplan MG, Douglas UI. Influence of parental loss in children with depressed mood. *J Child Psychol Psychiatry* 1969;**10**:225–232.
16. Tennant C, Bebbington P, Hurry J. Parental death in childhood and risk of adult depressive disorder: A review. *Psychol Med* 1980;**10**:289–299.
17. Gregory I. Anterospective data following childhood loss of a parent: I. Delinquency and high school dropout. *Arch Gen Psychiatry* 1965;**13**:99–109.
18. Markuson T, Fulton R. Childhood bereavement and behavioral disorders: A critical review. *Omega* 1971;**2**:107–117.
19. Bendickson R, Fulton R. Death and the child: An anterospective test of the childhood bereavement and later behavior disorder hypothesis. In: Fulton R (ed.) *Death and Identity*. Bowie, MD: Charles Press, 1976.
20. Arthur B, Kemme ML. Bereavement in childhood. *J Child Psychol Psychiatry* 1964;**5**:37–49.
21. Furman E. *A Child's Parent Dies*. New Haven, CT: Yale University Press, 1974.
22. Kliman G. *Psychological Emergencies of Childhood*. New York: Grune & Stratton, 1968.
23. Lifshitz M, Berman D, Galili A, *et al*. Bereaved children: The effect of mother's perception and social system organization on their short-range adjustment. *J Am Acad Child Psychiatry* 1977;**16**:272–284.
24. Van Eerdewegh MM, Bieri MD, Parilla RH, *et al*. The bereaved child. *Br J Psychiatry* 1982;**140**:23–29.
25. Elizur E, Kaffman M. Factors influencing the severity of childhood bereavement reactions. *Am J Orthopsychiatry* 1983;**53**:668–676.
26. Weller E, Weller R. Grief in children and adolescents. In: Garfinkel BD, Carlson GA, Weller EB (eds) *Psychiatric Disorders in Children and Adolescents*. Philadelphia: W.B. Saunders Co., 1990;37–47.
27. Weller RA, Weller EB, Fristad MA, *et al*. Depression in recently bereaved prepubertal children. *Am J. Psychiatry* 1991;**148**:536–540.
28. Sanchez L, Fristad M, Weller R, *et al*. Anxiety in acutely bereaved prepubertal children. *Ann Clin Psychiatry* 1994;**6**:39–42.
29. Cerel, J. et al. 2006. Childhood Bereavement: Psychopathology in the 2 years Postparental Death. *J. Am. Acad. Child Adolesc. Psychiatry* 45:6, 681–690.
30. Brent D, Melhem N, Donohoe MB, Walker M. The incidence and course of depression in bereaved youth 21 months after the loss of a parent to suicide, accident, or sudden natural death. *Am J Psychiatry* 2009;**166**:786–794.
31. Kaplow J, Saunders J, Angold A, Costello EJ. Psychiatric symptoms in bereaved versus nonbereaved youth and young adults: a longitudinal epidemiological study. *J Am Acad Child Adolesc Psychiatry* 2010;**49**:1145–1154.
32. Bowlby J. Grief and mourning in infancy and early childhood. *Psychoanal Study Child* 1960;**15**:9–52.
33. Bowlby J. Childhood mourning and its implications for psychiatry. *Am J Psychiatry* 1961;**118**:481–498.
34. Bowlby J. Pathological mourning and childhood mourning. *J Am Psychoanal* 1963;**11**:500–541.
35. Schuchter SR. *Dimensions of Grief: Adjusting to the Death of a Spouse*. San Francisco: Jossey-Bass, 1986.
36. Worden W. *Grief Counseling and Grief Therapy: A Handbook for the Mental Health Practitioner*. New York: Springer, 1982.
37. Baker J, Sedney M, Gross E. Psychological tasks for bereaved children. *Am J Orthopsychiat* 1992;**62**:105–116.
38. Glick IO, Weiss RS, Parkes CM. *The First Year of Bereavement*. New York: Wiley-Interscience, 1974.
39. Silverman PR, Nickman S, Worden JW. Detachment revisited: The child's reconstruction of a dead parent. *Am J Orthopsychiatry* 1992;**62**:494–503.

40. Mallouh SK, Abbey SE, Gillies LA. The role of loss in treatment outcomes of persistent somatization. *Gen Hosp Psychiatry* 1995;**17**:187–191.

41. Vélez C, Wolchik SA, Tein JY, Sandler I. Protecting children from the consequences of divorce: a longitudinal study of the effects of parenting on children's coping processes. *Child Dev* 2011;**82**:244–257.

42. Guidubaldi J, Perry JD. Divorce and mental health sequence for children: A two-year follow-up of a nationwide sample. *J Child Psychiatry* 1985;**24**:531–537.

43. Hetherington EM, Cox M, Cox R. Long-term effects of divorce and remarriage on the adjustment of children. *J Child Psychiatry* 1985;**24**:518–530.

44. Kalter N, Rembar J. The significance of a child's age at the time of parental divorce. *Am J Orthopsychiatry* 1981;**51**:85–100.

45. Wallerstein JS, Kelly JB. *Surviving the Break-up.* New York: Basic Books, 1980.

46. Wallerstein JS. Children of divorce: Preliminary report of a ten-year follow-up of older children and adolescents. *J Am Acad Child Psychiat* 1985;**24**:545–553.

47. Fergusson DM, Horwood LJ, Lynskey MT. Parental separation, adolescent psychopathology, and problem behaviors. *J Am Acad Child Adolesc Psychiatry* 1994;**33**:1122–1131.

48. Black AE, Pedro-Carroll J. Role of parent-child relationships in mediating the effects of marital disruption. *J Am Acad Child Adolesc Psychiatry* 1993;**32**:1019–1027.

49. Kurtz L. Psychosocial coping resources in elementary school-age children of divorce. *Am J Orthopsychiatry* 1994;**64**:554–563.

50. Bolgar R, Zweig-Frank H, Paris J. Childhood antecedents of interpersonal problems in young adult children of divorce. *J Am Acad Child Adolesc Psychiatry* 1995;**34**:143–150.

51. Radin R. The role of the father in cognitive, academic, and intellectual development. In: Lamb M (ed.) *The Role of the Father in Child Development.* New York: John Wiley & Sons, Ltd, 1985; pp. 237–276.

52. Kurdek LA. Children's reasoning about parental divorce. In: Ashmore JRD, Brodzinsky PM (eds) *Thinking About the Family: Views of Parents and Children.* Hillsdale, NJ: Lawrence Erlbaum Associates Inc., 1986; pp. 233–276.

53. Neal JH. Children's understanding of their parents' divorce. In: Kurdeck LA (ed.) *New Directions for Child Development, Vol 19. Children and Divorce.* San Francisco: Jossey-Bass, 1983; pp. 3–14.

54. Kalter N, Riemer B, Brickman A, Chen JW. Implications of parental divorce for female development. *J Am Acad Child Psychiatry* 1985;**24**:538–544.

55. Kalter N. Long-term effects of divorce on children: A developmental vulnerability model. *Am J Orthopsychiatry* 1987; **57**:587–599.

29

Foster Care and Adoption

Jill D. McCarley, Christina G. Weston

Foster Care

Until the mid- to late nineteenth century, the care of children who had no means of provision other than state custody was frequently dismal. Children who lost both parents due to illness or war were abandoned, and those whose parents simply had no means to care for them usually resided in custodial institutions such as infirmaries and almshouses. These institutions were the catchall placement for the poor and infirm of all ages, therefore it was not uncommon for orphaned and abandoned children to reside with the severely mentally ill, the aged, or the contagious.

The situation changed during the latter half of the nineteenth century, with the evolution of the orphanage. Here, an orphaned or abandoned youth could obtain adequate, if perhaps less than ideal, care. It was also during this same time that the concept of foster care evolved, furthered by the efforts of Charles Loring Brace, who began the movement to place children from large custodial institutions to live with Midwestern farm families. And so was born the idea of foster care although among much controversy at the time [1]. Foster care in the United States has become a system for placing children who are unable to live with their biological parents, with other families to live. These other families receive money to cover the cost of caring for these children. These children are considered to be in the custody of the county child welfare/children's services board.

Controversy at its inception and still today – foster care is much beleaguered by debate both about its concept and implementation. Foster care has long been a source of public policy debate over the role of child welfare agencies in determining when to remove a child, and more recently over the ever-increasing cost of paying for out-of-home placements and how to finance the additional services that these children often need. Current controversies concern gay and lesbian foster care,

custody relinquishment, multiple placements, and health-care delivery while in foster care. No matter the theoretical underpinnings of the current foster care system, there is no doubt that children in foster care face unique challenges, as do their guardians and health-care providers. As health-care providers, we can be strong advocates for these children and the families who care for them.

Entry into Foster Care

Death due to abuse or neglect affects approximately 2 of every 100 000 children in the United States each year, usually at the hands of adults who are responsible for their care [2]. Educators, health-care providers, relatives, and other concerned persons report their apprehensions about the well-being of a child to children's protective agencies, who in turn send out their caseworkers to investigate suspicions of abuse or neglect. During the course of the investigation, a caseworker will have to make the difficult choice of whether or not to remove a child from the custody of his or her parent(s) in order to assure the child's safety and well-being.

The decision to remove a child from his or her home for placement into foster care is never an easy one. Caseworkers for children's protective services often have to make the best possible selection from various seemingly disagreeable options. On the one hand they know the decision to remove a child will bring about emotional pain and conflict at the very least, on the other they are painfully aware of the risks involved in not being cautious.

Unfortunately, there is limited consensus on what criteria are used in determining when a child is to be removed and placed into foster care. As a result, there are wide variations in the rate of child removal among US states, with California (highest rate of removal) being 16 times more likely than Alabama (lowest rate of removal) to remove a child from his or her home for

Clinical Child Psychiatry, Third Edition. Edited by William M. Klykylo and Jerald Kay.
© 2012 John Wiley & Sons, Ltd. Published 2012 by John Wiley & Sons, Ltd.

suspected abuse or neglect. Multiple studies have suggested that the major determining factor in the decision to remove a child seems to be the socioeconomic status of the family involved [1]. As a result, a child entering foster care is much more likely to come from an impoverished background.

The latest available statistics indicate that over 400 000 children are currently in foster care, with about one-quarter of them being cared for in the homes of relatives (kinship care). Most children stay in custody for 2 years or less. About half of the children who leave foster care return to the care of their parents or former primary caretakers. About 40% are white, 30% are black, and 20% Hispanic [3]. Almost all children in foster care have endured either neglect or abuse. Most have also witnessed domestic violence and/or drug abuse in the home. These factors greatly increase the likelihood that a child will have a psychiatric diagnosis requiring treatment.

Vignette 1

Robert was brought to his doctor's appointment by his foster parent and caseworker from children's protective services. An 11-year-old boy, Robert had been diagnosed 3 years ago with ADHD but had received only intermittent treatment since the diagnosis was made. He has been living in foster care for the past 3 weeks after he and his brothers were found to be neglected by their biological mother, mostly due to her problems with substance dependence. Since the placement, Robert's behavior has become unmanageable and he has been suspended from school for fighting. The foster parent describes both impulsive behavior and irritability. Medical history is unknown, as is family history. Robert describes having been on several stimulant medications in the past but is unable to remember dosages or how he responded to any specific one, stating, "It doesn't matter, anyway. I'm going to act up until I get to go home."

The above vignette, while fictitious, illustrates several issues that are, unfortunately, commonly encountered by pediatricians, family practice, and emergency room physicians, as well as child and adolescent psychiatrists.

Delivery of health care to foster children is complicated by several factors, including but not limited to:

(1) Unexpected entry of the child into the foster care system.

(2) Lack of known medical or mental health history.
(3) Increased risk of chronic health, mental health, and developmental problems.
(4) Lack of a central care coordinator.
(5) Cost of care.
(6) Multiple placements.
(7) Severity of a child's social and psychological deficits.

Unexpected Entry

Children who enter foster care frequently do so on an emergent basis. Victims of abuse or neglect are commonly taken from a chaotic environment, perhaps after normal business hours. This precipitous transition, while no doubt difficult for the child, also creates difficulties when medical or mental health care is required immediately upon entry into foster care or shortly thereafter. There may be confusion as to issues of consent or confidentiality that need to be addressed, therefore delaying nonemergent care. In addition, health-care coverage may be unknown or not yet initiated, which may make finding a provider challenging. As a result, a foster child may be taken to an emergency room for nonemergent health or mental health issues that could be better addressed in a routine visit with a primary care physician. Besides increasing the cost of medical care dramatically, the trip to the emergency room has the potential of making an already stressful event much more difficult for the child involved.

Lack of Health History

Many children enter foster care from chaotic environments, and as a result will not often have had the usual well-child examinations or routine screenings. What medical care has been obtained may not be clear, as records may reside in various clinics or are lost by parents. Also, the sudden transfer of the child into foster care may not allow for the prompt possession of what medical records do exist. Important information regarding allergies, immunizations, medications, or medical conditions may be unknown or at the very least delayed in finding their way to new providers via the agency. Unfortunately, this leaves the next provider in the dark, as well as the foster parents. Often, this necessitates the repetition of testing and/or subspecialty referrals that may be unnecessary. In addition to a child's health history the family history of mental illness is important. Many psychiatric disorders can be difficult to diagnose in young children, and the knowledge of the parents' history can help to validate the diagnosis, or at least to narrow the differential.

Commonly, the early period of foster care is marked with much activity among agency representatives, and obtaining medical records may not be a high priority unless emphasized by a physician. It is more likely that existing records can be much more easily obtained earlier than later in the course of foster care. By strongly encouraging that every effort is made to obtain any available records, providers can make a positive influence on the short- and long-term care of a child. As electronic health records become more available and used, it is hoped that many of these issues will be resolved in the future.

Increased Probability of Chronic Health, Mental Health, and Developmental Problems

Children who enter foster care have much higher rates of chronic medical, mental, and developmental problems when compared to other children not in foster care. Many factors are thought to be related to this, including inadequate medical treatment or routine physical examinations and high rates of parental substance abuse.

Estimates for rates of emotional/behavioral problems range widely. Zima *et al.*, in 2000, found that 27% of 302 children in foster care exhibited at least one behavioral problem within a level of clinical significance [4]. Another study found that 13% had also taken psychotropic medication within the past year [5]. Stahmer *et al.*, in 2005, found that 41.8% of toddlers and 68.1% of pre-schoolers in foster care had developmental and behavioral issues, while only 22.7% were receiving services [6]. Comparison of foster children with children receiving other types of governmental aid, such as Supplemental Security Income (a US federal program that provides income for adults and children with physical or psychiatric disabilities), found that youths in foster care were twice more likely to have a mental disorder [7].

In another study, which used a national survey of children who had involvement with child welfare agencies, revealed that almost half scored within the clinical range for problems on the Child Behavior Checklist. Of those, adolescents were more likely to score in the clinical range as compared to younger children, as were children placed in nonrelative foster care. Although almost half of the children surveyed scored within the clinical range for emotional or behavioral difficulties, only 15.8% had obtained any mental health intervention within the year prior to the survey [8].

Perhaps connected to this increased rate of emotional and behavioral disorders is the significant amount of parental substance abuse. One source estimates that perhaps as many as 62% of children entering foster care have had prenatal exposure to drugs or alcohol and/or have experienced postnatal environmental deficits due to parental substance abuse [9].

Another risk factor associated with emotional disorders in children is a history of prior abuse. To this end, it is important to realize that at least half of children in foster care have been victims of some form of abuse [10]. While not all children who have been abused will meet full criteria for post-traumatic stress disorder (PTSD), a great many will and no doubt numerous others will display other sequelae related to the abuse experience that while not yet severe enough to meet criteria for full diagnosis, nevertheless will have significant impact on development and functioning.

Care Coordination

Medical care of children in foster care is also complicated by the lack of a central care coordinator. Under the best of circumstances, a child would have a defined primary care provider who, in concert with a guardian, would follow the care of a child for an extended period of time. Under this model, the primary provider would offer the usual basic care as well as arrange for subspecialty referral when required. Having a centralized locus of care also simplifies record-keeping and minimizes duplication of services that may be unnecessary.

Coordination of care within the foster care system creates its own challenges. Aside from the concerns already mentioned, there frequently are the additional complications of consent and confidentiality. For instance, the guardian of a child in foster care may not have the legal power to consent for treatment. It is also common that the child welfare agency itself is required to consent for medical or psychiatric treatment of a child in its custody, sometimes creating another barrier to timely care as the appropriate paperwork and signatures are sought. There are also instances where the biological parent retains the right to consent or refuse treatment of his/her child even while the child resides in foster care.

Because of these issues and those previously discussed, medical providers need to be acutely aware of who has the power to consent for treatment and who has legal access to the child's medical information in each case. Once the legality and appropriateness of information sharing is established, good communication and distribution of data may aid in filling the gap left by not having a dedicated central care coordinator.

Multiple Placements

It is not uncommon for a child in foster care to have a series of different placements for various reasons. Occasionally, foster families experience a change in situation resulting in the child's return to the agency for placement with another family. A child may be reunited with his or her family briefly, then return to state custody. At times, a child's behavior itself may be so unmanageable as to precipitate a move to another foster family. Additionally, a child with mental, medical, or developmental challenges is more likely to have multiple placements.

These multiple moves and placements create special problems for children. Although data and controlled studies are limited, it seems that multiple placements for children in foster care have negative consequences that get expressed via the health-care system. One study of Medicaid claims found that over 40% of children in foster care had had three or more placements within the past year [11]. The same study also indicated that multiple placements increased the probability of high mental health resource utilization.

Case Vignette 2

Seven-year-old twin boys present to a child and adolescent psychiatrist with their foster parents. They have been in foster care for the past 2 years and in this foster home for the past 4 months. This is their third foster home, chosen because these foster parents have had extra training to provide therapeutic foster care, as both boys have significant developmental delays as well as bipolar disorder. They have not had psychiatric treatment since the move into this foster home, but the parents present a thick packet of records from an assortment of previous providers. These records describe a lengthy history of partial responses to multiple medication trials and two previous hospitalizations for one of the boys due to his uncontrollable and occasionally dangerous behavior.

The children are loud and boisterous during the evaluation, at times requiring physical separation while arguing over toys. The foster parents handle each situation calmly and offer expert redirection and positive reinforcement for good behavior. They smile warmly at the boys and indicate a strong commitment to "hang on to these guys," expressing a desire to eventually adopt them.

A provider when faced with situations similar to the above vignette may have to decide to "start fresh" due to some of the unique situations that foster care introduces. Complicated medical and/or psychiatric histories, often incomplete or unclear, can be overwhelming. Multiple trials of medications in the past – sometimes inadequate in dosage or length of time attempted due to the movement of a foster child – may yield less than favorable results. This, combined with treatments attempted in the face of other, perhaps rather dramatic changes in a child's social or academic environment clouds the picture of what may or may not have been effective. For these reasons, it is not necessarily wise to dismiss or disregard a prior treatment as a universal failure for a child. It is plausible that an option that failed or met with limited success may have a vastly different outcome when paired with a stable environment and or other interventions.

A provider might feel a sense of dread when reviewing page after page of previous treatment failures for a particular child. However, when the commitment of the parent(s) is evident, that dread feeling conceivably could lead to hope when the stability of the home and positive regard for the child is present. These assets may just provide the child with the link that was previously missing for treatment to meet with success.

Grandparent/Kinship Care

In the United States there has been a dramatic increase in the number of grandparents raising their grandchildren. Some are in kinship care while others are in the full custody of their grandparents. Kinship care refers to the practice of placing foster care children with family members rather than non-biologically related foster parents. From 1990 to 1998 the number of custodial grandparents increased by 53% [12]. The structure of these homes with grandparents as head of household can be difficult to define. They can have both grandparents present, grandmother present, or grandfathers present. They can also have some of the parents present or no parents present. In their analysis of 1997 census data, Casper and Bryson found that 6.7% of families with children were maintained by grandparents; [12] 35% were both grandparents, with some parents present; 17% were both grandparents, with no parents present; 29% were grandmother only with some parents present; 14% were grandmother only, with no parents present; and 6% were grandfather only. From 1990 to 1997 the highest increase among these groups was among grandfather only – 39%; both grandparents, with no parents present – 31%; and grandmother only with no parents present – 27%. The very same factors that are contributing to increasing rates of foster care are creating custodial grandparents. Parental substance abuse, in-carceration, teenage pregnancy, divorce, the rapid rise of single parenthood, and increasing rates of child abuse are all believed to be contributing to this trend.

These grandparents and children in these homes are more likely to suffer economic hardships. Children in a grandparent's household without a parent were twice as likely to be below the poverty level when compared with children living with both grandparents and a parent [12]. They were also twice as likely to be uninsured when they lived with their grandparent's household without a parent present – 36% versus 15% of children living with grandparents in their parent's home. They were also more likely to be receiving public assistance. In custodial grandparent homes, significant health problems are found in both the grandparents and the grandchildren. The grandparents have been found to have high rates of depression, poor self-rated health, multiple chronic health problems, and a decreased ability to perform activities of daily living [13, 14]. The grandchildren raised by grandparents have higher rates of physical disabilities; hyperactivity, asthma, and poor sleeping and eating patterns [14, 15].

In addition to health effects the children in grandparent-headed homes are more likely to have caregivers who haven't graduated from high school. They are also more likely to be younger, have an older nonworking head of household, live in the South and inner city, and to be poor [11]. Over half of the children living in grandparents' homes are under 6 years old. When racial differences are examined, historically African-American grandmothers have acted as surrogate parents for their grandchildren when compared to white grandmothers [16]. In 2002, the largest ethnic group to live in their grandparents' household was African-American children at 9%, followed by 6% of Hispanic children, 4% of non-Hispanic white children, and 3% of Asian children. Two-thirds of the African-American children living in their grandparents' household were with only one grandparent. All other ethnic groups were more likely to have both grandparents present.

This trend toward grandparents as parents of their grandchildren creates many psychosocial issues. As discussed above many of these grandparents are less physically, emotionally, and financially able to support their grandchildren. In cases where their grandchildren were removed due to their children's substance abuse, incarceration, and/or abuse/neglect of the children, they may have the added emotional guilt of having failed to raise the children successfully. They may feel pressure to raise their grandchildren better the second time around.

They frequently are conflicted between helping their children or their grandchildren. As this trend has increased rapidly, there are several public policy implications. Some welfare reform rules designed for young parents unfairly punish retirement age custodial grandparents for not working. Foster care advocates have recommended that parity should be established between kinship foster care homes and nonrelative foster care payment rates. Currently nonrelative foster care homes receive higher reimbursement. Policies for securing adoption and guardianship can be made easier for grandparents to use.

With the increasing trend toward grandparents raising their grandchildren, there has been an interest in creating support programs for these grandparents. In a small pilot program with separate grandparent and child groups, participants found the experience helpful [17]. The grandparents even went to great lengths to attend sessions that they found helpful. While this pilot did not quantify how much families improved, it highlighted the need for longer-term group support and continued contact with social workers after an initial group as the families found the social interaction and support helpful. It identified ways to structure therapeutic interventions to grandparent-led families so they can be most beneficial.

Adoption

After World War II, adoption became more common and more widely accepted than it had been before. For the first time, a broad white middle-class consensus proclaimed adoption the 'best solution' to the 'problem' of pregnancy out of wedlock.

Barbara Melosh [18]

The face of adoption has changed significantly over time. The above quote marks one milestone of change, when during 1945–1965 there was a shift to a more uniform practice surrounding adoption policies. Specifically, children were matched to parents ethnically and only upon a confidential basis. These "closed" adoptions were the norm for many decades, where neither the child nor the biological parents knew the identity or whereabouts of the other. At times, even birth certificates were amended to reflect the identity of the adoptive parents. Children were often matched according to physical appearance and temperament, with the goal of affecting the equivalence of full kinship [18].

Starting in the 1980s, adoption agencies began to utilize the concept of "open" adoption. The concept was that birth mothers who were ambivalent about giving up their children into anonymity forever might be more willing to grant adoption if they knew more about where and with whom their children were placed. The term "open adoption" has since come to mean a spectrum of contact, from yearly reports all the way to active, regular participation of the biological parent with the adoptive family. Some agencies even allow the birth mother to choose which family her child will eventually go to.

Not surprisingly, this change from closed to open adoption has caused much heated debate. Both sides present sound arguments. Proponents of open adoption argue that the secretive nature of closed adoption creates psychological difficulties linked with a veil of shame or guilt about unknown backgrounds. They contend that an individual has a basic right to know his or her own history. Proponents of open adoption also point out that it may be important for older children in foster care to see their future adoptive parents welcomed into their current home by caretakers that they have grown to trust. In this way, it is less likely to be perceived by the child that he or she has been "snatched away" by a caseworker to be delivered to the adoptive family. Also, when a child begins to have positive feelings for his or her new adoptive family, he or she may feel less conflicted about being unfaithful to the former caretakers or loving them less.

Opponents of open adoption cite that the biological parents' involvement may confuse children and disrupt relationships or bonding with the adoptive parent. Ideological positions aside, research seems to indicate that there is not typically enough contact between the biological parent and adoptive family to make much difference, for good or ill, to the development of the child [18].

Nevertheless, there has been a movement among adopted adults to force open previously sealed documents about their own births and adoptions. This surge has been powerful enough to challenge state laws, establish adoption registries, and allow third-party delegates to read sealed adoption records. The drive of many adopted persons who take the time and effort to pursue these records likely means that many others, if not most, struggle less obviously with the ramifications of not knowing their own histories. In addition, they may be conflicted by even having the desire to uncover their pasts, feeling guilt over "betraying" the adoptive parents that they care deeply for.

Race, Age, and Adoption

In the United States, of the almost 424 000 children in foster care in 2009, 114 500 were awaiting adoption, and 57 500 were actually adopted from the public foster care system [19].Table 29.1 compares the race and age distribution of children awaiting adoption and those who were adopted.

Table 29.1 Race and age distribution of children awaiting adoption and those adopted.

	Awaiting adoption	Adopted
Race		
Black, non-Hispanic	30%	25%
White, non-Hispanic	38%	44%
Hispanic	22%	21%
Age (years)		
1–5	43%	25%
6–10	26%	44%
11–15	25%	21%
16–18	7%	3%

Source: US Department of Health and Human Services, Administration for Children and Families, Administration on Children, Youth and Families, Children's Bureau: Preliminary FY 2009 Estimates as of July 2010. http://www.acf.hhs.gov/programs/cb/stats_research/afcars/tar/report17.htm

These numbers indicate that there is a racial as well as an age discrepancy between children awaiting adoption and those who are adopted. Children aged 11–15 years are at a disadvantage for successful adoption compared to younger children who are available for adoption. Parents wishing to adopt are usually seeking younger children or infants, often working with the notion that a younger child is less likely to exhibit difficulties as they may have less of a "bad" history and therefore less "damage" has been done. Also, future adoptive parents may view an older child with some degree of skepticism, perhaps wondering if something was wrong with the child to prevent earlier adoption.

Another striking factor in adoption from foster care is the length of time the process itself takes. The mean number of months between termination of parental rights to adoption was 13.9 months, although 14% waited 2 years or more before adoption. However, 54% of those adopted were adopted by a foster parent. For those children who were awaiting adoption, the mean number of months in continuous foster care was 38 [19].

Understandably, children who are awaiting adoption from foster care may be quite conflicted about the possibility of adoption. Although parental rights may have been terminated, a great many children have difficulty accepting or understanding this fact and continue to express a hope to eventually return. Conversely, a child who is angry at his or her parents may openly express a desire to break all ties and see adoption as a way for this to occur. However, if this anger at parents is not reckoned with, relationships with alternate parental figures may be compromised. Encouraging open, honest exploration of a child's feelings about adoption may smooth the transition.

Vignette 3

A 4-year-old girl presents with her adoptive mother for evaluation. The mother expresses worry about her daughter's defiant behavior. The child often refuses to follow directions from her mother, frequently erupting into a tantrum, which usually results in the child getting her way. This pattern of behavior occurs only with the mother, as the child's father and preschool teacher have described her as "a little stubborn, but overall a good kid." When questioned about relenting to the child's wishes, the mother rather sheepishly defends her parenting style, stating, "Well, she had such bad luck before she came to us. What she went through was just awful and I want her to be happy."

Adoptive and foster parents may have conflicting feelings about disciplining their children. On the one hand, they realize that children need rules and consequences, yet on the other they may feel a need to "make up" for the child's bad experiences prior to entering their home. In addition, they may also try to hasten or aid the bonding relationship of the child to them by being excessively permissive. While parents may know logically that no amount of "Santa Claus" parenting will make up for the suffering the child endured, many parents experience a different affective state when disciplining their adopted child versus other children. As with any child, foster and adoptive children need firm rules and boundaries in order to meet developmental goals successfully. Emphasizing this to parents may relieve them of some of the guilt or anxiety they feel about disciplining their child.

Controversies in Foster Care and Adoption

Gay and Lesbian Foster/Adoptive Parents

In the United States, as more children are placed in the out-of-home care system, the available pool of prospective families has decreased. Caseworkers are frequently forced to seek more nontraditional families to care for and adopt these children. Single parents, transracial families, and most recently gay and lesbian couples are becoming options to meet the increased need. The placement of foster children with gay men and lesbians is controversial in some conservative parts of US society.

Research on gay and lesbian biological families has found that they are just as capable at raising children as heterosexual parents.

A common fear is that children raised by homosexual parents will have difficulty with gender identity, or are more likely to develop a homosexual sexual orientation. In fact these children have been found to develop appropriate gender roles and sexual orientation consistent with their biological gender [20, 21]. Additionally, a literature review of studies done in multiple countries from 1978 to 2000 revealed little to no statistical difference in several other outcome measures, including emotional functioning, stigmatization, behavioral adjustment, and cognitive functioning [22]. In a study of social work staff and homosexual foster and adoptive parents, Brooks and Goldberg made several findings that highlight the challenges in lesbian and gay placements. A bias toward extra scrutiny of homosexual prospective foster parents based only on their sexual orientation was found. Gay men and lesbians were more likely to accept children with special needs. A lack of clear local and state social service policy on gay and lesbian placements made agency decisions difficult. In most US states, two individuals cannot jointly adopt a child if they are not legally married, leading most children to be adopted by one primary parent of a homosexual couple [23].

Case Vignette 4

Gayle is a 14-year-old teenager who came to her first appointment with her child and adolescent psychiatrist. She was brought by her new foster mother. She had been neglected in her birth family and removed 3 years ago after it was determined that her older brother had sexually abused her. She had been in several foster homes since her removal and had placements changed mainly due to her outbursts and anger toward older men. The most recent change came when her custody status changed and she became eligible for adoption. She moved to her current foster to adoptive home 1 week ago. Her foster parents are a lesbian couple in their mid-50s who are professionals. One partner has adult biological children. Both the foster mom and child report that things are going well during the first week of placement. The child denies any difficulties with being placed with a lesbian home and replies that she tells her friends she has "many moms." Her foster mom discusses how they have prepared Gayle for possible teasing by her peers. Over the next several months of

---

visits Gayle and her mothers continue to do well. Her outbursts decrease and she is becoming academically successful for the first time in her life. After the 6-month waiting period she is adopted by one of her foster mothers as allowed by state law.

This case illustrates a successful placement with a lesbian couple. It also illustrates the need for preparation of children for possible expressions of homophobia and discrimination based on their parents' sexual orientation. Since foster children may already feel different from children raised in biological families, discussing sexual orientation well in advance can prepare them for possible teasing.

Custody Versus Care

Many parents of children with severe mental illness may have to make an agonizing choice to relinquish custody of their child in order to obtain adequate treatment for the child's mental illness. It is a choice far more common than once thought. A report of the General Accounting Office estimated that in 2001, over 12 700 children were placed in child welfare or juvenile justice agencies so as to procure treatment for mental disorders [24]. At the same time, the report cautions that this number is merely an *approximation*, as there is no formal tracking method for these placements and several states were unable to even provide estimates.

Families face this choice for several reasons. First, health insurance often does not cover, or has limited coverage, for mental health services, particularly those that require long-term treatments such as residential services. This often leaves a wide financial gap for families to fill. At the same time, care of the ill child may interfere significantly with the parents' ability to work in order to provide the coverage needed.

Other issues surround the availability of services. Mental health services for children are often in short supply, especially psychiatric services. Long waiting lists or distance to the service are commonplace. Even when resources happen to be available, children may not meet eligibility requirements for various agencies, or coordination between agencies is poor. As a result, parents stressed by the needs of their child and frustrated by the lack of care, or access to it, may see giving up custody as the only chance their child has for obtaining proper care.

Case Vignette 5

At an early age Joey's behavior was difficult for his mother to handle. His rages and violent actions threatened his own health and the health of his family. Trials of medication and outpatient counseling from 5–6 years old were unsuccessful in improving his behavior. When Joey was aged 6, his mother and stepfather decided to give up custody to the local county children's services board so he could be placed in a residential treatment center. He was placed in a series of residential treatment centers, foster homes, and juvenile detention facilities over a period of several years. At one point he was sexually abused by a peer and then began to act out sexually. His mother remained involved in his treatment and he was able to visit with his family regularly throughout his care. After 4 years, Joey was returned to his mother and stepfather when the residential treatment center he was at closed its doors due to lack of funding. His problems remain and he still has rage attacks and is violent and threatening to his family.

This case highlights some of the difficulties with treating severely mentally ill children. While giving up custody of a child is something parents would never want to do, some are forced to do so out of desperation when a child's behavior becomes dangerous.

To do so is to take on terrible risks, however. Parents who relinquish custody may also lose control over what treatment their child receives or where he/she is sent. In order to regain custody, parents may have to appeal to a court for a ruling. Custody relinquishment can be seen as unfairly biasing poor, minority, and single-parent families as they are more likely to have to relinquish their children to obtain services. It can be harmful for a parent's self-esteem and perception of family in society. It can lead to adversarial relationships between parents and agencies and further erode the relationship between parents and their children [25]. Sometimes, parents may lose track of their child altogether for a period of time.

The plight of these families has become more visible within the popular press, which may aid in prompting changes within the system of care delivery. Several states have either passed or are considering mental health parity laws, which would require insurance to provide equal coverage for mental health treatments on a par with other medical coverage. In 1993 Oregon passed the Voluntary Child Placement Agreement (VCPA) to allow caregivers to voluntarily place their child in out-of-home care without giving up custody. Parents who chose this also had to agree to having a certain amount of their income dedicated to the support of their child, which at times created conflict. In an evaluation of the first 5 years of the law it was discovered that VCPA children were not easily identified and were hard to track. A lack of knowledge among caseworkers about the law was found – only 3% of caseworkers could identify which hypothetical cases could qualify for the program [26]. While a step in the right direction, these laws are still a long way from correcting the problems faced by families of children with severe mental illness.

Intercountry (International) Adoption

The adoption of children from other countries presents unique challenges to families and the health-care providers who care for them. The US Department of State reveals that a total of 11 059 children from other countries were adopted in the United States in 2010 alone. The top three countries of origin were China (3401), Ethiopia (2513), and Russia (1082) [27]. This represents a significant proportion of children when aggregated over time, year-to-year. Each year increases the chance that health-care providers will need to care for and advocate on behalf of these families as they navigate through the difficulties adopted children commonly endure, plus the extra challenges that may stem from their journeys into a stable adopted home from abroad.

Cultural issues can be a concern, as families who participate in intercountry adoption only rarely share cultural or racial backgrounds with the children they adopt. There can be conflicts within a family, as there is within the adoption community at large, about what is more important: cultural identity or acculturation. It is encouraged that each case be treated individually, with extensive exploration into the beliefs and expectations of both the child and the family.

Despite the growing numbers for intercountry adoptions, data and research have been slow to accumulate. There is much we simply do not know for certain, but there are trends that bear watching, including the persistent finding that the longer a child has been institutionalized, the more likely that he/she will suffer psychiatric problems or social difficulties. A literature review by Weitzman and Albers bears this out, particularly with issues surrounding secure attachment, as institutionalization in orphanages before adoption frequently is characterized by fragmented caregiving and therefore less opportunity for secure or stable attachments [28].

Thus, what may be most important regarding the adopted child's country of origin may have less to do with cultural differences than the likelihood of institutionalization prior to adoption and immigration. This is of particular concern given that children adopted from the most common countries of origin described above are also very likely to have spent at least some time in an institutional setting. It is also telling that Hellerstedt et al., in their work with the International Adoption Project, discovered that the parents of children who had spent more time in an institutional setting prior to adoption were less likely than others to recommend international adoption [29]. To understand why some problems may be emerging in a family who has adopted internationally, we as clinicians cannot know too much. Exploring and knowing the child's background and experiences are essential to understanding what direction treatment should take.

In short, the topic of intercountry adoption is a complex and increasingly important consideration for the clinician. The more we learn about the special concerns of these families and children, the more we can help to ensure a happy, stable, and successful placement.

Conclusion

Children who are in foster care or who have been adopted often face uncommon challenges, as do their families and providers. In particular, child and adolescent psychiatrists have a unique role in aiding these children and their adult caretakers. Although child and adolescent psychiatrists are continually pushed to shorten visits and see more children in less time, a thoughtful and team-oriented approach is best when it comes to children and their families who are enmeshed in various social systems. A seemingly small investment by a child's physician to be present at a treatment team, a planning meeting, or just to write out clear recommendations/guidance in a child's case can make an enormous difference. If good communication and healthy give-and-take can be established with pivotal people in agencies within the community, all will benefit. It is encouraged that all physicians involved with these complex children take the time to build relationships and dialogue with these agencies, with a view for the long haul. Though at times the complexities may seem daunting, the reward of seeing a child improve while in a new, stable environment is well worth the endeavor.

Acknowledgement

Special thanks go to Lila Roberts, RN, for her invaluable insights as both a foster parent and mental health nurse.

References

1. Lindsey D. *The Welfare of Children.* New York, NY: Oxford University Press, 2004; pp. 12–13, 168–175.
2. National Adoption Information Clearinghouse (NAIC). *Child Abuse and Neglect Fatalities: Statistics and Interventions.* Washington, DC: Government Printing Office, 2004.
3. Child Welfare Information Gateway. *Foster Care Statistics 2009.* Washington, DC: U.S. Department of Health and Human Services, Children's Bureau, 2011.
4. Zima B, Bussing R, Freeman S, Yang X, Belin TR, Forness SR. Behavior problems, academic skill delays and school failure among school-aged children in foster care; their relationships to placement characteristics. *J Child Fam Studies* 2000;**9**:87–103.
5. Zima B, Bussing R, Crecelius M, Kaufman A, Belin TR. Psychotropic medication use among children in foster care: relationship to severe psychiatric disorders. *Am J Public Health* 1999;**89**:1732–1735.
6. Stahmer AC, Leslie LK, Hurlburt M, *et al.* Developmental and behavioral needs and service use for young children in child welfare. *Pediatrics* 2005;**116**;891–900.
7. dos Reis S, Zito JM, Safer DJ, Soeken KL. Mental health services for youths in foster care and disabled youths. *Am J Public Health* 2001;**91**:1094–1099.
8. Burns BJ, Phillips SD, Wagner HR, *et al.* Mental health need and access to mental health services by youths involved with child welfare: a national survey. *J Am Acad Child Adolesc Psychiatry* 2004;**43**:960–969.
9. US General Accounting Office. *Foster Care: Health Needs of Many Young Children are Unknown and Unmet.* Washington, DC: Government Printing Office, 1995.
10. Finch SJ, Fanshel D. Testing the equality of discharge patterns in foster care. *Soc Work Res Abstr* 1985;**21**:3–10.
11. Rubin D, Alessandrini EA, Feudtner C, Mandrell DS, Localio AR, Hadley T. Placement stability and mental health costs for children in foster care. *Pediatrics* 2004;**113**;1336–1341.
12. Casper LM, Bryson K. Co-resident grandparents and their grandchildren: Grandparent maintained families. Technical Working Paper No. 26. Washington, DC: U.S. Census Bureau. Population Division, 1998.
13. Minkler M, Fuller-Thomson E. The Health of Grandparents Raising Grandchildren: results of a national study *Am J Public Health* 1999;**89**:1384–1389.
14. Dowdell EB. Caregiver burden: grandparents raising their high risk children. *J Psychosoc Nurs* 1995;**33**:27–30.
15. Minkler M, Roe KM. Grandparents as surrogate parents. *Generations* 1996;**20**:34–38.
16. Thomas JL, Sperry L, Yarbrough MS. Grandparents as parents: research findings and policy recommendations. *Child Psychiat Hum Dev* 2000;**31**:3–22.
17. Dannison LL, Smith AB. Custodial Grandparents Community Support Program: lessons learned. *Children and Schools* 2003;**26**:87–95.
18. Carp W. *Adoption in America: Historical Perspectives.* Ann Arbor, MI: University of Michigan Press, 2002; pp. 17–18, 218–220.
19. U.S. Department of Health and Human Services, Administration for Children and Families, Administration on Children, Youth and Families, Children's Bureau: Preliminary FY 2009 Estimates as of July 2010. http://www.acf.hhs.gov/programs/cb/stats_research/afcars/tar/report17.htm
20. Tasker F, Golombok S. Adults raised as children in lesbian families. *Am J Orthopsychiatry* 1995;**65**:203–215.
21. Green R, Mandel JB, Hotvedt ME, Gray J, Smith L. Lesbian mothers and their children: a comparison with solo parent heterosexual mothers and their children. *Arch Sex Behav* 1986;**15**:167–184.
22. Anderseen N, Amlie C, Ytteroy EA. Outcomes for children with lesbian or gay parents. A review of studies from 1978 to 2000. *Scand J Psychol* 2002;**43**:335–351.
23. Brooks D, Goldberg S. Gay and lesbian adoptive and foster care placements: can they meet the needs of waiting children. *Social Work* 2001;**46**:147–157.
24. US General Accounting Office. *Child Welfare and Juvenile Justice: Federal Agencies Could Play a Stronger Role in Helping States Reduce the Number of Children Placed Solely to Obtain Mental Health Services.* Washington, DC: GAO, 2003, p. 14. Available at: http://www.gao.gov/new.items/d03397.pdf.
25. Friesen BJ, Giliberti M. Research in the service of policy change: the "custody problem". *J Emot Behav Disord* 2002;**11**:39–47.
26. Blankenship K, Pullmann M, Friesen BJ. *Keeping Families Together: Implementation of an Oregon Law Abolishing the Custody Relinquishment Requirement.* Portland, OR: Portland State University, Research & Training Center on Family Support and Children's Mental Health, 1999.
27. US Department of State. *FY 2010 Annual Report on Intercountry Adoptions.* Available at: http://adoption.state.gov/content/pdf/fy2010_annual_report.pdf.
28. Weitzman C, Albers L. Long-term developmental, behavioral, and attachment outcomes after international adoption. *Pediatr Clin N Am* 2005;**52**:1395–1419.
29. Hellerstedt WL, Madsen NJ, Gunnar MR, Grotevant HD, Lee RM, Johnson DE. The International Adoption Project: population-based surveillance of Minnesota parents who adopted children internationally. Rudd Adoption Research Program Publication Series, Paper 2. University of Massachusetts Amherst, 2008. Available at: http://scholarworks.umass.edu/rudd_publications/2.

30

Child Psychiatry and the Law

Douglas Mossman

Introduction

The idea that the legal system should treat children differently from adults and afford them special rights and protections is a recent historical phenomenon, one that coincides with what are, from a historical perspective, recent social developments in Western societies' views of children and their preparation for citizenship. Until well into the nineteenth century, most children in the Western nations lived in rural areas, attended school sporadically, and often started full-time employment in their early teens. The word "adolescence" was coined in 1890 [1], a scientific development that reflected broad social developments in the United States of the late nineteenthcentury. Urbanization, industrialization, and large-scale immigration helped to produce major changes in family structure and the workplace. The community at large responded to these social developments by requiring compulsory education, passing child labor laws, and creating a separate justice system to respond to teenagers who violated behavioral social norms of propriety and obedience [1, 2].

English common law traditionally regarded immaturity ("infancy") as a barrier to criminal prosecution, and children have long been barred from exercising many legal rights accorded to adults (e.g., voting). The development in the United States of special courts for children only began around 1900, coincident with the time when the socially constructed notion of adolescence had firmly taken hold in American thought. Ideas about the legal treatment of children that we now take for granted – that they are not the property of their parents, that they should attend school until adulthood, that they deserve special protection in employment settings, that society owes them protection from their parents' violence, and that special, "juvenile" courts should handle their lawbreaking– reflect distinctly modern views about and expectations of children [3].

Practicing child forensic psychiatry forces the clinician to confront the ever-changing clinical, social, and legal issues that reflect Americans' seemingly constant reconfiguration of their work habits, family life, and communities. Readers should therefore understand that this chapter does not provide an exhaustive treatment of issues related to children, child psychiatry, and the law. Rather, what follows is only basic background information about the legal matters that child psychiatrists commonly encounter in their practices.

Legal Issues in the Treatment of Minors

Competence and Consent for Treatment

Competence is the legal capacity to perform a legal function, such as getting married, writing a will, entering into a business contract, managing funds, or obtaining medical treatment. The law presumes that adults are competent for all such functions and that minors are incompetent. Some 16-year-olds can understand and reason about medical information better than many adults, but the law generally does not allow adolescents to give authorization for medical treatment. Before treating minors, clinicians usually must obtain express permission from the child's legal custodian, an adult with the right to make the major decisions about a child's life. In so-called "intact" families where both biological parents are married to each other, either biological parent can give permission for treatment. After married couples divorce, some US states still permit either biological parent to authorize treatment. In other jurisdictions, the child's custodial parent or other legal guardian does so.

Though there are exceptions to the "custodian-must-give-permission" rule, most do not involve circumstances where minors are obtaining psychiatric care. Child psychiatrists should be aware of the exceptions,

Clinical Child Psychiatry, Third Edition. Edited by William M. Klykylo and Jerald Kay.
© 2012 John Wiley & Sons, Ltd. Published 2012 by John Wiley & Sons, Ltd.

however, because fellow professionals may request their consultation on youths whose medical treatment was appropriately initiated without the legal custodian's consent, but whose receipt of psychiatric treatment would require such consent.

Emergencies

One may assume consent for a minor's treatment in situations where delaying treatment to obtain the appropriate adult's permission would jeopardize the life or health of the child. Most states have statutes that specify what constitutes an emergency exception to the normal requirement for adult consent, and what efforts (if any) physicians must make to contact the legal custodian before beginning urgently needed treatment. Clinicians who work in emergency settings should be familiar with local laws that address this issue. They should also be aware that federal law [4] entitles every patient presenting to the emergency room of a federal-funded hospital to a medical screening examination, regardless of capacity to consent.

Psychiatrists should realize that in many cases where emergency medical treatment has been appropriately rendered without an adult's consent, a psychiatrist should get express permission from the legal custodian before initiation of mental health care. For example, an adolescent brought to a hospital after an overdose may need medical treatment quickly to avert serious consequences. Once the child is stabilized, however, a psychiatric consultation to assess future suicide risk and any need for further treatment can usually wait until the appropriate adult has been contacted and has given permission for the evaluation.

Emancipated and Mature Minors

Children who are married, living independently, or supporting themselves and who can show that they can manage their own affairs may ask a court to recognize them as "emancipated." Emancipated minors are treated as adults for a variety of legal purposes, including consent to treatment. Because a child must petition a court to attain this status, clinicians rarely encounter patients who truly are emancipated. Interestingly, an adolescent mother generally may make medical treatment decisions for herself and her child (ren), but may or may not be regarded as legally competent to make other decisions. In many jurisdictions, "mature minor" statutes recognize that older adolescents can participate intelligently in medical treatment decisions, though they may still be living at home and are financially dependent on adults. These statutes specify minimum ages and circumscribed clini-cal contexts (such as drug/alcohol dependence, need for brief mental health outpatient treatment, and obtaining contraceptives) in which teenagers may receive care without an adult's permission.

Children of Divorced Parents

When the need arises, a biological parent who has physical custody of a child generally may authorize treatment for an acute pediatric problem, even if the parent is not the child's legal custodian. However, if the treatment is elective, ongoing, and/or nonroutine (as is much psychiatric treatment), the clinician may (in some states) need to obtain consent for treatment from the child's legal custodian [5]. When a divorced parent brings a child for nonemergency outpatient psychiatric care, the psychiatrist should make sure that the parent is the legal custodian; if not, the psychiatrist should await the custodial parent's express permission before initiating treatment. In some circumstances (e.g., where the psychiatrist wonders whether a noncustodial parent has kidnapped the child), the prudent psychiatrist may ask to see written proof of custody [6].

Reproductive and Gynecological Care

Reproductive Counseling and Abortion

The US Supreme Court's 1977 *Carey* decision [7] established minors' right to privacy in making decisions about use of contraceptives. In response, most states have recognized the right of teenagers to obtain reproductive counseling and contraceptive services without their parents' consent or knowledge. Most states, however, have passed laws requiring physicians to obtain permission from or at least notify parents or guardians of girls who seek abortions. In *Planned Parenthood v. Casey* (1992) [8], the US Supreme Court held that a Pennsylvania law requiring parental notification, but allowing pregnant girls to petition for a judicial bypass of this requirement, was constitutional. Minors may obtain family planning assistance without parental consent or knowledge under federal statutory provisions (the Social Security Act and the Family Planning Services and Population Research Act of 1970).

Sexually Transmitted Diseases (STDs)

Most states allow minors to obtain treatment for STDs without parental consent or knowledge, although state laws vary in the ages at which this may occur and in post-treatment notification requirements (to parents or guardians and/or public health officials).

Outpatient Substance Abuse and Mental Health Counseling

In most states, statutes expressly allow adolescents above a certain age (usually 12 to 14 years) to obtain information about and treatment for substance abuse without their legal custodian's consent. States vary about whether a clinician may or must inform the parent/guardian after contact with the minor has occurred. A minority of states expressly allow minors to obtain mental health treatment without the custodian's consent, and in many states, laws that govern provision of medical care to emancipated or mature minors would apply to physicians rendering psychiatric care.

Nevertheless, the *legality* of treating an adolescent without parental consent does not mean that treatment without parental involvement is necessarily *advisable*. Of course, mental health clinicians must respect their adolescent patients' legal rights and emotional needs for privacy. But clinicians should also recognize that parental involvement is usually crucial to the success of a child's therapy. Figuring out what and how to tell parents about what is going on in therapy is an important clinical aspect of most psychotherapeutic work with a teenage patient.

Psychiatric Hospitalization and Civil Commitment

US states vary considerably in their laws and rules concerning psychiatric hospitalization of minors. US constitutional law [9–11] gives adults a panoply of judicial protections and procedural rights before they undergo nonconsensual hospitalization. In *Parham v. J. R.* (1976) [12], however, the Supreme Court held that children do not have the same constitutional rights. According to *Parham*, the Constitution permits minors to undergo involuntary hospitalization without judicial review if the child's legal custodian consents, the treating clinicians concur, and the clinicians periodically review the need for continued inpatient treatment.

States may grant their citizens additional rights beyond those guaranteed by the federal constitution, however, and many states have enacted laws that accord children avenues for protesting admission or seeking release once hospitalized. In some states, these laws closely resemble adults' protections against involuntary hospitalization (e.g., right to notice, a hearing, and attorney representation). In other states, avenues for relief are not as formal as those that are available to adults. Clinicians who treat children as psychiatric inpatients thus must be aware of how their state's statutes or case law requirements affect procedures for involuntary psychiatric hospitalization: unlike most pediatric hospital treatment, the parent's or guardian's consent to inpatient treatment may not suffice.

Confidentiality of Records and Communications

The question of how to afford minors appropriate confidentiality in psychotherapy requires psychiatrists to recognize and sort through potential conflicts among treatment goals, ethical principles, state law, and federal law.

Intrafamilial Issues

Although some states that permit minors to consent to some forms of treatment also prohibit release of a minor's records for such treatment without the minor's consent, the minor's legal custodian usually decides who may have access to the minor's medical records. In theory, this implies that parents have broad rights to review information about their children's psychiatric treatment.

Despite parents' legal prerogatives, authorities who write about children's psychotherapy believe that mental health clinicians have ethical obligations that go beyond what the law allows or requires. For children and adults, the American Psychiatric Association's *Principles of Medical Ethics* tells psychiatrists to reveal only information that "is relevant to a given situation" and deems it "usually unnecessary" to reveal "sensitive information such as an individual's sexual orientation or fantasy material," even if psychiatrists have received a broader authorization (ref [13], p. 6). The *Principles* also recommends that psychiatrists exercise "careful judgment" about including parents or guardians in a child's treatment, while simultaneously assuring the child's "proper confidentiality" (ref. [13], p. 7).

These seemingly contradictory recommendations reflect the competing obligations that psychiatrists face in their work with children. The following paragraphs outline a scheme – consistent with the American Academy of Child and Adolescent Psychiatry (AACAP) Code of Ethics [14] – for balancing a child's needs for privacy with the therapeutic obligation to speak with parents/guardians and third parties involved in the child's daily life.

Ground Rules At the outset of treatment, the clinician should decide with the child and parents/guardians about how the clinician will handle the child's communications and keep adults informed. Exactly what and how the therapist informs adults will vary depending on the format and goals of treatment. For example, the therapist-to-parent communication in the family-centered treatment of a 7-year-old with encopresis will be very different from the communication to adults about therapy with 16-year-old who is dealing with issues of sexual identity. In all cases, however, minors should know that their parents or guardians must receive information about certain features of treatment, such as prescription of psychotropic medication (for which the adults must give consent), emergencies (e.g., possible suicide or behavior that threatens life and limb), the times of the child's appointments, and whether the child has attended appointments.

The Role of Confidentiality Some older published discussions of this topic often emphasized precautions to protect the child's privacy and to limit disclosure to absolutely necessary information. While these emphases reflected valid clinical concerns, they also might lead to misunderstanding by the naive therapist, to the detriment of a child patient's treatment. Confidentiality is not an end in itself; it serves therapy's larger goal of enhancing and respecting a patient's autonomy.

Value of Communication Adolescents may object to the therapist telling parents uncensored details of their sex lives, and psychiatrists may have to remind overcurious parents of their children's need for privacy. Yet, almost all minors *want* therapists to help them to communicate with the adults in their lives. Thus, a psychiatrist can often say to a minor patient, "Now that we see what's bothering you, how should we help your parents understand this?" When the psychiatrist and minor patient discuss what to tell adults, how the adults will be told, and who will say it, the patient learns that the psychiatrist respects his or her thoughts, feelings, and personhood. The minor patient also gets to communicate with adults in a way that enhances autonomy, and learns that adults are separate individuals who can provide support without compromising autonomy. A clinician's awareness of the autonomy-enhancing aspects of communication to parents is important whether the communication deals with an urgent issue (e.g., a suicide threat) or merely important but nonpressing material about developments in ongoing therapy.

Promoting Autonomy A psychiatrist who is treating a minor in individual psychotherapy should usually seek the child's *explicit* permission before revealing information to a parent or guardian. If information must be disclosed over the child's objection (again, e.g., a threat of suicide), the child should still get prior notice of the disclosure and an opportunity to discuss the matter with the therapist. The clinician can further convey respect for the objecting child's autonomy by explaining why

the communication must take place and by describing how the communication will include only that information necessary to allow adults to respond appropriately to the child's needs.

The Health Insurance Portability and Accountability Act (HIPAA) and Extrafamilial Disclosures

Rules about protecting information, releasing information, and what an authorization form must contain vary from state to state and are also subject to provisions of the (perhaps misnamed) Health Insurance Portability and Accountability Act (HIPAA) of 1996 [15]. In August 2002, the US Department of Health and Human Services issued the "Privacy Rule" to implement HIPAA's requirements concerning handling of "protected health information" (PHI). The Privacy Rule governs use and disclosure of individuals' PHI by so-called "covered entities," i.e., entities affected by the Rule. The Rule also sets standards for helping individuals to understand their privacy rights and control use of their health information. The following discussion is adapted from a summary and a synthesis of federal regulations prepared by the Department of Health and Human Services [16].

"*Covered Entities*" Under the Privacy Rule, "covered entities" are health plans, health-care clearinghouses, and health-care providers (including doctors and hospitals) that transmit health information in electronic form, for example, by electronically filing insurance claims or referral authorizations. The Rule governs handling and release of any "individually identifiable health information" that deals with a person's physical or mental health, providing the person with health care, or the paying for the person's health care.

Disclosures A major purpose of the Privacy Rule is to define and limit the circumstances in which covered entities may use or disclose an individual's PHI. A covered entity must disclose PHI to patients when they ask to see their own records or inquire about disclosures to others. Covered entities are allowed to disclose PHI for other reasons consistent with professional ethics. Examples of such reasons include obtaining payment, emergency situations, situations where the individual gives verbal consent (e.g., to discuss care with a relative), and writing a prescription that a pharmacist fills.

Covered entities also may disclose PHI without the individual's authorization when required by law to do so (e.g., pursuant to a statute or court order); they may also give information to police to permit criminal investigations. Covered entities also are allowed to report child abuse and certain communicable diseases, and they may release work-related PHI information so that employers can comply with state or federal law. Also permitted are *Tarasoff*-type disclosures to law enforcement agencies or other third parties to prevent harm.

In cases where disclosure is not permitted by the privacy rule, covered entities must get an individual's written authorization to release PHI. Authorization forms must use simple language and should state what specific PHI will be disclosed, who will disclose and receive the PHI, the expiration date, and the patient's right to revoke the authorization. A covered entity must get the patient's or legal representative's permission to disclose psychotherapy notes except for these purposes: (i) the notes are being used for training (e.g., resident supervision), (ii) the covered entity is being sued by the patient, (iii) a *Tarasoff*-type breach of confidentiality is needed, (iv) lawful oversight of the therapist, or (v) to assist lawful activities of a coroner or medical examiner. (For purposes of HIPAA, the term "psychotherapy notes" refers to records that document or analyze private counseling sessions and that are kept separate from the rest of the medical record. Records about medication, the frequency or times of counseling sessions, types of therapy, test results, diagnosis, functional status, treatment plans, symptoms, prognosis, and progress to date are not included within the HIPAA definition of "psychotherapy notes.")

Patients' Rights

- The Privacy Rule requires that patients receive notice of a covered entity's privacy practices, including how the covered entity uses and discloses PHI, patients' right to complain if their privacy is violated, and a point of contact for more information or to make complaints. Except in emergencies, covered entities must make good faith efforts to get a patient's written acknowledgment that he or she received the privacy practices notice and must document reasons for failing to get that acknowledgment.
- Patients also have the right to review their medical records, with these exceptions: psychotherapy notes; information compiled for legal proceedings; and certain laboratory results. Covered entities also may refuse to grant a patient access if doing so might harm the patient or someone else, though patients are entitled to have such denials reviewed via a second opinion.
- Patients have the right to request corrections in their medical records if the records are inaccurate or incomplete. Covered entities must make reasonable efforts to provide any corrected record to persons whom the patient believes needs the information or to other persons who might need the information. A covered entity may deny the patient's request for a correction but must give the patient a written explanation and allow the patient to place a statement of disagreement in the record.
- Patients have a right to find out to whom their PHI has been released over the previous 6 years. There are many exceptions to this rule, however, including disclosures: for treatment, payment, or health-care operations; to persons involved in an individual's health care; for payment for health care; or pursuant to an authorization.

Administrative Requirements Covered entities must have written privacy policies and procedures for implementing the Privacy Rule. They must have designated privacy officials responsible for developing and implementing privacy policies and procedures, and a contact person or office that receives complaints and gives patients information about privacy practices. Covered entities must train their staff members on privacy policies and procedures as is needed for them to carry out work functions, and must apply appropriate sanctions against staff members who violate policies, procedures, or the Privacy Rule. Finally, covered entities must develop reasonable procedures and safeguards to prevent improper use or disclosure of PHI. Examples of such safeguards include shredding documents that contain PHI before discarding them and keeping medical records in a locked area.

HIPAA and Parents The Privacy Rule acknowledges that parents usually are the "personal representatives" of their minor children for purposes of health care and, therefore, that parents may generally access medical records on behalf of their minor children. However, if a minor has consented to or obtained health-care services for which no adult's consent is legally required, parents or guardians may not access medical records without the minor's permission. When a parent is not the minor's representative, the Privacy Rule defers to state and other laws concerning the rights of parents to access and control PHI. Where state and other law is silent about parental access, covered entities may deny a parent access to the minor's health information when the decision to deny access is made by a licensed health-care professional utilizing professional judgment.

Penalties Covered entities may have to pay civil penalties of $100 per failure to comply with a Privacy Rule requirement. Such penalties may not be imposed if there was a reasonable cause for the failure, the failure did not involve willful neglect, and the covered entity corrected the violation within 30 days of learning about the violation. HIPAA provides for possible criminal sanctions as well: an individual who knowingly obtains or discloses PHI may be fined $50 000 and receive up to a year's imprisonment.

Comment Long before HIPAA, psychiatrists were sensitive and cautious about responding to outsiders' requests for information. In child psychiatric practice, legitimate but informally tendered requests for information about treatment will come from noncustodial parents or extrafamilial third parties (teachers, lawyers, courts, community agencies). Many states have laws that give noncustodial parents the same access to records that custodial parents enjoy. Except in an emergency, however, the psychiatrist should obtain appropriate *written* authorization for the disclosure before releasing information to other parties. The author's practice is to obtain the child's verbal permission as well, and, for children old enough to understand the procedure, to have children sign the consent form along with their parents or guardians. Some jurisdictions require the *consent* of minors older than a specific age for records concerning certain types of medical treatment (including mental health care) in addition to the legal guardian's consent.

Documents authorizing release of records should comply with HIPAA guidelines and those of one's own jurisdictions. Authorization forms must state explicitly whether the disclosure may include information about drug or alcohol treatment, HIV/AIDS, and other conditions. Any state laws that are contrary to the Privacy Rule are pre-empted by the federal requirements, which means that the HIPAA rules will apply.

Child Abuse and Neglect

Background

Following the 1962 publication of the landmark article "The battered child syndrome" by Kempe and colleagues [17], physicians and other health-care professionals lobbied legislatures across the country to create law requiring certain individuals to report child abuse to state authorities. As a result, laws in every state now command physicians and various other professionals who *know or suspect* that a child is being or has been abused or neglected to report their belief to a law enforcement office or the appropriate local social service agency.

Most states base their definition of neglect and abuse on wording in the federal Child Abuse Prevention and

Treatment Act of 1974, which defines abuse as "the physical and mental injuring, sexual abuse, negligent treatment or maltreatment of a child under the age of 18 by a person who is responsible for the child's welfare." [18] The obligation to report overrides clinicians' ordinary confidentiality obligations, and clinicians who make good-faith reports are immune from civil liability stemming from the reports.

Despite the nondiscretionary nature of state reporting requirements, mental health professionals who work with families may feel reluctant to report abuse to a social service or law enforcement agency. A professional might believe, for example, that making a report would be detrimental to the child or would disrupt therapy that will address the problem. Empirical evidence, however, suggests that although reporting abuse may temporarily injure a therapeutic relationship, it can lead to a subsequent strengthening of the treatment alliance [19]. Moreover, in most states, practitioners who do not report suspected or known abuse may face criminal prosecution and civil liability for damages stemming from their failure to report.

Signs of Physical Abuse

Child psychiatrists typically learn about abuse through a child's or adult's verbal reports, perhaps during discussions about parents' disciplinary practices or their responses when angry with a child. Many childhood behaviors and parental characteristics have been associated with abuse and/or neglect [20]. These suspicion-creating signs are nonspecific, however, and (out of fairness to parents) should not be occasions for reporting abuse to authorities unless they are confirmed by verbal reports.

Pediatricians, especially those working in emergency settings, are more likely than psychiatrists to encounter children with physical injuries that are suggestive of child abuse. These include:

- bruises or welts in nonbony areas with shapes that suggest an object was used to inflict them;
- cigarette burns;
- burns caused by immersion in hot water, which have sharp demarcation lines and appear on extensor surfaces of the limbs and torso;
- lacerations involving the anus or genitalia;
- spiral fractures of the lower limbs (caused by twisting), multiple fractures in several stages of healing, or periosteal elevation;
- head injuries such as linear skull fractures in infants, subdural hematomas and retinal hemorrhages (caused by blows or shaking), jaw fractures, and

scalp injuries (hemorrhages or missing hair caused by hair-pulling);
- abnormal vaginal flora and cultures positive for sexually transmitted diseases.

Encountering these injuries or findings obliges evaluating clinicians to rule out physical or sexual abuse. The likelihood that abuse has caused a physical injury is heightened by parental explanations that are inconsistent with the nature of the injury (e.g., a statement that a fall caused a welt that is shaped like an extension cord). Clinicians need to be aware, of course, that scientific controversy surrounds what kinds of physical findings are convincing evidence of abuse [21–23].

Interviewing Children for Suspected Sexual Abuse

Alleged sexual abuse is a common and contentious complaint encountered by psychiatrists in clinical contexts and forensic situations (e.g., child custody evaluations). The legal system may address this issue through criminal prosecution of an alleged perpetrator and/or through protective action by juvenile or family courts. Clinicians who participate in sexual abuse investigations must recognize that they may face complex legal issues involving the nature and presentation of courtroom evidence [24–26], and potentially vigorous cross-examination by the party that opposes their position.

The AACAP has promulgated guidelines for evaluating children who may have been sexually abused [27], to which readers who undertake such evaluations are referred. Key elements of the evaluation process are: establishing rapport; establishing the child's ability to recognize and report only the truth; allowing the child to give an uninterrupted report of the alleged abusive event; and avoiding leading questions. Interviewing children is just one part of an evaluation of alleged sexual abuse, however. Conducting such evaluations also involves receiving the request for an evaluation (which may come from a parent, attorney, or court), clarifying the social/legal situation (e.g., a divorcing couple battling for custody), and finding out what questions must be addressed. The child psychiatrist must then decide whether to accept the case (which includes deciding that one has the requisite expertise and emotional fortitude). Having accepted the case, the psychiatrist must then arrange to receive available appropriate records and establish conditions of the evaluation (who will be seen, appointment times, and payment procedures).

From a clinical standpoint, evaluating psychiatrists must take special precautions to ensure that they remain objective and must recognize their vulnerability to biases that might influence their evaluation procedures or conclusions [24, 27]. They should document their findings appropriately, and they should make sure that their opinions have a rational basis and are informed by the growing scientific literature in this area.

Child interviewers encounter several pitfalls on their way to completing evaluations. They can be tempted to adopt a therapeutic, rather than an evaluative, attitude. Seemingly innocuous comments ("I'm sorry this happened to you") convey a value judgment that may contaminate a child's recollections. Well-meant assurances or praise for talking about events risks encouraging a child whose immaturity limits ability to distinguish fact from fantasy to produce nonfactual material. Many readers will be familiar with notorious cases in which evaluators' and prosecutors' conscious or unconscious agendas led them to grosser interviewing errors: asking leading questions, asking the same question repeatedly until the desired answer is given, introducing information that the child has not uttered ("I know someone touched you; please tell me who?"), refusing to accept children's initial denials of abuse, or reinforcing children for "good" (accusation-confirming) answers.

A combination of "free play" and "structured" interview protocols may help evaluators to assess cognitive and developmental ability, level of sexual knowledge (which may be inappropriately high in abused children), and information specific to the allegation. Use of anatomically detailed dolls, once considered valuable tools in evaluating abused children, is a source of scientific and legal controversy, and for preschoolers may generate more problems than advantages [24, 28]. Audiorecording and videorecording allow interviewers more freedom to concentrate on their interaction with the child than does taking notes during interviews. Recordings also can provide evidence that a child's accusatory statements were not obtained through leading or contaminating interview techniques.

Termination of Parental Rights

The law and social traditions of the United States grant parents very broad discretion in how they rear their children. In *Smith v. OFFER* (1977) [29], the US Supreme Court held that parents have a "constitutionally recognized liberty interest" in maintaining custody of their children "that derives from blood relationship, state law sanction, and basic human right." This interest is not absolute, however, and is counterposed by the state's *parens patriae* duties to protect citizens who cannot fend for themselves.

The state may take steps to limit or end parent-child contact and make children eligible for permanent placement or adoption when the parents have (i) abused, neglected, or abandoned their children; (ii) become incapacitated in their ability to parent; (iii) refused or been unable to remedy serious identified problems in caring for their children; or (iv) experienced a severe breakdown in their relationship with their children (e.g., due to a lengthy prison sentence). Recognizing that severing the parent-child relationship is a dismal and serious measure, the Supreme Court held in *Santosky v. Kramer* (1982) [30] that a court may terminate parental rights only if the state shows by clear and convincing evidence that a parent has failed in one of these four ways. Most state statutes also contain provisions for parents to relinquish parental rights voluntarily.

Courts and child welfare agencies are guided by two complementary federal laws governing cases in which parents' capacities to care for their children come into question. Passed in 1984, the Family Preservation and Support Services Act [31] requires states, as a condition of receiving federal funds, to make "reasonable efforts" to obviate the need to remove a child from his or her home, or, once a child has been removed, to reunite the child with his or her family. The Adoption and Safe Families Act (ASFA) of 1997 [32] explicitly recognizes that reunification is not always advisable, and stresses that, "while reasonable efforts to preserve and reunify families are still required, the child's health and safety is [sic] the paramount concern in determining" what efforts at reunification should be made. Moreover, no such efforts need be made in certain circumstances, including those in which a parent has: committed a felony assault that caused serious injury to the child or sibling; killed or tried to kill a sibling; engaged in egregious mistreatment (including abandonment, torture, chronic abuse, or sexual abuse); or had parental rights to a sibling terminated involuntarily. The ASFA also requires that safety of children in foster care be considered during case planning, and allows "dual planning" (continuation of efforts at family reunification co-occurring with efforts to place a child with a legal guardian or to arrange an adoption).

Child psychiatrists may become involved with this issue as evaluators of parents who have come to a domestic court's attention. Termination requires a finding that a parent's actions or condition makes the parent unable to care for his or her child and unlikely to become able in the future. A court may request a clinician's assessment of an adult's capacity to parent, the relationship between the adult and child, and the child's special emotional needs. In doing such assessments, clinicians may discover that a psychiatric disorder is an important factor impairing parenting capacity. Courts will then need to know whether the psychiatric disorder is amenable to treatment, the time course of such treatment, and the parent's expected competence following treatment. Clinicians doing these evaluations should remember that their focus is the adequacy of parents, not the comparative benefits of the child's remaining with a parent versus an available alternative placement.

Disabled Children

Access to Education

Since the passage in 1975 of the Education for All Handicapped Children Act [33], all US states must provide disabled children aged 3 to 21 years a free public education in the least restrictive setting that is appropriate to the child's needs. In 1990, Congress passed the Individuals with Disabilities Education Act (IDEA, amended in 1997) [34], which gives states an affirmative responsibility to locate children who need special services and to inform parents about availability of special education programs. Because of this requirement, it is now difficult for schools to ignore referrals for assessment from psychiatrists, psychologists, and teachers who identify a student who may be a "child with a disability." As used in the IDEA (20 U.S.C. §1401(3) (A)), a "child with a disability" includes children "with mental retardation, hearing impairments (including deafness), speech or language impairments, visual impairments (including blindness), serious emotional disturbance, orthopedic impairments, autism, traumatic brain injury, other health impairments, or specific learning disabilities; and who, by reason thereof, needs special education and related services."

Children identified as disabled must undergo re-evaluation at least every 3 years and must have a written Individualized Education Program (IEP). Under Federal law (20 U.S.C. §1414(d)(1)(A)), IEPs must describe:

(i) the child's present levels of educational performance;

(ii) measurable annual goals for enabling the child to be involved and progress in school;

(iii) the special services to be provided to the child;

(iv) the extent of the child's participation in regular classes;

(v) any modifications in or exceptions from participating in state- or district-wide proficiency testing;

(vi) projected date for the beginning of the services;

(vii) for teenagers, plans for transitional services to more advanced studies (e.g., advanced placement courses or a vocational education); and

(viii) how progress will be measured and how parents will be informed about progress.

Federal law (20 U.S.C. §1414(d)(1)(B)) also requires that an IEP be crafted by an "IEP Team" that includes:

(i)   the disabled child's parents;

(ii)   the child's regular education teacher (if the child is in regular classes);

(iii)   a special education teacher;

(iv)   a representative of the local educational agency who can provide or supervise specially designed instruction;

(v)   someone who can interpret the instructional implications of evaluation results;

(vi)   at parents' or the agency's discretion, other individuals with special expertise concerning the child; and

(vii)   whenever appropriate, the child.

Once signed by parents and school personnel, the IEP becomes a legal contract, the conditions of which are enforceable through administrative hearings or state or federal court rulings.

Mental health professionals may be asked for their ideas either during the crafting of an IEP or during litigation concerning fulfillment of an IEP's conditions or the requirements of the IDEA itself. Disagreements about the precise limits of a school system's responsibilities under the IDEA often lead to litigation. One recurring and common area of contention is the school system's financial obligations for special (and often costly) services – including counseling or psychological services – within or outside the regular school setting.

Other commonly litigated issues deal with the expulsion of disabled children, which courts have construed as a change in education placement. Federal law states that disabled children may be suspended for no more than 10 consecutive school days without triggering an IEP meeting unless the child was suspended for carrying weapons or drugs, in which case suspensions up to 45 days are permitted. A key issue that arises in cases of serious misbehavior is whether the misbehavior is a manifestation of the child's disability. If not, schools may require the disabled child to submit to any disciplinary procedure they would use with a nondisabled child. However, because federal law entitles all children to a free, appropriate public education, even those children suspended or expelled must receive education in "an alternative setting."

If a child's misbehavior *is* deemed a manifestation of his or her disability, the IEP must re-evaluate his or her placement, determine whether additional supportive measures are needed, and develop or revise a behavioral intervention plan. This plan should include measures for monitoring progress in reducing the child's misbehavior. Parents have rights to appeal school decisions with which they disagree, including mediation and formal hearings.

Intellectual Disability (Formerly "Mental Retardation")

The American Psychiatric Association's *Diagnostic and Statistical Manual of Mental Disorders, Fourth Edition, Text Revision* (DSM-IV-TR) [35] describes "mental retardation" as disorder with age of onset before age 18 years, characterized by "significantly subaverage intellectual functioning" along with "concurrent deficits or impairments in adaptive functioning" that affect daily activities, such as communication, caring for oneself, school performance, and workplace functioning. Mental retardation is subclassified as "mild" (roughly, IQ = 50–55 to 70), "moderate" (IQ = 35–40 to 50–55), "severe" (IQ = 20–25 to 35–40), and "profound" (IQ below 20–25).

In future editions of the DSM, the condition historically called "mental retardation" will probably be termed "intellectual disability," defined as "a disorder that includes both a current intellectual deficit and a deficit in adaptive functioning with onset during the developmental period." [36] The subclassifications by IQ level will be dropped to be consistent with current practices of the American Association on Intellectual and Developmental Disability. Eliminating subclassifications will also address problems that arise from inaccuracies in testing of severely impaired persons and the failure of older criteria to consider adaptive behaviors in judging levels of severity.

Legal issues frequently addressed in the forensic evaluation of intellectually disabled children and adolescents include their need for involuntary hospitalization due to risk of harm to self or others, their ability to serve as witnesses or stand trial in juvenile or criminal courts, the ability of their parents to care for them, and their needs for special educational provisions under the IDEA. Following *Atkins v. Virginia* [37], a 2002 US Supreme Court decision outlawing execution of persons with "mental retardation," a mental health clinician's determination about a youthful defendant's level of mental functioning can have life-or-death implications [38].

In legal contexts, evaluations of intellectually disabled children – or for that matter, any child with below-average intelligence or a disability that impairs communication or verbal comprehension – pose special challenges for psychiatrists. Although the psycholegal questions (e.g., "Is this child competent to stand trial?") are often not fundamentally different from those asked concerning minors of average intelligence, forensic evaluations of children with intellectual disabilities must frequently take into account the complex interaction of the disability, coexisting mental illness, developmental immaturity, and simple ignorance arising from limited exposure to social expectations and legal proceedings.

Children with intellectual disabilities often arrive at evaluations with little understanding of why they are seeing the psychiatrist and are therefore prone to feeling frightened, overwhelmed, or perplexed. Complex and confusing legal processes only add to these feelings. The psychiatrist may need to take additional time to help the child understand his or her situation, to explain what the evaluation will consist of and why it is occurring, to gain his or her assent, and establish interpersonal rapport. The psychiatrist also should take extra care to make sure that the child understands questions and should make special allowances for limitations in communication. Obtaining factual background information from external sources – parents, schools, and medical records – is an important feature of most child psychiatric evaluations, but becomes even more critical when the evaluee has well-below-average communication or comprehension skills.

Children as Plaintiffs and Witnesses

Psychic Trauma

The typical context in which mental health professionals conduct forensic evaluation of children are those involving juvenile delinquency or domestic relations matters. However, mental health professionals occasionally receive requests to evaluate children who are plaintiffs in what the law terms "tort actions." In a tort action, one party (the plaintiff) sues another party (the defendant) in civil court, alleging that the defendant's willful or negligent behavior caused damages for which the plaintiff should receive compensation (i.e., cash). When the alleged tortious act is intentional – e.g., in an action alleging emotional harm stemming from sexual misconduct with a minor – the plaintiff must show that the defendant's intentional behavior caused the injury. In a negligence suit – e.g., a medical malpractice suit or an action alleging injury stemming from a car accident – the plaintiff must show that the defendant owed the plaintiff a "duty of care" (i.e., had a recognized social obligation to behave prudently), breached the duty through the negligent act, and thereby caused the plaintiff harm. These legal principles are the same for children as for adults. One difference involves the statute of limitations, that is, the time after discovery of the injury during which the plaintiff may sue. Because minors are techni-

cally incompetent, the statutory time limit is "tolled" (does not start) until a child reaches majority.

Many issues and pitfalls in evaluating tort plaintiffs are similar for children and adults. In both cases, the evaluating psychiatrist is expected to conduct a thorough, objective examination of the plaintiff. The psychiatrist often devotes considerable time to gathering and reviewing documents and information from third-party observers. The psychiatrist's goal is to learn whether the plaintiff has an emotional problem, the connection between the allegedly tortious act and the plaintiff's problem, the extent and impact of the impairment on the plaintiff's functioning, and the prognosis for recovery. In contrast to adults, however, evaluating and formulating opinions about children requires the psychiatrist to consider and comment about the effects of normal developmental trends on the injury. The psychiatrist also must attempt to weigh the impact of an emotional problem on educational attainment and subsequent psychosocial development.

A full description of the legal and clinical steps in such evaluations and in preparing for trial lies beyond the scope of this chapter, but readers seeking chapter- or article-length introductions to these topics will find several excellent resources available [39–41].

The Child as Witness

Children may need to testify in civil cases where they are plaintiffs, in domestic cases involving contested custody determinations, in juvenile court proceedings where they are defendants, or in criminal trials where they have witnessed allegedly illegal behavior. Although young children were once viewed as incompetent, Rule 601 of the Federal Rules of Evidence now states a presumption that "every person is competent to be a witness." Many states have similar rules; in the rest, only children above a certain age are presumed competent.

Competence to be a witness entails a capacity to observe, remember, and recount events and to understand the obligation to tell the truth. Though a child meets a jurisdiction's test for *presumed* competence, a judge may investigate a child's capacity before allowing him or her to testify. The judge may do this either by questioning the child in chambers or by having a mental health professional evaluate the child and submit a sealed report to the judge. Clinicians preparing such reports must address whether the child has a mental disorder or defect and whether that condition affects the powers needed to be a witness.

A child's *credibility* as witness is related to, but distinct from, his or her competence, and is influenced by age-appropriate developmental limitations and the way that the child is questioned. Young children have limited powers of free recall, and therefore will not do well if asked open-ended questions requiring lengthy, organized statements. Between ages 5 and 10, retrieval strategies become better developed, and children become able to give longer, discursive accounts of events. Prelatency children are quite suggestible, and their interlocutors must take care to avoid contaminating or influencing their responses by asking leading questions. Young children also lack the ability to describe event times or sequences accurately, and they may not have achieved other concrete operational milestones such as conservation. They thus may have difficulty identifying or recognizing a defendant who was casually dressed and had a beard at the time of an offense but who has shaved and put on a suit for the trial. Child psychiatrists can assist court personnel by helping them understand these limitations and teaching them about how to ask questions (e.g., to use simple words in short sentences; to avoid pronouns and passive voice).

Children may need special accommodations to testify effectively and to not be intimidated by the courtroom context. Such accommodations include having a support person present, altering the scheduling and timing of testimony, and special considerations concerning admissibility of evidence, particularly in criminal cases involving sexual abuse. Several state laws allow children to testify via videotape or closed-circuit television. Although the 6th Amendment establishes a defendant's right to confront witnesses, the US Supreme Court held in *Coy v. Iowa* (1987) [42] that "individualized findings that...particular witnesses needed special protection" might justify deviation from the customary requirement of face-to-face testimony. In a 1990 case (*Maryland v. Craig*) [43], the Supreme Court let stand a sexual assault conviction based on a 6-year-old's closed-circuit television testimony, holding that the purpose of the confrontation clause – insuring that evidence is reliable and subject to potentiallyrigorous cross-examination – was addressed by the closed-circuit arrangement.

Divorce and Child Custody

Background

Between 1950 and 1979, the US per capita divorce rate doubled. Since then, the per capita divorce rate has declined some, but the marriage rate has fallen too. Though several other countries have higher percentages of marriage that end in divorce, only in Russia is the per capita divorce rate higher than in the United States. Recent US Census Bureau projections suggest that half of couples who marry at child-bearing age will divorce,

and an estimated two-thirds of divorcing couples have minor children. Other estimates suggest that a child born to married parents currently has a 40–50% chance of seeing his or her parents divorce before he or she reaches adulthood.

Because parental divorce is a potent risk factor for a child's needing mental health services, a disproportionate fraction of the children seen for psychiatric treatment come from families where once-married parents no longer live together. About 20% of divorcing parents dispute custody, and courts frequently obtain the consultation of mental health professionals to help decide this issue. Child psychiatrists are thus very likely to be involved, either as therapist or custody evaluator, with children who are involved in custody disputes.

Historically, courts' resolution of these disputes has reflected the larger society's views about parental roles and functions. Before the nineteenth century, children – like wives – were deemed the property of adult men and were awarded to fathers after divorce. From the nineteenth century through the first two-thirds of the twentieth century, regard for the importance of maternal attention during a child's "tender years" led to a strong presumption favoring placement with the mother. Currently, every state directs its courts to assign custody based on a "best interests of the child" model most famously articulated by the Iowa Supreme Court in *Painter v. Bannister* (1966) [44]. The Uniform Marriage and Divorce Law, a model statute adopted by many states, directs courts to consider the wishes of the child (ren) and parents, interactions and relationships between the children and parents, siblings, and other involved persons, the child(ren)'s adjustment to school, home, and community, and the mental and physical health of all those involved. Courts are *not* to consider parental conduct (e.g., homosexuality or cohabitation) that does not affect the parent-child relationship.

Courts may award divorcing parents joint *legal* custody, in which both parents retain shared responsibility for major decisions affecting their child(ren), even when the child(ren) will live primarily with one parent. Since the late 1980s, many states have adopted legislation directing courts to view joint custody as the preferred or default arrangement for children of divorcing parents. The success of these arrangements varies with each parent's self-esteem, capacity to empathize, and respect for the bond between the child(ren) and the ex-spouse. Research suggests that children's outcomes depend less on the legal custody arrangements than the pre-divorce psychological functioning of parents and the post-divorce hostility between them. Continued, regular contact with the noncustodial parent is also associated with better post-divorce emotional adjustment.

Divorce *mediation* is a process that parents sometime use (and which, in some states is legally mandated) to reach a settlement without going to trial. Here, the divorcing parties meet without their attorneys in the presence of a neutral person (typically a lawyer or mental health professional who has undergone special training in divorce mediation) to examine areas of contention systematically. The goal of the process is to produce a voluntary agreement about issues such as property division and custody arrangements. This process offers the potential for helping families to avoid lengthy litigation and for developing a plan to which the sides will adhere. However, mediation is often unsuccessful – especially if it is imposed on parties who are already antagonized toward each other – and it can be negatively affected by the limitations of the mediator (e.g., bias, inexperience, lack of "clinical" skills).

Collaborative law, a more recent development, provides another avenue for parents who want to try to work out a divorce agreement. Like mediation, collaborative law is a form of "alternative dispute resolution," but unlike mediation, parents have the advantage of retaining and consulting with their lawyers throughout the negotiation process. Typically, the collaborative law process begins with a four-party "participation agreement" involving both parents and their two lawyers (who usually must have special training in collaboration) stating that they will not go to court before making every possible effort to negotiate a resolution. The agreement also has a disqualification provision saying that the lawyers who represent parents during collaboration may not represent them if the parents later take their dispute to court. Parents and their attorneys then engage in informal discussions, trying to resolve all issues. If the parents and their lawyers cannot resolve all matters this way, the collaboration process ends, and both parents must retain new attorneys for court proceedings.

Thus, under the collaborative law approach, parents do not relinquish their rights to court proceedings. However, collaborative lawyers have no incentive to encourage unreasonable, accusatory, or belligerent positions that might require court proceedings to resolve, nor do they reap the financial benefits of lengthy discovery processes or preparing and attending hearings. Instead, collaborative attorneys have an incentive to facilitate settlement of differences. As for parents, if collaboration fails, they both suffer the disadvantage (and expense) of having to hire new attorneys, which reduces the incentive to argue, accuse, and threaten ("I'll see you in Court!"). The experience of collaboration may also help the parent-clients communicate better, which would benefit their children following the divorce.

Involvement in Divorce Proceedings

Because divorce is so common, and because undergoing divorce is a common reason for seeking psychiatric treatment, clinicians stand a high likelihood of becoming involved in the legal proceedings of divorcing parents. It is unwise for a therapist who has been seeing a divorcing parent in individual treatment to attempt to do a custody evaluation: the therapist's obligations to the patient and greater familiarity with one side of the matter would preclude objectivity in the evaluation, while making an honest, objective appraisal of both parents might interfere with effective therapy for the patient who is in treatment.

Even without serving as custody evaluators, child psychiatrists may have their records subpoenaed and be called to testify in disputed custody cases. In such situations, clinicians should not release records or reveal information about patients without the patients' express written consent, unless the court commands them to do so. Courts regard the need to resolve legal issues as a higher priority than preserving doctor-patient confidentiality. A judge who finds that a psychiatrist has information needed to help decide what is in a child's best interest may therefore order the psychiatrist to produce records or testify despite a parent's objections. Clinicians must comply with such orders or risk being held in contempt of court.

Juvenile Courts and Juvenile Delinquency

Background

A "juvenile delinquent" – in the noncolloquial use of the term – is a minor (in most states, someone less than 18 years old) who has committed an act that would be a crime were it committed by an adult. Besides dealing with delinquent children, juvenile courts have jurisdiction over children who are "unruly" (i.e., who have committed prohibited but noncriminal acts, such as running away or being truant), and also children who have been found dependent, neglected, or abused and are thus entitled to state protection.

Juvenile courts form the vertex of a cultural funnel into which our society pours many problems affecting children and families, particularly those problems that stem from or are caused by the United States' comparatively high level of violence. Children and adolescents in the United States– especially, but not exclusively, those who live in impoverished conditions – are exposed to, are victims of, and commit violence far out of proportion to their representation in the population. US children spend more time watching television than they spend in school, and a huge fraction of television programs – especially so-called "children's programming" – depict violent acts [45]. Various entertainment media–e.g., video games and the internet – offer children graphic opportunities for exposure to violence. Many urban children witness knifings, shootings, and killings before they enter first grade, and each year, millions of children witness domestic violence. According to the National Center for Injury Prevention and Control, more than 675 000 persons aged 10–24 were injured in 2007 by nonfatal, violent acts serious enough to merit medical attention [46]. Homicide is the second leading cause of death among persons aged 15–24 years [47]. In a 2009 US survey, 17.5% of high school students said they had carried a weapon in the last 30 days; 31.5% of high school students reported having been in a physical fight during the 12 months preceding the survey [48].

In the latter third of the twentieth century, lethal violence by US juveniles escalated alarmingly. Between 1984 and 1994, the number of US juvenile homicide offenders nearly tripled, and the number of juvenile killings with firearms quadrupled [49]. After peaking in 1994, the juvenile arrest rate declined significantly. In 2002, there were 2.26 million arrests of young people for all crimes. These included 91 000 arrests for index violent crimes (murder, forcible rape, robbery, and aggravated assault), the lowest level since 1980 and about half the 1994 peak level. Though the once-feared "epidemic" of youth crime had subsided somewhat by the beginning of the twenty-first century, youths still account for roughly 16% of all arrests for violent crimes and 26% of all property crime arrests [50].

Juvenile Justice System

Until juvenile courts were established in most states in the early twentieth century, minors were subject to prosecution in the same fashion as adults, though from the mid-nineteenth century they might be housed separately once found guilty [51]. Juvenile courts' mission since then has reflected a social-parental role that mixes the urge to punish with a belief that delinquency implies that a child needs treatment and rehabilitation. Although juveniles now enjoy many of the formal legal protections accorded to adults accused of crimes, juvenile courts retain their informal and less adversarial character. Juvenile courts also use social service agencies in handling cases, and they frequently rely on mental health professionals' ideas in interpreting and understanding children's circumstances and behavior.

Special Terminology

Juvenile courts typically employ a distinct (and initially confusing) terminology for their proceedings that reflects their historically therapeutic posture. The first step is often called "intake," at which an official (often a probation officer) decides whether a "referral" (i.e., a report of a violation or crime) should be immediately dismissed or accepted for further action. A referral will often result in "diversion," that is, a decision, again often made by a probation officer, to handle an offense using an informal (nonlegal) response, such as a referral to another agency for treatment. Juvenile courts refer to subsequent judicial proceedings as "adjudication" (as opposed to "trial") and "disposition" (as opposed to "sentencing"). Post-sentencing monitoring is often referred to as "aftercare" (rather than "parole" or "community control").

Dispositions available to the juvenile court include probation (sometimes conditioned on school attendance and conforming to other adolescent social norms, sometimes accompanied by requirements for restitution and community service), residential placements (for non-dangerous children who can benefit from a structured, therapeutic community setting), psychiatric hospitalization (for mentally ill children), and "training school" (a euphemism for a juvenile prison for serious and/or repeat offenders). Juvenile courts' dispositional options include a wide range of community agencies – if appropriate services are available. Unlike adult sentencing, juvenile court dispositions may reflect therapeutic needs rather than mere considerations of proportionality and just desert, and may be directed toward people other than the offender (e.g., parents). Consistent with their original treatment-oriented posture, records of juvenile court proceedings are sealed, and conviction as a minor generally does not become part of one's adult criminal record. Federal law requires that minors be housed separately from adults before adjudication, and even those minors found delinquent of serious offenses must be held in special juvenile facilities separate from adult criminals. In 2003, more than 96 000 US teenagers – 307 per 100 000 population – were confined pursuant to court order in various facilities; 85% were boys [52].

Rights

Supreme Court rulings in the last third of the twentieth century established that minors charged with offenses in juvenile court enjoy some but not all of the constitutional protections accorded to adults charged with crimes. *In re Gault* (1967) [53] held that minors facing juvenile court charges have certain due process entitlements under the Fourteenth Amendment, including the right to written notice of charges, *Miranda* protections, and legal representation. *In re Winship* (1970) [54] extended the requirement for proof of guilt "beyond a reasonable doubt" to accusations raised in juvenile courts. *Breed v. Jones* (1975) [55] interpreted the Fifth Amendment's prohibition against double jeopardy to bar prosecution of a minor in both juvenile and adult criminal courts. However, juveniles are not constitutionally entitled to trial by jury in juvenile court (*McKeiver v. Pennsylvania*, 1971) [56]. Also, juveniles who pose serious risk of committing another offense may be subject to pre-trial preventive detention without possibility of bail (*Schall v. Martin*, 1984) [57].

Transfer of Jurisdiction, or "Waiver"

In the late twentieth century, as youth violence was increasing and as administering punishment replaced rehabilitation as the perceived *raison d'être* of US criminal courts, both the public and legal scholars argued for more severe and more adult-like handling of juvenile criminals. Recommended measures included minimizing therapeutic interventions, application of a "just deserts" punishment-oriented model, and – for repeat offenders and youths accused of violent crimes – developing ways to impose sentences beyond the usual maximum of the juvenile court's jurisdiction. One way to make a lengthy sentence possible is for the juvenile court to transfer its jurisdiction over an accused minor to an adult criminal court, where the minor can face trial and the potential for adult criminal sanctions. By the late 1990s, use of this last procedure (also called "waiver," "bindover," or "certification") had substantially increased. In several states, prosecutors had gained increased discretion to file certain cases in adult court. In other states, legislatures mandated adult criminal court prosecution for youths accused of certain crimes [51]. Though some scholars question whether transfers to the adult system reduce violence, and even suggest that such practices are counterproductive [58], laws permitting transfer remain in effect.

A 1966 US Supreme Court case [59] established minimal constitutional protections before a minor's transfer to adult court for prosecution, including a hearing, access to reports written for juvenile court, and statement of reasons for waiver. Beyond these basics, however, transfers of jurisdiction follow rules that vary across jurisdictions. Usually, state laws require that a youth be above a minimum age (typically 14, but lower in some states), be charged with a serious felony, and that there be "probable cause" (i.e., good reason) to believe the youth committed the act. In cases where transfer is optional, courts often must also find that the youth is not amenable to treatment or that placement in a juvenile facility would threaten the community's safety. When making this last determination, juvenile courts often request the opinion of mental health professionals, who then provide assessments and information that can have an enormous potential impact on a young person's future.

In addition to increased use of waivers, many states' statutes require mandatory minimum sentences for certain violent or serious offenders. States have also raised maximum ages for the juvenile court to retain jurisdiction over juvenile offenders, which permits juvenile courts to order dispositions that extend beyond the typical upper age of original jurisdiction, which in various states ranges from age 17 to 24 years. Finally, several states have created the possibility of "blended sentences," which allow courts to impose a combination of juvenile and adult criminal sanctions on certain minors.

Competence to Proceed with Adjudication

All jurisdictions recognize (either through judicial decision or statute) that a minor must be competent at a juvenile court hearing. Usually, competence to proceed in juvenile court is defined as is competence to stand trial for adults, in accordance with the Supreme Court's 1960 *Dusky v. U.S.* ruling [60]. *Dusky* requires that an accused person have "sufficient present ability to consult with his attorney with a reasonable degree of rational understanding" and "a rational as well as factual understanding of the proceedings against him." The legal and theoretical bases for requiring juveniles to be competent are summarized by Bonnie and Grisso [61], who suggest that those children whose cases remain in juvenile court may not need to have the same decision-making capacities as adult criminal court requires. Grisso [62] recommends that the question of a juvenile's competence to proceed with adjudication be raised whenever one or more of the following are the case:

- the child is younger than 13 years old;
- the minor has a history of mental illness or intellectual disability
- the minor has a history of cognitive deficits, such as borderline intellectual functioning or a learning disability;
- current contacts with the child suggest that he/she deviates from normal juveniles in his/her attentional abilities, memory, or capacity to recognize reality.

Despite what evaluators and judges sometimes assume, minors' prior contact with the juvenile justice system provides little assurance that they grasp legal issues related to adjudicatory competence. Previous arrests or delinquency findings do not correlate well with juveniles' ability to appreciate legal rights, the meaning of plea bargains, or trial proceedings.

Over the last four decades, psychologists have developed several structured instruments to aid in assessing adult defendants' competence to proceed with adjudication in a criminal court. Several of these instruments might be useful for assessing minors' competence to proceed in juvenile court [63], but one – the Juvenile Adjudicative Competence Interview (JACI) [64]– was developed with juveniles specifically in mind. Compared with instruments created primarily with adults' competence in mind, the JACI offers special advantages of developmental appropriateness, face validity, flexibility, and opportunities for exploring youths' abilities to grasp new information. The information elicited using the JACI consistently promotes a thorough evaluation that reflects the demands of the evaluee's particular charges and situation, and assists evaluators in formulating clinical findings for use in court [65].

Competence to Waive Miranda Rights

Confessions frequently play a crucial role as evidence supporting a criminal conviction, yet persons unfamiliar with the criminal justice system often do not appreciate the extent and intensity with which law enforcement personnel frequently try to obtain confessions from suspects. In a landmark 1966 decision, *Miranda v. Arizona* [66], the US Supreme Court held that to be valid, a suspect's waiver of the rights to remain silent and to have an attorney present during questioning must be made voluntarily, knowingly, and intelligently. Psychiatrists therefore may be asked (usually by defense counsel) to evaluate whether a minor's confession was made after a competent waiver.

Among the factors that could invalidate a minor's confession are immaturity (chronological or social), low intelligence, lack of familiarity with legal processes, and the length and style of the interrogation. Although several commentators (e.g., Grisso [67]) argue that a confession made by a minor without an attorney or supportive adult present should never be admissible, only a few jurisdictions have adopted this position. Instead, courts are governed by the Supreme Court's ruling in *Fare v. Michael C.* (1979) [68], which includes a rebuttable presumption of a juvenile's competence to confess. *Fare* directs a trial court to consider admissibility of a confession based on "the totality of circumstances" surrounding the confession, including the child's "age, experience, education, background, intelligence," the child's understanding of his or her *Miranda* rights, and his or her understanding of the consequences of waiving those rights. A research-based assessment tool [69, 70] can be used in evaluating *Miranda*-related competence, which allows comparison of a specific evaluee's performance with performances of children and adults.

The Insanity Defense

Insanity is a legal term implying that, at the time of an otherwise criminal act, a defendant's mental disorder or intellectual disability so impaired his or her rationality that he or she should not be held responsible [71]. Infrequently used in adult criminal proceedings, the insanity defense is even more rarely invoked in juvenile settings. One practical reason is that a successful defense would usually have little impact on the case's outcome: the usual disposition for minors with serious mental illness is treatment in a hospital, even when they have been adjudicated delinquent.

The insanity defense is most likely to be invoked when juveniles are tried as adults for serious offenses. States are free to define insanity as they see fit, or (as has happened in a few states) to abolish the insanity defense altogether. In states that allow an insanity defense in juvenile court, the criteria for a successful defense usually are the same as those used in adult criminal court. Most jurisdictions use a variation on one of two well-known definitions of insanity. The "McNaghten" standard, formulated in Great Britain in response to Daniel McNaghten's 1843 insanity acquittal, allows for a successful defense only if the defendant was so mentally impaired at the time of his otherwise criminal act that he could not grasp the nature or wrongfulness of the act charged. The American Law Institute (ALI) test is a more liberal standard. It allows for an insanity acquittal if, at the time of the allegedly criminal act, the defendant's mental impairment rendered him unable to appreciate the criminality of his behavior or "conform his conduct to the requirements of the law."

The Child Psychiatrist in Court

Some Basic Concepts

Many problems that child psychiatrists encounter in their clinical work – abuse and neglect, need for involuntary hospitalization, custody resolution during divorce, or the effects of psychic trauma – have legal as well as treatment implications. In addition, several strictly legal issues discussed earlier in this chapter, such as competence to stand trial and legal sanity, require the special knowledge and clinical expertise of professionals who inform courts and help them make legal judgments. Psychiatrists, who are socialized to seek consensus, generally find adversarial court proceedings, testifying, and (especially) being cross-examined unpleasant. Given the nature of our work, however, most psychiatrists probably cannot avoid making at-least-occasional courtroom appearances. In certain psychiatric practice settings (e.g., working at hospital where many patients undergo civil commitment), giving testimony can become a frequent feature of one's clinical work. Fortunately, many excellent books (e.g., refs [72]–[74]), articles, and continuing medical education offerings are available to help psychiatrists become more familiar and comfortable in their interactions with the legal system. The following paragraphs are just an introduction to courtroom matters, intended to encourage readers to explore more detailed treatments of the subject.

Fact Witnesses and Expert Witnesses

Courts hear testimony from two kinds of witnesses. Fact witnesses are persons who, by virtue of personal observation, have direct knowledge about events bearing on a legal issue. Fact witnesses must confine their testimony to what they have done or directly perceived. Expert witnesses are persons who, having shown to the court's satisfaction that they have specialized knowledge, are allowed to state *opinions* about issues within their areas of expertise. Physicians' specialized training and experience make them, in the eyes of courts, experts on issues related to medicine. Thus courts will allow a physician to testify about symptoms (observable facts) in a patient, plus the patient's diagnoses, which, in the law's view, is an opinion about the causes of symptoms.

Two Avenues to Becoming a Witness

As was suggested above, psychiatrists are at high risk for becoming witnesses because their clinical work is often intimately related to issues of concern to courts. However, their special expertise may lead attorneys to ask them to evaluate clients or otherwise become involved in legal matters not for any treatment purpose, but simply because a psychiatric opinion is needed to obtain an appropriate legal outcome. Examples include custody determinations, personal injury litigation, and criminal issues such as competence to stand trial and insanity. Here, psychiatrists have the opportunity to use their expertise in evaluating complex emotional issues to assist the legal system in ways that can profoundly affect the lives of persons involved.

When psychiatrists give testimony about matters where their knowledge is merely the result of their having undertaken the treatment of a patient, their observations and opinions naturally will reflect the exigencies and limitations of the clinical context. In these circumstances, a physician should attempt (and a court hearing the testimony should expect) no more than a conscientious effort to inform listeners about the

clinical data and how the physician interpreted those data. When psychiatrists evaluate individuals for the specific purpose of helping a court address a legal issue, however, they know that their work will be used for legal and not clinical purposes, that their data and opinions may be sharply critiqued, and that their courtroom testimony may be challenged vigorously during cross-examination. This knowledge requires evaluating psychiatrists to insure that their findings will reflect the efforts of an objective and thorough evaluation; that their written reports to court reflect careful attention to clarity, detail, and soundness of conclusions; and that any potential testimony will be grounded in clinical data and supported by current medical and scientific knowledge.

The Forensic Examination

Accepting a Referral

Although many referrals for child forensic evaluations come from a child's guardian *ad litem* or from a court, some will come from an attorney who represents one side in a legal case. Frequently, attorneys will not be sure what they want from the psychiatrist, and – as often happens in consultation-liaison psychiatry – the psychiatrist's first step will involve clarifying the legal purpose of, and questions to be addressed by, the evaluation.

With this accomplished, the psychiatrist should then ask him or herself:

- Do I feel comfortable undertaking this evaluation?
- Am I being asked to render an opinion on a matter about which psychiatrists truly have expertise?
- Do I have the relevant background and experience?
- Do I have enough time to complete a good evaluation?
- Given the nature of the case, can I remain objective and refrain from letting personal feelings about the issues or the persons affect my judgment?

If all these questions get affirmative answers, the psychiatrist may be willing to accept the case. Before doing so, however, she or he should clarify several other issues. The psychiatrist should make sure that the attorney will permit (and hopefully assist with obtaining) access to all relevant written records (e.g., from schools, social service agencies, and medical/psychological treatment). The psychiatrist should establish the need to speak with all relevant third parties (e.g., in a custody evaluation, both parents and other adults, such as relatives and schoolteachers, with pertinent information). The psychiatrist should also learn what deadlines are operative (e.g., a hearing date) and figure out whether he/she can complete a report in the time available.

Finally, psychiatrists should explain what their fees are and establish how they will be paid. In working with public agencies, one often may bill for services only after all work is completed. In working with private attorneys, however, requesting payment in advance is customary. Attorneys call such payment a "retainer." Advance payment should cover a substantial portion of the time that the expert expects to spend reviewing records, conducting interviews, and writing a report. Contingency fees – that is, fees dependent on the outcome of a case – are perfectly reasonable for attorneys to accept. But agreeing to payment on this basis is inappropriate for a psychiatrist because it may compromise or appear to compromise the psychiatrist's role of objective expert.

Conducting the Evaluation

The primary goal of most clinical encounters is to relieve suffering. The usual aim of forensic evaluations, however, is to discover the truth about why a psychiatric condition developed or how it influenced behavior. Ordinarily, when child psychiatrists conduct evaluations for treatment purposes, clinicians make the reasonable (if not always correct) assumption that informants are straightforward and honest. In forensic evaluations, where outcomes may affect substantial monetary gains or losses, custody arrangements, or incarceration, such an assumption is unreasonable and unwise. Forensic evaluators should treat their evaluees respectfully while remaining skeptical about what those evaluees say. Evaluators must pay careful attention to detail and carefully explore implausible statements, contradictions, or inconsistencies. Whenever possible, evaluators should compare interviewees' statements with independent observations or available records. These special requirements of a forensic evaluation often mean that the psychiatrist will spend much longer conducting interviews and reviewing documents than is ordinarily needed to formulate a clinical diagnosis and treatment plan.

In meeting with parents and children, the forensic evaluator should begin by stating who she or he is, why the interview is occurring, and what will be done with information obtained. Often, this information is presented in writing, which if signed by the evaluee(s) is a helpful way to document that the explanation occurred. Evaluees should be informed of the option not to answer some questions, along with consequences of not answering (e.g., not answering may be noted in reports or testimony). Evaluees should also know that taking short breaks is permitted and that truthful responses are expected.

Even when the evaluation context makes these matters seem obvious, forensic evaluees are frequently confused because of their mental impairments or the complexities of legal maneuvers. For example, evaluees may expect that, because they are talking to "a doctor," the purpose of the interview is to help them and its contents will remain confidential. One must make sure evaluees understand that exactly the opposite is the case. Before accepting the evaluee's verbal and/or written consent to participate, it is often useful to see whether the evaluee can paraphrase the evaluator's explanation about the interview's nature, purpose, and nonconfidentiality.

The Written Report

In some cases (especially civil litigation), attorneys will request that the psychiatric expert prepare only a limited report, leaving it to opposing counsel to learn about what the expert thinks during a deposition (explained further below). In other cases, however, the expert's written report is *the* crucial product of the forensic evaluation. Because most legal issues are resolved without trial, the written report – which will be reviewed by both sides as they think about a settlement – will count far more than any potential medical testimony offered by the evaluator. Also, judges give great weight to written reports, expecting that they represent the clinician's considerations reduced to thoughtful prose, in contrast with unprepared and less reflective statements made during testimony.

The length and structure of a report will vary greatly depending on a case's circumstances and complexity and on the retaining attorney's needs. A typical format includes: (i) an introduction stating the reason for the referral; (ii) a list of sources of information; (iii) history or background information about the evaluee; (iv) contents of the psychiatric interview(s), including the mental status evaluation; and (v) an "opinion" section, in which the evaluator addresses the legal question for which the evaluation was sought.

Ideally, a report should be a stand-alone document, that is, a document from which the reader can obtain a complete understanding of a case and the author's conclusions without reference to other documents. A report should present all the relevant information that formed the basis for the evaluator's conclusions and should outline clearly how the evaluator used available data to reach those conclusions. In their training, physicians learn to use the passive voice and a host of stock terms and phrases ("multiple" for "many," "symptomatology" for "symptoms," "secondary to" for "because of ") that help them allay anxiety, cope with uncertainty, and sound sophisticated. With assiduous practice, however, physicians can unlearn these bad habits and express themselves in prose that is simple, clear, and concise.

Because most readers of forensic reports are nonphysicians (i.e., judges and lawyers), psychiatrists should avoid using medical or psychiatric jargon and should explain technical terms. A short example: Instead of writing "he was treated with risperidone 2 mg b.i.d.," one can write, "he took risperidone (an antipsychotic medication) 2 mg twice a day." Experts should proofread their reports carefully. Minor errors can create misunderstanding, and opposing counsel can use them at trial to portray the expert as careless.

Child Custody Evaluations

Most child custody evaluations are requested in contentious and emotionally charged contexts. Because these evaluations are prone to several kinds of errors that can generate angry recriminations by losing parties, authorities have developed recommendations for clinicians willing to offer courts their assistance in this area. Clinicians with little experience doing such evaluations would be well advised to obtain the consultation of a more experienced mentor. The following paragraphs provide an introduction to appropriate procedures for a custody evaluation and the reasons for those procedures. Readers who intend to do such evaluations should refer to much more detailed discussions available elsewhere [75–77].

Accepting Referrals

A clinician should not agree to do a custody evaluation concerning a child or parent whom he has treated. As was stated earlier, to do so could disrupt needed therapy, lead to violations of confidentiality, and/or undermine the objectivity of the custody assessment. A clinician should not agree to do a partisan evaluation in which only one parent is evaluated at the request of that parent's attorney. Clinicians who do such work are often viewed as potentially biased "hired guns," and they can offer courts little of value where parents' comparative merits, and not their mental health per se, are at issue. Ideally, a clinician should do an evaluation as an agent of the court (i.e., as a court-appointed expert), or failing this, as an expert accepted and agreed upon by both sides. Before the psychiatrist accepts the referral, all parties should agree to the structure of the evaluation (who will be seen, for how many sessions, and

in what combinations) and to the fee arrangements (often being full payment in advance).

The Evaluation

Some evaluators prefer to begin by meeting with both parents to explain and clarify the purpose and nature of the assessment. In a subsequent series of interviews, evaluators will meet with each parent individually. The evaluator's goal is to understand the parents' reasons for wanting custody, how they themselves were raised, their reliability and consistency, their perception of themselves and the other spouse, and their disciplinary methods. Interviews with children assess levels of functioning, areas of special emotional or physical needs, attachments to each parent, and current and upcoming developmental tasks. Evaluators also make observations about parent–child interactions, sometimes having appointments take place around activities or tasks (e.g., a trip to a restaurant) where the evaluator can observe each parent's ability to get and stay organized, nurturing, and limit-setting in circumstances more natural and spontaneous than the office. Finally, and with the agreement of both parties, evaluators may speak with several "collateral sources" – grandparents, schoolteachers, future stepparents – who may have valuable information about parental behavior.

Issues to Consider

Several issues commonly arise in child custody evaluations. These include continuity (which arrangements would be conducive to the most stable living arrangement), major attachments (to parents, siblings, and others), children's preferences (especially for children over age 12 years), parents' attunement to special needs or handicaps (mental and physical), education opportunities, parents' mental and physical health, how well styles of parenting and discipline fit with children's emotional make-up, available social supports, religious differences between parents, and parents' ability to resolve conflicts. In addition, many child custody evaluations must take into account issues that reflect emerging social, political, and scientific developments. Such issues include parental kidnapping, gay and lesbian parents, rights of step-parents and/or grandparents, accusations of sexual molestation, and embryological technology (e.g., custody of frozen embryos).

The Report

Although written reports of custody evaluations may include diagnoses, the aim of the evaluation is not to reach a clinical diagnosis. Instead, the evaluator's report should give the court the evaluator's specific, factually buttressed views about the child(ren)'s special needs and how those needs interact with each parent's abilities and limitations. The report, which may take the form of a letter to the court, can be structured using the previously described forensic report format. Ample use of quoted statements may help convey the evaluator's sense of the evaluees and the tone of the meetings with them. An evaluator should avoid using judgmental language, recognizing that both parents will read the report. The report's final section (perhaps titled "Recommendations") need not address psychiatric diagnosis, since parenting, not clinical status, is at issue. The report should include the evaluator's specific views about custody and/or visitation arrangements.

Testifying

Testifying in court is a knowledge-based performance skill at which psychiatrists can develop varying degrees of proficiency. Psychiatrists who must frequently appear in the witness chair may want to expend some time and effort toward developing their ability to give effective and persuasive expert testimony. Several publications geared toward forensic mental health professionals (e.g., refs [72] and [74]) provide suggestions about presenting oneself in court and handling the challenges, barbs, and verbal ruses of opposing attorneys. For most child psychiatrists, however, spending extra time to develop courtroom skills is not necessary. Knowing the basics of courtroom procedure for handling experts is helpful, however.

Sequence of Testimony

The first part of an expert witness's testimony involves answering a series of attorney questions intended to establish the clinician's expertise, that is, the expert's qualifications to offer opinion testimony about his or her area of special knowledge. The next portion is termed the "direct" examination. Here, the attorney who called the expert asks questions that, from the court's standpoint, establish the "foundation" for the expert's testimony and opinion. During direct examination, the attorney will ask the witness to identify the person examined, to describe facts and findings, and to state and explain opinions. At certain points, the opposing attorney may object to questions, often for technical reasons related to proper legal procedure for presenting evidence. When this occurs, the witness should not respond until the judge rules on the objection. If the objection is overruled, the witness may answer; if the objection is sustained, the examining attorney must withdraw the question or rephrase it in a legally acceptable way.

Cross-examination follows the conclusion of direct examination. Its ostensible purpose is to further the court's efforts to seek the truth by pointing up the flaws or limitations in the expert's direct testimony. When an attorney's cross-examination exposes genuine limitations in the expert's knowledge, the witness should acknowledge them; doing so should not reduce the expert's general credibility if the expert has done a thorough evaluation and reached sensible conclusions.

In the author's experience, it is unusual to encounter the vigorous, incisive, highly critical cross-examination typically found in media depictions of trials (real or fictional). Occasionally, however, cross-examination gets nasty, insulting, or inappropriately personal. When this occurs, the witness should refrain from responding in kind (as difficult as this is); instead, the witness should respond patiently and politely, doing his or her best to explain points clearly, and keeping in mind that the judge and jury – not opposing counsel – are his or her real audience.

Following cross-examination, attorneys have the opportunity to do "redirect" and "recross" examinations aimed at challenging or bolstering points made during earlier direct testimony and cross-examination. Once such testimony is concluded, the judge may ask the expert a few questions. After this, the expert is "excused." The expert then should leave the courtroom, rather than linger to hear other witnesses' testimony.

A Few Tips

- Dress neatly in business attire. For men, this means wearing a suit and tie; for women, it means wearing a conservatively styled suit or dress.
- Try to maintain your professional demeanor. It's fine to appear confident, but is an error to appear smug or arrogant.
- Take time to think before giving answers, and if necessary elaborate briefly when asked questions that seem to call for a yes-or-no answer but really cannot be answered properly in that fashion. It helps (if you can) to try to think about where the attorney is heading. This lets you avoid getting trapped or boxed in by previous answers.
- Don't talk too much. If a question can be answered fully with a one-word response, do so.
- If asked about your fees for time in court, answer the questions nondefensively.
- Recognize that cross-examination may seem vicious and personal, but it's only part of the opposing attorney's job. Don't expect to escape the cross-examining attorney's jabs unscathed; be prepared to bleed a little bit.

- Finally, always bear in mind why you are testifying as an expert: to supply the court with information so it can decide a legal issue. Although you may have been retained by one side to a dispute or have an opinion about how the case should be resolved, the goal in testifying should be to explain the psychiatric findings succinctly, clearly, and honestly. Doing only this constitutes fulfillment of the psychiatrist's courtroom duty to provide information to help the judge or jury make its best decision.

References

1. Empey LT. Detention, discretion and history. *J Res Crime Delinq* 1977;**14**:173–176.
2. McDermott MJ, Laub JH. Adolescence and juvenile justice policy. *Crim Justice Policy Rev* 1986;**1**:438–454.
3. Ainsworth JE. Youth justice in a unified court: response to critics of juvenile court abolition. *Boston College L Rev* 1995;**36**:927–951.
4. Emergency Medical Treatment and Labor Act 42 USC §1395dd (1986).
5. Bernet W. The noncustodial parent and medical treatment. *Bull Am Acad Psychiatry Law* 1993;**21**:357–364.
6. Simon RI, Shuman DW. Psychiatry and the law. In: Hales RE, Yudovsky SC, Gabbard GO (eds) *The American Psychiatric Publishing Textbook of Psychiatry*, 5th edn. Arlington, VA: American Psychiatric Publishing, 2008; pp. 1555–1599.
7. *Carey v. Population Services International*, 431 U.S. 678 (1977).
8. *Planned Parenthood of Southeastern Pennsylvania v. Casey*, 505 U.S. 833 (1992).
9. *O'Connor v. Donaldson*, 422 U.S. 562 (1975).
10. *Addington v. Texas*, 441 U.S. 418 (1979).
11. *Zinermon v. Burch*, 494 U.S. 113 (1990).
12. *Parham v. J.R.*, 442 U.S. 584 (1979).
13. American Psychiatric Association. *The Principles of Medical Ethics with Annotations Especially Applicable to Psychiatry*, 2010 edition. Available at: http://www.psych.org/MainMenu/PsychiatricPractice/Ethics/ResourcesStandards.aspx [accessed 3 May 2011].
14. American Academy of Child and Adolescent Psychiatry. *Code of Ethics*. Adopted 30 January 2009. Available at: http://www.aacap.org/galleries/AboutUs/AACAP_Code_of_Ethics.pdf.pdf [accessed 12 May 2011].
15. Health Insurance Portability and Accountability Act of 1996 (Public Law 104–191).
16. United States Department of Health and Human Services, Office for Civil Rights. Summary of the HIPAA Privacy Rule (describing portions of 45 C.F.R. §160 and §164). Last revised May 2003. Available at: http://www.hhs.gov/ocr/privacy/hipaa/understanding/summary/index.html [accessed 3 May 2011].
17. Kempe H, Silverman F, Steele B, Proegemueller, Selver H. The battered child syndrome. *JAMA* 1962;**181**:17–24.
18. Child Abuse Prevention and Treatment Act (Public Law 93–247).
19. Alvarez K, Kenny M, Donohue B, Carpin K. Why are professionals failing to initiate mandated reports of child maltreatment, and are there any empirically based training programs to assist professionals in the reporting process? *Aggress Violent Behav* 2004;**9**:563–578.
20. DeAngelis C. Clinical indicators of child abuse. In: Schetky DH, Benedek EP (eds) *Child Psychiatry and the Law*. Baltimore: Williams & Wilkins, 1992; pp. 104–118.
21. Geddes JF, Plunkett J. The evidence base for shaken baby syndrome. *Brit Med J* 2004;**328**:719–720.
22. Reece RM. The evidence base for shaken baby syndrome. *Brit Med J* 2004;**328**:1316–1317.
23. Hornor G. Physical abuse: Recognition and reporting. *J Pediatr Health Care* 2005;**19**:4–11.
24. Quinn KM. Interviewing children for suspected sexual abuse. In: Benedek EP, Ash P, Scott CL (eds) *Principles and Practice of Child and Adolescent Forensic Mental Health*. Arlington, VA: American Psychiatric Publishing, 2010; pp. 229–240.
25. Brooks CM. The law's response to child abuse and neglect. In: Sales BD, Shuman DW (eds) *Law, Mental Health, and Mental Disorder*. Pacific Grove, CA: Brooks/Cole Publishing Co., 1996; pp. 464–486.
26. Leavitt WT, Armitage DT. The forensic role of the child psychiatrist in child abuse and neglect cases. *Child Adolesc Psychiatr Clin N Am* 2002;**11**:767–779.
27. Bernet W, Ayres W, Dunne JE, *et al.* Practice parameters for the forensic evaluation of children and adolescents who may have been physically or sexually abused. *J Am Acad Child Adolesc Psychiatry* 1997;**36**(10 Suppl):37S–56S.
28. Bruck M, Ceci SJ, Francoeur E. Children's use of anatomically detailed dolls to report genital touching in a medical examination: developmental and gender comparisons. *J Exp Psychol Appl* 2000;**6**:74–83.
29. *Smith v. Organization of Foster Families for Equality and Reform (OFFER)*, 431 U.S. 816 (1977).
30. *Santosky v. Kramer*, 455 U.S. 745 (1982).
31. Family Preservation and Support Services Act (Public Law 96–272).
32. Adoption and Safe Families Act (Public Law 105-89)
33. Education for All Handicapped Children Act (Public Law 94–142).
34. Individuals with Disabilities Education Act (Public Law 101–476, amended in Public Law 105–17).
35. American Psychiatric Association. *Diagnostic and Statistical Manual of Mental Disorders*, 4th edn, Text Revision. Washington, DC: American Psychiatric Association, 2000.
36. American Psychiatric Association. DSM-5 development, A 00 Intellectual Developmental Disorder. Available at: http://www.dsm5.org/ProposedRevision/Pages/proposedrevision.aspx?rid=384 [accessed 9 May 2011].
37. *Atkins v. Virginia*, 536 U.S. 304 (2002).
38. Mossman D. *Atkins v. Virginia*: A psychiatric can of worms. *New Mexico Law Review* 2003;**33**:255–291.
39. Hoffman BF, Spiegel H. Legal principles in the psychiatric assessment of personal injury litigants. *Am J Psychiatry* 1989;**146**:164–169.
40. Guyer MJ, Schetky DH, Ash P. Civil litigation and psychic trauma. In: Benedek EP, Ash P, Scott CL (eds) *Principles and Practice of Forensic Mental Health*. Arlington, VA: American Psychiatric Publishing, 2010; pp. 405–417.
41. Lubit R, Hartwell N, van Gorp WG, Eth S. Forensic evaluation of trauma syndromes in children. *Child Adolesc Psychiatr Clin N Am* 2002;**11**:823–57.
42. *Coy v. Iowa*, 487 U.S. 1012 (1988).
43. *Maryland v. Craig*, 497 U.S. 836 (1990).

44. *Painter v. Bannister*, 140 N.W.2d 152 (Iowa, 1966).

45. National Television Violence Study. Technical Reports 2 and 3. Thousand Oaks, CA: Sage, 1997, 1998.

46. Office of Statistics and Programming, National Center for Injury Prevention and Control, CDC.10 Leading Causes of Nonfatal Violence-Related Injury, United States (2007). Available at: http://www.cdc.gov/ncipc/wisqars/nonfatal/quickpicks/quickpicks_2007/violall.htm [accessed 9 May 2011].

47. Kochanek KD, Xu JQ, Murphy SL, Miniño AM, Kung HC. *Deaths: Preliminary Data for 2009. National Vital Statistics Reports*, vol. 59, no. 4. Hyattsville, MD: National Center for Health Statistics, 2011.

48. Eaton DK, Kann L, Kinchen S, *et al.* Youth risk behavior surveillance – United States, 2009. *MMWR SurveillSumm* 2010;**59**:1–142.

49. Gest T, Pope V. Crime time bomb. *U.S. News & World Report* 1996;**120**:28–36.

50. Puzzanchera C. *Juvenile Arrests 2008. Juvenile Justice Bulletin*. Washington, DC: Office of Juvenile Justice and Delinquency Prevention, 2009. Available from: www.ncjrs.gov.

51. Snyder HN, Sickmund M. *Juvenile Offenders and Victims: 1999 National Report*. Washington, DC: Office of Juvenile Justice and Delinquency Prevention, 1999.

52. Snyder HN, Sickmund M. *Juvenile Offenders and Victims: 2006 National Report*. Pittsburgh, PA: National Center for Juvenile Justice. Available at: http://www.ojjdp.gov/ojstatbb/nr2006/index.html [accessed 9 May 2011].

53. In re Gault, 387 U.S. 1 (1967).

54. In re Winship, 397 U.S. 358 (1970).

55. *Breed v. Jones*, 421 U.S. 519 (1975).

56. *McKeiver v. Pennsylvania*, 403 U.S. 528 (1971).

57. *Schall v. Martin*, 467 U.S. 253 (1984).

58. McGowan A, Hahn R, Liberman A, *et al.* Effects on violence of laws and policies facilitating the transfer of juveniles from the juvenile justice system to the adult justice system: a systematic review. *Am J Prev Med* 2007;**32**(4S):S7–S28.

59. *Kent v. United States*, 383 U.S. 541 (1966).

60. *Dusky v. United States*, 362 U.S. 402 (1960).

61. Bonnie RJ, Grisso T. Adjudicative competence and youthful offenders. In: Grisso T, Schwartz RG (eds) *Youth on Trial*. Chicago: University of Chicago Press, 2000; pp. 73–104.

62. Grisso T. *Forensic Evaluation of Juveniles*. Sarasota, FL: Professional Resource Press, 1998.

63. Kruh I, Grisso T. *Evaluation of Juveniles' Competence to Stand Trial*. New York: Oxford University Press, 2009.

64. Grisso T. *Evaluating Juveniles' Adjudicative Competence*. Sarasota, FL: Professional Resource Press, 2005.

65. Lexcen F, Heavin S, Redick C. A clinical application of the juvenile adjudicative competence interview (JACI). *Open Access J Forensic Psychol* 2010;**2**:287–305.

66. *Miranda v. Arizona*, 384 U.S. 436 (1966).

67. Grisso T. Juveniles' capacities to waive *Miranda* rights: an empirical analysis. *Calif Law Rev* 1980;**68**:1134–1166.

68. *Fare v. Michael C.*, 442 U.S. 707 (1979).

69. Grisso T. *Instruments for Assessing Understanding and Appreciation of Miranda Rights*. Sarasota, FL: Professional Resource Press, 1998.

70. Goldstein NE, Riggs Romaine CL, Zelle H, Kalbeitzer R, Mesiarik C, Wolbransky M. Psychometric properties of the Miranda Rights Comprehension Instruments with a juvenile justice sample. *Assessment* 2011; doi: 10.1177/1073191111400280 [epub ahead of print].

71. Moore MS. *Law and Psychiatry: Rethinking the Relationship*. Cambridge, MA: Cambridge University Press, 1984.

72. Gutheil TG, Simon RI. *Mastering Forensic Psychiatric Practice: Advanced Strategies for the Expert Witness*. Washington, DC: American Psychiatric Press, 2002.

73. Simon RI, Gold LH (eds). *The American Psychiatric Publishing Textbook of Forensic Psychiatry*, 2nd edn. Arlington, VA: American Psychiatric Publishing, 2010.

74. Gutheil TG. *The Psychiatrist as Expert Witness*, 2nd edn. Arlington, VA: American Psychiatric Publishing, 2009.

75. Herman SP, Bernet W. Practice parameters for child custody evaluation. *J Am Acad Child Adolesc Psychiatry* 1997;**36**(10Suppl):57S–68S.

76. Bernet W. Child custody evaluations. *Child Adolesc Psychiatric Clin N Am* 2002;**11**:781–804.

77. Ludolph PS. Child custody evaluation. In: Benedek EP, Ash P, Scott CL (eds) *Principles and Practice of Child and Adolescent Forensic Mental Health*. Arlington, VA: American Psychiatric Publishing, 2010; pp. 147–156.

Index

Clinical Child Psychiatry, Third Edition. Edited by William M. Klykylo and Jerald Kay.
© 2012 John Wiley & Sons, Ltd. Published 2012 by John Wiley & Sons, Ltd.